The GALE ENCYCLOPEDIA of CANCER

A GUIDE TO CANCER AND ITS TREATMENTS

FOURTH EDITION

The GALE ENCYCLOPEDIA *of* CANCER

A GUIDE TO CANCER AND ITS TREATMENTS

FOURTH EDITION

VOLUME

3

P–Z
ORGANIZATIONS
GLOSSARY
INDEX

KRISTIN FUST, EDITOR

GALE
CENGAGE Learning·

Farmington Hills, Mich • San Francisco • New York • Waterville, Maine
Meriden, Conn • Mason, Ohio • Chicago

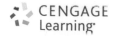

© 2015 Gale, Cengage Learning

WCN: 01-100-101

Gale Encyclopedia of Cancer: A Guide to Cancer and Its Treatments, Fourth Edition

Project Editor: Kristin Fust

Acquisitions Editor: Christine Slovey

New Product Manager: Douglas Dentino

Editorial Support Services: Andrea Lopeman

Indexing Services: Andriot Indexing, LLC

Rights Acquisition and Management:
  Moriam Aigoro

Composition: Evi Abou-El-Seoud

Manufacturing: Wendy Blurton

Imaging: John Watkins

Product Design: Pam Galbreath, Kris Julien

Vice President & Publisher, New Products &
  GVRL: Patricia Coryell

For product information and technology assistance, contact us at
Gale Customer Support, 1-800-877-4253.
For permission to use material from this text or product,
submit all requests online at **www.cengage.com/permissions.**
Further permissions questions can be emailed to
permissionrequest@cengage.com

While every effort has been made to ensure the reliability of the information presented in this publication, Gale, a part of Cengage Learning, does not guarantee the accuracy of the data contained herein. Gale accepts no payment for listing; and inclusion in the publication of any organization, agency, institution, publication, service, or individual does not imply endorsement of the editors or publisher. Errors brought to the attention of the publisher and verified to the satisfaction of the publisher will be corrected in future editions.

LIBRARY OF CONGRESS CATALOGING-IN-PUBLICATION DATA

The Gale encyclopedia of cancer : a guide to cancer and its treatments. -- Fourth edition / Kristin Fust, editor.
    p. ; cm.
  Encyclopedia of cancer
  Includes bibliographical references and index.
    ISBN 978-1-4103-1740-7 (hardback : set) -- ISBN 978-1-4103-1741-4 (vol. 1) -- ISBN 978-1-4103-1742-1 (vol. 2) -- ISBN 978-1-4103-1743-8 (vol. 3) -- ISBN 978-1-4103-1744-5 (e-book)
  I. Fust, Kristin, editor. II. Title: Encyclopedia of cancer. [DNLM:
  1. Neoplasms--Encyclopedias--English.   2. Medical Oncology--Encyclopedias--English. QZ 13]
  RC262
  616.99'4003--dc23
                        2014047836

Gale
27500 Drake Rd.
Farmington Hills, MI, 48331-3535

ISBN-13: 978-1-4103-1740-7 (set)
ISBN-13: 978-1-4103-1741-4 (vol. 1)
ISBN-13: 978-1-4103-1742-1 (vol. 2)
ISBN-13: 978-1-4103-1743-8 (vol. 3)

This title is also available as an e-book.
ISBN-13: 978-1-4103-1744-5
Contact your Gale, a part of Cengage Learning sales representative for ordering information.

Printed in China
1 2 3 4 5 6 7 19 18 17 16 15

ADVISORY BOARD

WITHDRAWN

CONTENTS

PLEASE READ—IMPORTANT INFORMATION

The *Gale Encyclopedia of Cancer: A Guide to Cancer and Its Treatments* is a health reference product designed to inform and educate readers about a wide variety of cancers; other diseases and conditions related to cancers; diagnostic tests and procedures; nutrition and dietary practices beneficial to cancer patients; and various cancer treatments, including drugs. Cengage Learning believes the product to be comprehensive, but not necessarily definitive. It is intended to supplement, not replace, consultation with a physician or other healthcare practitioner. While Cengage Learning has made substantial efforts to provide information that is accurate, comprehensive, and up to date, Cengage Learning makes no representations or warranties of any kind, including without limitation, warranties of merchantability or fitness for a particular purpose, nor does it guarantee the accuracy, comprehensiveness, or timeliness of the information contained in this product. Readers should be aware that the universe of medical knowledge is constantly growing and changing, and that differences of opinion exist among authorities. Readers are also advised to seek professional diagnosis and treatment for any medical condition, and to discuss information obtained from this book with their healthcare provider.

FOREWORD

Unfortunately, man must suffer disease. Some diseases are totally reversible and can be effectively treated. Moreover, some diseases with proper treatment have been virtually annihilated, such as polio, rheumatic fever, smallpox, and, to some extent, tuberculosis. Other diseases seem to target one organ, such as the heart, and there has been great progress in either fixing defects, adding blood flow, or giving medications to strengthen the diseased pump. Cancer, however, continues to frustrate even the cleverest of doctors or the most fastidious of health-conscious individuals. Why?

By its very nature, cancer is a survivor. It has only one purpose: to proliferate. After all, that is the definition of cancer: unregulated growth of cells that fail to heed the message to stop growing. Normal cells go through a cycle of division, aging, and then selection for death. Cancer cells are able to circumvent this normal cycle and escape recognition to be eliminated.

There are many mechanisms that can contribute to this unregulated cell growth. One of these mechanisms is inheritance. Some individuals can be programmed for cancer due to inherited disorders in their genetic makeup. In its simplest terms, a person can inherit a faulty gene or a missing gene whose role is to eliminate damaged cells or to prevent imperfect cells from growing. Without this natural braking system, the damaged cells can divide and lead to more damaged cells with the same abnormal genetic makeup as the parent cells. Given enough time, and our inability to detect them, these groups of cells can grow to a size that will cause discomfort or other symptoms.

Inherited genetics are obviously not the only source of abnormalities in cells. Humans do not live in a sterile world devoid of environmental attacks or pathogens. Humans must work, and working environments can be dangerous. Danger can come in the form of radiation, chemicals, or fibers to which we may be chronically exposed with or without our knowledge. Moreover, humans must eat, and if our food is contaminated with these environmental hazards, or if we prepare our food in

a way that may change the chemical nature of the food to hazardous molecules, then chronic exposure to these toxins could damage cells. Finally, humans are social. They have found certain habits that are pleasing because they are relaxing or help release inhibitions. Such habits, including smoking and alcohol consumption, can have a myriad of influences on the genetic makeup of cells.

Why the emphasis on genes in the new century? Because they are potentially the reason as well as the answer for cancer. Genes regulate our micro- and macrosopic events by eventually coding for proteins that control our structure and function. If environmental events cause errors in those genes that control growth, then imperfect cells can start to take root. For the majority of cases, a whole cascade of genetic events must occur before a cell is able to outlive its normal predecessors. This cascade of events could take years to occur, in a silent, undetected manner until the telltale signs and symptoms of advanced cancer are seen, including pain, lack of appetite, cough, loss of blood, or the detection of a lump. How did these cells get to this state where they are now dictating the everyday physical, psychological, and economic events for the person afflicted?

At this time, the sequence of genetic catastrophes is much too complex to comprehend or summarize, because it is only in the past decade that we have even been able to map what genes we have and where they are located in our chromosomes. We have learned, however, that cancer cells are equipped with a series of self-protection mechanisms. Some of the altered genes are actually able to express themselves more than in the normal situation. These genes could then code for more growth factors for the transforming cell, or they could make proteins that could keep our own immune system from eliminating these interlopers. Finally, these cells are chameleons: if we treat them with drugs to try to kill them, they can "change their colors" by mutation, and then be resistant to the drugs that may have harmed them before.

Then what do we do for treatment? Humans have always had a fascination with grooming, and grooming involves removal—dirt, hair, waste. The ultimate removal involves cutting away the spoiled or imperfect portion. An abnormal growth? Remove it by surgery ... make sure the edges are clean. Unfortunately, the painful reality of cancer surgery is that it is most effective when performed in the early stages of the disease. "Early stages of the disease" implies that there is no spread, or, hopefully, before there are symptoms. In the majority of cases, however, surgery cannot eradicate all the disease because the cancer is not only at the primary site of the lump, but also has spread to other organs. Cancer is not just a process of growth, but also a metastasizing process that allows for invasion and spread. The growing cells need nourishment so they secrete proteins that allow for the growth of blood vessels (angiogenesis); once the blood vessels are established from other blood vessels, the tumor cells can make proteins that will dissolve the imprisoning matrix surrounding them. Once this matrix is dissolved, it is only a matter of time before the cancer cells will migrate to other places, making the use of surgery fruitless.

Since cancer cells have a propensity to spread to other organs, therapies must be geared to treat the whole body and not just the site of origin. The problem with these chemotherapies is that they are not selective and wreak havoc on tissues that are not affected by the cancer. These therapies are not natural to the human host, and result in nausea, loss of appetite, fatigue, and a depletion in the cells that protect us from infection and those that carry oxygen. Doctors who prescribe such medications must walk a fine line between helping the patient (causing a "response" in the cancer by making it smaller) or causing "toxicity," which, due to effects on normal organs, causes the patient problems. Although these drugs are far from perfect, we are fortunate to have them because when they work, their results can be remarkable.

But that's the problem—"when they work." We cannot predict who is going to benefit from our therapies, and doctors must inform the patient and his/her family about countless studies that have been done to validate the use of these potentially beneficial/potentially harmful agents. Patients must suffer the frustration that oncologists have because each individual afflicted with cancer is different, and each cancer is different. This makes it virtually impossible to personalize an individual's treatment expectations and life expectancy. Cancer, after all, is a very impersonal disease, with little regard to sex, race, age, or any other "human" characteristics.

Cancer treatment is in search of "smart" options. Like modern-day instruments of war, successful cancer treatment necessitates the construction of therapies that can do three basic tasks: search out the enemy, recognize the enemy, and kill the enemy without causing "friendly fire." The successful therapies of the future will involve the use of "living components," "manufactured components," or a combination of both. Living components, white blood cells, will be educated to recognize where the cancer is, and help our own immune system fight the foreign cells. These lymphocytes can be educated to recognize signals on the cancer cell that make them unique. Therapies in the future will be able to manufacture molecules with these signature, unique signals that are linked to other molecules specifically for killing the cells. Only the cancer cells are eliminated in this way, hopefully sparing the individual from toxicity.

Why use these unique signals as delivery mechanisms? If they are unique and are important for growth of the cancer cell, why not target them directly? This describes the ambitious mission of gene therapy, whose goal is to supplement a deficient, necessary genetic pool or diminish the number of abnormally expressed genes fortifying the cancer cells. If a protein is not being made that slows the growth of cells, gene therapy would theoretically supply the gene for this protein to replenish it and cause the cells to slow down. If the cells can make their own growth factors that sustain them selectively over normal cells, then the goal is to block the production of this growth factor. There is no doubt that gene therapy is the wave of the future, and it is under intense investigation and scrutiny. The problem, however, is that there is no way to tell when this future promise will be fulfilled.

No book can fully describe the medical, psychological, social, and economic burden of cancer, and if this is your first confrontation with the enemy, you may find yourself overwhelmed with its magnitude. Books are only part of the solution. Newly enlisted participants in this war must seek proper counsel from educated physicians who will inform the family and the patient of the risks and benefits of a treatment course in a way that can be understood. Advocacy groups of dedicated volunteers, many of whom are cancer survivors, can guide and advise. The most important component, however, is an intensely personal one. The afflicted individual must realize that he/she is responsible for charting the course of his/her disease, and this requires the above described knowledge as well as great personal intuition. Cancer comes as a series of shocks: the symptoms, the diagnosis, and the treatment. These shocks can be followed by cautious optimism or profound disappointment. Each one of these shocks either reinforces or chips away at one's resolve, and how an individual reacts to these issues is as unique as the cancer that is being dealt with.

While cancer is still life-threatening, strides have been made in the fight against the disease. Thirty years ago, a young adult diagnosed with testicular cancer had few options for treatment that could result in cure. Now, chemotherapy for good-risk stage II and III testicular cancer can result in a complete response of the tumor in 98% of the cases and a durable response in 92%. Sixty years ago, there were no regimens that could cause a complete remission for a child diagnosed with leukemia, but now, using combination chemotherapy, complete remissions are possible in 96% of these cases. Progress has been made, but more progress is needed. The first real triumph in cancer care will be when cancer is no longer thought of as a life-ending disease, but as a chronic disease whose symptoms can be managed. Anyone who has been touched by cancer or who has been involved in the fight against it lives in hope that that day will arrive.

Helen A. Pass, MD, FACS
Director, Breast Care Center
William Beaumont Hospital
Royal Oak, MI

INTRODUCTION

The *Gale Encyclopedia of Cancer: A Guide to Cancer and Its Treatments* is a unique and invaluable source of information for anyone touched by cancer. This collection of more than 600 entries provides in-depth coverage of specific cancer types, diagnostic procedures, treatments, cancer side effects, and cancer drugs. In addition, entries have been included to facilitate understanding of related concepts, such as cancer biology, carcinogenesis, and cancer genetics, as well as cancer issues such as clinical trials, home health care, fertility issues, and cancer prevention. This easy-to-read encyclopedia defines medical concepts and terminology in language that general readers can understand while still providing thorough coverage.

SCOPE

Entries follow a standardized format to help users find information quickly. Rubrics include the following headings (as applicable):

Cancer types

- Definition
- Description
- Demographics
- Causes and symptoms
- Diagnosis
- Treatment team
- Clincial staging
- Treatment
- Prognosis
- Coping with cancer treatment
- Clinical trials
- Prevention
- Special concerns
- Resources

Drugs, herbs, and supplements

- Definition
- Description
- Recommended dosage
- Precautions
- Side effects
- Interactions
- Resources

Tests, treatments, and other procedures

- Definition
- Purpose
- Description
- Benefits
- Precautions
- Preparation
- Aftercare
- Risks
- Results
- Alternatives
- Health care team roles
- Research and general acceptance
- Caregiver concerns
- Training and certification

INCLUSION CRITERIA

A preliminary list of cancers and related topics was compiled from a wide variety of sources, including professional medical guides and textbooks as well as consumer guides and encyclopedias. The advisory board, made up of medical doctors and oncology pharmacists, evaluated the topics and made suggestions for inclusion. Final selection of topics to include was made by the advisory board in conjunction with the editor.

ABOUT THE CONTRIBUTORS

The essays were compiled by experienced medical writers, including physicians, pharmacists, nurses, and other healthcare professionals. Medical advisors reviewed the completed essays to ensure that they are appropriate, up to date, and accurate.

HOW TO USE THIS BOOK

The *Gale Encyclopedia of Cancer* has been designed with ready reference in mind.

• Straight **alphabetical arrangement** of topics allows users to locate information quickly.

• **Bold-faced terms** within entries indicate that full-length articles exist for those topics.

• **Cross-references** placed throughout the encyclopedia direct readers from alternate names and related topics to their intended entries.

• A list of **key terms** is provided in most entries to define unfamiliar or complicated terms or concepts.

• A **glossary**, located at the end of volume 3, contains a list of all key terms, arranged alphabetically.

• **Questions to Ask Your Doctor** sidebars are provided when appropriate to help facilitate patient discussions with physicians and other healthcare providers.

• **See also** suggestions at the end of some entries point readers toward similar or related topics.

• **Resources** sections at the end of entries direct readers to additional sources of information on a topic.

• Valuable **contact information** for organizations and support groups is included with most entries. All of the contact information is compiled in an appendix in the back of volume 3, arranged alphabetically.

• A comprehensive **general index** guides readers to all topics mentioned in the text.

• **Author and advisor bylines** provide information on who updated and reviewed the entries, including their credentials. Advisor bylines are new to this edition and are not yet present in every article, but the absence of an advisor byline does not mean that the entry was never reviewed.

A note about **drug entries**: Drug entries are listed in alphabetical order by common **generic names**. However, because many oncology drugs have more than one common generic name, and because the brand name may be used interchangeably with a generic name, drug entries may be located in three ways: The reader may find the intended entry under the generic drug name in alphabctical order; may be directed to the entry from an alternate name cross-reference; or may use the **index** to look up a **brand name**, which will direct the reader to the appropriate entry.

GRAPHICS

The *Gale Encyclopedia of Cancer* is enhanced by 275 color photographs, illustrations, and tables.

ALPHABETICAL LIST OF ENTRIES

A

Abarelix
Accelerated partial breast irradiation
Acoustic neuroma
Acute erythroblastic leukemia
Acute lymphocytic leukemia
Acute myelocytic leukemia
Adenocarcinoma
Adenoma
Adjuvant chemotherapy
Ado-trastuzumab emtansine
Adrenal fatigue
Adrenal tumors
Adrenocortical carcinoma
Adult cancer pain
Advance directives
Afatinib
AIDS-related cancers
Alcohol consumption and cancer
Aldesleukin
Alemtuzumab
Allopurinol
Alopecia
Altretamine
Amantadine
Amenorrhea
American Joint Committee on Cancer
Amifostine
Aminoglutethimide
Amitriptyline
Amputation
Amsacrine
Anagrelide
Anal cancer
Anemia

Angiogenesis
Angiogenesis inhibitors
Angiography
Anorexia
Anoscopy
Antiandrogens
Antibiotics
Anticancer drugs
Antidiarrheal agents
Antiemetics
Antiestrogens
Antifungal therapy
Antimicrobials
Antineoplastic agents
Antioxidants
Antiviral therapy
Aromatase inhibitors
Arsenic trioxide
Ascites
Asparaginase
Astrocytoma
Axillary dissection
Azacitidine
Azathioprine

B

Bacillus Calmette-Guérin
Barium enema
Barrett's esophagus
Basal cell carcinoma
BCR-ABL inhibitors
Bendamustine hydrochloride
Benzene
Benzodiazepines

Bevacizumab
Bexarotene
Bile duct cancer
Biological response modifiers
Biopsy
Bisphosphonates
Bladder cancer
Bleomycin
Body image/self image
Bone marrow aspiration and biopsy
Bone marrow transplantation
Bone pain
Bone survey
Bortezomib
Bowen disease
Brain and central nervous system
    tumors
BRCA1 and *BRCA2*
Breast cancer
Breast reconstruction
Breast self-exam
Breast ultrasound
Bronchoalveolar lung cancer
Bronchoscopy
Burkitt lymphoma
Buserelin
Busulfan

C

Calcitonin
Cancer
Cancer biology
Cancer cluster
Cancer diet

Cancer genetics
Cancer of unknown primary
Cancer predisposition
Cancer prevention
Cancer research
Cancer screening guidelines for men
Cancer screening guidelines for women
Cancer survivorship issues
Cancer therapy, palliative
Cancer vaccines
Cancer-fighting foods
Capecitabine
Capsaicin
Carbamazepine
Carboplatin
Carcinogenesis
Carcinogens
Carcinoid tumors, gastrointestinal
Carcinoid tumors, lung
Carcinoma
Carcinomatous meningitis
Cardiomyopathy
Carmustine
Cartilage supplements
Castleman disease
Central nervous system carcinoma
Central nervous system lymphoma
Cervical cancer
Cetuximab
Chemoembolization
Chemoprevention
Chemotherapy
Childhood cancers
Chlorambucil
Chondrosarcoma
Chordoma
Choroid plexus tumors
Chromosome rearrangements
Chronic lymphocytic leukemia
Chronic myelocytic leukemia
Cigarettes
Cisplatin
Cladribine
Clinical trials
Coenzyme Q10
Colectomy
Colon cancer

Colonoscopy
Colorectal surgery
Colostomy
Complementary cancer therapies
Computed tomography
Cone biopsy
Corticosteroids
Craniopharyngioma
Craniosynostosis
Craniotomy
Cryotherapy
CT-guided biopsy
Cushing syndrome
Cutaneous T-cell lymphoma
Cyclooxygenase 2 inhibitors
Cyclophosphamide
Cyclosporine
Cystectomy
Cystosarcoma phyllodes
Cystoscopy
Cytarabine
Cytogenetic analysis
Cytology

D

Dabrafenib
Dacarbazine
Daclizumab
Dactinomycin
Danazol
Dasatinib
Daunorubicin
Debulking surgery
Degarelix
Demeclocycline
Denileukin diftitox
Denosumab
Depression
Dexamethasone
Dexrazoxane
Diarrhea
Diazepam
Dietary factors and cancer risk
Diethylstilbestrol diphosphate
Digital rectal examination
Dilatation and curettage
Diphenhydramine

Disseminated intravascular coagulation
DNA flow cytometry
Docetaxel
Doxorubicin
Drug resistance
Ductogram
Dutasteride

E

Endocrine system tumors
Endometrial cancer
Endorectal ultrasound
Endoscopic retrograde cholangiopancreatography
Enteritis
Environmental factors in cancer development
Ependymoma
Epidermal growth factor receptor antagonists
Epirubicin
Epstein-Barr virus
Erlotinib
Erythropoiesis-stimulating agents
Esophageal cancer
Esophageal resection
Esophagogastrectomy
Essiac
Estramustine
Etoposide
Everolimus
Ewing sarcoma
Exenteration
Extracranial germ cell tumors
Extragonadal germ cell tumors

F

Familial cancer syndromes
Family and caregiver issues
Fanconi anemia
Fatigue
Fecal occult blood test
Fertility issues
Fever
Fibrocystic condition of the breast

Fibrosarcoma
Filgrastim
Flow cytometry
Floxuridine
Fludarabine
Fluorouracil
Fluoxymesterone
Folic acid

G

Gabapentin
Gallbladder cancer
Gallium nitrate
Gallium scan
Gastrectomy
Gastroduodenostomy
Gastrointestinal cancers
Gastrointestinal complications
Gefitinib
Gemcitabine
Gemtuzumab
Gene therapy
Genetic testing
Germ cell tumors
Gestational trophoblastic tumors
Giant cell tumors
Global cancer incidence and
   mortality
Glossectomy
Glutamine
Goserelin acetate
Graft-versus-host disease
Gynecologic cancers

H

Hairy cell leukemia
Hand-foot syndrome
Head and neck cancers
Health insurance
Hemolytic anemia
Hemoptysis
Heparin
Hepatic arterial infusion
Herpes simplex
Herpes zoster
Histamine 2 antagonists

Hodgkin lymphoma
Home health services
Horner syndrome
Hospice care
Human growth factors
Human papillomavirus
Hydroxyurea
Hypercalcemia
Hypercoagulation disorders
Hyperthermia
Hypocalcemia

I

Ibritumomab
Idarubicin
Ifosfamide
Imaging studies
Imatinib mesylate
Immune globulin
Immune response
Immunoelectrophoresis
Immunohistochemistry
Immunotherapy
Incontinence, cancer-related
Infection and sepsis
Intensity-modulated radiation
   therapy
Interferons
Interleukin 2
Intrathecal chemotherapy
Intravenous urography
Investigational drugs
Irinotecan
Itching

K

Kaposi sarcoma
Ki67
Kidney cancer

L

Lambert-Eaton myasthenic
   syndrome
Laparoscopy
Lapatinib

Laryngeal cancer
Laryngeal nerve palsy
Laryngectomy
Laryngoscopy
Late effects of cancer treatment
Laxatives
Leiomyosarcoma
Leucovorin
Leukemias, acute
Leukemias, chronic
Leukoencephalopathy
Leukotriene inhibitors
Leuprolide acetate
Levamisole
Li-Fraumeni syndrome
Limb salvage
Lip cancer
Liver biopsy
Liver cancer
Lobectomy
Lomustine
Lorazepam
Low molecular weight heparins
Lumbar puncture
Lumpectomy
Lung biopsy
Lung cancer, non-small cell
Lung cancer, small cell
Lymph node biopsy
Lymph node dissection
Lymphangiography
Lymphocyte immune globulin
Lymphoma

M

Magnetic resonance imaging
Male breast cancer
Malignant fibrous histiocytoma
MALT lymphoma
Mammography
Mantle cell lymphoma
Mastectomy
Matrix metalloproteinase inhibitors
Mechlorethamine
Meclizine
Mediastinal tumors
Mediastinoscopy

Medroxyprogesterone acetate
Medulloblastoma
Megestrol acetate
Melanoma
Melphalan
Memory change
Meningioma
Meperidine
Mercaptopurine
Merkel cell carcinoma
Mesna
Mesothelioma
Metastasis
Methotrexate
Methylphenidate
Metoclopramide
Micronutrients and cancer prevention
Mistletoe
Mitomycin-C
Mitotane
Mitoxantrone
Modified radical mastectomy
Mohs surgery
Monoclonal antibodies
Mucositis
Multiple endocrine neoplasia
Multiple myeloma
Myasthenia gravis
Mycophenolate mofetil
Mycosis fungoides
Myelodysplastic syndromes
Myelofibrosis
Myeloma
Myeloproliferative diseases
Myelosuppression

N

Nasal cancer
Nasopharyngeal cancer
National Cancer Institute
National Comprehensive Cancer
   Network
Nausea and vomiting
Nephrectomy
Nephrostomy
Neuroblastoma
Neuroendocrine tumors

Neuropathy
Neurotoxicity
Neutropenia
Night sweats
Nilotinib
Non-Hodgkin lymphoma
Nonsteroidal anti-inflammatory
   drugs
Nuclear medicine scans
Nutritional support

O

Obesity and cancer risk
Obinutuzumab
Occupational exposures and cancer
Ofatumumab
Oligodendroglioma
Omega-3 fatty acids
Ommaya reservoir
Oncologic emergencies
Oophorectomy
Opioids
Oprelvekin
Oral cancers
Orchiectomy
Oropharyngeal cancer
Osteosarcoma
Ovarian cancer
Ovarian epithelial cancer

P

Paget disease of the breast
Pain management
Pancreatectomy
Pancreatic cancer
Pancreatic cancer, endocrine
Pancreatic cancer, exocrine
Panitumumab
Pap test
Paracentesis
Paranasal sinus cancer
Paraneoplastic syndromes
Parathyroid cancer
PC-SPES
Pegaspargase
Pemetrexed

Penile cancer
Pentostatin
Percutaneous transhepatic
   cholangiography
Pericardial effusion
Pericardiocentesis
Peritoneovenous shunt
Pesticides
Peutz-Jeghers syndrome
Pharyngectomy
Phenytoin
Pheochromocytoma
Pheresis
Photodynamic therapy
Physical therapy
Pilocarpine
Pineoblastoma
Pituitary tumors
Plerixafor
Pleural biopsy
Pleural effusion
Pleurodesis
Plicamycin
Ploidy analysis
Pneumonectomy
Pneumonia
Polyomavirus hominis type 1 (BK
   virus) infection
Pomalidomide
Porfimer sodium
Positron emission tomography
Pregnancy and cancer
Primary site
Procarbazine
Prostate cancer
Prostatectomy
Protein electrophoresis
Proteomics
Psycho-oncology

Q

Quadrantectomy

R

Radiation dermatitis
Radiation therapy

Radical neck dissection
Radiofrequency ablation
Radiofrequency energy and cancer risk
Radiopharmaceuticals
Raloxifene
Ramucirumab
Receptor analysis
Reconstructive surgery
Rectal cancer
Rectal resection
Regorafenib
Renal pelvis tumors
Retinoblastoma
Rhabdomyosarcoma
Richter syndrome
Rituximab

S

Salivary gland tumors
Sarcoma
Sargramostim
Saw palmetto
Scopolamine
Screening test
Second cancers
Secondhand smoke
Second-look surgery
Segmentectomy
Semustine
Sentinel lymph node biopsy
Sentinel lymph node mapping
Sexual issues for cancer patients
Sézary syndrome
Sigmoidoscopy
Simple mastectomy
Sipuleucel-T
Sirolimus
Skin biopsy
Skin cancer
Skin cancer, non-melanoma
Skin check
Small intestine cancer
Smoking cessation
Soft tissue sarcoma
Sorafenib
Spinal axis tumors

Spinal cord compression
Spiritual and ethical concerns
Splenectomy
Squamous cell carcinoma of the skin
Stem cell transplantation
Stenting
Stereotactic needle biopsy
Stereotactic surgery
Stomach cancer
Stomatitis
Streptozocin
Substance abuse
Sunitinib
Superior vena cava syndrome
Supratentorial primitive neuroectodermal tumors
Suramin
Surgical oncology
Survivorship care plans
Syndrome of inappropriate antidiuretic hormone

T

Tacrolimus
Tamoxifen
Tanning
Taste alteration
Temozolomide
Temsirolimus
Teniposide
Testicular cancer
Testicular self-exam
Testolactone
Testosterone
Tetrahydrocannabinol
Thalidomide
Thioguanine
Thiotepa
Thoracentesis
Thoracic surgery
Thoracoscopy
Thoracotomy
Thrombocytopenia
Thrombopoietin
Thrush
Thymic cancer
Thymoma

Thyroid cancer
Thyroid nuclear medicine scan
Topotecan
Toremifene
Tositumomab
Tracheostomy
Trametinib
Transfusion therapy
Transitional care
Transitional cell carcinoma
Transurethral bladder resection
Transvaginal ultrasound
Transverse myelitis
Trastuzumab
Tretinoin
Trichilemmal carcinoma
Trimetrexate
Triple negative breast cancer
Triptorelin pamoate
Tube enterostomy
Tumor grading
Tumor lysis syndrome
Tumor markers
Tumor necrosis factor
Tumor removal
Tumor staging

U

Ultrasonography
Upper gastrointestinal endoscopy
Upper gastrointestinal series
Ureterosigmoidostomy
Ureterostomy, cutaneous
Urethral cancer
Urostomy

V

Vaginal cancer
Valrubicin
Vascular access
Vinblastine
Vincristine
Vindesine
Vinorelbine
Vitamins

Alphabetical List of Entries

CONTRIBUTORS

Margaret Alic, PhD
Science Writer
Eastsound, WA

Lisa Andres, MS, CGC
*Certified Genetic Counselor and
    Medical Writer*
San Jose, CA

Racquel Baert, MSc
Medical Writer
Winnipeg, Canada

Julia R. Barrett
Science Writer
Madison, WI

Nancy J. Beaulieu, RPh, BCOP
Oncology Pharmacist
New Haven, CT

Linda K. Bennington, CNS, MSN
Clinical Nurse Specialist
Department of Nursing
Old Dominion University
Norfolk, VA

Kenneth J. Berniker, MD
Attending Physician
Emergency Department
Kaiser Permanente Medical Center
Vallejo, CA

Olga Bessmertny, PharmD
Clinical Pharmacy Manager
Pediatric Hematology/Oncology/
    Bone Marrow Transplant
Children's Hospital of New York
Columbia Presbyterian Medical
    Center
New York, NY

Patricia L. Bounds, PhD
Science Writer
Zürich, Switzerland

Cheryl Branche, MD
Retired General Practitioner
Jackson, MS

Tamara Brown, RN
Medical Writer
Boston, MA

Diane M. Calabrese
*Medical Sciences and Technology
    Writer*
Silver Spring, MD

**Rosalyn Carson-DeWitt, BSN,
    MD**
Medical Writer
Durham, NC

Lata Cherath, PhD
Science Writer
Franklin Park, NY

Lisa Christenson, PhD
Science Writer
Hamden, CT

Rhonda Cloos, RN
Medical Writer
Austin, TX

David Cramer, MD
Medical Writer
Chicago, IL

L. Lee Culvert, PhD
Medical Writer
Portland, ME

Tish Davidson, AM
Medical Writer
Fremont, CA

Dominic DeBellis, PhD
Medical Writer and Editor
Mahopac, NY

Tiffani A. DeMarco, MS
Genetic Counselor
Cancer Control
Georgetown University
Washington, DC

Lori DeMilto
Medical Writer
Sicklerville, NY

Stefanie B. N. Dugan, MS
Genetic Counselor
Milwaukee, WI

Janis O. Flores
Medical Writer
Sebastopol, CA

Paula Ford-Martin
Medical Writer
Chaplin, MN

Rebecca J. Frey, PhD
*Research and Administrative
    Associate*
East Rock Institute
New Haven, CT

Jason Fryer
Medical Writer
Lubbock, TX

Jill Granger, MS
Senior Research Associate
University of Michigan
Ann Arbor, MI

David E. Greenberg, MD
Medicine Resident
Baylor College of Medicine
Houston, TX

Maureen Haggerty
Medical Writer
Ambler, PA

Contributors

Kevin Hwang, MD
Medical Writer
Morristown, NJ

Michelle L. Johnson, MS, JD
Patent Attorney and Medical Writer
Portland, OR

Paul A. Johnson, EdM
Medical Writer
San Diego, CA

Cindy L. A. Jones, PhD
Biomedical Writer
Sagescript Communications
Lakewood, CO

Crystal H. Kaczkowski, MSc
Medical Writer
Montreal, Canada

David S. Kaminstein, MD
Medical Writer
Westchester, PA

Beth Kapes
Medical Writer
Bay Village, OH

Janet M. Kearney
Writer
Gainesville, FL

Bob Kirsch
Medical Writer
Ossining, NY

Melissa Knopper
Medical Writer
Chicago, IL

Monique Laberge, PhD
Research Associate
Department of Biochemistry and Biophysics
University of Pennsylvania
Philadelphia, PA

Jill S. Lasker
Medical Writer
Midlothian, VA

G. Victor Leipzig, PhD
Biological Consultant
Huntington Beach, CA

Lorraine Lica, PhD
Medical Writer
San Diego, CA

John T. Lohr, PhD
Utah State University
Logan, UT

Warren Maltzman, PhD
Consultant, Molecular Pathology
Demarest, NJ

Richard A. McCartney MD
Fellow, American College of Surgeons
Diplomat, American Board of Surgery
Richland, WA

Sally C. McFarlane-Parrott
Medical Writer
Mason, MI

Monica McGee, MS
Science Writer
Wilmington, NC

Alison McTavish, MSc
Medical Writer and Editor
Montreal, Quebec

Molly Metzler, RN, BSN
Registered Nurse and Medical Writer
Seaford, DE

Beverly G. Miller, MT(ASCP)
Technical Writer
Charlotte, NC

Mark A. Mitchell, MD
Medical Writer
Seattle, WA

Laura J. Ninger
Medical Writer
Weehawken, NJ

Nancy J. Nordenson
Medical Writer
Minneapolis, MN

Melinda G. Oberleitner
Associate Dean and Professor
College of Nursing and Allied Health Professions
University of Louisiana at Lafayette
Lafayette, LA

Teresa G. Odle
Medical Writer
Albuquerque, NM

Lee Ann Paradise
Science Writer
Lubbock, TX

J. Ricker Polsdorfer, MD
Medical Writer
Phoenix, AZ

Elizabeth J. Pulcini, MS
Medical Writer
Phoenix, AZ

Kulbir Rangi, DO
Medical Doctor and Writer
New York, NY

Esther Csapo Rastegari, EdM, RN, BSN
Registered Nurse and Medical Writer
Holbrook, MA

Toni Rizzo
Medical Writer
Salt Lake City, UT

Martha Floberg Robbins
Medical Writer
Evanston, IL

Richard Robinson
Medical Writer
Tucson, AZ

Edward R. Rosick, DO, MPH, MS
University Physician and Clinical Assistant Professor
Student Health Services
Pennsylvania State University
University Park, PA

Nancy Ross-Flanigan
Science Writer
Belleville, MI

Belinda Rowland, PhD
Medical Writer
Voorheesville, NY

Andrea Ruskin, MD
Whittingham Cancer Center
Norwalk, CT

Laura Ruth, PhD
Medical, Science, and Technology Writer
Los Angeles, CA

Kausalya Santhanam, PhD
Technical Writer
Branford, CT

Marc Scanio
Doctoral Candidate in Chemistry
Stanford University
Stanford, CA

Joan Schonbeck, RN
Medical Writer
Massachusetts Department of
 Mental Health
Marlborough, MA

Kristen Mahoney Shannon, MS, CGC
Genetic Counselor
Center for Cancer Risk
 Analysis
Massachusetts General Hospital
Boston, MA

Judith Sims, MS
Science Writer
Logan, UT

Genevieve Slomski, PhD
Medical Writer
New Britain, CT

Anna Rovid Spickler, DVM, PhD
Medical Writer
Salisbury, MD

Laura L. Stein, MS
Certified Genetic Counselor
Familial Cancer Program-
 Department of Hematology/
 Oncology
Dartmouth Hitchcock Medical
 Center
Lebanon, NH

Phyllis M. Stein, BS, CCRP
Affiliate Coordinator
Grand Rapids Clinical Oncology
 Program
Grand Rapids, MI

Kurt Sternlof
Science Writer
New Rochelle, NY

Deanna M. Swartout-Corbeil, RN
Medical Writer
Thompsons Station, TN

Jane M. Taylor-Jones, MS
Research Associate
Donald W. Reynolds Department of
 Geriatrics
University of Arkansas for Medical
 Sciences
Little Rock, AR

Carol Turkington
Medical Writer
Lancaster, PA

Samuel Uretsky, PharmD
Medical Writer
Wantagh, NY

Marianne Vahey, MD
Clinical Instructor
Medicine
Yale University School of
 Medicine
New Haven, CT

Malini Vashishtha, PhD
Medical Writer
Irvine, CA

Ellen S. Weber, MSN
Medical Writer
Fort Wayne, IN

Ken R. Wells
Writer
Laguna Hills, CA

Barbara Wexler, MPH
Medical Writer
Chatsworth, CA

Wendy Wippel, MSc
*Medical Writer and Adjunct
 Professor of Biology*
Northwest Community College
Hernando, MS

Debra Wood, RN
Medical Writer
Orlando, FL

Kathleen D. Wright, RN
Medical Writer
Delmar, DE

Jon Zonderman
Medical Writer
Orange, CA

Michael V. Zuck, PhD
Writer
Boulder, CO

Contributors

ILLUSTRATIONS OF BODY SYSTEMS

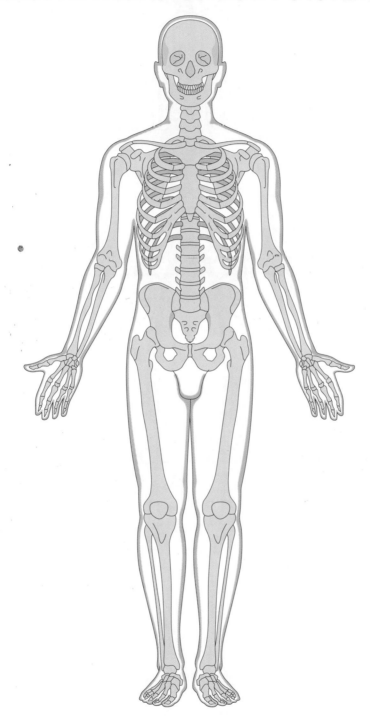

HUMAN SKELETON and SKIN. Some cancers that affect the skeleton are: Osteosarcoma; Ewing sarcoma; Fibrosarcoma (can also be found in soft tissues like muscle, fat, connective tissues, etc.). Some cancers that affect tissue near bones: Chondrosarcoma (affects joints near bones); Rhabdomyosarcoma (formed from cells of muscles attached to bones); Malignant fibrous histiocytoma (common in soft tissues, rare in bones). SKIN CANCERS: Basal cell carcinoma; Melanoma; Merkel cell carcinoma; Squamous cell carcinoma of the skin; and Trichilemmal carcinoma. Precancerous skin condition: Bowen disease. Lymphomas that affect the skin: Mycosis fungoides; Sézary syndrome. *(Illustration by Argosy Publishing. © Cengage Learning®.)*

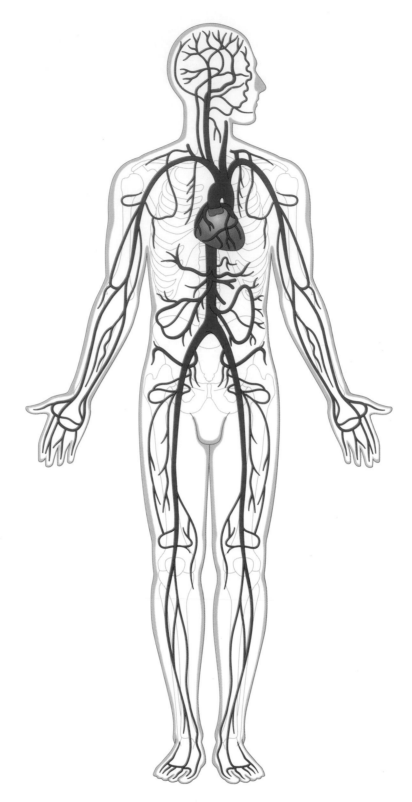

HUMAN CIRCULATORY SYSTEM. Some cancers of the blood cells are: Acute erythroblastic leukemia; Acute lymphocytic leukemia; Acute myelocytic leukemia; Chronic lymphocytic leukemia; Chronic myelocytic leukemia; Hairy cell leukemia; and Multiple myeloma. One condition associated with various cancers that affects blood is called Myelofibrosis. *(Illustration by Argosy Publishing. © Cengage Learning®.)*

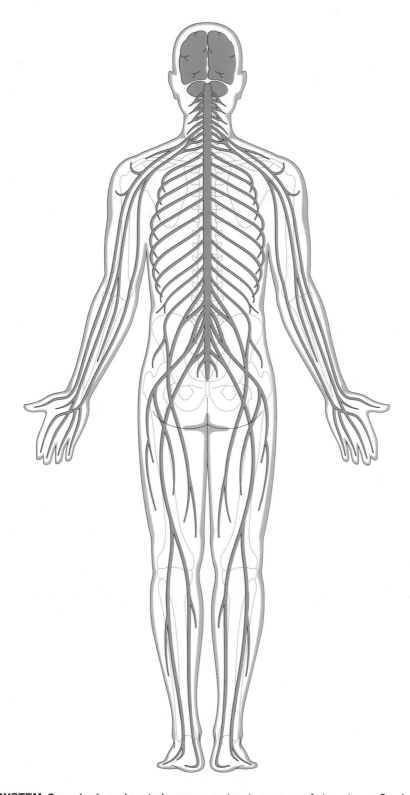

HUMAN NERVOUS SYSTEM. Some brain and central nervous system tumors are: Astrocytoma; Carcinomatous meningitis; Central nervous system carcinoma; Central nervous system lymphoma; Chordoma; Choroid plexus tumors; Craniopharyngioma; Ependymoma; Medulloblastoma; Meningioma; Oligodendroglioma; and Spinal axis tumors. One kind of noncancerous growth in the brain: Acoustic neuroma. *(Illustration by Argosy Publishing. © Cengage Learning®.)*

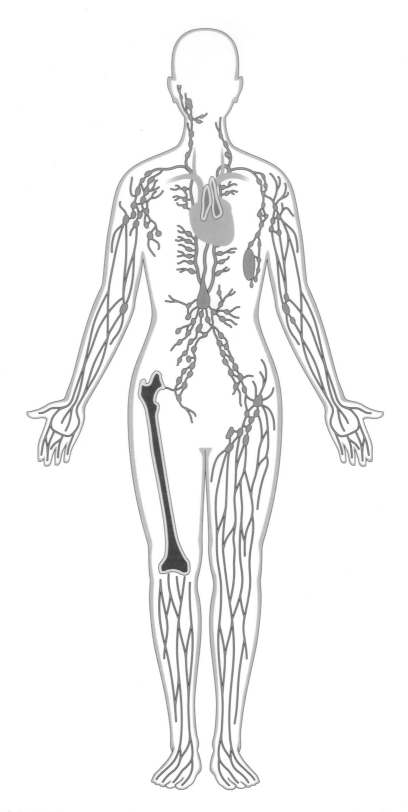

HUMAN LYMPHATIC SYSTEM. The lymphatic system and lymph nodes are shown here in pale green, the thymus in deep blue, and one of the bones rich in bone marrow (the femur) is shown here in purple. Some cancers of the lymphatic system are: Burkitt lymphoma; Cutaneous T-cell lymphoma; Hodgkin lymphoma; MALT lymphoma; Mantle cell lymphoma; Sézary syndrome; and Waldenström macroglobulinemia. *(Illustration by Argosy Publishing. © Cengage Learning®.)*

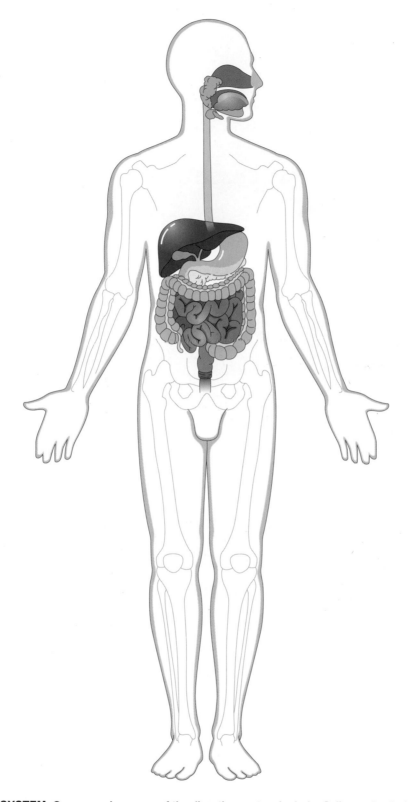

HUMAN DIGESTIVE SYSTEM. Organs and cancers of the digestive system include: Salivary glands (shown in turquoise): Salivary gland tumors. Esophagus (shown in bright yellow): Esophageal cancer. Liver (shown in bright red): Bile duct cancer; Liver cancer. Stomach (pale gray-blue): Stomach cancer. Gallbladder (bright orange against the red liver): Gallbladder cancer. Colon (green): Colon cancer. Small intestine (purple): Small intestine cancer; can have malignant tumors associated with Zollinger-Ellison syndrome. Rectum (shown in pink, continuing the colon): Rectal cancer. Anus (dark blue): Anal cancer.
(Illustration by Argosy Publishing. © Cengage Learning®.)

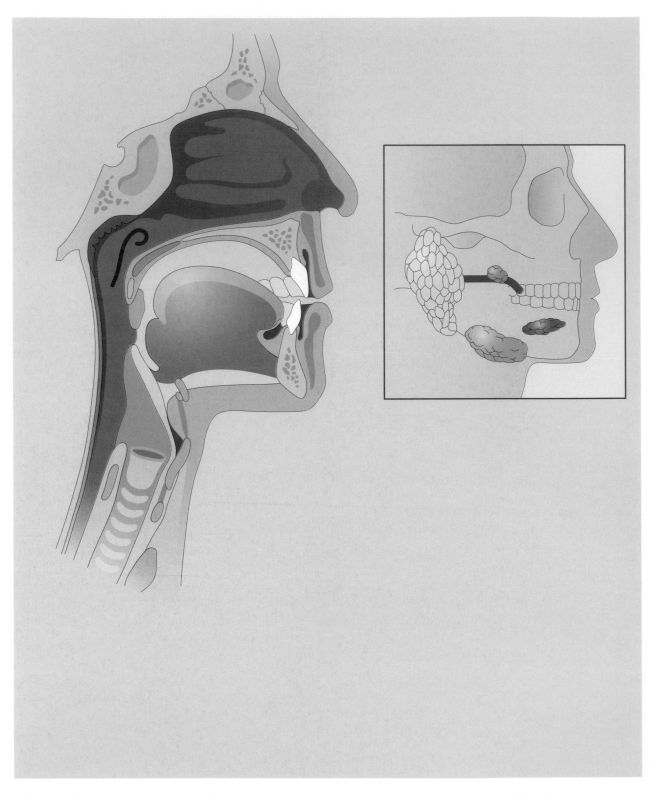

HEAD AND NECK. The pharynx, the passage that leads from the nostrils down through the neck, is shown in orange. This passage is broken into several divisions. The area behind the nose is the nasopharynx. The area behind the mouth is the oropharynx. The oropharynx leads into the laryngopharynx, which opens into the esophagus (still in orange) and the larynx (shown in the large image in medium blue). The cancers that affect these regions include: Nasopharyngeal cancer; Oropharyngeal cancer; Esophageal cancer; and Laryngeal cancer. Oral cancers can affect the lips, gums, and tongue (pink). Referring to the inset picture of the salivary glands, salivary gland tumors can affect the parotid glands (shown in yellow), the submandibular glands (turquoise), and the sublingual glands (purple). *(Illustration by Argosy Publishing. © Cengage Learning®.)*

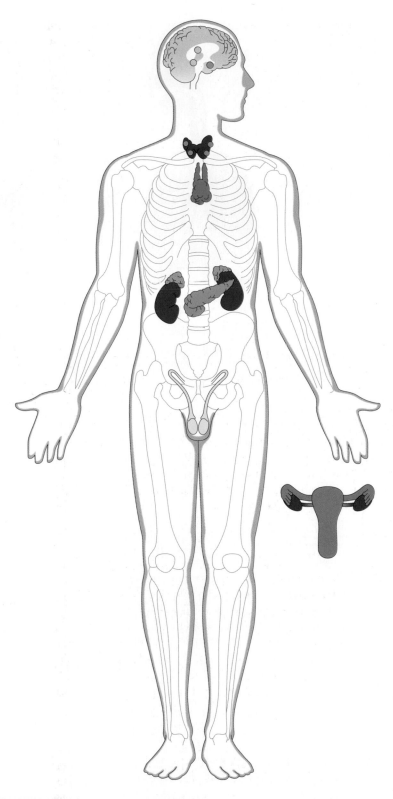

HUMAN ENDOCRINE SYSTEM. The glands and cancers of the endocrine system include (in the brain): the pituitary gland shown in blue (pituitary tumors), the hypothalamus in pale green, and the pineal gland in bright yellow. Throughout the rest of the body: Thyroid (shown in dark blue): Thyroid cancer. Parathyroid glands, adjacent to the thyroid: Parathyroid cancer. Thymus (green): Thymic cancer; Thymoma. Pancreas (turquoise): Pancreatic cancer; Zollinger-Ellison syndrome tumors can also be found in the pancreas. Adrenal glands (shown in apricot, above the kidneys): Neuroblastoma; Pheochromocytoma. Testes (in males, shown in yellow): Testicular cancer. Ovaries (in females, shown in dark blue in inset image): Ovarian cancer. *(Illustration by Argosy Publishing. © Cengage Learning®.)*

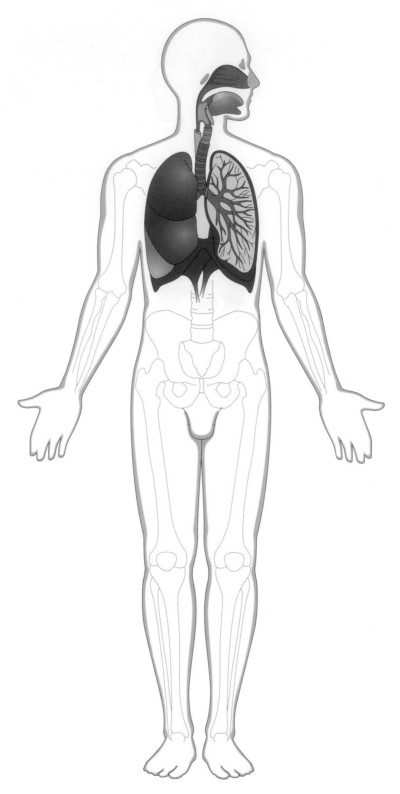

HUMAN RESPIRATORY SYSTEM. Air is breathed in through the nose or mouth, enters the pharynx (shown in orange), and passes through the larynx (shown as the green tube with a ridged texture; the smooth green tube is the esophagus, which is posterior to the larynx but is involved in digestion instead of breathing). The air then passes into the trachea (purple), which divides into two tubes called bronchi. One bronchus passes into each lung and continues to branch within the lung. These branches are called bronchioles, and each bronchiole leads to a tiny cluster of air sacs called alveoli. This is where the air and gases breathed in get diffused to the blood. The lungs (deep blue) are spongy and can be affected by Lung cancer, both the non-small cell and small-cell types. *(Illustration by Argosy Publishing. © Cengage Learning®.)*

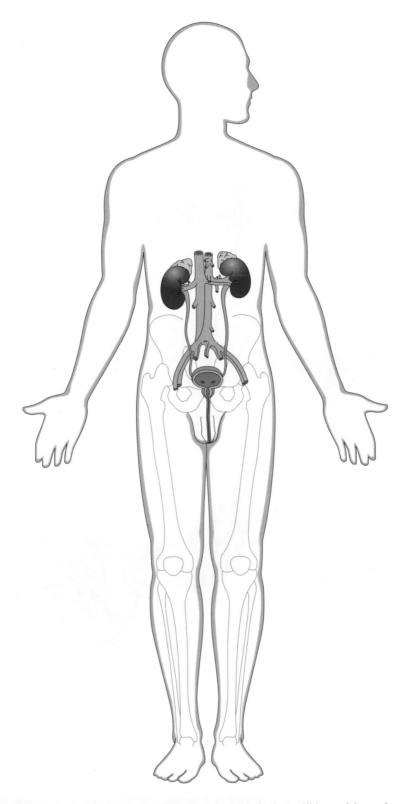

HUMAN URINARY SYSTEM. Organs and cancers of the urinary system include: Kidneys (shown in purple): Kidney cancer; Renal pelvis tumors; Wilms tumor. Ureters are shown in green. Bladder (blue-green): Bladder cancer. The kidneys, bladder, or ureters can be affected by Transitional cell carcinoma. *(Illustration by Argosy Publishing. © Cengage Learning®.)*

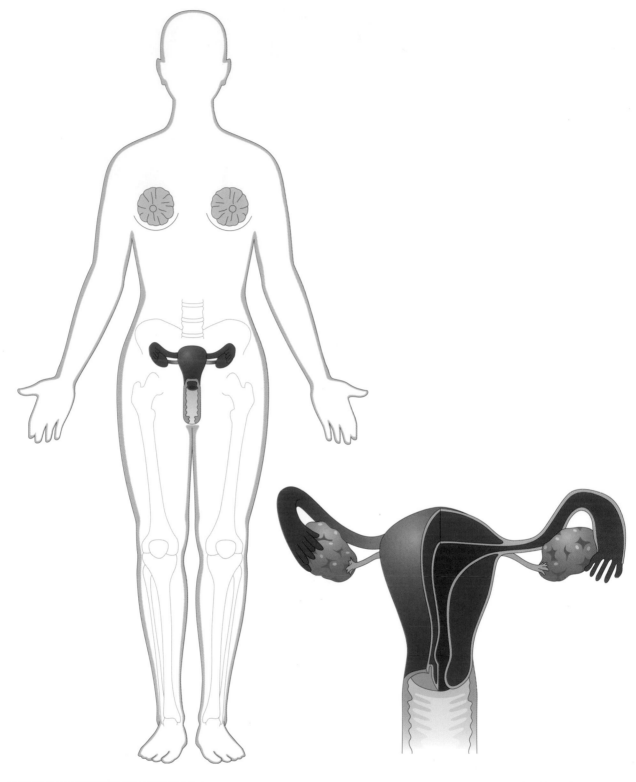

FEMALE REPRODUCTIVE SYSTEM. Organs and cancers of the female reproductive system include: Uterus, shown in red with the uterine or Fallopian tubes: Endometrial cancer. Ovaries (blue): Ovarian cancer. Vagina (shown in pink with a yellow interior or lining): Vaginal cancer. Breasts: Breast cancer; Paget disease of the breast. Shown in detailed inset only (in turquoise), Cervix: Cervical cancer. *(Illustration by Argosy Publishing. © Cengage Learning®.)*

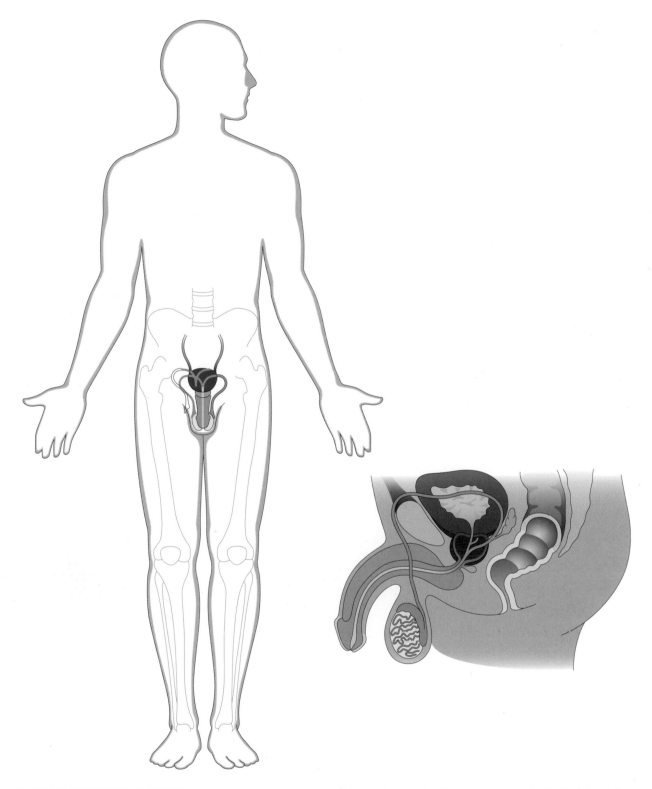

MALE REPRODCTIVE SYSTEM. Organs, glands, and cancers of the male reproductive system include: Penis (shown in pink): Penile cancer. Testes (shown in yellow): Testicular cancer. Prostate gland (shown in full-body illustration in a peach/apricot color, and in the inset as the dark blue gland between the bladder and the penis): Prostate cancer. *(Illustration by Argosy Publishing. © Cengage Learning®.)*

P

Paget disease of the breast

Definition

Paget disease of the breast is a rare type of **breast cancer** that is characterized by a red, scaly lesion on the nipple and surrounding tissue (areola).

Description

Paget disease of the breast, also called mammary Paget disease, is a rare breast condition that is often associated with underlying breast **cancer**. It is believed that Paget disease of the breast occurs when invasive **carcinoma** or intraductal carcinoma (cancer of the milk ducts) spreads through the milk ducts to the nipple.

Although in most cases the underlying breast cancer is extensive, in 10% of the cases, cancer affects only the nipple and surrounding tissue. Rarely, there is no detectable underlying breast cancer. Paget disease located elsewhere on the body (extramammary Paget disease) is rarely associated with an underlying invasive cancer. This type of Paget disease, most commonly found on and around the genitals, is believed to arise directly from the cells lining certain sweat gland ducts. The few cases of mammary Paget disease without an underlying breast cancer may have a similar origin.

Paget disease of the breast accounts for 2% of all breast cancers. On average, women are 62 years old and men are 69 years old at diagnosis. Breast cancer, however, rarely occurs in men.

Causes and symptoms

The causes of Paget disease of the breast are unknown. The most common signs and symptoms of Paget disease include redness, scaling, and flaking on and around the nipple and areola. Other symptoms include **itching**, tingling, burning, oversensitivity, or pain. The lesion may bleed or weep, and open sores (ulcers) may be present.

Diagnosis

A thorough breast examination would be performed. A breast mass can be felt (palpated) in about half of the women with Paget disease. **Mammography** and **ultrasonography** should be conducted to look for cancer within the breast that cannot be felt.

The definitive diagnosis of Paget disease is the presence of certain cells called Paget cells in the skin of the nipple. A tissue sample may be easily obtained by touching a microscope slide to a weeping lesion or by scraping a scaly or crusted lesion gently with a microscope slide. Alternatively, a sample of the lesion may be obtained by cutting out a small piece of nipple tissue (**biopsy**). The biopsy is performed with local anesthetic in the physician's office. If a mass was felt, a breast biopsy would be performed.

Treatment

The traditional treatment of Paget disease of the breast is to surgically remove the breast (**mastectomy**). Conservative surgery (nipple-areolar sacrificing **lumpectomy**), in which just the nipple, areola, and underlying tissue are removed, may be sufficient in some cases. The underarm (axillary) lymph nodes are rarely sampled or removed (lymphadenectomy) unless an underlying invasive cancer is a concern.

Radiation therapy may be used as adjuvant therapy to complement the surgical treatment; if a lumpectomy is performed, radiation must be employed. Radiation therapy uses high-energy radiation from x-rays and gamma rays to kill the cancer cells. The skin in the treated area may become red and dry; **fatigue** is also a common side effect.

Chemotherapy, also used as adjuvant therapy if an underlying invasive breast cancer is found, uses drugs to kill the cancer cells. The side effects of chemotherapy include stomach upset, vomiting, appetite loss (**anorexia**), hair loss (**alopecia**), mouth or vaginal sores, fatigue, menstrual cycle changes, premature menopause, and low white blood cell counts with an increased risk of infection.

Alternative and complementary therapies

Although alternative and complementary therapies are used by many cancer patients, very few controlled studies on the effectiveness of such therapies exist. Mind-body techniques such as biofeedback, visualization, meditation, and yoga have not shown any effect in reducing cancer, but they can reduce stress and lessen some of the side effects of cancer treatments.

A few studies found an association between longer survival time and a diet high in beta-carotene and fruits. Acupuncture has been found to relieve chemotherapy-induced **nausea and vomiting** and reduce pain. In some studies, **mistletoe** has been shown to reduce tumor size, extend survival time, and enhance immune function. Other studies have failed to show a response to mistletoe treatment.

Prognosis

As with other breast cancers, the prognosis of Paget disease depends on the extent of the cancer and whether it has spread to the lymph nodes and other organs.

Paget disease alone

The survival rate of women with Paget disease of the breast alone is 99.5%.

Paget disease with invasive breast cancer

The prognosis for Paget disease and invasive cancer is based on the stage of the underlying breast cancer. Staging for breast cancer is as follows:

• Stage 1—The cancer is no larger than 2 cm (0.8 in) and no cancer cells are found in the lymph nodes.

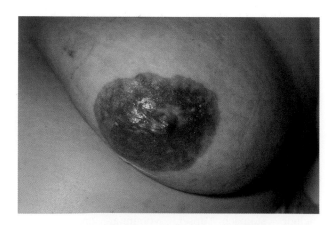

Nipple of a patient with Paget disease of the breast.
(Dr. M.A. Ansary/Science Source)

• Stage 2—The cancer is between 2 cm and 5 cm, and the cancer has spread to the lymph nodes.

• Stage 3A—Tumor is larger than 5 cm (2 in) or is smaller than 5 cm, but has spread to the lymph nodes, which have grown into each other.

• Stage 3B—Cancer has spread to tissues near the breast (local invasion) or to lymph nodes inside the chest wall along the breastbone.

• Stage 4—Cancer has spread to skin and lymph nodes beyond the axilla (regional lymph nodes) or to other organs of the body.

The prognosis depends on the type and stage of cancer. Over 80% of stage I patients are cured by current therapies. Stage II patients survive overall about 70% of the time, those with more extensive lymph nodal involvement having a poorer prognosis than those with disease confined to the breast. About 40% of stage III patients survive five years, and about 20% of stage IV patients do so.

Prevention

There are no specific factors that increase a person's risk of developing Paget disease. Men who are at an increased risk of developing breast cancer include those who have had radiation exposure and those with Klinefelter's syndrome. Women's risk factors for breast cancer include:

• a personal history of breast cancer

• a family history of breast cancer

• alterations in certain genes (e.g., *BRCA1* and *BRCA2*)

• changes in breast tissue (e.g., lobular carcinoma in situ or atypical hyperplasia)

QUESTIONS TO ASK YOUR DOCTOR

- What type of cancer do I have?
- What stage of cancer do I have?
- What is the five-year survival rate for women with this type and stage of cancer?
- Has the cancer spread?
- What are my treatment options?
- How much breast tissue will you remove?
- Where will the scars be?
- What will my breast look like after surgery?
- Should I have breast reconstruction?
- What are the risks and side effects of these treatments?
- What medications can I take to relieve treatment side effects?
- Are there any clinical studies under way that would be appropriate for me?
- What effective alternative or complementary treatments are available for this type of cancer?
- How debilitating is the treatment? Will I be able to continue working?
- Are there any local support groups for breast cancer patients?
- What is the chance that the cancer will recur?
- Is there anything I can do to prevent recurrence?
- How often will I have follow-up examinations?

- long-term exposure to estrogen (e.g., early age at first menstruation or late menopause), and possibly use of hormone replacement therapy
- exposure to diethylstilbestrol (DES) before birth
- first pregnancy after 30 years of age
- alcohol consumption

Regularly scheduled screening mammograms are recommended for all women over the age of 40 years. Those with a significant family history (one or more first-degree relatives who have been treated for breast cancer), should start annual mammograms 10 years younger than the youngest relative was when she was diagnosed, but not earlier than 35. Monthly breast self examinations and yearly clinical breast examinations are recommended for all women. Daily exercise, totalling two to four hours a week, decreases a woman's risk of breast cancer by 50% to 75%. Women with a high risk of breast cancer may take the drug **tamoxifen**, which has been shown to reduce the occurrence (or recurrence) of breast cancer. Women at a very high risk may choose to have a mastectomy to prevent breast cancer (prophylactic mastectomy).

Special concerns

Of special concern to the young woman with breast cancer is the impact that treatment will have on her fertility and **body image**. **Depression** is common. There is ongoing research investigating whether timing breast cancer surgery to coincide with the luteal phase (after ovulation) of the menstrual cycle leads to an increased survival rate.

Resources

PERIODICALS

Lim, H.S., Jeong, S.J., Lee, J.S., Park, M.H., Kim, J.W., Shin, S.S., Park, J.G., Kang, H.K. "Paget Disease of the Breast: Mammographic, US, and MR Imaging Findings With Pathologic Correlation." *Radiographics* 31, no. 7 (2011): 1973–87. http://pubs.rsna.org/doi/full/10.1148/rg.317115070 (accessed November 10, 2014).

WEBSITES

Cancer Research UK. "Paget's Disease of the Breast." http://www.cancerresearchuk.org/about-cancer/type/breast-cancer/about/types/pagets-disease (accessed November 10, 2014).

National Cancer Institute. "Paget Disease of the Breast." http://www.cancer.gov/cancertopics/factsheet/Sites-Types/paget-breast (accessed November 10, 2014).

ORGANIZATIONS

American Cancer Society, 250 Williams St. NW, Atlanta, GA 30303, (800) 227-2345, http://www.cancer.org.

Breastcancer.org, 7 E. Lancaster Ave., 3rd Fl., Ardmore, PA 19003, (610) 642-6550, Fax: (610) 642-6559, http://www.breastcancer.org.

National Cancer Institute, 9609 Medical Center Dr., BG 9609 MSC 9760, Bethesda, MD 20892-9760, (800) 4-CANCER (422-6237), http://www.cancer.gov.

Belinda Rowland, PhD

Pain management

Definition

Pain management in **cancer** care includes pharmacological, psychological, and spiritual approaches to prevent, reduce, or halt pain from cancer and its treatments.

KEY TERMS

Acute—Short-term pain in response to injury or other stimulus that resolves when the injury heals or the stimulus is removed.

Adjuvant—A treatment or therapy in addition to the primary treatment, such as other medications in addition to an opioid for cancer pain.

Analgesic—Any drug that provides pain relief without unconsciousness.

Central nervous system (CNS)—The brain and spinal cord.

Chronic—Pain that endures beyond the term of an injury or painful stimulus, including cancer pain.

Cytokines—Proteins that regulate immune responses and mediate intercellular communication.

Endorphins—A class of peptides in the brain that bind to opiate receptors, resulting in pleasant feelings and pain relief.

Hepatic capsule—The membranous bag enclosing the liver.

Metastasis—Spread of cancer from a primary tumor to other parts of the body.

Narcotic—A drug that dulls senses and relieves pain, but that in excessive doses causes stupor, coma, or convulsions.

Neuropathic—Referring to nerve pain.

Neurotransmitters—Nervous system chemicals that transmit information between nerve cells.

Nociceptor—A nerve cell that senses pain and transmits pain signals.

Nonpharmacological—Therapy that does not involve drugs.

Nonsteroidal anti-inflammatory drugs (NSAIDs)—Over-the-counter and prescription medications for reducing pain and inflammation.

Opioids—Natural, semi-synthetic, or synthetic narcotics for managing moderate to severe pain.

Palliative—Relieving or alleviating symptoms such as pain without curing the disease.

Peripheral nervous system (PNS)—Nerves outside the brain and spinal cord.

Pharmacological—Therapy that relies on drugs.

Prostaglandins—A group of fatty-acid metabolites that perform a variety of hormone-like functions, including augmenting pain perception.

Radiation—Cancer treatment with x-rays or other sources of ionizing radiation.

Somatic pain—Localized pain such as bone pain from cancer metastases.

Tolerance—The requirement for increasingly higher doses of a substance, such as an opioid, to achieve the same effect.

Virtual reality—The creation of a convincing visual and auditory environment by computer technology for pain management in children.

Visceral pain—Pain caused by activation of nociceptors in internal organs, such as those of the chest, abdomen, or pelvis.

Purpose

Pain is a localized sensation ranging from mild discomfort to an unbearable, excruciating experience. It is, in its origins, a protective mechanism, designed to alert the brain to injury or disease. Once the pain message has been received and interpreted by the brain, further pain can be counterproductive. Unfortunately, once the cause of the pain is identified, such as in diagnosed cancer, and treatment is initiated, pain often continues. Pain has a negative impact on quality of life, causing **depression** and impeding recovery. Unrelieved pain can become a syndrome in itself and cause a downward spiral in health and outlook. Proper pain management facilitates recovery, prevents additional health complications, and improves quality of life.

About 70% of cancer patients experience pain at some point during the course of their disease. Between 30% and 40% of patients undergoing cancer treatment report pain, and 70%–90% of patients with advanced cancer have pain. The U.S. Joint Commission on Accreditation of Healthcare Organizations and the American Pain Society have developed standards for proper pain management. However, fewer than 50% of cancer patients receive adequate pain management. U.S. studies have found that women and minorities are less likely than Caucasian males to receive adequate pain management. Studies have also shown that pain in cancer survivors often goes unreported, unrecognized, or inadequately managed. Furthermore, according to the World Health Organization (WHO), in most parts of the world, the majority of cancer patients are not presented for treatment until their cancers are advanced, and pain management is the only treatment possible. However, in most developing countries, cancer pain management is limited by national drug laws that severely restrict access to opioid pain medications. Cancer pain relief can also be limited by geographical barriers, medical infrastructure, and financial resources. The WHO estimates that more than 80% of the global population have little or no access to opioid analgesics (painkillers) to manage cancer pain.

Description

Pain management has been a major concern since ancient times. By 400 BCE, Hippocrates, the father of medicine, had theorized that the brain, not the heart, was the controlling center of the body, and Greek anatomists had begun to identify various nerves and their purposes. The pain-relieving properties of the opium poppy were utilized to relieve suffering. Two thousand years ago in China, acupuncture was used to treat pain.

What is pain?

Pain is the means by which the peripheral nervous system (PNS) warns the central nervous system (CNS) of injury or potential injury to the body. The CNS comprises the brain and spinal cord, and the PNS is composed of the nerves that stem from and lead into the CNS. Pain messages are transmitted to the CNS by special PNS nerve cells called nociceptors. Nociceptors are distributed throughout the body and respond to different stimuli depending on their location. For example, nociceptors that extend from the skin are stimulated by sensations such as pressure, temperature, and chemical changes. When a nociceptor is stimulated, neurotransmitters are released to transmit the signal to nerve cells within the spinal cord, which convey the pain message to the thalamus, a specific region in the brain.

Once the brain has received and processed the pain message and coordinated an appropriate response, pain has served its purpose. The body's natural painkillers, called endorphins, are meant to derail further pain messages from the same source. However, endorphins may not adequately dampen a continuing pain message. Furthermore, depending on how the brain has processed the pain information, certain hormones, such as prostaglandins, may be released. These hormones enhance the pain message and play a role in immune system responses to injury and inflammation. Certain neurotransmitters, especially substance P and **calcitonin** gene-related peptide, actively enhance the pain message at the injury site and within the spinal cord.

Researchers hypothesize that uninterrupted and unrelenting pain can induce changes in the spinal cord. Intractable pain that cannot be relieved or managed is sometimes treated by severing nerve connections to the CNS. However, the lack of sensory information from that nerve can cause pain transmission in the spinal cord to go into overdrive, as evidenced by phantom limb pain experienced by amputees. Evidence is accumulating that unrelenting pain or the complete lack of nerve signals increases the number of pain receptors in the spinal cord. Nerve cells in the spinal cord may also begin secreting pain-amplifying neurotransmitters independent of actual pain signals from the body. Immune chemicals, primarily cytokines, may play a prominent role in such changes.

What is cancer pain?

The majority of cancer pain results from a cancerous tumor pressing on organs, nerves, or bone. However, studies by pain pioneer Dr. John Bonica and others have shown that although 78% of all cancer pain is indeed related to the disease, 19% is caused by cancer treatment (3% of pain complaints were unrelated to either the disease or treatment).

Cancer pain is generally classified in three categories:

- *visceral pain*, usually caused by pressure resulting from the invasiveness of the tumor, expansion of the hepatic capsule, or injury caused by radiation or chemotherapy
- *somatic pain*, often resulting from bone metastasis
- *neuropathic pain* caused by the pressure of a tumor on nerves or trauma to nerves by radiation, chemotherapy, or surgery

Managing cancer pain

PHARMACOLOGICAL. The WHO has developed an "analgesic ladder" for cancer pain relief:

- Step 1 for patients with mild-to-moderate pain is a nonopioid analgesic, such as acetaminophen (Tylenol), or a nonsteroidal anti-inflammatory drug (NSAID), and an adjuvant drug if indicated. NSAIDs and acetaminophen are available in over-the-counter and prescription strengths and are frequently the initial pharmacological treatment. NSAIDs include aspirin, ibuprofen (Motrin, Advil), and naproxen (Aleve). NSAIDs treat pain from inflammation and block the production of pain-enhancing neurotransmitters, such as prostaglandins. Acetaminophen is effective against pain, but its ability to reduce inflammation is limited. NSAIDs and acetaminophen are effective for most forms of acute (sharp, short-lasting) pain. Adjuvant drugs for mild-to-moderate pain include a milder opioid medication combined with acetaminophen or an NSAID. Opioids include natural and semi-synthetic opiates, such as morphine and codeine, and synthetic drugs based on opium, including oxycodone (OxyContin) and methadone. Opioids provide pain relief by binding to specific opioid receptors in the brain and spinal cord to block pain perception.
- Step 2—for patients with moderate-to-severe pain or who failed to achieve adequate pain relief in step 1—is

an opioid typically used for moderate pain, a nonopioid analgesic, such as acetaminophen or an NSAID, and an adjuvant drug as indicated.

• Step 3—for patients with severe pain or who failed to achieve adequate pain relief in step 2—is an opioid typically used for severe pain and possibly a nonopioid analgesic and/or adjuvant drug.

Morphine is sometimes referred to as the "gold standard" of palliative care, because it is inexpensive, its dose can be gradually increased, and it is highly effective over a long period of time. It can be administered orally (by mouth), rectally, or by injection. Morphine and other **opioids** can also be administered by an implanted patient-controlled delivery system. By pressing a button, the patient releases a set dose of medication into an intravenous solution or an implanted catheter. Some implanted catheters deliver pain medication directly to the spinal cord. Implantable pumps have greatly improved pharmacological approaches to pain management. They not only provide more effective pain relief, but may actually reduce doses, as well as side effects and complications associated with long-term opioid use.

Antidepressant drugs can be effective in combating cancer pain, chronic headaches, and pain associated with nerve damage. Antidepressants that have analgesic properties include **amitriptyline**, trazodone, and imipramine. Anticonvulsants developed to treat epilepsy may also relieve pain. Drugs such as **phenytoin** (Dilantin) and **carbamazepine** are prescribed to treat pain associated with nerve damage.

Close monitoring is required to ensure adequate dosing for pain relief. Once a patient is comfortable with a certain dosage, oncologists typically convert to a long-acting version. Transdermal fentanyl patches are an example of a long-acting opioid commonly used for cancer pain management. A patch containing the drug is applied to the skin, and the drug is continuously absorbed by the body. Research is under way to develop substances that act selectively on nerve cells that carry pain messages to the brain.

NONPHARMACOLOGICAL. Pain treatment options that do not involve drugs are often used as adjuncts to, rather than replacements for, drug therapy. One of the benefits of nondrug therapies is that the patient has a more active role. Relaxation techniques, such as yoga and meditation, are used to shift the focus of the brain away from the pain, decrease muscle tension, and reduce stress. Tension and stress can also be reduced through biofeedback, in which the patient consciously attempts to modify skin temperature, muscle tension, blood pressure, and heart rate. Hypnosis-like approaches—particularly guided imagery, relaxation techniques, and hypnotic suggestion—

may be more effective in managing pain than other behavioral approaches.

Other approaches to pain management include:

• acupuncture—the insertion of small needles into the skin at key points, usually on the ear for treating cancer pain

• acupressure—applying pressure to the same key acupuncture points, perhaps causing the release of endorphins

• heat application and massage, which are relaxing and help reduce stress

• transcutaneous electrical nerve stimulation (TENS)—medically supervised application of a weak electric current to certain parts of nerves, potentially interrupting pain signals and inducing endorphin release

• virtual reality for managing cancer pain in children by diverting their attention from the pain and accompanying anxiety

Participating in normal activities and exercising can help control pain levels. **Physical therapy** can teach patients beneficial exercises for reducing stress, strengthening muscles, and staying fit. Regular exercise has also been linked to endorphin production.

Preparation

The U.S. Veterans Administration has called pain "the fifth vital sign" (after temperature, pulse, respiration, and blood pressure). Assessment of cancer pain is essential for pain management. Pain scales or questionnaires are sometimes used as an objective measure of a subjective experience. Objective measurements enable healthcare workers to better understand pain experienced by the patient. Pain evaluation also includes physical examinations and diagnostic tests to determine the underlying cause of pain. Some evaluations require assessments from several specialties, including neurology, psychiatry or psychology, and physical therapy.

Risks

Owing to their long-term toxicity, even nonprescription drugs must be carefully monitored in chronic pain management. NSAIDs can cause gastrointestinal bleeding, and long-term use of acetaminophen has been linked to kidney and liver damage. Other drugs, especially narcotics, have side effects such as constipation, drowsiness, and nausea. Sedation can often be reduced by medication timing, such as taking the drug at bedtime. Constipation can be reduced by increasing fruits, vegetables, and whole grains in the diet or by the use of **laxatives**, stool softeners, or enemas. Antidepressants and anticonvulsants may cause serious side effects, which may discourage or prevent their use. These side effects include mood swings, confusion, bone thinning, cataract formation, increased blood pressure, and other problems.

A traditional concern about narcotic use has been the risk of promoting tolerance or addiction. When narcotics are used over time, as for terminal cancer, the body becomes accustomed to the drug and adjusts normal functioning to accommodate the drug. As tolerance develops, the dosage must be increased to elicit the same degree of pain relief. Alternatively, a different medication or formulation can be prescribed. Proper dosage and prescribed uses of narcotic medications by cancer patients have been repeatedly shown to not cause addiction. However, abruptly stopping an opioid medication or reducing the dose can cause withdrawal—a potentially serious medical condition characterized by agitation, rapid heart rate, profuse sweating, and sleeplessness. Gradually reducing the dosage so that the body has time to adjust prevents withdrawal symptoms.

Of greater concern for cancer patients than tolerance or addiction to opioids is inadequate pain treatment. A survey published in 2012 of more than 3,000 patients with invasive breast, prostate, lung, and colorectal cancers, in both academic medical centers and community-based hospitals, reported that more than two-thirds reported pain or required analgesics at their first oncology appointments, and one-third were inadequately treated for their pain, including about 40% with moderate-to-severe pain. Furthermore, 20% of patients with severe pain received no pain medication at all. At four- to five-week follow-up visits with oncologists, patients reported little improvement in pain management. Minority patients were almost twice as likely as Caucasian patients to receive inadequate pain management. The study also found inadequate pain management in patients with earlier-stage cancer. Only one in six oncologists in the study reported that they frequently referred patients to pain-management or palliative-care specialists. The study concluded that physicians, nurses, and other healthcare staff require more training in pain management.

Nonpharmacological therapies are generally risk-free. However, patients recovering from serious illness or injury should consult with their healthcare providers or physical therapists before using adjunct therapies. Invasive procedures carry risks similar to other surgical procedures, such as infection, reaction to anesthesia, iatrogenic injury (injury as a result of treatment), and heart failure.

Results

Effective pain management techniques reduce or eliminate cancer pain, improve quality of life, and aid in recovery. The Bill of Rights for Cancer Pain includes:

QUESTIONS TO ASK YOUR DOCTOR

- Does my type of cancer usually cause pain? If so, how will my pain be treated?
- Will my radiation or chemotherapy treatments cause pain?
- What are the side effects of my pain medications?
- What can I do to help with my pain management?
- Does pain indicate that my cancer is progressing or responding to treatment?

- the right to be believed about the severity of pain
- the right to have pain controlled
- the right to have pain resulting from treatments and procedures prevented or minimized
- the right to be treated with respect at all times with regard to required medication and to not be regarded as a drug abuser

Resources

BOOKS

Bourke, Joanna. *The Story of Pain: From Prayer to Painkillers*. New York: Oxford University, 2014.

Colvin, Lesley, and Marie Fallon, eds. *ABC of Pain*. Hoboken, NJ: Wiley-Blackwell/BMJ, 2012.

Foltz-Gray, Dorothy. *Make Pain Disappear: Proven Strategies to Get the Relief You Need*. New York: Reader's Digest, 2012.

Gaguski, Michele E., and Susan D. Bruce. *Cancer Pain Management Scenarios*. Pittsburgh, PA: Oncology Nursing Society, 2013.

Hanna, Magdi, and Zbigniew Zylicz. *Cancer Pain*. London: Springer, 2013.

Hester, Joan, Nigel Sykes, and Sue Peat. *Interventional Pain Control in Cancer Pain Management*. New York: Oxford University, 2012.

Sharma, Manohar. *Practical Management of Complex Cancer Pain*. Oxford: Oxford University, 2014.

Washington, Tabitha A., Khalilah Brown, and Gilbert Fanciullo. *Pain*. New York: Oxford University, 2012.

PERIODICALS

Brody, Jane E. "The Treatment That Respects Pain." *New York Times* (December 3, 2013): D7.

Peterson, Mary Ann. "Should I Consider Acupuncture?" *Natural Solutions* 157 (October 2013): 54–55.

Schwartz, Saul. "Through Six Seasons, I Did What I Could for My Wife. It Wasn't Enough." *Washington Post* (February 18, 2014): E1.

OTHER

"Guide to Controlling Cancer Pain." American Cancer Society. June 10, 2014. http://www.cancer.org/acs/groups/cid/documents/webcontent/002906-pdf.pdf (accessed October 12, 2014).

WEBSITES

"Many Patients with Cancer Need Better Treatments for Pain." National Cancer Institute. May 9, 2012. http://www.cancer.gov/cancertopics/coping/physicaleffects/pain-mx-survey0412 (accessed October 12, 2014).

"Pain (PDQ)." National Cancer Institute. April 10, 2014. http://www.cancer.gov/cancertopics/pdq/supportivecare/pain/Patient (accessed October 12, 2014).

"Pain Control: Support for People with Cancer." National Cancer Institute. May 16, 2014. http://www.cancer.gov/cancertopics/coping/paincontrol (accessed October 12, 2014).

ORGANIZATIONS

American Cancer Society, 250 Williams Street NW, Atlanta, GA 30303, (800) 227-2345, http://www.cancer.org.

American Pain Society, 8735 West Higgins Road, Suite 300, Chicago, IL 60631, (847) 375-4715, info@americanpainsociety.org, http://www.americanpainsociety.org.

Joint Commission, 1 Renaissance Boulevard, Oakbrook Terrace, IL 60181, (630) 792-5000, Fax: (630) 792-5005, webmaster@jointcommission.org, http://www.jointcommission.org.

National Cancer Institute, 6116 Executive Boulevard, Suite 300, Bethesda, MD 20892-8322, (800) 4-CANCER (422-6237), http://www.cancer.gov.

Julia Barrett
Rebecca J. Frey, PhD
REVISED BY MARGARET ALIC, PhD
REVIEWED BY KEVIN GLAZA, RPh

Palliative cancer therapy *see* **Cancer therapy, palliative**

Pamidronate *see* **Bisphosphonates**

Pancreatectomy

Definition

A pancreatectomy is the surgical removal of the pancreas. A pancreatectomy may be total, in which case the entire organ is removed, usually along with the spleen, gallbladder, common bile duct, and portions of the small intestine and stomach. A pancreatectomy may also be distal, meaning that only the body and tail of the pancreas are removed, leaving the head of the organ attached. When the duodenum is removed along with all or part of the pancreas, the procedure is called a pancreaticoduodenectomy, which surgeons sometimes refer to as the **Whipple procedure**. Pancreaticoduodenectomies are increasingly used to treat a variety of malignant and benign diseases of the pancreas. This procedure often involves removal of the regional lymph nodes as well.

Purpose

A pancreatectomy is the most effective treatment for **cancer** of the pancreas, an abdominal organ that secretes digestive enzymes, insulin, and other hormones. The thickest part of the pancreas near the duodenum (a part of the small intestine) is called the head, the middle part is called the body, and the thinnest part adjacent to the spleen is called the tail.

While surgical removal of tumors in the pancreas is the preferred treatment, it is possible only in the 10%–15% of patients who are diagnosed early enough for a potential cure. Patients who are considered suitable for surgery usually have small tumors in the head of the pancreas (close to the duodenum, or first part of the small intestine), have jaundice as their initial symptom, and have no evidence of metastatic disease (spread of cancer to other sites). The stage of the cancer will determine whether the pancreatectomy to be performed should be total or distal.

A partial pancreatectomy may be indicated when the pancreas has been severely injured by trauma, especially injury to the body and tail of the pancreas. While such surgery removes normal pancreatic tissue as well, the long-term consequences of this surgery are minimal, with virtually no effects on the production of insulin, digestive enzymes, and other hormones.

Chronic pancreatitis is another condition for which a pancreatectomy is occasionally performed. Chronic pancreatitis—or continuing inflammation of the pancreas that results in permanent damage to this organ—can develop from long-standing recurrent episodes of acute (periodic) pancreatitis. This painful condition usually results from alcohol abuse or the presence of gallstones. In most patients with the alcohol-induced disease, the pancreas is widely involved; therefore, surgical correction is almost impossible.

Description

A pancreatectomy can be performed through an open surgery technique, in which case one large incision is made, or it can be performed laparoscopically, in which case the surgeon makes four small incisions to insert tube-like surgical instruments. The abdomen is filled with gas, usually carbon dioxide, to help the surgeon view the abdominal cavity. A camera is inserted

KEY TERMS

Chemotherapy—A cancer treatment that uses synthetic drugs to destroy the tumor either by inhibiting the growth of the cancerous cells or by killing the cancer cells.

Computed tomography (CT) scan—An imaging technique that creates a series of pictures of areas inside the body taken from different angles. The pictures are created by a computer linked to an x-ray machine.

Endoscopic retrograde cholangiopancreatography (ERCP)—A procedure to x-ray the ducts (tubes) that carry bile from the liver to the gallbladder and from the gallbladder to the small intestine.

Laparoscopy—A procedure in which a laparoscope (a thin, lighted tube) is inserted through an incision in the abdominal wall to determine whether the cancer is within the pancreas only or has spread to nearby tissues and whether it can be removed by surgery later. Tissue samples may be removed for biopsy.

Magnetic resonance imaging (MRI)—A procedure in which a magnet linked to a computer is used to create detailed pictures of areas inside the body.

Pancreas—A large gland located on the back wall of the abdomen, extending from the duodenum (first part of the small intestine) to the spleen. The pancreas produces enzymes essential for digestion and the hormones insulin and glucagon, which play a role in carbohydrate metabolism.

Pancreaticoduodenectomy—Removal of all or part of the pancreas along with the duodenum. Also known as Whipple's procedure or Whipple's operation.

Pancreatitis—Inflammation of the pancreas, either acute (sudden and episodic) or chronic, usually caused by excessive alcohol intake or gallbladder disease.

Positron emission tomography (PET) scan—An imaging system that creates a picture showing the location of tumor cells in the body. A substance called radionuclide dye is injected into a vein, and the PET scanner rotates around the body to create the picture. Malignant tumor cells appear brighter in the picture because they are more active and take up more dye than normal cells.

Radiation therapy—A treatment using high-energy radiation from x-ray machines, cobalt, radium, or other sources.

Ultrasonogram—A procedure in which inaudible high-frequency sound waves are bounced off internal organs and tissues. These sound waves produce a pattern of echoes that are then used by the computer to create sonograms, or pictures of areas inside the body.

through one of the tubes and displays images on a monitor in the operating room. Other instruments are placed through the additional tubes. The laparoscopic approach allows the surgeon to work inside the patient's abdomen without making a large incision.

If the pancreatectomy is partial, the surgeon clamps and cuts the blood vessels, and the pancreas is stapled and divided for removal. If the disease affects the splenic artery or vein, the spleen is also removed.

If the pancreatectomy is total, the surgeon removes the entire pancreas and attached organs. He or she starts by dividing and detaching the end of the stomach. This part of the stomach leads to the small intestine, where the pancreas and bile duct are both attached. In the next step, the surgeon removes the pancreas along with the connected section of the small intestine. The common bile duct and the gallbladder are also removed. To reconnect the intestinal tract, the stomach and the bile duct are then connected to the small intestine.

During a pancreatectomy procedure, several tubes are also inserted for postoperative care. To prevent tissue fluid from accumulating in the operated site, a temporary drain leading out of the body is inserted, as well as a gastrostomy or G-tube leading out of the stomach in order to help prevent **nausea and vomiting**. A jejunostomy or J-tube may also be inserted into the small intestine as a pathway for supplemental feeding.

Diagnosis

Patients with symptoms of a pancreatic disorder undergo a number of tests before surgery is even considered. These can include **ultrasonography**, x-ray examinations, **computed tomography** scans (CT scan), and **endoscopic retrograde cholangiopancreatography** (ERCP), a specialized imaging technique to visualize the ducts that carry bile from the liver to the gallbladder. Tests may also include **angiography**, another imaging technique used to visualize the arteries feeding the pancreas, and needle aspiration **cytology**, in which cells are drawn from areas suspected to contain cancer. Such tests are required to establish a correct diagnosis of the pancreatic disorder and in planning the surgery.

Preparation

If the patient has become undernourished, appropriate **nutritional support**—sometimes by tube feedings—may be required prior to surgery.

Some patients with pancreatic cancer deemed suitable for a pancreatectomy will also undergo **chemotherapy** and/or **radiation therapy**. This treatment is aimed at shrinking the tumor, which will improve the chances of successful surgical removal. Sometimes, patients who are not initially considered surgical candidates may respond so well to chemoradiation that surgical treatment becomes possible. Radiation therapy may also be applied during the surgery (intraoperatively) to improve the patient's chances of survival, but this treatment is not yet in routine use. Some studies have shown that intraoperative radiation therapy extends survival by several months.

Patients undergoing distal pancreatectomy that involves removal of the spleen may receive preoperative medication to decrease the risk of infection.

Aftercare

Pancreatectomy is major surgery. Therefore, extended hospitalization is usually required with an average hospital stay of two to three weeks.

Some pancreatic cancer patients may also receive combined chemotherapy and radiation therapy after surgery. This additional treatment has been clearly shown to enhance survival rates.

After surgery, patients may experience pain in the abdomen and will be prescribed pain medication. Follow-up exams are required to monitor the patient's recovery and remove implanted tubes.

A total pancreatectomy leads to a condition called pancreatic insufficiency, because food can no longer be processed with the enzymes normally produced by the pancreas. Insulin secretion is likewise no longer possible. These conditions are treated with pancreatic enzyme replacement therapy, which supplies digestive enzymes, and with insulin injections. In some cases, distal pancreatectomies may also lead to pancreatic insufficiency, depending on the patient's general health condition before surgery and on the extent of pancreatic tissue removal.

Risks

There is a fairly high risk of complications associated with any pancreatectomy procedure. A recent Johns Hopkins study documented complications in 41% of cases. The most devastating complication is postoperative bleeding, which increases the mortality risk to 20%–50%. In cases of postoperative bleeding, the patient may require another surgery to find the source of hemorrhage, or may undergo other procedures to stop the bleeding.

One of the most common complications from a pancreaticoduodenectomy is delayed gastric emptying, a condition in which food and liquids are slow to leave the stomach. This complication occurred in 19% of patients in the Johns Hopkins study. To manage this problem, many surgeons insert feeding tubes at the original operation site, through which nutrients can be fed directly into the patient's intestines. This procedure, called enteral nutrition, maintains the patient's nutrition if the stomach is slow to recover normal function. Certain medications called promotility agents can help move the nutritional contents through the gastrointestinal tract.

The other most common complication is pancreatic anastomotic leak. This is a leak in the connection that the surgeon makes between the remainder of the pancreas and the other structures in the abdomen. Most surgeons avoid this problem by checking the connection during surgery.

Results

After a total pancreatectomy, the body loses the ability to secrete insulin, enzymes, and other substances; therefore, the patient has to take supplements for the rest of his or her life.

Patients usually resume normal activities within a month after surgery, although they are asked to avoid heavy lifting for six to eight weeks and not to drive as long as they take narcotic medication.

When a pancreatectomy is performed for chronic pancreatitis, the majority of patients obtain some relief from pain. Some studies report that one-half to three-quarters of patients become free of pain.

Morbidity and mortality rates

The mortality rate for pancreatectomy has decreased in recent years to 5%–10%, depending on the extent of the surgery and the experience of the surgeon. A study of 650 patients at Johns Hopkins Medical Institution in Baltimore found that only nine patients, or 1.4%, died from complications related to surgery.

Unfortunately, pancreatic cancer is the most lethal form of gastrointestinal malignancy. However, for a

QUESTIONS TO ASK YOUR DOCTOR

- What do I need to do before surgery?
- What type of anesthesia will be used?
- How long will it take to recover from the surgery?
- When can I expect to return to work and/or resume normal activities?
- What are the risks associated with a pancreatectomy?
- How many pancreatectomies do you perform in a year?
- Will there be a scar?

highly selective group of patients, a pancreatectomy offers a chance for cure, especially when performed by experienced surgeons. The overall five-year survival rate for patients who undergo pancreatectomy for pancreatic cancer is about 10%; patients who undergo pancreatico-duodenectomy have a 4%–5% survival at five years. The risk of tumor recurrence is thought to be unaffected by whether the patient undergoes a total pancreatectomy or a pancreaticoduodenectomy, but it is increased when the tumor is larger than 1.2 in. (3 cm) and the cancer has spread to the lymph nodes or surrounding tissue.

Alternatives

Depending on the medical condition, a pancreas transplantation may be considered as an alternative for some patients.

Health care team roles

A pancreatectomy is performed by a surgeon trained in gastroenterology, the branch of medicine that deals with the diseases of the digestive tract. An anesthesiologist is responsible for administering anesthesia and the operation is performed in a hospital setting, with an oncologist on the treatment team if pancreatic cancer is present.

Resources

BOOKS

Bastidas, J. Augusto, and John E. Niederhuber. "The Pancreas." In *Fundamentals of Surgery*, edited by John E. Niederhuber. Stamford: Appleton & Lange, 1998.

Lillemoe, Keith D., and William R. Jarnagin, eds. *Hepatobiliary and Pancreatic Surgery*. Philadelphia: Lippincott Williams & Wilkins, 2013.

Longo, Dan, et al. *Harrison's Principles of Internal Medicine*. 18th ed. New York: McGraw-Hill, 2012.

PERIODICALS

Bhayani, Neil H., et al. "Morbidity of Total Pancreatectomy with Islet Cell Auto-Transplantation Compared to Total Pancreatectomy Alone." *HPB* (August 29, 2013): e-pub ahead of print. http://dx.doi.org/10.1111/hpb.12168 (accessed October 3, 2014).

Feng, W. M., et al. "Spleen-Preserving Distal Pancreatectomy: Perioperative and Long-Term Outcome Analysis." *Hepato-gastroenterology* 128, no. 60 (Nov–Dec 2013): 1881–84.

Kendal, Wayne S. "Pancreatectomy versus Conservative Management for Pancreatic Cancer: A Question of Lead-Time Bias." *American Journal of Clinical Oncology* (September 21, 2013): e-pub ahead of print. http://dx.doi.org/10.1097/COC.0b013e3182a533ea (accessed October 3, 2014).

WEBSITES

National Cancer Institute. "Pancreatic Cancer." http://www.cancer.gov/cancertopics/types/pancreatic (accessed October 3, 2014).

Pancreatic Cancer Action Network. "Learn about Pancreatic Cancer: Surgery." http://www.pancan.org/section_facing_pancreatic_cancer/learn_about_pan_cancer/treatment/surgery/index.php (accessed October 3, 2014).

ORGANIZATIONS

American College of Gastroenterology, 6400 Goldsboro Rd., Ste. 200, Bethesda, MD 20817, (301) 263-9000, info@acg.gi.org, http://gi.org.

American Gastroenterological Association, 4930 Del Ray Ave., Bethesda, MD 20814, (301) 654-2055, Fax: (301) 654-5920, member@gastro.org, http://www.gastro.org.

National Cancer Institute, 6116 Executive Blvd., Ste. 300, Bethesda, MD 20892-8322, (800) 4-CANCER (422-6237), http://cancer.gov.

Pancreatic Cancer Action Network, 1500 Rosecrans Ave., Ste. 200, Manhattan Beach, CA 90226, (310) 725-0025, (877) 272-6226, Fax: (310) 725-0029, info@pancan.org, http://www.pancan.org.

Caroline A. Helwick
Monique Laberge, PhD

Pancreatic cancer

Definition

There are two types of **cancer** of the pancreas. **Endocrine pancreatic cancer** is a disease in which cancerous cells originate within the tissues of the pancreas that produce hormones. **Exocrine pancreatic**

cancer is a disease in which cancerous cells originate within the tissues of the pancreas that produce digestive juices.

Description

The pancreas is a 6–8 in. (15–20 cm) long slipper-shaped gland located in the abdomen. It lies behind the stomach within a loop formed by the small intestine. Other nearby organs include the gallbladder, spleen, and liver. The pancreas has a wide end (head), a narrow end (tail), and a middle section (body). A healthy pancreas is important for normal food digestion and plays a critical role in the body's metabolic processes.

The pancreas has two main functions, each performed by distinct types of tissue. The exocrine pancreas secretes fluids into an intricate system of channels or ducts, which are tubular structures that carry pancreatic juices to the small intestine where they are used for digestion. The endocrine tissue secretes hormones and peptides (small protein molecules) that circulate in the bloodstream and affect other organs. The exocrine pancreas makes up the vast majority of the gland; it produces pancreatic juices containing enzymes that help break down proteins and fatty food. The endocrine tissue of the pancreas makes up only 2% of the gland's total mass. It consists of small patches of cells that produce hormones (such as insulin) that control how the body stores and uses nutrients. These patches are called islets (islands) of Langerhans or islet cells and are interspersed evenly throughout the pancreas. Each islet contains approximately 1,000 endocrine cells and a dense network of capillaries (tiny blood vessels) that allow immediate entry of hormones into the circulatory system.

Pancreatic tumors are classified as either exocrine or endocrine tumors depending on which type of tissue they arise from within the gland. Endocrine tumors of the pancreas are very rare, accounting for only 5% of all pancreatic cancers. The majority of endocrine pancreatic tumors are functional adenocarcinomas that overproduce a specific hormone. There are several types of islet cells, and each produces its own hormone or peptide (small protein molecule). Functional endocrine tumors are named after the hormone they secrete. Insulinoma is the most common tumor of the endocrine pancreas. Patients with this disease usually develop hypoglycemia due to increased insulin production that leads to abnormally low blood sugar levels. Gastrinoma, a disease in which gastrin (hormone that stimulates stomach acid production) is overproduced, causes multiple ulcers in the upper gastrointestinal (GI) tract. Gastrinoma was first described in patients with a rare form of severe peptic ulcer disease known as **Zollinger-Ellison syndrome** (ZES). The less common glucagonoma causes mild

diabetes due to excess glucagon (hormone that stimulates glucose production) secretion. Other rare islet cell tumors include vipoma (vasoactive intestinal peptide) and somatostatinoma. Nonfunctional pancreatic endocrine tumors are not associated with an excess production of any hormone and can be difficult to distinguish from exocrine pancreatic cancer. Cancers of the endocrine pancreas are relatively slow-growing compared to the more common ductal adenocarcinomas of the exocrine pancreas.

Ninety-five percent of pancreatic cancers occur in tissues of the exocrine pancreas. Ductal adenocarcinomas arise in the cells that line the ducts of the exocrine pancreas and account for 80%–90% of all tumors of the pancreas. Unless specified, nearly all reports on pancreatic cancer refer to ductal adenocarcinomas. Less common types of pancreatic exocrine tumors include acinar cell carcinomas, which are cystic tumors that are typically benign but may become cancerous, and papillary tumors that grow within the pancreatic ducts. Pancreatoblastoma is a very rare disease that primarily affects young children.

Two-thirds of pancreatic tumors occur in the head of the pancreas; tumor growth in this area can lead to the obstruction of the nearby common bile duct that empties bile fluid into the small intestine. When bile cannot be passed into the intestine, patients may develop yellowing of the skin and eyes (jaundice) due to the buildup of bilirubin (a component of bile) in the bloodstream. Tumor blockage of bile or pancreatic ducts may also cause digestive problems, because these fluids contain enzymes critical to the digestive process. Depending on their size, pancreatic tumors may cause abdominal pain by pressing on the surrounding nerves. Because of its location deep within the abdomen, pancreatic cancer often remains undetected until it has spread to other organs such as the liver or lung. Pancreatic cancer tends to spread rapidly to other organs, even when the primary (original) tumor is relatively small.

Risk factors

Although the exact cause for pancreatic cancer is not known, several risk factors have been shown to increase susceptibility to this particular cancer, the greatest of which is tobacco use, including smokeless tobacco. Approximately one-third of pancreatic cancer cases occur among smokers. In addition, people who have diabetes develop pancreatic cancer twice as often as nondiabetics. Numerous studies suggest that a family history of pancreatic cancer is another strong risk factor for developing the disease, particularly if two or more relatives in the immediate family have the disease. Other risk factors include chronic (long-term) inflammation of the pancreas (pancreatitis); diets high in fat; obesity; and occupational exposure to certain chemicals, such as petroleum.

Demographics

Exocrine cancer

Although pancreatic cancer accounts for only 3% of all cancers, it is the fourth most common cause of cancer deaths. The American Cancer Society estimated that approximately 42,420 cases of pancreatic cancer were diagnosed in the United States in 2014, and 39,590 people died from the disease.

Pancreatic cancer is primarily a disease associated with advanced age, with 80% of cases occurring between the ages of 60 and 80. Men are almost twice as likely to develop this disease as women. Countries with the highest frequencies of pancreatic cancer include the United States, New Zealand, Western European nations, and Scandinavia. The lowest occurrences of the disease are reported in India, Kuwait, and Singapore. African Americans have the highest rate of pancreatic cancer of any ethnic group worldwide. Whether this difference is due to diet, genetics, or environmental factors remains unclear.

Endocrine cancer

Between one and four cases of insulinoma occur per million people per year, and 90% of these tumors are benign (noncancerous). They occur mostly between the ages of 50 and 60 and affect men and women equally. Fewer than three cases of gastrinoma per million people are diagnosed each year, but gastrinomas are the most common functional islet cell tumor in patients with multiple endocrine tumors, a condition known as **multiple endocrine neoplasia** (MEN) syndrome. Vipoma and glucagonoma are even rarer, and they occur more frequently in women. Somatostatinoma is exceedingly uncommon; fewer than 100 cases have been reported worldwide. Nonfunctional islet cell cancers account for approximately one-third of all cancers of the endocrine pancreas, and the majority of these are malignant.

Causes and symptoms

The exact cause of most pancreatic cancers is unknown. Nevertheless, about 10% of cancers of the pancreas are attributable to specific gene mutations. These include:

- mutations in the *BRCA2* gene, which also predisposes women to breast and ovarian cancer
- mutations in the *CDKN2A* gene, which predisposes individuals to melanoma (aggressive skin cancer)

- mutations in the gene *PRSS1*, which predisposes individuals to pancreatitis
- mutations in multiple genes that predispose individuals to certain types of colorectal cancer
- mutations in the gene *STK1*, which predisposes individuals to digestive tract cancers

There are no known causes of islet cell cancer, but a small percentage of cases occur due to hereditary syndromes such as multiple endocrine neoplasia (MEN). This condition frequently causes more than one tumor in several endocrine glands, such as the parathyroid and pituitary, in addition to the islet cells of the pancreas. Twenty-five percent of gastrinomas and less than 10% of insulinomas occur in MEN patients. Von Hippel-Lindau (VHL) syndrome is another genetic disorder that causes multiple tumors; 10% to 15% of VHL patients will develop islet cell cancer.

Exocrine pancreatic cancer often does not produce symptoms until it reaches an advanced stage. Even then, many of the symptoms can also be caused by other diseases and disorders. Patients with exocrine pancreatic cancer may present with the following signs and symptoms:

- upper abdominal and/or back pain
- jaundice
- weight loss
- loss of appetite (anorexia)
- diarrhea
- weakness
- nausea

Symptoms of endocrine pancreatic cancer vary among the different islet cell cancer types. Insulinoma causes repeated episodes of hypoglycemia (low blood sugar), sweating, and tremors, while patients with gastrinoma have inflammation of the esophagus, epigastric pain, multiple ulcers, and possibly **diarrhea**. Symptoms of glucagonoma include a distinctive skin rash, inflammation of the stomach, glucose intolerance, **weight loss**, weakness, and **anemia** (less common). Patients with vipoma have episodes of profuse, watery diarrhea, even after fasting. Somatostatinoma causes mild diabetes, diarrhea/steatorrhea (fatty stools), weight loss, and gallbladder disease. Nonfunctional endocrine tumors frequently produce the same symptoms as cancer of the exocrine pancreas, such as abdominal pain, jaundice, and weight loss.

Diagnosis

Pancreatic cancer is difficult to diagnose, especially in the absence of symptoms, and as of 2014, there was no screening method sensitive enough for early detection. The most sophisticated techniques available often do not detect very small tumors that are localized (have not begun to spread). At advanced stages in which patients show symptoms, a number of tests may be performed to confirm a diagnosis and to assess the stage of the disease. Approximately half of all pancreatic cancers are metastatic (have spread to other sites) at the time of diagnosis.

The first step in diagnosing pancreatic cancer is a thorough medical history and complete physical examination. The abdomen will be palpated to check for fluid accumulation, lumps, or masses. If there are signs of jaundice, blood tests will be performed to rule out the possibility of liver diseases such as hepatitis. Urine and stool tests may be performed as well.

Tests

Noninvasive imaging tools such as high-resolution contrast-enhanced spiral **computed tomography** (CT) scans and **magnetic resonance imaging** (MRI) can be used to produce detailed pictures of the internal organs. CT is the tool most often used to diagnose pancreatic cancer, as it allows the doctor to determine whether the tumor can be removed by surgery. It is also useful in staging a tumor by showing the extent to which the tumor has spread. During a CT scan, patients receive an intravenous injection of a contrast dye so the organs can be visualized more clearly. MRI may be performed instead of CT if a patient has an allergy to the CT contrast dye. In some cases in which the tumor is impinging on blood vessels or nearby ducts, MRI may be used to generate an image of the pancreatic ducts.

If the doctor suspects pancreatic cancer and no visible masses are seen with a CT scan, a patient may undergo a combination of invasive tests to confirm the presence of a pancreatic tumor. Endoscopic ultrasound (EUS) involves the use of an ultrasound probe at the end of a long, flexible tube that is passed down the patient's throat and into the stomach. This instrument can detect a tumor mass through high-frequency sound waves and echoes. EUS can be accompanied by fine-needle aspiration (FNA), in which a long needle, guided by the ultrasound, is inserted into the tumor mass in order to take a **biopsy** sample. **Endoscopic retrograde cholangiopancreatography** (ERCP) is a technique often used in patients with severe jaundice because it enables the doctor to relieve blockage of the pancreatic ducts. The doctor, guided by endoscopy and **x-rays**, inserts a small metal or plastic stent into the duct to keep it open. During ERCP, a biopsy can be done by collecting cells from the pancreas with a small brush. The cells are then examined under the microscope by a pathologist, who determines the presence of any cancerous cells.

In some cases, a biopsy may be performed during a type of surgery called **laparoscopy**, which is done under general anesthesia. Doctors insert a small camera and instruments into the abdomen after a minor incision is made. Tissue samples are removed for examination under the microscope. This procedure allows a doctor to determine the extent to which the disease has spread and decide whether the tumor can be removed by further surgery.

An **angiography** is a type of test that studies the blood vessels in and around the pancreas. This test may be done before surgery so that the doctor can determine the extent to which the tumor invades and interacts with the blood vessels within the pancreas. The test requires local anesthesia due to the insertion of a catheter into the patient's upper thigh. A dye is then injected into blood vessels that lead into the pancreas, and x-rays are taken.

Functional endocrine tumors can occur in multiple sites in the pancreas and are often small, making them difficult to diagnose. Nonfunctional tumors tend to be larger, which makes them difficult to distinguish from tumors of the exocrine pancreas. Methods such as computed tomography (CT) scan and magnetic resonance imaging (MRI) are used to take pictures of the internal organs and allow the doctor to determine whether a tumor is present. Somatostatin receptor scintigraphy is an imaging system used to localize endocrine tumors, especially gastrinomas and somatostatinomas. Endoscopic ultrasound (EUS) is a more sensitive technique that may be used if a CT scan fails to detect a tumor. Endocrine tumors usually have many blood vessels, so angiography may be useful in the doctor's assessment and staging of the tumor. Surgical exploration is sometimes necessary in order to locate very small tumors that occur in multiple sites. These techniques also help the doctor evaluate how far the tumor has spread. A biopsy can be taken to confirm diagnosis, but more often, doctors look at the size and local invasion of the tumor in order to plan a treatment strategy.

Clinical staging

Exocrine cancer

After cancer of the pancreas has been diagnosed, doctors typically use a tumor/node/metastasis (TNM) staging system to classify the tumor based on its size and the degree to which it has spread to other areas in the body. T indicates the size and local advancement of the primary tumor. Since cancers often invade the lymphatic system before spreading to other organs, regional lymph node involvement (N) is an important factor in staging. M indicates whether the tumor has metastasized (spread) to distant organs. In stage I, the tumor is localized to the pancreas and has not spread to surrounding lymph nodes or other organs. Stage II pancreatic cancer has spread to nearby organs, such as the small intestine or bile duct, but not the surrounding lymph nodes. Stage III indicates lymph node involvement, regardless of whether the cancer has spread to nearby organs. Stage IVA pancreatic cancer has spread to organs near the pancreas such as the stomach, spleen, or colon. Stage IVB is a cancer that has spread to distant sites; for example, the liver and lungs. If pancreatic cancer has been treated with success and then appears again in the pancreas or in other organs, it is referred to as recurrent disease.

Endocrine cancer

The staging system for islet cell cancer is still evolving, but the tumors typically fall into three categories: cancers that arise in one location within the pancreas, cancers that arise in several locations within the pancreas, and cancers that have spread to nearby lymph nodes or to other organs in the body.

Treatment

Exocrine cancer

Treatment of pancreatic cancer will depend on several factors, including the stage of the disease and the patient's age and overall health status. A combination of therapies is often employed in the treatment of this disease to improve the patient's chances of survival.

SURGERY. Three types of surgery are used in the treatment of pancreatic cancer, depending on which section of the pancreas contains the tumor. A **Whipple procedure** removes the head of the pancreas, part of the small intestine, and some of the surrounding tissues. This procedure is the most common because the majority of pancreatic cancers occur in the head of the organ. A total **pancreatectomy** removes the entire pancreas and the organs around it. Distal pancreatectomy removes only the body and tail of the pancreas. **Chemotherapy** and radiation may precede surgery (neoadjuvant therapy) or follow surgery (adjuvant therapy). Surgery is also used to relieve symptoms of pancreatic cancer by draining fluids or bypassing obstructions. Side effects from surgery can include pain, weakness, **fatigue**, and digestive problems. Some patients may develop diabetes or malabsorption as a result of partial or total removal of the pancreas.

RADIATION THERAPY. Radiation therapy is sometimes used to shrink a tumor before surgery or to remove remaining cancer cells after surgery. Radiation may also be used to relieve pain or digestive problems caused by the tumor if it cannot be removed by surgery. External

radiation therapy refers to radiation applied externally to the abdomen using a beam of high-energy x-rays. High-dose intraoperative radiation therapy is sometimes used during surgery on tumors that have spread to nearby organs. Internal radiation therapy refers to the use of small radioactive seeds implanted in the tumor tissue. The seeds emit radiation over time to kill tumor cells. Radiation treatment may cause side effects such as fatigue, tender or itchy skin, nausea, vomiting, and digestive problems.

CHEMOTHERAPY. Chemotherapeutic agents are powerful drugs that are used to kill cancer cells. They are classified according to the mechanism by which they induce cancer cell death. Multiple agents are often used to increase the chances of tumor cell death. **Gemcitabine** is the standard drug used to treat pancreatic cancers; it can be used alone or in combination with other drugs, such as 5-fluorouracil (5-FU, or **fluorouracil**), oxaliplatin (Eloxatin), **irinotecan** (Camptosar) and albumin-bound paclitaxel (Abraxane). Chemotherapy may be administered orally or intravenously in a series of doses over several weeks. During treatment, patients may experience fatigue, nausea, vomiting, hair loss (**alopecia**), and mouth sores, depending on which drugs are used.

Endocrine cancer

Surgery is the only curative method for islet cell (endocrine) cancers, and studies have shown that an aggressive surgical approach can improve survival and alleviate symptoms of the disease. As with most forms of cancer, the earlier it is diagnosed, the greater the chance for survival. With the exception of insulinoma, the majority of islet cell tumors are malignant at the time of diagnosis, and more than half are metastatic. However, surgery and chemotherapy have been shown to improve the outcome of patients even if they have metastatic disease. Surgery may include partial or total removal of the pancreas; in patients with gastrinoma, the stomach may be removed as well. **Streptozocin, doxorubicin**, and 5-fluorouracil (5-FU, or fluorouracil) are chemotherapeutic agents commonly used in the treatment of islet cell cancer. Patients may experience **nausea and vomiting** as well as kidney toxicity from streptozocin, and bone marrow suppression from doxorubicin. Hormone therapy is used to relieve the symptoms of functional tumors by inhibiting excess hormone production. Other techniques may be used to block blood flow to the liver in an attempt to kill the cancer cells that have spread there. Abdominal pain, nausea, vomiting, and **fever** may result from this type of treatment. Radiation has little if any role in the treatment of islet cell cancer.

Alternative therapies

Acupuncture or hypnotherapy may be used in addition to standard therapies to help relieve the pain associated with pancreatic cancer. Because of the poor prognosis associated with pancreatic cancer, some patients may try special diets with vitamin supplements, certain exercise programs, or unconventional treatments not yet approved by the FDA. Patients should always inform their doctors of any alternative treatments they are using, as these could interfere with standard therapies.

Prognosis

Exocrine cancer

Cancer of the pancreas is often fatal; median survival from diagnosis is less than six months, while the overall five-year survival rate is 4%. The five-year survival rate by stage is as follows: stage IA, 37%; stage IB, 21%; stage IIA, 12%; stage IIB, 6%; stage III, 2%; stage IV, 1%. These statistics demonstrate the aggressive nature of most pancreatic cancers and their tendency to recur. Pancreatic cancers tend to be resistant to radiation and chemotherapy; these modes of treatment are mainly used to relieve pain and tumor burden (palliative care).

Endocrine cancer

Islet cell cancers overall have a more favorable prognosis than cancers of the exocrine pancreas, and the median survival from diagnosis is three-and-a-half years. This survival rate is mainly due to their slow-growing nature. Insulinomas have a five-year survival rate of 80% and gastrinomas have 65%. When malignant, islet cell cancers do not generally respond well to chemotherapy, and the treatment is mainly palliative. Most patients with **metastasis** do not survive five years. Islet cell cancer tends to spread to the surrounding lymph nodes, stomach, small intestine, and liver.

Prevention

Although the exact cause of pancreatic cancer is not known, there are certain risk factors that may increase a person's chances of developing the disease. Quitting smoking will certainly reduce the risk of pancreatic cancer and many other cancers. The American Cancer Society recommends a diet rich in fruits, vegetables, and dietary fiber in order to reduce the risk of pancreatic cancer. According to the **National Cancer Institute**, workers who are exposed to petroleum and other chemicals may be at greater risk of developing the disease and should follow their employer's safety precautions. People with a family history of pancreatic

---

QUESTIONS TO ASK YOUR DOCTOR

- What type of pancreatic cancer do I have?
- Do you have experience in treating this form of cancer?
- What is the standard course of treatment for my cancer at this stage?
- How long will the course of treatment take?
- What side effects will I experience?
- Am I at risk for developing other endocrine tumors?
- What can be done to relieve my abdominal pain?
- What should I do to prepare for surgery?
- Can you refer me to a nutritionist or dietitian?
- Are there any alternative therapies you would recommend?
- Am I eligible to participate in a clinical trial?
- Will my health insurance cover costs associated with a clinical trial?
- Are there any support groups I can join?

---

cancer are at greater risk than the general population, as a small percentage of pancreatic cancers are considered hereditary.

Special concerns

Pain control is probably the single greatest problem for patients with pancreatic cancer. As the cancer grows and spreads to other organs in the abdomen, it often presses on the surrounding network of nerves, which can cause considerable discomfort. In most cases, pain can be alleviated with analgesics or **opioids**.

Pancreatic cancer patients frequently have difficulty maintaining their weight because food may not taste good or the pancreas is not releasing enough enzymes needed for digestion. Therefore, supplements of pancreatic enzymes may be helpful in restoring proper digestion. Other nutritional supplements may be given orally or intravenously in an effort to boost calorie intake. However, cachexia (severe muscle breakdown) caused by certain substances that the cancer produces remains a significant problem to treat.

Patients with pancreatic cancer may experience anxiety and **depression** during their diagnosis and treatment. Statistics on the prognosis for the disease can be discouraging; however, there are many new treatments on the horizon that may significantly improve the outcome of this disease. Many patients find it helpful to join support groups where they can discuss their concerns with others who are also coping with the illness.

Resources

BOOKS

Ahuja, Nita, and Joanne Coleman. *Johns Hopkins Patients' Guide to Pancreatic Cancer.* Sudbury, MA: Jones & Bartlett Learning, 2010.

WEBSITES

American Cancer Society. "Pancreatic Cancer." http://www.ighome.com/?t=289192 (accessed September 1, 2014).

Dagovich. Tomislav. "Pancreatic Cancer." Medscape Reference, April 25, 2014. http://emedicine.medscape.com/article/280605-overview (accessed September 1, 2014).

National Cancer Institute. "Neuroendocrine Pancreatic Tumors (Islet Cell Tumors)." http://www.cancer.gov/cancertopics/pdq/treatment/isletcell/patient (accessed September 1, 2014).

"Pancreatic Cancer." MedlinePlus, June 6, 2014. http://www.nlm.nih.gov/medlineplus/pancreaticcancer.html (accessed September 1, 2014).

ORGANIZATIONS

American Cancer Society, 1599 Clifton Rd., NE, Atlanta, GA 30329, (404) 320-3333, (800) ACS-2345, http://www.cancer.org.

National Cancer Institute, BG 9609 MSC 9760, 9609 Medical Center Drive, Bethesda, MD 20892-9760, (800) 4-CANCER, TTY: (800) 332-8615, http://www.cancer.gov.

National Pancreas Center, 3 Bethesda Metro Center, Suite 700, Bethesda, MD 20814, (301) 961-1508, (866) 726-2737, Fax: (301) 657-9776, info@pancreasfoundation.org, http://www.pancreasfoundation.org.

Elizabeth Pulcini, MSc

REVISED BY TISH DAVIDSON, AM

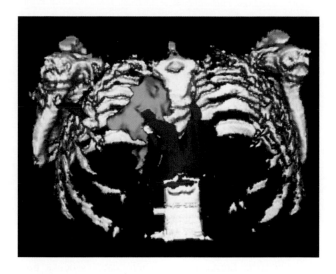

Colorized computed tomography (CT) scan showing the location of a cancerous tumor of the pancreas (green). *(CNRI/Science Source)*

Other nearby organs include the gallbladder, spleen, and liver. The pancreas has a wide end (head), a narrow end (tail), and a middle section (body). The pancreas contains two different types of tissue and has two main functions, each performed by one of the distinct tissue types. Exocrine tissue secretes fluids into the other organs of the digestive system. Endocrine tissue secretes hormones that circulate in the bloodstream and affect distant organs. The exocrine pancreas makes up the vast majority of the gland. It produces pancreatic juices containing enzymes that help break down proteins and fatty food. The endocrine tissue of the pancreas makes up only 2% of the gland's total mass. It consists of small patches of cells that produce hormones that control how the body stores and uses nutrients. These patches are called islets (islands) of Langerhans or islet cells, and they are interspersed evenly throughout the pancreas. Each islet contains approximately 1,000 endocrine cells and a dense network of capillaries (tiny blood vessels) that allow immediate entry of hormones into the circulatory system.

Pancreatic tumors are classified as either exocrine or endocrine tumors depending on which type of tissue they arise from within the gland. Endocrine tumors of the pancreas are very rare, accounting for only 5% of all pancreatic cancers.

There are a variety of different subtypes of endocrine cells, each producing a different hormone or peptide (small protein molecule): insulin, glucagon, gastrin, somatostatin, vasoactive intestinal peptide, and pancreatic polypeptide. Tumors are named for the type of cell that has become cancerous. For example, insulomas are tumors that arise from cells that make insulin.

Pancreatic cancer, endocrine

Definition

Endocrine **pancreatic cancer** is a disease in which cancerous cells originate within the tissues of the pancreas that produce hormones.

Description

The pancreas is a 6–8 in. (15–20 cm) long, slipper-shaped gland located in the abdomen. It lies behind the stomach within a loop formed by the small intestine.

Collectively, these tumors are known as **neuroendocrine tumors**.

The majority of endocrine pancreatic tumors are functional adenocarcinomas that overproduce a specific hormone. Insulinoma is the most common tumor of the endocrine pancreas. Patients with this disease usually develop hypoglycemia due to increased insulin production that leads to abnormally low blood sugar levels. Gastrinoma, a disease in which gastrin (the hormone that stimulates stomach acid production) is overproduced, causes multiple ulcers in the upper gastrointestinal (GI) tract. Gastrinoma was first described in patients with a rare form of severe peptic ulcer disease known as **Zollinger-Ellison syndrome** (ZES). The less common glucagonoma causes mild diabetes due to excess glucagon (the hormone which stimulates glucose production) secretion. Other rare islet cell tumors include vipoma (vasoactive intestinal peptide) and somatostatinoma. Nonfunctional pancreatic endocrine tumors are not associated with an excess production of any hormone and can be difficult to distinguish from **exocrine pancreatic cancer**. Cancers of the endocrine pancreas are relatively slow-growing compared to the more common ductal adenocarcinomas of the exocrine pancreas.

Demographics

Neuroendocrine tumors are rare. Between one and four cases of insulinoma occur per million people per year, and 90% of these tumors are benign (noncancerous). They occur mostly between the ages of 50 and 60 and affect men and women equally. Fewer than three cases of gastrinoma per million people are diagnosed each year, but gastrinomas are the most common functional islet cell tumor in patients with multiple endocrine tumors, a condition known as **multiple endocrine neoplasia** (MEN) syndrome. Vipoma and glucagonoma are even rarer, and they occur more frequently in women. Somatostatinoma is exceedingly uncommon; fewer than 100 cases have been reported worldwide. Nonfunctional islet cell cancers account for approximately one-third of all cancers of the endocrine pancreas, and the majority of these are malignant.

Causes and symptoms

There are no known causes of islet cell **cancer**, but a small percentage of cases occur due to hereditary syndromes such as MEN. This condition frequently causes more than one tumor in several endocrine glands (such as the parathyroid and pituitary), in addition to the islet cells of the pancreas. Twenty-five percent of gastrinomas and less than 10% of insulinomas occur in MEN patients. Von Hippel-Lindau (VHL) syndrome is another genetic disorder that causes multiple tumors, and 10% to 15% of VHL patients will develop islet cell cancer.

Symptoms vary among the different islet cell cancer types. Insulinoma causes repeated episodes of hypoglycemia, sweating, and tremor, while patients with gastrinoma have inflammation of the esophagus, epigastric pain, multiple ulcers, and possibly **diarrhea**. Symptoms of glucagonoma include a distinctive skin rash, inflammation of the stomach, glucose intolerance, **weight loss**, weakness, and **anemia** (less common). Patients with vipoma have episodes of profuse, watery diarrhea, even after fasting. Somatostatinoma causes mild diabetes, diarrhea/steatorrhea (fatty stools), weight loss, and gallbladder disease. Nonfunctional endocrine tumors frequently produce the same symptoms as cancer of the exocrine pancreas, such as abdominal pain, jaundice, and weight loss.

Diagnosis

A thorough physical exam is usually performed when a patient visits a doctor with the above symptoms; however, functional endocrine tumors of the pancreas tend to be small and are not detected by palpating the abdomen. Once other illnesses such as infection are ruled out, the doctor will order a series of blood and urine tests. The functional endocrine tumors can be identified through increased levels of hormones in the bloodstream.

Functional endocrine tumors can occur in multiple sites in the pancreas and are often small (less than 1 cm), making them difficult to diagnose. Nonfunctional tumors tend to be larger, which makes them difficult to distinguish from tumors of the exocrine pancreas. Methods such as **computed tomography** (CT) scan and **magnetic resonance imaging** (MRI) are used to take pictures of the internal organs and allow the doctor to determine whether a tumor is present. Somatostatin receptor scintigraphy is an imaging system used to localize endocrine tumors, especially gastrinomas and somatostatinomas. Endoscopic ultrasound (EUS) is a more sensitive technique that may be used if a CT scan fails to detect a tumor. Endocrine tumors usually have many blood vessels, so **angiography** may be useful in the doctor's assessment and staging of the tumor. Surgical exploration is sometimes necessary in order to locate very small tumors that occur in multiple sites. These techniques also help the doctor evaluate how far the tumor has spread. A **biopsy** can be taken to confirm diagnosis, but more often, doctors look at the size and local invasion of the tumor in order to plan a treatment strategy.

Treatment team

Patients with islet cell cancer are cared for by a number of specialists from different disciplines. Medical

KEY TERMS

Adenocarcinoma—A malignant tumor that arises within the tissues of a gland and retains its glandular structure.

Angiography—Diagnostic technique used to study blood vessels in a tumor.

Biopsy—Removal and microscopic examination of cells to determine whether they are cancerous.

Chemotherapy—Drug treatment administered to kill cancerous cells.

Endocrine—Refers to glands that secrete hormones directly into the bloodstream.

Endoscopic ultrasonography (EUS)—Diagnostic imaging technique in which an ultrasound probe is inserted down a patient's throat to determine whether a tumor is present.

Gastrinoma—Tumor that arises from the gastrin-producing cells in the pancreas.

Insulinoma—Tumor that arises from the insulin-producing cells in the pancreas.

Islets of Langerhans—Clusters of cells in the pancreas that make up its endocrine tissue.

oncologists, gastroenterologists, radiologists, and surgeons all interact with the patient to develop an appropriate treatment plan. Endocrinologists play an important role in helping patients with diabetes maintain steady blood sugar levels. Much of the treatment of islet cell cancer focuses on relieving symptoms of the tumor through medication that inhibits hormone overproduction. It is best for patients to work with doctors who are experienced in treating this rare form of cancer.

Clinical staging

The staging system for islet cell cancer is still evolving and is based on the type, size, and spread of the tumor. Tumors typically fall into three categories: cancers that arise in one location within the pancreas, cancers that arise in several locations within the pancreas, and cancers that have spread to nearby lymph nodes or to other organs in the body.

Treatment

Surgery is the only curative method for islet cell cancers; studies have shown that an aggressive surgical approach can improve survival and alleviate symptoms of the disease. As with most forms of cancer, the earlier it is diagnosed, the greater the chance for survival. With the exception of insulinoma, the majority of islet cell tumors are malignant at the time of diagnosis, and more than half are metastatic. However, surgery and **chemotherapy** have been shown to improve the outcome of patients even if they have metastatic disease.

Surgery may include partial or total removal of the pancreas, and in patients with gastrinoma, the stomach may be removed as well. Chemotherapy is individualized based on the type of tumor and the hormone produced. **Streptozocin**, **doxorubicin**, and 5-fluorouracil (5-FU, or **fluorouracil**) are the chemotherapeutic drugs commonly used. Patients may experience **nausea and vomiting** (as well as kidney toxicity) from streptozocin, and bone marrow suppression from doxorubicin.

Hormone therapy is used to relieve the symptoms of functional tumors by inhibiting excess hormone production. Other techniques may be used to block blood flow to the liver in an attempt to kill the cancer cells that have spread there. Abdominal pain, nausea, vomiting, and **fever** may result from this type of treatment. Radiation has little if any role in the treatment of islet cell cancer.

Prognosis

Islet cell cancers overall have a more favorable prognosis than cancers of the exocrine pancreas, and the median survival from diagnosis is three-and-a-half years. This survival rate is mainly due to their slow-growing nature. Insulinomas have a five-year survival rate of 80% and gastrinomas have a 65% survival rate. When metastasized, islet cell cancers do not generally respond well to chemotherapy, and the treatment is mainly palliative. Most patients with **metastasis** do not survive five years. Islet cell cancer tends to spread to the surrounding lymph nodes, stomach, small intestine, and liver.

Coping with cancer treatment

Patients should discuss with their doctors any side effects they experience from treatment. Many drugs are available to relieve the nausea and vomiting associated with cancer treatments and for combating **fatigue**. Insulin may be prescribed if patients develop diabetes as a result of partial or total removal of their pancreas. Special diets or fluids may be recommended if patients have more than one digestive organ removed. These patients may require intravenous feeding after surgery until they recover.

Clinical trials

Because this is such a rare disease, relatively few **clinical trials** are available to people with islet cell cancer. Nevertheless, patients and their families can search for new trials on the **National Cancer Institute** website at http://www.cancer.gov/clinicaltrials/search.

Prevention

There are no known risk factors associated with sporadic islet cell cancer; therefore, it is not clear how to prevent its occurrence. Individuals with MEN syndrome or VHL, however, have a genetic predisposition to developing islet cell cancer and should be screened regularly in an effort to detect the disease early.

Special concerns

Many patients find it helpful to join support groups after being diagnosed with cancer. Discussing the condition with others who are experiencing a similar situation may help to relieve anxiety and **depression**, which are often associated with cancer and its treatment. Medication may also be prescribed to alleviate depression. Patients should learn as much as they can about their illness and find out what their treatment options are. It is important for patients to remember that each cancer has unique characteristics and responds differently to treatment depending on those characteristics.

See also Carcinoid tumors, gastrointestinal; Chemoembolization; Complementary cancer therapies; Endocrine system tumors; Familial cancer syndromes; Pancreatic cancer, exocrine; Upper gastrointestinal endoscopy.

Resources

BOOKS

Ahuja, Nita, and Joanne Coleman. *Johns Hopkins Patients' Guide to Pancreatic Cancer*. Sudbury, MA: Jones & Bartlett Learning, 2010.

WEBSITES

American Cancer Society. "Pancreatic Cancer." http://www.ighome.com/?t=289192 (accessed August 25, 2014).
National Cancer Institute. "Neuroendocrine Pancreatic Tumors (Islet Cell Tumors)." http://www.cancer.gov/cancertopics/pdq/treatment/isletcell/patient (accessed August 25, 2014).
Ong, Evan S. "Neoplasms of the Endocrine Pancreas." Medscape Reference. http://emedicine.medscape.com/article/276943-overview (accessed August 25, 2014).
"Pancreatic Cancer." MedlinePlus. http://www.nlm.nih.gov/medlineplus/pancreaticcancer.html (accessed August 25, 2014).

ORGANIZATIONS

American Cancer Society, 1599 Clifton Rd., NE, Atlanta, GA 30329, (404) 320-3333, (800) ACS-2345, http://www.cancer.org.
National Cancer Institute, BG 9609 MSC 9760, 9609 Medical Center Drive, Bethesda, MD 20892-9760, (800) 4-CANCER, TTY: (800) 332-8615, http://www.cancer.gov.
National Pancreas Center, 3 Bethesda Metro Center, Suite 700, Bethesda, MD 20814, (301) 961-1508, (866) 726-2737, Fax: (301) 657-9776, info@pancreasfoundation.org, http://www.pancreasfoundation.org.
National Organization for Rare Disorders (NORD), 55 Kenosia Avenue, Danbury, CT 06810, (203) 744-0100, Fax: (203) 798-2291, http://www.rarediseases.org.

Elizabeth Pulcini, MSc
REVISED BY TISH DAVIDSON, AM

Pancreatic cancer, exocrine

Definition

Exocrine **pancreatic cancer** is a disease in which cancerous cells originate within the tissues of the pancreas that produce digestive juices.

Description

The pancreas is a 6–8 inch long, slipper-shaped gland located in the abdomen. It lies behind the stomach within a loop formed by the small intestine. Other nearby organs include the gallbladder, spleen, and liver. The pancreas has a wide end (head), a narrow end (tail), and a middle section (body). A healthy pancreas is important for normal food digestion and also plays a critical role in the body's metabolic processes. The pancreas has two main functions, and each are performed by distinct types of tissue. The exocrine tissue makes up the vast majority of the gland and secretes fluids into the other organs of the digestive system. The endocrine tissue secretes

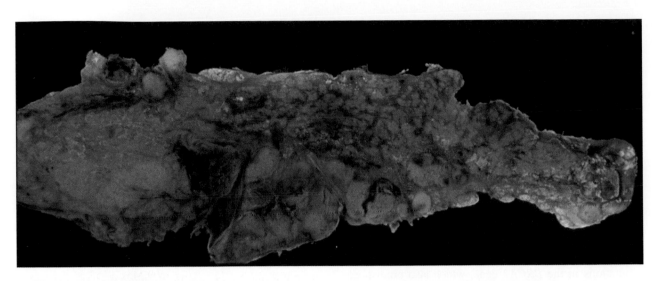

Carcinoma of the head of the pancreas. Tumors appear as gritty, gray, hard nodules, invading the adjacent gland. *(BIOPHOTO ASSOC/Science Source)*

hormones such as insulin that are circulated in the bloodstream and affect other organs. These substances control how the body stores and uses nutrients.

The exocrine tissue of the pancreas produces pancreatic (digestive) juices. These juices contain several enzymes that help break down proteins and fatty foods. The exocrine pancreas forms an intricate system of channels or ducts, which are tubular structures that carry pancreatic juices to the small intestine where they are used for digestion.

Pancreatic tumors are classified as either exocrine or endocrine tumors depending on which type of tissue they arise from within the gland. Ninety-five percent of pancreatic cancers occur in the tissues of the exocrine pancreas. Ductal adenocarcinomas arise in the cells that line the ducts of the exocrine pancreas and account for 80%–90% of all tumors of the pancreas. Unless specified, nearly all reports on pancreatic **cancer** refer to ductal adenocarcinomas. Less common types of pancreatic exocrine tumors include acinar cell **carcinoma**, cystic tumors that are typically benign but may become cancerous, and papillary tumors that grow within the pancreatic ducts. Pancreatoblastoma is a very rare disease that primarily affects young children.

Two-thirds of pancreatic tumors occur in the head of the pancreas; tumor growth in this area can lead to the obstruction of the nearby common bile duct that empties bile fluid into the small intestine. When bile cannot be passed into the intestine, patients may develop yellowing of the skin and eyes (jaundice) due to the buildup of bilirubin (a component of bile) in the bloodstream. Tumor blockage of bile or pancreatic ducts may also cause digestive problems, because these fluids contain

critical enzymes needed in the digestive process. Depending on their size, pancreatic tumors may cause abdominal pain by pressing on the surrounding nerves. Because of its location deep within the abdomen, pancreatic cancer often remains undetected until it has spread to other organs such as the liver or lungs. Pancreatic cancer tends to spread rapidly to other organs, even when the primary (original) tumor is relatively small.

Demographics

Although pancreatic cancer accounts for only 3% of all cancers, it is the fourth most common cause of cancer deaths. In 2014, the American Cancer Society estimated that about 42,420 new cases of pancreatic cancer would be diagnosed in the United States and 39,590 people would die of the disease.

Pancreatic cancer is primarily a disease associated with advanced age, with 80% of cases occurring between the ages of 60 and 80. Men are almost twice as likely to develop this disease as women. Countries with the highest frequencies of pancreatic cancer include the United States, New Zealand, Western European nations, and Scandinavia. The lowest occurrences of the disease are reported in India, Kuwait, and Singapore. African Americans have the highest rate of pancreatic cancer of any ethnic group worldwide. Whether this difference is due to diet, genetics, or environmental factors remains unclear.

Causes and symptoms

Several risk factors have been shown to increase susceptibility to this particular cancer, the greatest of which is tobacco use, including smokeless tobacco.

Approximately one-third of pancreatic cancer cases occur among smokers. People who have diabetes develop pancreatic cancer twice as often as nondiabetics. Obesity, especially beginning at a young age, is also a risk factor. There appears to be an inherited genetic component to pancreatic cancer, particularly if two or more relatives in the immediate family have the disease. Other risk factors include chronic (long-term) inflammation of the pancreas (pancreatitis); diets high in processed meat and low in fruits and vegetables; and occupational exposure to certain chemicals, such as petroleum.

The exact cause of most pancreatic cancers is unknown, but researchers have pinpointed several gene mutations that account for about 10% of cancers of the pancreas. These include:

- mutations in the *BRCA2* gene, which also predisposes women to breast and ovarian cancer.
- mutations in the *CDKN2A* gene, which predisposes individuals to melanoma (aggressive skin cancer)
- mutations in the gene *PRSS1*, which predisposes individuals to pancreatitis
- mutations in multiple genes that predispose individuals to certain types of colorectal cancer
- mutations in the gene *STK1*, which predisposes individuals to digestive tract cancers

Pancreatic cancer often does not produce symptoms until it reaches an advanced stage. Patients may then present with the following signs and symptoms:

- upper abdominal and/or back pain
- jaundice
- weight loss
- loss of appetite (anorexia)
- diarrhea
- weakness
- nausea

These symptoms may also be caused by other illnesses; therefore, it is important to consult a doctor for an accurate diagnosis.

Diagnosis

Pancreatic cancer is difficult to diagnose, especially in the absence of symptoms, and there is no current screening method for early detection. There is a blood test for a protein the cancer cells produce, but it is not sensitive enough to identify cancer in its early stages and often does not detect very small tumors that are localized (have not begun to spread). At advanced stages in which patients show symptoms, a number of tests may be performed to confirm the diagnosis and to assess the stage of the disease. Approximately half of all pancreatic cancers are metastatic (have spread to other sites) at the time of diagnosis.

The first step in diagnosing pancreatic cancer is a thorough medical history and complete physical examination. The abdomen will be palpated to check for fluid accumulation, lumps, or masses. If there are signs of jaundice, blood tests will be performed to rule out the possibility of liver diseases such as hepatitis. Urine and stool tests may be performed as well.

Noninvasive imaging tools such as **computed tomography** (CT) scans and **magnetic resonance imaging** (MRI) can be used to produce detailed pictures of the internal organs. CT may also be used to determine whether the tumor can be removed by surgery. It is also useful in staging a tumor by showing the extent to which the tumor has spread. During a CT scan, patients receive an intravenous injection of a contrast dye so the organs can be visualized more clearly. MRI may be performed instead of CT if a patient has an allergy to the CT contrast dye. In some cases in which the tumor is impinging on blood vessels or nearby ducts, MRI may be used to generate an image of the pancreatic ducts.

If the doctor suspects pancreatic cancer and no visible masses are seen with a diagnostic scan, a patient may undergo a combination of invasive tests to confirm the presence of a pancreatic tumor. Endoscopic ultrasound (EUS) involves the use of an ultrasound probe at the end of a long, flexible tube that is passed down the patient's throat and into the stomach. This instrument can detect a tumor mass through high-frequency sound waves and echoes. EUS can be accompanied by fine-needle aspiration (FNA), in which a long needle, guided by the ultrasound, is inserted into the tumor mass in order to take a **biopsy** sample. **Endoscopic retrograde cholangiopancreatography** (ERCP) is a technique often used in patients with severe jaundice, because it enables the doctor to relieve blockage of the pancreatic ducts. The doctor, guided by endoscopy and **x-rays**, inserts a small metal or plastic stent into the duct to keep it open. During ERCP, a biopsy can be done by collecting cells from the pancreas with a small brush. The cells are then examined under the microscope by a pathologist, who determines the presence of any cancerous cells.

In some cases, a biopsy may be performed during a type of surgery called **laparoscopy**, which is done under general anesthesia. Doctors insert a small camera and instruments into the abdomen after a minor incision is made. Tissue samples are removed for examination under the microscope. This procedure allows a doctor to determine the extent to which the disease has spread and decide whether the tumor can be removed by further surgery.

KEY TERMS

Acinar cell(s)—Cells that comprise small sacs terminating the ducts of some exocrine glands.

Acinar cell carcinoma—A malignant tumor arising from the acinar cells of the pancreas.

Angiography—Diagnostic technique used to study blood vessels in a tumor.

Biopsy—Removal and microscopic examination of cells to determine whether they are cancerous.

Cancer vaccine—A treatment that uses the patient's immune system to attack cancer cells.

Chemotherapy—Drug treatment administered to kill cancerous cells.

Ductal adenocarcinoma—A malignant tumor arising from the duct cells within a gland.

Endoscopic retrograde cholangiopancreatography (ERCP)—Diagnostic technique used to obtain a biopsy. Also a surgical method of relieving biliary obstruction caused by a tumor.

Endoscopic ultrasonography (EUS)—Diagnostic imaging technique in which an ultrasound probe is inserted down a patient's throat to determine whether a tumor is present.

Exocrine—Refers to glands that secrete their products through a duct.

Laparoscopic surgery—Minimally invasive surgery in which a camera and surgical instruments are inserted through a small incision.

Pancreatectomy—Partial or total surgical removal of the pancreas.

Radiation therapy—Use of radioisotopes to kill tumor cells; applied externally through a beam of x-rays, intraoperatively (during surgery), or deposited internally by implanting radioactive seeds in tumor tissue.

Whipple procedure—Surgical removal of the head of the pancreas, part of the small intestine, and some surrounding tissue.

An **angiography** is a type of test that studies the blood vessels in and around the pancreas. This test may be done before surgery so that the doctor can determine the extent to which the tumor invades and interacts with the blood vessels within the pancreas. The test requires local anesthesia due to the insertion of a catheter into the patient's upper thigh. A dye is then injected into blood vessels that lead into the pancreas, and x-rays are taken.

Treatment team

Pancreatic cancer is a complex disease that involves specialists from a variety of medical disciplines. Patients are likely to interact with medical oncologists, gastroenterologists, radiologists, and surgeons to develop a suitable treatment plan. Treatment plans vary depending on the stage of the disease and the overall health of the patient. Cancers of the pancreas frequently cause intense pain by pressing on the surrounding network of nerves in the abdomen; therefore, anesthesiologists who specialize in **pain management** may play a role in making a patient more comfortable. Obstruction of the intestine or bowel can also be a cause of pain, but is usually relieved through surgery. Patients receiving **chemotherapy** meet with oncologists who determine the dose schedule and oncology nurses who administer the chemotherapy. Patients who undergo partial or total removal of their pancreas may develop diabetes, and an endocrinologist will prescribe insulin or other medication to help them manage this condition. It is important for patients to get proper nutrition during any treatment for cancer. Patients may wish to consult a nutritionist or dietitian to assist them (their care may require oral replacement of digestive enzymes).

Clinical staging

After cancer of the pancreas has been diagnosed, doctors typically use a TNM staging system to classify the tumor based on its size and the degree to which it has spread to other areas in the body. T indicates the size and local advancement of the primary tumor. Because cancers often invade the lymphatic system before spreading to other organs, regional lymph node involvement (N) is an important factor in staging. M indicates whether the tumor has metastasized (spread) to distant organs.

In stage I, the tumor is localized to the pancreas and has not spread to surrounding lymph nodes or other organs. Stage II pancreatic cancer has spread to nearby organs such as the small intestine or bile duct, but not the surrounding lymph nodes. Stage III indicates lymph node involvement, regardless of whether the cancer has spread to nearby organs. Stage IVA pancreatic cancer has spread to organs near the pancreas such as the stomach, spleen, or colon. Stage IVB is a cancer that has spread to distant sites (liver, lungs). If pancreatic cancer has been treated with success and then appears again in the pancreas or in other organs, it is referred to as recurrent disease.

Treatment

Treatment of pancreatic cancer depends on several factors, including the stage of the disease and the patient's age and overall health status. A combination of therapies is often employed in the treatment of this disease to improve the patient's chances for survival. Surgery is used whenever possible and is the only means by which cancer of the pancreas can be cured. However, less than 15% of pancreatic tumors can be removed by surgery. By the time the disease is diagnosed (usually at stage III), therapies such as radiation and chemotherapy or both are used in addition to surgery to relieve a patient's symptoms and enhance quality of life. For patients with metastatic disease, chemotherapy and radiation are used mainly as palliative (pain-alleviating) treatments.

Surgery

Three types of surgery are used in the treatment of pancreatic cancer, depending on the tumor's location within the pancreas. A **Whipple procedure** removes the head of the pancreas, part of the small intestine, and some of the surrounding tissues. This procedure is most common since the majority of pancreatic cancers occur in the head of the organ. A total **pancreatectomy** removes the entire pancreas and the organs around it. Distal pancreatectomy removes only the body and tail of the pancreas. Chemotherapy and radiation may precede surgery (neoadjuvant therapy) or follow surgery (adjuvant therapy). Surgery is also used to relieve symptoms of pancreatic cancer by draining fluids or bypassing obstructions. Side effects from surgery can include pain, weakness, **fatigue**, and digestive problems. Some patients may develop diabetes or malabsorption as a result of partial or total removal of the pancreas.

Radiation therapy

Radiation therapy is sometimes used to shrink a tumor before surgery or to remove remaining cancer cells after surgery. Radiation may also be used to relieve pain or digestive problems caused by the tumor if it cannot be removed by surgery. External radiation therapy refers to radiation applied externally to the abdomen using a beam of high-energy x-rays. High-dose intraoperative radiation therapy is sometimes used during surgery on tumors that have spread to nearby organs. Internal radiation therapy refers to the use of small radioactive seeds implanted in the tumor tissue. The seeds emit radiation over a period of time to kill tumor cells. Radiation treatment may cause side effects such as fatigue, tender or itchy skin, nausea, vomiting, and digestive problems.

Chemotherapy

Chemotherapeutic agents are powerful drugs that are used to kill cancer cells. They are classified according to the mechanism by which they induce cancer cell death. Multiple agents are often used to increase the chances of tumor cell death. **Gemcitabine** is the standard drug used to treat pancreatic cancers; it can be used alone or in combination with other drugs, such as 5-fluorouracil (5-FU, or **fluorouracil**), oxaliplatin (Eloxatin), **irinotecan** (Camptosar), and albumin-bound paclitaxel (Abraxane). Chemotherapy may be administered orally or intravenously in a series of doses over several weeks. During treatment, patients may experience fatigue, nausea, vomiting, hair loss (**alopecia**), and mouth sores, depending on which drugs are used.

Alternative and complementary therapies

Many patients find that alternative and complementary therapies help to reduce the stress associated with illness, improve immune function, and boost spirits. While there is no clinical evidence that these therapies specifically combat disease, such activities as biofeedback, relaxation, therapeutic touch, massage therapy, and guided imagery have no side effects and have been reported to enhance well-being.

Several other healing therapies are sometimes used as supplemental or replacement cancer treatments, such as antineoplastons, Cancell, cartilage (bovine and shark), laetrile, and **mistletoe**. Many of these therapies have not been the subject of safety and efficacy trials by the **National Cancer Institute** (NCI). The NCI has conducted trials on Cancell, laetrile, and some other alternative therapies and found no anticancer activity. These treatments have varying effectiveness and safety considerations. Patients using any alternative remedy should first consult their doctors in order to prevent harmful side effects or interactions with mainstream cancer treatment.

Prognosis

Unfortunately, cancer of the pancreas is often fatal, and median survival from diagnosis is less than six months, while the five-year survival rate is 4%. This high mortality rate is mainly due to the lack of screening methods available for early detection of the disease. Yet even when localized tumors can be removed by surgery, patient survival after five years is only 10%–15%. These statistics demonstrate the aggressive nature of most pancreatic cancers and their tendency to recur. Pancreatic cancers tend to be resistant to radiation and chemotherapy, and these modes of treatment are mainly used to relieve pain and tumor burden.

Clinical trials

Clinical trials are government-regulated studies of new treatments and techniques that may prove beneficial in diagnosing or treating a disease. Participation is always voluntary and at no cost to the participant. Because the outcomes of exocrine pancreatic cancer are poor, most patients are advised to seek out clinical trials for treatment options. Clinical trials are conducted in three phases. Phase 1 tests the safety of the treatment and looks for harmful side effects. Phase 2 tests the effectiveness of the treatment. Phase 3 compares the treatment to other treatments available for the same condition.

The selection of clinical trials under way changes frequently. Patients and their families can search for new trials on the National Cancer Institute website at http://www.cancer.gov/clinicaltrials/search.

Coping with cancer treatment

Patients should discuss with their doctors any side effects they experience from treatment. Many drugs are available to relieve **nausea and vomiting** associated with cancer treatments and for combating fatigue. Special diets or supplements, including pancreatic enzymes, may be recommended if patients are experiencing digestive problems. Insulin or other medication may be prescribed if patients develop diabetes as a result of partial or total removal of their pancreas.

Prevention

Although the exact cause of pancreatic cancer is not known, there are certain risk factors that may increase a person's chances of developing the disease. Quitting smoking will certainly reduce the risk of pancreatic cancer and many other cancers. The American Cancer Society recommends a diet rich in fruits, vegetables, and dietary fiber in order to reduce the risk of pancreatic cancer. According to the NCI, workers who are exposed to petroleum and other chemicals may be at greater risk of developing the disease and should follow their employer's safety precautions. People with a family history of pancreatic cancer are at greater risk than the general population, as a small percentage of pancreatic cancers are considered hereditary.

Special concerns

Pain control is probably the single greatest problem for patients with pancreatic cancer. As the cancer grows and spreads to other organs in the abdomen, it often presses on the surrounding network of nerves, which can cause considerable discomfort. In most cases, pain can be alleviated with analgesics or **opioids**.

Pancreatic cancer patients frequently have difficulty maintaining their weight because food may not taste good or the pancreas is not releasing enough enzymes needed for digestion. Therefore, supplements of

---

QUESTIONS TO ASK YOUR DOCTOR

- What is my prognosis?
- What is the standard course of treatment for my cancer at this stage?
- How long will the course of treatment take?
- What side effects will I experience?
- What can be done to relieve my abdominal pain?
- What should I do to prepare for surgery?
- Can you refer me to a nutritionist or dietitian?
- Are there any alternative therapies you would recommend?
- Am I eligible to participate in a clinical trial?
- Will my health insurance cover costs associated with a clinical trial?
- Are there any support groups I can join?

---

pancreatic enzymes may be helpful in restoring proper digestion. Other nutritional supplements may be given orally or intravenously in an effort to boost caloric intake. However, cachexia (severe muscle breakdown) caused by certain substances that the cancer produces remains a significant problem to treat.

Patients with pancreatic cancer may experience anxiety and **depression** during their diagnosis and treatment. Statistics on the prognosis of the disease can be discouraging; however, there are many new treatments on the horizon that may significantly improve the outcome for this disease. Many patients find it helpful to join support groups where they can discuss their concerns with others who are also coping with the illness.

See also Cigarettes; Drug resistance; Gastrointestinal cancers; Immunologic therapies; Nutritional support; Pancreatic cancer, endocrine; Smoking cessation.

Resources

BOOKS

Ahuja, Nita, and Joanne Coleman. *Johns Hopkins Patients' Guide to Pancreatic Cancer*. Sudbury, MA: Jones & Bartlett Learning, 2010.

WEBSITES

American Cancer Society. "Pancreatic Cancer." http://www.ighome.com/?t=289192 (accessed September 24, 2014).

Dagovich, Tomislav. "Pancreatic Cancer." Medscape Reference April 25, 2014. http://emedicine.medscape.com/article/280605-overview (accessed September 24, 2014).

"Pancreatic Cancer." MedlinePlus June 6, 2014. http://www.nlm.nih.gov/medlineplus/pancreaticcancer.html (accessed September 24, 2014).

ORGANIZATIONS

American Cancer Society, 1599 Clifton Rd., NE, Atlanta, GA 30329, (404) 320-3333, (800) ACS-2345, http://www.cancer.org.

National Cancer Institute, BG 9609 MSC 9760, 9609 Medical Center Drive, Bethesda, MD 20892-9760, (800) 4-CANCER (422-6237), http://www.cancer.gov.

National Pancreas Center, 3 Bethesda Metro Center, Suite 700, Bethesda, MD 20814, (301) 961-1508, (866) 726-2737, Fax: (301) 657-9776, info@pancreasfoundation.org, http://www.pancreasfoundation.org.

Elizabeth Pulcini, MSc

REVISED BY TISH DAVIDSON, AM

Panitumumab

Definition

Panitumumab is an anticancer drug designed to treat colorectal **cancer**. Panitumumab inhibits tumor cellular signaling by antagonizing a signaling pathway affecting tumor cell development. The tumor cells panitumumab is used against have a receptor on their cell surface called the epidermal growth factor receptor (EGFR).

Purpose

Panitumumab is used to treat colorectal cancer that has high levels of the epidermal growth factor receptor. Panitumumab treats colorectal cancer that is metastatic (spread from other parts of the body) and has failed to respond to treatment with other drugs. Only colorectal cancer that has EGFR may be targeted by panitumumab. Patients in the **clinical trials** that evaluated panitumumab treatment were required to have immunohistochemical evidence (testing cancer cells viewed under a microscope) of EGFR expression.

Description

Panitumumab is manufactured by Amgen under the trade name Vectibix. Panitumumab is a type of monoclonal antibody used in the treatment of colorectal cancer. **Monoclonal antibodies** are produced in the laboratory as substances that can locate and bind to cancer cells to destroy them. Studies have shown that use of panitumumab increases progression-free survival compared to placebo. The term *progression-free survival*

describes the length of time during and after treatment in which a patient is living with a disease that does not get worse. In a clinical trial designed to test out a cancer drug in human, progression-free survival is a way to measure the effectiveness of a treatment.

Panitumumab specifically targets the EGFR expressed by cancer cells to prevent cancer cell growth and replication. The EGFR is a type of chemical receptor that sits on the outer membrane of both normal cells and cancer cells. Chemical receptors in the body activate a sequence of cellular events known as a chemical cascade or signaling pathway. It is these signaling pathways that are responsible for many normal body functions. Drugs or natural chemicals that bind to and activate the receptor signaling pathway are known as receptor agonists. Drugs that bind to the receptor and block them from creating a signaling pathway are known as receptor antagonists, because they antagonize the effects of that receptor. EGFRs are receptors that bind growth factors to create signaling cascades that are a natural part of cell development and necessary for normal cell growth. The agonist that normally binds to the EGFR is epidermal growth factor (EGF). When EGF binds to the EGFR, it initiates chemical signals that tell the cell how to grow and replicate. Some cancer cells have a mutated form of the EGFR that can be targeted by drugs that differentiate between the normal and mutated EGFRs. Panitumumab antagonizes the mutant EGFR by binding to it and blocking the signaling pathway for growth. Panitumumab mainly acts on cancer cells instead of normal cells because it targets the mutated form of the EGFR.

Panitumumab is a chimeric (fusion) mouse and human monoclonal antibody used to treat metastatic colorectal cancer and malignant head and neck cancer. Drugs like panitumumab are made in mice for experimental purposes but need to be humanized to eliminate or reduce the chance that patients will mount an immune reaction to the antibody when administered in therapy. Panitumumab binds to and blocks the EGFR to fight tumor cells, and in some cases has also been shown to be directly toxic to tumor cells. By blocking EGFR, panitumumab blocks the biological signal that promotes tumor growth and **metastasis**. The biological signal also promotes new blood vessel formation in the process of **angiogenesis**. Once a solid tumor reaches a certain size, it needs blood vessels in order for its cells to remain alive and continue to grow. Blood vessels that grow in tumors in the process called angiogenesis also contribute to its metastasis to other parts of the body. All of these components are critical to the ongoing survival of the tumor and blocked by panitumumab.

Recommended dosage

Panitumumab is administered intravenously. It is not given as a rapid infusion or as a bolus (one large dose at one time). Panitumumab is given as an infusion over 60 minutes if the dose is less than or equal to a total of 1 g. Panitumumab is given as an infusion over 90 minutes if the dose is greater than a total of 1 g. The dose chosen for use depends on the weight of the patient and the response to treatment with regard to both the development of side effects and therapeutic effect. A typical dosage for EGFR-expressing metastatic colorectal cancer that has not responded to other treatments is 6 mg/kg, given as a 60 minute infusion every 14 days.

While panitumumab is not frequently associated with the development of adverse reactions to drug infusions, intravenous drugs often cause serious medical conditions upon infusion. The infusion rate of panitumumab is altered in the case of infusion reactions, based on the presence and severity level. If the infusion reaction is considered mild or moderate, the infusion rate is decreased by 50%. If the infusion reaction is considered severe, therapy is discontinued permanently.

Precautions

Panitumumab is a pregnancy category C drug, and is used during pregnancy only when medically necessary. A pregnancy category C drug is one for which studies done in animals have shown potential harm to a fetus but there are not sufficient data in humans. If the potential benefits for the patient outweigh the potential risks to the fetus, the drug may be used during pregnancy. However, panitumumab may cause harm to or death of a fetus. Panitumumab is contraindicated for use during breastfeeding and cannot be used within 2 months of beginning breastfeeding. The safety and effectiveness of panitumumab has not been established in patients less than 18 years of age. Panitumumab may not be appropriate for use in patients with skin inflammation or infections, some types of lung disease, or septic blood.

Monoclonal antibody drugs have been associated with severe infusion reactions, such as breathing complications, heart attack, collapse of the blood vessels, shock, and death. Panitumumab has a very low rate of infusion reactions compared with other monoclonal antibody cancer drugs. In clinical trials, infusion reactions occurred in only 4% of patients with only 1% severe. No fatalities were reported. However, in patients who do develop infusion reactions the dosage may need to be decreased, infusion rate decreased, or therapy discontinued altogether.

Caution is used when dosing panitumumab due to toxic reactions. Skin-related toxicity is commonly

KEY TERMS

Abscess—Pocket of infection present in body tissues.

Angiogenesis—Physiological process involving the growth of new blood vessels from preexisting blood vessels; process used by some cancers to create their own blood supply.

B cell—Type of white blood cell that creates antibodies to fight infection.

Cytochrome P450—Enzymes present in the liver that metabolize drugs.

Epidermal growth factor—Natural body chemical involved in cellular processes of growth and development.

Epidermal growth factor receptor—Structure on the surface of cells that binds growth factors to allow them to effect growth via a chemical signaling cascade.

Metastasis—The process by which cancer spreads from its original site to other parts of the body.

Monoclonal antibody—Antibodies produced by one type of B cell that are all clones of the parent cell and so are identical.

Pulmonary thromboembolism—Formation in a blood vessel of a clot (thrombus) that breaks loose (embolus) and is carried by the bloodstream to plug a vessel in the lungs.

Septic blood—Blood that is infected with bacteria to the point of illness; may be fatal.

associated with panitumumab therapy. Toxicity may involve **itching**, redness and inflammation, rash, acne, peeling skin, inflammation of the inner lining of the mouth, and fissured skin. Skin reactions that are severe may develop into infections leading to septic blood and death. Eye toxicity involves inflammation and redness, tearing, and irritation. Many of these toxic reactions occur within the first 14 to 15 days of treatment and resolve approximately 84 days after the last dose.

Panitumumab is associated with the risk of photosensitivity and severe sunburn. Excessive sun exposure should be avoided and protective measures such as sunscreen are advised. Panitumumab may cause severe imbalances in blood chemicals called electrolytes, especially for magnesium. Blood is monitored to check for signs of toxicity or abnormality. Panitumumab may also cause severe lung disease in some patients, including

Pap test

QUESTIONS TO ASK YOUR DOCTOR

- How long will I need to take this drug before you can tell whether it helps me?
- How often must I have blood work and other laboratory tests done to check the effect the drug is having?
- Is this drug safe to take with the other drugs that I am currently taking?
- What side effects should I watch for? When should I call the doctor about them?
- Are there any clinical trials of this drug combined with other therapies that might benefit me?

permanent fibrous changes to lung tissue that interfere with breathing capacity. Panitumumab therapy may not be appropriate for patients with existing skin abscesses, skin inflammation, or lung disease.

Side effects

Panitumumab is used when the medical benefit is judged to be greater than the risk of side effects. Commonly seen side effects include abdominal pain and cramping, constipation, **diarrhea**, peeling skin infections, **fatigue**, blood chemistry imbalances in magnesium and calcium, nausea, vomiting, itchy skin, rash, fissured painful skin, and sun sensitivity. Other side effects include acne, eye inflammation, cough, dehydration, dry skin, and mouth sores. Rarely panitumumab may cause lung disease, **fever**, septic blood, severely low pressure, and pulmonary thromboembolism. These side effects are most commonly seen with toxic doses of panitumumab and avoided during therapy.

Interactions

Panitumumab may cause multiple different potentially serious adverse effects. Use of panitumumab in the same time period as other drugs that cause similar medical problems may cause an additive effect. An additive effect is seen with the drug **bevacizumab**, increasing risk of skin-related toxicity, severe diarrhea, and lung disease. Interactions may occur between panitumumab and the drug **erlotinib**, causing an increased risk of gastrointestinal perforation and toxicity. Combination of panitumumab and the drugs **fluorouracil** or **irinotecan** increases risk of severe diarrhea.

Most medications are metabolized by a set of liver enzymes known as cytochrome P450 (CYP450). There are

multiple subtypes of CYP450s, each responsible for metabolism of their own set of drugs. It is unknown which specific CYP450 subtypes metabolize panitumumab. However, other drugs that induce or activate the CYP450 enzyme subtype that acts on panitumumab would increase the metabolism of panitumumab. This activity may result in lower levels of therapeutic panitumumab, thereby having a negative effect on treatment. For this reason drugs that induce the panitumumab CYP450 subtype may interact with panitumumab, and any medications, herbs, or supplements taken during fertility treatment should be temporarily minimized if medically appropriate.

Resources

BOOKS

Brunton, Laurence, Bruce Chabner, and Bjorn Knollman. *Goodman and Gilman's The Pharmacological Basis of Therapeutics.* 12th ed. New York: McGraw-Hill Medical Publishing, 2012.

Hamilton, Richard J., ed. *Tarascon Pharmacopoeia 2015 Professional Desk Reference Edition.* Burlington, MA: Jones & Bartlett Learning, 2015.

WEBSITES

National Cancer Institute. "Panitumumab." http://www.cancer.gov/cancertopics/druginfo/panitumumab (accessed November 10, 2014).

ORGANIZATIONS

National Cancer Institute, 9609 Medical Center Dr., BG 9609 MSC 9760, Bethesda, MD 20892-9760, (800) 4-CANCER (422-6237), http://www.cancer.gov.

U.S. Food and Drug Administration, 10903 New Hampshire Ave., Silver Spring, MD 20993, (888) INFO-FDA (463-6332), http://www.fda.gov.

Maria Basile, PhD

Pap test

Definition

The Papanicolaou test is a procedure in which a physician scrapes cells from the cervix or vagina to check for **cervical cancer**, **vaginal cancer**, or abnormal changes that could lead to **cancer**. It is most often called a Pap smear or Pap test.

The Pap test is not a diagnostic test. It identifies women who are at increased risk of cervical dysplasia (abnormal cells) or cervical cancer, but only an examination of the cervix with a special lighted instrument (colposcopy) and samples of cervical tissue (biopsies) can actually diagnose these conditions.

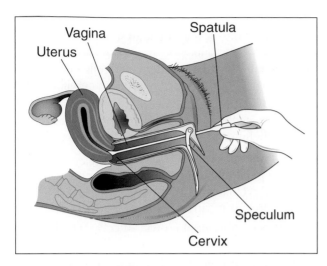

The Pap test is a procedure used to detect abnormal growth of cervical cells that may be a precursor to cancer of the cervix. It is administered by a physician, who inserts a speculum into the vagina to open and separate the vaginal walls. A spatula is then inserted to scrape cells from the cervix. These cells are transferred onto glass slides for laboratory analysis. The Pap test may also identify vaginitis, some sexually transmitted diseases, and cancers of the uterus and ovaries. *(Illustration by Electronic Illustrators Group. © Cengage Learning®.)*

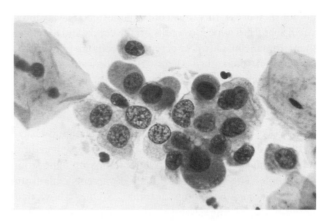

These malignant (cancerous) cells were taken from a woman's cervix during a Pap test. *(PARVIZ POUR/Science Source)*

Purpose

The Pap test is used to detect abnormal growth of cervical cells. The goal is to detect any abnormalities at an early stage, when the condition is easiest to treat. This microscopic analysis of cells can detect cervical cancer, precancerous changes, inflammation (vaginitis), infections, and some sexually transmitted diseases (STDs). The Pap test can also occasionally detect endometrial (uterine) cancer or **ovarian cancer**, even though it was not designed for this purpose.

Women should begin to have Pap tests at the age of 21 or within three years of becoming sexually active, whichever comes first. Young people are more likely to have multiple sex partners, which increases their risk of certain diseases that can cause cancer, such as **human papillomavirus** (HPV).

The American Congress of Obstetricians and Gynecologists (ACOG) recommends that women receive Pap smears every three years until age 30. From ages 30–65, women need to undergo testing every five years. The ACOG advises receiving an HPV test along with the Pap test. Once a woman reaches age 65, she can stop having a routine Pap test so long as her last three tests were negative and she does not have a history of cancer or dysplasia.

If a woman has any concerns, however, she can have the test done more frequently, and women with certain risk factors may need to have yearly tests. Women at highest risk of cervical cancer are those who started having sex before age 18; those with many sex partners (especially if they did not use condoms, which protect against STDs); those who have had STDs, such as genital herpes or genital warts; and those who smoke. Women who experience bleeding after menopause or who have had a positive test result in the past may need screening more frequently. Women who have been diagnosed with cervical cancer or precancer at any point in their lives should have regular Pap smears.

Description

The Pap test is an extremely cost-effective and beneficial exam. Cervical cancer used to be a leading cause of cancer deaths in the United States, but widespread use of this diagnostic procedure reduced the death rate from this disease by 74% between 1955 and 1992. A 2003 study reported that the test reduces rates of invasive cervical cancer by as much as 94%. In 2003, the FDA approved a new **screening test** that combined DNA testing for the HPV type that causes the most cases of cervical cancer with the standard Pap test, thus increasing its screening value.

The Pap test, sometimes called a cervical smear, is the microscopic examination of cells scraped from both the outer cervix and the cervical canal. The cervix is the opening between the vagina and the uterus, or womb. It is called the Pap test after its developer, Dr. George N. Papanicolaou. It is performed during a gynecologic examination and is usually covered by insurance. For those with coverage, Medicare will pay for one screening Pap smear every three years.

During the pelvic examination, an instrument called a speculum is inserted into the vagina to open it. The doctor then uses a tiny brush or a cotton-tipped swab and a small spatula to wipe loose cells off the cervix and to scrape them from the inside of the cervix. The cells are transferred, or smeared, onto glass slides. The slides are treated to stabilize the cells and are then sent to a laboratory for microscopic examination. The entire procedure is usually painless and takes less than ten minutes.

A newer method of testing, called liquid-based **cytology** or the liquid-based Pap test, involves spreading the cells more evenly on a slide after removing them from the sample. The liquid-based method prevents cells from drying out and becoming distorted. Studies show that liquid-based testing slightly improves cancer detection and greatly improves detection of precancers.

Precautions

The Pap test is usually not done during the menstrual period because of the presence of blood cells. The best time is in the middle of the menstrual cycle.

The Pap test may show abnormal results when a woman is healthy or normal results in women with cervical abnormalities as much as 25% of the time. It may even miss up to 5% of cervical cancers.

Preparation

Most women are not routinely advised to make any special preparations for a Pap test. However, some simple preparations may help to ensure that the test results are reliable. Measures women can take to help increase the test's reliability include:

• avoiding sexual intercourse for two days before the test

• not using douches for two or three days before the test

• avoiding tampons, vaginal creams, or birth control foams or jellies for two to three days before the test

• scheduling the Pap smear when not menstruating

Before the exam, the physician will take a complete sexual history to determine a woman's risk status for cervical cancer. Questions may include the date and results of the last Pap test, any history of abnormal Pap tests, date of last menstrual period and any irregularity, use of hormones and birth control, family history of gynecologic disorders, and any vaginal symptoms. These topics are relevant to the interpretation of the Pap test, especially if any abnormalities are detected. Immediately before the Pap test, the woman should empty her bladder to avoid discomfort during the procedure.

Aftercare

Harmless cervical bleeding is possible immediately after the test; a woman may need to use a sanitary napkin.

KEY TERMS

Carcinoma in situ—Malignant cells that are present only in the outer layer of the cervix.

Cervical intraepithelial neoplasia (CIN)—A term used to categorize degrees of dysplasia arising in the epithelium, or outer layer, of the cervix.

Dysplasia—Abnormal changes in cells.

Human papillomavirus (HPV)—The most common STD in the United States. Various types of HPV are known to cause cancer.

Neoplasia—Abnormal growth of cells, which may lead to a neoplasm, or tumor.

Squamous intraepithelial lesion (SIL)—A term used to categorize the severity of abnormal changes arising in the squamous, or outermost, layer of the cervix.

She should also be sure to comply with her doctor's orders for follow-up visits.

Risks

No appreciable health risks are associated with the Pap test. However, abnormal results (whether valid or due to technical error) can cause significant anxiety. Women may wish to have their sample double-checked, either by the same laboratory or by the new technique of computer-assisted rescreening; however, any abnormal Pap test should be followed by colposcopy, not by double-checking the Pap test.

Results

Normal (negative) results from the laboratory exam mean that no atypical, dysplastic, or cancer cells were detected, and that the cervix is normal.

Abnormal results

TERMINOLOGY. Abnormal cells found on the Pap test may be described using two different grading systems. Although this can be confusing, the systems are quite similar. The Bethesda system is based on the term "squamous intraepithelial lesion" (SIL). Precancerous cells are classified as atypical squamous cells of undetermined significance, low-grade SIL, or high-grade SIL. Low-grade SIL includes mild dysplasia (abnormal cell growth) and abnormalities caused by HPV; high-grade SIL includes moderate or severe dysplasia and **carcinoma** in situ (cancer that has not spread beyond the cervix).

Another term that may be used is "cervical intraepithelial neoplasia" (CIN). In this classification system, mild dysplasia is called CIN I, moderate is CIN II, and severe dysplasia or carcinoma in situ is CIN III.

Regardless of terminology, it is important to remember that an abnormal (positive) result does not necessarily indicate cancer. Results may be falsely abnormal after infection or irritation of the cervix. Up to 40% of mild dysplasia reverts to normal tissue without treatment, and only 1% of mild abnormalities ever develop into cancer.

CHANGES OF UNKNOWN CAUSE. ASCUS or LSIL cells are found in 5%–10% of all Pap tests. The most common abnormality is atypical squamous cells of undetermined significance, which are found in 4% of all Pap tests. Sometimes these results are described further as either reactive or precancerous. Reactive changes suggest that the cervical cells are responding to inflammation, such as from a yeast infection. These women may be treated for infection and then undergo repeat Pap testing in three to six months. If those results are negative, no further treatment is necessary. This category may also include atypical "glandular" cells, which could imply a more severe type of cancer and requires repeat testing and further evaluation.

DYSPLASIA. The next most common finding (in about 25 of every 1,000 tests) is low-grade SIL, which includes mild dysplasia or CIN I and changes caused by HPV. Unlike cancer cells, these cells do not invade normal tissues. Women are most susceptible to cervical dysplasia between the ages of 25 and 35. Typically, dysplasia causes no symptoms, although women may experience abnormal vaginal bleeding. Because dysplasia is precancerous, it should be treated if it is moderate or severe.

Treatment of dysplasia depends on the degree of abnormality. In women with no other risk factors for cervical cancer, mild precancerous changes may be simply observed over time with repeat testing, perhaps every four to six months. This strategy works only if women are diligent about keeping later appointments. Premalignant cells may remain that way without causing cancer for five to ten years, or may never become malignant.

Women with positive results or risk factors should undergo colposcopy and **biopsy**. A colposcope is an instrument with a light and a magnifier that is used to view the cervix. Biopsy, or removal of a small piece of abnormal cervical or vaginal tissue for analysis, is usually done at the same time.

High-grade SIL (found in 3 of every 50 Pap tests) includes moderate to severe dysplasia or carcinoma in situ (CIN II or III). After confirmation by colposcopy and biopsy, it must be removed or destroyed to prevent further growth. Several outpatient techniques are

---

QUESTIONS TO ASK YOUR DOCTOR

- When will I find out my results?
- What does an abnormal result mean?
- When should I schedule my next Pap test?

---

available: conization (removal of a cone-shaped piece of tissue), laser surgery, **cryotherapy** (freezing), or the loop electrosurgical excision procedure. Cure rates are nearly 100% after prompt and appropriate treatment of carcinoma in situ. Frequent checkups are then necessary.

CANCER. HPV may be responsible for many cervical cancers. Symptoms may include unusual vaginal bleeding or discharge, bowel and bladder problems, and pain. Women are at greatest risk of developing cervical cancer between the ages of 30 and 40 and between the ages of 50 and 60. Most new cancers are diagnosed in women between 50 and 55. Although the likelihood of developing this disease begins to level off for Caucasian women at the age of 45, it increases steadily for African Americans for another 40 years. The need for a biopsy is indicated when any abnormal growth is found on the cervix, even if the Pap test is negative.

Doctors have traditionally used **radiation therapy** and surgery to treat cervical cancer that has spread within the cervix or throughout the pelvis. In severe cases, postoperative radiation is administered to kill any remaining cancer cells, and **chemotherapy** may be used if cancer has spread to other organs. Recent studies have shown that giving chemotherapy and radiation at the same time improves a patient's chance of survival. The **National Cancer Institute** has urged physicians to strongly consider using both chemotherapy and radiation to treat patients with invasive cervical cancer. The five year survival rate of early-stage cervical cancer is as high as 93%; however, this number decreases significantly as the cancer progresses. Prevention and risk reduction are key to supporting a woman's gynecologic health.

Health care team roles

The Pap test is typically administered by either a physician, gynecologist, or nurse practitioner. The samples are sent to a laboratory for analysis.

Resources

BOOKS

Lentz, Gretchen, et al. *Comprehensive Gynecology*, 5th ed. St. Louis: Mosby/Elsevier, 2012.

PERIODICALS

Bakkum-Gamez, J., and S. Dowdy. "Retooling the Pap Smear for Ovarian and Endometrial Cancer Detection." *Clinical Chemistry* (September 16, 2013): e-pub ahead of print. http://dx.doi.org/10.1373/clinchem.2013.204933 (accessed August 26, 2014).

WEBSITES

American Cancer Society. "Survival Rates for Cancer of the Cervix." http://www.cancer.org/cancer/cervicalcancer/overviewguide/cervical-cancer-overview-survival-rates (accessed August 26, 2014).

American Congress of Obstetricians and Gynecologists. "New Guidelines for Cervical Cancer Screening." September 2013. http://www.acog.org/For_Patients/Search_FAQs/documents/New_Guidelines_for_Cervical_Cancer_Screening (accessed August 26, 2014).

Centers for Disease Control and Prevention. "Cervical Cancer Screening." http://www.cdc.gov/cancer/cervical/basic_info/screening.htm (accessed August 26, 2014).

National Cancer Institute. "Pap and HPV Testing." http://www.cancer.gov/cancertopics/factsheet/detection/Pap-HPV-testing (accessed August 26, 2014).

ORGANIZATIONS

American Cancer Society, 250 Williams St. NW, Atlanta, GA 30303, (800) 227-2345, http://www.cancer.org.

American Congress of Obstetricians and Gynecologists, 409 12th St. SW, Washington, DC 20024-2188, (202) 638-5577, (800) 673-8444, resources@acog.org, http://www.acog.org.

National Cancer Institute, 6116 Executive Blvd., Ste. 300, Bethesda, MD 20892-8322, (800) 4-CANCER (422-6237), http://cancer.gov.

Laura J. Ninger
REVISED BY TERESA G. ODLE

Paracentesis

Definition

Also known as peritoneal tap or abdominal tap, paracentesis consists of drawing fluid from the abdomen through a needle.

Purpose

Although little or no fluid is present in the abdominal (peritoneal) cavity of a healthy adult male, more than half an ounce may accumulate at certain times during a woman's menstrual cycle. Any **cancer** that originates in or spreads to the abdomen can result in fluid accumulation (malignant **ascites**).

Doctors remove fluid (ascites) from the abdomen to analyze its composition and determine its origin, to relieve the pressure and discomfort it causes, and to check for signs of internal bleeding This procedure should be performed whenever an individual experiences sudden or worsening abdominal swelling or when ascites is accompanied by **fever**, abdominal pain, confusion, or coma.

Paracentesis in cancer patients

When performed on a patient who has been diagnosed with cancer, paracentesis helps doctors determine the extent (stage) of the disease and whether conservative or radical treatment approaches would most effectively relieve symptoms or lengthen survival.

Precautions

Before undergoing paracentesis, the patient should advise the doctor of any allergies, bleeding problems or use of anticoagulants, or pregnancy or possibility of pregnancy.

Description

Paracentesis is performed in a doctor's office or a hospital. The puncture site is cleansed and if necessary, shaved. The patient may feel some stinging as a local anesthetic is administered, and pressure as the doctor inserts a special needle (tap needle) into the abdomen. Occasionally, guidance with CT or ultrasound may be used.

When paracentesis is performed for diagnostic purposes, less than an ounce of fluid is drawn from the patient's abdomen into a syringe. As much as 15 ounces may be needed to determine whether the ascites contains cancer cells. When the purpose of the procedure is to relieve pressure or other symptoms, many quarts of ascites may be drained from the abdomen. Because removing large amounts of fluid in a short time can cause dizziness, lightheadedness, and a sudden drop in blood pressure, the doctor may drain fluid slowly enough that the patient's circulatory system has time to adapt.

Laboratory analysis of abdominal fluid can detect blood, cancer cells, infection, and elevated protein levels often associated with malignant ascites. Results of these tests can help doctors determine the most appropriate course of treatment for a particular patient.

Preparation

No special preparations are required before this procedure. Patients should ask their doctors about special preparation requirements, but usually may eat, drink and take medications normally prior to paracentesis.

Aftercare

After removing the tap needle, the doctor may use a stitch or two to close any incision made (to ease the needle's entry into the abdomen) and apply an adhesive dressing to the puncture site.

Risks

Paracentesis occasionally causes infection. There is also a slight chance of the tap needle puncturing the bladder, bowel, or blood vessels in the abdomen. If large amounts of ascites are removed, the patient may need to be hospitalized and given intravenous (IV) fluids to prevent or correct severe fluid, protein, or electrolyte imbalances. A patient who has undergone extensive paracentesis should be warned about the possibility of fainting (syncope) episodes.

Results

Paracentesis is designed to establish the cause of, or to relieve symptoms associated with, an abnormal accumulation of fluid in the abdomen.

Abnormal results

Laboratory tests of ascites may indicate the presence of:

- appendicitis
- cancer
- cirrhosis
- damaged bowel
- disease of the heart, kidneys, or pancreas
- infection

Ascites that contains cancer cells is usually bloody. Cloudy abdominal fluid has been found in patients with extensive intraabdominal lymphomas. Ascites will continue to accumulate until its cause is identified and eliminated. Some patients need to undergo paracentesis repeatedly.

Resources

BOOKS

Irwin, Richard S., et al. *Procedures, Techniques, and Minimally Invasive Monitoring in Intensive Care Medicine.* 5th ed. Philadelphia: Wolters Kluwer Health/Lippincott Williams & Wilkins, 2011.

WEBSITES

Canadian Cancer Society. "Paracentesis." http://www.cancer.ca/en/cancer-information/diagnosis-and-treatment/tests-and-procedures/paracentesis/?region=on (accessed November 10, 2014).

Cancer Research UK. "Treating Fluid in the Abdomen." http://www.cancerresearchuk.org/about-cancer/coping-with-cancer/coping-physically/fluid-in-the-abdomen-ascites/treating-fluid-in-abdomen (accessed November 10, 2014).

Maureen Haggerty

Paranasal sinus cancer

Definition

Paranasal sinus **cancer** is the presence of a cancerous tumor in the mucus-producing tissues of the paranasal sinuses—the four hollow pockets of bone surrounding the nasal cavity.

Description

Paranasal sinus cancer is one of the major types of cancer in the head and neck region and belongs to a group of tumors collectively called head and neck cancer. The head and neck is an anatomically complex region in which tumors, including those in the paranasal sinuses, can easily invade a variety of structures even before symptoms appear. Structures that may be affected include the orbit of the eye (the bony cavity protecting the eyeball), the brain, the optic nerves, and the carotid arteries.

The paranasal sinuses are arranged symmetrically around the nasal cavity, which is the space just behind the nose through which air passes. The sinuses are air-filled areas within the cheeks, including the:

- frontal sinuses found in the forehead, directly above the nose

- ethmoid sinuses found on each side of the nasal cavity, just behind the upper part of the nose

- maxillary sinuses found on each side of the nasal cavity, in the upper region of the cheek bones

- sphenoid sinuses found behind the ethmoid sinuses, in the center of the skull

The paranasal sinuses are lined by mucus-producing tissues called mucous membranes that moisten the air entering the nose. Because the sinuses are air-filled, they allow the voice to echo and resonate.

The pharynx (throat) is divided into three sections: the nasopharynx, oropharynx, and laryngopharynx. The nasopharynx is the area behind (posterior to) the nose. The oropharynx is the area posterior to the mouth. The laryngopharynx opens into the larynx and esophagus. These areas contain several types of tissue that are each made up of different types of cells (squamous epithelial cells, salivary gland cells, nerve cells, infection-fighting cells, and blood vessel cells), which may lead to the development of various types of cancer. Usually, cancers of the paranasal sinuses originate in the lining of the nasopharynx or oropharynx, including squamous cell **carcinoma**, which is the most common type of paranasal sinus cancer, and **adenocarcinoma**, the second most common type, which begins in gland cells. More rarely (about 1% of cases), melanomas—a type of cancer arising from dark pigment-producing cells called melanocytes—may appear in the naso- or oropharynx. Another exceptionally rare malignant neoplasm (growth) known as an esthesioneuroblastoma, or olfactory **neuroblastoma**, may develop in an area of specialized sensory epithelium (surface layer of cells) through which the terminal branches of the olfactory nerve enter the roof of the nasal cavity.

Infrequently, a cancer may arise from the muscles or the soft tissues of the paranasal sinus region; these lesions are called sarcomas. Occasionally, lesions called midline granulomas (a granular-type tumor usually arising from lymphoid or epithelioid cells) occur; these lesions arise in the nose or paranasal sinuses and spread to surrounding tissues. Also rare are slow-growing benign wartlike growths called inverting papillomas, of which 10% to 15% may become cancerous.

Demographics

Malignant growths of the paranasal sinuses are uncommon in the general population, with only about 2,000 people in the United States diagnosed with these cancers annually. Paranasal sinus cancer represents 3% of all cancers in the upper aerodigestive tract (air and food passages) and less than 1% of all malignancies in the body. The incidence of paranasal sinus cancer is about one case per 100,000 people per year in the United States. Only about 200 new cases a year are diagnosed in the United States. The disease is more common in Asia Minor and China than in Western countries. The incidence of maxillary sinus cancer is highest among South African Bantus and in Japan.

Paranasal sinus tumors occur about two to three times more frequently in men than women, and diagnosis increases with age—80% of cases occur in people aged 55 and older. Cancers of the maxillary sinus are the most common of the paranasal sinus cancers, representing about 80% of all paranasal sinus cancers. Tumors of the ethmoid sinuses are less common (about 20%), and tumors of the sphenoid and frontal sinuses are rarest (less than 1%).

Squamous cell carcinoma, which originates in squamous cells in the top layer of the skin (epidermis) is the most common type of malignant tumor in the paranasal sinuses (about 80%). Adenocarcinomas (cancer that begins in glandular cells) constitute 15%, and the remaining 5% comprise all other types.

Causes and symptoms

Although the precise causes of paranasal sinus cancer are not known, the most significant risk factor is tobacco use, either smoked, snuffed, or chewed. Exposure to secondhand smoke and marijuana use has also been associated with the development of paranasal sinus cancer. Heavy alcohol use is associated with these cancers and is compounded when alcohol and tobacco are both used. In addition, several occupational groups are at increased risk of developing these tumors. These groups include leather and textile workers, nickel refiners, woodworkers, and manufacturers of isopropyl alcohol, chromium, and radium. Also, snuff (a form of tobacco that is inhaled) and thorium dioxide (a radiological contrast agent) have been associated with an increased incidence of paranasal sinus cancer. It has not been established whether these factors cause cancer by direct cancer production (**carcinogenesis**) or by altering the normal nasal epithelial physiology.

Nickel workers primarily develop squamous cell carcinomas, which usually arise in the nasal cavity. Woodworkers, however, usually develop adenocarcinomas that arise in the ethmoid sinuses. The incidence of adenocarinomas in these workers is 1,000 times higher than that of the general population. Air pollution exposure is also believed to increase the risk of paranasal sinus cancer. Viral agents, specifically the **human papillomavirus** (HPV), may also play a causative role.

In patients with cancer of the head and neck, the immune system is often not functioning properly. Malignant cells are not recognized as foreign, or when recognized, the immune system does not effectively destroy the cancer cells. Severe malnutrition, substances in the tumor that deactivate the immune system, and genetic predisposition are blamed for these immune system failures.

The symptoms of paranasal sinus cancer vary with the type, location, and stage of cancer. Symptoms typical of early lesions often resemble those of an upper respiratory tract infection and include nasal obstruction, facial pain, and thin, watery nasal discharge (rhinorrhea), which can at times be blood-tinged. The duration of symptoms differentiates an upper respiratory infection from a malignant lesion. An upper respiratory infection generally clears up or improves dramatically in several weeks with appropriate medical care, but symptoms associated with a malignancy typically persist.

The most common symptoms of paranasal sinus cancer include:

- persistently blocked nose
- recurrent "sinus infections"
- bleeding without apparent cause from the nose or the paranasal sinuses
- progressive pain and swelling of the upper region of the face or around the eyes
- closing up of one eye, blurred vision, or visual loss
- persistent pain in the forehead, the front of the skull, or over the cheekbones
- swelling in the roof of the mouth
- loosening of teeth, poorly fitting dentures, or bleeding from upper teeth sockets

Tumors in the nasal cavity and paranasal sinuses metastasize (spread) to the cervical lymph nodes (lymph nodes in the neck) in about 15% of individuals, which can lead to distant metastases in other organ systems.

Diagnosis

Diagnosis of paranasal sinus cancer entails several steps. The first step is a thorough medical history, followed by a physical examination. The physical

KEY TERMS

Adenocarcinoma—Cancer that begins in cells that line certain internal organs and that have glandular (secretory) properties.

Adenopathy—Large or swollen lymph glands.

Adjuvant therapy—Treatment (such as chemotherapy, radiation therapy, or hormone therapy) given after the primary treatment to increase the chances of a cure.

Angiogenesis inhibitor—A substance that prevents the growth of new blood vessels.

Antimetabolite—A chemical very similar to one required in normal biochemical reactions in cells; an antimetabolite can stop or slow down the reaction.

Antineoplaston—A substance isolated from normal human blood and urine and tested as a type of treatment for some tumors and AIDS.

Epithelium—A thin layer of tissue that covers organs, glands, and other structures within the body.

Monoclonal antibody—Laboratory-produced substance that can locate and bind to cancer cells.

Nasal cavity—The cavity between the floor of the cranium and the roof of the mouth.

Neoplasm—Any new and abnormal formation of tissue, as a tumor or growth.

Radiotherapy—Radiation treatment (external or internal).

examination may reveal a lesion in the nose or a submucosal (below the mucous membrane) mass arising in an adjacent sinus.

After the history and physical examination, a series of tests are performed to determine the precise nature of the suspicious growth and the extent of its spread. These tests may include:

- Biopsy (removal of a sample of tissue from a suspicious lesion) is performed after a lesion is identified. The tissue is studied microscopically by a pathologist.
- Computed tomography (CT) scan, which may be used to produce a series of detailed radiographic images with thin cross-sectional slices of the target area that can be interpreted using a computer.
- Nasoscopy, which utilizes an instrument called the nasoscope for examining the nasal cavity and the paranasal sinuses.

- Magnetic resonance imaging (MRI), which uses a powerful magnetic force to polarize electrons in the body and produce detailed images that are then interpreted by a computer.
- Posterior rhinoscopy, in which the nasopharynx and the rear portion of the nose are examined using a light and a special mirror.

Although endoscopic techniques (visualizing the nasal cavity with a tubelike fiberoptic device called an endoscope) have greatly improved the ability to examine the nasal cavities and the paranasal sinuses, radiographic studies are also necessary to complete the diagnostic evaluation. The most important radiographic studies include CT and MRI scans, usually used in combination. CT scans are preferred for evaluating the bony structures in the paranasal sinus area. MRI studies provide the most detailed information about soft-tissue differences, not only differentiating tumor tissue from inflammatory changes in the nose and sinuses, but also evaluating involvement of the soft tissues in, for example, the orbit, the brain, and the optic nerve. MRI has therefore become the essential radiographic test for accurate delineation of the pretreatment tumor and is also used for patient follow-up after treatment.

Obtaining a **biopsy** is crucial to diagnosis and is usually obtained during endoscopic sinus surgery. Combining endoscopic surgery with CT imaging, however, allows the surgeon to access small recesses of the nose and sinuses and areas along the base of the skull, making biopsy more accurate and safe.

Treatment team

Patients with paranasal sinus cancer are usually treated by a team of specialists with a multifaceted approach. Each patient receives a treatment plan that is tailored to fit his or her case, specifically the patient's overall health status, the tumor grade, and the disease stage. The treatment team usually includes:

- an otorhinolaryngologist (ear, nose, and throat specialist)
- an oncologist (cancer specialist)
- a radiotherapist (x-ray treatment specialist)

If extensive surgery is required, a plastic and reconstructive surgeon may also become part of the treatment team.

Clinical staging

Paranasal sinus cancer staging involves carefully establishing whether the cancer has spread, the extent of spread, and the involvement of lymph nodes and other organ systems.

Cancer grading is determined by the examination of cells from the tumor taken through biopsy either prior to or during surgery. The tumor tissue will be prepared in the laboratory and a pathologist will examine it microscopically to determine the type of cancer cell and the degree of aggressiveness of the cancer. The term *well-differentiated* means less aggressive; the terms *moderately differentiated*, *intermediately aggressive*, and *poorly differentiated* indicate increasing degrees of aggressiveness.

Both grading and staging help the physician establish the prognosis (degree of seriousness of the disease) and likely outcome.

Staging may involve additional imaging tests such as CT scan of the brain, abdominal ultrasound, bone scan, or chest x-ray. Although no clear-cut staging protocol exists for the relatively uncommon cancers of the paranasal sinuses, the following practical staging exists for cancer of the maxillary sinuses, the most common cancer of the nasal cavity/paranasal sinus area:

- Stage I: The cancer is confined to the maxillary sinus, with no bony erosion or spread to the lymph nodes.
- Stage II: The cancer has begun to destroy the surrounding bones but without spread to the lymph nodes.
- Stage III: The cancer has spread no further than the bones around the sinus and to one node on the same side of the neck and is no greater than 3 cm (1.1 in) in size, or has spread to the cheek, the rear portion of the sinus, the eye socket, or the ethmoidal sinus (spread to lymph nodes on the same side of the neck may or may not be present).
- Stage IV: The cancer has spread to the eye, other sinuses, or tissues adjacent to the sinuses (spread to lymph nodes on the same side of the neck may or may not be present). The cancer may have spread within the sinus itself or to surrounding tissues, to lymph nodes in the neck on one or both sides, to any node larger than 6 cm (2.3 in.), or to other parts of the body. Recurrent maxillary sinus cancer—either in the same location or in a different one after primary treatment has been completed—is also in this category.

Another staging system that may be applied to paranasal sinus cancer is the TNM system of the **American Joint Committee on Cancer**. The TNM system is based on three key factors: T represents tumor and how far it has grown into nearby structures; N represents lymph nodes in the head and neck, the number involved; and M stands for **metastasis** or spread to other organs. Numerical grades of 0-4 are assigned to each factor to obtain a TNM score. Higher scores correspond to higher stages as described above.

Treatment

The major treatment options for paranasal sinus cancer include:

- Surgery. May be necessary for the removal of a section of the nasal cavity or the paranasal sinus at any stage of the disease. Also, some lymph node dissection may be required in the neck, depending upon the staging and grading, or it may be combined with radiotherapy at any stage, depending on the type of cancer and its location. Depending on how extensive the surgery must be, reconstructive plastic surgery may also be required.

- Radiotherapy. Also called radiation therapy, radiotherapy is sometimes used alone in stage I and II disease or in combination with surgery in any stage of the disease. In the early stages of paranasal sinus cancer, radiotherapy is considered the alternative local therapy to surgery. Radiotherapy involves the use of high-energy, penetrative external beam treatment to destroy cancer cells in the area being treated. Radiation therapy is also employed to control symptoms and improve comfort (palliative care) in patients with advanced cancer. Teletherapy (external beam radiation) is administered via a machine remote from the body, while internal radiation (brachytherapy) is given by implanting a radioactive source into the cancerous tissues. Patients may or may not require both types of radiation. Radiotherapy usually takes just five to 10 minutes per day, five days a week for about six weeks, depending upon the type of radiotherapy used.

- Chemotherapy. Usually reserved for stage III and IV disease. In addition to local therapy, systemic therapy using chemotherapeutic agents is the best attempt to kill cancer cells that may be circulating in the body. Chemotherapy may be delivered intravenously or through oral medications. Chemotherapy is typically administered in weekly or biweekly cycles depending on the type of drug or combination of drugs. Targeted therapy for paranasal sinus cancer may include treatment with monoclonal antibodies such as cetuximab (Erbitux, which can be combined with radiotherapy for early-stage cancers and combined with chemotherapy drugs such as cisplatin for more advanced cancers. Chemotherapy may also be used in combination with surgery, radiotherapy, or both.

Molecular biology and **gene therapy** are the focus of ongoing research and are providing new insights into the basic mechanisms of cancer genesis and treatment. The detection of various oncogenes (genes that can induce tumor formation) in head and neck cancer is also progressing rapidly. Many **head and neck cancers** have been found to have gene mutations of a cancer suppressor gene called *TP53*. Although gene therapy trials are under way to introduce genetic material to help the immune system recognize cancer cells, results have not been encouraging so far.

Integrative therapies

Integrative therapies may be used at any stage of the disease either in place of conventional treatments or in addition to conventional treatments. Much anecdotal (nonscientific) evidence exists to suggest that integrative cancer therapies may be effective. Some therapies, such as acupuncture, may be covered by insurance plans, others are not.

Accepted integrative therapies include:

- acupuncture
- biofeedback
- dietary and nutritional guidelines that emphasize fresh whole fruits and vegetables and whole grains
- therapeutic massage
- guided meditation, prayer, or creative visualization
- nutritional supplements, including vitamins (especially antioxidants A, E, and C), minerals, and herbs

The National Center for Complementary and Alternative Medicine, part of the National Institutes of Health, describes some alternative and complementary cancer treatments on its website: http://www.nccam.nih.gov.

Prognosis

Paranasal sinus cancer has a high mortality rate (5-year survival and poor prognosis, primarily associated with its typical late diagnosis, as 75% of lesions are at an advanced stage at the time of definitive diagnosis. The American Cancer Society reports that 5-year survival rates are 65% for stage I, 61% for stage II, 50% for stage III, and 35% for stage IV. Survival rates, however, are generalizations based on previous cases and cannot predict the outcomes of individual cases. Surgical treatment alone may be sufficient for stage I or II lesions if adequate surgical margins are obtained. However, for advanced tumors, combined therapy with radical surgical excision and postoperative radiotherapy has been shown to improve the five-year survival rate.

The primary cause of death is failure of local control of tumor growth. Most paranasal sinus cancers grow rapidly and invade nearby tissues but are slow to spread to distant sites. Thus, patients with advanced disease usually die from a local recurrence of the tumor, even after aggressive treatment.

Coping with cancer treatment

Cancer treatments such as radiotherapy and **chemotherapy** not only destroy cancer cells but also damage healthy tissue. The effects of radiation depend upon the dose of radiation, the size of the area radiated, and the number and size of each fraction. When doses are fractionated, the total dose of **radiation therapy** is divided into several smaller, equal doses delivered over a period of several days.

The most common side effect of radiotherapy is extreme **fatigue**. Although rest is encouraged, most radiotherapists advise patients to move around as much as possible. Another common side effect is radiation dermatitis—the skin covering the radiated area becomes red, dry, itchy, and may show signs of scaling. This skin problem is associated only with teletherapy (external beam radiation therapy).

Radiation also may cause **nausea and vomiting**, **diarrhea**, and urinary discomfort. There may also be a decrease in white blood cells (leukopenia), which are needed to fight infection. Usually the radiotherapist or oncologist can suggest the drugs and diet necessary to alleviate these problems.

Chemotherapy drugs may cause a wide spectrum of side effects. The severity of these symptoms varies with each drug and with each individual. Some of the most common side effects of chemotherapy include:

• diarrhea

• hair loss (alopecia)

• hearing loss

• skin rashes

• tingling and numbness in the fingers and toes

• vomiting

Most of these side effects are treatable, temporary, and recede after therapy ends. However, the attitude of the patient is very important during cancer therapy. The more psychologically prepared the patient is for treatment, the higher the chances of experiencing fewer side effects.

If extensive surgery is required, reconstruction and rehabilitation by specialized physicians can improve the patient's quality of life.

Clinical trials

Ongoing **clinical trials** involving paranasal sinus cancer can be located on the website: http://www.clinicaltrials.gov, a service of the National Institutes of Health and the National Library of Medicine.

Some of the new drugs under investigation for advanced, recurrent, or metastatic head and neck cancer—either alone; in combination; with concurrent radiotherapy; or with standard chemotherapy drugs such as **fluorouracil** (5-FU), paclitaxel, or cisplatin—include:

• A10 and AS2-1 (antineoplastons)

• Dimesna (chemoprotective agent)

• Fenretinide (retinoid, or vitamin A derivative)

• Targeted therapies such as the monoclonal antibodies erlotinib, sunitinib, sorafenib, and lapatinib in combination with chemotherapy or radiation

• Flavopiridol (cyclin-dependent kinase [Cdk] inhibitor; kinases play a role in cell cycle regulation and tumor formation)

• Gemcitabine (antimetabolite)

• ONYX-015 (genetically engineered cold virus)

• Oxaliplatin (platinum compound; chemotherapeutic agent)

• SU5416 (angiogenesis inhibitor)

Prevention

The precise causes of paranasal sinus cancer are unknown. However, avoiding environmental risk factors such as heavy smoking or drinking, or inhalation of wood dust or other toxic substances (such as isopropyl alcohol, chromium, or radium) on a regular basis may help to decrease the chances of developing this form of cancer.

Special concerns

Although surgical treatment of squamous cell carcinoma of the head and neck offers the best chance for cure in many patients, the results of the surgery may be extremely disfiguring and functionally debilitating. The changes in facial appearance and loss of ability to speak, swallow, and breathe normally can be devastating, both physically and psychologically. In such cases, if the anticipated surgical defect is large, the reconstructive team will often harvest tissue from a distant site in the body to use as a graft once the oncology team has removed the cancer. Reconstructive teams were once solely concerned with simply closing the surgical defect and re-establishing a more natural form. Increasingly, the focus has turned to re-establishing normal function.

Resources

BOOKS

Abeloff, Martin D., James O. Armitage, Allen S. Licter, and John E. Niederhuber. "Paranasal Sinuses and Nose." In *Clinical Oncology.* 5th ed. New York: Churchill Livingstone, 2013.

Harrison, Louis B., Roy B. Sessions, and Merrill S. Kies, editors. *Head and Neck Cancer: A Multidiscplinary Approach.* 4th ed. Philadelphia: Lippincott Williams & Wilkins, 2013.

Niederhuber, J.E., et al. *Clinical Oncology.* 5th ed. Philadelphia: Elsevier, 2014.

PERIODICALS

Gelbard, A., K. S. Hale, and Y. Takahashi, et al. "Molecular Profiling of Sinonasal Undifferentiated Carcinoma." *Head & Neck* 36 (January 2014): 15–21.

Jegoux, F., A. Metreau, G. Louvel, and C. Bedfert. "Paranasal Sinus Cancer." *European Annals of Otorhinolayngology, Head & Neck Diseases* 130 (December 2013): 327–335.

Teudt, I. U., J. E. Meyer, and M. Ritter, et al. "Perioperative Image-Adapted Brachytherapy for the Treatment of Paranasal Sinus and Nasal Cavity Malignancies." *Brachytherapy* 13 (March April 2014): 178–186.

WEBSITES

American Cancer Society. "Nasal Cavity and Paranasal Sinuses Cancer." http://www.cancer.org/cancer/nasalcavityandparanasalsinuscancer/index (accessed November 17, 2014).

American Society of Clinical Oncology. "Nasal Cavity and Paranasal Sinus Cancer." http://www.cancer.net/cancer-types/nasal-cavity-and-paranasal-sinus-cancer (accessed October 14, 2014).

ORGANIZATIONS

American Cancer Society, 250 Williams St. NW, Atlanta, GA 30303, (800) 227-2345, http://www.cancer.org.

American Society of Clinical Oncology, 2318 Mill Rd., Ste. 800, Alexandria, VA 22314, (571) 483-1300, (888) 651-3038, contactus@cancer.net, http://www.cancer.org.

National Center for Complementary and Alternative Medicine, 9000 Rockville Pike, Bethesda, MD 20892, (888) 644-6226, TTY: (866) 464-3615, http://nccam.nih.gov.

Genevieve Slomski, PhD

REVISED BY L. LEE CULVERT

Paraneoplastic syndromes

Description

Paraneoplastic syndromes are rare disorders caused by substances that are secreted by a benign tumor, a malignant (cancerous) tumor, or a malignant tumor's metastases. The disturbances caused by paraneoplastic syndromes occur in body organs at sites that are distant or remote from the primary or metastatic tumors. Body systems that may be affected by paraneoplastic syndromes include neurological, endocrine, cutaneous, renal, hematologic, gastrointestinal, and other systems. The most common manifestations of paraneoplastic syndromes are cutaneous, neurologic, and endocrine disorders. An example of a cutaneous paraneoplastic disorder are telangiectasias, which can be caused by **breast cancer** and lymphomas. Lambert-Eaton myasthenic syndrome (LEMS, and also known as Eaton-Lambert syndrome) is a neurologic paraneoplastic syndrome that can be caused by a variety of tumors including **small-cell lung cancer**, **lymphoma**, breast, colon and other cancers. Syndrome of inappropriate antidiuretic hormone (SIADH) is an endocrine paraneoplastic syndrome, which is seen in as many as 40% of patients diagnosed with small-cell lung **cancer**.

Approximately 15% of patients already have a paraneoplastic disorder at the time of initial diagnosis with cancer. As many as 50% of all cancer patients will develop a paraneoplastic syndrome at some time during the course of their disease. Some clinicians categorize the **anorexia**, cachexia, and **fever** that occur as a result of cancer as metabolic paraneoplastic syndromes. Virtually all patients diagnosed with cancer are affected by at least one of these metabolic paraneoplastic syndromes.

Paraneoplastic syndromes can occur with any type of malignancy. However, they occur most frequently with lung cancer, specifically small-cell lung **carcinoma**. Other types of cancer that commonly cause paraneoplastic syndromes are breast cancer and **stomach cancer**. With the exception of **Wilms tumor** and **neuroblastoma**, paraneoplastic syndromes do not usually occur in children diagnosed with cancer.

In general, paraneoplastic syndromes may be present in the patient before a diagnosis of cancer is made, or, as stated earlier, may be present at the time the patient is first diagnosed with cancer. Most paraneoplastic syndromes appear in the later stages of the disease. Frequently, the presence of a paraneoplastic syndrome is associated with a poor prognosis. Paraneoplastic syndromes are difficult to diagnose and are often misdiagnosed. Some paraneoplastic syndromes may be confused with metastatic disease or spread of the cancer. The presence of the syndrome may be the only indication that a patient has a malignancy or that a malignancy has recurred. Paraneoplastic syndromes may be useful as clinical indicators to evaluate the response of the primary cancer to the treatment. Resolution of the paraneoplastic syndrome can be correlated with tumor response to treatment. That is, if the paraneoplastic syndrome resolves, the tumor has usually responded to the treatment.

Causes and symptoms

Paraneoplastic syndromes occur when the primary or original tumor secretes substances such as hormones, proteins, growth factors, cytokines, and antibodies. These substances are referred to as mediators. These mediators have effects on remote or distant body organs, which are termed target organs. Mediators interfere with communication between cells in the body. This miscommunication results in abnormal or increased activity of the cell's normal function. For example, a lung tumor may cause the paraneoplastic syndrome known as ectopic **Cushing syndrome**, which is the result of abnormal functioning of the pituitary gland located in the brain. In this example, the lung cancer is the primary tumor and the pituitary gland is the target organ. Ectopic Cushing syndrome is caused by overproduction of the mediator adrenocorticotropic hormone (ACTH).

Treatment

There are usually two approaches taken in the treatment of paraneoplastic syndromes. The first step is treatment of the cancer that is causing the syndrome. This treatment can be surgery, administration of **chemotherapy**, biotherapy, **radiation therapy**, or a combination of these therapies. The next approach is to suppress the substance or mediator causing the paraneoplastic syndrome. Often treatment targeted to the underlying cancer and to the paraneoplastic syndrome occur at the same time. However, even with treatment, irreversible damage to the target organ can occur.

Selected paraneoplastic syndromes

SYNDROME OF INAPPROPRIATE ANTIDIURETIC HORMONE (SIADH). SIADH is a common paraneoplastic syndrome that affects the endocrine system. This syndrome is most often associated with small-cell lung cancer; however, other cancers such as **brain tumors**, leukemia, lymphoma, colon, prostate, and **head and neck cancers** can lead to SIADH. SIADH is caused by the inappropriate production and secretion of arginine vasopressin or antidiuretic hormone (ADH) by tumor cells. Patients with SIADH may not have symptoms, especially in the early stages. When symptoms do occur, they are usually related to hyponatremia, which leads to central nervous system toxicity if left untreated. Signs and symptoms associated with hyponatremia include **fatigue**, anorexia, headache, and mild alteration in mental status in early stages. If SIADH remains untreated, symptoms can progress to confusion, delirium, seizures, coma, and death. Treatment approaches for SIADH are to treat the underlying tumor and restrict fluids. More severe cases may require the administration of medications.

LAMBERT-EATON MYASTHENIC SYNDROME. Lambert-Eaton myasthenic syndrome, also known as LEMS and Eaton-Lambert syndrome, has been associated with a number of cancers, including small-cell lung cancer, lymphoma, breast, stomach, colon, and prostate cancers. Potential mediators associated with paraneoplastic LEMS are antibodies that interfere with release of acetylcholine at the neuromuscular junction. This interference prevents the flow of calcium, which results in decreased or absent impulse transmission to muscle. The disruption in muscular impulse transmission leads to mild symptoms including weakness in the legs and thighs, muscle aches, muscle stiffness, and muscle fatigue. Treatment of LEMS includes administration of **corticosteroids**, intravenous immunoglobulin, and plasmapheresis. Depending on the extent of damage, irreversible loss of function may occur even with treatment.

ECTOPIC CUSHING SYNDROME. Cushing syndrome is most often associated with small-cell lung cancer, **ovarian cancer**, and medullary cancers of the thyroid. ACTH precursors are activated by tumor cells that result in overproduction of ACTH by the pituitary gland. Signs and symptoms of ectopic Cushing syndrome include hypertension, hyperglycemia, hypokalemia, edema, muscle weakness, and **weight loss**. The primary approach to treating ectopic Cushing syndrome is to treat the underlying cancer. In early stages, surgery is the treatment of choice. However, surgery is not usually an option for patients diagnosed with small-cell cancer of the lung. If the tumor cannot be removed or controlled, or if the patient has severe symptoms, then treatment targeted to the syndrome is initiated. Medical therapy is usually focused on inhibiting cortisol production and involves the use of medications such as ketoconazole and **aminoglutethimide**.

Resources

BOOKS

Winter, Lora H., ed. *Paraneoplastic Syndromes: Symptoms, Diagnosis and Treatment.* Hauppauge, NY: Nova Science Publishers, 2014.

PERIODICALS

Kanaji, N., Watanabe, N., Kita, N., Bandoh, S., Tadokoro, A., Ishii, T., Dobashi, H., and Matsunaga, T. "Paraneoplastic Syndromes Associated With Lung Cancer." *World Journal of Clinical Oncology* 5, no. 3 (2014): 197–223. http://www.ncbi.nlm.nih.gov/pmc/articles/PMC4127595/ (accessed November 10, 2014).

WEBSITES

Micromedex. "Paraneoplastic Syndrome of the Nervous System." Mayo Clinic. http://www.mayoclinic.org/diseases-conditions/paraneoplastic-syndromes/basics/definition/con-20028459 (accessed November 10, 2014).

Melinda Granger Oberleitner, R.N., D.N.S.

Paraplatin *see* **Carboplatin**

Parathyroid cancer

Definition

Parathyroid **cancer** is a rare, slow-growing tumor of one or more parathyroid glands in the neck.

Description

Cancer of the parathyroid glands is exceptionally rare. The four parathyroid glands in the human body are designated as the right superior, right inferior, left superior, and left inferior glands. They usually lie adjacent to the thyroid, but rarely can be found in the upper chest. The parathyroid glands secrete parathyroid hormone, which plays a central role in regulating calcium levels in the blood. In the condition called primary hyperparathyroidism, excess production of parathyroid hormone leads to abnormally high levels of calcium (**hypercalcemia**) mobilized from the bones into the blood circulation. Adenomas, or hyperplasias, of the parathyroid glands are responsible for about 99% of all cases of primary hyperparathyroidism. Parathyroid cancer accounts for the remaining 1%.

Demographics

Parathyroid cancer is found in about one patient in every 5,000 patients with parathyroid disease. Only a few hundred cases of parathyroid cancer have been described in clinical reports. It is more common in Asia, especially Japan, than in Western countries. Men and women are affected equally. Parathyroid cancer develops in adults aged 30 and older. The average age of patients at diagnosis is around 40.

Causes and symptoms

No predisposing factors have been found to clearly increase the risk of parathyroid cancer. However, the disease has occasionally been associated with a genetic defect called **multiple endocrine neoplasia** type I, which may increase risk in people with this defect. Parathyroid cancer also develops in patients with adenomas, autosomal dominant familial isolated hyperparathyroidism, or hyperplasia of the parathyroid.

Most parathyroid cancers are functioning tumors that overproduce parathyroid hormone. Thus, the signs and symptoms of parathyroid cancer are chiefly related to hyperparathyroidism and the resultant hypercalcemia. Common complaints are weakness, **fatigue**, insomnia, **weight loss**, **anorexia**, constipation, nausea, and vomiting. Patients may also report frequent urination and extreme thirst. Since excess parathyroid hormone causes bones to release too much calcium into the bloodstream, patients may experience **bone pain** and fractures. The

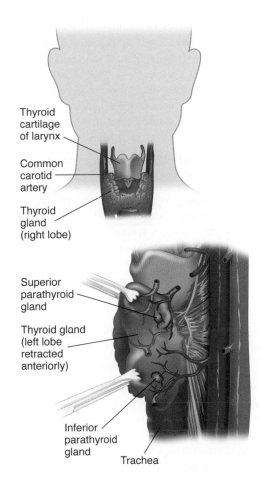

Illustration showing the location of the parathyroid glands.
(Illustration by Electronic Illustrators Group. © 2015 Cengage Learning®.)

extra calcium in the blood can be deposited in the kidneys, leading to the formation of painful kidney stones. Pancreatitis is another consequence of hypercalcemia, as are stomach and small intestine ulcers. The levels of parathyroid hormone and calcium in patients with parathyroid cancer are usually dramatically elevated compared to the levels in patients with benign causes of hyperparathyroidism.

Sometimes a parathyroid tumor may be large enough to form a mass in the neck that can be easily felt. If the mass is large enough, it can impinge upon a nerve that controls the vocal cords, leading to hoarseness and difficulty speaking. In contrast, these features are uncommon in benign hyperparathyroidism.

Diagnosis

The diagnosis of parathyroid cancer can be difficult because it produces symptoms similar to those of benign hyperparathyroidism due to adenomas or hyperplasia. However, the symptoms of parathyroid cancer are generally more severe, and the levels of parathyroid hormone and calcium are usually much higher than in benign **adenoma**. The presence of a neck mass or hoarseness also suggests cancer. Beyond this, no single biochemical test or diagnostic imaging examination is able to definitively diagnose parathyroid cancer; final diagnosis must rely on pathologic examination of tissue from **biopsy** or surgery.

Four somewhat different scenarios may be involved in the diagnosis of parathyroid cancer:

• Parathyroid cancer is first suspected on the basis of symptoms and signs. Surgery is performed with the intent to remove the cancer. A special radioactive scintigraphy scan called a sestamibi scan, which uses technetium (99mTc), may be done prior to surgery to precisely locate the lesion to be removed. Biopsy of a suspected tumor either prior to or during surgery may confirm the diagnosis of cancer.

• A patient with hyperparathyroidism undergoes surgery to remove one or more glands that are thought to contain an adenoma or hyperplasia. During surgery, the underlying lesion is judged to most likely be cancer, and a biopsy is done to confirm.

• Similarly, a patient with hyperparathyroidism undergoes surgery to remove one or more glands that are thought to contain an adenoma or hyperplasia. After the surgery is complete, the resected specimen is analyzed and found to contain cancer cells.

• Symptoms of hyperparathyroidism may reappear after surgery, which suggests an incompletely treated parathyroid cancer that may be localized in the neck or may have spread to distant organs. Several imaging examinations can be helpful in this situation. Scintigraphy and ultrasound are useful in detecting recurrent tumors in the neck. Computed tomography (CT scan) and magnetic resonance imaging (MRI) can detect cancer in distant organs, such as the lungs or liver. MRI is especially useful in visualizing details of soft tissue in the tumor area or possible distant metastases.

Clinical staging

Parathyroid cancer begins in the parathyroid gland and extends to adjacent structures. Late in the course of the disease, it spreads to lymph nodes and ultimately spreads to the lungs, liver, and sometimes bones through the lymphatic system.

Treatment

The preferred treatment for parathyroid cancer is surgical removal of the cancerous gland. This surgery is

---

KEY TERMS

Adenoma—Benign tumor derived from glandular structures.

Biopsy—Obtaining a piece of tissue from the body for diagnostic examination.

Computed tomography—A radiologic examination that uses x-rays to generate images of cross-sectional planes of the body.

Diuretic—A drug that promotes the excretion of urine.

Hyperplasia—Generalized overgrowth of body tissues or organs due to an excessive increase in the number of cells.

Magnetic resonance imaging—A diagnostic imaging examination that uses magnetic fields and radiowaves to reconstruct detailed images of the body, especially of soft tissue.

Pancreatitis—Inflammation of the pancreas.

Peptic ulcer—Distinct erosions of the inner layer of the stomach or small intestine.

Scintigraphy—A radiologic examination that involves the injection and detection of radioactive isotopes to obtain two-dimensional images of a body organ and which assists in evaluating organ system functioning.

Ultrasound—A diagnostic imaging procedure that uses high-frequency sound waves to create real-time images of specific body organs.

---

most often performed as a minimally invasive, radio-guided focused parathyroidectomy. **Stereotactic surgery** may be used to provide the best view of the tumor site and help to maintain the patient's position to allow complete removal of cancerous tissue. In order to assure complete resection of the cancer, part of the thyroid gland, nearby lymph nodes, and other adherent tissue must be removed with the specimen. Cancer that has spread to distant organs should be removed if possible.

Parathyroid hormone may be monitored during surgery, which has been shown to improve surgical outcomes. A gamma probe is sometimes used during the surgery to help guide the dissection and allow identification of abnormal tissue, as well as to confirm that the tissue being resected is definitely parathyroid tissue.

A few cases have been reported in which **radiation therapy** or **chemotherapy** have been used to partially control the growth and symptoms of parathyroid cancer.

However, these interventions have not been successful in the majority of patients, and surgery remains the mainstay of treatment for parathyroid cancer.

Surgical cure is often possible, but not if the cancer has spread too widely. Therapy then becomes focused on controlling hypercalcemia. General measures include infusing saline solution intravenously to restore lost fluid and to encourage urinary excretion of calcium. Diuretics are drugs that further stimulate urinary excretion of calcium. **Bisphosphonates** and **plicamycin** both inhibit the release of calcium from the bone. Other agents, such as **gallium nitrate**, have shown promise in the treatment of hypercalcemia associated with parathyroid cancer. However, further studies must be conducted to confirm their effectiveness and safety.

Prognosis

The prognosis of parathyroid cancer depends upon the stage of the cancer and the completeness of the surgical resection. If the cancer is detected early and completely removed, cure is possible and likely. However, parathyroid cancer has been reported to recur up to 20 years after surgery, and cure is unlikely after recurrence. Even so, survival can be significantly extended by surgery aimed at removing as much recurrent or distant cancer as possible. In general, parathyroid cancer grows and spreads so slowly that oversecretion of parathyroid hormone is more clinically evident than the actual growth of the cancer.

Severe hypercalcemia is the most serious complication of parathyroid cancer and, because it is difficult to control, is responsible for more deaths than parathyroid cancer itself.

Resources

BOOKS

Abeloff, Martin D., James O. Armitage, Allen S. Licter, and John E. Niederhuber. "Cancer of the Endocrine System" In *Clinical Oncology*. 5th ed. New York: Churchill Livingstone, 2013: 1112–1131.

Harrison, Louis B., Roy B. Sessions, and Merrill S. Kies, eds. *Head and Neck Cancer: A Multidiscplinary Approach*. 4th ed. Philadelphia: Lippincott Williams & Wilkins, 2013.

Niederhuber, J. E., et al. *Clinical Oncology*. 5th ed. Philadelphia: Elsevier, 2014.

PERIODICALS

Kolluri, S., K. Lai, R. Chang, and N. Mandava. "Parathyroid Carcinoma: A Silent Presentation." *Glandular Surgery* 3 (August 2014): 211–14.

Mohebati, A., A. Shaha, and J. Shah. "Parathyroid Carcinoma: Challenges in Diagnosis and Treatment." *Hematology and Oncology Clinics of North America* 26 (December 2012): 1221–38.

WEBSITES

National Cancer Institute. "Parathyroid Cancer Treatment (PDQ®)." http://www.cancer.gov/cancertopics/pdq/treatment/parathyroid/patient (accessed October 22, 2014).

ORGANIZATIONS

American Cancer Society, 250 Williams St. NW, Atlanta, GA 30303, (800) 227-2345, http://www.cancer.org.

National Cancer Institute, 9609 Medical Center Dr., BG 9609 MSC 9760, Bethesda, MD 20892-9760, (800) 4-CANCER (422-6237), http://www.cancer.gov.

L. Lee Culvert
Kevin O. Hwang, MD

PC-SPES

Definition

PC-SPES is an herbal mixture of eight botanical compounds adapted from traditional Chinese medicine that is used to treat **prostate cancer**, particularly the forms that do not respond to antiandrogen (hormone) therapy.

As PC-SPES is considered an alternative treatment for **cancer**, the National Center for Complementary and Alternative Medicine (NCCAM) began to conduct four separate **clinical trials** of the compound in the early 2000s. These studies were put on hold in June 2002 after the U.S. Food and Drug Administration (FDA) determined that samples of PC-SPES were contaminated with "undeclared prescription drug ingredients that could cause serious health effects if not taken under medical supervision." The California distributors of the product voluntarily recalled it, and closed their business at the end of 2002.

Because the early trials of PC-SPES gave promising results, NCCAM is interested in funding newer studies of the product, but will not do so until a fully standardized and uncontaminated product using the original formulation becomes available.

Purpose

PC-SPES is an herbal remedy that has been marketed as an over-the-counter drug for the treatment of prostate cancer. Anecdotal evidence of greatly reduced prostate-specific antigen (PSA) levels in patients taking this preparation prompted more formal testing of its effect. Laboratory studies show that PC-SPES has the ability to slow growth of both hormone-sensitive and hormone-insensitive prostate cancer cell lines in the test tube. Studies done with mice that have been implanted with prostate cancer cells indicate that the treatment triggers apoptosis (programmed cell death) in the artificially created hormone-insensitive tumors.

PC-SPES was shown in three clinical studies to reduce the serum prostate-specific antigen (PSA) levels in the overwhelming majority of patients suffering from prostate cancer that is unresponsive to androgen therapy. The treatment also reduces prostate acid phosphatase (PAP) levels, an enzyme often elevated with hormone-resistant disease. Treatment with the mixture has been shown to decrease pain, decrease narcotic use, and increase perceived quality of life. Researchers noted bone scan improvements, indicating a reduction in the size of cancer metastases to the bone. The majority of the work with this treatment has been done with patients having advanced disease, characterized by elevated PSA values and Gleason tumor scores.

According to one Japanese study, PC-SPES also shows promise in treating leukemia.

Description

PC-SPES is a mixture of eight herbs used in Chinese medicine: *Ganoderma lucidum*, *Scutellaria baicalensis*, *Rabdosia (Isodon) rubescens*, *Isatis indigotica*, *Dendranthema morifolium*, *Seronoa repens* (**saw palmetto**), *Panax pseudoginseng*, and *Glycyrrhiza uralensis* (licorice). The PC portion of the name stands for prostate cancer, while SPES is Latin for "hope." It has been commercially available since 1996. Manufacturers claim it stimulates the immune system and has antitumor activity. The mixture appears to act like estrogen against the tumors, and the side effects are very similar for the two therapies. Yet an analysis using liquid chromatography shows that diethylstilbestrol (DES), estrone, or estradiol are all absent. Additionally, some patients who did not respond to traditional estrogen therapy and alkylating agents did respond to PC-SPES, suggesting the mechanism may be different from that used by DES or **estramustine** (nitrogen mustard, an alkylating agent). Researchers plan a clinical trial that will directly compare the action of DES and PC-SPES in an effort to compare and contrast the two treatment methods.

Recommended dosage

In the clinical trials, PC-SPES was given either in a dosage of nine tablets per day, three before each mealtime; or six tablets a day, three before breakfast and three before dinner. As there was essentially no difference in the antitumor effect for the studies, six tablets a day might be a recommended starting dosage.

With herbal medications, such as PC-SPES, potency of herb per tablet and recommended dosage may vary from manufacturer to manufacturer.

Precautions

As PC-SPES has been used only in relatively small clinical trials, the full spectrum of precautions has yet to be determined. The clinical trials required taking the tablets on an empty stomach. Furthermore, despite the small sample size, experience does suggest that patients with known heart disease or stroke tendencies should take this medicine with caution, as it might aggravate these conditions.

Side effects

The side effects for PC-SPES are relatively mild and include, from most frequent to least frequent, nipple tenderness, **nausea and vomiting**, **diarrhea**, **fatigue**, gynecomastia (swelling of the male breast), leg cramps or swelling, angina, increased hot flashes, and blood clots. The incidence of angina occurred in a patient with pre-existing coronary disease and was treated by altered heart medications and a reduction in the amount of PC-SPES administered.

Interactions

There have been no studies of drug interactions between PC-SPES and other medications. The lack of information about potential adverse interactions suggests caution in adding PC-SPES to other more traditional treatment methods for prostate cancer.

Resources

WEBSITES

American Cancer Society. "PC-SPES, PC-HOPE, and PC-CARE." http://www.cancer.org/treatment/treatmentsandsi deeffects/complementaryandalternativemedicine/herbsvi taminsandminerals/pc-spes-pc-hope-and-pc-care (accessed November 10, 2014).

Cancer Research UK. "PC-SPES, PC-HOPE, PC-CARE and PC-PLUS." http://www.cancerresearchuk.org/about-can cer/cancers-in-general/cancer-questions/pcspes-and-pchope (accessed November 10, 2014).

Johns Hopkins Medicine. "Herbal Remedies for Prostate Cancer." http://www.hopkinsmedicine.org/healthlibrary/ conditions/prostate_health/herbal_remedies_for_prostate_ cancer_85,P01253/ (accessed November 10, 2014).

ORGANIZATIONS

National Center for Complementary and Alternative Medicine, 9000 Rockville Pike, Bethesda, MD 20892, (888) 644-6226, TTY: (866) 464-3615, http://nccam.nih.gov.

U.S. Food and Drug Administration, 10903 New Hampshire Ave., Silver Spring, MD 20993, (888) INFO-FDA (463-6332), http://www.fda.gov.

Michelle Johnson, M.S., J.D.
Rebecca J. Frey, PhD

Pegaspargase

Definition

Pegaspargase (also known as PEG-L-asparaginase and Oncaspar) is a modified enzyme used to stop growth of **cancer** and formation of new cancer cells.

Purpose

Pegaspargase is used as part of the induction regimen for the treatment of **acute lymphocytic leukemia** (ALL) in children who developed an allergy to **asparaginase**.

Description

Pegaspargase is a slightly changed version of the native form of asparaginase (*E. coli* asparaginase), an enzyme that is linked to a polyethylene glycol (PEG) molecule. This medicine was made available in 1994 under the brand name Oncaspar. It is more expensive than the native form and is mainly used in patients who developed an allergy to the native form. The advantage of pegaspargase over asparaginase is that it is less likely to cause an allergic reaction, has a longer duration in the body, and can be given less frequently. Pegaspargase kills cancer cells by depleting a certain amino acid in the blood (L-asparagine), which is needed for survival and growth of tumor cells in patients with acute lymphocytic leukemia. Fortunately, normal cells can make their own L-asparagine and are not dependent on L-asparagine from the blood for survival.

Pegaspargase is mainly given in combination with other drugs, usually **vincristine** (a vinca alkaloid anticancer drug) and steroids (either prednisone or **dexamethasone**). Other **chemotherapy** medicines are added to this regimen if a patient is at a high risk of disease recurrence.

Recommended dosage

Adults and children with body surface area greater than 0.6 square meters

In induction chemotherapy for acute lymphocytic leukemia, doses vary between different chemotherapy protocols. The usual dose is 2,500 international units (IU) per square meter of body surface area, given every 14 days.

Children with body surface area less than 0.6 square meters

In induction chemotherapy for acute lymphocytic leukemia, the usual dose is 82.5 IU per kg given every 14 days.

Administration

This medicine can be given directly into the muscle (intramuscular) or into the vein (intravenous). Intramuscular injection of pegaspargase is preferred over the intravenous route because of the lower risk of liver disease, blood clotting problems, stomach, and kidney problems. When used intramuscularly, it must be administered as deep injection into a large muscle. When given intravenously, it must be infused over one to two hours. Patients will be monitored closely by a physician for 30 to 60 minutes.

Precautions

The use of this medication should be avoided in patients with active pancreatitis (inflammation of the pancreas) or history of pancreatitis, and in patients who have had a serious allergic reaction to pegaspargase in the past.

Pegaspargase should only be administered in a hospital, and a patient will need to be observed by a physician for the first hour.

This medication can lower the body's ability to fight infections. Patients should avoid contact with any individuals who may have a cold, flu, or other infection.

Pegaspargase should be used with caution in the following populations:

- People with gout (it may increase uric acid levels and worsen gout).
- People with diabetes (it may increase blood sugar levels).
- Breast-feeding mothers (it is not known whether asparaginase crosses into breast milk).
- Women who are pregnant or may become pregnant (unless benefits to the mother outweigh the risks to the baby).

Patients should contact a doctor immediately if any of these symptoms develop:

- fever, chills, sore throat
- chest pain or heart palpitations
- yellowing of the skin or eyes
- puffy face, skin rash, trouble breathing, joint pain
- drowsiness, confusion, hallucinations, convulsions
- unusual bleeding or bruising
- stomach pain with nausea and vomiting, and loss of appetite (anorexia)

A physician will perform blood tests before starting therapy and during therapy to monitor complete blood count, blood sugar, pancreas, kidney, and liver functions.

Side effects

Pegaspargase is a very potent medicine that can cause serious side effects. An allergic reaction with skin rash, **itching**, joint pain, puffy face, and difficulty breathing is a side effect that happens very quickly after the drug is injected. The allergic reaction to pegaspargase is, however, less common than with asparaginase. The severe type of this allergic reaction (anaphylaxis) can result in death. Other common side effects include nausea, vomiting, **diarrhea**, loss of appetite, stomach cramps, yellowing of the eyes or skin, swelling of hands or feet, and pain at the injection site. Less frequent side effects include high blood sugar, chest pain, heart palpitations, headache, chills, **night sweats**, convulsions,

decreased kidney function, increased blood clotting, mouth sores, and decreased ability to fight infections. Usually the side effects of pegaspargase are more severe in adults than in children.

Interactions

Pegaspargase can decrease effectiveness of **methotrexate** (an antimetabolite, or compound that prevents the synthesis and utilization of normal cellular metabolites) in killing cancer cells when given right before and together with methotrexate. The use of these two medicines together should be avoided.

Pegaspargase can decrease the breakdown and increase toxicity of **cyclophosphamide**, a DNA alkylating anticancer drug.

Risk of liver disease may be increased in patients receiving both pegaspargase and **mercaptopurine**, a purine analog antimetabolite anticancer drug.

This medicine can increase blood sugar levels, especially when given with steroids.

Pegaspargase should be given after vincristine instead of before or with vincristine because it can increase the risk of numbing, tingling, and pain in hands and feet.

People taking blood thinners (**warfarin**, **heparin**, or its derivatives), aspirin, and nonsteroidal anti-inflammatory drugs (ibuprofen, naproxen) may be at increased risk of bleeding. A physician and a pharmacist must be informed about any prescription or over-the-counter medications the patient is taking.

Resources

BOOKS

Chu, Edward, and Vincent T. DeVita, Jr. *Physicians' Cancer Chemotherapy Drug Manual 2014*. Burlington, MA: Jones & Bartlett Learning, 2014.

WEBSITES

AHFS Consumer Medication Information. "Pegaspargase Injection." American Society of Health-System Pharmacists. Available from: http://www.nlm.nih.gov/medlineplus/druginfo/meds/a695031.html (accessed November 11, 2014).

American Cancer Society. "Pegaspargase." http://www.cancer.org/treatment/treatmentsandsideeffects/guidetocancerdrugs/pegaspargase (accessed November 11, 2014).

Olga Bessmertny, Pharm.D.

PEG-I-asparaginase *see* **Pegaspargase**

Pelvic exenteration *see* **Exenteration**

Pemetrexed

Definition

Pemetrexed is an anticancer drug that is used to treat malignant pleural **mesothelioma** and **non-small cell lung cancer**.

Purpose

Malignant pleural mesothelioma (MPM) is a rare type of **cancer** of the mesothelium (the lining of the chest cavity around the lungs and the abdomen). About 2,000–2,500 new cases of MPM are diagnosed in the United States annually. Twice that many cases occur in Europe. MPM usually is caused by exposure to asbestos. Inhaled asbestos fibers attach to the outer lining of the lung and the chest wall, causing tumor growth. The disease takes years to develop after asbestos exposure. Symptoms of MPM usually are not apparent or are misdiagnosed until after the disease is well advanced and difficult to treat with surgery or **radiation therapy**. Average survival time is nine to 13 months after diagnosis. Pemetrexed is used for patients with MPM that cannot be treated surgically.

Lung cancer—usually caused by smoking—is the most common cause of cancer death in the United States. Almost 174,000 people develop lung cancer each year

and more than 160,000 die from it annually. Non-small cell lung cancer (NSCLC) accounts for about 80% of all lung cancers and includes squamous cell **carcinoma**, **adenocarcinoma**, and large-cell carcinoma. Pemetrexed is used to treat stage III or IV NSCLC in patients whose cancer has recurred following **chemotherapy** and is advancing or has spread (metastasized). Pemetrexed does not improve rates of survival over the standard second-line treatment drug **docetaxel**, but pemetrexed has fewer side effects and thus may improve the patient's quality of life. Neither drug cures recurrent lung cancer.

Description

During the 1980s a new class of drugs called multitargeted anti-folates (MTA) were developed. These drugs limit the ability of cancer cells to obtain **folic acid**, a member of the B-vitamin complex that is required for cell growth and reproduction. However, these drugs were considered too toxic to use until pemetrexed was discovered by a Princeton University biochemist in the 1990s.

Pemetrexed disodium heptahydrate (Alimta), manufactured by Eli Lilly, was approved by the U.S. Food and Drug Administration (FDA) in February 2004 for use in combination with the anticancer drug **cisplatin** to treat MPM. Pemetrexed, also known as LY231514, was the first drug for treating this type of cancer and, as an orphan drug for a rare disease, received priority review from the FDA. The Orphan Drug Act granted Eli Lilly seven years of exclusive marketing. In August 2004, the FDA approved pemetrexed for the treatment of NSCLC.

Pemetrexed is a member of a large group of chemotherapy drugs known as antineoplastics or anti-metabolites; it sometimes is referred to as an antifolate antineoplastic agent. It inhibits three folate-dependent enzymes that mesothelioma and lung cancer cells need for the synthesis of the nucleotides that make up DNA and RNA. Fast-growing cancer cells have a much higher requirement for nucleotides than normal cells.

Effectiveness

The effectiveness of pemetrexed for treating MPM was established in a single clinical trial with 448 patients, comparing combined treatment with pemetrexed and cisplatin to treatment with cisplatin alone. Patients receiving the combined treatment lived 3 months longer than those receiving cisplatin alone—12 months versus 9 months. The patients receiving the combination also had improved lung function. Tumors shrank in 41% of the patients treated with the combined drugs, compared with 17% of those treated with cisplatin alone.

In an earlier clinical trial, pemetrexed combined with the chemotherapy drug **carboplatin**, which is similar to cisplatin, increased the average survival time of mesothelioma patients to 15 months; some patients were still alive after nearly three years. More than two-thirds of the treated patients had reduced pain and improvement in other symptoms. Tumors shrank in almost one-third of the patients.

In a clinical trial of 571 patients with recurrent NSCLC, those treated with either pemetrexed or docetaxel had a one-year survival rate of 30%; however, those receiving pemetrexed were significantly less likely to experience the following:

• fever
• infections
• hospitalizations
• hair loss
• numbness in the arms and legs

Recommended dosage

Pemetrexed is supplied as a sterile powder in single-dose vials of 500 mg pemetrexed and 500 mg mannitol. Pemetrexed is given in a single 10-minute intravenous infusion once every three weeks. The dose depends on body size and may be adjusted or delayed depending on the patient's blood counts, kidney and liver function, and general condition.

For treating MPM, cisplatin is infused for two hours, beginning about 30 minutes after the end of the pemetrexed infusion. As much fluid as possible is taken before and after treatment with cisplatin to keep the kidneys functioning properly. Intravenous fluids usually are given during cisplatin infusion.

Since pemetrexed interferes with both folic acid and vitamin B_{12}, these nutrients are always taken as supplements to prevent severe side effects. Folic acid—350–1,000 micrograms—is taken every day for at least five out of seven days prior to pemetrexed treatment. It is continued daily until 21 days after the final treatment. Folic acid is available as an over-the-counter supplement as well as in many multivitamins. Vitamin B_{12} is injected during the week before the first pemetrexed treatment and once every nine weeks during treatment.

Patients also take a corticosteroid such as **dexamethasone** twice a day for three days, beginning the day before pemetrexed infusion, to lower the risk of skin reactions.

Precautions

Pemetrexed causes birth defects if administered to a woman during the conception period or during pregnancy, or to a man near the time of conception. Birth control must be used by patients while they receive pemetrexed treatment. Women should not breastfeed while being treated with pemetrexed. Like many other chemotherapy drugs, pemetrexed may cause sterility.

Medical conditions that may interfere with the use of pemetrexed include the following:

• chicken pox or exposure to chicken pox
• gout
• heart disease
• congestive heart failure
• shingles
• kidney stones or kidney disease
• liver disease
• third-space fluid (extra body fluid such as ascites in the stomach area or pleural effusion in the lungs and chest)
• other types of cancer

Other precautions during pemetrexed treatment include avoiding the following:

- touching the eyes or inside of the nose without first washing the hands
- cuts or bleeding
- contact sports, bruising, or injury

It is important to avoid vaccinations during and after pemetrexed treatment. It also is important to avoid contact with those who have taken oral polio vaccine within the past several months. A protective face mask that covers the nose and mouth may be used if contact is unavoidable. If possible, people with any infection should be avoided.

Side effects

Pemetrexed has fewer side effects than many **anticancer drugs**; however, the most common side effects are as follows:

- anemia (low red blood cell count) that may cause fatigue, paleness, or shortness of breath
- a temporary decline in white blood cells, particularly during the first 10–14 days after each treatment
- a decline in blood platelets
- nausea and vomiting
- diarrhea
- constipation
- loss of appetite
- weight loss
- heartburn
- dry mouth
- redness or sores in the mouth or throat or on the lips a few days after treatment
- rash or itching between treatments
- wrinkled or peeling skin
- burning, tingling, numbness, or pain in the extremities
- muscle aches, cramping, stiffness, or pain
- joint swelling or pain
- difficult or rapid breathing
- pain or burning in the throat
- difficult or painful swallowing
- stuffy or runny nose
- sunken eyes
- irritability
- mood swings or depression
- lightheadedness or dizziness
- confusion
- insomnia

- difficulty concentrating
- hair loss
- increased heart rate
- decreased urination
- severe weakness and fatigue for a few days after treatment
- liver problems, as indicated by fluctuating liver function blood tests

Blood counts are taken before and after each pemetrexed treatment. Rare side effects of pemetrexed include a severe allergic reaction or blood clots.

Pemetrexed suppresses production of blood cells in the bone marrow and decreases the white blood cell count. Symptoms of infection caused by decreased white blood cells include the following:

- fever above 100.5°F (38°C)
- chills
- cough
- hoarseness
- lower back or side pain
- difficult or painful urination

Pemetrexed can reduce the number of blood platelets, thereby increasing the risk of the following:

- unusual bleeding or bruising
- nosebleeds
- bleeding gums when teeth are cleaned
- black, tarry stools
- tiny red spots on the skin
- blood in the urine or stool

Other serious side effects of pemetrexed can include:

- swollen glands
- increased thirst
- swelling of the eyes, face, fingers, or lower legs
- pain in the chest, groin, or legs, especially in the calves
- sudden severe headaches
- sudden changes in vision
- sudden slurred speech
- fast or irregular breathing
- chest tightness or wheezing
- increased blood pressure
- loss of coordination
- fainting or loss of consciousness
- weight gain

Interactions

Known interactions of pemetrexed with other drugs include:

- oral contraceptives

- vitamins and herbal supplements

- nonsteroidal anti-inflammatory drugs (NSAIDs), including aspirin, ibuprofens such as Motrin, naproxens such as Aleve, and celecoxib (Celebrex)

Resources

BOOKS

Chu, Edward, and Vincent T. DeVita Jr. *Physicians' Cancer Chemotherapy Drug Manual 2014*. Burlington, MA: Jones & Bartlett Learning, 2014.

WEBSITES

American Cancer Society. "Pemetrexed." http://www.cancer. org/treatment/treatmentsandsideeffects/guidetocancer-drugs/pemetrexed (accessed Novemer 11, 2014).

Cancer Research UK. "Pemetrexed (Alimta)." http://www. cancerresearchuk.org/about-cancer/cancers-in-general/ treatment/cancer-drugs/pemetrexed (accessed November 11, 2014).

Margaret Alic, PhD

Penile cancer

Definition

Penile **cancer** is the growth of malignant cells on the external skin and in the tissues of the penis.

Description

The penis (plural, penes) is the external sexual organ in males that conveys sperm into the female vagina during sexual intercourse. Its name is derived from the Latin word for tail. The male urethra, which carries urine to the outside of the body during urination, is also contained in the penis. In 95% of adult males, the erect penis ranges in size from 4.2 to 7.5 inches in length. At birth, the glans penis (sometimes simply called the glans), which is the bulb of sensitive skin at the lower end of the penis, is covered by a ring of smooth tissue called the foreskin. The foreskin may be surgically removed shortly after birth for cultural or religious reasons; this practice is called circumcision.

Penile cancer is a disease in which cancerous cells appear on the penis. It is almost always a primary cancer;

it is rare for cancers that start elsewhere in the body to metastasize to the penis. If left untreated, this cancer can grow and spread from the penis to the lymph nodes in the groin and eventually to other parts of the body. Most cases of penile cancer (about 95%) are squamous cell carcinomas or SCCs. The other 5% are verrucous (wartlike) carcinomas, basal cell carcinomas (BCCs), melanomas, and adenocarcinomas, which start in the sweat glands in the skin of the penis.

Risk factors

There are a number of risk factors for penile cancer:

- Age. Although penile cancer is rare, a man's risk of developing this cancer increases sharply after age 50.

- Long-term heavy smoking.

- HIV infection. Men who are HIV-positive are eight times more likely to develop penile cancer than men who are HIV-negative.

- Human papillomavirus (HPV) infection. About 40% of men diagnosed with penile cancer are found to be infected with HPV. The types of HPV most likely to cause cancer are HPV16, HPV18, and HPV31.

- A large number of sexual partners.

- Genital warts. About 50% of men diagnosed with penile cancer also have genital warts, which are caused by the human papillomavirus.

- Poor personal hygiene. Smegma, a whitish substance produced from dead skin cells and skin oils, may accumulate beneath the foreskin. While smegma is not in itself carcinogenic, its excessive accumulation may irritate the skin of the glans and cause chronic inflammation.

- Balanitis. Balanitis is inflammation of the glans resulting from bacterial, viral, or fungal infection; poorly controlled diabetes; or allergic reactions to some types of soap. Chronic balanitis increases the risk of developing penile cancer by a factor of 3.9.

- Repeated injuries (abrasions and small cuts) to the skin of the penis.

- Phimosis. Phimosis is a medical condition in which the foreskin cannot be completely retracted. It is linked to a threefold increase in the risk of developing penile cancer. Circumcision is thought to reduce the risk of penile cancer because it eliminates the development of phimosis and heavy accumulation of smegma, and reduces the risk of HPV infection.

Demographics

Penile cancer is a rare form of cancer that develops in about one out of 100,000 men per year in the United States. The lifetime risk for American men is estimated to be about 1 in 1,437. It is primarily a disease of older men, with 80% of cases diagnosed in men over 55. According to the American Cancer Society (ACS), about 0.2% of cancers in men in the United States are penile cancers. The ACS predicted that 1,640 new cases of penile cancer would be diagnosed in the United States in 2014 and that 320 men would die from the disease. Race or ethnicity does not appear to be a risk factor for this type of cancer.

Penile cancer is more common in other parts of the world, particularly in underdeveloped countries in Africa and South America, particularly Paraguay and Uruguay. The American Cancer Society reports that up to 10% of cancer in men in these areas is penile cancer. In Uganda, penile cancer is the most common form of cancer in men.

Causes and symptoms

The cause of penile cancer is unknown. The most common symptoms of penile cancer include:

- a tender spot, an open sore, or a wart-like lump on the penis
- unusual, bad-smelling liquid discharges from the penis
- pain or bleeding in the genital area

Other symptoms of penile cancer may include:

- swelling at the end of the penis
- changes in the color of the skin of the penis
- a velvety red rash on the penis
- swellings in the groin area

Diagnosis

In order to diagnose penile cancer, the doctor takes a thorough patient history to evaluate the presence of any risk factors and then examines the patient's penis for lumps or other abnormalities. A tissue sample (**biopsy**) may be ordered to distinguish cancerous cells from syphilis and penile warts. If the results confirm a diagnosis of cancer, additional tests are done to determine whether the disease has spread to other parts of the body. These tests may include a fine-needle aspiration biopsy (FNAB) of lymph nodes in the groin area and **imaging studies**, such as CT scans, MRI, or ultrasound.

Treatment team

A doctor who specializes in the genitourinary tract (urologist) is usually the first point of contact for the patient and makes the diagnosis of penile cancer. Once the urologist diagnoses the cancer, a specialist in cancer (oncologist) will become involved to determine the stage of the cancer and recommend appropriate treatments. Other members of the treatment team may include a radiation oncologist, nurse practitioner, and psychologist.

Clinical staging, treatments, and prognosis

In Stage I penile cancer, malignant cells are found only on the surface of the head (glans) and on the foreskin of the penis. If the cancer is limited to the foreskin, treatment may involve wide local excision and circumcision. Wide local excision is a form of surgery that removes only cancer cells and a small amount of normal tissue adjacent to them. Circumcision is removal of the foreskin.

If the Stage I cancer is on the glans only, treatment may involve the use of a topical medication, usually a **fluorouracil** cream (Adrucil, Efudex) or imiquimod, and/or Mohs microsurgery. **Mohs surgery** is a technique that removes cancerous tissue layer by layer, which allows removal of only the smallest possible amount of normal tissue. This surgery requires specialized training. The doctor uses an instrument that provides a comprehensive view of the area where the cancer cells are located and helps to determine that all malignant cells have been removed during surgery. Another treatment for Stage I cancers is cryosurgery, in which a probe cooled with liquid nitrogen is used to freeze the cancer cells.

In Stage II, the penile cancer has spread to the surface of the glans, tissues beneath the surface, and the shaft of the penis. The treatment recommended may be **amputation** of all or part of the penis (total or partial penectomy). If the disease is diagnosed in its earliest stages, surgeons are often able to preserve enough of the organ for urination and sexual activity. Treatment may also include microsurgery and external **radiation therapy**, in which a machine provides radiation to the affected area. Laser surgery is an experimental treatment for Stage II cancers. Laser surgery uses an intense, precisely focused beam of light to dissolve or burn away cancer cells.

In Stage III, malignant cells have spread to lymph nodes in the groin, where they cause swelling. The recommended treatment may include amputation of the penis and removal of the lymph nodes on both sides. Radiation therapy may also be suggested, administered either as external beam radiation therapy; or brachytherapy, in which hollow needles filled with radioactive pellets are inserted into the penis. More advanced disease requires systemic treatments that use drugs (**chemotherapy**). In chemotherapy, medicines are administered intravenously or taken by mouth. These drugs enter the bloodstream and kill cancer cells that have spread to other parts of the body. Chemotherapy drugs used to treat penile cancer include **ifosfamide**, **vincristine**, **cisplatin**, **methotrexate**, **bleomycin**, and paclitaxel.

In Stage IV, the disease has spread throughout the penis and lymph nodes in the groin, or has traveled to other parts of the body, such as the lungs or liver. These cancers are very difficult to treat. Treatments are similar to those for Stage III cancer. The patient may be given chemotherapy prior to surgery in order to shrink the tumor and make it easier to remove; this approach is called neoadjuvant therapy.

Recurrent penile cancer is disease that recurs in the penis or develops in another part of the body after treatment has eradicated the original cancer cells.

In addition to the treatments previously described, biological therapy is another treatment that is currently being studied. Biological therapy is a type of treatment that is sometimes called biological response modifier (BRM) therapy. It uses natural or artificial substances to boost, focus, or reinforce the body's disease-fighting resources.

Alternative and complementary therapies

The term "alternative therapy" refers to therapy used instead of conventional treatment. By definition, these treatments have not been investigated as thoroughly and with the same standards as conventional treatments. The terms "complementary" or "integrative therapy" denote practices used in conjunction with rather than instead of conventional treatment. Patients should inform their doctors of any alternative or complementary therapies they are using or considering using, as some alternative and complementary therapies have adverse effects on the conventional treatments prescribed by physicians. Some common complementary and alternative medicine therapies include:

- prayer and faith healing

- meditation

- mind/body techniques: support groups, visualization, guided imagery, hypnosis

- energy work: therapeutic touch, Reiki

- acupuncture and traditional Chinese medicine

- body work: yoga, massage, t'ai chi

- vitamin, mineral, and/or herbal supplements

- special diets: vegetarian, vegan, macrobiotic

Prognosis

Cure rates are high for cancers diagnosed in Stage I or II (about 85% as of 2014), but lower for Stages III and IV (about 59%), since these stages indicate that cancer cells have spread to the lymph nodes. If the cancer has spread to distant sites, the 5-year survival rate drops to 11%. Prognosis depends on the type of cancer, the stage of the cancer, and the parts of the body to which the cancer has spread.

Coping with cancer treatment

Physical side effects of treatments may include constipation, **fatigue**, and sleep disorders. These effects are manageable through a combination of diet and environment as well as supplemental drug treatments. Psychological side effects sometimes result as well. They include **depression**, decreased sexuality, anxiety, and feelings of grief. Patients should seek support if they experience any of these symptoms.

Prevention

There is no known prevention for penile cancer. However, it is possible to take steps to reduce the risk. These steps include:

- Quit smoking.

- Circumcise male infants.

- Limit the number of sexual partners.

- Practice good genital hygiene; retract the entire foreskin if uncircumcised and wash the entire penis.

- Use condoms during sex.

- Get vaccinated against HPV. Of the two vaccines recommended for use in females, only Gardasil has been approved for use in males. The Advisory Committee on Immunization Practices (ACIP) recommended Gardasil in 2011 for routine use in boys aged 11 or 12 years. The committee also recommends giving the vaccine to males aged 13 through 21 years who have not been vaccinated or have not completed the three-dose series.

Resources

BOOKS

Culkin, Daniel J., ed. *Management of Penile Cancer*. New York: Springer, 2014.

Munir, Asif, Manit Arya, and Simon Horenblas, eds. *Textbook of Penile Cancer*. New York: Springer, 2012.

Spiess, Philippe E. *Penile Cancer: Diagnosis and Treatment*. New York: Springer, 2013.

PERIODICALS

Clark, P.E., et al. "Penile Cancer: Clinical Practice Guidelines in Oncology." *Journal of the National Comprehensive Cancer Network* 11 (May 1, 2013): 594–615.

Gupta, S., and A. Rajesh. "Magnetic Resonance Imaging of Penile Cancer." *Magnetic Resonance Imaging Clinics of North America* 22 (May 2014): 191–199.

Hernandez, B.Y., et al. "Human Papillomavirus Genotype Prevalence in Invasive Penile Cancers from a Registry-based United States Population." *Frontiers in Oncology* 4 (February 5, 2014): 9.

Mooney, D., et al. "Update in Systemic Therapy of Urologic Malignancies." *Postgraduate Medicine* 126 (January 2014): 44–54.

Moses, K.A., et al. "Contemporary Management of Penile Cancer: Greater Than 15 year MSKCC Experience." *Canadian Journal of Urology* 21 (April 2014): 7201–7206.

Spiess, P.E., and the National Comprehensive Cancer Network. "New Treatment Guidelines for Penile Cancer." *Journal of the National Comprehensive Cancer Network* 11 (May 2013) (5 Suppl.): 659–662.

Zukiwskyj, M., P. Daly, and E. Chung. "Penile Cancer and Phallus Preservation Strategies: A Review of Current Literature." *BJU International* 112 (November 2013): Suppl. 2: 21–26.

WEBSITES

American Cancer Society (ACS). "Penile Cancer." http://www.cancer.org/cancer/penilecancer/detailedguide/index (accessed July 29, 2014).

MedicineNet. "Penis Cancer." http://www.medicinenet.com/penis_cancer/article.htm (accessed May 18, 2014).

National Cancer Institute (NCI). "Penile Cancer." http://www.cancer.gov/cancertopics/types/penile (accessed May 18, 2014).

ORGANIZATIONS

American Cancer Society (ACS), 250 Williams Street NW, Atlanta, GA 30303, (800) 227-2345, http://www.cancer.org/aboutus/howwehelpyou/app/contact-us.aspx, http://www.cancer.org/index.

American Urological Association (AUA), 1000 Corporate Boulevard, Linthicum, MD 21090, (410) 689-3700, (866) 746-4282, Fax: (410) 689-3800, aua@AUAnet.org, http://www.auanet.org/.

National Cancer Institute (NCI), BG 9609 MSC 9760, 9609 Medical Center Drive, Bethesda, MD 20892-9760, (800) 4-CANCER (422-6237), http://www.cancer.gov/global/contact/email-us, http://www.cancer.gov/.

Maureen Haggerty
REVISED BY TISH DAVIDSON, A.M.
REVISED BY REBECCA J. FREY, PhD

Pentamidine *see* **Antibiotics**

Pentostatin

Definition

Pentostatin is an anticancer (antineoplastic) agent belonging to the class of drugs called antimetabolites (compounds that prevent the synthesis and utilization of normal cellular metabolites). It is a natural product

KEY TERMS

Antineoplastic—A drug that prevents the growth of a neoplasm by interfering with the maturation or proliferation of the cells of the neoplasm.

Hairy cell leukemia—A rare form of cancer in which hairy cells grow out of control in the blood, liver, and spleen.

Lymphoma—A malignant tumor of the lymphatic system.

Neoplasm—New abnormal growth of tissue.

isolated from *Streptomyces antibioticus*. It also acts as a suppressor of the immune system. It is available under the brand name Nipent. Other common names for pentostatin include 2'-deoxycoformycin and 2'DCF.

Purpose

Pentostatin is primarily used to treat a particular type of **cancer** of the blood called **hairy cell leukemia**. It is also used in the treatment of low-grade lymphomas. **Clinical trials** are under way to determine the effectiveness of pentostatin in fighting **cutaneous T-cell lymphoma** (CTCL), **chronic lymphocytic leukemia** (CLL), non-Hodgkin lymphomas (NHL), and prolymphocytic leukemia.

Description

Pentostatin chemically interferes with the synthesis of the genetic material (DNA and RNA) of cancer cells, which prevents these cells from being able to reproduce and continue the growth of the cancer.

Recommended dosage

Pentostatin may be taken only as an injection. It is generally given once every two weeks. A typical dosage is 4 mg per square meter of body surface area. However, the dosage prescribed can vary widely depending on the patient, the cancer being treated, and whether other medications are also being taken.

Precautions

Pentostatin should be taken on an empty stomach. If stomach irritation occurs, it should be taken with small amounts of food or milk. Pentostatin should always be taken with plenty of fluids.

Pentostatin can cause an allergic reaction in some people. Patients with a prior allergic reaction to pentostatin should not take pentostatin.

Pentostatin can cause serious birth defects if either the man or the woman is taking this drug at the time of conception or if the woman is taking this drug during pregnancy.

Because pentostatin is easily passed from mother to child through breast milk, breast-feeding is not recommended while pentostatin is being taken.

Pentostatin suppresses the immune system and interferes with the normal functioning of certain organs and tissues. For these reasons, it is important that the prescribing physician is aware of any of the following pre-existing medical conditions:

• a current case of or recent exposure to chicken pox

• herpes zoster (shingles)

• a current case or history of gout or kidney stones

• all current infections

• kidney disease

• liver disease

Also, because pentostatin is such a potent immunosuppressant, patients taking this drug must exercise extreme caution to avoid contracting any new infections. They should do their best to:

• avoid any person with any type of infection

• avoid bleeding injuries, including those caused by brushing or flossing the teeth

• avoid contact of the hands with the eyes or nasal passages (inside of the nose) unless the hands have just been washed and have not touched anything else since this washing

• avoid contact sports or any other activity that could cause a bruising or bleeding injury

Side effects

The most common side effects of pentostatin are cough, extreme **fatigue**, increased susceptibility to infection, loss of appetite (**anorexia**), skin rash or **itching**, nausea, temporary hair loss (**alopecia**), vomiting, and **weight loss**.

Less common side effects include anxiety or nervousness; changes in vision; nosebleed; sores in the mouth or on lips; sore, red eyes; trouble sleeping (insomnia); numbness or tingling in the hands and/or feet; and swelling in the feet or lower legs.

A doctor should be consulted immediately if the patient experiences shortness of breath, chest or abdominal pain, persistent cough, **fever** and chills, pain in the lower back or sides, painful or difficult urination, unusual bleeding or bruising, blood in the urine or stool, or tiny red dots on the skin.

Interactions

Pentostatin should not be taken in combination with any prescription drug, over-the-counter drug, or herbal remedy without prior consultation with a physician. It is particularly important that the prescribing physician be aware of the use of any of the following drugs or any **radiation therapy** or **chemotherapy** medicine:

- amphotericin B
- antithyroid agents
- azathioprine
- chloramphenicol
- colchicine
- flucytosine
- fludarabine
- ganciclovir
- interferon
- plicamycin
- probenecid
- sulfinpyrazone
- vidarabine
- zidovudine

Resources

BOOKS

Chu, Edward, and Vincent T. DeVita Jr. *Physicians' Cancer Chemotherapy Drug Manual 2014*. Burlington, MA: Jones & Bartlett Learning, 2014.

WEBSITES

American Cancer Society. "Pentostatin." http://www.cancer.org/treatment/treatmentsandsideeffects/guidetocancer-drugs/pentostatin (accessed November 11, 2014).

Cancer Research UK. "Pentostatin (Nipent)." http://www.cancerresearchuk.org/about-cancer/cancers-in-general/treatment/cancer-drugs/pentostatin (accessed November 11, 2014).

Paul A. Johnson, EdM

Percutaneous transhepatic cholangiography

Definition

Percutaneous transhepatic cholangiography (PTHC) is an x-ray test used to identify obstructions either in the liver or bile ducts that slow or stop the flow of bile from the liver to the digestive system.

KEY TERMS

Ascites—Abnormal accumulation of fluid in the abdomen.

Bile ducts—Tubes that carry bile, a thick yellowish-green fluid that is made by the liver, stored in the gallbladder, and helps the body digest fats.

Cholangitis—Inflammation of the bile duct.

Fluoroscope—An x-ray machine that projects images of organs.

Granulomatous disease—Disease characterized by growth of tiny blood vessels and connective tissue.

Jaundice—Disease that causes bile to accumulate in the blood, causing the skin and whites of the eyes to turn yellow. Obstructive jaundice is caused by blockage of bile ducts, while nonobstructive jaundice is caused by disease or infection of the liver.

Purpose

Because the liver and bile ducts are not normally seen on x-rays, the doctor injects the liver with a special dye that will appear on the resulting picture. This dye distributes evenly to fill the whole liver drainage system. If the dye does not distribute evenly, it indicates a blockage, which may caused by a gallstone or a tumor in the liver, bile ducts, or pancreas.

Precautions

Patients should report allergic reactions to:

- anesthetics
- dyes used in medical tests
- iodine
- shellfish

PTHC should not be performed on anyone who has cholangitis (inflammation of the bile duct), massive **ascites**, a severe allergy to iodine, or a serious uncorrectable or uncontrollable bleeding disorder. Patients who have diabetes should inform their doctors.

Description

PTHC is performed in a hospital, doctor's office, or outpatient surgical or x-ray facility. The patient lies on a movable x-ray table and is given a local anesthetic. The patient will be told to hold his or her breath, and a doctor, nurse, or laboratory technician will inject a special dye into the liver as the patient exhales.

The patient may feel a twinge when the needle penetrates the liver, a pressure or fullness, or brief discomfort in the upper right side of the back. Hands and feet may become numb during the 30–60 minute procedure.

The x-ray table will be rotated several times during the test, and the patient helped to assume a variety of positions. A special x-ray machine called a fluoroscope will track the dye's movement through the bile ducts and show whether the fluid is moving freely or whether its passage is obstructed.

PTHC costs about $1,600. The test may have to be repeated if the patient moves while x-rays are being taken.

Preparation

An intravenous antibiotic may be given every four to six hours during the 24 hours before the test. The patient will be told to fast overnight. Having an empty stomach is a safety measure in case of complications, such as bleeding, that might require emergency repair surgery. Medications such as aspirin or nonsteroidal anti-inflammatory drugs that thin the blood should be stopped for some three to seven days prior to taking the PTHC test. Patients may also be given a sedative a few minutes before the test begins.

Aftercare

A nurse will monitor the patient's vital signs and watch for:

• itching

• flushing

• nausea and vomiting

• sweating

• excessive flow of saliva

• possible serious allergic reactions to contrast dye

The patient should stay in bed for at least six hours after the test, lying on the right side to prevent bleeding from the injection site. The patient may resume normal eating habits and gradually resume normal activities. The doctor should be informed right away if pain develops in the right abdomen or shoulder or in case of **fever**, dizziness, or a change in stool color to black or red.

Risks

Septicemia (blood poisoning) and bile peritonitis (a potentially fatal infection or inflammation of the membrane covering the walls of the abdomen) are rare but serious complications of this procedure. Dye occasionally leaks from the liver into the abdomen, and there is a slight risk of bleeding or infection.

Results

Normal x-rays show dye evenly distributed throughout the bile ducts. Obesity, gas, and failure to fast can affect test results.

Abnormal results

Enlargement of bile ducts may indicate:

• obstructive or nonobstructive jaundice

• cholelithiasis (gallstones)

• hepatitis (inflammation of the liver)

• cirrhosis (chronic liver disease)

• granulomatous disease

• pancreatic cancer

• bile duct or gallbladder cancers

Resources

WEBSITES

A.D.A.M Medical Encyclopedia. "Percutaneous Transhepatic Cholangiography." MedlinePlus. http://www.nlm.nih.gov/medlineplus/ency/article/003820.htm (accessed November 11, 2014).

Harvard Health Publications. "Percutaneous Transhepatic Cholangiography (PTCA)." Harvard Medical School. http://www.health.harvard.edu/diagnostic-tests/percutaneous-transhepatic-cholangiography.htm (accessed November 12, 2014).

Johns Hopkins Medicine. "PTC (also called Percutaneous Transhepatic Cholangiography)." http://pathology.jhu.edu/pancreas/ptc.php (accessed November 11, 2014).

Maureen Haggerty

Pericardial effusion

Definition

A pericardial effusion is a fluid collection that develops between the pericardium, the lining of the heart, and the heart itself. Pericardial effusions can be found in up to 20% of **cancer** patients at autopsy, but of those, only about 30% would have had symptoms from their effusions.

Description

Most of the organs of the body are covered by thin membranes. The membrane that surrounds the heart is called the pericardium. Normally, only a few milliliters of fluid lie between the pericardium and the muscle of the

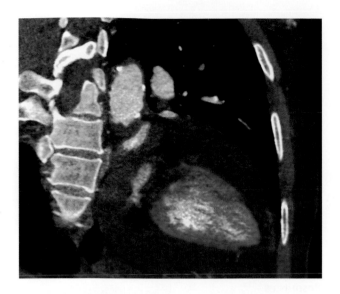

Computed tomography (CT) scan of the heart revealing pericardial effusion, or excess fluid surrounding the heart. *(Zephyr/Science Source)*

heart. Any larger, abnormal collection of fluid in that space is called a pericardial effusion.

A pericardial effusion can interfere with the normal contraction and expansion of the heart muscle, which decreases the heart's ability to pump blood effectively. A large or rapidly developing effusion can cause a condition called cardiac tamponade. Tamponade is a medical emergency and can be fatal if not diagnosed and treated promptly.

Causes and symptoms

Causes

A pericardial effusion in a cancer patient is caused either by the disease itself or by the treatment for the disease.

Many cancers can metastasize or spread to the pericardium or the heart itself. They include cancers of the:

- lung
- breast
- thyroid
- esophagus
- kidney
- pancreas
- endometrium
- larynx
- cervix
- stomach
- mouth
- liver
- ovary
- colon
- prostate
- leukemia
- melanoma
- lymphoma
- sarcoma
- myeloma

The presence of the cancerous cells on the pericardium is an irritant and causes a reactive fluid buildup, much as a blister forms under the skin due to irritation. Some cancers cause less fluid buildup, instead thickening the pericardium and making it less elastic. This process can also cause symptoms of tamponade.

Another cause of pericardial effusion in a cancer patient is previous **radiation therapy** to the chest, especially in the case of lung cancer or **lymphoma**. While such effusions are less likely to produce tamponade, it is possible.

Many of the drugs that are used to treat cancer can cause pericardial disease and thus potentially cause pericardial effusions. Some of the chemotherapeutic drugs that can affect the pericardium are **cytarabine**, **fluorouracil**, **cyclophosphamide**, **doxorubicin**, and **daunorubicin**. Granulocyte-macrophage colony-stimulating factor (**sargramostim**), often given to help increase the population of white blood cells during intensive **chemotherapy**, is also a pericardial irritant.

Other causes of pericardial effusions are heart failure, liver disease, and kidney disease. Any of these can also affect cancer patients.

Symptoms

Symptoms of tamponade include shortness of breath, rapid pulse, cough, and chest discomfort. As tamponade progresses, low blood pressure and shock develop, and cardiac arrest can follow. A smaller or more slowly developing pericardial effusion also causes chest discomfort. Other symptoms, such as shortness of breath, difficulty swallowing, hoarseness, or hiccups result from pressure from the enlarged, fluid-filled pericardium pressing against nearby organs. Although chronic or smaller effusions are not emergencies, they do cause discomfort and can become more serious.

Diagnosis

The diagnosis of pericardial effusion is made on the basis of patient history, physical examination and appropriate laboratory studies. Heart sounds can be muffled, the veins in the neck engorged, and the pulse rapid. A chest x-ray shows enlargement of the silhouette of the heart. An echocardiogram or cardiac ultrasound will show the fluid surrounding the heart, as will CT and MRI scans.

Treatment

Treatment of pericardial effusion depends on the presence or absence of cardiac tamponade. Tamponade is a medical emergency; symptoms such as cyanosis, a blue tinge to the lips and skin, shock, or a change in mental status require urgent drainage of the fluid. This drainage is accomplished with a procedure called **pericardiocentesis**, in which a needle is inserted into the pericardial space and the fluid withdrawn into a large syringe. Chronic effusions can be drained electively, and some need not be drained at all. If a patient's prognosis is poor and the pericardial effusion is not compromising the function of the heart, the risks of a drainage procedure may outweigh its benefits and the effusion may be left alone. Effusions caused by lymphoma often resolve after aggressive chemotherapy and need no further treatment.

Elective drainage of a pericardial effusion is done by one of several surgical procedures. The surgeon might open the chest, make a small incision under the bottom of the breastbone, or use a video-assisted technique called **thoracoscopy**. In addition to permitting drainage of the pericardial fluid, these procedures permit the surgeon to take a pericardial **biopsy**, which can confirm the diagnosis of metastatic cancer.

Sometimes a catheter is placed in the pericardium and connected to an external drainage system to collect any fluid that might reaccumulate.

Occasionally, sclerosing agents—drugs that cause scarring—are infused into the pericardium through a catheter. These agents, such as tetracycline, minocycline or **bleomycin**, irritate the pericardium, causing it to thicken and adhere to the heart muscle. This scarring prevents the further accumulation of fluid. Some malignant pericardial effusions resolve after the instillation of chemotherapeutic drugs such as **thiotepa** or platinum directly into the pericardial cavity. Others resolve after radiation therapy directed at the pericardium.

Alternative and complementary therapies

No complementary or alternative treatments are aimed specifically at treating pericardial effusions, but practitioners of acupressure and acupuncture designate a pressure point for the pericardium at two and a half finger breadths above the wrist crease on the inner aspect of the arm. Acupressure and acupuncture do offer some relief of symptoms to those suffering from shortness of breath and might offer benefit to those with pericardial effusions.

See also Pericardiocentesis.

KEY TERMS

Pericardium—The thin membrane that surrounds the heart.

Sclerosing agents—Drugs that are instilled into parts of the body to deliberately induce scarring.

Tamponade—A medical emergency in which fluid or other substances between the pericardium and heart muscle compress the heart muscle and interfere with the normal pumping of blood.

Thoracoscopy—Chest surgery done with the guidance of special video cameras that permit the surgeon to see inside the chest.

Resources

PERIODICALS

Klein, A.L., et al. "American Society of Echocardiography Clinical Recommendations For Multimodality Cardiovascular Imaging of Patients With Pericardial Disease: Endorsed By the Society For Cardiovascular Magnetic Resonance and Society of Cardiovascular Computed Tomography." *Journal of the American Society of Echocardiography* 26, no. 9 (2013): 965–1012. http://www.onlinejase.com/article/S0894-7317(13)00533-6/abstract (accessed November 14, 2014).

WEBSITES

Micromedex. "Pericardial Effusion." http://www.mayoclinic.org/diseases-conditions/pericardial-effusion/basics/definition/con-20034161 (accessed November 11, 2014).

National Cancer Institute. "Malignant Pericardial Effusion." http://www.cancer.gov/cancertopics/pdq/supportivecare/cardiopulmonary/Patient/page5 (accessed November 12, 2014).

Marianne Vahey, M.D.

Pericardiocentesis

Definition

Pericardiocentesis is a therapeutic and diagnostic procedure in which fluid is removed from the pericardium, the sac that surrounds the heart.

Purpose

The pericardium normally contains only a few milliliters (less than a teaspoon) of fluid to cushion the heart. Many illnesses cause larger volumes of fluid, called pericardial effusions, to develop. Spread of **cancer** to the pericardium is a frequent cause of pericardial effusions. If an effusion is too large, pressure develops within the sac that can interfere with the normal pumping action of the heart. Should that interference become severe, a life-threatening condition called cardiac tamponade can develop, which can lead to shock or death.

Pericardiocentesis is a procedure to remove the excess fluid, which allows the heart to pump normally again. The fluid is analyzed for the presence of cancer cells or microorganisms. If cardiac tamponade is present, pericardiocentesis must be done on an urgent basis. If tamponade is not present, an elective pericardial drainage procedure can be scheduled.

Precautions

The presence of tamponade is a medical emergency and requires urgent treatment. The blood pressure can be low and breathing compromised. Fluids and intravenous medications might be needed to raise the blood pressure until the pericardiocentesis can be performed.

Description

When possible, pericardiocentesis is performed in the cardiac catheterization laboratory of the hospital, but it can be done at the bedside or in the emergency department. The patient lies on his or her back with the head elevated at about 45 degrees. The skin is sterilized and local anesthetic given. A long needle attached to a large sterile syringe is inserted under the breastbone into the pericardium. If available, an echocardiogram or cardiac ultrasound is done to guide the physician to the pericardium. Once the needle is in the pericardium, the doctor withdraws the pericardial fluid into the syringe. The fluid can then be tested for cancer cells. If the

volume of the fluid is large or likely to reaccumulate, a catheter or drain is placed with one end in the pericardial space and the other outside the chest attached to a collecting bag. This catheter can stay in place for several days, until there is no more fluid to drain. After withdrawing either the needle or the catheter, the doctor will apply direct pressure to the site.

If a pericardiocentesis is unsuccessful in draining the **pericardial effusion**, other procedures are available such as percutaneous balloon pericardiotomy, in which a balloon-tipped catheter is inserted through the skin and then used to puncture a hole in the pericardium. This is a painful procedure and should be done under anesthesia. The pericardial fluid is allowed to drain into the chest cavity into the pleural space, the area between the pleurae, the membranes that line the lungs, and the lungs themselves. The pleural space can accommodate more fluid than the pericardium without significant discomfort.

Alternatively, if emergent pericardiocentesis is unsuccessful, the patient can be taken to the operating room for a surgical procedure that will drain the fluid. These elective surgical procedures are similar to pericardiocentesis; however, for open surgical procedures, image guidance is not necessary. These procedures are typically performed under general anesthesia. They present the surgeon with the opportunity to perform a **biopsy** of the pericardium to confirm the suspicion that the patient's cancer has metastasized there. The operation can also be performed as a thoracoscopic procedure.

Finally, if necessary, a pericardiectomy, sometimes called a pericardial stripping, can be performed. This is a surgical procedure to remove the pericardium and is reserved for the most refractory cases. Pericardiectomy tends to carry more risk than other procedures.

Preparation

For a scheduled pericardiocentesis, a patient will take nothing by mouth for several hours before the procedure. The patient will undergo preoperative blood tests, an electrocardiogram, and an echocardiogram or ultrasound of the heart.

Aftercare

Most patients are admitted to an intensive care unit for monitoring after a pericardial drainage procedure. Frequent checks of blood pressure and pulse will be done, and the neck veins will be examined for bulging. Such bulging might indicate a bleeding complication. If a drain has been placed, the fluid collected will be measured and the site checked for signs of bleeding or infection. Most patients spend several days in the hospital after pericardial drainage, but a few who do not have drains placed can go home the next day.

Risks

There is about a 5% risk of complications with a pericardiocentesis. These risks include:

• cardiac arrest

• myocardial infarction or heart attack

• abnormal heart rhythms

• laceration or puncture of the heart muscle

• laceration of the coronary arteries

• laceration of the lungs

• laceration of the stomach, colon, or liver

• air embolism, in which a pocket of air becomes trapped in a blood vessel, blocking blood flow

When a pericardial effusion is caused by the presence of cancer cells, there is also a risk that the fluid might reaccumulate. Injecting irritants into the pericardial sac can initiate scarring of the pericardium. This scarring causes it to adhere to the surface of the heart and prevents fluid from collecting there again. The irritating or sclerosing agents that are instilled into the pericardial space through a catheter include tetracycline, minocycline, and **bleomycin**. The injection of these drugs into the pericardium can cause pain. Sometimes, the simple presence of a drainage catheter will induce the desired scarring, and this method is preferred, when possible, to the use of the irritant drugs.

Results

The most important result is the relief of tamponade or other symptoms of heart failure from excess pericardial fluid. The blood pressure should return to normal, chest pain should be relieved, and breathing should become easier.

The fluid will be analyzed. Normal pericardial fluid is clear, has no cancer cells, no evidence of infection, and fewer than 1,000 white blood cells.

Abnormal results

On rare occasions, the pressure changes surrounding the heart that occur after pericardial drainage can cause temporary worsening of symptoms. This condition is called pericardial shock.

The most likely cause of a pericardial effusion in a person with cancer is spread of cancer to the pericardium. Thus, the fluid might, upon analysis, contain cancerous cells, high levels of protein, and many white blood cells. These materials can make the fluid thick and viscous. If the pericardial biopsy is performed, as can be done with a

---

QUESTIONS TO ASK YOUR DOCTOR

• What is a pericardiocentesis?

• Why do I need this procedure?

• What are the risks?

• What are the risks of not having a pericardiocentesis?

• What sort of anesthesia will I have?

• What do you expect to find?

• What can I expect after the test?

• How long will I need to stay in the hospital?

---

surgical drainage procedure, that biopsy might also reveal the presence of cancer cells.

Resources

BOOKS

Tubaro, Marco, et al. *The ESC Textbook of Acute and Intensive Cardiac Care.* New York: Oxford University Press, 2011.

WEBSITES

A.D.A.M Medical Encyclopedia. "Pericardiocentesis." Medline Plus. http://www.nlm.nih.gov/medlineplus/ency/article/003872.htm (accessed November 11, 2014).

University of Ottawa Heart Institute. "Pericardiocentesis." http://www.ottawaheart.ca/patients_family/pericardiocentesis.htm (accessed Novmeber 14, 2014).

Marianne Vahey, M.D.

Peripheral neuropathy *see* **Neuropathy**

Peritoneovenous shunt

Definition

A peritoneovenous shunt (PVS) is a device that is inserted surgically into the body to create a passage between the peritoneum (abdominal cavity) and the jugular vein to treat refractory cases of peritoneal **ascites**. Ascites is a condition in which an excessive amount of fluid builds up within the abdominal cavity.

Purpose

The abnormal buildup of fluid in the spaces found between the tissues and organs of the abdominal cavity is

KEY TERMS

Abdomen—The part of the body which lies between the diaphragm and the rim of the pelvis.

Circulatory system—The circulatory system consists of the heart and blood vessels. It serves as the body's transportation system.

Esophagus—The part of the digestive tract that carries food from the mouth to the stomach.

Jugular veins—Large veins returning the blood from the head to the heart into two branches (external and internal) located on each side of the neck.

Lymph—Colorless liquid that carries the white blood cells in the lymphatic vessels.

Lymphatic system—A subsystem of the circulatory system that consists of lymphatic fluid, lymphatic vessels, and lymphatic tissues (lymph nodes, tonsils, spleen, and thymus). It returns excess fluid to the blood and defends the body against disease.

Peritoneum—Smooth membrane that lines the cavity of the abdomen and surrounds the viscera (large interior organs), forming a nearly closed bag.

Peritonitis—Inflammation of the peritoneum.

Venae cavae—Very large veins. There are two venae cavae in the body. The superior vena cava returns blood from the upper limbs, head, and neck to the heart, and the inferior vena cava returns blood from the lower limbs to the heart.

a common symptom of liver disease such as cirrhosis of the liver, but approximately 10% of the diagnosed cases occur as a side effect of several types of cancers, such as ovarian, gastric, exocrine pancreatic, and colorectal cancers, and **lymphoma**. This condition is known as ascites, and it causes pain and discomfort in patients. When doctors cannot treat advanced ascites with medication, they recommend an operation such as the PVS procedure as a means to empty the abdomen of the accumulated fluid.

The ascites that results from **cancer** contains high levels of proteins. It occurs because of functional imbalances in the cells of the organs affected by the cancer and because the walls of the capillaries containing the normal abdominal fluid start leaking. Depending on the type of cancer, there may also be a decrease in the ability of the lymphatic system of the body to absorb fluids.

Description

The most common PVS device is the LeVeen shunt, used since the 1970s to relieve ascites due to liver disease and since the 1980s for cancer-related ascites. It consists of a plastic or silicon rubber tube fitted with a pressure-activated one-way polypropylene valve that connects the peritoneal space where the fluid is collecting to a large vein located in the neck called the jugular vein. The tube enters the jugular vein and terminates in another large vein called the superior vena cava that returns blood to the heart. Thus, the fluid goes from the abdominal cavity into the venous blood circulatory system and is then eliminated by the kidneys. The function of the one-way valve is to prevent blood from flowing back into the peritoneal space.

The PVS is inserted under the skin of the chest under local or general anesthesia, depending on the general health of the patient.

An alternative option to treat ascites due to cirrhosis is to use a transjugular intrahepatic portosystemic shunt (TIPS). This shunt is also a tube that is passed through the skin of the neck and into the jugular vein, but it is pushed all the way through the liver and into the portal vein, which drains into the liver. It thus creates a shunt of blood across the liver in an attempt to reduce pressure and fluid formation.

Precautions

The PVS procedure is restricted to patients with livers that function normally. Additionally, the required veins must be healthy so as to allow the insertion of the shunt device. The PVS insertion is not performed in the following cases:

- patients having undergone previous extensive abdominal surgery
- patients diagnosed with bacterial peritonitis
- patients with diseased veins in the esophagus
- patients with heart disease
- patients with a diseased major organ

In cases of ascites due to cancer (malignant ascites), there is a concern that the use of a PVS could facilitate the spread of the cancer. In evaluating a cancer patient as a candidate for a PVS, the risk of cancer spread must be balanced against pain/discomfort relief, quality of life issues, and the expected survival period.

Preparation

Abdominal **computed tomography** (CT) scans are used to determine the extent of the ascites. Lab tests are usually performed to determine whether the excess abdominal fluid is infected and other **imaging studies** such as ultrasound may be performed to assess the general condition of the veins selected for insertion of the PVS tube. For the operation, the patient is usually injected with a mild sedative and local anesthetic. The surgeon uses a puncture needle to create the opening required for insertion of the PVS device so as to avoid surgical incisions that take longer to heal.

Aftercare

Antibiotics are usually prescribed for approximately four days after surgery. Any **fever** or chills that the patient experiences should be reported to the doctor without delay.

Risks

Complications following PVS insertion are very common and include infection, leakage of fluid, fluid buildup in the lungs, problems with blood coagulation, heart failure, and blockage of the PVS device.

Results

The PVS insertion is considered successful when the excess abdominal fluid gradually disappears after the operation.

Abnormal results

The most common complication resulting from PVS insertion is obstruction of the valve or tube, which can be due to a blood clot or to scar tissue forming around the shunt and eventually blocking it. This complication occurs in approximately 60% of cases during the first year of follow-up.

Resources

PERIODICALS

Inoue, Y., Hayashi, M., Hirokawa, F., Takeshita, A., Tanigawa, N. "Peritoneovenous Shunt For Intractable Ascites Due to Hepatic Lymphorrhea After Hepatectomy." *World Journal of Gastrointestinal Surgery* 3, no. 1 (2011): 16–20. http://www.ncbi.nlm.nih.gov/pmc/articles/PMC3030739/ (accessed November 14, 2014).

Nitta, H., Okamura, S., Mizumoto, T., Matsushita, H., Nishimura, T., Shimokawa, Y., Kimura, M., Baba, H. "Prognosis Assessment of Patients With Refractory Ascites Treated With a Peritoneovenous Shunt." *Hepato-Gastroenterology* 60, no. 127 (2013): 1607–10. http://www.ncbi.nlm.nih.gov/pubmed/24634930 (accessed November 14, 2014).

WEBSITES

National Cancer Institute. "Shunt." http://www.cancer.gov/dictionary?cdrid=46579 (accessed November 14, 2014).

Monique Laberge, PhD

Pesticides

Definition

Pesticides are chemicals used to kill or control destructive or disease-carrying insects (insecticides), ticks and mites (acaricides), animals (rodenticides), fungi (fungicides), or weeds (herbicides). Some pesticides are known or suspected **carcinogens**, and occupational exposure to various agricultural pesticides has been linked to some cancers.

Description

An estimated 5.1 billion lb. (2.3 billion kg) of pesticides are applied to U.S. crops every year. Several factors have significantly increased the use of agricultural pesticides, including multiple harvests, the introduction of genetically modified crops (GMOs) that are resistant to high levels of herbicides, and rising pesticide and herbicide resistance among insects and weeds. Pesticides are also used to control disease. For example, following Hurricane Katrina much of the Gulf Coast was sprayed with the insecticides Naled and Anvil to control flies and mosquitoes. Consumers use pesticides on their lawns and gardens—up to ten times more per acre than farmers, according to the U.S. Fish and Wildlife Service. Household pesticides include cockroach sprays, rat poison, ant traps, and pet flea and tick treatments and collars. Stronger indoor formulations are used by professional pest controllers.

Types of pesticides

Many more pesticides are used worldwide. The majority fall into four main categories:

- Organophosphates, such as malathion and Naled, are nerve toxins that are among the most commonly used insecticides. Chlorpyrifos is an insecticide used on grains, fruits, nuts, and vegetable crops, as well as lawns and ornamental plants. Glyphosate, the active ingredient in Roundup, is the most widely used herbicide in the United States—about 100 million lb. (45 million kg) are applied to U.S. farms and lawns each year. Glyphosate has been linked to some cancers.

- Organochlorines include 2,4-D, one of the most widely used herbicides worldwide and the most common herbicide used on residential lawns in the United States. Its use has increased with the introduction of 2,4-D-resistant GMO crops. Occupational use of 2,4-D has been associated with certain cancers. Organochlorine insecticides were commonly used in the past, but many—such as DDT and chlordane—have been outlawed.

- Pyrethroids, such as Anvil, are synthetic versions of the naturally occurring insecticide pyrethrin, derived from chrysanthemum flowers. Permethrins are broad-spectrum neurotoxic insecticides used widely on crops and are the most common ingredient in indoor/outdoor insect sprays. They are classified by the U.S. Environmental Protection Agency (EPA) as likely human carcinogens.

- Carbamates are nerve toxins that include carbaryl, an insecticide used on a wide variety of crops.

Benzene is a human carcinogen and one of the 20 most widely used chemicals in the United States. It is a starting material for many products, including pesticides.

Dioxins are toxic and carcinogenic contaminants in some insecticides and herbicides, including 2,4-D. Industrial releases of dioxins have declined 80–90% since the 1980s, and levels in the general population are very low. Nevertheless, dioxins will persist in the environment long into the future.

Banned pesticides

Pesticides that are banned in the United States and other Western countries often remain in wide use in developing countries. Furthermore, although DDT was banned in the United States in 1972, DDT and its breakdown product DDE remain in agricultural soils and the bodies of all Americans as well as most farm animals and wildlife. DDE builds up in body fat, tends to increase throughout life, and is rarely excreted except in human and cow's milk. DDT, DDE, and chlordane, another environmentally persistent insecticide that was widely used on food crops until 1978, are possible human carcinogens. The insecticide aldrin was completely banned by 1987, but its degradation product dieldrin, a possible carcinogen, persists in the environment.

Lindane is a neurotoxic insecticide that was widely used in the 1960s and 1970s. Agricultural uses have now been outlawed in most of the world, but it continues to be used pharmaceutically to treat lice and scabies. A lindane by-product, beta-HCH, persists in soil and water and accumulates in and is magnified by biological systems.

Inorganic arsenic—a known carcinogen—was banned from agricultural pesticides in 1993, but treated soils may still be contaminated.

Pesticide exposure

Pesticides can enter the body through the skin, by inhalation, or through food or drink. Workers who manufacture, mix, load, or apply pesticides; clean or repair application equipment; or work in fields, nurseries, or greenhouses, as well as home gardeners, are at risk of exposure. Workers are at added risk from using defective or inadequate protective gear, eating contaminated produce or eating with contaminated hands, or drinking or washing with water from irrigation canals or holding ponds where pesticides accumulate.

Most crops are sprayed with pesticides using ground-based equipment or aircraft. Sprayed pesticides can be carried on the wind to other areas and then washed by rainwater into streams, lakes, and rivers or absorbed into groundwater. Pesticides are found in nearly every stream and fish and in many wells. People are exposed to low levels of pesticides through normal daily activities, including residues on foods, especially fruits and vegetables, in groundwater, and on contaminated surfaces. Dioxin exposure occurs most often through animal fats from meat and dairy products and fatty fish. Current evidence suggests that the trace amounts of pesticides found in food and water do not increase **cancer** risk, although their effects may be cumulative.

Pesticides currently used in the United States are generally assumed to present few dangers to humans if used correctly. However, their improper use in agriculture, industry, and other occupations, as well as in the home, can present a serious risk to human health.

Exposure in children

Rapidly growing children take in more pesticides than adults from food, water, and air, and their smaller bodies accumulate higher levels. Children also have increased exposure from playing on pesticide-treated lawns and putting objects or their fingers in their mouths. Outdoor pesticides are tracked into homes and blown in through windows and vents. Indoor exposure of young children to 2,4-D has been estimated to increase tenfold

KEY TERMS

2,4-D—2,4-dichlorophenoxyacetic acid; one of the most commonly used herbicides worldwide, and the most common lawn herbicide in the United States.

Aldrin—An organochlorine insecticide that breaks down to dieldrin, a possible carcinogen. Although aldrin was banned by 1987, dieldrin persists in the environment and is associated with cancer.

Arsenic—A poisonous element and known carcinogen that was a common pesticide ingredient prior to 1993.

Benzene—A toxic and carcinogenic hydrocarbon used in pesticide manufacture.

Beta-HCH—Beta-hexachlorocyclohexane; a lindane by-product that persists in the soil and water and accumulates in biological systems.

Carbamates—Neurotoxic insecticides such as carbaryl (1-naphthyl methylcarbamate); used on a wide variety of crops.

Carcinogen—A substance or agent that promotes cancer, either directly or following activation in the body.

Chlordane—A banned organochlorine insecticide that persists in the environment.

DDE—Dichlorodiphenyldichloroethylene; a common breakdown product of DDT that remains in agricultural soils and the body fat of all Americans and most animals.

DDT—Dichlorodiphenyltrichloroethane; a toxic organochlorine insecticide widely used for mosquito control but banned in the United States since 1972.

Dioxins—Toxic, environmentally persistent contaminants from pesticides and other chemicals.

Endocrine disrupters—Environmental chemicals, including some pesticides, that interfere with the function of hormones and may increase the risk of hormone-sensitive cancers.

Genetically modified (GM or GMO) crops—Crops that contain genes from other organisms that confer resistance to herbicides.

Leukemia—A cancer of the blood; the most common childhood cancer. Acute myeloid leukemia (AML) is the most common leukemia in adults.

Lindane—Gamma-hexachlorocyclohexane; a neurotoxic insecticide that was widely used on crops in the 1960s and 1970s and is still used to treat lice and scabies.

Monoclonal gammopathy of undetermined significance (MGUS)—A precancerous condition that often progresses to myeloma, a bone marrow cancer.

Organochlorines—A large class of pesticides that includes 2,4-D and the discontinued insecticides DDT, chlordane, and aldrin.

Organophosphates—A large class of pesticides including the neurotoxic insecticides malathion, Naled, and glyphosate (N-[phosphonomethyl]glycine), the most widely used herbicide in the United States.

Permethrin—A common neurotoxic insecticide and insect repellent.

Pyrethroids—Synthetic insecticides that resemble pyrethrins from chrysanthemums.

---

during the week after lawn treatment. Indoor sprays and foggers leave pesticide residues on eating utensils, toys, furniture, floors, carpets, and bedding, as well as on dust. Pesticides are used frequently in many childcare centers.

Higher rates of leukemia and brain cancer in children of farmworkers have been attributed to pesticides. Various studies have found disturbing patterns of exposure:

• A 2013 EPA study of urine from 135 preschool children reported that 99% tested positive for chlorpyrifos, 92% for 2,4-D, and 64% were positive for permethrins.

• A 2013 Canadian study found permethrins in 97% of children's urine samples.

• All of the children in a 2012 California study exceeded cancer benchmark levels for DDE, dieldrin, dioxins, and arsenic, solely on the basis of the food they ate.

Common diseases and disorders

Pesticides can have a wide range of health effects—including nerve damage, birth defects, and cancer—depending on the type of pesticide and the degree and frequency of exposure. Some effects, especially cancers, may not become evident until many years after exposure. Many common pesticides, such as 2,4-D, are also endocrine disrupters that affect the hormones that control most bodily functions. Among other health effects, endocrine disrupters may increase the risk of hormone-sensitive cancers such as breast and prostate cancers.

Agricultural Health Study (AHS)

The AHS is an ongoing project conducted by a consortium of U.S. Government agencies. Since 1993, the AHS has followed the health of almost 90,000 men and women who live and/or work on farms in Iowa and North Carolina. The AHS also includes about 5,000 commercial pesticide applicators in Iowa. As of 2014, more than 20 pesticides had been investigated for associations with cancer, Parkinson's disease, and other conditions.

In 2003, an AHS study reported an association between specific pesticides and **prostate cancer** in farmers with a family history of the disease. An analysis of 2,000 men completed in 2013 found some evidence of an overall association between specific pesticides and prostate cancer. Furthermore, a strong link was found between frequent users of malathion and terbufos (an organophosphate insecticide and acaricide) and a fast-growing, aggressive type of prostate cancer. Fonofos (an organophosphate insecticide used on corn and lawns) and aldrin were also linked to increased risk of aggressive prostate cancer.

In 2009, AHS researchers reported that users of the weed killer imazethapyr were at increased risk of bladder and colon cancers. Imazethapyr is one of the most common herbicides used on dry beans, soybeans, alfalfa, and other crops. People with the highest cumulative exposure had more than twice the risk of **bladder cancer** compared with people with no exposure. They also had a 78% increased risk of **colon cancer**, primarily cancer in the upper part of the colon. Based on animal studies, the EPA had previously classified imazethapyr as unlikely to be a human carcinogen.

Researchers from the **National Cancer Institute** previously established an association between pesticide exposure and increased risk of **multiple myeloma**. Using AHS data, they subsequently reported that farmers and others with occupational exposure to pesticides were at almost twice the risk of a multiple **myeloma** precursor known as monoclonal gammopathy of undetermined significance (MGUS). MGUS risk was associated with the use of dieldrin, a carbon tetrachloride/carbon disulfide fumigant mixture, the fungicide chlorothalonil, and possibly other pesticides.

Other studies

Studies have found high rates of blood and lymphatic cancers—including leukemia, myeloma, and non-Hodgkin lymphoma—melanoma and other skin cancers, and cancers of the lip, stomach, lung, brain, and prostate among people with high pesticide exposure, including farmers, crop dusters and other pesticide applicators, and workers in pesticide manufacturing. More research is needed to confirm these potential associations. Workers manufacturing arsenic-containing pesticides inhaled very high levels and had increased risk of lung cancers; the risk increased with higher and more prolonged exposure. Higher rates of leukemia, especially acute myeloid leukemia (AML), have been reported among workers exposed to high levels of benzene. An association between exposure to a DDT by-product and increased risk of **testicular cancer** has also been reported. Numerous studies have failed to find a direct link between pesticide exposure and **breast cancer**.

Some studies have associated pesticide exposure during pregnancy with increased risk of **childhood cancers**, but other studies have found no association. Such studies are difficult because the degree of maternal pesticide exposure is usually unknown. A 2013 Australian study found that exposure of either parent to certain pesticides during the year before a child's birth increased the risk of childhood brain cancer. Some studies have suggested possible links between childhood leukemia, especially AML, and exposure to household pesticides during pregnancy and early childhood or maternal workplace exposure during pregnancy.

As of 2014, researchers were conducting a large controlled study comparing childhood leukemia rates in the San Francisco Bay area and in the agricultural counties of California's Central Valley, where much of the population works in agriculture or lives near pesticide-sprayed fields. This is the first large-scale childhood leukemia study to target both Hispanic and agricultural populations. In addition to assessing exposure to agricultural pesticides, researchers are measuring exposure to home and garden pesticides by analyzing household dust.

Public health role and response

EPA

The EPA is responsible for approving pesticides for specific uses. Every 15 years, the agency reevaluates pesticides for acute and chronic toxicity, carcinogenicity, and environmental persistence. EPA regulations require that pesticides be properly labeled with rules for use, the training of handlers and workers in safe use, protective clothing and gear, available decontamination supplies and emergency medical assistance, notification of pesticide application, and restricted entry following application. However in many cases, neither safe exposure limits nor the combined effects of chemical mixtures are known.

In February 2014, the EPA proposed revisions to its 22-year-old standards to better protect America's two million farmworkers and their families. The proposed changes include:

• pesticide protection training annually rather than every five years

• no-entry buffer zones of 25–100 feet around pesticide-treated fields

• expanded posted warnings against entering newly treated fields

• prohibiting children under 16 from handling pesticides unless they are part of a family farm

The EPA limits the amount of pesticides that can be used on food crops and the amount that can remain on food sold to consumers. Nevertheless, fruits and vegetables should be scrubbed under running water, skins peeled, and outer leaves trimmed to reduce remaining pesticides. Trimming fat from meat can also reduce exposure. Consuming a variety of foods may prevent excessive exposure to a single pesticide. According to the EPA, snap beans, watermelon, tomatoes, and potatoes are likely to have higher pesticide residues than other produce.

Other responses

The U.S. government's Healthy People 2020 program targets call for reducing concentrations of banned pesticides in the general population. The specific goals for blood and urine concentrations of pesticides or their metabolites are:

• DDT (as DDE) reduction from 1860 nanograms per gram (ng/g) to 1303 ng/g of lipid (fat)

• chlordane (oxychlordane) reduction from 37.7 ng/g of lipid to 26.3 g/ng

• beta-HCH from 56.5 ng/g to 39.55 ng/g of lipid

States and counties differ greatly in rules governing the use of pesticides and the posting of warnings; in addition, warning signs are often ignored. Although chemical companies tell consumers to avoid sprayed surfaces for six to 24 hours, many experts believe that two to three days are necessary to avoid overexposure. For years, various consumer and environmental groups have called for stricter pesticide regulations and enforcement.

Preventing exposure

Organic foods grown without synthetic pesticides, although not free from pesticide residues, have lower levels and fewer chemicals. Currently, no research indicates that organically grown foods can reduce cancer risk. The American Academy of Pediatrics—in addition

---

QUESTIONS TO ASK YOUR DOCTOR

• Is my family at risk from pesticide spraying of neighboring fields?

• Is it safe to use weed killer on my lawn?

• Is it safe to use indoor insecticides?

• Can I safely use lindane to treat my child's lice?

• Should I feed my children organic foods?

---

to calling for more research about associations between pesticide exposure and birth defects, childhood cancers, behavior disorders, and asthma—recommends feeding children organic foods.

Pest control services should be open about the chemicals they use and all safety concerns and precautions. Household and garden pesticides should be used with care, including:

• using only the least toxic pesticide possible

• carefully reading warnings and following all instructions

• never exceeding recommended amounts

• storing pesticides safely in their original containers and disposing of them properly

• never reusing empty pesticide containers

• keeping pesticides locked up and out of children's reach

• never using outdoor pesticides on windy days or indoors

• indoor spraying only with doors and windows closed

• treating infested areas only

• not treating entire floors, walls, or ceilings

• never spraying in food preparation or storage areas

• keeping people and pets away from treated areas

• immediately washing any body parts or clothing that come in contact with a pesticide

There are various alternatives to chemical pesticides for controlling pests and preventing infestations indoors and out:

• Water and food should not be left out to attract pests.

• Areas where pests hide should be destroyed, and entry holes sealed.

• Biological control methods include attracting birds and bats that eat insects.

• Manual control methods include pulling weeds or setting traps, baits, or gels.

- Natural pesticides are available that do not contain synthetic chemicals.
- Integrated pest management combines nonchemical controls with less toxic pesticides.

Resources

BOOKS

Magner, Mike. *A Trust Betrayed: The Untold Story of Camp Lejeune and the Poisoning of Generations of Marines and Their Families.* Boston: Da Capo, 2014.

Stewart, B. W., and C. P. Wild. *World Cancer Report 2014.* Geneva: World Health Organization, 2014.

PERIODICALS

Harvey, Bethany. "Protecting Farming Families & Field-Workers." *Professional Safety* 59, no. 3 (March 2014): 68–70.

Hudson, Gwendolyn, Gregory G. Miller, and Kathy Seikel. "Regulations, Policies, and Guidelines Addressing Environmental Exposures in Early Learning Environments: A Review." *Journal of Environmental Health* 76, no. 7 (March 2014): 24–34.

Lewis, Diane. "The Toxic Brew in Our Yards." *New York Times* (May 11, 2014): SR4.

Mitra, Maureen Nandini. "Trouble in Paradise." *Earth Island Journal* 29, no. 1 (Spring 2014): 18–23.

Moore, Anna Blackmon. "My Friend Melanie Has Breast Cancer." *American Scholar* (Winter 2014): 39–47.

Pleasant, Barbara. "Pesticides and Kids." *Mother Earth News* 264 (June/July 2014): 13.

OTHER

National Institute of Environmental Health Sciences. "The New Environmental Health." http://www.niehs.nih.gov/health/assets/docs_p_z/the_new_environmental_health.pdf (accessed July 10, 2014).

WEBSITES

Gillam, Carey. "U.S. Proposes New Safety Rules for Farm Pesticide Use." Reuters Health Information, February 24, 2014. http://www.medscape.com/viewarticle/820924 (accessed July 10, 2014).

National Cancer Institute. "Pesticides." *Cancer Trends Progress Report—2011/2012 Update*, June 20, 2012. http://progressreport.cancer.gov/doc_detail.asp?pid=1&did=2007&chid=71&coid=713&mid= (accessed July 10, 2014).

National Institutes of Health. "2014 Study Update." NIH Agricultural Health Study. http://aghealth.nih.gov/news/2014.html (accessed July 10, 2014).

U.S. Environmental Protection Agency. "Effective Control of Household Pests: How to Reduce Exposure to Pesticide Hazards." http://www.epa.gov/research/aging/factsheets/echp-rd.html (accessed July 10, 2014).

ORGANIZATIONS

American Cancer Society, 250 Williams Street NW, Atlanta, GA 30303, (800) 227-2345, http://www.cancer.org.

National Cancer Institute, 6116 Executive Boulevard, Suite 300, Bethesda, MD 20892-8322, (800) 4-CANCER (422-6237), http://www.cancer.gov.

National Institute of Environmental Health Sciences, PO Box 12233, MD K3-16, Research Triangle Park, NC 27709, (919) 541-3345, Fax: (919) 541-4395, webcenter@niehs.nih.gov, http://www.niehs.nih.gov.

U.S. Environmental Protection Agency, 4601M, Ariel Rios Building, 1200 Pennsylvania Avenue, NW, Washington, DC 20460, (202) 564-3750, ogwdw.web@epa.gov, http://www.epa.gov.

Margaret Alic, PhD

PET scan *see* **Positron emission tomography**

Peutz-Jeghers syndrome

Definition

Peutz-Jeghers syndrome (PJS) is a rare familial **cancer** syndrome that causes intestinal polyps, skin freckling, and an increased risk of cancer.

Description

Peutz-Jeghers syndrome affects both males and females. The characteristic, or pathognomonic, features of PJS are unusual skin freckling and multiple polyps in the small intestine. The skin freckles, which are bluish to brown to black in color, can be found on the lips, inside the mouth, around the eyes, on the hands and feet, and on the genitals. The freckles are called benign hyperpigmented macules and do not become cancerous. The polyps in PJS are called hamartomatous polyps, and are found in the small intestine, small bowel, stomach, colon, and sometimes in the nose or bladder. Hamartomatous polyps are usually benign (not cancerous), but they occasionally become malignant (cancerous). A person with PJS is at increased risk of cancer of the colon, small intestine, stomach, and pancreas. Women with PJS are also at increased risk of breast and **cervical cancer**, and a specific type of benign ovarian tumor called SCTAT (sex cord tumors with annular tubules). Men with PJS are also at increased risk of benign testicular tumors.

Risk factors

Hamartomatous polyps may be diagnosed from early childhood to later in adulthood. On average, a person with PJS develops polyps by his or her early 20s. The lifetime risk of cancer is greatly increased over that of the general population, and cancer may occur at an earlier

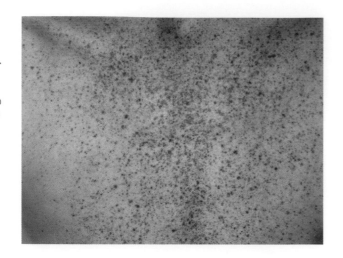

The unusual skin freckling of Peutz-Jeghers syndrome. Here, the freckles are shown on the chest. *((c) Logical Images, Inc.)*

age. Early and regular screening is important to try to detect any cancers at an early stage. The benign ovarian tumors in women with PJS may cause early and irregular menstruation. The benign testicular tumors in men may cause earlier growth spurts and gynecomastia (development of the male breasts).

Causes and symptoms

Causes

PJS is a genetic disease caused by a mutation of a tumor suppressor gene called *LKB1* (or *STK11*) on chromosome 19. The exact function of *LKB1* is unknown at this time. PJS is inherited as an autosomal dominant condition, which means that a person with PJS has a 50% chance of passing it on to each of his or her children. Screening and/or **genetic testing** of family members can help sort out who has PJS or who is at risk of developing PJS. Identification of a person with PJS in a family may result in other family members with more mild symptoms being diagnosed, and then receiving appropriate screening and medical care.

Symptoms

Dozens to thousands of hamartomatous polyps may develop in an affected person. A person with PJS with benign hamartomatous polyps can have abdominal pain, blood in the stool, or complications such as colon obstruction or intussusception (a condition in which one portion of the intestine telescopes into another). Surgery may be required to remove the affected part of the colon.

About half of all persons with PJS will have family members with symptoms of PJS. Symptoms can vary between families and between members of the same family. Some family members may have just freckling, while others may have more serious medical problems such as bowel obstruction or cancer diagnosis. The freckles in PJS usually appear in childhood and fade as a person gets older, so it may be necessary to look at childhood photos in an adult who is being examined for signs of PJS.

Diagnosis

The diagnosis of Peutz-Jeghers syndrome can be made clinically in a person with the characteristic freckles and at least two hamartomatous polyps. A pathologist needs to confirm that the polyps are hamartomatous instead of another type of polyp. If a person has a family history of PJS, the diagnosis can be made in a person who has either freckles or hamartomatous polyps. When someone is the first person in his/her family to be diagnosed with PJS, it is important for all first-degree relatives to be carefully examined for clinical signs of PJS.

Fifty percent of people clinically diagnosed with PJS will have a mutation in the *LKB1/STK11* gene detected in the lab. The other half will not have a detectable mutation at that time, but may have other PJS-causing genetic mutations discovered in the future. In families with a known mutation, family members can be tested for the same mutation. A person who tests positive for the family mutation will be diagnosed with PJS (even if he or she does not currently show signs of PJS), will need to have the recommended screening evaluations, and is able to pass on the mutation to his or her children. A person who tests negative for a known family mutation will be spared from screening, and his or her children will not be at risk of PJS. When the mutation cannot be found in a family, genetic testing is not useful, and all persons at risk of inheriting PJS will need to have screening for PJS throughout their life spans.

Treatment

Regular medical examinations and special screening tests are needed in people with PJS. The age at which screening begins and the frequency of the tests is best determined by a physician familiar with PJS. Screening schedules depend on symptoms and family history. **Colonoscopy**, used to search for polyps in the colon, usually begins in adolescence. X-rays and/or **upper gastrointestinal endoscopy** are used to screen for polyps in the stomach and small intestine. The goal of screening is to remove polyps before they cause symptoms or become cancerous. Surgery may be necessary to remove the polyps. Females with PJS

KEY TERMS

Gynecomastia—Overdevelopment of the mammary glands in males; male breast development.

Intussusception—The folding of one segment of the intestine into another segment of the intestine.

Pathognomonic—Characteristic of a disease; a pattern of symptoms not found in any other condition.

Polyp—A mushroom-like growth that may be a precursor to cancer.

need to have annual gynecologic examinations by age 18, and breast **mammography** starting between the ages of 25 and 35. Males with PJS need to have annual testicular examinations. If a person with PJS develops cancer, it is treated as it would be in the general population.

See also Cancer genetics; Familial cancer syndromes.

Resources

PERIODICALS

Tomas C., Soyer P., Dohan A., Dray X., Boudiaf M., Hoeffel C. "Update on Imaging of Peutz-Jeghers Syndrome." *World Journal of Gastroenterology.* 20, no. 31 (2014): 10864–75. http://www.ncbi.nlm.nih.gov/pmc/articles/PMC4138465/ (accessed November 12, 2014).

ORGANIZATIONS

Genetic Alliance, 4301 Connecticut Ave. NW, Ste. 404, Washington DC, 20008–2304, (202) 966-5557, info@geneticalliance.org.

Laura L. Stein, M.S., C.G.C

Pharyngectomy

Definition

A pharyngectomy is the total or partial surgical removal of the pharynx, the cavity at the back of the mouth that opens into the esophagus at its lower end. The pharynx is cone-shaped, has an average length of about 3 in. (76 mm), and is lined with mucous membrane.

Purpose

A pharyngectomy is performed to treat cancers of the pharynx, including:

- Throat cancer, which occurs when cells in the pharynx or larynx (voice box) begin to divide abnormally. A total or partial pharyngectomy is usually performed for cancers of the hypopharynx (lowest part of the throat, also known as the laryngopharynx), in which all or part of the hypopharynx is removed.

- Hypopharyngeal carcinoma, a form of cancerous tumor that may develop in the pharynx or adjacent locations and for which surgery may be indicated.

Description

Whether a pharyngectomy is performed in total or with only partial removal of the pharynx depends on the localized amount of **cancer** found. The procedure may also involve removal of the larynx, in which case it is called a laryngopharyngectomy. Well-localized, early-stage HPC tumors can be amenable to a partial pharyngectomy or a laryngopharyngectomy, but laryngopharyngectomy is more commonly performed for more advanced cancers. It can be total, involving removal of the entire larynx, or partial, and may also involve removal of part of the esophagus (esophagectomy). Patients undergoing laryngopharyngectomy will lose some speaking ability and require special techniques or reconstructive procedures to regain the use of their voice.

Following a total or partial pharyngectomy, the surgeon may also need to reconstruct the throat so that the patient can swallow. A tracheotomy is used when the tumor is too large to remove. In this procedure, a hole is made in the neck to bypass the tumor and allow the patient to breathe.

For this type of surgery, patient positioning requires access to the lower part of the neck for the surgeon. This is achieved by placing the patient on a table fitted with a head holder, allowing the head to be bent back but well supported.

If a laryngopharyngectomy is performed, the surgeon starts with a curved horizontal incision in the skin of the neck. The **laryngectomy** incision is usually made from the breastbone to the lowermost of the laryngeal cartilages, leaving a 1–2 in. (2.54–5.08 cm) bridge of skin preserved. Once the incision is deepened, flaps are elevated until the larynx is exposed. The anterior jugular veins and strap muscles are left undisturbed. The sternocleidomastoid muscle is then identified. The layer of cervical fibrous tissue is cut (incised) longitudinally from the hyoid (the bony arch that supports the tongue) to the clavicle (collarbone). Part of the hyoid is then divided, which allows the surgeon to enter the loose compartment bounded by the sternomastoid muscle and carotid sheath (which covers the

KEY TERMS

Anesthesia—A combination of drugs administered to provide sedation, amnesia, analgesia (pain relief), and immobility adequate for the accomplishment of a surgical procedure with minimal discomfort and without injury to the patient.

Biopsy—Procedure that involves obtaining a tissue specimen for microscopic analysis to establish a precise diagnosis.

Carcinoma—A malignant growth that arises from epithelium, found in skin or, more commonly, the lining of body organs.

Computed tomography (CT) scan—An imaging technique that creates a series of pictures of areas inside the body, taken from different angles. The pictures are created by a computer linked to an x-ray machine.

Dysphagia—Difficulty in eating as a result of disruption in the swallowing process. Dysphagia can be a serious health threat because of the risk of aspiration pneumonia, malnutrition, dehydration, weight loss, and airway obstruction.

Esophagectomy—Surgical removal of the esophagus.

Esophagus—A long hollow muscular tube that connects the pharynx to the stomach.

Fine-needle aspiration (FNA)—Use of a very thin type of needle to withdraw cells and body fluid for examination.

Fistula—An abnormal passage or communication, usually between two internal organs or leading from an internal organ to the surface of the body.

Hypopharynx—The lowest part of the throat or the pharynx; also called the laryngopharynx.

Laryngectomy—Surgical removal of the larynx.

Laryngopharyngectomy—Surgical removal of both the larynx and the pharynx.

Laryngoscopy—The visualization of the larynx and vocal cords. This procedure may be done directly with a fiber-optic scope (laryngoscope) or indirectly with mirrors.

Larynx—Voice box.

Magnetic resonance imaging (MRI)—A procedure in which a magnet linked to a computer is used to create detailed pictures of areas inside the body.

Pharynx—The cavity at the back of the mouth. It is cone-shaped and has an average length of about 3 in. (76 mm) and is lined with mucous membrane. The pharynx opens into the esophagus at the lower end.

Tracheotomy—Surgical opening of the trachea (windpipe) to the outside through a hole in the neck.

---

carotid artery) and by the pharynx and larynx in the neck. The pharyngectomy incisions and laryngeal removal are performed, and a view of the pharynx is then possible. Using scissors, the surgeon performs bilateral (on both sides) direct cuts, separating the pharynx from the larynx. If a preliminary tracheotomy has not been performed, the oral endotracheal tube is withdrawn from the tracheal stump and a new cuffed flexible tube is inserted for connection to new anesthesia tubing. The wound is thoroughly irrigated (flushed), all clots are removed, and the wound is closed. The pharyngeal wall is closed in two layers. The muscle layer closure always tightens the opening to some extent and is usually left undone at points where narrowing may be excessive. In fact, studies show that a mucosal (inner layer) closure alone is sufficient for proper healing.

Diagnosis

The initial physical examination for a pharyngectomy usually includes examination of the neck, mouth, pharynx, and larynx. A neurologic examination is sometimes also performed. **Laryngoscopy** is the examination of choice, performed with a long-handled mirror or with a lighted tube called a laryngoscope. A local anesthetic may be used to ease discomfort. An MRI of the oral cavity and neck may also be performed.

If the physician suspects throat cancer, a **biopsy** will be performed—this procedure involves removing tissue for examination in the laboratory under a microscope. Throat cancer can only be confirmed through a biopsy or using fine-needle aspiration (FNA). The physician also may use an imaging test called a **computed tomography** (CT) scan. This is a special type of x-ray that provides images of the body from different angles, allowing a cross-sectional view. A CT scan can help to find the location of a tumor, to judge whether a tumor can be removed surgically, and to determine the cancer's stage of development.

Preparation

Before surgery, the cancer is carefully staged to determine its severity and spread within the body. The patient is also examined for nutritional assessment and supplementation, and surgical airway management is planned with the anesthesiologist and surgeon to determine the timing of tracheotomy and intubation. The anesthesiologist may elect to use an orotracheal (through the mouth and trachea) tube with anesthetic, which can be removed if a subsequent tracheotomy is planned.

Aftercare

After undergoing a pharyngectomy, special attention is given to the patient's pulmonary function and fluid/nutritional balance, as well as to local wound conditions in the neck, thorax, and abdomen. Regular postoperative checks of calcium, magnesium, and phosphorus levels are necessary; supplementation with calcium, magnesium, and 1,25-dihydroxycholecalciferol is usually required. A patient may be unable to take in enough food to maintain adequate nutrition and experience difficulty eating (dysphagia). Sometimes it may be necessary to have a feeding tube placed through the skin and muscle of the abdomen directly into the stomach to provide extra nutrition. This procedure is called a gastrostomy.

Reconstructive surgery is also required to rebuild the throat after a pharyngectomy in order to help the patient with swallowing after the operation. Reconstructive surgeries represent a great challenge because of the complex properties of the tissues lining the throat and underlying muscle that are so vital to the proper functioning of this region. The primary goal is to re-establish the conduit connecting the oral cavity to the esophagus, thus retaining the continuity of the alimentary tract. The two main techniques used are:

- Myocutaneous flaps. Sometimes a muscle and area of skin may be rotated from an area close to the throat, such as the chest (pectoralis major flap), to reconstruct the throat.
- Free flaps. With the advances of microvascular surgery (sewing together small blood vessels under a microscope), surgeons have many more options to reconstruct the area of the throat affected by a pharyngectomy. Tissues from other areas of the patient's body, such as a piece of intestine or a piece of arm muscle, can be used to replace parts of the throat.

Risks

Potential risks associated with a pharyngectomy include those associated with any head and neck surgery, such as excessive bleeding, wound infection, wound slough, fistula (abnormal opening between organs or to the outside of the body) formation, and, in rare cases, blood vessel rupture. Specifically, the surgery is associated with the following risks:

- Drain failure. Drains unable to hold a vacuum represent a serious threat to the surgical wound.
- Hematoma. Although rare, blood clot formation requires prompt intervention to avoid pressure separation of the pharyngeal repair and compression of the upper windpipe.
- Infection. A subcutaneous infection after total pharyngectomy is recognized by increasing redness and swelling of the skin flaps three to five days after surgery. Associated odor, fever, and elevated white blood cell count will occur.
- Pharyngocutaneous fistula. Patients with poor preoperative nutritional status are at significant risk of fistula development.
- Narrowing. This is more common at the lower esophageal end of the pharyngeal reconstruction than at the upper end, where the recipient lumen of the pharynx is wider.
- Functional swallowing problems. Dysphagia is also a risk that depends on the extent of the pharyngectomy.

Results

Oral intake is usually started seven days after surgery, although it may be delayed if the patient has had preoperative **radiation therapy**. Mechanical voice devices are sometimes useful in the early postoperative phase until the pharyngeal wall heals. Results are considered normal if there is no recurrence of the cancer at a later stage.

Morbidity and mortality rates

Smokers are at high risk of throat cancer. According to Harvard Medical School, throat cancer is associated closely with other cancers: 15% of throat cancer patients also are diagnosed with cancer of the mouth, esophagus, or lung. Another 10%–20% of throat cancer patients develop these cancers later in life. Other people at risk include those who drink a lot of alcohol, especially if they also smoke. Vitamin A deficiency and certain types of **human papillomavirus** (HPV) infection also have been associated with an increased risk of throat cancer.

Surgical treatment for hypopharyngeal carcinomas is difficult, as most patients are diagnosed with advanced disease; five-year disease-specific survival is only 30%. Cure rates have been the highest with surgical resection followed by postoperative radiotherapy. Immediate reconstruction can be accomplished with regional and free tissue transfers. These techniques have greatly

QUESTIONS TO ASK YOUR DOCTOR

- How will the surgery affect my ability to swallow and to eat?
- What type of anesthesia will be used?
- How long will it take to recover from the surgery?
- When can I expect to return to work and/or resume normal activities?
- To what extent will my ability to speak be affected?
- What are the risks associated with a pharyngectomy?
- How many pharyngectomies do you perform in a year?

reduced morbidity and allow most patients to successfully resume an oral diet.

Health care team roles

A pharyngectomy is major surgery performed by a surgeon trained in otolaryngology. An anesthesiologist is responsible for administering anesthesia, and the operation is performed in a hospital setting. Otolaryngology is the oldest medical specialty in the United States. Otolaryngologists are physicians trained in the medical and surgical management and treatment of patients with diseases and disorders of the ear, nose, throat (ENT), and related structures of the head and neck. They are commonly referred to as ENT physicians.

With cancer involved in pharyngectomy procedures, the otolaryngologist usually works with radiation and medical oncologists in a treatment team approach.

Resources

BOOKS

Harrison, Louis B., Roy B. Sessions, and Merrill S. Kies. *Head and Neck Cancer: A Multidisciplinary Approach*. Philadelphia: Wolters Kluwer Health/Lippincott Williams & Wilkins, 2013.

Judd, Sandra J. *Ear, Nose, and Throat Disorders Sourcebook*. 2nd ed. Detroit, MI: Omnigraphics, 2007.

PERIODICALS

Chung, Eun-Jae, et al. "Alternative Treatment Option for Hypopharyngeal Cancer: Clinical Outcomes after Conservative Laryngeal Surgery with Partial Pharyngectomy." *Acta Oto-laryngologica* 133, no. 8 (2013): 866–73. http://

dx.doi.org/10.3109/00016489.2013.785018 (accessed October 3, 2014).

Genden, Eric M., et al. "The Role of Reconstruction for Transoral Robotic Pharyngectomy and Concomitant Neck Dissection." *JAMA Otolaryngology—Head & Neck Surgery* 137, no. 2 (2011): 151–56. http://dx.doi.org/10.1001/archoto.2010.250 (accessed October 3, 2014).

WEBSITES

American Cancer Society. "Surgery for Laryngeal and Hypopharyngeal Cancers." http://www.cancer.org/cancer/laryngealandhypopharyngealcancer/detailedguide/laryngeal-and-hypopharyngeal-cancer-treating-surgery (accessed October 3, 2014).

ORGANIZATIONS

American Academy of Otolaryngology—Head and Neck Surgery, 1650 Diagonal Rd., Alexandria, VA 22314-2857, (703) 836-4444, http://www.entnet.org.

American Cancer Society, 250 Williams St. NW, Atlanta, GA 30303, (800) 227-2345, http://www.cancer.org.

Monique Laberge, PhD

Phenytoin

Definition

Phenytoin is an anticonvulsant, a drug that acts to prevent seizures. In the United States, phenytoin is sold under the brand name Dilantin.

Purpose

Phenytoin helps prevent some types of seizure activity. It is often used to aid in controlling nerve pain associated with some cancers and **cancer** treatments. Nerve pain causes a burning, tingling sensation. Phenytoin also may be ordered to control a rapid or irregular heart rate. Phenytoin may be given to stop uncontrolled seizures. It may be used during brain surgery to prevent seizure activity. In 2003, a group of researchers in California reported that phenytoin is effective in controlling the acute mania associated with bipolar disorder. Additional uses are under study.

Description

Phenytoin works on areas of the brain to limit electrical discharges and stabilize cellular activity. Like many drugs that control seizures, it also has proven helpful in managing nerve pain.

KEY TERMS

Anticonvulsant—A type of medication given to prevent seizures. Phenytoin is an anticonvulsant.

Bipolar disorder—A mood disorder in which the patient experiences both periods of mania and periods of depression.

Epilepsy—Disorder of the nervous system that causes seizures.

Lymphatic system—A part of the immune system that includes lymph nodes and tissue.

Mania—The phase of bipolar disorder in which the patient is easily excited, hyperactive, agitated, and unrealistically cheerful. Phenytoin appears to be a useful treatment for mania.

Recommended dosage

The dose ordered depends on blood levels of the drug determined during routine monitoring. For pain, doctors usually order 200–500 mg per day, either at bedtime or in divided doses. Patients usually start on a low dose. Depending on the patient's response and drug blood levels, the dose may be increased. For seizures, patients are usually started at 100 mg, three times per day. Blood is drawn to check the level of phenytoin in seven to 10 days. The dose is adjusted accordingly. The doctor may prescribe a dose based on an older person's weight. A child's dose also is based on his or her weight.

It is very important that this drug be used exactly as directed. This medication should be taken at the same time every day. Patients should take a missed dose as soon as it is noted but should not take two doses within four hours of each other. This medication should be stored in a dry place, not in the bathroom.

Precautions

Patients should not suddenly stop taking this medication. The abrupt withdrawal of phenytoin could trigger seizures. Patients should not crush or break extended-release drugs. Chewable tablets should be chewed before swallowing. Other pills should be swallowed whole. Older adults may be more prone to adverse effects than younger people. Patients should not change brands without approval of the doctor.

Phenytoin should not be taken by patients who are allergic to this drug. People with slow heart rates, certain other heart conditions, or a flaking, broken skin condition also should not take it. Phenytoin may be used cautiously in patients with asthma, allergies, limited kidney or liver function, heart disease, and blood disorders. It also should be used with caution in those with alcoholism, diabetes mellitus, lupus, poor thyroid function, or porphyria, a rare metabolic disorder. Pregnant women should discuss the risks and benefits of this medication with the doctor. It has been associated with birth defects and possibly cancer in children born to women taking the drug; one study done in 2003 suggested that phenytoin interferes with the normal development of the baby's blood circulation. Expectant mothers who are taking it to prevent seizures should not abruptly stop the drug. Those using it for pain control should discuss its continued use with the doctor. Patients on this drug should not breast feed.

Side effects

Drowsiness is a common side effect of phenytoin. Patients should exercise caution when driving or operating machinery. Alcohol may increase drowsiness. Patients should not consume alcoholic beverages while taking this drug. Other less frequent effects related to the central nervous system include an unsteady gait, slurred speech, confusion, and dizziness. Patients may experience **depression**, difficulty sleeping, nervousness, irritability, tremor, and numbness. Twitching, headache, mental health problems including psychotic episodes, and more seizure activity may occur. This medication may also cause **nausea and vomiting**, stomach upset, **diarrhea**, constipation, and swollen gum tissue. Side effects also include a rash, hair loss (**alopecia**) or excessive hair growth, vision changes, uncontrolled eye movements, and inflammation of the surface of the eye. Patients may develop chest pain, swelling, **fever**, increase in weight, enlarged lips, or joint or muscle pain. Patients should practice good dental hygiene to decrease the risk of gum disease. With the doctor's approval, phenytoin may be taken with food to decrease stomach upset.

Phenytoin may produce changes in the normal makeup of the blood, including high blood sugar levels and **anemia**. It may trigger disorders of the lymphatic system and cause liver damage. If the liver is not able to properly break down phenytoin, it can produce toxic effects even at low doses. Doctors typically assess kidney and liver function prior to ordering it. The tests are repeated at regular intervals. Patients should notify the doctor promptly of any side effects. If a skin rash develops, the doctor will instruct the patient to taper off and stop the drug.

Interactions

Many drugs interact with phenytoin and may increase or decrease its blood levels. Phenytoin may alter the effectiveness of other drugs. The list of interactions is long and varied. Drugs that interfere with phenytoin include anticoagulants (blood thinners), sulfa and other **antibiotics**, antifungal agents, drugs used to treat ulcers, methadone, antidepressants, and disulfiram, which is used to treat alcoholism. It also interacts with **corticosteroids**, estrogen hormones, birth control pills and injections, drugs to treat hypoglycemia, asthma drugs, such other anticonvulsants as **carbamazepine**, lidocaine, heart medications, Parkinson's disease drugs, anti-inflammatory drugs, narcotic pain relievers, and **anticancer drugs**. Additionally, taking phenytoin with certain antidepressants may cause seizures in some patients.

Phenytoin has also been reported to interact with certain herbs, including evening primrose (*Oenothera biennis*), ginkgo (*Ginkgo biloba*), wormwood (*Artemisia pontica*), and an Ayurvedic preparation known as Shankapushpi. Patients should always tell their doctors about any herbal preparations they may be taking as well as other prescription medications.

Alcohol ingestion can interfere with maintaining proper blood levels of phenytoin. Patients should not drink alcoholic beverages while taking this medication, as phenytoin can accumulate to toxic levels in the body of noncompliant patients. Antacids and calcium can lower the effectiveness of phenytoin. These drugs should be taken two to three hours apart from phenytoin. Tube feeding may decrease the amount of phenytoin absorbed. Patients should not have tube feedings for two hours before and after taking this drug. Patients should talk to the doctor before taking **folic acid**. It may interfere with this drug.

Resources

WEBSITES

AHFS Consumer Medication Information. "Phenytoin." http://www.nlm.nih.gov/medlineplus/druginfo/meds/a682022.html (accessed November 12, 2014).

Cancer Research UK. "Epilepsy Drugs and Lymphoma." http://www.cancerresearchuk.org/about-cancer/cancers-in-general/cancer-questions/epilepsy-drugs-and-lymphoma (accessed November 12, 2014).

U.S. Food and Drug Administration. "Safety Information: Dilantin (Phenytoin)." http://www.fda.gov/safety/medwatch/safetyinformation/ucm243476.htm (accessed November 12, 2014).

ORGANIZATIONS

U.S. Food and Drug Administration, 10903 New Hampshire Ave., Silver Spring, MD 20993, (888) INFO-FDA (463-6332), http://www.fda.gov.

Debra Wood, R.N.
Rebecca J. Frey, PhD

Pheochromocytoma

Definition

Pheochromocytoma is a tumor of special cells (called chromaffin cells), most often found in the middle of the adrenal gland.

Description

Because pheochromocytomas arise from chromaffin cells, they are occasionally called chromaffin tumors. Most (90%) are benign tumors and do not spread to other parts of the body. However, these tumors can cause many problems and may result in death if they are not treated.

Pheochromocytomas can be found anywhere chromaffin cells are found. They may be found in the heart and in the area around the bladder, but most (90%) are found in the adrenal glands. Every individual has two adrenal glands that are located above the kidneys in the back of the abdomen. Each adrenal gland is made up of two parts: the outer part (called the adrenal cortex) and the inner part (called the adrenal medulla). Pheochromocytomas are found in the adrenal medulla. The adrenal medulla normally secretes two substances, or hormones, called norepinephrine and epinephrine. These two substances considered together are known as adrenaline. Adrenaline is released from the adrenal gland, enters the bloodstream, and helps to regulate many functions in the body, including blood pressure and heart rate. Pheochromocytomas cause the adrenal medulla to secrete too much adrenaline, which in turn causes high blood pressure. The high blood pressure usually causes the other symptoms of the disease.

Demographics

Pheochromocytomas are rare tumors. They have been reported in babies as young as five days old as well as adults as old as 92 years. Although they can be found at any time during life, they usually occur in adults between 30 and 40 years of age. Pheochromocytomas are somewhat more common in women than in men.

Causes and symptoms

The cause of most pheochromocytomas is not known. A small minority (about 10–20%) of pheochromocytomas arise because a person has an inherited susceptibility to them. Inherited pheochromocytomas are associated with four separate syndromes: **multiple endocrine neoplasia, type 2A** (MEN2A), multiple endocrine neoplasia, type 2B (MEN2B), **von Hippel-Lindau disease** (VHL), and neurofibromatosis type 1 (NF1).

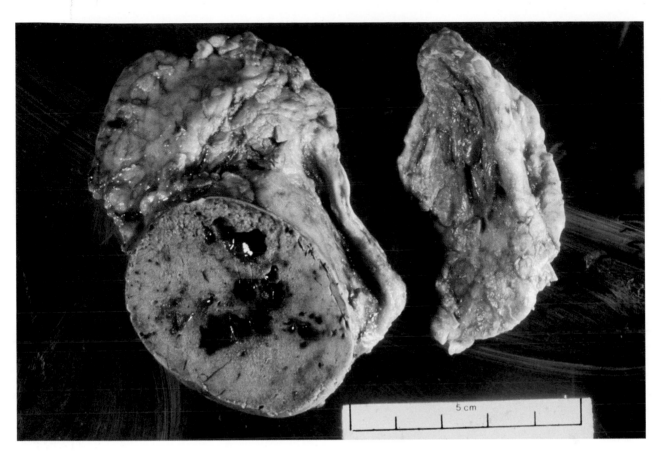

Pheochromocytoma. *(Biophoto Associates/Science Source)*

Individuals with pheochromocytomas as part of any of these four syndromes usually have other medical conditions as well. People with MEN2A often have **cancer** (usually **thyroid cancer**) and other hormonal problems. Individuals with MEN2B can also have cancer and hormonal problems, but also have other abnormal physical features. Both MEN2A and MEN2B are due to genetic alterations or mutations in a gene called *RET*, found at chromosome 10q11.2. Individuals with VHL often have other benign tumors of the central nervous system and pancreas, and can sometimes have renal cell cancer. This syndrome is caused by a mutation in the *VHL* gene, found at chromosome 3p25-26. Individuals with NF1 often have neurofibromas (benign tumors of the peripheral nervous system). NF1 is caused by mutations in the *NF1* gene, found at chromosome 17q11.

All of these disorders are inherited in an autosomal dominant inheritance pattern. With autosomal dominant inheritance, men and women are equally likely to inherit the syndrome. In addition, children of individuals with the disease arc at 50% risk of inheriting it. **Genetic testing** is available for these four syndromes (MEN2A, MEN2B, VHL, and NF1), but due to their complexity, genetic counseling should be considered before testing.

Most people (90%) with pheochromocytoma have hypertension, or high blood pressure. The other symptoms of the disease are extremely variable. These symptoms usually occur in episodes (or attacks) called paroxysms, and include:

- headaches
- excess sweating
- racing heart
- rapid breathing
- anxiety/nervousness
- nervous shaking
- pain in the lower chest or upper abdomen
- nausea
- heat intolerance

The episodes can occur as often as 25 times a day or, as infrequently as once every few months. They can last a few minutes, several hours, or several days. Usually, the attacks occur several times a week and last for about 15 minutes. After the episode is over, the person feels exhausted and fatigued.

Between the attacks, people with pheochromocytoma may experience the following:

- increased sweating
- cold hands and feet
- weight loss
- constipation

Diagnosis

If a pheochromocytoma is suspected, urine and/or a blood tests are usually recommended. A test called 24-hour urinary catecholamines and metanephrines will be done. This test is designed to look for adrenaline and the breakdown products of adrenaline. Since the body excretes these hormones in the urine, patients being tested will need to collect their urine for 24 hours. The laboratory will determine whether the levels of hormones are too high. This test is very good at making the diagnosis of pheochromocytoma. Another test called serum catecholamines measures the level of adrenaline compounds in the blood. It is not as sensitive as the 24-hour urine test, but can still provide some important information if it shows that the level of adrenaline compounds is too high.

One of the difficulties with these tests is that a person needs to have an attack of symptoms either during the 24-hour urine collection time period or shortly before the blood is drawn for a serum test to ensure the test's accuracy. If a person did not have an episode during that time, the test may yield a false negative. If a doctor suspects the patient has gotten a false negative result, additional tests called pharmacologic tests can be ordered. During these tests, a specific drug is given to the patient (usually through an IV), and the patient's hormone levels are monitored. These types of tests are only done rarely.

Once a person has been diagnosed with a pheochromocytoma, he or she will undergo tests to identify exactly where in the body the tumor is located. The imaging techniques used are usually **computed tomography** scan (CT scan) and **magnetic resonance imaging** (MRI). A CT scan creates pictures of the interior of the body from computer-analyzed differences in x-rays passing through the body. CT scans are performed at a hospital or clinic and take only a few minutes. An MRI is a computerized scanning method that creates pictures of the interior of the body using radio waves and a magnet. An MRI is usually performed at a hospital and takes about 30 minutes.

Treatment team

A pheochromocytoma will usually be treated by an internist (general medical doctor), an anesthesiologist (doctor who administers anesthesia for surgery), and a specialized surgeon (doctor who removes the tumor from the body). If the tumor is found to be malignant, a radiation oncologist (doctor who specializes in radiation treatment for cancer) and medical oncologist (doctor who specializes in **chemotherapy** treatment for cancer) may be consulted.

Clinical staging, treatments and prognosis

Once a pheochromocytoma is found, more tests will be done to see whether the tumor is benign (not cancer) or malignant (cancer). If the tumor is malignant, tests will be done to see how far the cancer has spread. There is no accepted staging system for pheochromocytoma; but an observation of the tumor may provide one of these four indications:

- Localized benign pheochromocytoma means that the tumor is found in only one area, is not cancer, and cannot spread to other tissues of the body.
- Regional pheochromocytoma means that the tumor is malignant and has spread to the lymph nodes around the original cancer. Lymph nodes are small structures that are found all over the body that make and store infection-fighting cells.
- Metastatic pheochromocytoma means that the tumor is malignant and has spread to more distant parts of the body.
- Recurrent pheochromocytoma means that a malignant tumor that was removed has regrown.

Treatment in all cases begins with surgical removal of the tumor. Before surgery, medications such as alpha-adrenergic blockers are given to block the effect of the hormones and normalize blood pressure. These medications are usually started seven to 10 days prior to surgery. The surgery of choice is laparoscopic laparotomy, which is a minimally invasive outpatient procedure performed under general or local anesthesia. A small incision is made in the abdomen, the laparoscope is inserted, and the tumor is removed. The patient can usually return to normal activities within two weeks. If a laparoscopic laparotomy cannot be done, a traditional laparotomy will be performed. This is a more invasive surgery done under spinal or general anesthesia and requires five to seven days in the hospital. Usually patients are able to return to normal activities after four weeks. After surgery, blood and urine tests will be done to make sure hormone levels return to normal. If the hormone levels are still above normal, it may mean that some tumor tissue was not removed. If the entire tumor cannot be removed (as in malignant pheochromocytoma, for example) drugs will be given to control high blood pressure.

If a pheochromocytoma is malignant, **radiation therapy** and/or chemotherapy may be used. Radiation therapy uses high-energy x-rays to kill cancer cells and shrink tumors. Because there is no evidence that radiation therapy is effective in the treatment of malignant pheochromocytoma, it is not often used for treatment. However, it is useful in the treatment of painful bone metastases if the tumor has spread to the bones. Chemotherapy uses drugs to kill cancer cells. Like radiation therapy, it has not been shown to be effective in the treatment of malignant pheochromocytoma. Chemotherapy, therefore, is used only in rare instances.

Untreated pheochromocytoma can be fatal due to complications of high blood pressure. In the vast majority of cases, when the tumor is surgically removed, pheochromocytoma is cured. In the minority of cases (10%) in which the pheochromocytoma is malignant, prognosis depends on how far the cancer has spread and the patient's age and general health. The overall median five-year survival from the initial time of surgery and diagnosis is approximately 43%.

Coping with cancer treatment

If laparoscopic laparotomy is done and no further treatment is necessary, patients usually return to normal activity within two weeks. If more extensive surgery is performed, normal activity is delayed for a few weeks and can be emotionally difficult. In rare cases in which radiation and/or chemotherapy are needed, coping can be very difficult. Consultation with physicians, nurses, social workers, and psychologists may be beneficial.

Prevention

Unfortunately, little is known about environmental and other causes of pheochromocytoma. Some of these tumors are due to inherited predisposition. Because of these factors, pheochromocytoma cannot be prevented.

Special concerns

Pheochromocytoma in children

Pheochromocytoma is rare in children, but occurs most commonly between the ages of 8 and 14 years. Diagnosis of pheochromocytoma can be more difficult at this age, because other **childhood cancers** (e.g., **neuroblastoma**)

can also elevate adrenaline compounds in the body. Pheochromocytomas in children are more likely to be bilateral (on both the left and right sides of the body) and outside the adrenal glands. For this reason, transabdominal surgery is usually performed to remove the tumor.

Pheochromocytoma in pregnancy

Although rare, pheochromocytoma in pregnancy can be very dangerous. Because x-rays should be avoided in pregnancy, MRI and/or ultrasound is used to locate the tumor. Alpha-adrenergic blocking agents to reduce blood pressure are given to the woman as soon as the diagnosis is made. If the woman is in the first two trimesters of pregnancy, most often the tumor is removed. In the third trimester, the woman usually remains on alpha-adrenergic blocking agents until a cesarean section can be safely performed.

See also Multiple endocrine neoplasia syndromes; von Recklinghausen's neurofibromatosis.

Resources

BOOKS

Pacek, Karel, and Graeme Eisenhofer, eds. *Pheochromocytoma: First International Symposium*. Boston, MA: Blackwell, 2006.
Sturgeon, Cord, ed. *Endocrine Neoplasia*. New York: Springer, 2010.

PERIODICALS

Santos P., Pimenta T., Taveira-Gomes A. "Hereditary Pheochromocytoma." *International Journal of Surgical Pathology* 22, no. 5 (2014): 393–400.

WEBSITES

National Cancer Institute. "Pheochromocytoma and Paraganglioma." http://www.cancer.gov/cancertopics/types/pheochromocytoma (accessed November 12, 2014).

Lori De Milto
Kristen Mahoney Shannon, M.S., C.G.C.

Pheresis

Definition

Pheresis is a blood purification process that consists of:

- drawing blood
- separating red cells, plasma, platelets, and cryoprecipitated antihemophilic factor
- isolating the blood component needed to diagnose a suspected abnormality or treat a known disease
- returning the remaining blood to the donor

KEY TERMS

Babesiosis—Infection transmitted by the bite of a tick and characterized by fever, headache, nausea, and muscle pain.

Blood typing—Technique for determining compatibility between donated blood products and transfusion recipients.

Chagas disease—Acute or chronic infection caused by the bite of a tick and characterized by fever, swollen glands, rapid heartbeat, and other symptoms.

Purpose

Because most of the blood is returned to the donor, pheresis enables an individual to donate more of a specific component. The two main types of pheresis are removal of platelets (plateletpheresis) and removal of plasma (plasmapheresis).

Plateletpheresis

Cancer and cancer treatments can deplete the body's supply of platelets, the colorless particles that stick to the lining of blood vessels and make it possible for blood to clot. Patients who have leukemia or aplastic **anemia**, are receiving **chemotherapy**, or undergoing **bone marrow transplantation** need platelets donated by healthy volunteers to prevent potentially fatal bleeding problems.

Plasmapheresis

Also known as therapeutic plasma exchange, plasmapheresis removes cells from the straw-colored liquid portion of the blood, which contains clotting factors, infection-fighting antibodies, and other proteins. Plasma regulates blood pressure and maintains the body's mineral balance.

Frozen immediately after collection and thawed when needed for transfusion, fresh frozen plasma is sometimes given to control **disseminated intravascular coagulation** (DIC). A particular problem for cancer patients, this rare condition causes large numbers of blood clots to form, then dissolve.

Leukapheresis

Also known as apheresis, leukapheresis may be used to treat certain leukemias and to collect cells for autologous stem cell transplant. Performed before chemotherapy is administered, leukapheresis increases the treatment's effectiveness by reducing the number of cancer cells in the bloodstream and permitting the medication to circulate more freely.

Description

Throughout the procedure, which lasts between 90 minutes and three hours, the pheresis donor relaxes in a specially contoured chair and watches movies or listens to music. A flexible tube inserted into the donor's arm slowly draws blood into a sophisticated machine (centrifuge) that separates the various blood components, collects whichever component is being donated, and returns the remaining blood through a vein in the donor's other arm. Each pheresis donation is typed and designated for a specific patient.

Inserting the needle can cause mild momentary discomfort. Some pheresis donors feel a slight tingling around the lips and nose, but this sensation disappears as soon as the procedure is completed.

Plasmapheresis and plateletpheresis can be performed in a hospital or blood collection center. Leukapheresis should be performed in a hospital where bone marrow transplantation is frequently performed.

Precautions

The American Red Cross will not accept blood or blood products from anyone who is:

- less than 17 years old
- not in good health
- taking antibiotics or insulin
- unable to meet other requirements established to ensure the safety of donated blood

In general, cancer survivors who were treated surgically or with radiation and have been cancer-free for at least five years may donate blood. Because of the remote danger of contracting cancer as the result of a transfusion, blood donations are not accepted from cancer survivors who have been treated with chemotherapy or hormonal therapy or were diagnosed with leukemia or **lymphoma**.

The U.S. Food and Drug Administration (FDA) requires every blood donor to provide a detailed health history and have a physical examination. All donated blood is tested for babesiosis, bacterial infections, Chagas disease, human immunodeficiency virus (HIV), Lyme disease, malaria, syphilis, and viral hepatitis.

Preparation

Before undergoing pheresis, a donor should get a good night's sleep, eat a well-balanced meal, and drink plenty of caffeine-free liquids. A donor should not take aspirin within 72 hours or ibuprofen within 24 hours before undergoing plateletpheresis, because these medications would make the platelets less beneficial to the patient receiving the transfusion. The donor's physician will determine whether any other medications should be discontinued in preparation for the procedure.

Aftercare

A pheresis donor may feel tired for a few hours and should not plan on driving home after the procedure. Although the donor may resume normal activities right away, heavy lifting or strenuous exercise should be avoided until the following day.

Resources

PERIODICALS

Damato, E.M., Moriarty, J.T., Harper, S.J., Dick, A.D., Bailey, C.C. "Plasmapheresis in the Management of Choroidal Vasculitis Associated with C-ANCA Positive Renal Vasculitis." *Retinal Cases and Brief Reports* 4, no. 4 (2010): 356–360. http://www.ncbi.nlm.nih.gov/pubmed/25390916 (accessed November 14, 2014).

WEBSITES

American Cancer Society. "Plasmapheresis (Plasma Exchange) for Waldenström Macroglobulinemia." http://www.cancer.org/cancer/waldenstrommmacroglobulinemia/detailedguide/waldenstrom-macroglobulinemia-treating-plasmapheresis (accessed November 14, 2014).
Johns Hopkins Medicine. "Plasmapheresis." http://www.hopkinsmedicine.org/transplant/programs/kidney/incompatible/plasmapheresis.html (accessed November 14, 2014).

Maureen Haggerty

Photodynamic therapy

Definition

Photodynamic therapy (PDT) is a form of nonsurgical **cancer** treatment that combines a photosensitizing drug with exposure to a laser beam or other specific light wavelength to kill cancer cells. It is often admnistered as an outpatient procedure. It can be used before or after surgery or in combination with **chemotherapy** or radiation treatments. In some cases, PDT is administered during surgery to kill any cancer cells that were not removed by tumor and lymph node excision. PDT is a promising therapeutic approach to treating solid tumors. The photosensitizer drugs are minimally toxic and the photoactivating light is nonionizing, providing a safe, novel way to stop tumor growth without affecting healthy tissues.

Purpose

Photodynamic therapy, also called phototherapy or light therapy, involves the administration of an orally or intravenously administered drug that renders cells or body tissue sensitive to long-wave ultraviolet light (UVA). Photosensitizing drugs are pharmacologically inactive and become active only when exposed to ultraviolet radiation or sunlight. After the cancer cells are sensitized, treatment continues, using controlled exposure to a specific source of light. When photosensitizers are exposed to specific wavelengths of light, they are activated to produce a form of oxygen that destroys cells near the targeted area. While photosensitizing drugs are absorbed by all cells in the body, they disappear within 24–72 hours in normal cells but remain longer in cancer cells. That selective process allows photodynamic therapy to target the malignant tumor or lesion. Besides activating the form of oxygen that kills cells, PDT shrinks or destroys tumors by damaging blood vessels in the tumor, thus preventing the cancer from receiving essential nutrients. Phototherapy also activates the immune system to destroy tumor cells.

The use of photodynamic therapy is still evolving, both in terms of the types of cancer it is approved to treat and the specific drugs that are used. Some cancer centers in the United States administer PDT using **porfimer sodium** (Photofrin) for the treatment of certain types of **skin cancer** (squamous cell **carcinoma**, **basal cell carcinoma**, and **Bowen disease**), recurrent **breast cancer** following **mastectomy**, colorectal cancer, cancers of the vulva and cervix, **small-cell lung cancer**, and symptoms of **esophageal cancer** when the cancer blocks the esophagus or laser therapy alone is not effective. Another photosensitizing drug called aminolevulinic acid

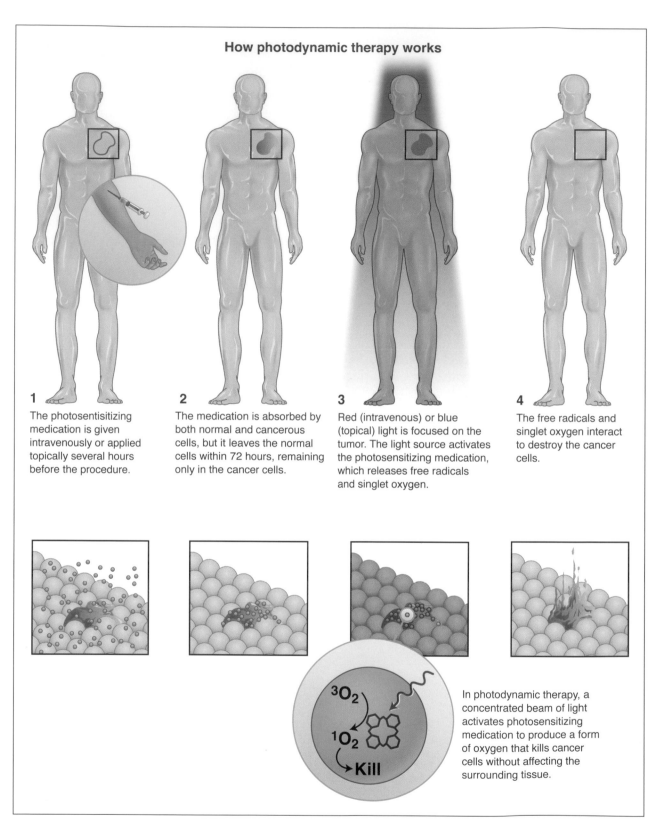

How photodynamic therapy works

1 The photosentisizing medication is given intravenously or applied topically several hours before the procedure.

2 The medication is absorbed by both normal and cancerous cells, but it leaves the normal cells within 72 hours, remaining only in the cancer cells.

3 Red (intravenous) or blue (topical) light is focused on the tumor. The light source activates the photosensitizing medication, which releases free radicals and singlet oxygen.

4 The free radicals and singlet oxygen interact to destroy the cancer cells.

$^3O_2$
$^1O_2$
→ Kill

In photodynamic therapy, a concentrated beam of light activates photosensitizing medication to produce a form of oxygen that kills cancer cells without affecting the surrounding tissue.

Photodynamic therapy uses concentrated beams of light to kill cancer cells. *(Illustration by Electronic Illustrators Group. © Cengage Learning®.)*

Actinic keratosis (plural, keratoses)—A type of precancerous skin growth with a scaly or bumpy surface caused by overexposure to the sun.

Barrett's esophagus—A precancerous condition of the esophagus that may develop as a complication of gastroesophageal reflux disease (GERD).

Bronchi (singular, bronchus)—The larger air passages inside the lungs.

Fiberoptics—Bundles of specially treated glass or plastic fibers that intensify light from a light source by internal reflection. Fiberoptics can be attached to lasers for use in PDT.

Free radicals—Highly reactive molecules that contain at least one unpaired electron. Free radicals are thought to destroy cells by disrupting their normal biological processes. Free radicals are released during PDT and help to kill tumor cells.

Hematoporphyrin—A dark reddish-purple pigment found in blood. A purified form of hematoporphyrin is used in the compounding of porfimer sodium.

Nanometer—A measurement of length equal to 10^{-9} meters, or one billionth of a meter, used as the unit of measurement for light waves.

Orphan drug—A one-of-a-kind drug that treats a rare disease—"rare disease" defined by the Food and Drug Association as one affecting fewer than 200,000 Americans. The category of orphan drug includes experimental as well as approved medications. Certain photosensitizing drugs used in Europe are considered orphan drugs in the United States.

Palliative—Referring to relief of symptoms of a disease or disorder rather than treatment to cure it.

Singlet oxygen—A highly reactive form of the oxygen molecule (O_2) formed during PDT that helps to destroy cancer cells by attacking the cell membranes.

(ALA, or Levulan Kerastick) is used to treat actinic keratosis, a precancerous skin disorder caused by sun exposure. ALA is also used for treatment of **mycosis fungoides** and other cancerous tumors on the surface of the skin.

Porfimer sodium and ALA are the only photosensitizing agents approved by the FDA for use in the United States; however, newer photosensitizing agents are being tested in cancer centers in the United States and Europe. The most important of these are described below.

In addition to cancer therapy, PDT is used to treat wet macular degeneration, an eye disorder that can lead to blindness, and also as treatment for benign skin conditions such as psoriasis, acne, and skin disorders caused by the **human papillomavirus**. In addition, PDT is under investigation as a possible treatment for certain forms of coronary artery disease.

Precautions

Precautions for this procedure are related to the use of photosensitizing drugs. Precautions for porfimer sodium (Photofrin) are as follows:

• Cannot be used in patients who are allergic to hematoporphyrin, a blood pigment used to make the drug.

• Cannot be used in pregnant or nursing women because its safety during pregnancy or lactation has not been established.

• Cannot be used to treat children.

• Lung tumors treated with Photofrin must be located in an airway where they can be accessed with a bronchoscope.

• Cannot be used to treat tumors in the esophagus or bronchi that are beginning to break into the patient's windpipe or a major blood vessel. The drug is used cautiously in treating bronchial tumors that could block the airway if PDT results in inflammation.

• Patients receiving radiotherapy cannot have PDT with porfimer sodium until four weeks after their last radiation treatment. Conversely, radiotherapy can only be given two to four weeks after a PDT treatment.

Precautions for aminolevulinic acid (ALA):

• Patients being treated with ALA are advised to protect their skin from exposure to sunlight or bright indoor light in the short time period between application of the drug to the skin and the PDT treatment.

• ALA is used cautiously or not at all in pregnant women or nursing mothers.

• If a second treatment is necessary, it is typically performed eight weeks after the first treatment.

Description

How PDT works

Photodynamic therapy is based on a series of chemical reactions that involve a specific wavelength of visible light, a photosensitizing drug, and oxygen. There is no standard wavelength of light, light source, exposure period, or method of administering the medication that covers all forms of PDT. The light source for PDT can be lasers or other sources, including light-emitting diodes (LEDs) for treating skin diseases. Most photosensitizing drugs are given intravenously, but some are applied to the skin or taken by mouth. Photosensitizers given by injection are activated by light in the red portion of the visible light spectrum, around 630–700 nanometers (nm; a nanometer is a measure of length, one billionth of a meter), while those applied to the skin are usually activated by blue light.

In general, cancerous tumors inside the body need more concentrated doses of light than abnormal growths on the body surface. Lasers are usually used to deliver highly concentrated light at one specific wavelength, while light sources that provide a larger area of illumination, such as LEDs, are more efficient for treating skin tumors. In general, PDT is able to treat tumors on the skin or on the surfaces of specific organs, but deeper tumors or lesions do not respond to PDT.

In contrast to their uses in surgery, lasers are not used in PDT to remove tissue or seal blood vessels with heat; rather they are used to start a chemical reaction. As a result, they do not become hot enough to burn tissue. The burning or stinging sensation that some patients experience during PDT is caused by the release of oxygen stimulating nearby nerve endings rather than heat from the laser itself.

Lasers can be used with fiberoptic cables for treating tumors inside the body. Fiberoptics are thin strands of plastic or glass with special optical properties that transmit light directly to a designated site. This transmission can be accomplished using a thin, lighted fiberoptic instrument called an endoscope or bronchoscope, used especially to treat cancer in the lungs or esophagus. Light from the laser is transmitted along the special fibers directly to the tumor, allowing the light to activate photosensitized cells in a very small area of tissue without damaging nearby normal tissue.

PDT is carried out in two steps. First, the photosensitizing drug is injected into a vein or applied to the skin several days or hours before the light treatment is scheduled. The drug is absorbed by all cells in the body but remains in cancer cells longer than in normal cells because the cancer cells are multiplying faster and do not die off as normal cells do. After the photosensitizing drug has had enough time to collect in the malignant cells, the light source of the proper wavelength is directed to the targeted area. When the light source strikes tissue containing the photosensitizing drug in the presence of oxygen, the drug is activated and produces free radicals and a highly reactive form of oxygen called singlet oxygen. The free radicals and singlet oxygen interact with the cell membranes of the cancer cells to destroy the energy-producing structures inside the cancer cells. In addition to killing the cancer cells directly, PDT works by damaging blood vessels inside the tumor, thereby shutting off the supply of nutrients, and by stimulating the immune system to produce interleukins (nonantibody proteins) and other substances that destroy the cancer.

Photosensitizing drugs

PORFIMER SODIUM. Porfimer sodium is a purified derivative of hematoporphyrin, a dark reddish-purple pigment found in blood. It is activated by red light at a wavelength of 630 nm; one disadvantage of this short wavelength is that it cannot penetrate tissue deeper than about a third of an inch, thus making porfimer sodium unsuitable for treating tumors that lie deep beneath the surface. The light used to activate this drug is usually generated by a laser.

Porfimer sodium has several other disadvantages for PDT. It is a complex chemical mixture that tends to break down over time; it has limited ability to penetrate tissue; and it takes four to six weeks to be cleared from the skin, thus leaving patients susceptible to a photosensitivity reaction for a long period of time following the PDT treatment. A photosensitivity reaction occurs when sensitized skin is exposed to sunlight or other bright light and is characterized by redness, swelling, and blistering of the exposed skin. Researchers are studying other photosensitizers with the following characteristics:

• Single compounds rather than mixtures of chemicals.
• More effective in absorbing the red region of the visible light spectrum to help reach deep or large tumors.
• More selective in targeting malignant tissue.
• More efficient in generating singlet oxygen.

AMINOLEVULINIC ACID. Aminolevulinic acid, or ALA, is a short-lived photosensitizer that is applied to the skin as a 5–20% oil-in-water mixture. It is activated by either a special blue light illuminator or by light at 630–635 nm. A newer skin cream formulation of ALA is called methyl ester of ALA (Metvixia cream). The formulation using esters is reportedly absorbed more readily into cancer cells than the original ALA.

SECOND-GENERATION PHOTOSENSITIZERS. Newer photosensitizing agents still being tested in **clinical trials** include:

- HPPH (2-[1-hexyloethyl]-2-devinyl-pyropheophorbide-a (Photochlor). HPPH is a photosensitizer that is activated by light more efficiently than porfimer sodium. In addition, patients treated with HPPH do not experience long-term photosensitivity reactions.

- Verteporfin or BPD-MA [benzoporphyrin derivative monoacid ring A] (Visudyne) is a second-generation photosensitizer with short-term skin photosensitivity. It is used primarily to treat cancer of the esophageal mucosa as well as eye disorders, including age-related macular degeneration, abnormal formations of blood vessels within the eye, and histoplasmosis (an eye infection caused by a fungus). Verteporfin is also being investigated as a possible treatment for skin cancer and psoriasis.

- Temoporfin (Meta-tetra hydroxyphenyl chlorin). Temoporfin (Foscan) is a chlorin-type photosensitizer developed in the United Kingdom. The FDA lists temoporfin as an orphan drug for the palliative treatment of inoperable head and neck cancers. Temocene is a porphycene analogue of temoporfin that is reported to have a 2.5-fold greater absorption in the red part of the light spectrum while maintaining excellent singlet oxygen photosensitization.

- Motexafin lutetium (brand name Lu-Tex). Lu-Tex is an injectable dye that has been used in clinical trials to treat malignant melanoma. It has a high degree of selectivity for cancer cells. It also shows promise as a treatment for recurrent breast cancer and atherosclerosis.

- Talaporfin sodium has been tested using a diode laser device in patients with early lung cancer and complete response was obtained in the majority of patients. Sensitivity disappeared with two weeks after treatment.

Clinical trials

Several cancer centers in the United States and Canada are investigating HPPH and other second-generation photosensitizers. Clinical trials are also under way to evaluate PDT for treatment of deeper cancers, such as those of the brain, prostate, intestines, stomach and liver.

Preparation

PDT for skin conditions

A patient receiving PDT for skin cancer or a precancerous skin disorder will have ALA applied to the affected area three to six hours before the scheduled treatment. The skin may or may not be covered with a dressing. The patient does not need to fast or make any other special preparations. If the affected area of skin is on the face, the patient may be given goggles to wear to protect the eyes from the blue light used to activate the drug.

PDT for internal cancers

The photosensitizing agents used for PDT or palliative treatment of esophageal or lung cancers are injected, usually two to three days before treatment. The patient may return home after the injection but must avoid sunlight and bright light indoors before the light treatment. The patient does not need to fast or discontinue other medications but is advised to cover the windows and skylights in his or her home before receiving the light treatment to prevent exposure to bright light.

Patients undergoing PDT for esophageal or lung cancers receive a local or general anesthetic before the doctor inserts the bronchoscope or endoscope. They may also be given a mild tranquilizer to relieve anxiety.

Aftercare

Aftercare following PDT with porfimer sodium involves four to six weeks of protection from sunlight and other sources of bright light, including **tanning** lamps or the examination lamps found in doctors' and dentists' offices. During this period, the patient should wear dark glasses; long-sleeved shirts made of light-colored, tightly woven fabric; long pants or slacks; and a wide-brimmed hat to protect the skin and eyes outdoors for at least 30 days after treatment. Sunscreen creams and lotions do not provide enough protection. It is best to run necessary errands after sundown or ask someone else in the household to drive the car. Women should not use helmet-type hair dryers or handheld dryers on a high setting, as the drug remains in the scalp for several weeks and may cause burns if exposed to high heat. Exposure to low levels of indoor light is necessary, however, in order to break down the Photofrin remaining in the skin. After 30 days, the doctor will give the patient instructions about how to test the skin for remaining light sensitivity.

Patients who have received PDT for cancers in the lining of the bronchi are advised to return two days after the treatment for a follow-up **bronchoscopy**, in which dead tumor cells and other pieces of tissue will be removed from the treated area. This follow-up procedure is necessary to prevent inflammation and possible blockage of the patient's airway. Treated tumor sites require between four and eight weeks for complete healing.

Patients who receive PDT with ALA do not need to take special precautions regarding sun exposure after treatment because the drug is short-lived. The treated

QUESTIONS TO ASK YOUR DOCTOR

- Is photodynamic therapy a possible treatment option for my cancer?
- Are you experienced in treating patients with PDT?
- How long is the course of treatment with phototherapy?
- What effects, if any, might I experience after undergoing phototherapy treatment?
- Should I consider enrolling in a clinical trial of a new PDT drug?

skin will usually form a crust or scale for several days before healing completely.

Risks

Porfimer sodium

Risks of PDT with porfimer sodium include photosensitivity reactions if the patient fails to observe the guidelines for aftercare; chest pain or a burning sensation in the chest or throat when the treatment is applied for lung or esophageal cancer; difficulty swallowing; **itching**; the formation of ulcers or scar tissue; and discomfort in the eyes when exposed to sunlight, bright lights, or car headlights. Most side effects are temporary. Breast cancer and lung cancer patients who experience severe chest pain after PDT may be given medications to control the pain.

Aminolevulinic acid

Some patients experience a stinging or burning sensation in the skin during the blue light treatment, but this usually disappears as soon as the light is turned off. Some patients also report temporary swelling or redness of the skin in the treated areas or minor changes in the pigmentation of their skin.

Results

Normal results of PDT include shrinkage of the tumor and destruction of cancer cells. Normal results of palliative treatment for cancer of the esophagus are sufficient tumor shrinkage to allow the patient to swallow.

Normal results for PDT of the skin include shrinkage and destruction of the tumor, although large skin tumors may require a second treatment for complete removal.

Abnormal results

Abnormal results include allergic reactions to the photosensitizing medication or failure of the tumor to respond to PDT.

Resources

PERIODICALS

Lim, C. K., J. Heo, and S. Sin, et al. "Nanophotosensitizers toward Advanced Photodynamic Therapy of Cancer." *Cancer Letter* 334 (July 2013): 176–87.

Master, A., M. Lingston, and A. Sen Gupta. "Photodynamic Nanomedicine in the Treatment of Solid Tumors: Perspectives and Challenges." *Journal of Controlled Release* 168 (May 2013): 88–102.

Schmitt, F., and L. Juillerat-Jeanneret. "Drug Targeting Strategies for Photodynamic Therapy." *Anticancer Agents in Medicinal Chemistry* 12 (June 2012): 500–525.

WEBSITES

American Cancer Society. "Photodynamic Therapy." http://www.cancer.org/treatment/treatmentsandsideeffects/treatmenttypes/photodynamic-therapy (accessed August 27, 2014).

Roswell Park Cancer Institute. "Photodynamic Therapy Center." https://www.roswellpark.org/specialized-services/photodynamic-therapy (accessed August 27, 2014).

ORGANIZATIONS

Roswell Park Cancer Institute, Elm and Carlton Streets, Buffalo, NY 14263, (877) ASK-RPCI (275-7724), askrpci@roswellpark.org, http://www.roswellpark.org.

L. Lee Culvert
Rebecca Frey, PhD

Photofrin *see* **Porfimer sodium**

Physical therapy

Definition

Physical therapy, also called physiotherapy, is the prevention and treatment of medical conditions by physical and mechanical means, including exercise, body manipulation, water, light, heat, and electricity.

Purpose

The purpose of physical therapy is to restore function, improve mobility, relieve pain, and prevent or limit permanent physical disabilities, with the goal of improving a patient's functioning at school or work and in daily life. Physical therapists treat patients with a variety of conditions and diseases, including injuries or pain. In oncology, or **cancer** care, physical therapists treat patients to help ease symptoms of their cancer or cancer treatment and to help maintain or restore physical function.

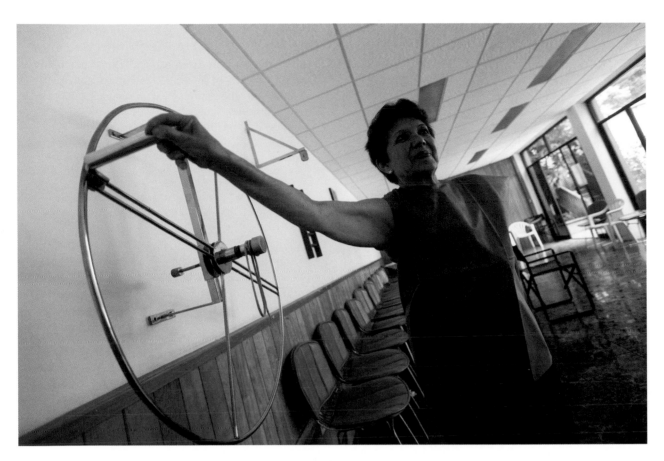

Breast cancer patient undergoing physical therapy. *(© EDGARD GARRIDO/Reuters/Corbis)*

A cancer patient may need help with physical function because of a cancer itself. For example, some **brain tumors** can cause problems such as weakness, balance problems, or paralysis. Treatment of brain cancers can also cause problems that require physical therapy. **Breast cancer** patients have often had problems with edema and lymphedema following removal of lymph nodes in their underarm areas for **biopsy**. New **sentinel lymph node biopsy** techniques have improved biopsy procedures and led to fewer effects, but some women still need some help following surgery for breast cancer and removal of affected lymph nodes.

Certain **chemotherapy** drugs can cause a condition called peripheral **neuropathy**, which damages nerves in the peripheral nervous system, the nerves around the body that affect senses and other functions. The condition can make cancer patients more vulnerable to injury and cause pain. Physical therapists can assess the extent of the damage and develop exercises for patients to help lessen symptoms.

Common applications of physical therapy for cancer patients may include:

• retraining muscles and adjusting them to the use of artificial joints or prostheses

• strengthening muscles and ligaments following fractures or surgery

• treating pain to minimize or avoid the use of prescription pain medications

• rehabilitating patients who need help regaining balance or mobility following surgery or aggressive cancer treatment

• helping patients develop strategies to cope with treatments before treatments begin so that the patients can better tolerate treatment effects

Description

Physical therapy is performed by physical therapists, physical therapy assistants, and physical therapy aides. Physical therapists take medical histories, perform physical exams, and assess the ability of patients to function independently. They use a variety of tests and measurements for evaluation. Range of motion is determined using a goniometer—an instrument that measures the largest angle through which a joint can move. The therapist determines whether restricted motion is due to tight muscles or tight ligaments and tendons. The therapist also evaluates:

KEY TERMS

Ambulation—Moving from place to place.

Goniometer—An instrument for measuring angles of a joint.

Lymphedema—Swelling (edema) due to damaged lymphatic drainage.

Orthotics—Support or bracing of weak or ineffectual muscles or joints.

Prosthesis—An artificial device that replaces or augments a body part.

Repetitive stress injury; repetitive strain injury (RSI)—Any of various musculoskeletal disorders—such as tendinitis or carpal tunnel syndrome—that are caused by cumulative damage to muscles, tendons, ligaments, nerves, or joints from highly repetitive movements, such as of the hand, wrist, arm, or shoulder.

Stroke—A sudden diminishing or loss of consciousness, sensation, or voluntary movement from a rupture or obstruction of a blood vessel in the brain.

Tilt table; tiltboard—An apparatus for rotating a person from a horizontal to an oblique or vertical position.

Traction—Pulling force exerted on a skeletal structure by a special device or piece of equipment.

• strength

• coordination and balance

• posture

• motor function

• muscle performance

• respiration

Based on these evaluations, physical therapists develop treatment plans, including purpose, strategy, and anticipated outcomes. During the course of physical therapy, a patient's progress is tracked with periodic examinations and tests.

Cancer patients often have treatment that removes a tumor, and at times, a limb. Examples include **osteosarcoma**, a type of bone cancer. These patients may need help adjusting to new mobility equipment, such as limb prostheses or wheelchairs. Some cancer patients undergo lengthy or extensive procedures that keep them bedridden for long periods of time and cause them to lose weight and muscle tone. A physical therapist can help the patient regain strength and physical function.

Physical therapy exercises are aimed at improving flexibility, range of motion, muscle strength, balance, coordination, ambulation (walking), and/or endurance. Patients are often taught exercises to perform at home. Activities can include water walking and swimming. Physical therapy also teaches patients to use assistive and adaptive devices such as crutches, wheelchairs, and prostheses.

For range-of-motion stretches, the muscles are often first warmed with heat to improve effectiveness and reduce pain. Tight ligaments or tendons require gentle stretching, whereas the joint can be stretched more vigorously if tight muscles are causing poor range of motion. An affected joint must be moved beyond the point of pain, but should not cause residual pain after the movement is stopped. Sustained moderate stretching may be applied with weights and pulleys. There are three types of range-of-motion exercises:

• active exercise for patients who can move their limbs and exercise a muscle or joint without assistance

• active-assistive exercise for patients who need some help moving their limbs and exercising muscles or for whom moving joints is painful

• passive exercise in which the therapist moves the limbs

There are a variety of other physical therapy exercises:

• There are many muscle-strengthening exercises, all of which progressively increase resistance. Muscle-strengthening exercises also increase muscle mass and endurance. Movement against gravity is used for very weak muscles; the resistance is gradually increased using stretchy bands or weights.

• Rehabilitation from a stroke or brain damage often requires coordination exercises that involve specific tasks that work multiple joints and muscles, such as picking up an object.

• Rehabilitation may also require balance exercises, beginning with shifting one's weight from side to side and front to back using parallel bars.

• Once a patient can balance while standing, ambulation exercises begin with walking using parallel bars and progressing to a walker, crutches, or a cane, possibly wearing a brace or assistive belt to prevent falls.

• Once a patient can walk on a level surface, ambulation exercises involve stepping over curbs or climbing stairs. These exercises may include teaching family members and caregivers how to correctly support the patient.

• General conditioning exercises combine range-of-motion, muscle-strengthening, and ambulation exercises to counter the effects of prolonged bed rest or immobilization, improve cardiovascular fitness, and maintain flexibility and muscle strength.

Transfer training—moving safely and independently from bed to chair, chair to toilet, or chair to standing—is a critical component of physical therapy. It is often required for patients who have had a hip fracture, **amputation**, or stroke. Transfer training techniques depend on whether the patient:

- can bear weight on one or both legs
- can balance well
- is paralyzed on one side
- can use assistive devices

Tilt tables are used for patients who have had strict bed rest for several weeks or have had a spinal cord injury, since they can become dizzy when standing up. Tilt tables retrain blood vessels to narrow and widen appropriately with changes in posture. The patient lies face-up on a padded table with a footboard and is held in place with a safety belt as the table is slowly tilted.

To decrease lower back pain and restore mobility, physical therapy utilizes:

- manual therapies, including spinal manipulation, to improve the mobility of joints and soft tissues
- specific strengthening and/or flexibility exercises
- training for sitting, sleeping, bending, lifting, and performing chores
- education about back care

Physical therapy uses a variety of techniques to reduce swelling and relieve pain, including:

- hot and cold packs
- paraffin baths
- electrical stimulation
- ultrasound
- massage, including deep-tissue massage
- traction

Physical therapy for children uses many of the same evaluation and therapeutic techniques as adult physical therapy, but often includes toys and pediatric therapy gyms with balls, benches, swings, and slides. Pediatric physical therapy may also include:

- identifying existing and potential problems
- developmental activities such as crawling and walking
- adaptive play
- aquatic therapy
- recommending safe sports and other activities

- consulting with medical, psychiatric, and school personnel on individual education plans

Benefits

Physical therapy can help patients gain and maintain mobility, independence, and quality of life. It can help prevent and manage medical conditions and motivate patients to improve on their own. Physical therapy can prevent loss of mobility by utilizing specific exercise programs based on individual characteristics. Physical therapy often can eliminate the need for prescription drugs or surgery.

Precautions

Physical therapy can be painful, and patients often must do much of the hard work on their own. For some conditions, such as tight ligaments or tendons, range of motion often cannot be increased by gentle stretching until after surgical intervention.

Preparation

Patient attitude and cooperation are central to successful physical therapy. Patients must be active participants in their treatment, aware of the short-term and long-term goals of their therapy, and able to communicate with their therapists.

Aftercare

Physical therapy often requires patients to follow a specially designed exercise program. Practicing on one's own can be an essential component of successful physical therapy.

Risks

Risks of physical therapy can include pain, falls, bruising, or injury.

Training and certification

Physical therapists have master's degrees or clinical doctorates in physical therapy. The programs include basic medical and clinical coursework and supervised clinical experience. Physical therapists are required to pass a national licensure exam and must be licensed in each state in which they practice. Physical therapists participate in continuing education courses and workshops.

The need for physical therapy is evident throughout health care. The American Physical Therapy Association represents nearly 90,000 physical therapists, assistants, and students around the country. APTA has a special Oncology Section dedicated to improving the knowledge

QUESTIONS TO ASK YOUR DOCTOR

- How will physical therapy help me heal from my cancer surgery?
- Does the physical therapist have experience working with cancer survivors?
- Will physical therapy hurt?
- Will I do therapy only at the office or in my home as well?

and skills of physical therapists who work with patients who have cancer or HIV/AIDS. It is increasingly common for large cancer centers to incorporate their own rehabilitation services department that includes physical therapy.

Resources

BOOKS

Jewell, Dianne V. *Guide to Evidence-Based Physical Therapist Practice*. 3rd ed. Burlington, MA: Jones and Bartlett, 2015.

Tecklin, Jan Stephen. *Pediatric Physical Therapy*. 4th ed. Philadelphia: Lippincott Williams & Wilkins, 2008.

PERIODICALS

Groopman, Jerome. "Robots That Care." *New Yorker* 85, no. 35 (November 2, 2009): 66.

Jamtvedt, Gro, et al. "Physical Therapy Intervention for Patients With Osteoarthritis of the Knee: An Overview of Systematic Reviews." *Physical Therapy* 88, no. 1 (January 2008): 123-136.

WEBSITES

American Physical Therapy Association. "Oncology Section." *Move Forward*.http://www.oncologypt.org/consumer-resources/index.cfm (accessed September 24, 2014).

American Society of Clinical Oncology. "Spotlight on Physical Therapists in Oncology." http://www.cancer.net/blog/2014-09/spotlight-physical-therapists-oncology (accessed September 24, 2014).

MD Anderson Cancer Center. "Rehabilitation Services." http://www.mdanderson.org/patient-and-cancer-information/care-centers-and-clinics/clinics/rehabilitation-services/index.html (accessed September 24, 2014).

"Physical Therapy (PT)." *The Merck Manuals Online Medical Library*. http://www.merck.com/mmhe/sec01/ch007/ch007c.html

ORGANIZATIONS

American Physical Therapy Association, 1111 North Fairfax Street, Alexandria, VA 22314-1488, (703) 684-2782, (800) 999-APTA (2782), Fax: (703) 684-7343, http://www.apta.org.

National Rehabilitation Information Center, 8201 Corporate Drive, Suite 600, Landover, MD 20785, (301) 459-5900, (800) 346-2742, Fax: (301) 459-4263, naricinfo@heitech services.com, http://www.naric.com/.

Margaret Alic, PhD
REVIEWED BY BRENDA W. LERNER
REVISED BY TERESA G. ODLE

PICC lines *see* **Vascular access**

Pilocarpine

Definition

Pilocarpine is a medicine used to treat **xerostomia**, or dryness of the mouth, caused by a decrease in saliva production following radiation or due to Sjögren's syndrome, a disorder of the immune system characterized by the failure of the exocrine glands. Pilocarpine is also known as pilocarpine hydrochloride or Salagen.

Purpose

Pilocarpine is used to treat side effects arising from radiation treatment for **head and neck cancers**. It alleviates dryness of the mouth and throat, and aids in chewing, tasting, and swallowing. It may also be given to treat dryness of the eyes resulting from **cancer** treatment.

Pilocarpine is also used in the form of eye drops or eye gel to treat glaucoma; it works by lowering the pressure of the fluid inside the eye.

Description

Pilocarpine is a naturally occurring substance found in the leaflets of *Pilocarpus jaborandi*, a South American shrub.

Pilocarpine works by stimulating the function of the exocrine glands, including the glands that produce saliva, sweat, tears, and digestive secretions. It also stimulates smooth muscles, such as those found in the bronchus, gallbladder, bile ducts, and intestinal and urinary tracts.

Pilocarpine was approved by the U.S. Food and Drug Administration as a sialogogue, or medication to increase the flow of saliva, in 1994. Pilocarpine was effective in relieving xerostomia symptoms after twelve weeks in over half the patients studied; however, the medication may not work for everyone.

Recommended dosage

Pilocarpine is taken orally. It is available in round white tablets containing 5 mg. Different patients may require different dosages of the drug. The usual dose for adults is five milligrams taken three times a day. If necessary, the physician may increase the dosage to 10 mg, three times a day. Because increasing the dose increases the likelihood of side effects, the lowest dose that is effective should be used for treatment.

Pilocarpine begins to act 20 minutes after ingestion. It will continue to act for three to five hours, with the maximum effect taking place one hour after ingestion. Twelve weeks of regular use may be required for improvement of symptoms.

If a dose is missed, it should be taken as soon as possible; however, if it is almost time for the next dose, only the next dose should be taken.

Precautions

Patients may wish to take this medication with a meal to avoid stomach upset; however, pilocarpine will have reduced effectiveness if it is taken with a meal that is high in fat. Patients should drink plenty of water to avoid dehydration due to increased sweating. Alcohol and antihistamines should not be used while taking pilocarpine. Due to the possibility of visual disturbances or dizziness, people using this medication should avoid driving or operating machinery, particularly at night. Patients should continue to see a dentist regularly during treatment even though symptoms may improve, since xerostomia may increase the likelihood of tooth decay and other dental problems.

Studies have not been done to test the safety of pilocarpine use in pregnant or nursing women; very high doses of the drug may cause birth defects in animals. Studies have also not been done to test the use of pilocarpine in children.

Pilocarpine should not be taken by people who are sensitive to it or who have uncontrolled asthma, or such eye problems as inflammation of the iris or angle-closure glaucoma. It should be used with caution by people with breathing problems, gallbladder disease, kidney problems, peptic ulcer, psychological disturbances, retinal disease, or heart or blood vessel disease.

Side effects

The most common side effect of pilocarpine use is increased sweating. Other less common side effects are as follows: **nausea and vomiting**, irritated nose, chills, flushing, frequent urination, dizziness, weakness, headache, difficulty with digestion, increased tear production, **diarrhea**, bloating, abdominal pain, and visual problems.

Symptoms of overdose include irregular heartbeat, chest pain, fainting, confusion, stomach cramps or pain, and trouble breathing. Unusually severe or continuing side effects such as diarrhea, headache, weakness, trembling, visual difficulties, nausea, and vomiting may also indicate overdose.

Interactions

Pilocarpine may interact with other medications, reducing or increasing their effects or, sometimes, increasing the side effects of the other medications.

Pilocarpine may also be less effective as a result of interaction with other medications. The following drugs may cause interactions:

- amantadine
- anticholinergics
- antidepressants
- antidyskinetics
- antihistamines
- antimyasthenics
- antipsychotics
- beta-adrenergic blocking agents
- bethanechol
- buclizine
- carbamazepine
- cyclizine
- cyclobenzaprine
- disopyramide
- flavoxate
- glaucoma medications
- ipratropium
- meclizine
- methylphenidate
- orphenadrine
- oxybutynin

- physostigmine
- procainamide
- promethazine
- quinidine

Pilocarpine may also interact with alcohol, cocaine, and marijuana.

Resources

BOOKS

Beers, Mark H., MD, and Robert Berkow, MD, editors. "Dentistry in Medicine." In *The Merck Manual of Diagnosis and Therapy*. Whitehouse Station, NJ: Merck Research Laboratories, 2007.

WEBSITES

AHFS Consumer Medication Information. "Pilocarpine." American Society of Health-System Pharmacists. Available from: http://www.nlm.nih.gov/medlineplus/druginfo/meds/a608039.html (accessed November 12, 2014).

Norris Cotton Cancer Center, Dartmouth. "Pilocarpine." http://cancer.dartmouth.edu/pf/health_encyclopedia/d04031a1 (accessed November 12, 2014).

Racquel Baert, M.Sc.
Rebecca J. Frey, PhD

Pineoblastoma

Definition

A pineoblastoma is an aggressive primary brain tumor typically found in young children that develops in the pineal body (sometimes called the epiphysis cerebri or pineal gland), which is a small cone-shaped organ located in the midbrain. The pineal body secretes melatonin, a hormone that regulates moods and the sleep-wake cycle in humans. Pineoblastomas are also known as pinealoblastomas.

Description

Pineoblastomas are rapidly growing tumors, and thereby distinguished from pineocytomas, which grow relatively slowly. They are defined by the World Health Organization (WHO) as primitive neuroectodermal tumors (PNETs) in the pineal gland; the word *primitive* in this context means that these tumors are composed of cells that have not yet separated into more specialized types of cells. The word *neuroectodermal* means that these tumors develop out of a layer of cells in the embryo that eventually gives rise to the baby's nervous system.

KEY TERMS

Blastoma—An abnormal growth of embryonic cells. A pineoblastoma is a blastoma that develops in the pineal body.

Endocrinologist—A doctor who specializes in diagnosing and treating disorders that affect the balance of hormones in the body or the organs that produce these hormones.

Melatonin—A hormone that regulates moods and the sleep-wake cycle in humans. It is produced by the pineal body.

Pineal body—A small cone-shaped endocrine gland attached to the roof of the third ventricle of the brain. The pineal body, which is also known as the pineal gland or epiphysis, secretes melatonin.

Pineocytoma—A slower-growing tumor of the pineal body found more commonly in adults.

Primary brain tumor—A tumor that starts in the brain, as distinct from a metastatic tumor that begins elsewhere in the body and spreads to the brain. A pineoblastoma is one type of primary brain tumor.

Primitive—Simple or undifferentiated. Pineoblastomas are classified as primitive tumors because they arise from cells that have not yet separated into groups of more specialized cells.

Shunt—A tube inserted by a surgeon to relieve pressure on the brain from blocked cerebrospinal fluid. The tube allows the fluid to bypass the tumor that is blocking its flow.

Ventricle—One of the small cavities located within the brain. The pineal body is attached to the roof of the third ventricle.

Pineoblastomas are considered highly malignant. They may invade nearby areas of brain tissue as well as spread into the cerebrospinal fluid, although they rarely metastasize to other parts of the body. In addition, pineoblastomas sometimes cause bleeding into the ventricles of the brain. The child's radiologist may be able to see areas of dying tissue in the brain when **imaging studies** are performed.

Demographics

Pineoblastomas are extremely rare, accounting for only 0.5–2% of childhood tumors of the central nervous system (CNS). About 2,200 children below the age of 15 are diagnosed with malignant tumors of the brain and spinal cord each year in the United States; between 10 and 40 of these children will be diagnosed with pineoblastomas. Research is studying some genetic changes (in particular, one called the RB-1 mutation) that predispose people to the development of pineoblastomas.

It is difficult to evaluate the statistical significance of racial or gender differences in such a small group; however, the available evidence from American **cancer** registries suggests that these cancers occur more frequently in Caucasian children than in African Americans, and more frequently in males than in females.

Pineoblastomas occur almost exclusively in younger children, with very few cases reported in adolescents or adults. A similar tumor called pineal parenchymal tumor of intermediate differentiation mostly occurs in adults. The slower-growing pineocytomas are most likely to develop in adults between the ages of 25 and 35.

Causes and symptoms

The cause of pineoblastomas is unknown, but may be associated with gene mutations. A group of British radiologists reported in 2004 that the chances of survival in children diagnosed with pineoblastoma who had inherited a mutation of the **retinoblastoma** (RB) gene are much lower than the chances of children who did not inherit the RB mutation. The researchers suggested that this mutation may cause pineoblastomas, as well as reduce or inhibit their response to therapy. Genetic research continues, and in 2014, authors reported on a mutation called RB-1 that puts infants at higher risk of pineoblastoma. Still, inheritance of the genetic mutation alone does not mean a child will develop pineoblastoma.

The symptoms of a pineoblastoma result from blockage of the flow of cerebrospinal fluid and increased pressure on the brain. Depending on the size of the tumor and the child's age, symptoms may include the following:

- headache
- double vision
- nausea and vomiting
- weakness, balance problems, or loss of sensation on one side of the body
- seizures
- developmental delays or failure to thrive (in younger children)
- lowered energy level or unusual need for sleep
- personality changes
- unexplained changes in weight or appetite

Parents should note, however, that these symptoms are not unique to pineoblastomas; they may be produced by other types of **brain tumors**, head trauma, meningitis, migraine headaches, or several other medical conditions. In any event, a child with these symptoms should be seen by a doctor at once.

Diagnosis

The diagnosis of a pineoblastoma begins with a review of the child's medical history and a thorough physical examination. The child may be given several vision tests if he or she is seeing double or having other visual disturbances. The child's doctor will then order both laboratory tests and imaging studies. The laboratory tests are done to rule out such diseases as meningitis and to see whether the child's liver and other organs are functioning normally. The imaging studies are performed to determine the extent of the cancer and to assign the child to a risk group.

Unless surgical removal of the tumor is considered too risky, a neurosurgeon will perform what is known as an open **biopsy** to confirm the diagnosis of pineoblastoma. He or she will remove a small piece of the tumor for examination by a pathologist.

Laboratory tests

Standard laboratory tests for children with brain tumors include a complete blood count (CBC); electrolyte analysis; tests of kidney, liver, and thyroid function; and tests that determine whether the child has been recently exposed to certain viruses. In addition, a **lumbar puncture** will be performed to look for cancer cells in the child's spinal fluid.

Imaging tests

Imaging tests for pineoblastomas include **magnetic resonance imaging** (MRI) or magnetic resonance spectroscopy of the spinal cord and brain because pineoblastomas are more likely than other PNETs to spread into the cerebrospinal fluid. MRI uses high-frequency radio waves and magnets instead of x-rays to create detailed images. The child may receive an injection of a contrast agent to better display cancer cells. A chest x-ray or bone scan may be performed to determine whether the cancer has spread to other areas of the body.

Treatment team

Since the 1960s, most children diagnosed with brain tumors have been treated in specialized children's cancer centers. A child with pineoblastoma will usually have a pediatric oncologist as his or her primary doctor, along with one or more specialists. These specialists may include a neurosurgeon, pathologist, neuroradiologist, radiation oncologist, medical oncologist, endocrinologist, nutritionist, physical therapist or rehabilitation specialist, and psychologist or psychiatrist. The team will also include social workers, clergy, and other professionals to help the parents cope with the stresses of their child's illness and treatments.

Clinical staging

Pineoblastomas are not staged in the same way as cancers elsewhere in the body. As of 2014, children with these tumors are instead divided into two risk groups, average risk and poor risk. Assignment to these groups is based on the following factors:

• child's age
• whether the child is older or younger than age three
• whether the tumor has spread to other parts of the body
• whether the tumor was completely removed by surgery

The risk of recurrence, or return of the cancer, is higher for children in the high-risk group.

Treatment

Treatments for pineoblastoma depend on the child's age and his or her risk group. Children younger than three years are not usually given **radiation therapy** because it can affect growth and normal brain development; they are usually treated with surgery to remove as much of the tumor as possible, followed by **chemotherapy** if they are considered high-risk patients. The drugs most often used to treat brain and spinal cord tumors in children include **lomustine**, **cisplatin**, **carboplatin**, and **vincristine**.

In addition to removing the tumor, the surgeon may also place a shunt to reduce pressure on the child's brain if the tumor is blocking the flow of cerebrospinal fluid. The shunt is a plastic tube with one end placed within the third ventricle of the brain. The rest of the shunt is routed under the skin of the head, neck, and chest with the other end placed in the abdomen or near the heart. Shunts are used very conservatively in children with pineoblastomas, however, because there have been reports of these tumors spreading into the abdomen via the shunt.

Children three years and older are treated with surgery first, followed by radiation treatment of the entire brain and spinal cord. Those considered at high risk may also be given chemotherapy. Recurrent pineoblastomas are treated with further surgery and an additional course of chemotherapy. Stereotactic radiation therapy, also called stereotactic radiosurgery, is a technique that delivers precise radiation to a tumor in the brain, sparing normal brain tissue.

Some children may receive high-dose chemotherapy with stem cell rescue. The child's stem cells are removed from the blood or bone marrow and returned after giving the child high doses of chemotherapy.

Alternative and complementary therapies

Some complementary therapies that are reported to help children with pineoblastomas cope with their treatment include pet therapy, humor therapy, and music therapy. All of these can be pleasurable for the child as well as relaxing. Ginger or peppermint may help to relieve the **nausea and vomiting** associated with chemotherapy.

Prognosis

The prognosis for children with pineoblastomas depends largely on their risk group. In general, however, these tumors have a poorer prognosis than other types of brain tumors, in part because of the difficulty of removing the complete tumor due to the location of the pineal body deep within the brain. The overall five-year survival rate of children with pineoblastoma is reported to be 50%–60%, but is much lower in children younger than three years and in older children who do not respond to radiation therapy.

Recurrent pineoblastomas are almost always fatal; a child who has a recurrent tumor usually is best served by enrollment in a clinical trial testing new therapies. Doctors continue to research more information about the genes behind these tumors so that they can develop drugs to target the cancer cells responsible for pineoblastomas and spare healthy cells, thereby creating more effective treatments with less severe side effects.

Coping with cancer treatment

Children can be given additional medications to treat nausea and other side effects of chemotherapy. With regard to homesickness and other emotional reactions to being away from home, children's cancer centers have social workers and child psychologists who can educate the child's family about the cancer as well as help the child deal with separation issues.

The side effects of radiation therapy in children with brain tumors may include the formation of dead tissue at the site of the tumor. This formation is known as radiation necrosis. It occurs in about 5% of children who receive radiation therapy and may require surgical removal. Radiation necrosis, however, is not as serious as recurrence of the tumor.

Children who have difficulty speaking after brain surgery, or who experience physical weakness, difficulty walking, visual impairment, or other sensory problems,

QUESTIONS TO ASK YOUR DOCTOR

- Which risk group has my child been assigned to?
- What treatments would you recommend for a child in that group, and why would you recommend them?
- Is my child eligible for any current clinical trials for children with pineoblastoma?
- Would you recommend any of the treatments currently considered experimental?
- What is my child's life expectancy? What can I do to make the remaining time as pain-free and enjoyable as possible?

are given **physical therapy** and/or speech therapy on either an inpatient or outpatient basis.

Clinical trials

Because pineoblastomas are so rare, the American Cancer Society recommends that children diagnosed with these tumors be enrolled in an appropriate clinical trial. **Clinical trials** as of 2014 included ways to control nausea in children having aggressive chemotherapy, the use of proton beam radiation therapy for pineoblastoma, and use of a new drug in children with recurrent pineoblastoma or tumors that are resistant to other treatment. The **National Cancer Institute** has information on clinical trials at 800-422-6237 or at http://www.cancer.gov/clinicaltrials.

Special concerns

Children diagnosed with pineoblastomas, like children with other long-term illnesses, may develop emotional problems in reaction to restrictions on their activities, uncomfortable treatments, or being treated in a cancer center away from home. These children may withdraw from others, become angry or bitter, or feel inappropriately guilty about their illness. It is important to reassure the child that he or she did not cause the cancer or deserve it as a punishment for being "bad." Parents may benefit from consulting a child psychiatrist about these and other emotional problems.

Another special concern is the task of explaining the child's illness and treatments to other family members and friends in ways that they can understand. Members of the child's treatment team can be helpful in providing simplified descriptions for siblings or schoolmates.

A third area of concern with **childhood cancers** is the parents' relationships with their other children and with each other. Siblings may resent the amount of time and attention given to the child with cancer, or they may fear that they too will develop a brain tumor. Support groups for families of children with cancer can help by sharing strategies for coping with these problems as well as allowing members to express anxiety and other painful feelings in a safe setting.

See also Brain and central nervous system tumors; Supratentorial primitive neuroectodermal tumors.

Resources

BOOKS

Abeloff, M. D., et al. *Clinical Oncology.* 5th ed. New York: Churchill Livingstone, 2013.

American Brain Tumor Association (ABTA). *A Primer of Brain Tumors.* Des Plaines, IL: ABTA, 2004.

"Intracranial Neoplasms (Brain Tumors)." Section 14, Chapter 177 in *The Merck Manual of Diagnosis and Therapy,* edited by Mark H. Beers and Robert Berkow. Whitehouse Station, NJ: Merck Research Laboratories, 2004.

Niederhuber, J. E., et al. *Clinical Oncology.* 5th ed. Philadelphia: Elsevier, 2014.

PERIODICALS

Bruce, J. N., and A. T. Ogden. "Surgical Strategies for Treating Patients with Pineal Region Tumors." *Journal of Neurooncology* 69 (August–September 2004): 221–36.

Farnia, B., et al. "Clinical Outcomes and Patterns of Failure in Pineoblastoma: A 30-Year Single Institution Retrospective Review." *World Neurosurgery* (July 18, 2014): e-pub ahead of print. http://dx.doi.org/10.1016/j.wneu.2014.07.010 (accessed November 10, 2014).

Plowman, P. N., B. Pizer, and J. E. Kingston. "Pineal Parenchymal Tumours: II. On the Aggressive Behaviour of Pineoblastoma in Patients with an Inherited Mutation of the RB1 Gene." *Clinical Oncology* 16 (June 2004): 244–47.

OTHER

American Cancer Society. *Brain and Spinal Cord Tumors in Children.* http://documents.cancer.org/acs/groups/cid/documents/webcontent/003089-pdf.pdf (accessed November 10, 2014).

WEBSITES

National Cancer Institute. "Childhood Central Nervous System Embryonal Tumors Treatment (PDQ®)." http://www.cancer.gov/cancertopics/pdq/treatment/childCNSembryonal/patient/page4 (accessed November 10, 2014).

ORGANIZATIONS

American Brain Tumor Association, 8550 W. Bryn Mawr Ave., Ste. 550, Chicago, IL 60631, (773) 577-8750, (800) 886-2282, Fax: (773) 577-8738, info@abta.org, http://www.abta.org.

Rebecca Frey, PhD

REVISED BY TERESA G. ODLE

REVIEWED BY ROSALYN CARSON-DEWITT, MD

Pituitary tumors

Definition

Pituitary tumors are a growth of abnormal cells in the pituitary gland.

Description

Located in the center of the brain, the pea-sized pituitary gland is often referred to as the "master endocrine gland" because it makes and releases (secretes) at least nine distinct hormones (including oxytocin, antidiuretic hormone [ADH], prolactin, thyroid-stimulating hormone [TSH], adrenocorticotropic hormone [ACTH], follicle-stimulating hormone [FSH], luteinizing hormone [LH], and human growth hormone [HGH]). These hormones regulate the activities of several other endocrine glands and influence a number of physiological processes, including growth, sexual development and functioning, and the body's fluid balance. The pituitary gland is divided into the front or anterior part and the rear or posterior part. Each half of the pituitary gland secretes specific hormones. Tumors in the anterior part are common and are usually noncancerous (benign). Tumors rarely develop in the posterior portion. Between 10% and 15% of all tumors in the skull are pituitary tumors, which makes them the third most common type of brain tumor.

Virtually all pituitary tumors arise from a single cell type that is growing and dividing uncontrollably. Tumors that have originated from a single cell type are called monoclonal. The tumors themselves sometimes secrete hormones normally made by the pituitary gland and, because tumor cell growth is uncontrolled, they secrete large amounts of the hormones. Tumors that secrete hormones are called functional tumors and those that do not secrete hormone are called nonfunctional tumors. When a tumor produces and secretes hormones excessively, hormone imbalances will occur, along with related symptoms. The symptoms caused by a hormone imbalance are often the first signs of a pituitary tumor.

Several different types of pituitary tumors can develop. Pituitary adenomas (tumors that grow from glandular tissue) are the most common type. Most pituitary adenomas are benign, although they may spread to nearby tissues. Pituitary adenomas can be further classified based on which, if any, hormones are secreted by the tumor. Thirty-five percent of pituitary adenomas do not secrete hormones, 27% secrete prolactin (prolactinomas), and 21% secrete growth hormone. The remaining pituitary adenomas secrete sex hormones (6%), thyroid hormones (1%), or adrenal (adrenocorticotropic) hormones (8%). Plurihormonal adenomas secrete more than one type of hormone. Tumors that secrete

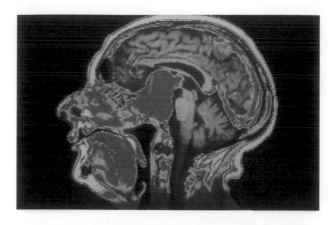

This colored magnetic resonance imaging (MRI) scan of a sagittal section of the brain reveals a large pituitary tumor (pink mass in center) located to the left of the brainstem. *(CMSP/Custom Medical Stock Photography)*

adrenocorticotropic hormone can cause **Cushing syndrome** and Nelson syndrome.

Craniopharyngiomas are benign tumors that originate in tissues next to the pituitary gland. Although they are not technically pituitary tumors, they do affect the pituitary gland. They are extremely difficult to remove, and radiation does not stop craniopharyngiomas from spreading throughout the pituitary gland. Craniopharyngiomas account for less than 5% of all **brain tumors**.

Pituitary **carcinoma** is an exceptionally rare condition. Fewer than 100 cases have ever been reported. It is usually diagnosed when a pituitary tumor that was believed to be an **adenoma** spreads (metastasizes) to distant organs. These pituitary tumors may or may not release hormones. Because pituitary carcinoma is often diagnosed late, it has a high death rate.

Demographics

About 10,000 pituitary tumors are diagnosed in the United States annually and almost all of them are benign adenomas. However, the actual number of pituitary tumors may be higher, because many are small without symptoms and go undiagnosed. Pituitary tumors occur more frequently in women than in men. They can occur at any age, even in children, but most are found in older adults. Half of all craniopharyngiomas occur in children, with symptoms most often appearing between the ages of five and ten. Pituitary tumors are rarely associated with a family history of the disease.

Causes and symptoms

The cause of pituitary tumors is not known. Most pituitary tumors are believed to result from changes to the DNA of one type of cell, leading to uncontrolled cell

KEY TERMS

Adenoma—A tumor that is derived from glandular tissue.

Agonist—A drug that increases the effectiveness of another drug or chemical.

Benign—A term used to describe a noncancerous growth.

Carney complex—A genetic disorder characterized by myxomas, spotty pigmentation of the skin and mucous membranes, and endocrine overactivity.

Dopamine—A neurotransmitter that is a chemical messenger in the brain.

Hormone—A chemical that is produced and released by one organ to regulate the function of another organ.

Invasive—A descriptive term for tumors that spread to nearby structures.

McCune-Albright syndrome—A genetic disorder that includes bone, endocrine, and skin abnormalities. Some individuals with this syndrome show the effects of excessive secretion of pituitary growth hormone.

Multiple endocrine neoplasia syndrome type I—An inherited disorder that affects the endocrine glands. The pituitary gland becomes overactive in about one-sixth of the individuals with this syndrome.

Nelson's syndrome—An endocrine disorder characterized by increase secretion of ACTH and melanocyte stimulating hormone by the pituitary gland.

growth. The genetic defects, **multiple endocrine neoplasia** syndrome type I (MEN I or Wermer syndrome), McCune-Albright syndrome, and the Carney complex, are associated with pituitary tumors. However, these defects account for only a small percentage of the cases of pituitary tumors. Also, a malignant pituitary tumor may be a secondary tumor resulting from the spread (**metastasis**) of **cancer** from another site. **Breast cancer** in women and lung cancer in men are the most common cancers to spread to the pituitary gland. Other cancers that spread to the pituitary gland include **kidney cancer**, **prostate cancer**, **melanoma**, and **gastrointestinal cancers**.

Symptoms related to tumor location, size, and pressure on neighboring structures include:

- persistent headache on one or both sides, or in the center of the forehead

- blurred or double vision; loss of side (peripheral) vision
- drooping eyelid (ptosis) caused by pressure on nerves leading to the eye
- numbness on the face
- dementia
- drowsiness
- enlarged head
- eating excessive (hyperphagia) or abnormally small (hypophagia) amounts of food
- seizures

The specific symptoms associated with hormone-secreting tumors (functioning tumors) will vary depending on which hormones are overproduced. Symptoms related to hormonal imbalance include:

- excessive sweating
- loss of appetite
- loss of interest in sex
- inability to tolerate cold temperatures
- nausea
- menstrual problems
- excessive thirst
- frequent urination
- dry skin
- constipation
- premature or delayed puberty
- delayed growth in children
- milk secretion in the absence of pregnancy or breast feeding (galactorrhea)
- reduced strength
- mood alterations (depression, anxiety, unstable emotions)
- muscle pain
- low blood glucose (sudden occurrence of shakiness and sweating)

Patients who have sudden pituitary failure caused by bleeding or tissue death (pituitary apoplexy, also known as Sheehan syndrome) may experience severe headaches, confusion, vision loss, and drowsiness. This condition is considered an emergency.

Tumors that secrete growth hormone may cause a condition called acromegaly. This long-term complication of hormone-secreting tumors is characterized by enlargement of the nose, ears, jaws, toes, and fingers. Joint pain, abnormal blood glucose metabolism, high blood pressure, carpal tunnel syndrome, and airway blockages can result.

Diagnosis

As many as 40% of all pituitary tumors do not release excessive quantities of hormones into the blood. Known as clinically nonfunctioning, these tumors are difficult to distinguish from tumors that produce similar symptoms. They may grow to be quite large before they are diagnosed.

The diagnosis of pituitary tumors is based on:

- the patient's own observations and medical history
- physical examination
- laboratory studies of the patient's blood and brain/spinal fluid (cerebrospinal fluid)
- x-rays of the skull, and diagnostic imaging studies that provide images of the inside of the brain (CT, MRI); MRI is the imaging method of choice for evaluating pituitary tumor spread.
- vision tests
- urinalysis

Treatment team

The treatment team for pituitary tumors may include a neuroendocrinologist, endocrinologist, neurosurgeon, oncologist, radiation oncologist, nurse oncologist, psychiatrist, psychological counselor, and social worker.

Clinical staging

As with other **central nervous system tumors**, no tumor-node-metastasis classification system exists for pituitary tumors, and there is no standard clinical staging system because most tumors found are benign. Instead, the pituitary adenomas are classified according to their size (0–5 cm), endocrine activity (hormone producing or not), cell characteristics, and growth patterns. The radiology classification for pituitary adenomas assigns grades of 0, normal appearance; I, microadenoma smaller than 10 mm and enclosed within the sella turcica (bone at the base of the skull); II, macroadenoma 10 mm or larger and enclosed within the sella turcica; III, invasive locally into the sella; IV, invasive diffusely into the sella.

Treatment

Treatment is determined by the type of tumor, the type of hormone released by the tumor, whether vision is affected, and whether the tumor has invaded tissues next to the pituitary gland. The goals of treatment are to normalize hormone levels and reduce the size of (or remove) the tumor. Treatment options include surgery, radiation, and/or medication. Some pituitary tumors stabilize without treatment. Small tumors that are not causing significant symptoms may be watched only.

Surgery is usually used to remove all or part of a tumor within the gland or the area surrounding it. Surgery may be combined with **radiation therapy** to treat tumors that extend beyond the pituitary gland. A neurosurgeon will operate immediately to remove the tumor or pituitary gland (hypophysectomy) of a patient whose vision is deteriorating rapidly. Approximately 96% of the surgeries are performed through the nose (transsphenoidal). If the tumor is large, the skull may be opened (**craniotomy**) for **tumor removal**. Removal or destruction of the pituitary gland requires lifelong hormone replacement therapy. The most common complications of surgery are leakage of cerebrospinal fluid through the nose and inflammation of the membranes that surround the brain and spinal column (meningitis).

Radiation therapy is not as effective as surgery and is usually reserved for tumors that have not responded to other treatments and those that recur. Radioactive pellets can be implanted in the brain to treat the tumor. Selected patients are treated with proton beam radiosurgery that uses high-energy particles in the form of a beam to destroy an overactive pituitary gland. **Fatigue**, upset stomach, **diarrhea**, and nausea are common complaints of patients undergoing radiation therapy. Radiation therapy to the brain can damage certain brain tissues.

Dopamine agonists, drugs that increase the effect of the brain chemical dopamine, are effective in treating tumors that release hormones. These drugs can reduce symptoms caused by a pituitary tumor and reduce the size of the tumor. Commonly used dopamine agonists include bromocriptine, pergolide, and cabergoline. Cabergoline is the most effective and produces fewer side effects than the other two drugs. Side effects associated with dopamine agonists include nausea, vomiting, and lightheadedness when rising (postural hypotension). Acromegaly may be treated with somatostatin and other drugs derived from somatostatin (analogues). Tumors and the symptoms they are causing return when drug use is stopped. Patients should wear medical identification tags identifying their condition and prescribed hormonal replacement medicines.

The common treatments for specific pituitary tumors are:

- Prolactin-secreting adenoma. Prolactinomas are treated with a dopamine agonist. Surgical treatment is used if the drug fails or causes intolerable side effects.
- Gonadotropin-secreting adenoma. Small tumors are not treated unless they cause symptoms. Large tumors and small tumors that are causing symptoms are treated surgically. Radiation therapy may be used.
- Adrenocorticotropic hormone-secreting adenoma. Surgery is the treatment of choice. Medications that

prevent adrenal hormone production or radiation therapy may be used if surgery fails.

- Growth hormone-secreting adenoma. Surgery is the treatment of choice. Medications (dopamine agonists, somatostatins) or radiation therapy may be used.

- Thyroid-stimulating hormone-secreting adenoma. Surgery, with or without radiation therapy, is the preferred treatment. Although somatostatin treatment may reduce hormone levels, it fails to shrink the tumor.

- Nonsecreting adenoma. Surgery is the treatment of choice. In general, medications are not effective for this type of tumor. Radiation therapy may be used to prevent tumor recurrence.

- Pituitary carcinoma. Carcinoma is treated with standard cancer radiation therapy and chemotherapy.

- Craniopharyngioma. These tumors are difficult to treat. Due to the nature of craniopharyngiomas, surgery is often incomplete and needs to be complemented by radiation therapy.

Prognosis

Pituitary tumors are usually curable. Pituitary adenomas that secrete adrenocorticotropic hormone are frequently persistent and have a high rate of recurrence. Approximately 5% of pituitary adenomas invade nearby tissues and grow to large sizes, making them more difficult to treat and subject to frequent recurrences. Metastasis of most pituitary tumors is very rare. However, pituitary carcinomas can metastasize and are associated with a poor prognosis.

Coping with cancer treatment

Patients are advised to consult with members of their treatment team regarding any side effects or complications of treatment. Patients may want to consult a psychotherapist and/or join a support group to deal with the emotional consequences of cancer and its treatment.

Clinical trials

Clinical trials are under way studying the safety and effectiveness of antineoplastons, drugs shown to be effective in treating serious or life-threatening brain tumors. Research is also focused on the modification of gene expression; this approach means turning genes on or off by manipulating the DNA. The use of epigenetic or "epi-drugs" has been shown to inhibit the uncontrolled cell growth of pituitary tumors, which may lead to effective therapies. The **National Cancer Institute** website has information on current clinical trials and their locations. Patients are advised to consult with their treatment teams to determine whether they are candidates for any ongoing studies.

QUESTIONS TO ASK YOUR DOCTOR

- Is my pituitary tumor cancerous? Is it invasive?
- What are my treatment options?
- What are the risks and side effects of these treatments?
- Is surgery really necessary?
- Which surgical approach will you use?
- How many pituitary surgeries have you performed?
- How will I feel immediately following surgery?
- Will I need to take medication for the rest of my life?
- How long will it take for my symptoms to go away?
- Will I be able to have children?
- Is it safe to become pregnant while taking this medication?
- How will pregnancy affect my tumor?
- What medications can I take to relieve treatment side effects?
- Are any clinical studies under way that would be appropriate for me?
- What is the chance that the tumor will recur?
- How will recurrence be detected?
- How often will I have follow-up examinations?

Special concerns

Long-term low levels of sex hormones (hypogonadism) can have negative effects on bone density and the cardiovascular system in men and women. The effect that a pituitary tumor has on fertility is a concern for both men and women. Women taking medications to treat pituitary tumors need to question their physicians regarding the potential effects the medications may have on an unborn baby.

See also Multiple endocrine neoplasia syndromes.

Resources

BOOKS

Edge, S. B., D. R. Byrd, and C. C. Compton, et al, eds. "Brain and Spinal Cord." In *AJCC Cancer Staging Manual*, 7th ed. New York: Springer, 2010.

Melmed, Shlomo, Kenneth S. Polonsky, P. Reed Larsen, and Henry M. Kronenberg. "Pituitary Masses and Tumors." In *Williams Textbook of Endocrinology: Expert Consult*, 12th ed. Elsevier Saunders, 2011.

PERIODICALS

Beck-Peccocz, P., A. Lania, A. Beckers, K. Chatterjee, and J. L. Wemeau. "2013 European Thyroid Association Guidelines for the Diagnosis and Treatment of Thyrotropin-Secreting Pituitary Tumors." *European Thyroid Journal* 2 (Jun 2013): 76–82.

Clarke, M. J., D. Erickson, M. R. Castro, and J. L. Atkinson. "Thyroid-Stimulating Hormone Pituitary Adenomas." *Journal of Neurosurgery* 109 (July 2008): 17–22.

Farrell, W. E. "Epigenetics of Pituitary Tumours: An Update." *Current Opinion in Endocrinology, Diabetes, and Obesity* 21 (June 2014): 299–305.

ORGANIZATIONS

American Brain Tumor Association, 8550 W. Bryn Mawr Ave., Ste. 550, Chicago, IL 60631, (773) 577-8750, (800) 886-2282, Fax: (773) 577-8738, info@abta.org, http://www.abta.org.

American Cancer Society, 250 Williams St. NW, Atlanta, GA 30303, (800) 227-2345, http://www.cancer.org.

National Brain Tumor Society, 55 Chapel St., Ste. 200, Newton, MA 02458, (617) 924-9997, http://www.braintumor.org.

National Cancer Institute, 9609 Medical Center Dr., BG 9609 MSC 9760, Bethesda, MD 20892-9760, (800) 4-CANCER (422-6237), http://www.cancer.gov.

L. Lee Culvert
Maureen Haggerty
Belinda Rowland, PhD

Plasma cell neoplasms *see* **Multiple myeloma; Waldenström macroglobulinemia**

Plasmacytoma *see* **Multiple myeloma**

Plasmapheresis *see* **Pheresis**

Platinol-AQ *see* **Cisplatin**

Plenaxis *see* **Abarelix**

Plerixafor

Definition

Plerixafor (Mozobil) is a hematopoietic stem cell mobilizing drug manufactured by Genzyme Corporation. It is used in combination with granulocyte-colony stimulating factor (G-CSF) to increase the number of hematopoietic stem cells in the bloodstream as part of treatment for **non-Hodgkin lymphoma** and **multiple myeloma**.

Purpose

High doses of **chemotherapy** drugs kill large numbers of healthy blood cells as well as killing cancerous (malignant) cells. To function well, the body needs to replace these healthy cells. Hematopoietic stem cells are undifferentiated cells that can become red blood cells, which carry oxygen and remove wastes throughout the body; white blood cells, which help fight infection; or platelets, which help the blood to clot. Plerixafor, when used in combination with G-CSF, stimulates the body to release hematopoietic stem cells from the bone marrow into the bloodstream. These stem cells can then be harvested through a process called apheresis.

Apheresis works by removing the blood from an individual and passing it through special filters that remove the desired component, in this case the hematopoietic stem cells, and then returning the blood to the individual. The hematopoietic stem cells are stored and later can be reinfused into the individual after high doses of chemotherapy. This process is called an autologous peripheral blood **stem cell transplantation**. The transfused stem cells settle into the bone marrow and begin differentiating into new blood cells. For an autologous peripheral blood stem cell transplantation to be successful, many millions of hematopoietic stem cells must be collected. Treatment with the combination of plerixafor and G-CSF stimulates the bone marrow to release these cells into the bloodstream and substantially reduces the number of days and apheresis sessions needed to collect enough for successful transplantation.

Description

Plerixafor injection, sold under the brand name Mozobil, is a sterile, preservative-free clear liquid that is intended for injection under the skin (subcutaneous injection). The U.S. Food and Drug Administration approved the drug for use in the United States on December 15, 2008; plerixafor holds orphan drug status in the United States and in the European Union. It was approved for use in Canada in 2011. Plerixafor continues to be tested in **clinical trials** in the United States for use against other cancers and in combination with other therapies. A list of clinical trials currently enrolling volunteers can be found at http://www.clinicaltrials.gov.

Recommended dosage

Plerixafor comes in single-use vials that should be stored at room temperature. First, the patient receives G-CSF once daily for four days. Following that, plerixafor is injected under the skin 11 hours before apheresis is to begin. Dosage is based on body weight, with a recommended dose of 0.24 mg/kg body weight, and may be repeated for up to four consecutive days. There are no data on overdosage.

KEY TERMS

Apheresis—The practice of removing blood from an individual and separating out certain components, returning the blood to the individual and storing the separated component in order to later transfuse it back into the same individual (autologous transplantation).

Autologous transplantation—Transplantation in which the individual's own stem cells or bone marrow are removed and then transplanted back into the individual later. Autologous transplantation removes the risk of rejection of the transplanted material.

Granulocyte-colony stimulating factor (G-CFS)—A genetically produced form of a naturally occurring hormone that stimulates the production of infection-fighting white blood cells called granulocytes in the bone marrow.

Hematopoietic stem cells—Cells that have the potential to differentiate into red blood cells, white blood cells, or platelets.

Leukocytes—Also called white blood cells, leukocytes fight infection and boost the immune system.

Lymphoma—A type of cancer that originates in the cells of the lymphatic system (lymph nodes, thymus, spleen, adenoids, tonsils and bone marrow). It is one of the four major types of cancer.

Multiple myeloma—Cancer of the plasma cells of the bone marrow.

Orphan drug—One that provides a significant benefit in treating a rare disease. Generally these drugs are not financially worthwhile for drug companies to produce despite their benefit to patients. If a drug is given orphan drug status in the United States or European Union, it may receive fast-track approval or extra research money, making it more economically viable for manufacturers.

Platelet—A small, disk-shaped cell in the blood that has an important role in blood clotting. Platelets form the initial plug at the rupture site of a blood vessel.

Pregnancy category—A system of classifying drugs according to their established risks for use during pregnancy. Category A: Controlled human studies have demonstrated no fetal risk. Category B: Animal studies indicate no fetal risk, but no human studies; or adverse effects in animals, but not in well-controlled human studies. Category C: No adequate human or animal studies; or adverse fetal effects in animal studies, but no available human data. Category D: Evidence of fetal risk, but benefits outweigh risks. Category X: Evidence of fetal risk. Risks outweigh any benefits.

Plerixafor is removed from the body by the kidneys. The recommended dosage for individuals with moderate to severe kidney (renal) impairment is reduced to 0.16 mg/kg body weight, not to exceed 27 mg/day. There are no other special recommendations for dosage.

The safety and effectiveness of this drug in children has not been established.

Precautions

The following precautions should be observed.

• Plerixafor should not be used in patients with leukemia because it may mobilize leukemia cells for release from bone marrow.

• A decrease in the number of blood platelets (thrombocytopenia) may reduce the ability of the blood to clot. An increase in the number of leukocytes also may occur. Blood count should be monitored.

• An increased number of tumor cells may be released from the bone marrow as a result of G-CSF/plerixafor stimulation. Some of these tumor cells may be unintentionally collected along with the hematopoietic stem cells harvested for transfusion. The effect of re-infusing these tumor cells is unknown.

• This drug may cause enlargement and rupture of the spleen. Symptoms of spleen enlargement should be evaluated promptly.

• Individuals with renal failure should receive reduced dosage (see recommended dosage above).

Pregnant or breastfeeding women

Plerixafor is a pregnancy category D drug. Woman who are pregnant or who might become pregnant should not use plerixafor. It is not known whether the drug is excreted in breast milk. Women taking this drug who are or who want to breastfeed should discuss the risks and benefits with their doctor and err on the side of caution,

QUESTIONS TO ASK YOUR DOCTOR

- Why do you believe the benefits outweigh the risks of using this drug?
- Is this drug safe to take with the other drugs that I am currently taking?
- What side effects should I watch for? When should I call the doctor about them?
- Are there any clinical trials of this drug combined with other therapies that might benefit me?

as there is the potential for this drug to cause serious adverse effects in nursing infants.

Side effects

The most serious side effects seen in clinical trials were the potential for tumor cell mobilization in leukemia patients, increased leukocytes and decreased platelets in the blood, and enlargement of the spleen.

Side effects that occurred in more than 10% of individuals given plerixafor during clinical trials included:

- diarrhea
- nausea and vomiting
- fatigue
- reactions at the injection site
- headache
- joint pain (arthralgia)
- dizziness

Interactions

Plerixafor is not known to interact with any drugs, herbs, or supplements. Individuals should check with their oncologist for changes in this information as more people are treated with plerixafor and information about the drug is collected.

Resources

WEBSITES

AHFS Consumer Medication Information. "Plerixafor Injection." American Society of Health-System Pharmacists. Available from: http://www.nlm.nih.gov/medlineplus/druginfo/meds/a609018.html (accessed November 12, 2014).

Pazdur, Richard. "FDA Approval for Plerixafor." National Cancer Institute. http://www.cancer.gov/cancertopics/druginfo/fda-plerixafor (accessed October 15, 2014).

U.S. Food and Drug Administration. "Mozobil (plerixafor) Injection, Subcutaneous." http://www.fda.gov/safety/med
watch/safetyinformation/ucm359917.htm (accessed November 12, 2014).

ORGANIZATIONS

American Cancer Society, 250 Williams St. NW, Atlanta, GA 30303, (800) 227-2345, http://www.cancer.org.

Leukemia & Lymphoma Society, 1311 Mamaroneck Avenue, Suite 310, White Plains, NY 10605, (800) 955-4572, http://www.leukemia-lymphoma.org.

National Cancer Institute, 9609 Medical Center Dr., BG 9609 MSC 9760, Bethesda, MD 20892-9760, (800) 4-CANCER (422-6237), http://www.cancer.gov

Tish Davidson, A.M.

Pleural biopsy

Definition

The pleurae are the membranes that line the lungs and chest cavity. A pleural **biopsy** is the removal of pleural tissue for examination and eventual diagnosis.

Purpose

Pleural biopsy is performed to differentiate between benign (noncancerous) and malignant (cancerous) disease; to diagnose viral, fungal, or parasitic diseases; and to identify a condition called collagen vascular disease of the pleurae. It is also ordered when a chest x-ray indicates a pleural-based tumor, reaction, or thickening of the pleura.

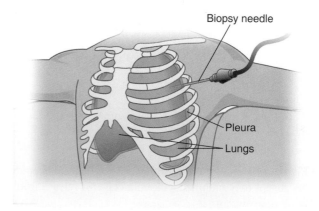

Illustration of a pleural biopsy. A biopsy needle is inserted into the pleurae, the membranes that line the lungs and chest cavity. *(Illustration by Electronic Illustrators Group. © 2015 Cengage Learning®.)*

KEY TERMS

Aspiration—Withdrawal of fluid from a cavity by suction.

Endotracheal—Referring to placement within the trachea, also known as the windpipe.

Pulmonary—Pertaining to the lungs.

Description

Pleural biopsy is usually ordered when pleural fluid obtained by another procedure called **thoracentesis** (aspiration of pleural fluid) suggests infection, signs of **cancer**, or tuberculosis. However, the procedure is most successful in diagnosing pleural tuberculosis (with a sensitivity up to 75%) rather than pleural malignancy (40–50% sensitivity).

The procedure most often performed for pleural biopsy is called a percutaneous (passage through the skin by needle puncture) needle biopsy or closed needle biopsy. This procedure can sample only the outer pleural membrane (parietal pleura), and the size of the tissue sample obtained is relatively small.

Although the biopsy needle itself remains in the pleura for less than one minute, the procedure takes 30–45 minutes. This type of biopsy is usually performed by a physician at the bedside if the patient is hospitalized or in an outpatient setting under local anesthesia.

The actual procedure begins with the patient in a sitting position, shoulders and arms elevated and supported. The skin overlying the biopsy site is anesthetized, and a small incision is made to allow insertion of the biopsy needle. This needle is inserted with a cannula (a plastic or metal tube) until fluid is removed. Then the inner needle is removed and a trocar (an instrument for withdrawing fluid from a cavity) is inserted to obtain the actual biopsy specimen. As many as three separate specimens are taken from different sites during the procedure. These specimens are then placed into a fixative solution and sent to the laboratory for tissue (histologic) examination.

Although used less frequently than the closed needle biopsy, an open pleural biopsy may be performed surgically in the operating room when a larger tissue sample is required. The incision is larger than that required for a closed needle biopsy, and an endotracheal tube is inserted through the windpipe to assure proper breathing during the procedure. The procedure takes two to three hours, is more invasive, and requires general anesthesia and hospitalization for one or more days.

Open biopsy is sometimes performed when there is no **pleural effusion** (an accumulation of fluid between the pleural layers) or when a direct view of the pleura and lungs is required.

Another procedure called **thoracoscopy** involves pleural biopsy under direct visualization through a thoracoscope. This procedure is highly accurate (sensitivity as high as 91%) in diagnosing both benign and malignant pleural disease. As in open needle biopsy, however, it requires general anesthesia and is usually used only after other diagnostic procedures fail.

Precautions

Because pleural biopsy—especially open pleural biopsy—is an invasive procedure, it is not recommended for patients with severe bleeding disorders.

Preparation

Preparations for this procedure vary, depending on the type of procedure requested. Closed needle biopsy requires little or no preparation. Open pleural biopsy, which is performed in a hospital, requires fasting (no solids or liquids) for 8 to 12 hours before the procedure because the stomach must be empty before general anesthesia is administered.

Aftercare

Potential complications of this procedure include bleeding or injury to the lung, or a condition called pneumothorax, in which air enters the pleural cavity (the space between the two layers of pleura lining the lungs and the chest wall). Because of these possibilities, a chest x-ray is always performed after the procedure (closed or open biopsy). Also, it is important for the patient to report any shortness of breath and for the nurses to note any signs of bleeding, decreased blood pressure, or increased pulse rate during the recovery period.

Risks

Risks for this procedure include respiratory distress on the side of the biopsy, as well as bleeding, possible shoulder pain, infection, pneumothorax (immediate), or **pneumonia** (delayed). Risk increases with stress, obesity, smoking, chronic illness, and the use of some medications (such as insulin, tranquilizers, and antihypertensives).

Results

Normal findings indicate no evidence of any pathologic or disease conditions in the pleural cavity.

QUESTIONS TO ASK YOUR DOCTOR

- What is the purpose of this test?
- Is the test dangerous?
- How do I prepare for the test?
- How long will the test take?
- How soon will I get my test results?

Abnormal results

Abnormal findings include tumors called neoplasms (any new or abnormal growth) that can be either benign or malignant. Pleural tumors are divided into two categories: primary (**mesothelioma**), or metastatic (spreading to the pleural cavity from a site elsewhere in the body). These tumors are often associated with pleural effusion, which itself may be caused by pneumonia, heart failure, cancer, or blood clot in the lungs (pulmonary embolism).

Other causes of abnormal findings include viral, fungal, or parasitic infections, and tuberculosis.

Resources

PERIODICALS

Koegelenberg, C. F., and A. H. Diacon. "Image-Guided Pleural Biopsy." *Current Opinion in Pulmonary Medicine* 19, no. 4 (2013): 368–73.

WEBSITES

A.D.A.M. Medical Encyclopedia. "Open Pleural Biopsy." MedlinePlus. http://www.nlm.nih.gov/medlineplus/ency/article/003863.htm (accessed November 12, 2014).

Johns Hopkins Medicine. "Pleural Biopsy." http://www.hop kinsmedicine.org/healthlibrary/test_procedures/pulmo nary/pleural_biopsy_92,P07757/ (accessed November 12, 2014).

ORGANIZATIONS

American Cancer Society, 250 Williams St. NW, Atlanta, GA 30303, (800) 227-2345, http://www.cancer.org.

American College of Chest Physicians, 2595 Patriot Boulevard, Glenview, IL 60026, (224) 521-9800, (800) 343-2227, Fax: (224) 521-9801, http://www.chestnet.org.

American Lung Association, 55 W. Wacker Dr., Ste. 1150, Chicago, IL 60601, (800) LUNG-USA (586-4872), Fax: (202) 452-1805, http://www.lung.org.

Lung Cancer Alliance, 888 16th St. NW, Ste. 150, Washington, DC 20006, (202) 463-2080, (800) 298-2436, info@lung canceralliance.org, http://www.lungcanceralliance.org.

Janis O. Flores

Pleural effusion

Definition

Pleural effusion is the accumulation of fluid in the pleural space. The pleural space is the region between the outer surface of each lung (visceral pleurae) and the membrane that surrounds each lung (parietal pleurae). Under normal conditions, the pleurae are kept wet with pleural fluid to allow movement of the lungs within the chest. The pleural fluid comes from cells that make up the pleurae. Pleural fluid is continuously produced and removed, a process that is precisely controlled by many factors. **Cancer** can interfere with this delicate balance within the pleural space, causing fluid to accumulate.

Description

Cancer is responsible for 40% of all pleural effusions, which are then called malignant pleural effusions. Pleural effusion is the first symptom of cancer for up to 50% of the patients. Thirty-five percent of the cases of malignant pleural effusion are caused by lung cancer, 23% by **breast cancer**, and 10% by **lymphoma**.

Causes and symptoms

Causes

Malignant pleural effusions are most often associated with lymphomas, leukemia, breast cancer, gastrointestinal cancer, lung cancer, and **ovarian cancer**. For the majority of patients, pleural effusion occurs in the lung on the same side as the cancer. For one-third of the patients, pleural effusion occurs in both lungs.

Pleural effusion in cancer patients can be caused by several different conditions. Blockage of the lymphatic system, a series of channels for drainage of body fluids, interferes with the removal of pleural fluid. Blockage of the veins of the lungs increases the pressure on the pleurae, which causes fluid accumulation. Cancerous cells may seed onto the pleurae and cause inflammation, which increases fluid in the pleural space. High numbers of cancerous cells may collect in the pleural space (tumor cell suspensions), which also causes extra fluid to be released. Accumulation of fluid in the abdominal cavity may cross over to the pleural space.

Symptoms

Pleural effusion can hinder the normal function of the lungs. Symptoms of pleural effusion include chest pain, chest heaviness, breathing difficulties, and a dry cough.

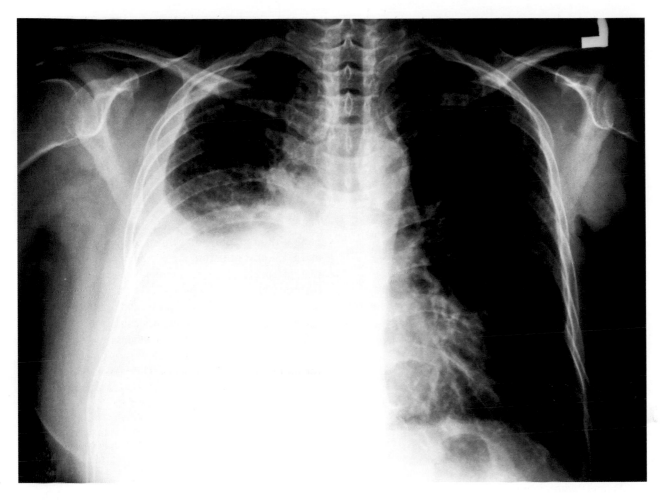

Chest x-ray revealing pleural effusion, or excess fluid in the pleural space in the chest and lungs. *(Puwadol Jaturawutthichai/ Shutterstock.com)*

Diagnosis

Chest x-rays and **computed tomography** scans may be performed to diagnose pleural effusion. **Thoracentesis**, the removal of pleural fluid through a long needle, is usually performed for diagnostic purposes. Fluid removed by thoracentesis will be sent to the lab to be thoroughly evaluated. **Thoracoscopy**, in which a wandlike lighted camera (endoscope) is inserted through the chest, may be conducted to diagnose pleural effusion. During thoracoscopy, samples (**biopsy**) of pleurae may be taken.

Treatment

Management of pleural effusion strives to relieve symptoms and improve quality of life. Cure is not always possible. The treatment method depends on the patient's age, prognosis, and location of the first tumor. Treatment for patients with pleural effusion who are asymptomatic (do not have symptoms) consists solely of observation.

Treatment options for pleural effusion include:

- Thoracentesis. Removal of the excess pleural fluid often relieves the symptoms of pleural effusion. However, effusion usually recurs within a few days. Repeat thoracentesis is not recommended unless the patient has end-stage disease.

- Tube thoracostomy. A tube is inserted through the chest and into the pleural space to drain pleural fluid. When used alone, recurrence is very common.

- Indwelling pleural catheters. A thin flexible tube (catheter) is placed between the pleural cavity and the chest skin to allow drainage of pleural fluid. This method allows for continual drainage of pleural fluid without much pain.

- Pleurodesis. After tube thoracostomy, one of any number of chemicals (sclerosing agents) is put into the pleural space to cause the visceral and parietal pleurae to stick together. Chemical pleurodesis is considered to be the treatment of choice for patients with malignant pleural effusion.

- Pleurectomy. Surgical removal of the parietal pleura through an incision in the chest wall (thoracotomy) is nearly 100% effective. Pleurectomy is not routinely performed and is reserved for patients for whom other treatments have failed. To be eligible for pleurectomy, the patient must have a long life expectancy and be able to tolerate major surgery.

- Pleuroperitoneal shunt. This procedure places a rubber tube between the pleural space and the abdominal cavity. A pump is used to move excess fluid out of the pleural space and into the abdominal cavity, where it would be absorbed. The patient must press the pump for several minutes four times daily. Although not frequently used, this is an effective treatment for cases that failed tube thoracostomy and pleurodesis.

- External radiation. Patients who have pleural effusion caused by blockage of a lymph duct may be treated by radiation therapy. External radiation therapy is successful for patients with pleural effusion related to lymphoma.

- Supportive care. Patients with end-stage cancer may not receive treatment for pleural effusion. Pain medications and oxygen therapy can be provided to keep the patient comfortable.

Prognosis

Patients with malignant pleural effusions tend to be weak and have a short-span life expectancy. The prognosis depends on the type of cancer. Sixty-five percent of patients with malignant pleural effusions die within three months, and 80% die within six months. However, patients with pleural effusion related to breast cancer have a longer life expectancy.

Resources

WEBSITES

A.D.A.M. Medical Encyclopedia. "Pleural Effusion." Medline Plus. http://www.nlm.nih.gov/medlineplus/ency/article/000086.htm (accessed November 12, 2014).

Canadian Cancer Society. "Pleural Effusion." http://www.cancer.ca/en/cancer-information/diagnosis-and-treatment/managing-side-effects/pleural-effusion/?region=bc (accessed November 12, 2014).

Micromedex. "Complications." Mayo Clinic. http://www.mayoclinic.org/diseases-conditions/lung-cancer/basics/complications/con-20025531 (accessed November 12, 2014).

Belinda Rowland, PhD

Pleural fluid analysis *see* **Thoracentesis**

Pleurodesis

Definition

Pleurodesis is the adherence of the outer surface of a lung to the membrane surrounding that lung, which is performed to treat the buildup of fluid around the lung.

Purpose

The pleural space is the region between the outer surface of each lung (visceral pleurae) and the membrane that surrounds each lung (parietal pleurae). Under normal conditions, the pleurae are kept wet with pleural fluid to allow movement of the lungs within the chest. **Pleural effusion**, the accumulation of fluid in the pleural space, is most commonly caused by **cancer**. Pleurodesis causes the pleurae to stick together, thereby eliminating the pleural space and preventing fluid accumulation. Chemical pleurodesis is considered to be the standard of care for patients with malignant pleural effusion.

Description

Before pleurodesis is conducted, all pleural fluid must be removed. This is achieved by inserting a chest tube through the skin and into the pleural space (thoracostomy). Insertion of the chest tube is carried out in the hospital. The patient is awake during the procedure. The skin is sterilized and a local pain killer is injected into the skin and underlying tissue. A small cut is made into the skin and a tube is placed into the pleural space. Fluid is withdrawn and the tube remains in place until all pleural fluid is drained, which usually takes two to five days. After the chest tube is inserted, the patient may either remain in the hospital or be allowed to return home with instructions on how to care for the tube. A chest x-ray may be taken to ensure that all the fluid has been drained.

Pleurodesis is achieved by putting one of any number of chemicals (sclerosing agents or sclerosants) into the pleural space. The sclerosant irritates the pleurae, which results in inflammation (pleuritis) and causes the pleurae to stick together. The patient is given a narcotic pain reliever; and lidocaine, a local pain killer, is added to the sclerosant. A variety of different chemicals are used as sclerosing agents. There is no one sclerosant that is more effective or safer than the others. Commonly used sclerosants and their success rates are:

- Talc: 90–96%
- Nitrogen mustard: 52%
- Doxycycline: 90%

- Bleomycin: 84%
- Quinacrine: 70% to 90%

After the sclerosant has been introduced through the chest tube, the tube is closed. The patient may be asked to change position every 15 minutes for a two-hour time period. This was believed to be necessary to achieve an even distribution of sclerosant in the pleural space. However, recent evidence suggests that the sclerosant spreads throughout the pleural space immediately. Afterward, the chest tube is reopened and the sclerosant is sucked out of the pleural space. The tube remains in place for several days to allow all fluid to drain. Once drainage slows down, the chest tube is removed and the wound edges stitched (sutured) back together.

Aftercare

The patient should keep the wound from the chest tube clean and dry until it heals. Also, the patient should watch for signs of wound infection such as redness, swelling, and/or drainage, and be alert to symptoms indicating that the effusion has recurred.

Risks

Complications of pleurodesis are uncommon but include infection, bleeding, acute respiratory distress syndrome, collapsed lung (pneumothorax), and respiratory failure. Other complications may be specific to the sclerosant used. Talc and doxycycline can cause **fever** and pain. Quinacrine can cause low blood pressure, fever, and hallucination. **Bleomycin** can cause fever, pain, and nausea. Severe respiratory complications can be fatal.

Results

Tube thoracostomy with pleurodesis is the most effective method to treat malignant pleural effusion. Successful pleurodesis prevents the recurrence of pleural effusion, which relieves symptoms and thereby improves quality of life.

Abnormal results

If drainage of sclerosant from the chest tube exceeds approximately one cup, the pleurodesis was unsuccessful and must be repeated. Pleurodesis may fail because of:

- trapped lung, in which the lung is enclosed in scar or tumor tissue
- formation of isolated pockets (loculation) within the pleural space
- loss of lung flexibility (elasticity)
- production of large amounts of pleural fluid
- extensive spread (metastasis) of pleural cancer
- improper positioning of the tube
- blockage or kinking of the tube

Resources

PERIODICALS

Rafiei, R., Yazdani, B., Ranjbar, S.M., Torabi, Z., Asgary, S., Najafi, S., Keshvari, M. "Long-Term Results of Pleurodesis in Malignant Pleural Effusions: Doxycycline vs Bleomycin." *Avanced Biomedical Research* 3, no. 149 (2014). http://www.ncbi.nlm.nih.gov/pmc/articles/PMC4162080/#__ffn_sectitle (accessed November 14, 2014).

WEBSITES

American Cancer Society. "Surgery and Other Procedures for Lung Carcinoid Tumors." http://www.cancer.org/cancer/

lungcarcinoidtumor/detailedguide/lung-carcinoid-tumor-treating-surgery (accessed November 14, 2014).

Cancer Research UK. "Treatment For Fluid on the Lung" http://www.cancerresearchuk.org/about-cancer/cancers-in-gen eral/cancer-questions/pleurodesis-treatment (accessed November 14, 2014).

Belinda Rowland, PhD

Plicamycin

Definition

Plicamycin is an antibiotic also known as mithramycin; it was sold under the trade name Mithracin. The drug was used to treat **testicular cancer** but was discontinued by the manufacturer in 2000.

Purpose

Plicamycin was used to treat testicular **cancer** in patients who were not good candidates for either surgery or **radiation therapy**. It was first approved for this use by the U.S. Food and Drug Administration (FDA) in May 1970.

Description

Plicamycin is produced by a bacterium known as *Streptomyces argillaceus*. It interacts chemically with the DNA in cells. It was thought that plicamycin also made tumor cells more sensitive to **tumor necrosis factor** (TNF), a nonantibody protein secreted by cells in the immune system that kills tumor cells.

Recommended dosage

For testicular cancer, some doctors gave 25 micrograms per kilograms (mcg/kg) of body weight every two to four days to start. However, if the patient had kidney or liver problems, the dose was decreased to 12.5 mcg/kg. Other doctors administered 25 to 30 mcg/kg every eight to ten days, and some gave as much as 50 mcg/kg per dose for approximately eight doses every other day.

Precautions

This medication was not given to patients with problems with blood clotting or with the bone marrow. Plicamycin was not given to pregnant women, nursing mothers, or children younger than 15 years of age.

People taking plicamycin were at increased risk of developing an infection and of having bleeding problems.

Doctors carefully monitored blood counts, liver function, and kidney function in patients who received more than one dose of plicamycin.

Side effects

The side effects of plicamycin included a tendency for abnormal bleeding; low levels of calcium, potassium, and phosphorus in the blood, as well as other blood problems; and kidney or liver problems. Other side effects included **diarrhea**, loss of appetite (**anorexia**), **nausea and vomiting**, soreness of the mouth, muscle and abdominal cramps, pain, soreness at the injection side, **fever**, weakness, headache, depressed mood, **fatigue**, and drowsiness. Incidence of side effects increased with doses over 30 mcg/kg.

Resources

WEBSITES

Micromedex. "Plicamycin (Intravenous Route)." Mayo Clinic. http://www.mayoclinic.org/drugs-supplements/plicamycin-intravenous-route/description/drg-20065552 (accessed October 9, 2014).

Bob Kirsch
Rebecca J. Frey, PhD

Ploidy analysis

Definition

Ploidy analysis is a test that measures the amount of DNA in tumor cells. It is also called DNA ploidy analysis.

Purpose

DNA ploidy analysis is used in addition to the traditional grading system as another way to evaluate the malignancy of a tumor. The advantage of this test is that it provides a numeric and therefore objective evaluation of how aggressive the **cancer** might be. This test has not yet replaced traditional systems of **tumor grading**. It is used only to supplement those tests in order to give the doctor as much information about the nature of the tumor as possible. Doctors may also use this test to help predict how a tumor may respond to the planned therapy.

Precautions

This test requires a certain sample size in order to be performed; the specimens acquired in some biopsies may

KEY TERMS

Aneuploid—Any number of chromosomes except the normal two sets.

Diploid—Two sets of 23 chromosomes; the normal number in a human cell.

Ploidy—The number of sets of 23 chromosomes in a human cell.

Tetraploid—Four sets of chromosomes; the normal number in a human cell that is about to divide to form two new cells.

not provide enough material to run the test. It is also important in this test that only tumor material is used to create the population of cells that are analyzed, as any healthy tissue included can significantly affect the results. Interpretation of the numeric results of this test is still somewhat controversial. There is no commonly accepted system for interpreting the results; in addition, the results of the test can vary greatly from one part of a tumor to another.

The way the test should be used for optimum results in the management of cancer patients remains questionable due to many unexplored issues, and results due to the lack of data accumulated so early into its history. Although research has shown that in general, patients whose tumors have lots of cells with abnormal amounts of DNA have shorter survival times, the results of the test have not for the most part been that successful in predicting how an individual patient will do.

Description

Ploidy analysis is performed on a sample of the tumor to determine how many of the cells have the normal number of chromosomes and how many have more or less than the normal number (called aneuploid). Cancerous cells are rapidly dividing cells. When cells divide, there is a period before the actual division during which the cells have twice the normal number of chromosomes. Tumors with higher proportions of aneuploid cells are generally considered to be more aggressive tumors.

Taking a sample of a tumor is called a **biopsy**. How and where that is done depends on where the tumor is located. Tissue from the surface of body cavities like the mouth or the vagina can be easily sampled from a simple scraping in a doctor's office. For some types of tumors (such as in **breast cancer**), it is possible to extract

enough cells with a needle and syringe. Often, however, a surgical biopsy will need to be performed in the hospital. The tissue removed will be taken to a laboratory and analyzed.

Preparation

Patient preparation for the collection of a tumor sample through biopsy will vary depending on the site of the tumor. Most biopsies call for little preparation on the patient's part. For biopsies of internal organs, the patient may need to avoid eating after midnight before the test, in case a complication occurs and surgery may be necessary. Patients should try not to be fearful of the collection of the sample. Doctors will make the procedure as painless as possible by using appropriate anesthesia.

Aftercare

There may be a little soreness at the biopsy site for a few days following the procedure; acetaminophen or another over-the-counter painkiller can be used if the patient feels a need for pain relief. If the site becomes swollen, red, or hot to the touch, it may be infected and the patient should contact a physician.

Risks

The risks involved in this test are only the risks inherent in having a biopsy. Since this procedure uses tissue obtained through a biopsy already being performed for the purpose of grading the tumor, there are no additional risks to the patient involved as a result of the test. This test can also be performed on stored biopsy tissues that were obtained at some previous time.

Results

Normal human cells, most of the time, have two sets of 23 chromosomes, one from each parent, for a total of 46 chromosomes. Normal cells contain four sets—or 92 total chromosomes—for a very brief time right before they divide. Normal tissues have a largely homogeneous population of cells containing 46 chromosomes, with a very small percentage of dividing cells that contain 92.

Abnormal results

Tumors have many cells that are in the process of reproducing, so tumor tissues typically have a significant population of cells containing four sets of chromosomes that are about to divide, in addition to the large population of normal cells containing two sets of chromosomes. Tumor cells can also contain numerous other variations of the normal number. Any tissue comprising significant numbers of cells that have anything but two sets of chromosomes would be considered abnormal.

See also DNA flow cytometry.

Resources

BOOKS

Pollack, Jonathan R., ed. *Microarray Analysis of the Physical Genome: Methods and Protocols*. New York: Humana, 2009.

PERIODICALS

Kenney, B., Zieske, A., Rinder, H., Smith, B. "DNA Ploidy Analysis as an Adjunct for the Detection of Relapse in B-Lineage Acute Lymphoblastic Leukemia." *Leukemia & Lymphoma* 49, no. 1 (2008): 42–48. http://informahealthcare.com/doi/abs/10.1080/10428190701760052 (accessed November 14, 2014).

Wendy Wippel, M.S.

Pneumonectomy

Definition

Pneumonectomy is the medical term for the surgical removal of a lung.

Purpose

A pneumonectomy is most often used to treat lung **cancer** when less radical surgery cannot achieve satisfactory results. It may also be the most appropriate treatment for a tumor located near the center of the lung that affects the pulmonary artery or veins, which transport blood between the heart and lungs. In addition, pneumonectomy may be the treatment of choice when the patient has a traumatic chest injury that has damaged the main air passage (bronchus) or the lung's major blood vessels so severely that they cannot be repaired.

Description

In a conventional pneumonectomy, the surgeon removes the entire diseased lung. In a partial pneumonectomy, one or more lobes of a lung are removed. In an extrapleural pneumonectomy, the surgeon removes the lung, part of the membrane covering the heart (pericardium), part of the diaphragm, and the membrane lining the chest cavity (parietal pleura). Each type of operation is extensive and requires that the patient be given general anesthesia. An intravenous line inserted into one arm supplies fluids and medication throughout the operation, which usually lasts one to three hours.

The surgeon begins the operation by cutting a large opening on the same side of the chest as the diseased lung. This posterolateral **thoracotomy** incision extends down the side of the patient's body from a point below the shoulder blade, following the curvature of the ribs at the front of the chest. Sometimes the surgeon removes part of the fifth rib in order to provide a clearer view of the lung and greater ease in removing the diseased organ.

Once the patient is open, the surgeon performing a traditional pneumonectomy then:

- orders the anesthesia personnel to deflate (collapse) the diseased lung

- dissects and divides the major blood vessels, bronchus, pulmonary artery, superior pulmonary vein, and inferior pulmonary veins

- identifies and preserves the vagus, phrenic, and recurrent laryngeal nerves

- ligates or ties off the lung's major blood vessels to prevent bleeding into the chest cavity

- clamps the main bronchus to prevent fluid from entering the air passage

- cuts through the bronchus

- removes the lung

- staples or sutures the end of the bronchus that has been cut

- makes sure that air is not escaping from the bronchus

- inserts a temporary drainage tube known as a chest tube between the layers of the pleura (pleural space) to draw air, fluid, and blood out of the surgical cavity

- closes the chest incision

Demographics

Approximately 400,000 Americans die of lung disease every year. Lung disease is responsible for one in six deaths in the United States, according to

Types of pneumonectomies

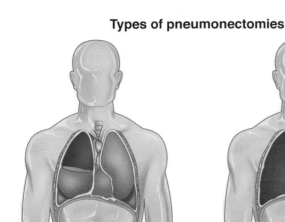
Partial pneumonectomy
(Lobectomy)

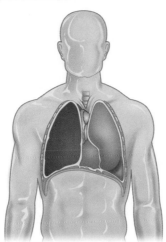
Pneumonectomy

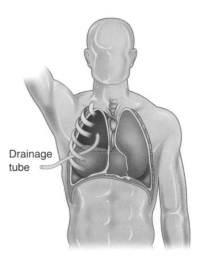
Drainage
tube

After a pneumonectomy, a
drainage tube is inserted in the
chest and the patient is closed
up. The drainage tubes drain
any fluids that may build up in
the chest.

A pneumonectomy is the removal of all or part of a lung. *(Illustration by Electronic Illustrators Group. © Cengage Learning®.)*

the American Lung Association. This statistic makes lung disease America's number three killer. More than 35 million Americans are now living with chronic lung disease. Lung disease costs the U.S. economy a total of $154 billion every year in direct health care expenditures and indirect costs.

Lung cancer

Lung cancer is the leading cause of cancer-related deaths in the United States. The American Cancer Society estimated that approximately 228,190 new cases of lung cancer were diagnosed in 2013, with lung cancer accounting for approximately 28% of all cancer deaths in 2012. It is the second most common cancer among both men and women and is the leading cause of death from cancer in both sexes. The five-year survival rate for all stages of lung cancer is only 16%; it was projected to claim more than nearly 159,480 lives in 2013. Lung cancer kills more people than cancers of the breast, prostate, colon, and pancreas combined.

Tobacco use is a major cause of lung cancer, and an estimated 438,000 Americans die each year from diseases directly related to cigarette smoking. **Second-hand smoke** contributes to the development of lung cancer among nonsmokers, and exposure to asbestos and other hazardous substances is also known to cause lung

cancer. Air pollution is another probable cause, but it makes a relatively small contribution to incidence and mortality rates. Indoor exposure to radon may also make a small contribution to the total incidence of lung cancer in certain geographic areas of the United States.

In each of the major racial/ethnic groups in the United States, the rates of lung cancer are higher among men than women. In 2009, African American males had the highest incidence of lung cancer, followed by Caucasian, Asian/Pacific Islander, American Indian/Alaska Native, and Hispanic men. Among women, Caucasian women had the highest rate followed by African American, American Indian/Alaska Native, Asian/Pacific Islander, and Hispanic women.

Diagnosis

In some cases, the diagnosis of a lung disorder is made when the patient consults a physician about chest pains or other symptoms. In cases involving direct trauma to the lung, the decision to perform a pneumonectomy may be made in the emergency room.

Lung cancer

The symptoms of lung cancer vary somewhat according to the location of the tumor; they may include

KEY TERMS

Bronchodilator—A drug that relaxes bronchial muscles, resulting in expansion of the bronchial air passages.

Bronchopleural fistula—An abnormal connection between an air passage and the membrane that covers the lungs.

Emphysema—A chronic disease characterized by loss of elasticity and abnormal accumulation of air in lung tissue.

Empyema—An accumulation of pus in the lung cavity, usually as a result of infection.

Pleural space—The small space between the two layers of the membrane that covers the lungs and lines the inner surface of the chest.

Pulmonary embolism—Blockage of a pulmonary artery by a blood clot or foreign matter.

Pulmonary rehabilitation—A program to treat COPD, which generally includes education and counseling, exercise, nutritional guidance, techniques to improve breathing, and emotional support.

persistent coughing, coughing up blood, wheezing, **fever**, and **weight loss**. Blood tests, a bone scan, and **computed tomography** scans of the head and abdomen will indicate whether the cancer has spread beyond the lungs. **Positron emission tomography** (PET) scanning is also used to help stage the disease.

Chronic obstructive pulmonary disease (COPD)

Chronic obstructive pulmonary disease (COPD) is one of the most common types of lung disease. Its primary symptoms include cough accompanied by phlegm or sputum and shortness of breath. COPD is most often caused by smoking, but other risk factors include:

• employment that requires working around dust and irritating fumes

• long-term exposure to secondhand smoke

• a family history of early COPD (before age 45)

Preparation

Before scheduling a pneumonectomy, the surgeon reviews the patient's medical and surgical history and orders a number of tests to help predict the surgery's success. Cardiac screening tests indicate how well the patient's heart will tolerate the procedure, and extensive pulmonary testing (e.g., breathing tests and quantitative

ventilation/perfusion scans) helps predict whether the remaining lung will be able to make up for the patient's diminished ability to breathe.

A patient who smokes must stop as soon as a lung disease is diagnosed. Patients should not take aspirin or ibuprofen for seven to ten days before surgery. Patients should also consult their physician about discontinuing any blood-thinning medications such as **warfarin** (Coumadin). The night before surgery, patients should not eat or drink anything after midnight.

Aftercare

Chest tubes drain fluid from the incision site, and a respirator helps the patient breathe for at least 24 hours after the operation. The patient may be fed and medicated intravenously. If no complications arise, the patient is transferred from the surgical intensive care unit to a regular hospital room within one to two days.

A patient who has had a conventional pneumonectomy will usually leave the hospital within ten days. Aftercare during hospitalization is focused on:

• relieving pain

• monitoring the patient's blood oxygen levels

• encouraging the patient to walk in order to prevent formation of blood clots

• encouraging the patient to cough productively in order to clear accumulated lung secretions

If the patient cannot cough productively, the doctor uses a flexible tube (bronchoscope) to remove the lung secretions and fluids.

Recovery is usually a slow process, with the remaining lung eventually taking on the work of the lung that has been removed. The patient may gradually resume normal non-strenuous activities. A pneumonectomy patient who does not experience postoperative problems may be well enough within eight weeks to return to a job that is not physically demanding; however, 60% of all pneumonectomy patients continue to struggle with shortness of breath six months after having surgery.

Risks

The risks for any surgical procedure requiring anesthesia include reactions to the anesthetic and breathing problems. The risks for any surgical procedure include bleeding and infection.

Between 40% and 60% of pneumonectomy patients experience such short-term postoperative difficulties as:

• prolonged need for a mechanical respirator

- heart problems, including abnormal heart rhythm (cardiac arrhythmia) or heart attack (myocardial infarction)
- pneumonia
- infection at the site of the incision
- a blood clot in the remaining lung (pulmonary embolism)
- an abnormal connection between the stump of the cut bronchus and the pleural space due to a leak in the stump (bronchopleural fistula)
- accumulation of pus in the pleural space (empyema)
- kidney or other organ failure

Over time, the remaining organs in the patient's chest may move into the space left by the surgery. This condition is called postpneumonectomy syndrome; the surgeon can correct it by inserting a fluid-filled prosthesis into the space formerly occupied by the diseased lung.

Results

The doctor will probably advise the patient to refrain from strenuous activities for a few weeks after the operation. The patient's rib cage will remain sore for some time.

A patient whose lungs have been weakened by noncancerous diseases like emphysema or chronic bronchitis may experience long-term shortness of breath as a result of this surgery. On the other hand, a patient who develops a fever, chest pain, persistent cough, or sudden shortness of breath, or whose incision bleeds or becomes inflamed, should notify his or her doctor immediately.

Morbidity and mortality rates

In the United States, the immediate survival rate for patients who have had the left lung removed is between 96% and 98%. Due to the greater risk of complications involving the stump of the cut bronchus in the right lung, between 88% and 90% of patients survive removal of this organ. Following lung volume reduction surgery, most investigators now report mortality rates of 5%–9%.

Alternatives

Lung cancer

The treatment options for lung cancer are surgery, **radiation therapy**, and **chemotherapy**, either alone or in combination, depending on the stage of the cancer.

After the cancer is found and staged, the cancer care team discusses the treatment options with the patient. In choosing a treatment plan, the most significant factors to consider are the type of lung cancer (small-cell or non-small cell) and the stage of the cancer. It is very important that the doctor order all the tests needed to determine the stage of the cancer. Other factors to consider include the patient's overall physical health; the likely side effects of the treatment; and the probability of curing the disease, extending the patient's life, and relieving his or her symptoms.

Chronic obstructive pulmonary disease

Although surgery is rarely used to treat COPD, it may be considered for people who have severe symptoms that have not improved with medication therapy. A significant number of patients with advanced COPD are at high risk of death despite advances in medical technology. This group includes patients who remain symptomatic despite the following:

- smoking cessation
- use of inhaled bronchodilators
- treatment with antibiotics (for acute bacterial infections) and inhaled or oral corticosteroids
- use of supplemental oxygen with rest or exertion
- pulmonary rehabilitation

After the severity of the patient's airflow obstruction has been evaluated and the foregoing interventions implemented, a pulmonary disease specialist should examine the patient, with consideration given to surgical treatment.

Surgical options for treating COPD include laser therapy or the following procedures:

- Bullectomy removes the part of the lung that has been damaged by the formation of large air-filled sacs called bullae.
- Lung volume reduction surgery removes a portion of one or both lungs, making room for the remaining lung tissue to work more efficiently. Its use is considered experimental, although it has been used in select patients with severe emphysema.
- Lung transplant replaces the diseased lung in a person with COPD with a healthy lung from a donor who has recently died.

Health care team roles

Pneumonectomies are performed in a hospital by a thoracic surgeon, who is a physician specializing in chest, heart, and lung surgery. Thoracic surgeons may further specialize in one area, such as heart surgery or lung surgery. They are board certified through the Board of **Thoracic Surgery**, which is recognized by the American Board of Medical Specialties. A general surgeon with specialized training in thoracic procedures may also perform pneumonectomies. A doctor becomes board certified by completing training in a specialty area and passing a rigorous examination.

QUESTIONS TO ASK YOUR DOCTOR

- Why is it necessary to remove the whole lung?
- What benefits can I expect from my pneumonectomy?
- What are the risks of this operation?
- What are the normal results?
- How long will my recovery take?
- What types of activities will be restricted after this surgery?
- What kind of pain and pain control is associated with this surgery?
- Are there any alternatives to this surgery?

Resources

BOOKS

Argenziano, Michael, and Mark E. Ginsburg, eds. *Lung Volume Reduction Surgery*. Totowa, NJ: Humana Press, 2002.

Khatri, V. P., and J. A. Asensio. *Operative Surgery Manual*. Philadelphia: Saunders, 2003.

Mason, Robert J., et al, eds. *Murray & Nadel's Textbook of Respiratory Medicine*. 5th ed. Philadelphia: Saunders/Elsevier, 2010.

Townsend, Courtney M., et al. *Sabiston Textbook of Surgery*. 19th ed. Philadelphia: Saunders/Elsevier, 2012.

PERIODICALS

Hu, Xue-fei, et al. "Risk Factors for Early Postoperative Complications After Pneumonectomy for Benign Lung Disease." *Annals of Thoracic Surgery* 95, no. 6 (2013): 1899–904. http://dx.doi.org/10.1016/10.1016/j.athoracsur.2013.03.051 (accessed October 3, 2014).

Philippakis, George E., and Marios Moustardas. "'Near Total' Pneumonectomy: Is It Feasible?" *International Journal of Surgery Case Reports* 4, no. 4 (2013): 422–24. http://dx.doi.org/10.1016/j.ijscr.2013.02.004 (accessed October 3, 2014).

Puri, Varun, et al. "Completion Pneumonectomy: Outcomes for Benign and Malignant Indications." *Annals of Thoracic Surgery* 95, no. 6 (2013): 1885–91. http://dx.doi.org/10.1016/j.athoracsur.2013.04.014 (accessed October 3, 2014).

Shah, A. A., et al. "Does Pneumonectomy Have a Role in the Treatment of Stage IIIA Non-Small Cell Lung Cancer?" *Annals of Thoracic Surgery* 95, no. 5 (2013): 1700–1707. http://dx.doi.org/10.1016/j.athoracsur.2013.02.044 (accessed October 3, 2014).

Slinger, Peter. "Update on Anesthetic Management for Pneumonectomy." *Current Opinion in Anaesthesiology* 22, no. 1 (2009): 31–37. http://dx.doi.org/10.1097/ACO.0b013e32831a4394 (accessed October 3, 2014).

Yunpeng, Liu, et al. "Right Lower Lobectomy Eight Years after Left Pneumonectomy for a Second Primary Lung Cancer." *Journal of Cardiothoracic Surgery* 8, no. 46 (2013). http://dx.doi.org/10.1186/1749-8090-8-46 (accessed October 3, 2014).

WEBSITES

A.D.A.M. Medical Encyclopedia. "Lung Surgery." MedlinePlus. http://www.nlm.nih.gov/medlineplus/ency/article/002956.htm (accessed October 3, 2014).

Aetna InteliHealth. "Lung Cancer." http://www.intelihealth.com/IH/ihtIH/WSIHW000/21827/24755/283984.html?d=dmtHealthAZ (accessed October 3, 2014).

American Lung Association. "Surgery." http://www.lung.org/lung-disease/copd/living-with-copd/surgery.html (accessed October 3, 2014).

American Thoracic Association. "Surgery in the COPD Patient." http://www.thoracic.org/clinical/copd-guidelines/for-health-professionals/management-of-stable-copd/surgery-in-and-for-copd/surgery-in-the-copd-patient.php (accessed October 3, 2014).

Cleveland Clinic. "Lung Volume Reduction Surgery." https://www.clevelandclinic.org/thoracic/Airway/Diagnosis_airway_Reduction.htm (accessed October 3, 2014).

Institute for Quality and Efficiency in Health Care. "Chronic Coughing and Breathing Difficulties: Chronic Obstructive Pulmonary Disease (COPD)." PubMed Health. http://www.ncbi.nlm.nih.gov/pubmedhealth/PMH0005192 (accessed October 3, 2014).

ORGANIZATIONS

American Association for Thoracic Surgery, 500 Cummings Ctr., Ste. 4550, Beverly, MA 01915, (978) 927-8330, http://aats.org.

American Cancer Society, 250 Williams St. NW, Atlanta, GA 30303, (800) 227-2345, http://www.cancer.org.

American Lung Association, 1301 Pennsylvania Ave. NW, Ste. 800, Washington, DC 20004, (202) 785-3355, (800) LUNG-USA (586-4872), http://www.lung.org.

American Thoracic Society, 25 Broadway, New York, NY 10004, (212) 315-8600, Fax: (212) 315-6498, atsinfo@thoracic.org, http://www.thoracic.org.

National Cancer Institute, 6116 Executive Blvd., Ste. 300, Bethesda, MD 20892-8322, (800) 4-CANCER (422-6237), http://cancer.gov.

National Comprehensive Cancer Network (NCCN), 275 Commerce Dr., Ste. 300, Fort Washington, PA 19034, (215) 690-0300, Fax: (215) 690-0280, http://www.nccn.org.

National Heart, Lung, and Blood Institute Information Center, PO Box 30105, Bethesda, MD 20824-0105, (301) 592-8573, Fax: (240) 629-3246, nhlbiinfo@nhlbi.nih.gov, http://www.nhlbi.nih.gov.

Maureen Haggerty
Crystal H. Kaczkowski, MSc
REVISED BY ROSALYN CARSON-DEWITT, MD
REVISED BY TAMMY ALLHOFF, CST/CSFA, AAS

Pneumonia

Definition

Pneumonia is a potentially life-threatening infection of one or both lungs. It is one of the most common pulmonary complications affecting **cancer** patients.

Description

Pneumonia is a serious inflammatory lung disorder in which the alveoli—tiny air-filled sacs in the lungs that ordinarily absorb oxygen from the air—fill with fluid or pus. As a result of this inflammation, the person cannot get enough oxygen into the bloodstream to meet the needs of body tissues. In addition, the disease organisms responsible for most cases of pneumonia can spread from the lungs into the bloodstream and infect other vital organs, resulting in death. Lobar pneumonia is a form of pneumonia that affects one section, or lobe, of the lung; bronchial pneumonia, or bronchopneumonia, affects scattered areas of either lung.

Pneumonia is not a single disease; it has at least 30 different causes. Although most cases of pneumonia are caused by bacteria, viruses, or other disease organisms, the illness can also be caused by chemical injuries to the lungs, food or saliva accidentally getting into the airway, or even by dust. It is possible for a patient to have bacterial and viral pneumonia at the same time.

Risk factors

Both cancer and the therapies used to treat it can injure the lungs or weaken the immune system, making cancer patients more susceptible to developing pneumonia. Tumors and infections can block the patient's airway or limit the lungs' ability to rid themselves of fluid and other accumulated secretions that make breathing difficult. Other factors that increase a cancer patient's risk of developing pneumonia (due to their impact on the immune system) include:

- radiation therapy
- chemotherapy
- surgery
- depressed white blood cell count (neutropenia)
- antibiotics
- steroids
- malnutrition
- limited mobility
- splenectomy-immune system deficits

Causes and symptoms

The risk of developing pneumonia is greatest for a cancer patient who has one or more additional health problems. Some patients who have pneumonia have few respiratory symptoms. Normally, however, a person with pneumonia has a high **fever**, chills, a cough with phlegm (productive cough), and chest pain.

In addition to the risk of pneumonia for cancer patients, a 2014 report showed that having a history of pneumonia may increase a person's risk of lung cancer. The risk was particularly high if the pneumonia had been diagnosed recently, or within the past two years.

Diagnosis

If pneumonia is suspected, the doctor will use a flexible tube (bronchoscope) to examine the lungs and airway (**bronchoscopy**) for inflammation, swelling, obstruction, and other abnormalities. The doctor may also remove a small piece of lung tissue (transbronchial **biopsy**) for microscopic examination and cultures and may prescribe medication to combat any fungal and viral organisms that may be responsible for the patient's symptoms. If the patient's condition continues to worsen, the doctor may remove additional lung tissue (thoracic needle biopsy or open **lung biopsy**) for microscopic analysis and cultures.

Treatment

Pneumonia in cancer patients must be treated promptly to speed the patient's recovery and prevent complications. To determine which course of treatment would be most appropriate, a doctor considers when symptoms first appeared, what pattern the illness has followed, and whether cancer or its treatments have diminished the patient's infection-fighting ability (**immune response**).

A doctor generally prescribes broad-spectrum oral **antibiotics** if:

- The patient has had a fever for less than a week.
- The pneumonia has not spread beyond the lung area where it originated.
- The patient's cancer is responding to treatment.
- The patient is otherwise in good health.

Although it is rarely used, a procedure called bronchoalveolar lavage, in which the lungs are washed out with a mucus-dissolving solution, may be performed if:

- The pneumonia is extensive, aggressive, or severe.
- Antibiotics do not clear the infection.
- The patient is very ill.

Alternative and complementary therapies

Nonmedical treatments will not cure pneumonia but may relieve symptoms and make the patient more comfortable. All of these therapies require the treating doctor's approval.

ACUPUNCTURE. Acupuncture may relieve congestion and reduce **fatigue**.

ESSENTIAL OILS. Added to a warm bath or vaporizer, essential oils of eucalyptus (*Eucalyptus globus*), lavender (*Lavandula officinalis*), or pine (*Abies sibirica*) can create a fragrant steam that may help the patient breathe more easily. Because steam inhalations can irritate the lungs, however, individuals who have asthma should not use them.

POSTURAL DRAINAGE. Postural drainage is a strenuous exercise that can help clear phlegm from the lungs. It should be practiced only with a doctor's approval and in the presence of a person who can provide support for a patient who becomes tired or weak.

Leaning over the side of the bed with forearms braced on the floor, the patient coughs up phlegm and spits it into a container. If the patient cannot cough productively enough to dislodge phlegm, the support person can help clear lung secretions by pounding gently on the patient's upper back. Postural drainage should be performed three times a day. Each session should last between five and fifteen minutes, unless the patient tires or weakens sooner.

MASSAGE. After the patient's fever has broken, gently massaging the upper back may relieve congestion and encourage productive cough.

HERBAL REMEDIES. Homemade cough medicines (expectorants) containing licorice (*Glycyrrhiza glabra*), black cherry (*Prunus serotina*) bark, raw onions, honey, and other natural ingredients may relieve congestion and encourage productive cough. Because natural substances can be poisonous, they should be used only with a doctor's approval and according to label directions.

Eating raw garlic (*Allium sativum*) or taking garlic supplements is believed to strengthen the immune system. Echinacea, brewed as tea or taken in liquid or capsule form, may help some patients recover more quickly.

VITAMINS. Zinc supplements and large doses of **vitamins** A, C, and E may strengthen the patient's immune system. Because large doses of some vitamins can cause **diarrhea** and other serious side effects, they should not be taken without a doctor's approval. Additionally, large doses of vitamins and herbal remedies may interfere with the primary cancer treatment programs. Approval from the treating physician is imperative.

Prevention

Cancer patients should work with their treatment team to prevent infections such as pneumonia. Those at particularly high risk of pneumonia may receive antibiotics while undergoing treatment to prevent pneumonia and other infections. Meanwhile, physicians and researchers continue to explore ways to prevent pneumonia related to cancer and cancer treatment. For example, doctors have found that performing minimally invasive lung surgery for lung cancer can reduce pain and risk of pneumonia. Minimally invasive surgery uses a few small incisions to allow surgeons to reach organs inside the body, guided by cameras on thin instruments and monitors.

See also Infection and sepsis.

Resources

BOOKS

Schmidt-Hieber, C., Daniel N. Ginn, and John N. Greene. "Pneumonia in Cancer Patients." In *Medical Care of Cancer Patients*. Shelton, CT: People's Medical Publishing House, 2009.

PERIODICALS

Denholm, Rachel, et al. "Is Previous Respiratory Disease a Risk Factor for Lung Cancer?" *American Journal of Respiratory and Critical Care Medicine* 190, no. 5 (2014): 549–59. http://dx.doi.org/10.1164/rccm.201402-0338OC (accessed November 5, 2014).

WEBSITES

American Lung Association. "Pneumonia Fact Sheet." http://www.lung.org/lung-disease/influenza/in-depth-resources/pneumonia-fact-sheet.html (accessed November 5, 2014).
The Scott Hamilton CARES Initiative. "Pneumonia." Chemocare.com. http://chemocare.com/chemotherapy/side-effects/pneumonia.aspx (accessed November 5, 2014).

ORGANIZATIONS

American Lung Association, 55 W. Wacker Dr., Ste. 1150, Chicago, IL 60601, (800) LUNG-USA (586-4872), Fax: (202) 452-1805, http://www.lung.org.

Maureen Haggerty
REVISED BY TERESA G. ODLE

Polyomavirus hominis type 1 (BK virus) infection

Definition

Infection with polyomavirus hominis type 1—commonly called BK virus or BKV—is ubiquitous in human populations. This pathogen normally causes problems only in immunocompromised individuals, primarily organ transplant recipients. However, a possible association between BKV and various cancers is the subject of ongoing research.

Description

As BKV is a so-called emerging virus, there remains a great deal to be learned about it. It was first isolated in 1971 from the urine of a Sudanese kidney transplant patient who was suffering from acute kidney failure and ureteral stenosis (constriction of the ureters—the ducts that carry urine from the kidney to the bladder). The virus was named with the patient's initials, B.K. There are two known species of polyomavirus that infect humans: BK (hominis 1) and JC (hominis 2). In healthy people BKV establishes a lifelong subclinical or latent infection, primarily in the kidneys and urinary tract. BKV replicates (reproduces itself) in the nuclei of proximal tubular cells of the human kidney, and the daughter viruses then spread to other cells.

Organ transplant recipients are treated with drugs that suppress their immune systems to prevent rejection of the transplanted organs. This immunosuppression can allow BKV to reactivate, causing severe disease in the kidney (nephropathy) and/or urinary bladder. In addition to reactivation of the latent virus, transplant patients may contract a primary BKV infection from the donor kidney or blood transfusions. Severe BKV nephritis (inflammation) or other BK virus-associated nephropathy (BKVAN) is a major cause of graft loss in kidney transplant recipients.

BKV has emerged as a major pathogen in bone marrow transplant recipients. It is associated with late-onset hemorrhagic cystitis (inflammation and bleeding of the urinary bladder), a rare but serious complication of **bone marrow transplantation** in children. BKV also can cause hemorrhagic cystitis in HIV/AIDS patients and kidney disease in other organ transplant recipients, such as liver transplant patients.

It has been known for some time that BKV, as well as some other primate polyomaviruses, can cause tumors in experimental animals. Infection of rodents with BKV often results in tumor formation. BKV DNA encodes two oncoproteins, large tumor (T) antigen and small tumor (t) antigen. When these oncoproteins are co-expressed (produced) along with activated oncogenes (human genes that have the potential to cause **cancer**), cultured human cells can be transformed into cancer cells. Specifically, BKV large T antigen appears to interact with the human tumor suppressor gene *TP53* to deregulate the control of cell growth.

BKV gene sequences and proteins have been found in a variety of human tumors. It has been suggested that BKV is associated with the development of:

- bladder cancers, especially in transplant patients
- urinary tract cancer
- chronic lymphocytic leukemia
- neuroblastomas, the most common malignancy in infants
- brain cancer
- colorectal cancer
- prostate cancer

Although BKV has been detected in both normal and abnormal prostate cells, large T antigen is detected much more frequently in cancerous prostates than in normal prostates. One suggestion is that BKV interferes with tumor suppression by protein p53 in the early stages of cancer development. Nevertheless, no clear relationship has been established between BKV infection and any human cancer.

Risk factors

The primary risk factor for active BKV infection is immune system suppression due either to immunosuppressive drugs administered to transplant recipients or to diseases such as HIV/AIDS.

Demographics

The vast majority of people become infected with BKV in early childhood, usually between the ages of four and five. Between 65% and 90% of all people are thought to be infected with BKV by the age of ten. The virus is found in humans throughout the world, except in a few very isolated communities. One study published in 2009 found that 92% of 451 control subjects had antibodies against BKV. Another 2009 study found that 82% of healthy blood donors tested positive for BKV.

BKV infection usually becomes symptomatic only in patients with suppressed immune systems. It has been estimated that the virus causes polyomavirus-associated nephropathy (PVAN) in 1–10% of kidney transplant recipients. Other researchers have estimated that up to 10% of kidney transplants fail because of BKV infection. Following the first identification of BKV in 1971, there were very few additional reports until 1995, when it was identified in about 1% of kidney transplant recipients. By 2001 the incidence had risen to 5% of kidney transplant recipients. BKV infection can be a serious problem for other transplant recipients as well. A 2009 study found that 42% of lung transplant recipients excreted BKV in their urine, an indication of active infection.

There have been occasional reports of reactivated BKV infection and viral shedding in the urine of patients who are not immunosuppressed. There also have been reports of PVAN arising in nontransplanted kidneys.

Causes and symptoms

Most people become infected with BKV in early childhood and perhaps even before birth. BKV is shed in saliva and may be transmissible through oral fluids. BKV can also be detected in 18% of stool samples from healthy adults and 46% of stool samples from hospitalized children. This finding suggests that BKV may be present in the gastrointestinal tract as well as the kidneys, and that it may be transmitted through feces. Initial infection with BKV rarely causes symptoms. When they do occur, symptoms are a mild **fever** or similar to those of a respiratory flu infection.

Symptoms of active BKV infection include:

• fever

• kidney problems or renal failure following an organ transplant

• interstitial nephritis following a kidney transplant

• narrowed ureters following a kidney transplant

• hemorrhagic cystitis following bone marrow transplantation

The major symptom of hemorrhagic cystitis is painful urination. Symptoms of kidney disease may include:

• changes in urine or patterns of urination

• swelling in the legs, ankles, feet, face, and/or hands from the failure of the kidneys to remove excess fluid

• fatigue due to anemia

• skin rash or itching from the buildup of waste products in the blood

• a metallic taste in the mouth and bad breath

• nausea and vomiting

• shortness of breath

• chills

• dizziness and difficulty concentrating

• pain in the back or leg

Diagnosis

Examination

A complete medical history and physical examination will be performed.

Tests

The presence of BKV in the urine or blood serum indicates an active BKV infection.

Procedures

Diagnosis of PVAN requires a renal biopsy—the removal of a small amount of tissue from the kidney. The

pathologist examines the tissue cells for changes that indicate polyomavirus activity. Immunohistochemical techniques are used to confirm infection with BKV.

Treatment

The primary treatment for active BKV infection is the reduction of immunosuppressive therapy in transplant recipients. Following renal graft loss to PVAN, retransplantation is an option.

Drugs

BKV infection may be treated with the antiviral drugs vidarabine and cidofovir and the anti-inflammatory drug leflunomide.

Prognosis

Untreated PVAN has a poor prognosis. The more advanced the kidney damage at the time of diagnosis, the poorer the prognosis. Although antiviral drugs have been used successfully to treat BKV infection, organ failure is common in BKV-infected transplant patients. In one study, BKV infection was associated with poorer survival among lung transplant patients.

Prevention

There is no known prevention for BKV infection. However, it is recommended that kidney transplant recipients be screened for the presence of BKV prior to the onset of kidney disease.

Resources

BOOKS

Ahsan, Nasimul. *Polyomaviruses and Human Diseases.* New York: Springer Science, 2006.

PERIODICALS

Abend, J. R., M. Jiang, and M. J. Imperiale. "BK Virus and Human Cancer: Innocent Until Proven Guilty." *Seminars in Cancer Biology* 19, no. 4 (August 2009). 252–60.

Egli, Adrian, et al. "Prevalence of Polyoma Virus BK and JC Infection and Replication in 400 Healthy Blood Donors." *Journal of Infectious Diseases* 199, no. 6 (March 15, 2009): 837–46.

WEBSITES

"Polyomaviruses." *MicrobiologyBytes*. http://www.microbiolo gybytes.com/virology/Polyomaviruses.html (accessed October 15, 2014).

"Polyomaviruses." *virology-online*. http://virology-online.com/ viruses/polyomaviruses.htm (accessed October 15, 2014).

ORGANIZATIONS

National Institute of Diabetes and Digestive and Kidney Diseases (NIDDK),Bethesda, MD 20892-2560, (301) 496-3583, http://www.niddk.nih.gov.

National Kidney Foundation, 30 E. 33rd St., New York, NY 10016, (800) 622-9010, info@kidney.org, http://www.kidney.org.

Margaret Alic, PhD

Pomalidomide

Definition

Pomalidomide (Pomalyst) is used to treat advanced **multiple myeloma**, a **cancer** of the bone marrow. Pomalidomide is a type of drug known as an immunomodulating agent.

Purpose

Pomalidomide is used alone or in combination with low-dose **dexamethasone** to treat multiple **myeloma** that has been treated with at least two other drugs, including lenalidomide (Revlimid) and **bortezomib** (Velcade), and that has progressed during treatment or within 60 days of the last treatment. The U.S. Food and Drug Administration (FDA) granted accelerated approval to pomalidomide in 2013. The approval was based on overall response rates of 7% in patients treated with pomalidomide alone and 20% in patients treated with a combination of pomalidomide and dexamethasone. Patients receiving the combination treatment had a median response duration of 7.4 months. As of 2014, improvement in symptoms or survival had not been demonstrated. Pomalidomide is also being studied for the treatment of other cancers and medical conditions.

Description

Pomalidomide is a derivative of a drug called **thalidomide** (Thalomid). Pomalidomide has potential

KEY TERMS

Angiogenesis—Blood vessel formation that is necessary for tumor growth and metastasis.

Dexamethasone—A corticosteroid that may be prescribed in combination with pomalidomide.

Immunomodulating—Affecting the immune response or immune-system functioning.

Multiple myeloma—A bone marrow cancer affecting multiple bones.

Natural killer (NK) cells—Lymphocytes that destroy tumor cells.

T cells—Immune-system cells that originate in the thymus gland; killer or cytotoxic T cells can destroy cancer cells.

Thalidomide—A drug similar to pomalidomide that was widely prescribed in the 1950s and caused severe fetal malformations and death.

Tumor necrosis factor (TNF)-alpha—A protein that activates immune system cells and induces the destruction of some tumor cells.

effects on immune system function (immunomodulating activity), the potential to block or slow tumor angiogenesis—the process by which cancers develop their own blood supply that enables them to survive, grow, and spread (metastasize)—and the potential to kill cancer cells in the bone marrow (antineoplastic activity). Pomalidomide also appears to stimulate the production of normal red blood cells by the bone marrow (erythropoiesis). It is not precisely clear how pomalidomide exerts its effects. It appears to inhibit the production of the immune system protein **tumor necrosis factor** (TNF)-alpha, as well as to enhance the activity of immune system T cells and natural-killer (NK) cells and the ability of the immune system to destroy cancer cells. It may also promote cell-cycle arrest in some tumor cell populations, so that the cells do not continue to grow and divide.

U.S. brand names

Pomalidomide, manufactured by Celgene Corporation, is marketed in the United States as Pomalyst capsules. It is also known as CC-4047.

Canadian brand names

Pomalidomide is marketed in Canada as Pomalyst.

International brand names

Pomalidomide was approved by the European Commission in August 2013 and is marketed in Europe as Imnovid. It is marketed in other countries as Pomalyst.

Recommended dosage

Pomalidomide is supplied as 1 milligram (mg), 2 mg, 3 mg, or 4 mg capsules. The usual dosage is one 4 mg capsule daily at least two hours before or two hours after a meal. It is taken at about the same time each day. It is taken daily for 21 days and then not taken for seven days. This 28-day cycle may be repeated. Pomalidomide should be taken exactly as prescribed—no more and no less. A missed dose should be taken as soon as possible, but if it is less than 12 hours before the next scheduled dose, the missed dose should be skipped and the regular schedule resumed. The capsule should be swallowed whole with water. Capsules should not be opened or handled more than necessary. If skin comes in contact with a broken capsule or the powder, the exposed area should be washed with soap and water. Serious side effects, including abnormal blood tests, may require delaying or lowering the dosage.

Precautions

Pomalidomide comes with a boxed warning concerning the risk of severe or life-threatening birth defects or fetal death if taken during pregnancy. The drug cannot be taken by patients who are pregnant or may become pregnant. The Pomalyst REMS program requires registration by all pomalidomide patients, even men and women who cannot become pregnant. The prescribing doctor and the pharmacy that fills the prescription must also be registered with Pomalyst REMS. This precaution is because a similar drug—thalidomide—that was widely prescribed in the 1950s for morning sickness during pregnancy led to the death or severe malformation of thousands of babies. Patients are given information about the risks of pomalidomide and must sign an informed consent stating that they understand the information. In addition:

- Women who could become pregnant—even women who have had tubal ligation (surgery to prevent pregnancy)—must use two methods of birth control approved by their doctor for four weeks before beginning pomalidomide, throughout treatment (even if treatment is temporarily halted), and for four weeks after treatment. These birth control methods must be used at all times unless the woman promises not to have any sexual contact with a male for four weeks before treatment, throughout treatment, and for four weeks afterwards. Women who have not menstruated for 24 consecutive months and have been declared by their doctor as postmenopausal or have had their uterus and/or both ovaries surgically removed may be excused from the birth control requirements.

- Women must have two negative pregnancy tests prior to starting pomalidomide. They will also have laboratory pregnancy tests during treatment.

- Because pomalidomide is present in semen, males taking the drug must use a latex or synthetic condom every time they have sexual contact with a female who is pregnant or could become pregnant. They must use a condom throughout the duration of their pomalidomide treatment and for four weeks after treatment, even if they have had a vasectomy.

- Males cannot donate sperm while taking pomalidomide and for four weeks after treatment ends.

- Patients cannot donate blood while taking pomalidomide and for four weeks after treatment ends.

- Pomalidomide must never be shared with anyone else.

It is not known whether pomalidomide affects fertility. It may affect blood cell counts, so blood tests are usually performed weekly for the first two months of treatment and at least once a month thereafter. Abnormal test results may require other medications or reducing, delaying, or halting pomalidomide treatment. Pomalidomide affects the immune system. Patients should not get any immunizations during or after treatment without their doctor's consent, as the drug could make the vaccine ineffective or cause a serious infection. Patients should avoid contact with anyone who has recently received a live virus vaccine, such as oral polio or smallpox. Pomalidomide also may:

- cause dizziness or confusion, so patients should not drive a car, operate machinery, or perform other tasks that require full alertness until they know how the drug affects them

- cause an allergic reaction in some people who have previously taken the similar drugs thalidomide or lenalidomide

- increase the risk of a blood clot in a leg that could move through the bloodstream to the lungs—patients may be prescribed medication, such as aspirin or warfarin (Coumadin), to reduce this risk

- lower white blood cell counts, increasing the risk of infection

- lower platelet counts, increasing the risk of bleeding

- lower red blood cell counts (anemia), usually a few weeks after starting treatment—this condition may require additional medications or even blood transfusions

- cause nerve damage (neuropathy)

- increase the risk of later developing leukemia

- increase the risk of developing other cancers

Pediatric

The safety and effectiveness of pomalidomide has not been evaluated in children under age 18.

Geriatric

In **clinical trials**, 41% of patients were 65 and older, and 12% were 75 and older. No overall differences in effectiveness were observed between older and younger patients; however, patients aged 65 and older were more likely than those aged 65 and younger to develop **pneumonia**. No dosage adjustment is required based on patient age.

Pregnant or breastfeeding

It is essential that women avoid pregnancy during and for four weeks after they or their partners take pomalidomide. Women must not breastfeed while taking pomalidomide.

Other conditions and allergies

Patients should inform their doctors if they have or have ever had any type of kidney or liver disease. These might interfere with clearing the drug from the body and cause side effects. Blood tests for kidney and liver function are performed before beginning treatment with pomalidomide. Patients should also inform their doctors if they:

- are allergic to anything, including medications, dyes, additives, or foods
- have ever had any major blood clots or bleeding problems
- have any other medical conditions, such as heart disease, diabetes, high blood pressure, gout, or infections

Side effects

The most common adverse reactions, affecting at least 30% of patients, are:

- weakness
- fatigue
- constipation
- nausea
- diarrhea
- low neutrophils (a type of white blood cell)
- anemia
- breathing difficulty
- upper respiratory tract infections
- back pain
- elevated body temperature

Other common side effects are:

- loss of appetite
- rash
- dizziness
- low platelet count with increased risk of bleeding
- swelling (edema) in the arms or legs
- pneumonia
- chest pain

Less common side effects include:

- fever, sometimes with chills
- muscle spasms
- joint or muscle pain
- itching
- dry skin
- vomiting
- cough
- nosebleeds
- headache
- weight loss
- bone pain
- anxiety
- confusion
- numbness or tingling in the hands or feet
- tremor
- urinary tract infections
- trouble sleeping
- excess sweating, especially at night
- high blood sugar levels
- blood tests showing abnormal levels of certain minerals
- kidney failure or blood test results showing kidney damage

Rare side effects include a(n):

- allergic reaction
- blood clot in the deep veins of the leg or in the lungs
- infection in the blood (sepsis)
- change in heart rhythm
- second cancer such as acute leukemia

Interactions

Pomalidomide may interact with many drugs and supplements. Patients should tell their doctors about any prescription or over-the-counter medicines, supplements, **vitamins**, and herbs that they are taking or intend to take. Patients should talk to their doctors before taking any drugs or supplements that could affect the ability to halt bleeding. These include aspirin and any medicines that contain aspirin, **warfarin** (Coumadin), any blood thinners, **heparin**, or vitamin E.

Drugs and supplements that may cause pomalidomide to build up in the blood and worsen side effects or cause other problems include:

- some antibiotics, such as erythromycin, clarithromycin, telithromycin, ciprofloxacin, and similar drugs

- antifungal medicines, such as ketoconazole, itraconazole, and voriconazole

- some antidepressants, such as nefazodone and fluvoxamine

- some HIV drugs, such as indinavir, ritonavir, nelfinavir, atazanavir, saquinavir, and others

- certain blood pressure medicines, such as diltiazem and verapamil

Smoking can lower the amount of pomalidomide in the blood and make it less effective. Drugs and supplements that can lower pomalidomide levels include:

- antiseizure drugs, such as carbamazepine, phenobarbital, and phenytoin

- tuberculosis drugs, such as rifampin, rifabutin, and rifapentine

- St. John's wort, an herbal supplement

Alcohol and some drugs that cause drowsiness—including tranquilizers, sleep aids, antidepressants, antihistamines, and muscle relaxants—may exacerbate pomalidomide side effects such as drowsiness, dizziness, and confusion. Grapefruit, grapefruit juice, or grapefruit extract could change the level of pomalidomide in the blood and may need to be avoided.

Resources

PERIODICALS

Bhogaraju, Sagar, and Ivan Dikic. "A Peek into the Atomic Details of Thalidomide's Clinical Effects." *Nature Structural & Molecular Biology* 21, no. 9 (September 2014): 739–40.

WEBSITES

Pazdur, Richard. "FDA Approval for Pomalidomide." July 3, 2013. http://www.cancer.gov/cancertopics/druginfo/fda-pomalidomide (accessed October 20, 2014).

"Pomalidomide." American Cancer Society. February 13, 2013. http://www.cancer.org/treatment/treatmentsandsideeffects/guidetocancerdrugs/pomalidomide (accessed October 20, 2014).

"Pomalidomide." MedlinePlus. July 15, 2013. http://www.nlm.nih.gov/medlineplus/druginfo/meds/a613030.html (accessed October 20, 2014).

ORGANIZATIONS

American Cancer Society, 250 Williams Street NW, Atlanta, GA 30303, (800) 227-2345, http://www.cancer.org.

National Cancer Institute, 6116 Executive Boulevard, Suite 300, Bethesda, MD 20892-8322, (800) 4-CANCER (422-6237), http://www.cancer.gov.

U.S. Food and Drug Administration, 10903 New Hampshire Avenue, Silver Spring, MD 20993-0002, (800) INFO-FDA (463-6332), http://www.fda.gov.

Margaret Alic, PhD

Pomalyst *see* **Pomalidomide**

Porfimer sodium

Definition

Porfimer sodium (trade name Photofrin) is a photosensitizing agent that belongs to a group of medicines known as antineoplastics. Porfimer sodium is sometimes called a hematoporphyrin derivative.

Purpose

Porfimer is used in a treatment called **photodynamic therapy** (PDT). This form of **cancer** treatment is for patients presenting with obstructing or partially obstructing esophageal and endobronchial non-small cell lung cancers (NSCLC) and early-stage radiologically occult endobronchial cancer. It is also approved for use in treating **Barrett's esophagus**, a condition that can lead to **esophageal cancer**.

Porfimer is sometimes prescribed to treat certain types of biliary tract cancer (cholangiocarcinoma), but it is not approved by the U.S. Food and Drug Administration (FDA) for this purpose.

Description

The FDA granted its original approval to porfimer sodium in December 1995. Porfimer is a chemical mixture of up to eight porphyrin units. The freeze-dried compound exists as a dark red to reddish-brown cake or powder and is typically reconstituted with 5% dextrose or 0.9% sodium chloride. Porfimer sodium's antitumor effects are dependent upon its activation by a specific wavelength of light that results in the subsequent release of highly toxic oxygen free radicals. Additionally, PDT using porfimer produces a significant decrease in blood flow to the treatment area that enhances necrosis in certain tumor cells. Clinical test results suggest that use of porfimer sodium for the palliative management of esophageal cancer and NSCLC yields a statistically significant improvement after a single course of therapy. Porfimer sodium and the associated laser treatment have not been formally tested in conjunction with other photosensitizing compounds; however, it may be speculated that an increase in the photosensitive reaction would result.

Recommended dosage

The dose of porfimer sodium will vary among patients. The oncologist will make a final dose determination based on a number of factors, including body weight. An appropriate starting regimen for adults would be:

- 2 mg porfimer per kg of body weight injected into a vein.
- Approximately 48 hours post injection, tumor illumination with a laser light source set at 630 nm wavelength.
- Two to three days post tumor illumination, the physician will remove the destroyed cancer cells.
- If prescribed, a second laser treatment may be given 96–120 hours after the initial porfimer injection followed by subsequent removal of destroyed cancer cells.
- Patients may receive a second dose of porfimer at a minimum of 30 days from the initial treatment for up to three cycles, each 30 days apart.

Precautions

All patients who have received PDT must avoid exposure of the skin and eyes to direct sunlight and bright indoor lighting for a minimum of 30 days. In July 2000, the FDA added the following to patient information labeling of Photofrin: "Some patients may remain photosensitive for up to 90 days or more." Sensitivity results from the residual porfimer that has not cleared the patient's system; therefore, ambient indoor lighting will help to gradually quench the photosensitive effect. Intermittent exposure trials of a small patch of skin to direct sunlight should be conducted in 10-minute segments beginning 30 days after PDT, and before returning to normal outdoor activities. If no photosensitive reaction (redness, edema, blistering) is apparent 24 hours after exposure, cautious and gradually increased exposure may continue. If the test results are positive, patients should continue precautions for an additional two weeks before repeating the exposure test. Over-the-counter sunscreens are of no use because the photoactivation of porfimer occurs in the visible light range. Patient eye sensitivity should be guarded for a minimum of 30 days by wearing dark sunglasses that allow for no greater than 4% of available white light to pass through the lenses. PDT treatment scheduling before or after **radiation therapy** should be properly spaced to avoid any cumulative inflammatory response from one treatment regimen to the next. A two- to four-week recovery phase between treatment types is recommended. Careful monitoring of endobronchial lesion patients is required to reduce the risk of respiratory distress caused by necrotic tissue obstructing the airway. These patients are also at risk of bleeding problems associated with erosion into a major blood vessel. As with all **antineoplastic agents**, pregnancy should be avoided. If the patient is pregnant, PDT should be used only if the potential benefits outweigh the risks to the fetus.

Side effects

Side effects are associated with all antineoplastic drugs, and patients should be instructed to discuss any concerns. Side effects seen with porfimer that may engender patient concern but do not typically require medical attention include mild **diarrhea** or constipation, mild **nausea and vomiting**, blistering, redness or swelling of the skin, difficulty sleeping, weakness, and vision changes. These conditions usually subside as the body adjusts to the porfimer. Side effects associated with porfimer sodium that do require immediate medical attention include:

- shortness of breath or trouble breathing
- fast or irregular heartbeat
- high or low blood pressure
- spitting blood
- severe stomach, abdominal, or chest pain
- chills or fever
- dizziness or fainting
- coughing or wheezing
- unusual weight gain
- excessive fatigue or weakness
- swelling in the face, feet, neck, or lower legs
- white patches in the mouth
- tightness in the chest
- yellow coloration of the eyes or skin

Interactions

There have been no formal interaction studies between porfimer and other drugs. One may speculate, however, on the possible synergistic effects of porfimer in conjunction with other photosensitizing agents, such as phenothiazines, chlorpropamide, **demeclocycline**, doxycycline, and tetracycline. Animal research studies suggest that certain compounds decrease the effectiveness of porfimer used in PDT. These inhibitors include drug compounds such as dimethyl sulfoxide (DMSO) and ethanol, which act by inhibiting the formation of free radicals. Other drug groups, such as thromboxane A_2 inhibitors, inhibit by decreasing clotting, vasoconstriction, or platelet aggregation. Other preclinical trial data suggest a decrease in porfimer efficacy in PDT in response to glucocorticoid hormones, calcium channel blockers, and prostaglandin synthesis inhibitors. As with any course of treatment, patients should first notify their doctors of any medications they are taking.

Resources

BOOKS

Beers, Mark H., MD, and Robert Berkow, MD, editors. "Tumors of the Gastrointestinal Tract." Section 3, Chapter 34 In *The Merck Manual of Diagnosis and Therapy*. Whitehouse Station, NJ: Merck Research Laboratories, 2004.

Gomer, Charles J., ed. *Photodynamic Therapy: Methods and Protocols*. New York: Springer, 2010.

PERIODICALS

Chan, H. H., N. S. Nishioka, M. Mino, et al. "EUS-Guided Photodynamic Therapy of the Pancreas: A Pilot Study." *Gastrointestinal Endoscopy* 59 (January 2004): 95–99.

Cuenca, R. E., R. R. Allison, C. Sibata, and G. H. Downie. "Breast Cancer with Chest Wall Progression: Treatment with Photodynamic Therapy." *Annals of Surgical Oncology* 11 (March 2004): 322–327.

Schmidt, M. H., G. A. Meyer, K. W. Reichert, et al. "Evaluation of Photodynamic Therapy Near Functional Brain Tissue in Patients with Recurrent Brain Tumors." *Journal of Neurooncology* 67 (March-April 2004): 201–207.

WEBSITES

U.S. National Library of Medicine. "PHOTOFRIN—Porfimer Sodium Injection, Powder, for Solution." http://dailymed. nlm.nih.gov/dailymed/drugInfo.cfm?setid=f5fdda24-da7d-4e61-936e-9d1a55056b82 (accessed November 18, 2014).

ORGANIZATIONS

U.S. Food and Drug Administration, 10903 New Hampshire Ave., Silver Spring, MD 20993, (888) INFO-FDA (463-6332), http://www.fda.gov.

Jane Taylor-Jones, MS
Rebecca J. Frey, PhD

Positron emission tomography

Definition

Positron emission tomography (PET) is a noninvasive scanning/imaging technique that utilizes small amounts of radioactive positrons (positively charged particles; also called antielectrons) to visualize body function and metabolism. The PET scan uses a special camera and tracer (such as glucose with an added radioactive chemical) to take images of organs and tissues within the body. The camera records the position of the tracer, and the resulting data are then sent to a computer for analysis.

When higher levels of chemical activity occur in the body, the radioactive chemical within the tracer will accumulate in such areas. These areas show up as brighter spots on a PET scan and are useful for evaluating

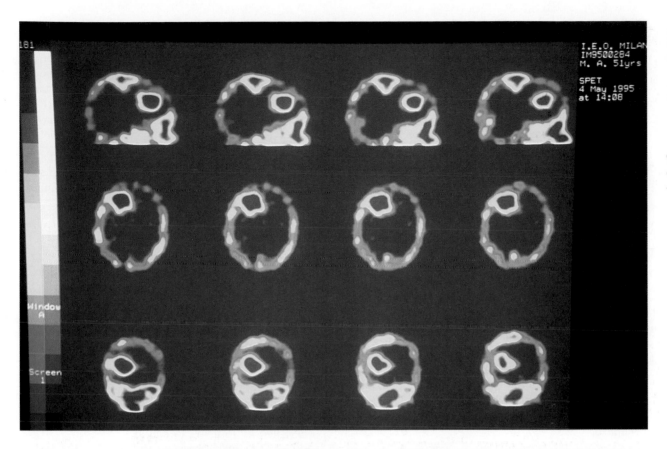

Positron emission tomography (PET) images of an oncology patient's brain. PET imaging can be used to differentiate between malignant (cancerous) and benign (noncancerous) cell growths, assess the spread of malignant tumors, and detect recurrent brain tumors. *(Marka/Custom Medical Stock Photography)*

problems within the body. The resulting image is used to evaluate for disorders such as **cancer**, neurological problems, and heart disease, as well as the flow of blood and the function of organs. PET scans are especially useful to study brain activity in patients with mental illness and the ways in which mental illness can change activity within the brain.

Purpose

PET is the fastest-growing nuclear medicine tool in terms of increasing acceptance and applications. It is useful in the diagnosis, staging, and treatment of cancer because it provides information that cannot be obtained by other techniques, such as **computed tomography** (CT) and **magnetic resonance imaging** (MRI).

PET scans are performed at medical centers equipped with a small cyclotron. Smaller cyclotrons and increasing availability of certain **radiopharmaceuticals** are making PET a more widely used imaging modality.

Physicians first used PET to obtain information about brain function and to study brain activity in various

neurological diseases and disorders, including stroke, epilepsy, Alzheimer's disease, Parkinson's disease, and Huntington's disease, and in psychiatric disorders such as schizophrenia, **depression**, obsessive-compulsive disorder (OCD), attention-deficit hyperactivity disorder (ADHD), and Tourette syndrome. PET is now used to evaluate patients for types of cancer, including head and neck, brain, **lymphoma**, **melanoma**, lung, colorectal, breast, prostate, and esophageal. Cancer is more likely to show up on a PET scan than on a CT or MRI scan, and PET imaging is very accurate in differentiating malignant from benign growths.

Because of the clarity of a PET scan, doctors can better see how advanced a cancer is at its place or origin and whether it has spread to other parts of the body. It may also be used to help physicians design the most beneficial therapies—for example, it may be used to assess a patient's response to **chemotherapy**.

Description

Whether the test is done in a nuclear medicine department of a hospital or a specialized PET center, the

PET involves injecting a patient with a radiopharmaceutical similar to glucose, a form of sugar. Often fludeoxyglucose (FDG), which contains a radioactive isotope (such as fluorine-18), is used as the trace material. The tracer is a liquid that is placed into the body, usually through an intravenous injection into a vein on the arm. The substance may also be inhaled or swallowed. While the patient lies very still on a table, the tracer moves through the body, collecting in specific organs or tissues. An hour after injection of this tracer, a PET scanner images a specific metabolic function by measuring the concentration and distribution of the tracer throughout the body. The scanner, which is shaped like a doughnut, moves around the patient. The complete test usually takes from one to three hours.

When it enters the body, the tracer courses through the bloodstream to the target organ, where it emits positrons. The positively charged positrons collide with negatively charged electrons, producing gamma rays (a type of electromagnetic radiation). The positrons are absorbed to a different extent by cells varying in their metabolic rate. The gamma rays are detected by photomultiplier-scintillator combinations positioned on opposite sides of the patient. These signals are processed by the computer, and images are generated.

PET scans do not show as much detail as CT scans or MRI scans. However, PET scans provide an advantage over CT and MRI because they can determine whether a lesion is malignant. The two other modalities provide images of anatomical structures but often cannot provide a determination of malignancy. CT and MRI show structure, while PET shows function. PET has been used in combination with CT and MRI to identify abnormalities with more precision and indicate the areas of most active metabolism. This additional information allows for more accurate evaluation of cancer treatment and management.

Precautions

Several precautionary factors may cause the PET scan to be canceled or invalidated. Three factors that might cancel the test are using alcohol, caffeine, or tobacco within 24 hours of the test; using sedatives before the test; or taking medicines such as insulin (which can change a body's metabolism). Two conditions that may invalidate the test include not lying still during the test or being too anxious or nervous during the test. In addition, a PET scan may have to be delayed if a patient recently had a **biopsy** taken from the body, chemotherapy, **radiation therapy**, or any type of surgery.

Preparation

Before having or scheduling a PET scan, patients should inform the referring doctor if they have diabetes, are pregnant, or are breast-feeding. The dosage of any diabetic medicine on the day of the scan may be reduced or eliminated to accommodate the PET procedure. Nursing mothers should not breast-feed for at least one day before having a PET scan and should discuss this with their physician before having the test. In addition, tell the referring doctor about any other medicines or herbal remedies being taken. Such substances may be stopped before the PET test. Do not smoke tobacco products, consume caffeinated beverages or foods, or drink alcoholic beverages for at least 24 hours before the test. Do not eat or drink for at least 6 hours before the test. Discuss the PET scan with the referring doctor or the attending medical team for other such considerations. Inform the referring doctor if a fear of enclosed spaces is a problem or of any concerns regarding anxiety or panic attacks while undergoing the test.

During the test, a small prick or sting may be felt at the injection site. When the tracer liquid is inserted into the body, it may initially make the patient feel warm and slightly flushed. In a small number of instances, patients feel sick to their stomach or may develop a headache. Always inform the medical staff if this reaction occurs.

Aftercare

Resume a normal schedule and level of activity after the scan is complete. Drink plenty of water or other fluids throughout the rest of the day to flush the tracer out of the body.

Risks

A consent form may be required to be signed before the test. Discuss any potential risks of the PET scan with the referring physician or other medical professional. Risk of slight damage to cells or tissue is possible but minimal from the low levels of radiation used for the test. Most of the radioactive tracer is flushed out of the body within 6 to 24 hours. The tracer may cause an allergic reaction, but such incidents are rare. The injection site of the tracer may become sore or swell. If so, the medical staff will apply a warm, moist compress and check the area from time to time for any other medical needs. Benefits usually are considered when talking with a medical professional about this test, and whether they outweigh the risks.

Results

The images produced during these scans are normally sent to the attending physician. Make an appointment with this medical professional to discuss the results of the scan. Results normally are available to the doctor within one to two days. A normal result means that blood flow is normal, and the organs and tissues examined are operating as they should. With this result, the tracer has flowed through the body in a normal distribution.

An abnormal result means different things depending on the portion of the body scanned. If the heart has been scanned, then a decreased flow of blood into or out of the heart and increased glucose metabolism may indicate that blood vessels are blocked. One possible diagnosis may be the presence of coronary artery disease; however, a medical professional is best prepared to make that determination. If the brain was scanned, and a decreased flow of blood and oxygen and an increased glucose metabolism were found, then epilepsy is one of several possible diagnoses. If only a decreased flow of blood and oxygen was found, then one probable diagnosis is a stroke. On the other hand, if only a decreased glucose metabolism was discovered, then dementia may be a possible diagnosis. In all cases, doctors will thoroughly review the results to make a determination as to why this abnormal result occurred. In

---

QUESTIONS TO ASK YOUR DOCTOR

- How long will the examination take?
- What may prevent me from having a PET scan?
- Is PET the best option for visualizing my condition?
- When will the results be provided to me?
- Will I need to have someone with me during the imaging study? Will this person need to drive me home?
- What special precautions should be taken with a child?
- Should I expect any side effects?
- How many scans should I have in any one year? How far apart should they be spaced?

---

many cases, further tests will be performed to validate the results of the PET scan.

Resources

BOOKS

Armstrong, Peter, Martin L. Wastie, and Andrea G. Rockall. *Diagnostic Imaging.* Chichester, UK: Wiley-Blackwell, 2009.

Granov, A. M., L. A. Tiutin, and Thomas Schwarz. *Positron Emission Tomography.* New York: Springer, 2013.

Lin, Eugene, and Abass Alavi. *PET and PET/CT: A Clinical Guide.* New York: Thieme, 2009.

Lynch, T. B., J. Clarke, and G. Cook. *PET/CT in Clinical Practice.* London: Springer-Verlag, 2007.

Valk, Peter P., et al, eds. *Positron Emission Tomography: Clinical Practice.* London: Springer, 2006.

PERIODICALS

Ko, Ji Hyun, Chris C. Tang, and David Eidelberg. "Brain Stimulation and Functional Imaging with fMRI and PET." *Handbook of Clinical Neurology* 116 (2013): 77–95. http://dx.doi.org/10.1016/B978-0-444-53497-2.00008-5 (accessed October 3, 2014).

WEBSITES

Cancer Research UK. "PET Scan." http://www.cancerresearchuk.org/cancer-help/about-cancer/tests/pet-scan (accessed October 3, 2014).

Radiological Society of North America. "Positron Emission Tomography—Computed Tomography (PET/CT)." RadiologyInfo.org. http://www.radiologyinfo.org/en/info.cfm?pg=pet (accessed October 3, 2014).

Society of Nuclear Medicine and Molecular Imaging. "Fact Sheet: What is PET?" http://www.snm.org/index.cfm?PageID=11123 (accessed October 3, 2014).

ORGANIZATIONS

American College of Radiology, 1891 Preston White Dr., Reston, VA 20191, (703) 648-8900, info@acr.org, http://www.acr.org.

National Cancer Institute, 6116 Executive Blvd., Ste. 300, Bethesda, MD 20892-8322, (800) 4-CANCER (422-6237), http://cancer.gov.

National Institute of Biomedical Imaging and Bioengineering, 9000 Rockville Pike, Bldg. 31, Rm. 1C14, Bethesda, MD 20892-8859, (301) 469-8859, info@nibib.nih.gov, http://www.nibib.gov.

Radiological Society of North America (RSNA), 820 Jorie Blvd., Oak Brook, IL 60523-2251, (630) 571-2670, (800) 381-6660, http://www.rsna.org.

Society of Nuclear Medicine and Molecular Imaging, 1850 Samuel Morse Dr., Reston, VA 20190, (703) 708-9000, feedback@snm.org, http://www.snm.org.

Dan Harvey
Lee A. Shratter, MD
REVISED BY WILLIAM A. ATKINS

Predisposition of cancer *see* **Cancer predisposition**

Prednisone *see* **Corticosteroids**

Pregnancy and cancer

Definition

Cancer during pregnancy is uncommon, occurring in approximately one in 1,000 pregnancies. When cancer does occur, it is usually unrelated to the pregnancy; the exception is choriocarcinoma, which occurs only in conjunction with pregnancy. The most common cancers during pregnancy are those that more often affect younger women—breast cancer, **cervical cancer**, **Hodgkin lymphoma**, **thyroid cancer**, and **melanoma**. The cancer rarely harms the fetus, and some cancer treatments are safe during pregnancy.

Description

For pregnant women who have not had regular medical exams, prenatal visits and screenings can be an opportunity for detecting hidden cancer. However, cancer diagnosis creates a complicated dilemma for the pregnant woman and her healthcare providers. Although rarely the cause of maternal mortality, there are always two patients to consider when cancer is diagnosed during pregnancy—the mother and the fetus—and the health of the mother may be pitted against fetal well-being. Although some cancers may spread to the placenta, most cancers

---

KEY TERMS

Cesarean delivery—Infant delivery through an incision in the abdominal wall and uterus.

Choriocarcinoma—A malignant tumor that typically develops in the uterus following pregnancy, miscarriage, or abortion, especially in association with a hydatidiform mole.

Colposcopy—A procedure in which a lighted instrument with magnifying lenses (a colposcope) is used to visualize and examine the vagina and cervix, and biopsy suspicious cells for examination by a pathologist.

Ectopic pregnancy—A pregnancy that occurs outside the uterus, most commonly in a fallopian tube.

Gestational trophoblastic disease (GTD)—A group of related rare tumors that arise during pregnancy or after childbirth from embryonic tissue and include hydatidiform mole, choriocarcinoma, and placental-site trophoblastic tumors.

Hydatidiform mole—Multiple cysts arising from the degeneration of chorionic villi—early fetal tissue that is imbedded into the uterine lining—and characterized by an enlarged uterus and vaginal bleeding.

Microcephaly—A congenital anomaly in which the head is small in proportion to the body, the brain is underdeveloped, and there is some degree of mental retardation.

Molar pregnancy—A complete or partial hydatidiform mole, in which the ovum is fertilized but lacks genetic material or the fetus has multiple anomalies and eventually dies; complete evacuation of the uterus is necessary to avoid the development of choriocarcinoma.

Placenta—The organ that develops in the uterus during pregnancy and connects the mother's blood supply with that of the fetus.

Teratogenic—Affecting normal fetal development, leading to congenital malformations; teratogens include alcohol, certain medications, and radiation.

---

cannot spread to the baby, and pregnant women with cancer can give birth to healthy babies.

Gestational trophoblastic disease (GTD)

GTD is a group of rare, related tumors that arise during pregnancy or after childbirth from embryonic tissue called the chorion and chorionic villi. Signs of GTD include vaginal bleeding and high levels of human chorionic gonadotropin (hCG). The incidence of GTD increases with maternal age. There are three main types of GTD.

A hydatidiform mole or molar pregnancy arises from an abnormally fertilized egg cell. It occurs in one of every 1,000–1,200 pregnancies in the United States. A complete molar pregnancy is a fertilized egg cell that lacks the mother's genetic material, so that there is no fetal tissue; rather, small cysts fill the uterus. A partial molar pregnancy results from more than one sperm fertilizing the egg, so that the placenta consists of both normal tissue and cysts. Molar pregnancies are diagnosed by ultrasound, and the tissue is evacuated and examined for cancerous cells. Most molar pregnancies are not cancerous and are simply removed from the uterus. However, about 20% of complete molar pregnancies and 1–4% of partial hydatidiform moles are cancerous, spreading within the uterine wall or metastasizing to other parts of the body, especially the lungs. More than 98% of women who have a molar pregnancy have future successful pregnancies.

Choriocarcinoma, which occurs in only one out of every 20,000–40,000 pregnancies, is a malignant type of GTD that spreads rapidly through the mother's body and requires aggressive treatment. It can arise from a molar pregnancy or from tissue remaining in the uterus after a miscarriage or normal childbirth. **Chemotherapy** is very effective in treating choriocarcinoma.

A placental-site trophoblastic tumor is a very rare type of GTD that occurs at the site of placental attachment in the uterus. It does not usually spread beyond the uterus.

Breast cancer

As the second most common cancer in women after **skin cancer**, **breast cancer** is also the most common cancer during pregnancy, affecting approximately one in 3,000 pregnant women. In women who are pregnant or have just given birth, breast cancer is most common between the ages of 32 and 38. Infiltrating ductal **carcinoma** is the most prevalent type of breast cancer in both pregnant and non-pregnant women. Pregnancy-related breast enlargement and tenderness can make it difficult to detect small tumors, and most women do not have screening mammograms while pregnant. Pregnancy also increases the density of the breasts and makes **mammography** less sensitive. As a result, breast cancer in women who are pregnant or have just given birth is often diagnosed two to six months later than in other women. Therefore, pregnant women should perform breast self-exams and have clinical breast exams during routine prenatal and postnatal visits.

QUESTIONS TO ASK YOUR DOCTOR

- What type and stage is my cancer?
- How do my treatment options differ because of my pregnancy?
- What is your experience in treating pregnant women with cancer?
- Could delaying treatment affect my prognosis?
- What are the possible effects on my baby from the proposed treatment?

Ultrasound can be used to differentiate between a fluid-filled lump and a solid tumor. Breast tumors are evaluated as estrogen receptor (ER)-positive or ER-negative. Pregnancy hormones accelerate the growth of ER-positive tumors. Pregnancy hormones can also alter test results and increase the risk of false negatives. About 67% of pregnant women with breast cancer have positive lymph nodes, as compared with 38% of non-pregnant women. The five-year survival for pregnant women with positive lymph nodes is also lower than that for non-pregnant women with positive nodes. Pregnant women may have bleeding from any procedures performed on the breast due to increased vascularization.

Pregnancy also helps protect against breast cancer. Full-term pregnancy in younger women lowers their lifetime risk of the disease.

Cervical cancer

Approximately 0.5%–5.0% of cervical cancers occur in pregnant women. Survival rates are similar for pregnant and non-pregnant women with cervical cancer. A **Pap test** performed as part of standard prenatal care can detect cervical cancer. Suspicious findings may lead to a colposcopy and **biopsy**. There may be increased bleeding from the biopsy site during pregnancy. If the cancer is early-stage, the pregnancy is usually carried to term, and treatment, usually a hysterectomy, is performed several weeks after childbirth. If the cancer is at a later stage and the pregnancy is advanced, a cesarean delivery is performed as soon as the baby is mature enough, and cancer treatment is initiated immediately.

Hodgkin lymphoma

The average age for a diagnosis of Hodgkin lymphoma is 30. Hodgkin occurs in about one in 6,000 pregnancies. Signs such as **fever**, **night sweats**, and unexplained **weight loss** indicate a later stage of disease.

A nodal biopsy can be safely performed during pregnancy, but pregnancy can alter the test results. The prognosis for a pregnant woman is about the same as for other women. Treatment may include a short course of chemotherapy and radiation to the affected nodal area if the fetus can be adequately shielded. Otherwise, radiation may be postponed until after delivery. **Non-Hodgkin lymphoma** usually occurs after the childbearing years.

Melanoma

Since the average age for diagnosis of malignant melanoma is 45, about 30–40% of cases develop during the childbearing years, and about 8% of women are pregnant at the time of diagnosis. During pregnancy, the thickness of the lesion is greater, and nodal metastases occur more frequently. If there has been nodal **metastasis**, survival may be less than three years. Because most lesions occur on the extremities, treatment may begin during pregnancy. Melanoma can spread to the placenta and fetus. However, the prognosis is better if the pregnancy is carried to term: there is a five-year survival rate of 66.5% versus 33.5% if the pregnancy is terminated.

Ovarian cancer

Ovarian cancer is extremely rare during pregnancy, occurring in only one in 10,000–100,000 full-term pregnancies. It is usually a low-grade and early-stage cancer (stage 1). Germ-cell malignancies are the most common form of ovarian cancer in young women. Prenatal ultrasound may provide the first sign of ovarian cancer. Ovarian tumors can undergo torsion or twisting, creating extreme pain that may be mistaken for appendicitis or an ectopic pregnancy.

Colorectal cancer

Colorectal cancer is the third most common cancer in women. About 10% of cases occur in patients under age 40 and about 2% under the age of 30. Early occurrence is associated with high risk. Signs of colorectal cancer include nausea, abdominal bloating, backache, rectal bleeding, pain, and a change in bowel habits. There can be a delay in diagnosis, since some of these symptoms coincide with pregnancy symptoms. Because of this delay, the disease may be more advanced at diagnosis. Women considering pregnancy may request colorectal screening prior to becoming pregnant.

Leukemia

Leukemia is very rare during pregnancy, occurring in one woman out of 75,000. Acute myelocytic leukemia is the most common type during pregnancy. If treatment is initiated immediately, the prognoses and complete remission rates for pregnant women are similar to those for other women. Untreated, the disease can quickly become fatal. Women with leukemia are at greater risk of miscarriage, fetal growth retardation, premature birth, and stillbirth.

Causes

As more women delay childbearing, the incidence of cancer during pregnancy is increasing, as childbearing age overlaps with the age of occurrence of certain cancers. The exact cause of most cancers is not known. However, estrogen plays a role in the development of breast, endometrial, and ovarian cancers. Smoking increases the risk of cervical and certain other cancers.

Treatment

Cancer treatment usually involves some combination of surgery, radiation, and chemotherapy. Treatment options during pregnancy depend on the gestational stage and the type, size, and stage of the cancer. If possible, treatment may be delayed until after the baby is born, but this delay may be dangerous for the mother or make the cancer more difficult to treat. During the first trimester (first 12 weeks of gestation), fetal organs are developing and are very susceptible to teratogenic substances that cause birth defects. Therefore, treatment is commonly delayed until at least the second trimester. Cancers diagnosed late in pregnancy may not be treated until after delivery. Labor may be induced early. A recent Israeli study indicated that a diagnosis of leukemia or **lymphoma** during the first trimester may require terminating the pregnancy to save the mother's life.

Surgery

Surgical risks for both mother and fetus must be considered. Surgery is possible during the second trimester, but there remains a risk of preterm labor, intrauterine growth retardation, and fetal death. **Mastectomy** is often recommended for breast cancer during pregnancy, although breast-conserving surgery may be an option. Abdominal surgery poses the greatest risk to the pregnancy, although it is possible to have an ovary removed and still bring a healthy fetus to term. Ovary removal cannot be performed until after the first trimester, when the placenta has taken over production of progesterone from the corpus luteum.

Radiation

During the first ten days following conception, radiation can cause fetal death or may have no effect on the fetus. Between 10 days and 14 weeks, a fetus exposed to radiation is at risk of:

- intrauterine growth retardation
- central nervous system (CNS) abnormalities
- microcephaly
- severe mental retardation
- eye anomalies

The fetus remains at risk of CNS abnormalities and milder forms of microcephaly and mental retardation from radiation throughout gestation. High doses of radiation can cause intrauterine death. The safe or threshold radiation dose is unknown, and the possibility of cancers developing during childhood, later in life, or in future generations are of concern. Research on children exposed to radiation *in utero* during the World War II bombing of Japan indicates that effects of radiation exposure may show up even after five generations.

Chemotherapy

Several recent European studies suggest that chemotherapy in the second or third trimester may be preferable to early delivery. However, chemotherapy is rarely administered near term when the placenta is less able to effectively remove the drugs. Congenital malformations and miscarriage are the most common adverse consequences of chemotherapy. Several factors must be considered when choosing chemotherapy during pregnancy:

- chemotherapy drugs that are both effective for the type of cancer and safe for the developing fetus
- stage of fetal development, with the first trimester presenting the greatest risk
- length and frequency of chemotherapy
- whether the chemotherapeutic agent crosses the placental barrier to the fetus
- effects on drug concentrations of increased blood volume and cardiac output during pregnancy
- effects of maternal obesity on lipid-soluble drugs

Chemotherapy drugs that appear to be well-tolerated by the fetus during the second and third trimesters include **fluorouracil**, **doxorubicin**, **bleomycin**, **vinblastine**, **dacarbazine**, and **cyclophosphamide**, although there is still risk of miscarriage, premature birth, and low birth weight. Drugs that may not harm the fetus may be harmful if consumed via breast milk, so breastfeeding is usually discouraged during chemotherapy. **Methotrexate** is teratogenic and is not administered during pregnancy. **Daunorubicin** and **cytarabine** are teratogenic in the first trimester. Other chemotherapy drugs are not used because their effects on the fetus are unknown.

Alternative and complementary therapies

Prescription, over-the-counter, and alternative medications that may help with side effects of cancer treatment may be harmful to the fetus. A practitioner experienced in the safe use of complementary therapies for cancer during pregnancy can be helpful. Mind/body techniques such as guided imagery and meditation can help decrease stress. Acupuncture may effective in dealing with nausea associated with chemotherapy. Support groups can be a good source of information and strength.

Prognosis

The prognosis for pregnant women with cancer is often the same as for other women of the same age with the same type and stage of cancer. However, if diagnosis or treatment is delayed during pregnancy, the cancer may become more extensive with a poorer prognosis. Furthermore, pregnancy hormones can potentially adversely affect the growth and spread of some types of cancer.

Special concerns

Pregnancy often delays a cancer diagnosis because some cancer symptoms—such as abdominal bloating, frequent headaches, or rectal bleeding—are common during pregnancy and are not considered suspicious. Pregnancy can also sometimes reveal cancers that were previously undetected.

Radiation from diagnostic x-rays is too low to harm the developing fetus. **Computed tomography** (CT) scans also use ionizing radiation. CT scans of the head or chest are usually considered safe during pregnancy because the fetus is not directly exposed. A lead shield can cover the abdomen during x-rays or CT scans. Other diagnostic tests for cancer— including ultrasound, **magnetic resonance imaging** (MRI), and biopsies—are considered safe during pregnancy.

A cancer diagnosis requires deciding whether to initiate or delay treatment, or whether to terminate the pregnancy if gestation is less than 24 weeks. Accurate staging of the tumor is critical. Depending on the type and stage of the cancer, a delay in treatment may not affect the prognosis. Fetal lung maturity may be monitored so that a safe early delivery can be planned. Oncologists experienced in treatment during pregnancy may be able to offer treatment while maintaining a viable pregnancy. They must also be experienced in managing treatment side effects in ways that are safe for the fetus. For example, **corticosteroids** can increase the incidence of cleft palate and affect maternal glucose tolerance.

A desire for future pregnancies is an important consideration when choosing a treatment plan.

See also Fertility issues.

Resources

BOOKS

Hartmann, Lynn C., and Charles L. Loprinzi. *The Mayo Clinic Breast Cancer Book*. Intercourse, PA: Good Books, 2012.

Perry, Michael C., Donald C. Doll, and Carl E. Freter. *Chemotherapy Source Book*. 5th ed. Philadelphia: Wolters Kluwer/Lippincott Williams & Wilkins, 2012.

Sutton, Amy L. *Breast Cancer Sourcebook*. 4th ed. Detroit: Omnigraphics, 2012.

PERIODICALS

Amant, Frédéric, et al. "Breast Cancer in Pregnancy." *The Lancet* 379, no. 9815 (February 11, 2012): 570–9.

Brenner, Benjamin, Irit Avivi, and Michael Lishner. "Haematological Cancers in Pregnancy." *The Lancet* 379, no. 9815 (February 11, 2012): 580–7.

Morice, Philippe, Catherine Uzan, and Serge Uzan. "Cancer in Pregnancy: A Challenging Conflict of Interest." *The Lancet* 379, no. 9815 (February 11, 2012): 495–6.

Morice, Philippe, et al. "Gynaecological Cancers in Pregnancy." *The Lancet* 379, no. 9815 (February 11, 2012): 558–69.

Schmidt, Charlie. "Pregnancy Options Expand for Women with Cancer." *Journal of the National Cancer Institute* 105, no. 21 (November 6, 2013): 1589.

WEBSITES

American Cancer Institute. "General Information About Breast Cancer and Pregnancy." Breast Cancer Treatment and Pregnancy (PDQ). May 23, 2014. http://www.cancer.gov/cancertopics/pdq/treatment/breast-cancer-and-pregnancy/Patient (accessed June 18, 2014).

"Cancer During Pregnancy." Cancer.Net. January 2013. http://www.cancer.net/coping-and-emotions/sexual-and-reproductive-health/cancer-during-pregnancy (accessed June 18, 2014).

"Gestational Trophoblastic Disease (GTD)." Foundation for Women's Cancer. http://www.foundationforwomenscancer.org/types-of-gynecologic-cancers/gestational-trophoblastic-disease-gdt (accessed June 18, 2014).

Simon, Stacy. "Cancer Can Be Treated During Pregnancy." American Cancer Society. May 31, 2012. http://www.cancer.org/cancer/news/news/cancer-can-be-treated-during-pregnancy (accessed June 19, 2014).

"Tumors and Pregnancy." MedlinePlus. June 16, 2014. http://www.nlm.nih.gov/medlineplus/tumorsandpregnancy.html (accessed June 18, 2014).

ORGANIZATIONS

American Cancer Society, 250 Williams Street NW, Atlanta, GA 30303, (800) 227-2345, http://www.cancer.org.

Foundation for Women's Cancer, 230 West Monroe, Suite 2528, Chicago, IL 60606-4902, (312) 578-1439, Fax: (312) 578-9769, (800) 444-4441, info@foundationforwomenscancer.org, http://www.foundationforwomenscancer.org.

Hope for Two . . . The Pregnant with Cancer Network, P.O. Box 253, Amherst, NY 14226, (800) 743-4471, info@hopefortwo.org., http://www.pregnantwithcancer.org.

National Cancer Institute, 6116 Executive Boulevard, Suite 300, Bethesda, MD 20892-8322, (800) 4-CANCER (422-6237), http://www.cancer.gov.

Esther Csapo Rastegari, R.N., B.S.N., Ed.M.
Teresa G. Odle
Margaret Alic, PhD

Prevention of cancer *see* **Cancer prevention**
Primary liver cancer *see* **Liver cancer**

Primary site

Definition

The area in which a **cancer** originates in the body. Once cancer spreads (metastasizes), the new tumors are called secondary tumors, or metastases.

Resources

WEBSITES

American Cancer Society. "What is a cancer of unknown primary?" http://www.cancer.org/cancer/cancerofunknownprimary/detailedguide/cancer-unknown-primary-cancer-of-unknown-primary (accessed November 12, 2014).

American Society of Clinical Oncology. "Types of Cancer." Cancer.net http://www.cancer.net/cancer-types/unknown-primary/overview (accessed November 12, 2014).

Cancer Research UK. "What is cancer of unknown primary (CUP)?" http://www.cancerresearchuk.org/about-cancer/type/unknown-primary-cancer/about/what-is-unknown-primary-cancer#primary (accessed November 12, 2014).

Kate Kretschmann

Procarbazine

Definition

Procarbazine is an anticancer agent that kills **cancer** cells, also known by the brand name Matulane. It is approved by the U.S. Food and Drug Administration (FDA) for the treatment of advanced **Hodgkin lymphoma** in combination with other **anticancer drugs**.

KEY TERMS

Cytotoxic drug—An anticancer drug that acts by killing or preventing the division of cells.

DNA (deoxyribonucleic acid)—An acid found in all living cells that contains tiny bits of genetic information.

Platelets—Components of the blood involved in clotting.

RNA (ribonucleic acid)—A type of nucleic acid that transmits genetic information from DNA to proteins produced by the cell.

Purpose

Procarbazine is used in the treatment of various cancers, although the best-established usage is with Hodgkin **lymphoma**. Other cancers in which procarbazine is sometimes used include other lymphomas, **brain tumors**, **skin cancer**, lung cancer, and **multiple myeloma**.

Description

Procarbazine is a cytotoxic drug, which means that it kills cancer cells. Procarbazine works by interfering with the way in which the DNA and RNA in cells produce proteins by binding to them in the cells.

Recommended dosage

Procarbazine is often given at a dose of 60 to 100 mg per square meter of body surface area for ten to fourteen days of each course of therapy. In addition, patients who have had pre-existing problems with liver, kidney, or bone marrow function may receive reduced doses.

Precautions

While on therapy with procarbazine, patients should not drink alcohol because it may interact with the drug to cause a flushed and hot sensation. Certain foods such as chocolate, fava beans, imported beer, Chianti wines, and ripe cheeses (Camembert, cheddar, Emmenthaler, Stilton), caviar, pickled herring, fermented sausages (bologna, pepperoni, salami, summer sausage), should be avoided as they may cause a dangerous increase in blood pressure if eaten while receiving procarbazine.

Side effects

A carefully monitored side effect of procarbazine is a decrease in the white blood cells that fight infection and the platelet cells that prevent bleeding. The most severe side effect is **nausea and vomiting**. Patients should adhere to the antiemetic regimen prescribed for them to prevent this side effect. There may be neurologic side effects such as confusion, sleepiness, **depression**, nightmares, agitation, and nervousness. Patients may have reproductive dysfunction.

Interactions

Procarbazine has numerous drug interactions, particularly with acetaminophen, aspirin, codeine, and other opioid pain relievers, as well as vaccines made with live viruses. Therefore, it is important that patients alert their physicians to all medications they are taking (prescription, over-the-counter, or herbal) prior to starting treatment with procarbazine or any other drug.

Resources

BOOKS

Chu, Edward, and Vincent T. DeVita Jr. *Physicians' Cancer Chemotherapy Drug Manual 2014*. Burlington, MA: Jones & Bartlett Learning, 2014.

WEBSITES

AHFS Consumer Medication Information. "Procarbazine." American Society of Health-System Pharmacists. Available from: http://www.nlm.nih.gov/medlineplus/druginfo/meds/a682094.html (accessed November 12, 2014).

Cancer Research UK. "Procarbazine." http://www.cancerresearchuk.org/about-cancer/cancers-in-general/treatment/cancer-drugs/procarbazine (accessed November 12, 2014).

Bob Kirsch

Prochlorperazine *see* **Antiemetics**

Prograf *see* **Tacrolimus**

Prokine *see* **Sargramostim**

Proleukin *see* **Aldesleukin**

Promethazine *see* **Antiemetics**

Prostate cancer

Definition

Prostate **cancer** is a disease in which cells in the prostate gland become abnormal and start to grow uncontrollably, forming tumors. Most prostate cancers are adenocarcinomas, which means that they begin in the glandular tissue of the prostate.

Description

Prostate cancer is a malignancy of one of the major male sex glands. Along with the testicles and the seminal vesicles, the prostate secretes the fluid that makes up semen. The prostate is about the size of a walnut and lies just behind the urinary bladder. A tumor in the prostate interferes with proper control of the bladder and normal sexual functioning. Often the first symptom of prostate cancer is difficulty in urinating, but because a very common noncancerous condition of the prostate known as benign prostatic hyperplasia (BPH) also causes the same problem, difficulty in urination is not necessarily due to cancer.

Cancerous cells within the prostate itself are generally not deadly on their own. As the tumor grows, however, some of the cells break off and spread to other parts of the body through the lymph or the blood—a process known as **metastasis**. The most common sites for prostate cancer to metastasize are the seminal vesicles, the lymph nodes, the lungs, and the bones around the hips and the pelvic region. These new tumors are the usual cause of death from prostate cancer.

Demographics

Prostate cancer is the most commonly diagnosed non-skin malignancy among adult males in Western countries. The **National Cancer Institute** (NCI) estimates that 233,000 men in the United States were diagnosed with prostate cancer in 2014, with 29,480 deaths. One in seven American men will be diagnosed with prostate cancer in the course of his lifetime. Although prostate cancer is often very slow-growing, it

Most common cancers in the United States, 2014

		Estimated number of new cases
1.	Prostate cancer	233,000
2.	Breast cancer (female)	232,670
3.	Lung and bronchial cancers	224,210
4.	Colorectal cancer	136,830
5.	Melanoma	76,100
6.	Bladder cancer	74,690
7.	Non-Hodgkin lymphoma	70,800
8.	Kidney cancer (including renal pelvis)	63,920
9.	Thyroid cancer	62,980
10.	Endometrial cancer	52,630

SOURCE: National Cancer Institute, Surveillance, Epidemiology, and End Results Program (SEER), "SEER Stat Fact Sheets: Prostate Cancer," http://seer.cancer.gov/statfacts/html/prost.html.

Prostate cancer is the most common cancer in the United States. (Table by Lumina Datamatics Ltd. © 2015 Cengage Learning®.)

can be aggressive, especially in younger men. Given its slow-growing nature, many men with the disease die of causes other than the cancer itself.

Prostate cancer is primarily a disease of older men; about 60% of cases are diagnosed in men over 50. It is rare in men younger than 40. Prostate cancer affects African American men twice as often as Caucasian men, and the mortality rate among African Americans is also two times higher. African Americans have the highest rate of prostate cancer of any population group in the world. On the other hand, Hispanic and Asian American men have relatively low rates of prostate cancer. The reasons for these racial and ethnic differences are not fully known as of 2014; however, researchers are investigating the possibility that unique mutations in the androgen receptor gene are responsible for the increased risk of prostate cancer in African Americans.

Causes and symptoms

The precise cause of prostate cancer is not known. However, there are several known risk factors for disease, including:

- being over 55 years old
- being of African American descent
- having a family history of the disease (particularly in a brother or father)
- experiencing occupational exposure to cadmium or rubber
- consuming a high-fat diet

Men with high plasma **testosterone** levels may also have an increased risk of developing prostate cancer.

Additional factors that are currently being investigated as possibly increasing a man's risk of prostate cancer include obesity, smoking, personal history of sexually transmitted diseases, having a vasectomy, and chronic inflammation of the prostate. None of these factors, however, have been proven to have a definite link to prostate cancer as of 2014. Although a few genes are being studied as possible risk factors, most prostate cancers are thought to arise from DNA mutations acquired during a man's lifetime rather than inherited mutations.

Prostate cancer often has no symptoms and the disease is diagnosed when the patient has a routine screening examination. When the tumor has grown, however, or the cancer has spread to the nearby tissues, the following symptoms may be seen:

- weak or interrupted flow of urine
- frequent urination (especially at night)
- difficulty starting urination
- inability to urinate

KEY TERMS

Adenocarcinoma—A type of cancer that begins in glandular tissue. Most prostate cancers are adenocarcinomas.

Antiandrogen—A substance that blocks the action of androgens, the hormones responsible for male characteristics. Used to treat prostate cancers that require male hormones for growth.

Benign prostatic hyperplasia (BPH)—Noncancerous swelling of the prostate.

Brachytherapy—A method of treating cancers that involves implanting radioactive pellets or rods near the tumor.

Gleason grading system—A method of predicting the tendency of a tumor in the prostate to metastasize based on the tumor's similarity to normal prostate tissue.

Granulocyte/macrophage colony stimulating factor (GM-CSF)—Also known as sargramostim, a substance produced by cells of the immune system that stimulates the attack upon foreign cells. Used to treat prostate cancers as a genetically engineered

component of a vaccine that stimulates the body to attack prostate tissue.

Histopathology—The study of diseased tissues on the microscopic level.

Luteinizing hormone-releasing hormone (LHRH) agonist—A substance that blocks the action of LHRH, a hormone that stimulates the production of testosterone (a male hormone) in men. Used to treat prostate cancers that require testosterone for growth.

Orchiectomy—Surgical removal of the testes, done to eliminate the production of testosterone.

Prostate-specific antigen (PSA)—A protein made by the cells of the prostate that is increased by both BPH and prostate cancer.

Radical prostatectomy—Surgical removal of the entire prostate, a common method of treating prostate cancer.

Transurethral resection of the prostate (TURP)—Surgical removal of a portion of the prostate through the urethra, a method of treating the symptoms of an enlarged prostate, whether from BPH or cancer.

- pain or burning sensation when urinating
- hematuria (blood in the urine)
- persistent pain in lower back, hips, or thighs (bone pain)
- painful seminal ejaculation

Diagnosis

Prostate cancer is curable when detected early. Yet the early stages of prostate cancer are often asymptomatic, so the disease often goes undetected until the patient has a routine physical examination. Diagnosis of prostate cancer can be made using some or all of the following tests.

Digital rectal examination (DRE)

In order to perform this test, the doctor puts a gloved and lubricated finger (digit) into the rectum to feel for any lumps in the prostate. The rectum lies just behind the prostate gland, and a majority of prostate tumors begin in the posterior region of the prostate. If the doctor does detect an abnormality, he or she may order more tests in order to confirm these findings.

Blood tests

Blood tests are used to measure the amounts of certain protein markers, such as prostate-specific antigen

(PSA), found circulating in the blood. The cells lining the prostate generally make this protein, and a small amount can be detected normally in the bloodstream. Prostate cancers produce higher amounts of this protein, significantly raising the circulating levels. A finding of a PSA level higher than normal for the patient's age group suggests that cancer is present.

As of 2014, there is some concern about routine PSA screening of men at only average risk of prostate cancer. One reason is that the PSA test is not 100% accurate, so men who receive false positive results may end up having unnecessary biopsies, which carry risks of bleeding and infection. A second reason for a conservative approach to PSA screening is that prostate cancer is not always dangerous. Some prostate cancers never produce any symptoms; however, patients may feel that they should be treated for them anyway, and their quality of life may be seriously affected by the side effects of surgery or **radiation therapy**. The American Cancer Society (ACS) recommends that men at age 50 (or 45 for African American men and men with first-degree relatives with prostate cancer) have a discussion with their doctor about the benefits and risks of PSA screening. The ACS asserts that men should not be screened without having this conversation. The American Urological Association (AUA) has issued guidelines about the use of PSA screening in asymptomatic men, men at only average risk of prostate cancer, and elderly patients. Given the fact that men in the United States have at most a 3% lifetime risk of dying from prostate cancer as of 2014, the AUA agrees with the ACS about avoiding unnecessary screening. The age group that appears to benefit most from routine PSA screening is men between the ages of 55 and 69.

Transrectal ultrasound

In a transrectal ultrasound (TRUS), a small probe is placed in the rectum and sound waves are released from the probe. These sound waves bounce off the prostate tissue and create an image. Since normal prostate tissue and prostate tumors reflect the sound waves differently, the test is an efficient and accurate way to detect tumors. Though the insertion of the probe into the rectum may be slightly uncomfortable, the procedure is generally painless and takes only about 20 minutes.

Prostate biopsy

If cancer is suspected from the results of any of the above tests, the doctor will remove a small piece of prostate tissue with a hollow needle. This sample is then checked under the microscope for the presence of cancerous cells. Prostate **biopsy** is the most definitive diagnostic tool for prostate cancer, and this procedure is done quickly and with little pain or discomfort.

Prostate cancer can also be diagnosed based on the examination of the tissue removed during a transurethral resection of the prostate (TURP). This procedure is performed to help alleviate the symptoms of BPH, a benign (noncancerous) enlargement of the prostate. Like a biopsy, TURP is a definitive diagnostic test of prostate cancer.

X-rays and imaging techniques

A chest x-ray may be ordered to determine whether the cancer has spread to the lungs. Such imaging techniques as **computed tomography** (CT) and **magnetic resonance imaging** (MRI), in which a computer is used to generate a detailed picture of the prostate and areas nearby, may be done to get a clearer view of the internal organs. A bone scan may be used to check whether the cancer has spread to the bones. ProstaScint, a scan that uses a radioactive material injected into the body, may be used to determine whether the cancer has spread to lymph nodes and other non-bony tissues. The ProstaScint test is not usually used for men who have been diagnosed with prostate cancer only recently.

Treatment team

Prostate cancer is often treated by a team of specialists, including a urologist (who may or may not

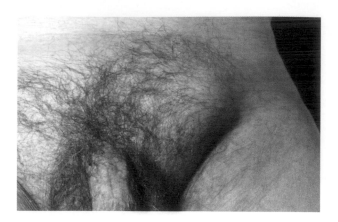

This patient's prostate cancer has metastasized (spread), causing swollen lymph nodes in the left groin. *(DR. MARAZZI/Science Source)*

perform surgery), a surgeon (if surgical treatment is used and it is not performed by the urologist), a medical oncologist, oncology nurses, and a radiation oncologist (if radiation therapy is used). A social worker and dietitian may also be part of the treatment team. The dietitian can help plan a nutritious diet if the patient suffers from nausea or loss of appetite as a side effect of radiation therapy or **chemotherapy**.

Clinical staging

Once cancer is detected during the microscopic examination of the prostate tissue during a biopsy or TURP, doctors will determine two different numerical scores that will help define the patient's treatment and prognosis.

Tumor grading

Initially, the pathologist will grade the tumor based on his or her examination of the biopsy tissue. The pathologist scores the appearance of the biopsy sample using the Gleason system. This system uses a scale of 1 to 5 based on the sample's similarity or dissimilarity to normal prostate tissue. If the tissue is very similar to normal tissue, it is still well differentiated and given a low grading number, such as 1 or 2. As the tissue becomes more and more abnormal (less and less differentiated), the grading number increases, up to 5. Less differentiated tissue is considered more aggressive and more likely to be the source of metastases.

The Gleason grading system is most predictive of the prognosis of a patient if the pathologist gives two scores to a particular sample—a primary and a secondary pattern. The two numbers are then added together and that is the Gleason score reported to the patient. Thus, the lowest Gleason score available is two (a primary and secondary pattern score of one each). A typical Gleason score is 5 (which can be a primary score of two and a secondary score of three or vice versa). The highest score available is 10, with a pure pattern of highly undifferentiated tissue; that is, of grade 5. The higher the score, the more abnormal the tissue, the greater the likelihood of metastases, and the more serious the prognosis after surgical treatment. A study found that the ten-year cancer survival rate without evidence of disease for grades 2, 3, and 4 cancers is 94% of patients. The rate is 91% for grade 5 cancers, 78% for grade 6, 46% for grade 7, and 23% for grades 8, 9, and 10 cancers.

Cancer staging

The second numeric score determined by the doctor will be the stage of the cancer, which takes into account the grade of the tumor determined by the pathologist. Based on the recommendations of the **American Joint Committee on Cancer** (AJCC), two kinds of data are used for staging prostate cancer. Clinical data are based on the external symptoms of the cancer, while histopathological data are based on surgical removal of the prostate and examination of its tissues. Clinical data are most useful in making treatment decisions, while pathological data are the best predictor of prognosis. For this reason, the staging of prostate cancer takes into account both clinical and histopathologic information. Specifically, doctors look at tumor size (T), lymph node involvement (N), the presence of visceral (internal organ) involvement (metastasis = M), and the grade of the tumor (G).

The classification of a tumor as T1 means that the cancer is confined to the prostate gland and the tumor is too small to be felt during a DRE. T1 tumors are often found after examination of tissue removed during a TURP. The T1 definition is subdivided into those cancers that show less than 5% cancerous cells in the tissue sample (T1a) or more than 5% cancerous cells in the tissue sample (T1b). T1c means that the biopsy was performed on the basis of an elevated PSA result. The second tumor classification is T2, in which the tumor is large enough to be felt during the DRE. T2a indicates that only the left or the right side of the gland is involved, while T2b means that both sides of the prostate gland have the tumor.

With a T3 tumor, the cancer has spread to the connective tissue near the prostate (T3a) or to the seminal vesicles as well (T3b). T4 indicates that cancer has spread within the pelvis to such tissues next to the prostate as the bladder's sphincter, the rectum, or the wall of the pelvis. Prostate cancer tends to spread next into the regional lymph nodes of the pelvis, indicated as N1. Prostate cancer is said to be at the M1 stage when it has metastasized outside the pelvis in distant lymph nodes (M1a), bone (M1b), or such organs as the liver or the brain (M1c). Pain, **weight loss**, and **fatigue** often accompany the M1 stage.

The grade of the tumor (G) can be assessed during a biopsy, TURP surgery, or after removal of the prostate. There are three grades recognized: G1, G2, and G3, indicating that the tumor is well, moderately, or poorly differentiated, respectively. The G, LN, M descriptions are combined with the T definition to determine the stage of the prostate cancer.

- Stage I prostate cancer comprises patients who are T1a, N0, M0, G1. The tumor has not spread beyond the prostate and might be too small to feel during a DRE. If known, the Gleason score is 6 or less, and the PSA level is under 10.
- Stage II encompasses a variety of condition combinations, including T1a, N0, M0, G2, 3 or 4; T1b, N0, M0, any G; T1c, N0, M0, any G; T1, N0, M0, any G; or T2, N0, M0, any G. The tumor is more advanced or is a higher grade than a Stage I tumor but has not spread beyond the prostate. The Gleason score is 7 and the PSA is less than 20.
- Stage III prostate cancer occurs when conditions are T3, N0, M0, any G. The tumor extends beyond the prostate but has not yet spread into the lymph nodes. The patient may have any Gleason score and any PSA level.
- Stage IV is T4, N0, M0, any G; any T, N1, M0, any G; or any T, any N, M1, any G. The tumor has spread beyond the prostate; it may have invaded the bladder or rectum, or spread to distant sites. Stage IV cancers also may be Gleason score and any PSA level.

Treatment

The doctor and the patient will decide on the treatment mode after considering many factors; for example, the patient's age, the stage of the disease, his general health, and the presence of any coexisting illnesses. In addition, the patient's personal preferences and the risks and benefits of each treatment protocol are also taken into account before any decision is made.

SURGERY. For stage I and stage II prostate cancer, surgery is the most common method of treatment because it offers the chance of completely removing the cancer from the body. Radical **prostatectomy** involves complete removal of the prostate. The surgery can be done using a perineal approach, in which the incision is made between the scrotum and the anus, or using a retropubic approach, in which the incision is made in the lower abdomen. The perineal approach is also known as nerve-sparing prostatectomy, as it is thought to reduce the effect on the nerves and thus reduce the side effects of impotence and incontinence. The retropubic approach, however, allows for the simultaneous removal of the pelvic lymph nodes, which can reveal important information about the tumor spread. A newer approach is robotic surgery, in which the surgeon sits at a computer console and uses a robot to remove the prostate through small incisions in the patient's abdomen.

The drawback to surgical treatment for early prostate cancer is the significant risk of side effects that may impact the patient's quality of life. Even using nerve-sparing techniques, studies by the National Cancer Institute (NCI) found that 60%–80% of men treated with radical prostatectomy reported themselves as impotent (unable to achieve an erection sufficient for sexual intercourse) two years after surgery. This side effect can be sometimes countered by prescribing sildenafil citrate (Viagra). Other options include penile implants or vacuum devices. Furthermore, 8%–10% of patients were incontinent (unable to control bladder and/or bowel function) in that time span. Despite the side effects, the majority of men were reported as satisfied with their treatment choice. In addition, there is some evidence that the skill and experience of the surgeon are central factors in the ultimate side effects seen.

A second method of surgical treatment of prostate cancer is cryosurgery, or **cryotherapy**. Guided by ultrasound, surgeons insert up to eight cryoprobes through the skin and into close proximity with the tumor. Liquid nitrogen (temperature of −320.8°F, or −196°C) is circulated through the probe, freezing the tumor tissue. In prostate surgery, a warming tube is also used to keep the urethra from freezing. Cryosurgery for prostate cancer can be performed as an outpatient procedure, and recovery time is about one week. Side effects have been reduced in recent years, although impotence still affects almost all men who have had cryosurgery for prostate cancer. Cryosurgery is considered a good alternative for people who are unable to have traditional surgery or radiation treatments, or when these more traditional treatments are unsuccessful. There is a limited amount of information about the long-term efficacy of this treatment for prostate cancer.

Another surgical alternative is high-intensity focused ultrasound therapy (HIFU), in which the surgeon inserts an ultrasound probe in the patient's rectum. The probe emits high-intensity ultrasound waves that heat the tumor to about 80°C and kill the cancer cells. HIFU is still considered experimental in the United States as of 2014, but it has been found to have the advantages of less blood loss and pain for the patient.

RADIATION THERAPY. Radiation therapy involves the use of high-energy **x-rays** to kill cancer cells or to shrink tumors. It can be used instead of surgery for Stage I and

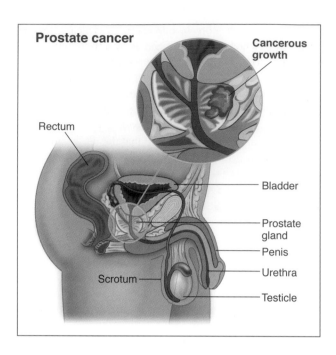

This illustration shows the anatomy of the prostate and surrounding organs, with a cancerous growth on the prostate. *(Illustration by Electronic Illustrators Group. © Cengage Learning®.)*

II cancer. The radiation can either be administered from a machine outside the body (external beam radiation), or small radioactive pellets can be implanted in the prostate gland in the area surrounding the tumor, called brachytherapy or interstitial implantation. Pellets containing radioactive iodine (I-125), palladium (Pd-103), or iridium (Ir-192) can be implanted on an outpatient basis, where they remain permanently. The radioactive effect of the seeds lasts only about a year.

The side effects of radiation can include inflammation of the bladder, rectum, and small intestine, as well as disorders of blood clotting (coagulopathies). Impotence and incontinence are often delayed side effects of the treatment. A study indicated that bowel control problems were more likely after radiation therapy when compared to surgery, but impotence and incontinence were more likely after surgical treatment. Long-term results with radiation therapy are dependent on the tumor's stage. A review of almost 1,000 patients treated with megavoltage irradiation showed 10-year survival rates to be significantly different by T-stage: T1 (79%), T2 (66%), T3 (55%), and T4 (22%). There does not appear to be a large difference in survival between external beam or interstitial treatments.

HORMONE (ANDROGEN DEPRIVATION) THERAPY. Hormone therapy is commonly used when the cancer is in an advanced stage and has spread to other parts of the body, such as stage III or stage IV. Prostate cells need the male hormone testosterone to grow. Decreasing the levels of this hormone or inhibiting its activity will cause the cancer to shrink. Hormone levels can be decreased in several ways. **Orchiectomy** is a surgical procedure that involves complete removal of the testicles, leading to a decrease in the levels of testosterone. Antiandrogen drugs may be given in addition to orchiectomy; these include drugs like flutamide (Eulexin), bicalutamide (Casodex), and nilutamide (Nilandron). Another type of hormone therapy is the use of luteinizing hormone-releasing hormone (LHRH) analogs. These drugs are given as implants under the skin and work by lowering the amount of testosterone produced by the testicles. They include leuprolide (Lupron), goserelin (Zoladex), and triptorelin (Trelstar). The LHRH analogs are expensive, but unlike orchiectomy, they offer the patient the advantage of allowing the testicles to remain in place. Antiandrogen hormone therapy may be given either continuously or intermittently.

Another approach to hormone therapy involves administering the female hormone estrogen. When estrogen is given, the body senses the presence of a sex hormone and stops making the male hormone testosterone. There are, however, some unpleasant side effects to estrogen hormone therapy. Men may have "hot flashes," enlargement and tenderness of the breasts (gynecomastia), or impotence and loss of sexual desire, as well as blood clots, heart attacks, and strokes, depending on the dose of estrogen. Another side effect is osteoporosis, or loss of bone mass leading to brittle and easily fractured bones. For this reason, as of 2014 the LHRH analogs are used more often than estrogen therapy.

CHEMOTHERAPY. Chemotherapy is not usually used to treat early-stage prostate cancer, but it may be used to treat metastatic cancer when hormone therapy stops working. Chemotherapy drugs are usually given one at a time rather than in combination to treat prostate cancer. Drugs that may be used include **docetaxel**, **estramustine**, **doxorubicin**, cabazitaxel, **etoposide**, and **vinblastine**. Side effects of chemotherapy for prostate cancer include loss of appetite, nausea, fatigue, hair loss, mouth sores, lowered resistance to infections, and a tendency to bruise easily.

VACCINE THERAPY. A vaccine called **Sipuleucel-T** (Provenge) became available in 2014 to treat advanced-stage prostate cancer that is not responding to hormone therapy but is producing few symptoms. This vaccine is not mass-produced but is made from the patient's own white blood cells. It works by boosting the patient's immune system to attack prostate cancer cells. The vaccine does not cure prostate cancer, but it does appear to extend the patient's survival time. Tests are still being done to determine whether the vaccine may benefit patients with less advanced cancer. Common side effects of vaccine therapy may include high blood pressure, **fever**, chills, fatigue, back and joint pain, nausea, and headaches. Other vaccines for prostate cancer were in **clinical trials** as of mid-2014.

ACTIVE SURVEILLANCE AND OBSERVATION. Active surveillance means that no immediate treatment is recommended, but doctors keep the patient under careful observation. Active surveillance is often done by using periodic PSA tests and DREs every 3 to 6 months; it is preferred for older patients with nonaggressive tumors and a life expectancy of 20 years or fewer. Observation entails less frequent exams and is performed in patients expected to live no more than 10 years. Prostate cancer in older men tends to be slow-growing; therefore, the risk of the patient's dying from prostate cancer, rather than from other causes, is relatively small. Studies have found active surveillance and observation to be equal to surgery in terms of outcomes, and traditional treatment options are pursued if the disease worsens.

Alternative and complementary therapies

Alternative treatments that have been found helpful in coping with the emotional stress associated with prostate cancer include meditation, guided imagery, and relaxation techniques. Acupuncture is effective in relieving pain in some patients.

A variety of herbal products have been used to treat prostate cancer, including various compounds used in traditional Chinese medicine, as well as single agents like Reishi mushrooms (*Ganoderma lucidum*). The benefits of these products are unproven, however, and patients should not use any herbal products or traditional folk medicines without consulting their treatment teams. Some herbal products can mask high PSA levels.

Prognosis

The prognosis for cancers detected and treated at Stages I and II is very good. For men treated with stage I or stage II disease, over 99% are alive after five years. Although the cancers of Stage III are more advanced, the five-year prognosis is still good, with 70% of men diagnosed at this stage still living. The spread of the cancer into the pelvis (T4), lymph (N1), or distant locations (M1) are very significant events, as the five-year survival rate drops to 28% for Stage IV.

Coping with cancer treatment

The treatment process for prostate cancer can be a physically and emotionally exhausting time. Suggestions that may help make the process easier include:

- Trust the treatment team once a treatment course has been chosen
- Remember that a patient is never without power and rights during the course of treatment.
- Put practical affairs in order.
- Closely monitor each step of the treatment.
- Keep close family and friends informed and delegate responsibilities as necessary.
- Try to make visits pleasant and comfortable.
- Be careful to eat, sleep, exercise, and conduct daily activities in a healthful manner.

Clinical trials

In 2014, there were 488 open clinical trials for prostate cancer in the United States. Studies included:

- research into genetic factors for the high risk of prostate cancer in African Americans
- the effect of diet and nutrition in halting the progression of prostate cancer
- various combinations of radiation therapy or chemotherapy with androgen-deprivation hormone therapy
- the effectiveness of pomegranate extract in preventing tumor growth in patients with localized prostate cancer
- various experimental drugs for the treatment of metastatic prostate cancer

Prevention

Because the cause of prostate cancer is not known, there is no definite way to prevent prostate cancer. Given its common occurrence and the low cost of screening, the American Cancer Society (ACS) and the **National Comprehensive Cancer Network** (NCCN) recommend that all men over age 40 have an annual rectal exam and that men have an annual PSA test beginning at age 50. African American men and men with a family history of prostate cancer should begin annual PSA testing even earlier, starting at age 45.

A low-fat diet may slow the progression of prostate cancer. To reduce the risk or progression of prostate cancer, the American Cancer Society recommends a diet rich in fruits, vegetables, and dietary fiber, and low in red meat and saturated fats.

Special concerns

The availability of an early detection system for prostate cancer with the development of the PSA serum test has complicated the treatment of this disease. Early detection of an often slow-growing cancer, where treatment can significantly impact the quality of life of the patient, can be complicated. Long-term studies are currently in progress that should provide the first real quantitative information about the relative efficacy of the different treatment options, the actual occurrence of side effects, and the comparative benefits of watchful waiting treatment compared with more aggressive action.

See also Antiandrogens.

Resources

BOOKS

Centeno, Arthur. *Prostate Cancer: A Man's Guide to Treatment.* 2nd ed. Omaha, NE: Addicus Books, 2014.

Ellsworth, Pamela. *100 Questions and Answers about Prostate Cancer.* 4th ed. Burlington, MA: Jones and Bartlett Learning, 2015.

Klein, Eric A., and J. Stephen Jones, eds. *Management of Prostate Cancer.* 3rd ed. Totowa, NJ: Humana Press, 2013.

Sciarra, Alessandro, ed. *Multidisciplinary Management of Prostate Cancer: The Role of the Prostate Cancer Unit.* New York: Springer, 2014.

PERIODICALS

Chang, S. L., et al. "The Impact of Robotic Surgery on the Surgical Management of Prostate Cancer in the United States." *BJU International* (June 24, 2014): e-pub ahead of print. http://dx.doi.org/10.1111/bju.12850 (accessed September 23, 2014).

Gulley, J. L., et al. "Immune Impact Induced by PROSTVAC (PSA-TRICOM), a Therapeutic Vaccine for Prostate Cancer." *Cancer Immunology Research* 2 (February 2014): 133–41.

Halabi, S., et al. "Updated Prognostic Model for Predicting Overall Survival in First-line Chemotherapy for Patients with Metastatic Castration-resistant Prostate Cancer." *Journal of Clinical Oncology* 32 (March 1, 2014): 671–77.

Hurwitz, M., and D. P. Petrylak. "Sequencing of Agents for Castration-Resistant Prostate Cancer." *Oncology (Williston Park)* 27 (November 2013): 1144–49, 1154–58.

Hussain, M., et al. "Intermittent versus Continuous Androgen Deprivation in Prostate Cancer." *New England Journal of Medicine* 368 (April 4, 2013): 1314–25.

Kim, S. P., et al. "Perceptions of Active Surveillance and Treatment Recommendations for Low-Risk Prostate Cancer: Results from a National Survey of Radiation Oncologists and Urologists." *Medical Care* 52 (July 2014): 579–85.

Koochekpour, S., et al. "Androgen Receptor Mutations and Polymorphisms in African American Prostate Cancer." *International Journal of Biological Sciences* 10 (June 5, 2014): 643–51.

Schlom, J., et al. "Therapeutic Cancer Vaccines." *Advances in Cancer Research* 121 (2014): 67–124.

Tsao, C. K., et al. "The Role of Cabazitaxel in the Treatment of Metastatic Castration-Resistant Prostate Cancer." *Therapeutic Advances in Urology* 6 (June 2014): 97–104.

Ukimura, O., et al. "Cryosurgery for Clinical T3 Prostate Cancer." *BJU International* 113 (May 2014): 684–85.

OTHER

American Cancer Society (ACS). "Prostate Cancer." http://www.cancer.org/acs/groups/cid/documents/webcontent/003134-pdf.pdf (accessed September 3, 2014).

WEBSITES

American Urological Association (AUA). "Early Detection of Prostate Cancer: AUA Guideline." http://www.auanet.org/education/guidelines/prostate-cancer-detection.cfm (accessed September 3, 2014).

MedicineNet. "Prostate Cancer." http://www.medicinenet.com/prostate_cancer/article.htm (accessed September 3, 2014).

National Cancer Institute (NCI). "What You Need to Know about Prostate Cancer." http://www.cancer.gov/cancertopics/wyntk/prostate/page1/AllPages (accessed September 3, 2014).

Simon, Stacy. "Study: Surgery No Better Than Observation for Localized Prostate Cancer." American Cancer Society. http://www.cancer.org/cancer/news/news/study-surgery-no-better-than-observation-for-localized-prostate-cancer (accessed September 3, 2014).

ORGANIZATIONS

American Cancer Society (ACS), 250 Williams Street NW, Atlanta, GA 30303, (800) 227-2345, http://www.cancer.org/aboutus/howwehelpyou/app/contact-us.aspx, http://www.cancer.org/index.

American Urological Association (AUA), 1000 Corporate Boulevard, Linthicum, MD 21090, (410) 689-3700, (866) 746-4282, Fax: (410) 689-3800, http://www.auanet.org/.

National Cancer Institute (NCI), BG 9609 MSC 9760, 9609 Medical Center Drive, Bethesda, MD 20892-9760, (800) 4-CANCER (422-6237), http://www.cancer.gov/global/contact/email-us, http://www.cancer.gov/.

Office of Cancer Complementary and Alternative Medicine (OCCAM), 9609 Medical Center Dr., Room 5-W-136, Rockville, MD 20850, (240) 276-6595, Fax: (240) 276-7888, ncioccam1-r@mail.nih.gov, http://cam.cancer.gov/.

Prostate Cancer Foundation (PCF), 1250 Fourth Street, Santa Monica, CA 90401, (310) 570-4700, (800) 757-CURE, Fax: (310) 570-4701, info@pcf.org, http://www.pcf.org/site/c.leJRIROrEpH/b.5699537/k.BEF4/Home.htm.

Lata Cherath, PhD
Michelle Johnson, MS, JD
Rebecca J. Frey, PhD

Prostatectomy

Definition

Prostatectomy is a medical procedure that involves the surgical removal of all or part of the prostate gland. It is commonly used to treat benign prostatic hyperplasia (BPH, also known as benign prostatic hypertrophy), a condition in which benign or noncancerous nodules grow in the prostate gland. Removal of the entire prostate is performed to treat **prostate cancer**.

Purpose

Prostate **cancer** is the single most common form of non-skin cancer in the United States and the most common cancer in men over 50. This condition does not always require surgery. In fact, many elderly men adopt a policy of watchful waiting, especially if their cancer is growing slowly. Younger men often elect to have their prostate gland totally removed along with the cancer it contains—an operation called radical prostatectomy. The two main types of this surgery, radical retropubic prostatectomy and radical perineal prostatectomy, are performed only on patients whose cancer is limited to the prostate. If cancer has broken out of the capsule surrounding the prostate gland and spread within the area or to distant sites, removing the prostate will not prevent the cancer from continuing to grow and spread throughout the body.

BPH, or enlargement of the prostate, is present in more than half of men in their 60s and as many as 90% of those over 90. An operation called transurethral resection of the prostate (TURP) relieves symptoms of BPH by removing prostate tissue that is blocking the urethra; it may also help alleviate symptoms related to prostate cancer.

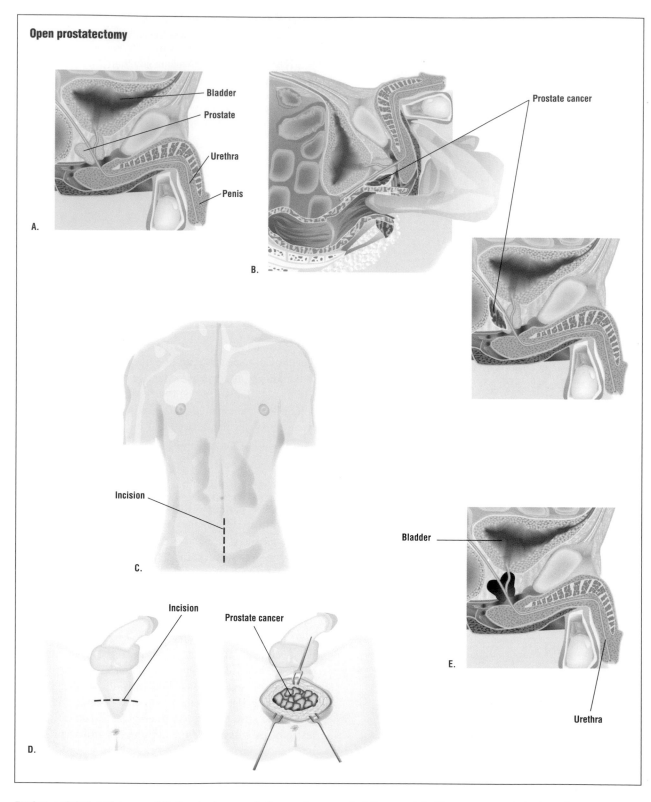

Open prostatectomy

A.
- Bladder
- Prostate
- Urethra
- Penis

B.
- Prostate cancer

Incision

C.

Incision

Prostate cancer

D.

Bladder

E.

Urethra

During a digital rectal exam (B), the doctor may feel an enlargement of the prostate. If an open prostatectomy is needed, an incision may be made the lower abdomen (C) or the perineal area (D). *(Illustration by GGS Information Services. © Cengage Learning®).*

Description

The two most common procedures performed to treat prostate cancer are radical retropubic prostatectomy and radical perineal prostatectomy.

Radical retropubic prostatectomy (RRP)

Abbreviated RRP, this surgical approach involves making a horizontal incision in the lower abdomen, with the patient under general or spinal anesthesia or an epidural. Some surgeons begin the operation by removing pelvic lymph nodes to determine whether cancer has invaded them, but recent findings suggest that there is no need to sample them in patients whose likelihood of lymph node metastases is less than 18%. A doctor who removes the lymph nodes for examination will not continue the operation if they contain cancer cells, because this finding means the chancer has spread. Other surgeons remove the prostate gland before examining the lymph nodes. The prostate is removed by going behind the pubic bone (retropubic).

The advantages of retropubic prostatectomy include:

- direct visualization of the prostatic tumor
- visualization to control bleeding after tumor removal
- exact incisions in the urethra, which will minimize the complication of urinary continence
- excellent anatomic exposure and visualization of the prostate
- little or no surgical trauma to the urinary bladder

Radical perineal prostatectomy (RPP)

RPP consists of an incision made by the surgeon in the perineum, approximately halfway between the rectum (anus) and scrotum (perineum). The prostate is removed through this incision. This procedure is less common than it used to be due to difficulties with circumventing the nerves and inadequate access of the lymph nodes. RPP is commonly performed when dealing with early-stage prostate cancer, when the cancer is confined to the prostate. RPP allows for reduced blood loss during the operation and a quicker recovery time than RRP due to the absence of an abdominal incision.

Laparoscopic radical prostatectomy (LRP)

This procedure, abbreviated LRP, consists of four small incisions in the abdomen that are used to remove the entire prostate for treatment of prostate cancer. LRP is an updated version of traditional forms of prostatectomy because it does not make large incisions in the patient. Instead, LRP is minimally invasive, using technology such as fiber optics and miniaturization. Because of these technological advances, little bleeding occurs with LRP,

---

KEY TERMS

BPH—Benign prostatic hypertrophy, a very common noncancerous cause of prostatic enlargement in older men.

Catheter—A tube placed through the urethra into the bladder in order to provide free drainage of urine and blood following either TUR or open prostatectomy.

Cryosurgery—In prostatectomy, the use of a very low-temperature probe to freeze and thereby destroy prostatic tissue.

Incontinence—The inability to retain urine or bowel movements until a person is ready to expel them voluntarily.

Prostate gland—The gland surrounding the male urethra just below the base of the bladder. It secretes a fluid that constitutes a major portion of the semen.

Urethra—The tube running from the bladder to the tip of the penis that provides a passage for eliminating urine from the body.

---

and with less bleeding, the number of risks during surgery and complications after surgery are reduced.

Robot-assisted laparoscopic radical prostatectomy (RALP)

Scientists from the Vattikuti Urology Institute at Henry Ford Hospital in Detroit, Michigan, are responsible for the development and popularization of robot-assisted laparoscopic radical prostatectomy (RALP). The first reported RALP, which used the da Vinci Surgical System (developed by Intuitive Surgical, Inc.), was performed in 2001. Robot-assisted laparoscopic radical prostatectomy involves the same type of keyhole incisions as LRP, but the surgeon is seated at a robotic console that controls the movement of the miniature instruments. This approach allows for an even higher degree of precision and for smaller incisions, resulting in less pain, bleeding, and risk of infection, as well as faster healing times and shorter hospital stays.

Transurethral resection of the prostate

Abbreviated TURP, transurethral resection of the prostate is a urological operation that is typically used to treat BPH. TURP was developed for this purpose in the mid-1900s. It is also used for symptomatic relief from prostate cancer. The operation is performed by visualizing the prostate through the urethra. Tissue is excised by sharp dissection or electrocautery. A resecto-scope (or resection cystoscope)—an instrument with a wide-angle telescope and an electrically activated wire loop—is moved up the urethra to the prostate. The surrounding tissue is then removed. Transurethral resection of the prostate is also sometimes called plural TURPs.

Preparation

Men must have a blood test called the prostate-specific antigen (PSA) test and routine **digital rectal examination** (DRE) before surgery. If the PSA levels and DRE are suspiciously indicative of prostate cancer, a transrectal ultrasound-guided needle **biopsy** of the prostate must be performed before open prostatectomy, to detect the presence of prostate cancer.

Additionally, preoperative patients should have lower urinary tract studies, including urinary flow rate and post void residual urine in the bladder. Because most patients are age 60 or older, preoperative evaluation should also include a detailed history and physical examination, standard blood tests, chest x-ray, and electrocardiogram (EKG) to detect any possible preexisting conditions.

Aftercare

Open prostatectomy is a major surgical operation requiring an inpatient hospital stay of four to seven days. Blood transfusions are generally not required due to improvements in surgical technique. Immediately after the operation, the surgeon must closely monitor urinary output and fluid status. On the first day after surgery, most patients are given a clear liquid diet and asked to sit up four times. Morphine sulfate, given via a patient controlled analgesic pump (IV), is used to control pain.

On the second postoperative day, the urethral catheter is removed if the urine does not contain blood. Oral pain medications are begun if the patient can tolerate a regular diet.

On the third postoperative day, the pelvic drain is removed if drainage is less than 75 milliliters (mL) in 24 hours. The patient should gradually increase activity. Follow-up with the surgeon is necessary following discharge from the hospital. Full activity is expected to resume within four to six weeks after surgery.

Laparoscopic radical prostatectomy may allow the patient to go home the day after surgery. It is usually advisable to stay in bed until the morning after surgery. Afterward, it is recommended to move about as much as possible. Other recommendations include:

- Change positions in bed every three to four hours to keep blood flowing.
- Cough or perform deep breathing exercises every three to four hours to prevent pneumonia.
- Wear special stockings on the legs to prevent blood clots.
- Take pain medicine as needed.

Risks

Improvements in surgical technique with open prostatectomy have lowered blood loss to a minimal level. For several weeks after open prostatectomy, patients may have urgency and urge incontinence. The severity of bladder problems depends on the patient's preoperative bladder status. Erectile dysfunction occurs in 3% to 5% of patients undergoing this procedure. Retrograde (backward flow) ejaculation occurs in approximately 50% to 80% of patients after open prostatectomy. The most common nonurologic risks include:

- pulmonary embolism
- myocardial infarction (heart attack)
- deep vein thrombosis
- cerebrovascular accident (stroke)

The incidence of any one of these potentially adverse effects is less than 1%.

For laparoscopic radical prostatectomy, the risks include:

- bowel incontinence (difficulty controlling bowel movements)
- impotence (erection problems)
- rectal injury
- urethral stricture (a tightening of the urinary opening due to scar tissue)
- urinary incontinence (difficulty controlling urine)

Results

In patients having radical prostatectomy for cancer, a successful operation will remove the tumor and prevent its spread to other areas of the body (**metastasis**). If examination of lymph nodes shows that cancer already had spread beyond the prostate at the time of surgery, other measures are available—such as **chemotherapy** or radiation therapy—to control the tumor.

Alternatives

Cryosurgery—also called **cryotherapy** or cryoablation—is a minimally invasive procedure that uses very low temperatures to freeze and destroy cancer cells in and

QUESTIONS TO ASK YOUR DOCTOR

- Why is a specific prostatectomy procedure recommended for me? Are others also recommended?

- What are the advantages and disadvantages of the various prostatectomy procedures?

- What forms of anesthesia and pain relief will be given?

- Where will the incision be located?

- What are the risks of the various procedures?

- Is the surgeon performing the procedure a board-certified urologist?

- Is there an alternative to the surgery selected for me?

- What are the chances of aftereffects, including erectile problems?

around the prostate gland. A catheter circulates warm fluid through the urethra to protect it from the cold. When used in connection with ultrasound imaging, cryosurgery permits very precise tissue destruction. Cryosurgery is most effective in patients with early-stage prostate cancer. It may also be used when other treatments, such as **radiation therapy**, are unsuccessful; to treat recurrent disease; or in patients who are not in good enough general health to undergo radical prostatectomy.

Health care team roles

Prostatectomy procedures are performed by a urological surgeon, who typically completes one year of general surgery training and four to five years of urology training. The procedures are usually performed in a large hospital.

Resources

BOOKS
Dasgupta, Prokar, and Roger S. Kirby, eds. *ABC of Prostate Cancer.* Chichester, U.K.: Blackwell, 2012.

Hubert, John, Peter Wiklund, and Jorn H. Witt, eds. *Atlas of Robotic Prostatectomy.* Berlin: Springer, 2013.

Klein, Eric A., and J. Stephen Jones, eds. *Management of Prostate Cancer.* New York: Humana Press, 2013.

Polascik, Thomas J., ed. *Imaging and Focal Therapy of Early Prostate Cancer.* New York: Humana Press, 2013.

Sutton, Amy L., ed. *Surgery Sourcebook.* Detroit: Omnigraphics, 2013.

WEBSITES
A.D.A.M. Medical Encyclopedia. "Radical Prostatectomy." MedlinePlus. http://www.nlm.nih.gov/medlineplus/ency/article/007300.htm (accessed August 20, 2014).

A.D.A.M. Medical Encyclopedia. "Transurethral Resection of the Prostate." MedlinePlus. http://www.nlm.nih.gov/medlineplus/ency/article/002996.htm (accessed August 20, 2014).

American Cancer Society. "Cryosurgery for Prostate Cancer." http://www.cancer.org/cancer/prostatecancer/detailed-guide/prostate-cancer-treating-cryosurgery (accessed August 20, 2014).

American Cancer Society. "Surgery for Prostate Cancer." http://www.cancer.org/cancer/prostatecancer/detailedguide/prostate-cancer-treating-surgery (accessed August 20, 2014).

Fulmer, Brant R. "Laparoscopic and Robotic Radical Prostatectomy." Medscape Reference. http://emedicine.medscape.com/article/458677-overview (accessed August 20, 2014).

ORGANIZATIONS
American Cancer Society, 250 Williams St. NW, Atlanta, GA 30303, (800) 227-2345, http://www.cancer.org.

American College of Physicians, 190 N. Independence Mall West, Philadelphia, PA 19106-1572, (215) 351-2400, (800) 523-1546, http://www.acponline.org.

American Medical Association, 515 N. State St., Chicago, IL 60654, (800) 621-8335, http://www.ama-assn.org/ama.

Prostate Cancer Foundation, 1250 Fourth St., Santa Monica, CA 90401, (310) 570-4700, Fax: (310) 570-4701, (800) 757-2873, info@pcf.org, http://www.pcf.org.

Laith Farid Gulli, MD, MS

REVISED BY TISH DAVIDSON, AM

REVISED BY WILLIAM A. ATKINS, BB, BS, MBA

Protein electrophoresis

Definition

Protein electrophoresis is a technique used to separate the different component proteins (fractions) in a mixture of proteins, such as a blood sample, on the basis of differences in how the components move through a fluid-filled matrix under the influence of an applied electric field.

Purpose

Protein electrophoresis is a **screening test** used to evaluate, diagnose, and monitor a variety of diseases and conditions through examination of the amounts and types of protein in a blood, urine, or cerebrospinal fluid (CSF) specimen.

KEY TERMS

Acute-phase proteins—Proteins produced during the acute-phase response, a set of physiological changes that occur in response to a biologic stressor such as trauma or sepsis.

Albumin—A blood protein produced in the liver that helps to regulate water distribution in the body.

Antibodies—Immunoglobulin protein molecules produced by B cells during the immune response. Each antibody recognizes an individual antigen to trigger immune defenses.

Antigen—Foreign body that triggers immune response.

Bence-Jones protein—The Ig light chain, part of an immunoglobulin detected by urine protein electrophoresis in the case of multiple myeloma.

Complement—A group of complex proteins of the beta-globulin type in the blood that bind to antibodies during anaphylaxis. In the complement cascade, each complement interacts with another in a pattern that causes fluid buildup in cells, leading to lysis (cell destruction).

Electrophoresis—A technique used to separate the proteins in a biological sample on the basis of differences in how the components move through a fluid-filled matrix under the influence of an applied electric field.

Globulins—A group of proteins in blood plasma whose levels can be measured by electrophoresis in order to diagnose or monitor a variety of serious illnesses.

Hemolysis—Also called hematolysis, the breakage of red blood cells and concomitant liberation of hemoglobin.

Lumbar puncture—Also called spinal tap, a procedure for the withdrawal of spinal fluid from the lumbar region of the spinal cord for diagnosis, for injection of a dye for imaging, or for administering medication or an anesthetic.

Paraprotein—An immunoglobulin produced by a clone of identical B cells.

Protein—Biologically important molecules made of long chains of connected amino acids that contain the elements carbon, hydrogen, nitrogen, and oxygen. Certain proteins may also contain sulfur, phosphorus, iron, iodine, selenium, or other trace elements.

Description

Proteins—long chains of connected amino acids—are biologically important building-block chemicals that contain the elements carbon, hydrogen, nitrogen, and oxygen. Some proteins also contain sulfur, phosphorus, iron, iodine, selenium, or other trace elements. There are 22 amino acids commonly found in all proteins. The human body is capable of producing fourteen of these amino acids; the remaining eight are called essential amino acids, and must be obtained from food. Proteins are found in muscles, blood, skin, hair, nails, and the internal organs and tissues. Enzymes and antibodies are proteins, and many hormones are proteinlike. Electrophoresis is one of a variety of techniques that can be used to fractionate (separate) protein mixtures into individual component proteins.

The serum protein electrophoresis test requires a blood sample drawn by venipuncture (having blood drawn from a vein) performed in the doctor's office or on site at a medical laboratory. The urine protein electrophoresis test requires either an early-morning urine sample or a 24-hour urine sample, according to the physician's request. A CSF specimen must be collected by **lumbar puncture** (spinal tap), generally performed by a physician as an outpatient procedure in a hospital. Because of risks associated with the lumbar puncture procedure, the patient must sign a consent form, and should be prepared to remain for six to eight hours under observation.

Precautions

Certain other diagnostic tests or prescription medications can affect the protein electrophoresis results. The administration of a contrast dye used in some other tests may falsely elevate apparent protein levels. Drugs that can alter results include aspirin, bicarbonates, chlorpromazine (Thorazine), **corticosteroids**, isoniazid (INH), and neomycin (Mycifradin). The total serum protein concentration may also be affected by changes in the patient's posture or by the use of a tourniquet during the drawing of blood.

Because there is less protein in urine and CSF samples than in blood, these samples often must be concentrated before analysis. The added sample handling can lead to contamination and erroneous results. In collection of a CSF specimen, it is important that the sample not be contaminated with blood proteins that would invalidate the CSF protein measurements.

Preparation

It is usually not necessary for the patient to restrict food or fluids before blood is drawn for a serum protein electrophoresis test; a four-hour fast is requested before drawing blood for lipoprotein testing. For protein electrophoresis on all types of samples, any factors that might affect test results, such as whether the patient is taking any medications, should be noted.

Aftercare

After a blood sample is drawn, a small bandage may be applied to the puncture site, and the patient may be cautioned about the possibility of fainting or of lightheadedness. Following lumbar puncture for the collection of CSF, the patient must be kept lying flat in the hospital under observation for at least six to eight hours.

Risks

Risks posed by the venipuncture are minimal but may include slight bleeding from the puncture site, the development of a small bruise at the puncture site, or both. Other risks include fainting or lightheadedness after the sample is drawn. Lumbar puncture can lead to leakage of CSF from the puncture site, headache, infection, symptoms of meningitis, nausea, vomiting, or difficulty urinating. Rarely, preexisting intracranial pressure can lead to brain herniation, resulting in brain damage or death.

Results

Blood proteins

Serum protein electrophoresis is used to determine the total serum protein concentration, which is an indication of the patient's hydration state: dehydration leads to high total serum protein concentration. Further, the levels of different blood proteins rise or fall in response to such disorders as **cancer** and associated protein-wasting syndromes, immune system disorders, liver dysfunction, impaired nutrition, and chronic fluid-retaining conditions. The different types of blood proteins are separated into fractions of five distinct classes: albumin, alpha$_1$-globulins, alpha$_2$-globulins, beta-globulins, and gamma-globulins (immunoglobulins). In addition to standard protein electrophoresis, **immunoelectrophoresis** may be used to assess the blood levels of specific immunoglobulins. Immunoelectrophoresis is usually ordered when the serum protein electrophoresis test shows an unusually high amount of protein in the gamma-globulin fraction.

ALBUMIN. Albumin, which is produced in the liver, is the most abundant blood protein. It makes a major contribution to the regulation of water movement between the tissues and the bloodstream. Albumin binds calcium, thyroid hormones, fatty acids, and many drugs, keeping them in the blood circulation and preventing them from being filtered out by the kidneys. Albumin levels can play a role in the effectiveness and toxicity of therapeutic drugs and in drug interactions.

GLOBULINS. Serum globulins are separated in protein electrophoresis as four main fractions: alpha$_1$-, alpha$_2$-, beta-, and gamma-globulins.

- The major alpha$_1$-globulin is alpha$_1$-antitrypsin, produced by the lungs and liver. Alpha$_1$-antitrypsin deficiency is a marker of an inherited disorder characterized by an increased risk of emphysema.

- Alpha$_2$-globulins include serum haptoglobin, alpha$_2$-macroglobulin, and ceruloplasmin. Haptoglobin binds to hemoglobin, released from damaged red blood cells during hemolysis, to prevent its excretion by the kidneys. Alpha$_2$-macroglobulin accounts for about one-third of the alpha$_2$-globulin fraction. Ceruloplasmin is involved in the storage and transport of copper and iron in the body.

- Beta-globulins include transferrin, low-density lipoprotein (LDL), and complement components. Transferrin transports dietary iron to the liver, spleen, and bone marrow. Low-density lipoprotein is the major carrier of cholesterol in the blood. Complement is a system of blood proteins involved in inflammatory response.

- The gamma-globulin fraction contains the immunoglobulins, a family of proteins that function as antibodies. Antibodies, in response to infection, allergic reactions, and organ transplants, recognize and bind foreign bodies, or antigens, to facilitate their destruction by the immune system. The immune response is regulated by a large number of antigen-specific gamma-globulins that fall into five main classes, called IgG, IgA, IgM, IgB, and IgE. When the serum protein electrophoresis test demonstrates a significant deviation from the normal gamma-globulin levels, a supplemental test, immunoelectrophoresis, should be ordered to identify the specific globulin(s) involved.

The following serum protein electrophoresis reference values are representative; some variation among laboratories and specific methods is to be expected. (1 gm = approximately 0.02 pt and 1 dL = approximately 0.33 fluid oz.)

- Total protein: 6.4–8.3 g/dL
- Albumin: 3.5–5.0 g/dL
- Alpha$_1$-globulin: 0.1–0.3 g/dL

- Alpha$_2$ globulin: 0.6–1.0 g/dL
- Beta-globulin: 0.7–1.2 g/dL
- Gamma-globulin: 0.7–1.6 g/dL

Urinary proteins

Protein electrophoresis is performed on urine samples to classify disorders that cause protein loss via the kidneys. In urine, normally no globulins and less than 0.050 g/dL albumin are present.

Cerebrospinal fluid (CSF) proteins

In CSF, the total protein concentration is normally 0.015–0.045 g/dL, with gamma-globulin accounting for 3% to 12%. The main use of CSF protein electrophoresis testing is in the diagnosis of central nervous tumors and multiple sclerosis.

Abnormal results

Deviations in serum protein levels from reference levels are considered in conjunction with symptoms and results from other diagnostic procedures.

Albumin levels are increased in dehydration and decreased in malnutrition, pregnancy, liver disease, inflammatory diseases, and protein-losing states such as malabsorption syndrome and certain kidney disorders. Low serum albumin levels can indicate disease and can influence analysis of thyroid hormones and calcium.

Alpha$_1$-globulins are increased in inflammatory diseases and decreased or absent in juvenile pulmonary emphysema, a hereditary disease.

Alpha$_2$-globulins are increased in acute and chronic inflammation and nephrotic syndrome. Decreased values may indicate hemolysis (the release of hemoglobin from red blood cells). Low haptoglobin can indicate tumor **metastasis**, severe sepsis, or chronic liver disease. The concentration of macroglobulin is increased during nephrosis. Ceruloplasmin concentration is increased during pregnancy and decreased in Wilson's disease, a rare inherited condition that leads to accumulation of copper in the liver.

Beta-globulin levels are increased in **multiple myeloma** and also in conditions of high cholesterol (hypercholesterolemia), such as in atherosclerosis, and in iron deficiency **anemia**. Levels are decreased in coagulation disorders.

Gamma-globulin levels are increased in multiple **myeloma**. The levels are increased as well in chronic inflammatory disease and autoimmune conditions such as rheumatoid arthritis and systemic lupus erythematosus, cirrhosis, and acute and chronic infection. The gamma-globulins are decreased in leukemia, in a variety of genetic immune disorders, and in secondary immune deficiency related to steroid use or to severe infection. Immunoglobulin deficiency due to inherited disorders can range from partial or complete loss of a single immunoglobulin class to complete absence of all immunoglobulins.

Finding an individual (oligoclonal) band in the gamma fraction of the electrophoresis result indicates the presence of a paraprotein. Type IgG or IgA paraproteins associated with multiple myeloma may be found by serum protein electrophoresis testing; however, the tumor may also produce only Ig light chains that are removed from the blood by the kidneys. This Ig light chain (also known as the Bence-Jones protein) is detected by urine protein electrophoresis and is found nearly exclusively in patients with multiple myeloma.

In urine samples, abnormal results other than the presence of the Bence-Jones protein indicate disruption of kidney function or acute inflammation. Hemoglobin and myoglobin are found in the urine of patients with infection or hemolysis.

An increase in total protein concentration in the CSF is often found with central nervous system (CNS) tumors and in meningitis.

Resources

PERIODICALS

Dash N.R., Mohanty B. "Multiple Myeloma: A Case of Atypical Presentation on Protein Electrophoresis." *Indian Journal of Clinical Biochemistry* 27, no. 1 (2012): 100–102. http://www.ncbi.nlm.nih.gov/pmc/articles/PMC3286584/ (accessed November 12, 2014).

WEBSITES

A.D.A.M. Medical Encyclopedia. "Protein Electrophoresis - Serum." Medline Plus. http://www.nlm.nih.gov/medlineplus/ency/article/003540.htm (accessed November 14, 2014).

Healthwise. "Serum Protein Electrophoresis (SPEP)." Norris Cotton Cancer Center, Dartmouth. http://cancer.dartmouth.edu/pf/health_encyclopedia/hw43650 (accessed November 14, 2014).

Patricia L. Bounds, PhD

Proteomics

Definition

Proteomics is the systematic study of all of the proteins in a given cell, tissue, or organism—referred to as the proteome. **Cancer** cells express different proteins than normal cells of the same cell type and different amounts of some proteins. Proteomics is a major area of

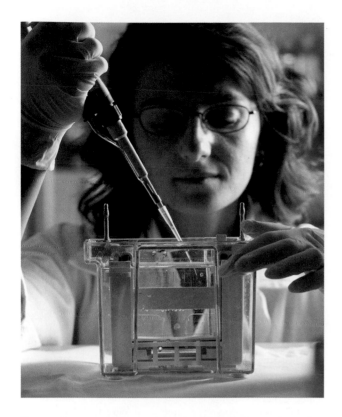

Researcher preparing a polyacrylamide gel electrophoresis (PAGE) machine to study the structure and function of proteins within an organism (proteomics). *(Mauro Fermariello/Science Source)*

cancer research, with great potential for cancer diagnosis and treatment. Although clinical use of cancer proteomics is in its infancy, it may someday lead to true personalized medicine.

Description

The term "proteome" was coined in 1994 to describe all of the proteins in a given cell, tissue, or organism. Proteomes are extremely complex. They differ among individuals, cell types, and within the same cell depending on cell activity, stimuli, and disease. In May 2014, two studies published in the journal *Nature* announced the identification of 17,000–18,000 proteins encoded by the estimated 21,000 genes that make up the human genome. This publicly available map of the human proteome is expected to accelerate the development of molecular diagnostics, which identifies cancer cells on the basis of: their genes and the proteins expressed by those genes, rather than their pathology; their appearance under the microscope; and the abnormal interactions among genes and proteins in cancerous and precancerous cells. These patterns of gene and protein expression are known as molecular signatures and are already improving cancer diagnosis. Eventually, all cancers may be diagnosed by their molecular signatures.

Proteomics is even more complicated than genomics—the DNA sequences of all the genes that encode proteins and regulate the expression of other genes and proteins.

- Whereas the genome has about 21,000 protein-encoding genes, there are estimated to be between 250,000 and one million different proteins in the human body. In part, this is because some genes encode multiple proteins, and proteins are rearranged and recombined to make different proteins.

- Whereas the genome is relatively stable, proteins are constantly changing. They are continually: being made and broken down; activated and deactivated; bound to cellular membranes; moved to different parts of the cell or the cell surface; formed into complexes with other proteins; and secreted to communicate with other cells or tissues in the body.

- After proteins are synthesized according to the DNA sequences of their genes, they can undergo a variety of chemical modifications that regulate their activities.

- Whereas some proteins are present in the body in very high amounts, others are present only in minuscule amounts and are difficult to detect among all the other proteins in blood and tissue. Some of these proteins that are present in tiny amounts are among the most important for cancer.

Cancer proteomics

The changes that occur in genes that precipitate the development of cancer affect the proteins that are made by cancer cells. Cancer proteomics is the study of how cellular pathways are switched in malignancy because critical proteins are produced, absent, damaged, inactive, or overactive. Different cellular pathways and communications are often affected in different types of cancers and may even differ among individuals with the same type of cancer.

Proteins that are expressed in cancer cells but not in normal cells of the same type or are present in much higher amounts in cancer cells are called biomarkers. Biomarkers may be detectable in blood, urine, or tissues from cancer patients. Biomarkers are useful not only for diagnosing cancer, but also for understanding the processes affected when a cell becomes malignant and for developing new targets for therapeutic intervention. Proteomics has led to the identification of many more biomarker proteins and the discovery of many new proteins in the blood. Proteomics has been used to identify hundreds of proteins in the ovary, breast, prostate, and esophagus that increase or decrease as cells begin to grow abnormally. Scientists are systematically linking changes in genes with changes in the types and amounts of proteins in order to develop genome and proteome maps for different types of cancer.

Phosphoproteomics is an emerging specialized field of proteomics that concentrates on identifying phosphorylated proteins. Small molecules called phosphates are commonly added to or removed from proteins to change their activity or function. Cellular signaling pathways that are activated or disrupted in cancer often involve protein phosphorylation and dephosphorylation. For example, specific changes in phosphorylated proteins are believed to be important for **prostate cancer** progression. Phosphoproteomics may help to not only classify cancers, but also to identify new drug targets and predict drug responses.

Proteomics is expected to lead to:

- identification of new biomarkers and protein patterns for detecting early cancers
- better cancer treatments
- better predictions of responses to treatments and the likelihood of relapse after treatment
- therapies individualized for each patient

Procedures

Cancer proteomics uses several different techniques to identify and quantify the proteins in cancer cells from a blood or **biopsy** sample. Blood or biopsy samples are immediately treated with enzymes that block dephosphorylation, so that the activation state of proteins in the cancer cells is preserved. Laser-capture microdissection microscopes use low-energy laser beams and special transfer film to lift single cells from a tissue, so that all of the proteins in a cell can be collected and analyzed. Pure samples of normal cells, precancerous cells, and tumor cells can be removed from a patient's biopsy tissue. The samples are treated in various ways to reduce their complexity and isolate particular protein fractions of interest.

Mass spectrometry (MS)

High-resolution MS can sort out the thousands of proteins and protein fragments in a sample on the basis of their molecular weight and electrical charge. A mass spectrometer consists of:

- an ionization source that removes electrons from (ionizes) the proteins and protein fragments in a sample so that they all have a positive charge
- a mass analyzer that measures the mass-to-charge ratio (m/z) of the ionized (charged) proteins and fragments, as gases under a vacuum

- a detector that determines the number of ions present at each m/z value

The result is a mass spectrum or chart with a series of spikes or peaks, each representing a charged protein fragment from the sample. The height of each peak represents the amount of that particular protein or fragment that is present in the sample. The sizes of the peaks and the distances between them constitute the protein pattern or array. Each spectrum may have more than 15,000 data points—one for every protein and protein fragment—with their molecular weights and intensity values reflecting their relative abundance in the sample. MS can distinguish proteins that differ in only a single hydrogen atom, which is the smallest atom.

Computers rapidly analyze the MS data, searching for subtle differences among multiple protein patterns and for proteins that might serve as biomarkers. Once potential biomarkers are identified, the computer is trained to sort through the patterns of thousands of proteins for the few small protein biomarkers that can distinguish between cancer and control samples or between cancer protein patterns before and after treatment.

MS-based proteomic analysis is very fast. The entire process—from collecting a few drops of blood to the spectral analysis—can occur in less than one minute. Extremely small amounts of protein can be detected, and hundreds of samples can be analyzed sequentially.

Other proteomics techniques

Protein microarrays are another tool for identifying and quantifying proteins in a sample. A protein microarray is typically a small piece of glass or plastic coated with thousands of molecules that each bind to a specific protein. Microarrays can be used to identify multiple biomarkers in a single sample.

Nanotechnologies are being developed that will further advance proteomics by being able to detect proteins in living cells and identify proteins that are present in very small amounts. Nanotechnologies are already being used therapeutically, and they have the potential to greatly enhance cancer diagnosis.

Clinical applications

The application of clinical cancer proteomics is dependent on further collection and analysis of large numbers of cancer specimens. It is also dependent on the development of new reagents for identifying proteins, including antibodies and other molecules that bind to specific proteins and reporter molecules that detect a target or modifications to a target protein. Finally, clinical applications depend on the further development

KEY TERMS

Antibodies—Immune system proteins that recognize specific antigens, such as disease-causing organisms or proteins on tumor cells.

Autoantibodies—Antibodies that the immune system produces against the body's own proteins.

Bioinformatics—Mathematical, statistical, and computer science methods for solving biological problems and analyzing data; it includes the collection, storage, analysis, and interpretation of DNA and protein sequence information; collection and analysis of patient statistics; data from tissue specimens; and results of clinical trials.

Biomarker—A protein or other molecule that is indicative of a process, condition, or disease, such as a protein secreted by a tumor.

Biopsy—The removal of a small piece of tissue for examination.

Genomics—The science of mapping genes and sequencing the DNA of an organism, collecting the results in a database, and analyzing and applying those results.

Laser-capture microdissection microscope—An instrument that uses low-energy laser beams and special transfer film to lift single cells from a tissue.

Mass spectroscopy (MS)—A technique that separates mixtures of substances, such as proteins, on the basis of molecular weight and electrical charge.

Mass-to-charge ratio (m/z)—The ratio of the molecular mass of a substance to its electrical charge; used for protein separation by mass spectroscopy.

Microarray—A glass or plastic slide with attached proteins that specifically bind to other proteins in a mixture for identification and proteomic analysis.

Personalized medicine—Medical care based on the specific genome and proteome of an individual patient's cancer cells.

Phosphoproteomics—The study of the subset of proteins in a cell or blood or tissue that are phosphorylated.

Phosphorylation—The addition of a phosphate molecule to a protein, usually to regulate its activity; dephosphorylation is the removal of a phosphate molecule.

Prostate-specific antigen (PSA)—A biomarker used as a preliminary screen for prostate cancer.

Protein array—The pattern of proteins in blood, tissue, or a cell as determined by mass spectrometry.

Proteome—The collection of all of the proteins in a cell, tissue, or organism.

---

of bioinformatics—systems for handling massive amounts of gene and protein data and analyses.

Proteomics should eventually lead to:

- the development of cancer screenings based on the relative amounts of different proteins in the blood, or even in exhaled breath for lung cancer screening

- identification of protein patterns that predict early-stage cancer

- methods for distinguishing more aggressive and less aggressive cancers

- predictions of how a particular treatment or drug will affect the network of proteins in a cell

- predictions of which patients are likely to have an early toxic response to a treatment, so that doses can be lowered or a different treatment can be chosen

- detecting early signs of cancer drug toxicity

- means for reducing side effects of treatment

- identifying mechanisms of cancer drug resistance

- identification of changes in protein patterns during tumor recurrence

Cancers

Much of early cancer proteomics has focused on ovarian and prostate cancers—cancers that usually progress without symptoms so that they are not detected in early stages when they are most treatable. By using proteomics for early detection, tumors may be treated before they spread (metastasize) to other parts of the body. Proteomic scientists also are studying other solid human tumors, including breast, colon, lung, and pancreatic cancers.

Ovarian cancer

More than 80% of ovarian cancers are not diagnosed until they have reached an advanced stage when the five-year-survival rate is 20% or less. However, in the 20% of women whose ovarian cancers are diagnosed at an early stage, the prognosis is excellent, with a five-year survival rate of over 95%. Thus, early detection could have a huge impact on cure rate.

The pattern of proteins in the blood is one method that is being tested for identifying early ovarian cancers. Although the protein CA-125 in the blood is considered a biomarker of **ovarian cancer**, it is not sensitive enough to detect early cancers and is not specific to ovarian cancer. Two large studies that used CA-125 in the blood along with ultrasound to screen for ovarian cancer found more cancers, including some at an early stage, but the screened women did not live longer and were no less likely to die from ovarian cancer than unscreened women. A 2013 proteomics study identified high-frequency autoantibodies that appear to be much more sensitive and specific for early-stage ovarian cancer than CA-125 levels.

Some companies have been overzealous in capitalizing on proteomics. As of 2014, the U.S. Food and Drug Administration (FDA) had requested the removal from the market of two different proteomics tests for ovarian cancer because they were ineffective.

Other cancers

Prostate-specific antigen (PSA) levels are used as a preliminary screen for prostate cancer. However, 70–75% of men who undergo biopsies because of abnormal PSA levels do not have cancer. Unfortunately, it has been difficult to rule out prostate cancer without a biopsy in patients with slightly elevated PSA levels (4–10 nanograms per milliliter). Scientists are continuing to search for blood protein patterns that may predict a person's risk of prostate cancer, **pancreatic cancer**, and **melanoma**.

As of 2014, recent advances in cancer proteomics included:

• protein patterns in lung and bladder tumors that may be useful for discriminating between cancerous and healthy tissues

• promising new biomarkers for pancreatic cancer

• novel proteins associated with colorectal cancer progression

• an 11-protein signature for aggressive triple-negative breast cancer (breast cancers that lack all three biomarkers that can be treated with targeted therapies)

Resources

BOOKS

Abeloff, M. D., et al. *Clinical Oncology*, 5th ed. New York: Churchill Livingstone, 2014.

Ferri, Fred. *Ferri's Best Test*, 3rd ed. Philadelphia: Saunders, 2015.

LaFond, Richard E., ed. *Cancer: The Outlaw Cell*, 3rd ed. New York: American Chemical Society/Oxford University, 2012.

McPherson, R. A., et al. *Henry's Clinical Diagnosis and Management by Laboratory Methods*, 22nd ed. Philadelphia: Saunders, 2011.

Niederhuber, J. E., et al. *Clinical Oncology*, 5th ed. Philadelphia: Elsevier, 2014.

Veenstra, Timothy Daniel. *Proteomic Applications in Cancer Detection and Discovery*. Hoboken, NJ: John Wiley & Sons, 2013.

PERIODICALS

Ballehaninna, Umashankar K., and Ronald S. Chamberlain. "Biomarkers for Pancreatic Cancer: Promising New Markers and Options Beyond CA 19-9." *Tumor Biology* 34, no. 6 (December 2013): 3279–3292.

Gan Yi, Daojin Chen, and Xiaorong Li. "Proteomic Analysis Reveals Novel Proteins Associated with Progression and Differentiation of Colorectal Carcinoma." *Journal of Cancer Research and Therapeutics* 10, no. 1 (January–March 2014): 89–96.

Karabudak, Aykan A., et al. "Autoantibody Biomarkers Identified by Proteomics Methods Distinguish Ovarian Cancer from Non-Ovarian Cancer with Various CA-125 Levels." *Journal of Cancer Research & Clinical Oncology* 139, no. 10 (October 2013): 1757–1770.

Khan, Amina. "Researchers Map Human Proteins; Understanding the Proteome May Someday Help Doctors Identify Damaged Tissues, Treat Cancers." *Los Angeles Times* (May 31, 2014): AA2.

Liu, Zexian, Yongbo Wang, and Yu Xue. "Phosphoproteomics-Based Network Medicine." *FEBS Journal* 280, no. 22 (November 2013): 5696–5704.

Yuan, Yuan, et al. "Assessing the Clinical Utility of Cancer Genomic and Proteomic Data Across Tumor Types." *Nature Biotechnology* 32, no. 7 (July 2014): 644–652.

WEBSITES

"Cancer in the Twenty-First Century." American Cancer Society. June 12, 2014. http://www.cancer.org/cancer/cancerbasics/

thehistoryofcancer/the-history-of-cancer-twenty-first-century-and-beyond (accessed October 22, 2014).

Hillis, Danny. "Understanding Cancer through Proteomics." Filmed October 2010. TED video, 19:55. http://www.ted.com/talks/danny_hillis_two_frontiers_of_cancer_treatment (accessed February 5, 2015).

Liu, Ning Qing, et al. "Comparative Proteome Analysis Revealing an 11-Protein Signature for Aggressive Triple-Negative Breast Cancer." *Journal of the National Cancer Institute* 106, no. 2 (February 2014). http://www.ncbi.nlm.nih.gov/pmc/articles/PMC3952199 (accessed October 22, 2014).

Office of Cancer Clinical Proteomics Research. "What is Cancer Proteomics?" National Cancer Institute. http://proteomics.cancer.gov/whatisproteomics (accessed October 22, 2014).

ORGANIZATIONS

American Cancer Society, 250 Williams Street NW, Atlanta, GA 30303, (800) 227-2345, http://www.cancer.org.

National Cancer Institute, 6116 Executive Boulevard, Suite 300, Bethesda, MD 20892-8322, (800) 4-CANCER (422-6237), http://www.cancer.gov.

Margaret Alic, PhD

REVISED BY MARGARET ALIC, PHD

Provenge *see* **Sipuleucel-T**

Pruritus *see* **Itching**

Psycho-oncology

Definition

Psycho-oncology is a broad-based approach to **cancer** therapy that treats the emotional, social, and spiritual distress that often accompanies a diagnosis of cancer, its treatment, and aftereffects.

Description

According to Dr. Jimmie Holland, the founder of psycho-oncology, the field has two major emphases: the first is the study of cancer patients' psychological reactions to their illness at all stages of its course; the second is analysis of the emotional, spiritual, social, and behavioral factors that influence the risk of developing cancer and long-term survival following treatment. Some psycho-oncologists consider their field a subspecialty of psychiatry, while others emphasize its multidisciplinary aspects. In addition to psychiatrists, psycho-oncology departments in major cancer centers may include psychologists, surgeons, nurses, bioethicists,

---

KEY TERMS

Bioethicist—A professional concerned with the moral and societal implications of medical research and treatments.

Distress—In general, an acute feeling of pain, anxiety, or sadness; in psycho-oncology, any unpleasant emotion that interferes with a cancer patient's ability to cope with symptoms and treatment.

Oncology—The medical specialty that deals with the development, diagnosis, and treatment of cancer.

Palliative—Relieving or alleviating symptoms such as pain without curing the disease.

Visualization—A technique for forming mental images or pictures of the healing process as a means of strengthening the immune system and/or fighting disease agents such as cancer cells.

---

social workers, clergy, palliative care specialists, and volunteers.

Origins

Psycho-oncology is a relatively new addition to cancer care. It began in the mid-1970s when Dr. Holland returned to her psychiatry practice after her children entered school. Married to an oncologist, she noted that her husband's colleagues focused on the physical effects of **chemotherapy** while failing to acknowledge its emotional and psychological effects on their patients. To some extent, this oversight was part of the medical culture of the 1950s and 1960s, at a time when cancer was stigmatized by low survival rates. In fact, many doctors had been taught in medical school to withhold a diagnosis of cancer from patients on the grounds that the disease was essentially a death sentence, and the truth would be unbearable. Such highly regarded newspapers as *The New York Times* even refused to print the words "breast cancer" when the founders of the Reach to Recovery program first wanted to insert notices of their meetings.

In the 1970s, however, this attitude of shame and secrecy was reversed, in part due to the patients' rights movement, but also because newer and more effective treatments for cancer began increasing the population of long-term survivors: as of 2014, 14 million Americans were living with or had survived cancer. In 1977, Dr. Holland founded the first full-time psychiatric service within a **cancer research** center for the study and treatment of emotional and psychological crises in cancer patients. She conducted some of the earliest research studies on the emotional impact of cancer on patients and their families.

By the early 2000s, psycho-oncology had become an established aspect of cancer treatment, with psycho-oncology departments in most major cancer centers in the United States and Canada, as well as the specialized journal *Psycho-Oncology*, and national and international professional societies. As of 2014, Dr. Holland had been caring for cancer patients for more than 30 years and held the Wayne E. Chapman Chair in Psychiatric Oncology at Memorial Sloan-Kettering Cancer Center in New York.

Psychological and emotional issues

A diagnosis of cancer is always a stressful and upsetting event. The distress felt by patients and their families and loved ones may include feelings of sadness, hopelessness, powerlessness, anxiety, fear, **depression**, vulnerability, and even panic. These feelings can make it difficult to cope with life changes dictated by a cancer diagnosis and can affect thoughts, behaviors, and relationships with others. Psychological and emotional issues can be particularly acute while awaiting surgery or other treatments. Patients may be concerned about their work and home lives and financial issues and can have psychological as well as physical difficulties in dealing with the side effects of treatment. For cancers that may have a genetic basis and could affect other family members, issues surrounding genetic counseling and testing can increase anxiety. For some people, the most difficult psychological issues arise after treatment and can last a lifetime, as most patients fear that their cancer will recur at some point.

Events that can worsen distress in cancer patients include:

- a new symptom
- waiting for a diagnosis or treatment
- returning home from the hospital
- finishing treatment and returning to "normal" life
- treatment failures
- worsening or advancing cancer
- follow-up visits to the doctor
- cancer recurrence
- approaching the end of life
- entering hospice care

Risk factors

Memories of past experiences can increase feelings of distress. These include serious illnesses or deaths of loved ones, previous depression or suicidal thoughts or attempts, and nightmares or panic attacks over painful past events. Other risk factors for more serious distress include:

- being female
- high stress levels before cancer diagnosis
- previous drug or alcohol abuse
- past mental health problems
- other serious medical problems in addition to cancer
- communication problems, such as speaking another language or difficulty reading or hearing
- social or family problems
- previous physical or sexual abuse
- living alone
- limited access to health care
- having young children
- financial problems
- religious or spiritual conflicts
- uncontrolled symptoms

Diagnosis

Signs and symptoms of serious psycho-oncological problems may include:

- overwhelming sense of dread
- panic
- unwillingness to undergo treatment because of anxiety or depression
- feelings of defeat or inability to continue
- unusual irritability or anger
- inability to cope with pain, fatigue, or nausea
- poor concentration, memory problems, or confused thinking ("chemo brain")
- inability to make even small decisions
- insomnia
- loss of appetite
- family conflicts
- constant thoughts of cancer or death
- questioning of religious faith that once provided comfort
- low self-esteem, feelings of worthlessness
- poor body image

There are several screening and diagnostic tools for assessing psycho-oncology issues. The American Cancer Society website offers two self-screening tools—the Thermometer and the Problem List—to help patients decide whether professional counseling might be helpful.

In addition to the above tools, psycho-oncologists use a pain scale or other tools for monitoring distress. These include: the Mental Adjustment to Cancer (MAC) scale, first published in the United Kingdom in 1987; the Brief Symptom Inventory (BSI); and the Distress Management Screening Measure (DMSM).

Treatment

Patients in distress are usually first referred to a social worker to determine whether their problems are practical issues that the social worker can help with, or psychosocial or psycho-oncological problems—such as major depression or anxiety, panic attacks, mood disorders or substance abuse—that may require a mental health professional.

Psycho-oncologists emphasize the importance of treating cancer patients as individuals with unique patterns of emotional responses to their disease, as well as unique physical responses to the disease and its treatments. Consequently, psycho-oncologists tailor their treatments to the needs and concerns of each patient, while monitoring their emotional distress levels. Treatments may include:

- individual psychotherapy or counseling
- support groups for patients and family members
- referrals to counseling in the patient's faith or tradition
- medication management
- strategies for dealing with pain and other physical symptoms
- specialized counseling or referrals to specialists in sex therapy or death and bereavement
- crisis intervention

Dr. Holland's recommendations for coping with cancer emphasize flexibility:

- Using coping techniques or patterns that the patient has found helpful in the past for dealing with stress; for example, people who have been helped in the past by talking through problems with trusted friends or family members should not suddenly keep problems to themselves when coping with cancer.
- Using techniques such as relaxation, meditation, listening to music, or other calming activities that have helped them in the past.
- Taking a "one-day-at-a-time" approach to dealing with symptoms and other problems. This approach, sometimes called "chunking it down," helps keep the focus on the present and makes large-scale worries about the future more manageable.
- Using support or self-help groups that improve feelings—and leaving any group that worsens feelings.

- Seeking out a doctor with whom the patient feels comfortable. A doctor/patient relationship based on trust and mutual respect makes it easier to ask appropriate questions and participate fully in treatment planning. Knowing what side effects or other problems to expect makes it easier to cope with these when and if they occur.
- Continuing to draw on religious or spiritual beliefs and practices that have been helpful in the past. Patients who do not consider themselves religious or spiritual may find comfort in activities that they find meaningful or inspiring, such as the performing arts or nature walks.
- Keeping a notebook for recording dates of treatments, medication side effects, laboratory test results, x-ray findings, and other information. This record can be valuable for monitoring or evaluating emotional ups and downs as well as changes in physical health.
- Keeping a journal or diary for expressing feelings and emotional reactions. This record may also be useful in providing perspective.
- Having a close friend or family member accompany the patient to medical appointments, tests, and procedures for support; to help hear and absorb information; and for practical assistance in keeping appointments and providing transportation.
- Finding complementary therapies approved by one's doctor to supplement regular treatment and improve quality of life.
- Participating in moderate exercise that can improve feelings, strength, and fitness, and lessen fatigue and anxiety.

Dr. Holland's list of "don'ts" include:

- believe that cancer means death
- blame oneself
- feel guilty for not having a constantly positive attitude
- suffer silently and alone
- feel embarrassed or ashamed for seeking professional help from a mental health expert
- keep anxieties or symptoms from closest friends or family members
- abandon regular treatment for an alternative therapy

Alternative and complementary therapies

Most psycho-oncologists support patients' use of alternative and complementary therapies that do not interfere with their mainstream treatments. These include yoga, Reiki, acupuncture, massage therapy (for cancer-related **fatigue**), and hyperbaric oxygen therapy.

Research

Areas of particular concern to psycho-oncologists include cultural differences that affect people's patterns of coping with cancer and the long-term psychological effects of cancer survivorship. For example, European studies have suggested that English-speaking patients and patients from southern Europe have different styles of coping with cancer diagnosis and treatment, even though both groups have similar percentages of highly distressed patients. The Behavioral Research Center of the American Cancer Society is conducting a long-term study of cancer survivors' quality of life, with a special focus on psychological adjustments and family relationships.

Special concerns

Special concerns of psycho-oncology include feelings of guilt or anxiety among many cancer patients that they cannot adopt or maintain the positive attitudes that some people believe are essential to fighting cancer. Such patients feel burdened by the notion—sometimes voiced by family members—that their survival depends on visualizations (usually visualizations of their immune system defeating the cancer) or otherwise acting cheerful and upbeat. Some extreme forms of "New Age" thought lead to "blaming the victim" with statements such as: "You must have subconsciously wanted this cancer" or "It is your bad karma—you must have done something in a previous existence to deserve this disease." Psycho-oncologists do not regard mental attitudes toward cancer as the sole factor affecting long-term survival, and they do not insist that patients adopt a one-size-fits-all approach to coping with cancer.

Psycho-oncologists can help patients deal with the increasing complexity of cancer therapy. Many patients have treatment teams that include several physicians in different subspecialties, as well as nurses, social workers, clergy, and other professionals. The sheer number of caregivers can be an additional source of stress.

Psycho-oncologists have found that psychological distress is a significantly greater issue in adolescent and young adult (AYA) cancer patients than among younger children and older adults. AYA patients often have more issues surrounding potential loss of fertility, educational or career disruptions, and social interactions. Psycho-oncologists have found that these issues and resulting isolation can affect AYAs for many years after surviving cancer. Psycho-oncology treatment for AYA cancer patients can be particularly challenging and requires a trained healthcare team. The **National Comprehensive Cancer Network** (NCCN) has issued guidelines for addressing AYA issues.

QUESTIONS TO ASK YOUR DOCTOR

- How do you feel about my use of complementary or alternative therapies as part of my treatment program? Are there any therapies that you would advise against?
- How do my emotional, psychological, and spiritual concerns fit into my treatment regimen?
- What professional counseling or other resources are available to me?
- What reading materials or other resources do you recommend for helping me cope with my symptoms and the side effects of cancer treatment?
- Do you recommend that I consult a psycho-oncologist?

See also Depression; Posttraumatic stress disorder.

Resources

BOOKS

Abeloff, M.D., et al. *Clinical Oncology*, 5th ed. New York: Churchill Livingstone, 2014.

Carr, Brian I., and Jennifer Steel. *Psychological Aspects of Cancer: A Guide to Emotional and Psychological Consequences of Cancer, Their Causes and Their Management*. New York: Springer, 2013.

Kreitler, S., M. W. Ben-Arush, and A. Martin, eds. *Pediatric Psycho-Oncology: Psychosocial Aspects and Clinical Interventions*, 2nd ed. Hoboken, NJ: John Wiley & Sons, 2012.

Niederhuber, J. E., et al. *Clinical Oncology*, 5th ed. Philadelphia: Elsevier, 2014.

Noggle, Chad A., and Raymond S. Dean, eds. *The Neuropsychology of Cancer and Oncology*. New York: Springer, 2013.

Stern, T. A., et al. *Massachusetts General Hospital Comprehensive Clinical Psychiatry*, 1st ed. Philadelphia: Mosby Elsevier, 2008.

Wise, Thomas N., Massimo Biondi, and Anna Costantini, eds. *Psycho-Oncology*. Arlington, VA: American Psychiatric, 2013.

PERIODICALS

Bauwens, Sabien, et al. "Systematic Screening for Distress in Oncology Practice Using the Distress Barometer: The Impact on Referrals to Psychosocial Care." *Psycho-Oncology* 23, no. 7 (July 2014): 804.

Carpenter, Kelly M., et al. "An Online Stress Management Workbook for Breast Cancer." *Journal of Behavioral Medicine* 37, no. 3 (June 2014): 458–468.

Costantini, Anna, et al. "Psychiatric Pathology and Suicide Risk in Patients with Cancer." *Journal of Psychosocial Oncology* 32, no. 4 (2014): 383.

Dilworth, Sophie, et al. "Patient and Health Professional's Perceived Barriers to the Delivery of Psychosocial Care to Adults With Cancer: A Systematic Review." *Psycho-Oncology* 23, no. 6 (June 2014): 601.

Fingeret, Michelle Cororve, et al. "Body Image Screening for Cancer Patients Undergoing Reconstructive Surgery." *Psycho-Oncology* 23, no. 8 (August 2014): 898.

Forsythe, Laura P., et al. "Social Support, Self-Efficacy for Decision-Making, and Follow-Up Care Use in Long-Term Cancer Survivors." *Psycho-Oncology* 23, no. 7 (July 2014): 788.

Gómez-Campelo, Paloma, et al. "Psychological Distress in Women with Breast and Gynecological Cancer Treated with Radical Surgery." *Psycho-Oncology* 23, no. 4 (April 2014): 459.

Oancea, S. Cristina, et al. "Emotional Distress Among Adult Survivors of Childhood Cancer." *Journal of Cancer Survivorship* 8, no. 2 (June 2014): 293–303.

Sveen, Josefin, et al. "They Still Grieve—A Nationwide Follow-Up of Young Adults 2–9 Years After Losing a Sibling to Cancer." *Psycho-Oncology* 23, no. 6 (June 2014): 658.

van der Geest, Ivana M., et al. "Parenting Stress as a Mediator of Parents' Negative Mood State and Behavior Problems in Children with Newly Diagnosed Cancer." *Psycho-Oncology* 23, no. 7 (July 2014): 758.

OTHER

"Distress in People With Cancer." American Cancer Society. August 13, 2014. http://www.cancer.org/acs/groups/cid/ documents/webcontent/002827-pdf.pdf (accessed October 22, 2014).

WEBSITES

"Cancer and Complementary Health Approaches." National Center for Complementary and Alternative Medicine. May 2013. http://nccam.nih.gov/health/cancer/camcancer.htm (accessed October 22, 2014).

ORGANIZATIONS

American Cancer Society, 250 Williams Street NW, Atlanta, GA 30303, (800) 227-2345, http://www.cancer.org.

American Psychosocial Oncology Society, 154 Hansen Road, Suite 201, Charlottesville, VA 22811, (434) 293-5350, Fax: (434) 977-1856, (866) APOS-4-HELP (276-7443), info@apos-society.org, http://www.apos-society.org.

National Cancer Institute, 6116 Executive Boulevard, Suite 300, Bethesda, MD 20892-8322, (800) 4-CANCER (422-6237), http://www.cancer.gov.

National Center for Complementary and Alternative Medicine, 9000 Rockville Pike, Bethesda, MD 20892, (888) 644-6226, http://www.nccam.nih.gov/.

National Comprehensive Cancer Network, 275 Commerce Drive, Suite 300, Fort Washington, PA 19034, (215) 690-0300, Fax: (215) 690-0280, http://www.nccn.org.

Rebecca Frey, PhD
Margaret Alic, PhD

Pulmonary carcinoid tumors *see* **Carcinoid tumors, lung**

Purinethol *see* **Mercaptopurine**

Quadrantectomy

Definition

Quadrantectomy is a surgical procedure in which a quadrant (approximately one-fourth) of the breast, including tissue surrounding a cancerous tumor, is removed. It is also called a partial or segmental **mastectomy**.

Purpose

Quadrantectomy is a type of breast-conserving surgery used as a treatment for **breast cancer**. Prior to the advent of breast-conserving surgeries, total mastectomy (complete removal of the breast) was considered the standard surgical treatment for breast **cancer**. Procedures such as quadrantectomy and **lumpectomy** (removing the tissue directly surrounding the tumor) have allowed doctors to treat cancer without sacrificing the entire affected breast.

Description

The patient is usually placed under general anesthesia for the duration of the procedure. In some instances, a local anesthetic may be administered with sedation to help the patient relax.

During quadrantectomy, a margin of normal breast tissue, skin, and muscle lining is removed around the periphery of the tumor. This removal decreases the risk of any abnormal cells being left behind and spreading locally or to other parts of the body (a process called **metastasis**). The amount removed is generally about one-fourth of the size of the breast (hence, the "quadrant" in quadrantectomy). The remaining tissue is then reconstructed to minimize any cosmetic defects, and then sutured closed. Temporary drains may be placed through the skin to remove excess fluid from the surgical site.

Some patients may have the lymph nodes removed from under the arm (called the axillary lymph nodes) on the same side as the tumor. Lymph nodes are small oval- or bean-shaped masses found throughout the body that act as filters against foreign materials and cancer cells. If cancer cells break away from their **primary site** of growth, they can travel to and begin to grow in the lymph nodes first, before traveling to other parts of the body. Removal of the lymph nodes is therefore a method of determining whether a cancer has begun to spread. To remove the nodes, a second incision is made in the area of the armpit, and the fat pad that contains the lymph nodes is removed. The tissue is then sent to a pathologist, who extracts the lymph nodes from the fatty tissue and examines them for the presence of cancer cells.

Demographics

The American Cancer Society estimates that approximately 232,600 new cases of breast cancer are diagnosed annually in the United States, and 39,600 women die as a result of the disease. Approximately one in eight women will develop breast cancer at some point in her life. The risk of developing breast cancer increases with age: women ages 30–40 have a one in 252 chance; ages 40–50 have a one in 68 chance; ages 50–60 have a one in 35 chance; and ages 60–70 have a one in 27 chance.

In the 1990s, the incidence of breast cancer was higher among Caucasian women (113.1 cases per 100,000 women) than African American women (100.3 per 100,000). The death rate associated with breast cancer, however, was higher among African American women (29.6 per 100,000) than Caucasian women (22.2 per 100,000). Rates were lower among Hispanic women (14.2 per 100,000), Native American women (12.0 per 100,000), and Asian women (11.2 per 100,000).

Diagnosis

Breast tumors may be found during self-examination or an examination by a health care professional. In other cases, they are visualized during a routine mammogram. Symptoms such as breast pain, changes in breast size or shape, redness, dimpling, or irritation may be an indication that medical attention is warranted.

Preparation

Prior to surgery, the patient is instructed to refrain from eating or drinking after midnight on the night before the operation. The physician will tell the patient what will take place during and after surgery, as well as expected outcomes and potential complications of the procedure.

Aftercare

The patient may return home the same day or remain in the hospital for one to two days after the procedure. Discharge instructions will include how to care for the incision and drains, which activities to restrict (e.g., driving and heavy lifting), and how to manage postoperative pain. Patients are often instructed to wear a well-fitting support bra for at least a week following surgery. A follow-up appointment to remove stitches and drains is usually scheduled 10–14 days after surgery.

If lymph nodes are removed, specific steps should be taken to minimize the risk of developing lymphedema of the arm, a condition in which excess fluid is not properly drained from body tissues, resulting in chronic swelling. This swelling can sometimes become severe enough to interfere with daily activity. Prior to being discharged, the patient will learn how to care for the arm, and how to avoid infection. She will also be told to avoid sunburn, refrain from heavy lifting, and to be careful not to wear tight jewelry and elastic bands.

Most patients undergo **radiation therapy** as part of their complete treatment plan. The radiation usually begins immediately or soon after quadrantectomy, and involves a schedule of five days of treatment a week for five to six weeks. Other treatments, such as **chemotherapy** or hormone therapy, may also be prescribed depending on the size and stage of the patient's cancer.

Risks

Risks associated with the surgical removal of breast tissue include bleeding, infection, breast asymmetry, changes in sensation, reaction to the anesthesia, and unexpected scarring.

Some of the risks associated with removal of the lymph nodes include excessive bleeding, infection, pain, excessive swelling, and damage to nerves during surgery. Nerve damage may be temporary or permanent, and may result in weakness, numbness, tingling, and drooping. Lymphedema is also a risk whenever lymph nodes have been removed; it may occur immediately following surgery or months to years later.

Results

Most patients will not experience recurrences of the cancer following a treatment plan of quadrantectomy and radiation therapy. One study followed patients for a period of 20 years after breast-conserving surgery, and found that only 9% experienced recurrence of the cancer.

Morbidity and mortality rates

Following removal of the axillary lymph nodes, there is approximately a 10% risk of lymphedema and a 20% risk of abnormal skin sensations. Approximately 17% of women undergoing breast-conserving surgery have a poor cosmetic result (e.g., asymmetry or distortion of shape). The risk of complications associated with general anesthesia is less than 1%.

Alternatives

A full mastectomy, in which the entire affected breast is removed, is one alternative to quadrantectomy. A **simple mastectomy** removes the entire breast, while a radical mastectomy removes the entire breast plus parts of the chest muscle wall and the lymph nodes. In terms of recurrence and survival rates, breast-conserving surgery has been shown to be equally effective as mastectomy in treating breast cancer.

A new technique that may eliminate the need for removing many axillary lymph nodes is called sentinel node **biopsy**. When lymph fluid moves out of a region, the sentinel lymph node is the first node it reaches. The theory behind **sentinel lymph node biopsy** is that if cancer is not present in the sentinel node, it is unlikely to have spread to other nearby nodes. This procedure may allow individuals with early-stage cancers to avoid the complications associated with partial or radical removal of lymph nodes if there is little or no chance that cancer has spread to them.

Health care team roles

Quadrantectomy is usually performed by a general surgeon, breast surgeon, or surgical oncologist. Radiation therapy is administered by a radiation oncologist, and chemotherapy by a medical oncologist. The surgical procedure is frequently done in a hospital setting (especially

QUESTIONS TO ASK YOUR DOCTOR

- Why is quadrantectomy recommended?
- What methods of anesthesia and pain relief will be used?
- Where will the incision be located, and how much tissue will be removed?
- Will a lymph node dissection be performed?
- Is sentinel node biopsy appropriate in this case?
- Is postsurgical radiation therapy recommended?

when lymph nodes are to be removed at the same time), but specialized outpatient facilities are sometimes preferred.

Resources

BOOKS

Townsend, Courtney M., et al. *Sabiston Textbook of Surgery*. 19th ed. Philadelphia: Saunders/Elsevier, 2012.

PERIODICALS

Magno, Stefano, et al. "Accessory Nipple Reconstruction following a Central Quadrantectomy: A Case Report." *Cases Journal* 2, no. 1 (2009): 32. http://dx.doi.org/10.1186/1757-1626-2-32 (accessed October 3, 2014).

Pusiol, T., et al. "Middle Ear Metastasis from Dormant Breast Cancer as the Initial Sign of Disseminated Disease 20 Years after Quadrantectomy." *Ear, Nose & Throat Journal* 92, no. 3 (2013): 121–24.

WEBSITES

American Cancer Society. "Surgery for Breast Cancer." http://www.cancer.org/cancer/breastcancer/detailedguide/breast-cancer-treating-surgery (accessed October 3, 2014).

ORGANIZATIONS

American Cancer Society, 250 Williams St. NW, Atlanta, GA 30303, (800) 227-2345, http://www.cancer.org.

Society of Surgical Oncology, 9525 W. Bryn Mawr Ave., Ste. 870, Rosemont, IL 60018, (847) 427-1400, info@surgonc.org, http://surgonc.org.

Stephanie Dionne Sherk

R

Radiation dermatitis

Definition

Radiation dermatitis, also called radiodermatitis or radiation-induced dermatitis, is injury to the skin from radiation, most often from **radiation therapy** for treating **cancer**.

Description

The most common radiation-induced injuries are to the skin. Radiation dermatitis has been associated with radiation exposure since the discovery of **x-rays** in 1895. Now used almost exclusively for the treatment of cancer, in the past radiation therapy was used to treat a variety of conditions, including acne, eczema, excessive hair growth, and ringworm, frequently resulting in radiation dermatitis. In the past, when x-ray machines and other radiation sources were less well-shielded, chronic radiation dermatitis frequently occurred among radiologists and technicians who were constantly exposed to ionizing radiation.

Although radiation dermatitis is common after any radiation treatment, it is particularly common after **breast cancer** therapy. Radiation dermatitis can occur immediately upon treatment or not develop until months after treatment is concluded. It can be very painful, and it is not uncommon for breast cancer patients to temporarily halt radiation therapy because of the pain from dermatitis. Both the pain and disfigurement from radiation dermatitis can adversely affect quality of life. Radiation dermatitis can also give rise to basal cell and squamous cell carcinomas, the most common types of **non-melanoma skin cancer**.

There are several types of radiation dermatitis:

• Acute radiation dermatitis is a reddening of the skin called erythema, which can occur up to 24 hours after treatment with an "erythema dose" to the skin, defined as 2 gray (Gy) or more of ionizing radiation. It can occur with the very first radiation treatment.

• Chronic radiation dermatitis occurs from exposure to lower doses of radiation over a longer period, with varying degrees of damage to the skin and underlying layers. Chronic dermatitis becomes apparent after a latent period lasting from several months to decades.

• Eosinophilic, polymorphic, and pruritic (itching) eruption is a radiation dermatitis that occurs most often in women receiving internal cobalt radiotherapy for cancer.

• A radiation recall reaction is radiation dermatitis that occurs on a previously irradiated area of skin following the administration of a chemotherapy drug. It can occur months or years after radiation treatment.

Demographics

About 95% of cancer patients treated with radiation therapy develop some degree of radiation dermatitis. The high incidence of radiation dermatitis includes more than 90% of women treated with radiation for breast cancer and 20% to 25% of patients undergoing radiotherapy for locally advanced **head and neck cancers**. Other cancer patients who experience severe radiation dermatitis include those being treated for lung cancer or **sarcoma**. Most often, the dermatitis is mild to moderate, but about 20% to 25% of patients will have moist destruction of tissue (desquamation) and crusty sores that do not heal easily (ulcerations).

Risk factors

The risk of radiation dermatitis depends on the type of cancer, the amount and location of skin exposed to radiation, and the radiation regimen. Different areas of the body have different levels of sensitivity to the effects of radiation. The most sensitive areas are the face, the front of the neck and chest, breast tissue, arms and legs, and the abdomen. Hair follicles of the scalp are also

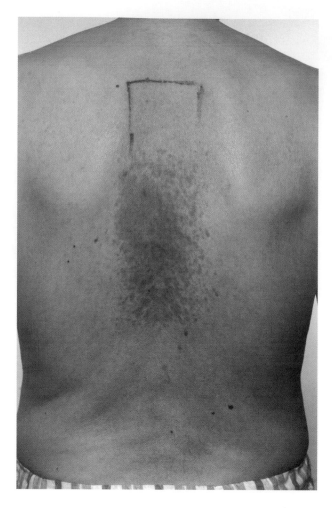

Rash caused by radiation therapy. *(Mediscan/Alamy)*

especially sensitive to radiation. The risk of severe radiation dermatitis depends on:

- the total radiation dose

- the dose per treatment

- the total duration of treatment

- the type of radiation beam and its energy

- the surface area of skin exposed to radiation

- the area of the body receiving radiation

Other factors also increase the risk of radiation dermatitis. Smoking, obesity, and previous or concurrent **chemotherapy** all increase the risk. There is some evidence that genetic factors play a role in the development of acute radiation dermatitis following radiotherapy for breast cancer. Breast reconstructions (transposed flaps or **mastectomy** flaps) and implants are also associated with increased risk of radiation injury because the reconstructed skin is not able to dissipate heat.

Causes and symptoms

Although radiation dermatitis is almost always caused by radiation therapy for treating cancer, other sources of radiation may also be a cause:

- Radiation dermatitis can be caused by fluoroscopy, a technique that is used in an increasing number of diagnostic procedures. Fluoroscopy-induced radiation dermatitis usually appears within 7–14 days of exposure and may be acute or chronic. However, the onset of symptoms is unpredictable, and it can develop months or years after radiation exposure.

- Very rarely, deep radiation sensitizes the skin in such a way that subsequent exposure to x-rays (radiation recall) may trigger acute radiation dermatitis.

- Occupational whole-body radiation exposure exceeding 100 rem (roentgen-equivalent-man) can cause radiation dermatitis.

Skin irradiation has complex effects involving direct tissue injury and the recruitment of inflammatory immune system cells to the damaged sites. Several different types of skin cells and vascular components may be damaged. Massive cell death occurs in severe radiation dermatitis. Tissue healing is reduced or prevented by the successive radiation doses used in many radiotherapy regimes.

Radiation dermatitis usually occurs within a few weeks to 90 days after the start of radiation therapy, depending on the intensity of the dose and the sensitivity of the patient's tissue. Transient erythema may redden the skin within hours of the initial radiation. Within 10–14 days the erythema may become persistent. As the cumulative radiation dose increases, damage to the basal cell layer in the deeper epidermis of the skin, and injury to the oil (sebaceous) and sweat glands causes the skin to become dry. During the third to sixth week of therapy, skin cells start peeling off in scales, a process called desquamation. These scales can be dry or moist.

Symptoms of acute radiation dermatitis include:

- red patches of inflamed itchy skin

- blistering of the skin

- hair loss

- decreased sweating

- dry desquamation

- wet desquamation

- swelling (edema)

- ulcerations

- bleeding

- skin cell death

These acute symptoms can cause considerable pain, limit daily activities, and may even interrupt or delay radiation treatment. Severe acute dermatitis leads to more severe late complications. These late complications can include hypopigmentation or hyperpigmentation of the skin resulting from damage to melanocytes (the cells that produce skin color), atrophy of the skin, and abnormally dilated capillaries.

Chronic radiation dermatitis usually occurs after second- or third-degree acute radiation dermatitis, but may not become apparent until years after radiotherapy. Symptoms include:

- damage to or loss of hair follicles
- development of hard atrophied plaques that are often whitish or yellowish
- increased collagen (the fibrous protein of connective tissue)
- damage to the elastic fibers of the dermis (an inner layer of skin)
- fragility of the outer skin
- patchy discoloration of the skin
- ulcers that do not heal well
- overgrowth of horny tissue (keratosis)
- cancer

Diagnosis

Examination

A history of radiation exposure and physical examination are the primary tools for diagnosing radiation dermatitis.

Procedures

Various histological and immunological methods may be used to analyze a **skin biopsy** sample to diagnose radiation dermatitis. The results vary depending on the length of time that has elapsed since the radiation exposure. Although chronic radiation dermatitis usually is readily identified, it is much more difficult to distinguish subacute radiation dermatitis from other skin conditions.

Grading

A number of different systems have been developed for grading radiation dermatitis. The National Cancer Institute's toxicity grading is as follows:

- grade 1: faint erythema or dry desquamation
- grade 2: moderate to brisk erythema; patchy moist desquamation, mostly confined to skin folds and creases; moderate swelling

- grade 3: moist desquamation beyond skin folds and creases; bleeding induced by minor trauma or abrasion
- grade 4: skin necrosis or ulceration throughout the dermis; spontaneous bleeding from involved site
- grade 5: death

Treatment

Conventional treatment

No effective treatment to prevent or ameliorate radiation skin injury has become the standard of care. The aim of radiation dermatitis treatment is to relieve discomfort and pain, help avoid further trauma, and restore skin integrity, if possible. For minor (grade 1) dermatitis, water-soluble lotions and topical corticosteroid creams may be used to reduce **itching** and skin irritation.

For grades 2 and 3, the focus is on preventing infection through the use of nonadherent dressings or silicone foam bandages. Topical wound gels such as RadiaPlex may be used directly on the skin before dressings are applied.

Treatment for grade 4 dermatitis is determined by the specific patient's needs. Treatment options may include stopping therapy or reducing the dosage, surgically removing damaged tissue (debridement), and/ or utilizing skin grafts.

Phototherapy

Studies have shown that the application of a low-power laser promotes tissue repair by reducing inflammation and restoring the production of collagen. Therefore, research is ongoing to determine whether this type of phototherapy may be an ideal treatment to prevent and to treat radiodermatitis in cancer patients receiving radiation therapy. No other clinically applicable preventive treatment is available, so this approach holds promise, especially for women undergoing radiation therapy after breast cancer surgery.

Drug therapy

A wide range of prescription and over-the-counter products are available that can be used to prevent and treat radiation dermatitis. However, little or no scientific evidence supports the effectiveness of most of these products. Softening agents (emollients) and hydrating or hydrophilic lotions are generally used for the early stages of radiation dermatitis.

Trolamine ointment is one of the most widely used treatments; however, studies have not found it useful in reducing the incidence of radiation dermatitis. Biafine is a topical emulsion containing trolamine and sodium alginate. Studies have indicated that patients find Biafine soothing. It may enhance healing by recruiting macrophages (immune system cells) to affected areas and providing a protective barrier against environmental contaminants, thus reducing the risk of secondary infection.

Other topical skin and mucous membrane agents used to treat radiation dermatitis include:

• fluorouracil (Efudex, Fluoroplex, Carac)

• VitE-Allant-MannPly-Hyalr Acid

• RadiaPlex

• Xclair cream

More severe radiation dermatitis is treated by topical and intralesional corticosteroid administration. Evidence indicates that preventive and ongoing use of a topical corticosteroid or a dexpanthenol-containing emollient ameliorates but does not prevent radiation dermatitis.

Alternative

Various alternative commercial treatments have been studied in preventing radiation dermatitis, including calendula (*Calendula officinalis* L.), petroleum-based ointment, almond oil, ascorbic acid, and silver sulfadiazine, but none have been found to be effective in preventing severe radiation dermatitis.

Aloe vera gel has long been reported to help heal burns, but no scientific evidence supports its specific use for burns typical of radiation dermatitis.

Home remedies

Home remedies for treating radiation dermatitis include:

• bathing

• applying saline compresses to alleviate discomfort

• avoiding shaving the affected area

Prognosis

Severe acute radiation dermatitis often leads to a chronic condition and eventually may lead to cancer. Although radiation dermatitis itself is not associated with shortened survival, it is associated with poor quality of life. Without treatment, radiation dermatitis can result in discontinuation or delay of subsequent radiation therapy sessions.

Prevention

Ointments applied at least twice a day beginning with the first radiation treatment and continuing throughout radiation therapy may help prevent more serious

---

QUESTIONS TO ASK YOUR DOCTOR

• Is my radiation dermatitis likely to get worse as my radiation treatments continue?

• Is there anything I can do to prevent radiation dermatitis?

• What treatment do you recommend?

• Should I delay my radiation therapy?

---

dermatitis. Researchers have suggested that exposing women to low-energy, nonthermal, light-emitting diode (LED) photomodulation following radiotherapy for breast cancer may reduce painful skin reactions and reduce the need to postpone radiation treatments. An ongoing clinical trial is also investigating the use of phototherapy for the prevention of radiodermatitis in breast cancer patients receiving radiation therapy.

Additional preventive measures that patients may take to help reduce the severity of radiation dermatitis include:

• Keep the skin clean and dry.

• Avoid using scented or alcohol-containing soaps, lotions, and other skin products, including perfumes.

• Wear loose clothing to avoid further irritation.

• Avoid using items that contain metals, such as deodorants made with aluminum.

• Avoid being outside in the sun.

• Do not apply any topical products to the skin prior to treatment.

Resources

BOOKS

Haller, D. G., L. D. Wagman, K. A. Camphausen, and W. J. Hoskins, eds. "Radiation Oncology" *Cancer Management: A Multidisciplinary Approach*, 14th ed. Philadelphia: Karger, 2012.

PERIODICALS

"A Fresh Look at Post-Procedural Wound Care & Radiation Dermatitis." *Dermatology Times* 29, no. 6 (June 2008): S1-7.

Costa, M. M., S. B. Silva, A. L. Quinto, et al. "Phototherapy 660 nm for the Prevention of Radiodermatitis in Breast Cancer Patients Receiving Radiation Therapy: Study Protocol for a Randomized Controlled Trial." *Trials* 15 (Aug 2014): 330–335.

Okunieff, P., J. Xu, and D. Hu, et al. "Curcumin Protects Against Radiation-induced Acute and Chronic Cutaneous

---

Toxicity in Mice and Decreases mRNA Expression of Inflammatory and Fibrogenic Cytokines." *International Journal of Radiation Oncology, Biology, and Physics* 65 (July 2006): 890–898.

"Radiation Dermatitis; Radiation Dermatitis in Head and Neck Cancer Patients Not Improved by Trolamine." *Science Letter* (July 18, 2006): 1126.

Ryan, J. L. "Ionizing Radiation: The Good, the Bad, and the Ugly." *Journal of Investigative Dermatology* 132 (March 2012): 985–993.

WEBSITES

Bernier, J., et al. "Consensus Guidelines for the Management of Radiation Dermatitis and Coexisting Acne-Like Rash in Patients Receiving Radiotherapy Plus EGFR Inhibitors for the Treatment of Squamous Cell Carcinoma." *Annals of Oncology.* http://www.ncbi.nlm.nih.gov/pubmed/17785763 (accessed October 2, 2014).

Henry, Michelle F., et al. "Fluoroscopy-Induced Chronic Radiation Dermatitis: A Report of Three Cases." *Dermatology Online Journal.* http://www.ncbi.nlm.nih.gov/pubmed/19281708 (accessed October 2, 2014).

National Research Standard Collaboration. "Calendula (*Calendula officinalis* L.)." *MedlinePlus.* http://www.nlm.nih.gov/medlineplus/druginfo/natural/patient-calendula.html (accessed October 2, 2014).

ORGANIZATIONS

American Academy of Dermatology, PO Box 4014, Schaumburg, IL 60168, (847) 240-1280, (866) 503-SKIN (7546), Fax: (847) 240-1859, http://www.aad.org.

National Cancer Institute, NCI Public Inquiries Office, 6116 Executive Boulevard, Room 3036A, Bethesda, MD 20006, (800) 4-CANCER, http://www.cancer.gov.

L. Lee Culvert
Margaret Alic, PhD

Radiation enteritis *see* **Enteritis**

Radiation therapy

Definition

Radiation therapy, sometimes called radiotherapy, x-ray therapy, radiation treatment, cobalt therapy, electron beam therapy, or irradiation, uses high-energy penetrating waves or particles such as **x-rays**, gamma rays, proton rays, or neutron rays to destroy **cancer** cells or keep the cells from reproducing.

Purpose

The purpose of radiation therapy is to destroy or damage cancer cells. Radiation therapy is a common

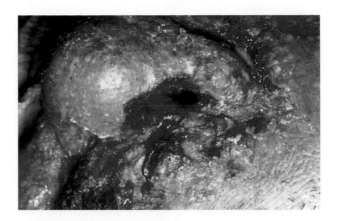

(SPL/Science Source)

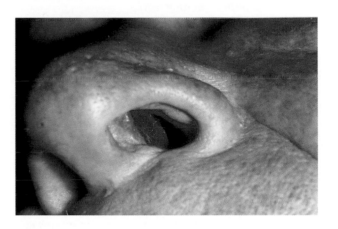

Two weeks after (l) and six months after (r) radiation therapy to treat squamous cell carcinoma inside the left nostril. *(DR. MARAZZI/Science Source)*

form of cancer therapy used in more than half of all cancer cases. Radiation therapy can be used:

- alone to kill cells

- before surgery to shrink a tumor and make it easier to remove

- during surgery to kill cancer cells that may remain in surrounding tissue after the surgery (intraoperative radiation)

- after surgery to kill cancer cells remaining elsewhere in the body

- to shrink an inoperable tumor in order to reduce pain and improve the patient's quality of life

- in combination with chemotherapy either before, during, or after chemotherapy treatments

For certain kinds of cancers such as early-stage **Hodgkin lymphoma**, non-Hodgkin lymphomas, and certain types of prostate or brain cancer, radiation therapy alone may cure the disease. In other cases, radiation therapy used in conjunction with **chemotherapy**, surgery, or both, increases survival rates over any of these therapies used alone. Sometimes both internal and external radiation therapy will be given.

Description

Radiation therapy is a painless localized treatment. The radiation can be directed from an external or an internal source. External-beam radiation therapy directs a beam of radiation from outside the body to the cancer site. Internal radiation therapy, called brachytherapy or implant therapy, places a source of radioactivity inside the body near the cancer site.

How radiation therapy works

High-energy radiation kills cells by damaging their DNA. DNA, or deoxyribonucleic acid, is present in each cell in the body, including cells that have become cancerous (malignant). It is a protein that carries the code for controlling most cellular activities and, as such, it is involved in cell growth (replication). When radiation damages the DNA in cancer cells, it blocks their ability to grow and multiply. Radiation also damages normal cells, but because normal cells tend to grow more slowly, they are better able to repair radiation damage than are cancer cells. In order to give normal cells time to heal and to reduce the side effects of radiation, the radiation treatments are often given in small doses over a six- or seven-week period. If radiation is the only treatment for a specific type of cancer, larger doses may be given.

External-beam radiation therapy

External-beam radiation therapy is the most common type of radiation therapy. It is usually done during outpatient visits to either a hospital radiology department or non-affiliated radiation center and is usually covered by insurance.

A treatment team comprising a radiation oncologist, a medical physicist, and a medical dosimetrist confer to determine the proper dose of radiation for a particular cancer. The dose is then divided into smaller doses called fractions. One fraction is usually given each day, five days a week for six to seven weeks. However, each radiation plan is individualized depending on the type and location of the cancer and what other treatments are also being given. The actual administration of the therapy usually takes about half an hour daily, although radiation is administered for only one to five minutes at each session. To get the most benefit from radiation therapy, individuals are advised to attend every scheduled treatment.

Radiology machines used to administer external-beam radiation therapy and the radioactive material that provides the radiation vary according to the type and location of the cancer. Generally, the patient lies down on the x-ray table or sits in a special chair. Parts of the body not receiving radiation are protected by covering them with special shields that block the rays. A radiologic technician then directs the prescribed beam of radiation to a predetermined spot on the body where the cancer is located. The targeted spot is marked on the body prior to the treatment. The patient must remain still during the administration of the radiation so that no other parts of the body are affected. As an extra precaution in some treatments, special molds are made to make sure the body is in the same position for each treatment. However, the treatment itself is painless, much like taking an x-ray of a bone.

Newer methods of more targeted radiotherapy aim to deliver radiation fractions so that they kill more cancer cells and fewer normal cells. These newer techniques give higher doses directly to the cancer with greater accuracy and less damage to surrounding cells and tissue, which reduces the side effects. Examples of these techniques include intensity-modulated radiotherapy (IMRT), image-guided radiotherapy (IGRT), and volumetric-modulated arc radiotherapy (VMAT). Another type of external-beam radiotherapy called stereotactic body radiotherapy (SBRT) delivers the external beam to the tumor from many different directions.

Internal radiation therapy

Internal radiation therapy is called brachytherapy, implant therapy, interstitial radiation, or intracavitary radiation. In one type of internal radiation therapy, a bit of solid radioactive material is sealed in a small implantable capsule. Radioactive seeds or ribbons can also be implanted. The implant is then placed as close as possible to the cancer site, usually by passing it through a small, stretchy tube called a catheter. Other types of applicators may also be used to deliver the implant to the cancer site. Another type of internal radiation uses a liquid form of radioactive material, which the patient will drink, swallow as a pill, or receive through an intravenous catheter (IV). Liquid radiation travels throughout the body seeking and destroying cancer cells. One advantage of solid internal radiation therapy is that it concentrates the radiation near the tumor and reduces the chance of damaging normal cells. Many different types of radioactive material can be implanted, including cesium, iridium, iodine, phosphorus, and palladium.

The size and location of the cancer determine how and where the implant is placed. Internal radiation therapy is used for tumors or lesions of the head, neck, eyes, esophagus, breast, female reproductive system, gall bladder, lung, and prostate. Liquid radiation therapy is used for **thyroid cancer** or Hodgkin **lymphoma**. Sometimes internal radiation will be combined with external-beam radiation or chemotherapy. Most people will have the radioactive capsule, seed, or ribbon implanted by a surgeon while under either general or local anesthesia at a hospital or surgical clinic. The liquid form is also typically given in the hospital setting because the patient will be radioactive for a few days after the treatment.

Patients receiving internal radiation therapy do become temporarily radioactive. They may need to limit their contact with others while the implant is in place, and patients undergoing high-dose treatment may need to remain in the hospital. The length of time is determined by the type of cancer and the dose of radioactivity to be delivered. Lower-dose implants are typically left in place for a few days; higher-dose implants are removed after approximately 10 20 minutes. During the time the implant is in place, the patient will have to stay in bed and remain reasonably still.

In some cases, an implant is left permanently inside the body. People who have permanent implants must stay in the hospital and away from other people for the first few days while they are radioactive. Gradually the radioactivity of the implant decreases, and it is safe to be around other people.

Radioimmunotherapy

Radioimmunotherapy is a form of selective targeting of cancer cells. Because it targets specific types of cells, it is an effective way to treat cancer that has spread (metastasized) to multiple locations throughout the body, and is also used to treat some lymphomas. Antibodies are immune system proteins that recognize and bind to specific corresponding antigens on the surface of only one type of cell. Therefore, they can be designed to bind with only one specific type of cancer cell. To carry out radioimmunotherapy, antibodies with the ability to bind specifically to a patient's cancer cells are attached to radioactive material and injected into the patient's bloodstream. When these synthetic antibodies find a cancer cell, they bind to it, allowing the radiation to kill the cancer cell. Radioimmunotherapy is often used in conjunction with chemotherapy.

Radiation used to treat cancer

IONIZING RADIATION. The radiation therapy used for treating cancer is called ionizing radiation because it forms electrically charged ions in the cells it passes through. The two major types of ionizing radiation are photon radiation (x-rays and gamma rays) and particle radiation (electrons, protons, neutrons, carbon ions, and alpha and beta particles). The different types of ionizing radiation vary in their energy levels; those with higher energy are able to penetrate more deeply into body tissue. The radiation oncologist will select the radiation therapy and energy level that is most appropriate for a specific type of cancer and specific location.

X-rays and gamma rays are high-energy rays composed of massless particles of energy (like light) called photons. Gamma rays originate from the decay of radioactive substances (such as radium and cobalt-60), while x-rays are generated by devices that excite electrons (such as cathode ray tubes and linear accelerators). These high-energy rays remove electrons from atoms within the molecules inside cells, either killing the cells or altering genes so that the cells lose their ability to divide and make new cells.

Particle radiation is radiation delivered by particles that have mass. Proton therapy uses proton rays or positively charged atomic particles rather than photons, which have neither mass nor charge. Like x-rays and gamma rays, proton rays disrupt cellular activity. The advantage of using proton rays is that they can be shaped to conform to the irregular shape of the tumor more precisely than x-rays and gamma rays. They allow delivery of higher radiation doses to tumors without increasing damage to the surrounding tissue.

Neutron therapy is another type of particle radiation that applies very high-energy neutron rays. These rays are composed of neutrons, which are particles with mass but no charge. The type of damage they cause to cells is much less likely to be repaired than that caused by x-rays, gamma rays, or proton rays. Neutron therapy can treat larger tumors than conventional radiation therapy. While conventional radiation therapy depends on the presence of oxygen to work, neutron radiation works in the absence of oxygen, making it especially effective for the treatment of inoperable **salivary gland tumors**, bone cancers, and some kinds of advanced cancers of the pancreas, bladder, lung, prostate, and uterus.

Carbon ion radiation, or heavy ion radiation, uses a particle heavier than either photons or neutrons. Carbon ions can do much more damage to targeted cancer cells than other types of radiation, but this treatment is only available in a few medical centers worldwide. It is only used for cancers that do not respond (are resistant) to other forms of radiation therapy.

Alpha and beta particles are produced by certain radioactive substances that can be injected, swallowed, or put into the body. Often called **radiopharmaceuticals**, these particles are more often used in enhanced imaging tests than in treating cancer.

Advances in radiation therapy

Stereotactic radiosurgery is a highly accurate form of radiation therapy that was originally limited to treating malignant and benign **brain tumors**. It is not actually a surgical procedure, despite its name. Stereotactic radiosurgery allows the doctor to deliver a single maximum dose of precisely directed radiation to the tumor without damaging nearby healthy tissue. The treatment is carried out with the help of three-dimensional computer-aided analysis of CT and MRI scans, systems to immobilize and position the patient, and image-guided radiation therapy to confirm the tumor location before the procedure and improve precision during the procedure. Gamma knife radiosurgery is done using a stationary machine that is applicable to small tumors, blood vessels, or similar targets. It is usually performed in one day on an outpatient basis. Another type of radiosurgery uses a movable linear accelerator-based machine that is preferred for larger tumors. This treatment is delivered in several small doses given over several weeks. The total dose of radiation is higher with a linear accelerator-based machine than with gamma knife treatment. Radiosurgery that is performed with divided doses is known as fractionated radiosurgery. Stereotactic radiosurgery can be used in addition to standard surgery to treat a recurrent brain tumor, or in place of surgery if the tumor cannot be reached by standard surgical techniques. It is used for many types of head and neck tumors. It is being investigated for use in treating small- to medium-size tumors in other areas of the body such as the lungs, liver, abdomen, spine and prostate.

Stereotactic body radiotherapy (SBRT) delivers an external beam at the tumor from many different directions. SBRT consists of one to five treatments over a period of weeks using the linear accelerator and an immobilization device as with stereotactic radiosurgery. X-rays or CT scans will be used to create images of the tumor area prior to and sometimes during the delivery of the radiation. The treatment takes about one hour and the patient will not feel pain or discomfort.

Intraoperative radiotherapy (IORT) refers to the use of mobile devices that allow the surgeon to use radiotherapy in early-stage disease and to operate in locations where it would be difficult to transport the patient during surgery for radiation treatment. Mobile IORT units have been used successfully in treating early-stage **breast cancer** and **rectal cancer**.

Hyperbaric oxygen therapy is not new, but it is newly being used in conjunction with radiation therapy. Hyperbaric treatments consist of breathing pure oxygen while in a special sealed, pressurized chamber. It has been found to increase the sensitivity of certain cancers to radiation and may help to reverse radiation damage to normal tissues.

Radiosensitizers are another recent innovation in radiation therapy. Sensitizers are medications that protect normal cells from radiation while making cancer cells easier to kill. These drugs may be given to patients receiving radiation therapy in areas where it is especially difficult not to expose normal tissues to radiation when treating a tumor, such as in the head and neck region. **Gemcitabine** (Gemzar) and **amifostine** (Ethyol) are already in use, and other sensitizers are being tested in **clinical trials**.

Precautions

Radiation therapy does not usually make the patients receiving the treatments radioactive, but patients receiving certain types of internal radiation therapy may become radioactive for the duration of the treatment. In almost all cases, the benefits of this therapy outweigh the risks. However, radiation therapy can have serious consequences, so it is important for patients to understand why their treatment team believes that radiotherapy is the best possible treatment option for their specific type of cancer. Radiation therapy is often not appropriate for pregnant women, because radiation can damage cells of the developing fetus. Women who think they might be pregnant should discuss treatment with their doctor.

Preparation

Before radiation therapy, the size and location of the patient's tumor are determined very precisely using **magnetic resonance imaging** (MRI) and/or **computed tomography** scans (CT scans). The correct radiation dose, the number of sessions, the interval between sessions, and the method of application are calculated by a radiation oncologist based on the tumor type, its size, and the sensitivity of the nearby tissues. Planning will include coordinating radiation therapy with other treatments such as chemotherapy or surgery.

The patient's skin is marked with a semi-permanent ink to help the radiation technologist achieve correct positioning for each treatment. Molds may be built to hold tissues in exactly the right place each time.

Aftercare

Many patients experience skin changes, **fatigue**, nausea, and vomiting after radiation therapy regardless of where the radiation is applied. After treatment, the skin around the site of the treatment may also become sore. Affected skin should be kept clean. Patients should avoid perfume and scented skin products and protect affected areas from the sun. Nothing should be applied to the affected area without first consulting with the treating physician.

Nausea and vomiting are most likely to occur when the radiation dose is high, if the abdomen or another part of the digestive tract is irradiated, or if the brain is within the treatment field. Sometimes nausea and vomiting occur after radiation to other regions, but in these cases the symptoms usually disappear within a few hours after treatment. Nausea and vomiting can be treated with antacids or the antiemetic ondansetron (Zofran).

Fatigue frequently starts after the second week of therapy and may continue until about two weeks after the therapy is finished. Patients may need to limit their activities, take naps, and get extra sleep at night.

Patients are encouraged to see their oncologist (cancer doctor) at least once within the first few weeks after their final radiation treatment and every six to

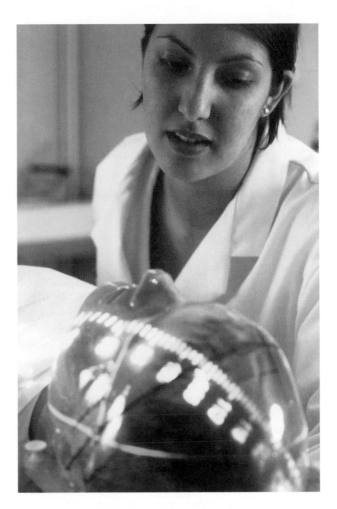

A radiographer prepares a patient for radiation therapy. She is aiming laser cross-hairs onto the site of a brain tumor. The patient's head is protected and held in place by a plastic mask. *(SIMON FRASER/Science Source)*

twelve months thereafter to make sure the tumor has not recurred or developed in another area of the body.

Risks

Radiation therapy can cause **anemia**, nausea, vomiting, **diarrhea**, hair loss (**alopecia**), skin changes, sterility, and rarely death. However, the benefits of radiation therapy almost always exceed the risks. Patients are advised to discuss the risks with their doctor and get a second opinion about their treatment plan.

Results

The outcome of radiation treatment varies depending on the type, location, and stage of the cancer. For some cancers such as Hodgkin lymphoma, about 75% of patients are cured. **Prostate cancer** also responds well to radiation therapy. Radiation to painful bony metastases may provide a dramatically effective form of pain control. Other cancers may be less sensitive to the benefits of radiation; in these cases, chemotherapy and/or surgery may also be recommended.

Resources

BOOKS

Pazdur, Richard, Lawrence D. Wagman, and Kevin A. Camphausen. *Cancer Management: A Multidisciplinary Approach*. 13th ed. Norwalk, CT: UBM Medica, 2010.

PERIODICALS

Ahmed, Z., et al. "Postoperative Stereotactic Radiosurgery for Resected Brain Metastases." *CNS Oncology* 3 (May 2014): 199–207.

Coleman, C. Norman, Theodore S. Lawrence, and David G. Kirsch. "Enhancing the Efficacy of Radiation Therapy:Premises, Promises, and Practicality." *Journal of Clinical Oncology* (August 11, 2014): e-pub ahead of print. http://dx.doi.org/10.1200/JCO.2014.57.3865 (accessed August 14, 2014).

Fisher, Christine M., and Rachael Rabinovitch. "Frontiers in Radiotherapy for Early-Stage Invasive Breast Cancer." *Journal of Clinical Oncology* (August 11, 2014): e-pub ahead of print. http://dx.doi.org/10.1200/JCO.2014.55.1184 (accessed August 14, 2014).

Lutz, S. T., J. Jones, and E. Chow. "Role of Radiation Therapy in Palliative Care of the Patient With Cancer." *Journal of Clinical Oncology* (August 11, 2014): e-pub ahead of print. http://dx.doi.org/10.1200/JCO.2014.55.1143 (accessed August 14, 2014).

Ozyigit, G., and M. Gultekin. "Advances in Radiation Therapy: Conventional to 3D, to IMRT, to 4F, and Beyond." *World Journal of Clinical Oncology* 5, no. 3 (2014): 425–39.

Teoh, M., et al. "Volumetric Modulated Arc Therapy: A Review of Current Literature and Clinical Use In Practice." *British Journal of Radiology* 84, no. 1007 (2011): 967–96. http://dx.doi.org/10.1259/bjr/22373346 (accessed September 29, 2014).

WEBSITES

American Society of Clinical Oncology. "Radiation Therapy: What to Expect." Cancer.Net podcast, 7:42. http://cancer.net/radiation-therapy-what-expect (accessed September 29, 2014).

Mayo Clinic staff. "Intensity-Modulated Radiation Therapy." MayoClinic.org. http://www.mayoclinic.org/tests-procedures/intensity-modulated-radiation-therapy/basics/definition/PRC-20013330 (accessed September 29, 2014).

Radiological Society of North America. "Image-Guided Radiation Therapy (IGRT)." RadiologyInfo.org. http://www.radiologyinfo.org/en/info.cfm?pg=IGRT (accessed September 29, 2014).

ORGANIZATIONS

American Cancer Society, 1599 Clifton Rd. NE, Atlanta, GA 30329-4251, (800) ACS-2345 (227-2345), http://www.cancer.org.

American College of Radiology, 1891 Preston White Dr., Reston, VA 20191, (703) 648-8900, info@acr.org, http://www.acr.org.

International Radiosurgery Support Association (IRSA), 3005 Hoffman Street, Harrisburg, PA 17110, (717) 260-9808, http://www.irsa.org.

National Association for Proton Therapy, 7910 Woodmont Ave., Suite 1303, Bethesda, MD 20814, (301) 913-9360, http://www.proton-therapy.org.

Radiological Society of North America, 820 Jorie Blvd., Oak Brook, IL 60523-2251, (800) 381-6660, Fax: (630) 571-7837, http://www.rsna.org.

L. Lee Culvert
Rebecca J. Frey, PhD

Radical neck dissection

Definition

Radical neck dissection is a surgical operation used to remove cancerous tissue in the head and neck.

Purpose

The purpose of radical neck dissection is to remove lymph nodes and other structures in the head and neck that are likely or known to be malignant. Variations on neck dissections depend on the extent of the **cancer**. A radical neck dissection removes the most tissue. It is performed when the cancer has spread widely in the neck. A modified neck dissection removes less tissue, and a selective neck dissection even less.

Description

Cancers of the head and neck often spread to nearby tissues and into the lymph nodes. Removing these structures is one way to control the cancer.

Of the 600 lymph nodes in the body, approximately 200 are in the neck. Only a small number of these are removed during a neck dissection. In addition, other structures such as muscles, veins, and nerves may be removed during a radical neck dissection. These include the sternocleidomastoid muscle (one of the muscles that functions to flex the head), internal jugular (neck) vein, submandibular gland (one of the salivary glands), and the spinal accessory nerve (a nerve that helps control speech, swallowing, and certain movements of the head and neck). The goal is always to remove all the cancer, but also to save as many components surrounding the nodes as possible.

An incision is made in the neck, and the skin is pulled back (retracted) to reveal the muscles and lymph nodes.

KEY TERMS

Barium swallow—A procedure in which barium is used to coat the throat to highlight the tissues lining the throat, allowing them to be visualized using x-ray pictures.

Computed tomography (CT or CAT) scan—Using x-rays taken from many angles and computer modeling, CT scans help locate and estimate the size of tumors and provide information on whether they can be surgically removed.

Lymph nodes—Small, bean-shaped collections of tissue found in lymph vessels. They produce cells and proteins that fight infection and filter lymph. Nodes are sometimes called lymph glands.

Magnetic resonance imaging (MRI)—An imaging modality that uses magnetic fields and computers to create detailed cross-sectional pictures of the interior of the body.

Malignant—Cancerous. Malignant cells tend to reproduce without normal controls on growth and form tumors or invade other tissues.

Metastasis—Spread of cells from the original site of a cancer to other parts of the body where secondary tumors are formed.

The surgeon is guided regarding which tissues to remove by tests performed prior to surgery and by examination of the size and texture of the lymph nodes.

Demographics

Experts estimate that there are approximately 5,000–10,000 radical neck dissections in the United States each year. Men and women undergo radical neck dissections at about the same rate.

Precautions

This operation should not be performed if the cancer has metastasized (spread) beyond the head and neck, or if the cancer has invaded the bones of the cervical vertebrae (the first seven bones of the spinal column) or the skull. In these cases, the surgery will not effectively contain the cancer.

Preparation

Radical neck dissection is a major operation. Extensive tests are performed before the operation to try to determine where and how far the cancer has spread.

These tests may include lymph node biopsies, **computed tomography** (CT) scans, **magnetic resonance imaging** (MRI) scans, and barium swallows, as well as standard preoperative blood and liver function tests. The candidate may meet with various health care professionals, including an anesthesiologist, nutritionist, and speech therapist, before or shortly after the operation. The candidate should tell the anesthesiologist about any drug allergies and all medications (including over-the-counter drugs, **vitamins**, and supplements) that are presently being taken.

Aftercare

A person who has had a radical neck dissection will stay in the hospital for up to one week after the operation. Drains are inserted under the skin to remove fluid that accumulates in the neck area. The patient may need to retain at least one drain for a short period of time after being discharged from the hospital. After the surgery, the patient will find it painful to swallow and may need to follow a liquid or soft-food diet while the neck heals. Follow-up doctor visits are required. Depending on how many structures are removed, a person who has had a radical neck dissection may require **physical therapy** to regain use of the arm and shoulder.

Risks

The greatest risk in a radical neck dissection is damage to the nerves, muscles, and veins in the neck. Nerve damage can result in numbness (either temporary or permanent) in different regions on the neck and loss of function (temporary or permanent) in parts of the neck, throat, and shoulder. The more extensive the neck dissection, the more function a person is likely to lose. It is common following radical neck dissection for people to have stooped shoulders, limited ability to lift one or both arms, and limited head and neck rotation and flexion due to the removal of nerves and muscles. Other risks are the same as for all major surgery: potential bleeding, infection, and allergic reaction to anesthesia.

Results

Normal lymph nodes are small and show no cancerous cells under a microscope. Abnormal lymph nodes may be enlarged and show malignant cells when examined under a microscope.

Morbidity and mortality rates

The mortality rate for radical neck dissection can be as high as 14%. Morbidity rates are somewhat higher and are due to bleeding, postsurgical infections, and medical errors.

QUESTIONS TO ASK YOUR DOCTOR

- Which tests will be performed to determine whether the cancer has spread?
- Which parts of the neck will be removed?
- How will a radical neck dissection affect my daily activities after recovery?
- What is the likelihood that the entire cancer can be removed with a radical neck dissection?
- Are the involved lymph nodes on one or both sides of the neck?
- What will be my resulting appearance after the surgery?
- How will my speech and breathing be affected?
- Is my surgeon board-certified in otolaryngology/head and neck surgery?
- How many radical neck procedures has my surgeon performed?
- What is my surgeon's complication rate?

Alternatives

Alternatives to radical neck dissection depend on the reason for the proposed surgery. Most alternatives are far less acceptable. Radiation and **chemotherapy** may be used instead of or in addition to a radical neck dissection in the case of cancer. Alternatives for some surgical procedures may reduce scarring but are not as effective in the removal of all pathological tissue. Chemotherapy and radiation or altered fractionated radiotherapy are reasonable alternatives.

Health care team roles

A radical neck dissection is usually performed by a surgeon with specialized training in otolaryngology/head and neck surgery. Occasionally, a general surgeon will perform a radical neck dissection. The procedure is performed in a hospital under general anesthesia.

Resources

BOOKS

Goldman, Lee, and Andrew I. Schafer. *Goldman's Cecil Medicine.* 24th ed. Philadelphia: Saunders/Elsevier, 2012.

Lucioni, Marco. *Practical Guide to Neck Dissection: Focusing on the Larynx.* 2nd ed. New York: Springer, 2013.

Townsend, Courtney M., et al. *Sabiston Textbook of Surgery.* 19th ed. Philadelphia: Saunders/Elsevier, 2012.

PERIODICALS

Dautremont, J. F., et al. "Planned Neck Dissection Following Radiation Treatment for Head and Neck Malignancy." *International Journal of Otolaryngology*, art. ID no. 954203 (September 24, 2012). http://dx.doi.org/10.1155/2012/954203 (accessed October 3, 2014).

Ferlito, A., et al. "Is the Standard Radical Neck Dissection No Longer Standard?" *Acta Otolaryngolica* 122, no. 7 (2002): 792–95.

Lango, Miriam N., et al. "Impact of Neck Dissection on Long-Term Feeding Tube Dependence in Head and Neck Cancer Patients Treated with Primary Radiation or Chemoradiation." *Head & Neck* 32, no. 3 (2010): 341–47. http://dx.doi.org/10.1002/hed.21188 (accessed October 3, 2014).

Nobis, J. F., et al. "Head and Neck Salivary Gland Carcinomas—Elective Neck Dissection, Yes or No?" *Journal of Oral and Maxillofacial Surgery* (July 25, 2013): e-pub ahead of print. http://dx.doi.org/10.1016/j.joms.2013.05.024 (accessed October 3, 2014).

Popescu, B., et al. "Functional Implications of Radical Neck Dissection and the Impact on the Quality of Life for Patients with Head and Neck Neoplasia." *Journal of Medicine and Life* 5, no. 4 (2012): 410–13.

Seethala, Raja R. "Current State of Neck Dissection in the United States." *Head and Neck Pathology* 3, no. 3 (2009): 238–45. http://dx.doi.org/10.1007/s12105-009-0129-y (accessed October 3, 2014).

WEBSITES

A.D.A.M. Medical Encyclopedia. "Neck Dissection." MedlinePlus. http://www.nlm.nih.gov/medlineplus/ency/article/007573.htm (accessed October 3, 2014).

MedStar Georgetown University Hospital. "Neck Dissection Patient Information." http://www.georgetownuniversity-hospital.org/body_dept.cfm?id=1016 (accessed October 3, 2014).

National Cancer Institute. "Metastatic Squamous Neck Cancer with Occult Primary Treatment (PDQ)." http://www.cancer.gov/cancertopics/pdq/treatment/metastatic-squamous-neck/Patient (accessed October 3, 2014).

ORGANIZATIONS

American Academy of Otolaryngology—Head and Neck Surgery, 1650 Diagonal Rd., Alexandria, VA 22314-2857, (703) 836-4444, http://www.entnet.org.

American Cancer Society, 250 Williams St. NW, Atlanta, GA 30303, (800) 227-2345, http://www.cancer.org.

American College of Surgeons, 633 N. Saint Clair St., Chicago, IL 60611-3211, (312) 202-5000, (800) 621-4111, Fax: (312) 202-5001, postmaster@facs.org, http://www.facs.org.

American Osteopathic Colleges of Otolaryngology—Head and Neck Surgery, 4764 Fishburg Rd., Ste. F, Huber Heights, OH 45424, (800) 455-9404, info@aocoohns.org, http://www.aocoohns.org.

National Cancer Institute, 6116 Executive Blvd., Ste. 300, Bethesda, MD 20892-8322, (800) 4-CANCER (422-6237), http://cancer.gov.

L. Fleming Fallon, Jr, MD, DrPH

Radiofrequency ablation

Definition

Radiofrequency ablation (RFA), or radiofrequency thermal ablation, is a minimally invasive treatment that uses radio waves to create heat that is directed through a probe to destroy tumors.

Purpose

Because it is less invasive than major surgery and destroys **cancer** cells with heat at a specific location, RFA is a good choice for localized treatment of many types of cancer, depending on the type, characteristics, and location of the cancer. RFA is also an alternative for patients who cannot undergo surgery or other cancer treatments, or for whom other treatments have failed. For example, some patients are unsuitable candidates for surgery because of heart or lung conditions that render a long procedure under general anesthesia too risky. Needle-based RFA can be performed through the skin, thereby avoiding open surgery. RFA is also used as an adjuvant to other treatments. In addition to treating cancers, RFA is used as a palliative treatment to relieve cancer pain from incurable disease, to treat recurrent tumors, and to treat some noncancerous conditions.

Although thermal ablation can also be performed with microwaves, lasers, high-intensity focused ultrasound, and **cryotherapy** or freezing below −4°F (−20°C), radiofrequency ablation is the most common technology for thermal ablation of cancers in the liver, lung, kidney, and

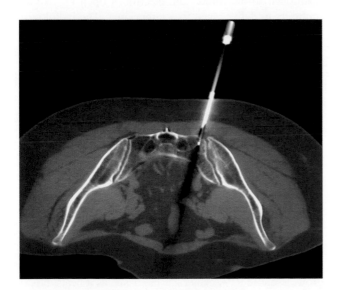

Computed tomography (CT) scan displaying radiofrequency ablation in progress. A probe is inserted directly into the tumor and emits radio waves to heat and destroy the cancerous cells with minimal damage to surrounding healthy tissue. *(Zephyr/Science Source)*

bone, as well as the breast, lymph nodes, nerve ganglia, and soft tissues.

Liver tumors

Liver tumors are the cancers most often treated with RFA. In many cases, liver tumors are either difficult to reach surgically or their surgical removal does not leave enough healthy tissue for the liver to function. Primary liver tumors, in particular, are usually not diagnosed until they are too large to remove surgically. Secondary liver tumors are often metastases that have migrated from cancers elsewhere in the body, with several tumors spread out across the organ, making surgery impossible. After smaller tumors that are too spread out or too difficult to remove surgically have been eliminated by RFA, it is sometimes possible to operate on the larger remaining tumor. RFA is also used when other treatments, such as **chemotherapy**, have failed, or when a liver tumor has recurred, which is very common. Local treatment with RFA is not a substitute for surgery, but it does preserve healthy liver tissue without the complications and side effects of systemic treatments such as chemotherapy and the morbidity and mortality of major liver surgery. RFA can also be used as an adjuvant to chemotherapy or **radiation therapy**. It is most effective for liver tumors of less than 3.8 cm (1.5 in.) in diameter.

Lung tumors

RFA is used to treat early-stage lung cancer and for patients who have a small number of lung metastases that have spread from elsewhere in the body, such as the kidney, intestine, or breast. It is also used for lung cancers in patients who are too ill for conventional surgery or want to avoid the long recovery and possible complications of surgery. RFA may be used to debulk or reduce the size of tumors that are too large to remove surgically, so that they can then potentially be eliminated with chemotherapy or radiation. RFA is also used to relieve pain caused by a lung tumor that has invaded the chest wall.

Kidney tumors

Although kidney (renal) cancer is generally treated with surgery, RFA is preferred for patients who have only one remaining kidney. It is also an alternative for patients with medical conditions that may prevent them from having surgery or for whom recovery from surgery would be difficult. RFA is a good choice for patients with more than one renal tumor, as long as the tumors are smaller than about 4–5 cm (1.6–2 in.).

Bone cancer and pain

RFA is used to relieve the pain of cancer that has spread to the bone. It is also used as palliative treatment

KEY TERMS

Adjuvant—A treatment or therapy in addition to the primary treatment, such as radiofrequency ablation in addition to chemotherapy, surgery, or radiation.

Cauterize—To burn, sear, or otherwise destroy tissue.

Debulking—Removal of a major portion of a tumor by surgery or radiofrequency ablation so that the remainder can be treated more effectively.

Laparoscopy—A visual examination of the inside of the body with an instrument called a laparoscope.

Lumpectomy—Surgical removal of a breast tumor and a limited amount of surrounding breast tissue.

Metastases—Tumors that have arisen from cancer cells that migrated from a primary cancer elsewhere in the body.

Palliative—Relieving or alleviating symptoms such as pain without curing the disease.

Percutaneous—Performed through the skin.

Recur, recurrence—Cancer that comes back after treatment.

Systemic—Having effects throughout the body.

to shrink other types of tumors that are causing pain and have not responded to other treatments or cannot be reached or treated with surgery.

Other cancers

Because RFA is fast, easy, predictable, safe, and relatively inexpensive compared to many other therapies, it is sometimes used to treat other cancers. For example, RFA can be used as adjuvant treatment to lumpectomies for **breast cancer** to help prevent recurrence and improve cosmetic results.

Description

Heat has been used as a treatment since ancient times. RFA uses radio waves, a form of electromagnetic energy, produced by an electrical generator. Electromagnetic energy includes visible light, microwaves, radio waves, and **x-rays**. The energy from radiofrequency is safer than that from x-rays because it is absorbed by living tissue as simple heat that does not change the structure of the cells.

Procedure

RFA procedures are most often performed by interventional radiologists. These are medical doctors who specialize in radiologic procedures for diagnosing and treating disease. RFA procedures are usually performed on an outpatient basis in hospitals, imaging centers, and physician offices. Because there can be some pain with RFA, an intravenous (IV) line is usually inserted to administer anesthesia that causes drowsiness. This type of anesthesia is known as conscious sedation. For complex procedures, general anesthesia may be required, with an anesthesiologist or nurse anesthetist to monitor the patient's vital signs. The patient lies on a table in an examination room or surgical suite and becomes part of the electrical circuit through which the radio waves pass. Grounding pads are placed on the patient's back or thighs. The radiologist uses real-time imaging with ultrasound, **computed tomography** (CT), or **magnetic resonance imaging** (MRI) equipment and video monitors to guide the needle or probe into the tumor and throughout the procedure.

Most often, a small needle or probe that transmits the current is passed through the patient's skin and directly into the tumor. This is called the percutaneous method and makes for an easier recovery. The 14–17.5-gauge needle electrode has an insulated shaft and noninsulated tip. The active tip is of varying lengths and configurations. Sometimes a single needle electrode is used. Alternatively, a straight needle contains numerous curved needles that are retracted inside the main probe until the tip is positioned within the tumor. Once the tip is positioned in the tumor, the electrodes open up like an umbrella to deliver heat to a larger area. The radiologist can accurately predict the required volume and shape of the ablation to destroy the tumor and margins of healthy tissue. Sometimes a laparoscope is used to introduce the probe. Although **laparoscopy** requires only a tiny incision, it still is considered surgery, and sometimes RFA is performed as a part of a general surgery.

The energy at the exposed tip is controlled by the physician. At temperatures above 113°F (45°C), RFA "cooks" the tumor and kills the cells. A small needle can accurately destroy a precise area. For a large tumor, the radiologist may have to guide and reposition the probe several times to destroy the entire tumor. The probe is also used to heat and destroy a small margin or rim of healthy tissue around the cancerous tumor. This technique helps ensure that no single cancerous cells are left behind to re-grow. Because RFA cauterizes the tissue as it heats, blood loss and bleeding risk are minimized.

Each RFA treatment takes 15–30 minutes, but the entire procedure can take longer, depending on the number of tumors, tumor size, and location. For example, the radiologist may have to reposition the probe several times for one liver mass and then move it to a second smaller mass, for a total procedure time of 90 minutes. Some procedures can take up to three hours. However, a single session involves only 10–60 minutes of active ablation.

Precautions

RFA is safe for most patients, including patients who cannot withstand longer surgical procedures, complications, and recovery times. The physician will discuss the benefits and risks with patients in advance of RFA. The procedure usually requires some anesthesia. A medical history and blood tests may rule out some patients or require that they adjust certain of their medications. Some tumors or cancers are not considered treatable with RFA, and the number and size of tumors that can be treated in a particular organ may be limited.

Preparation

Before an RFA procedure, patients will typically have blood drawn for routine blood tests. The physician, nurse, or scheduler will provide preparation instructions that will include concerns about eating or drinking before the procedure, depending on the type of planned anesthesia. Normally, patients will be told not to eat or drink eight hours (or after midnight) before RFA. Certain medications may need to be changed or stopped before the procedure to avoid complications; for example, blood thinners and aspirin may cause excessive bleeding. A patient should mention all current medications to the interventional radiologist.

Aftercare

After the treatment is completed, a small bandage is placed over the probe insertion site. The patient is removed to a recovery room to allow the anesthesia to wear off. Pain medication is administered as needed. Patients will remain in bed for the first few hours following the procedure, but seldom have to stay overnight. Some patients experience nausea and will receive medications and instructions for nausea and pain care before leaving the facility. Patients having RFA with surgery may require a hospital stay.

Once they return home, patients will be instructed to drink plenty of fluids and to take a prescription narcotic for the first day or two if pain continues. They likely will be instructed not to drive or make important decisions for 24 hours after the procedure because of anesthesia side effects. Excessive physical activity also is discouraged. However, most patients can resume their normal diets and physical and sexual activities within a few days of RFA.

Risks

RFA is a complicated procedure that should be performed only by specially trained physicians.

Most interventional radiologists have extensive experience with RFA and similar procedures, but patients can check with accrediting societies, local medical societies, and their primary care physicians and ask questions of the physician who will perform the procedure.

Risks associated with RFA are relatively minor compared to those associated with many other cancer treatments, especially surgery. However, no procedure is risk-free. Although rare, there is a risk of serious injury if the needle makes a hole in (perforates) a nearby organ. If this happens, the patient may require surgery to repair the injury. There also is a minor risk of infection at the site where the probe is inserted. Patients may experience bruising or bleeding. If air or gas enters the chest cavity (pneumothorax), a chest tube may be required for a few days to drain it.

Results

RFA results vary, depending on the location, type, and size of the tumor. It is a safe and effective local treatment for some cancers. Complication rates are very low. Survival rates are similar to those for surgery for hepatocellular carcinomas of less than 5 cm (2 in.) and liver metastases of less than 4 cm (1.6 in.) from colorectal carcinomas. RFA may also increase the cure rate for liver surgeries and can provide palliative relief. Fibrosis and scar tissue gradually replace the dead tumor tissue destroyed by RFA, and the scar tissue normally shrinks over time. After a few days, patients should experience no further pain from the procedure.

Abnormal results

If pain continues for more than a few days, the patient should contact the physician. Some patients develop flu-like symptoms and **fever** that can last for a few weeks. Bleeding also has been reported. If severe symptoms continue, the patient may need an additional RFA procedure or surgery to control bleeding. Any local recurrence of the cancer is usually at the margin of the tumor and can sometimes be re-treated with RFA.

Resources

PERIODICALS

Ni, Jia-yan, et al. "Percutaneous Ablation Therapy Versus Surgical Resection in the Treatment for Early-Stage Hepatocellular Carcinoma: A Meta-Analysis of 21,492 Patients." *Journal of Cancer Research & Clinical Oncology* 139, no. 12 (December 2013): 2012–33.

Phoa, K. Nadine, et al. "Radiofrequency Ablation vs Endoscopic Surveillance for Patients With Barrett Esophagus and Low-Grade Dysplasia: A Randomized Clinical Trial." *Journal of the American Medical Association* 311, no. 12 (March 26, 2014): 1209–17.

OTHER

National Institutes of Health Clinical Center. "Radiofrequency Ablation: Patient Information." http://www.cc.nih.gov/drd/rfa/pdf/patients.pdf (accessed August 25, 2014).

WEBSITES

Radiological Society of North America. "Radiofrequency Ablation (RFA) of Liver Tumors." RadiologyInfo.org. March 7, 2013. http://www.radiologyinfo.org/en/info.cfm?pg=rfalung (accessed August 25, 2014).

Radiological Society of North America. "Radiofrequency Ablation (RFA) of Lung Tumors." RadiologyInfo.org. March 7, 2013. http://www.radiologyinfo.org/en/info.cfm?pg=rfaliver (accessed August 25, 2014).

ORGANIZATIONS

American College of Radiology, 1891 Preston White Drive, Reston, VA 20191, (70) 648-8900, (800) 227-5463, http://www.acr.org.

Radiological Society of North America, 820 Jorie Boulevard, Oak Brook, IL 60523-2251, (630) 571-2670, Fax: (630) 571-7837, (800) 381-6660, http://www.rsna.org.

Society of Interventional Radiology, 3975 Fair Ridge Drive, Suite 400 North, Fairfax, VA 22033, (703) 691-1805, Fax: (703) 691-1855, (800) 488-7284, http://www.sirweb.org.

Teresa G. Odle

REVISED BY MARGARET ALIC, PhD

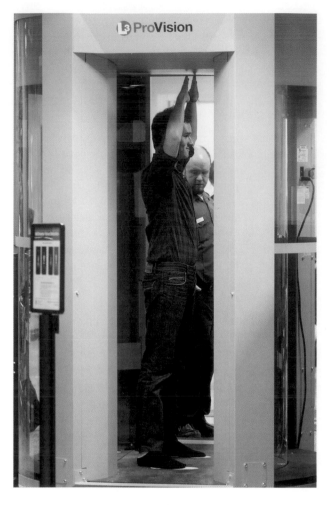

Body scanners at airports are a source of radiofrequency energy; although the dose of radiation is low, some people may not feel comfortable passing through the scanner. *(Bloomberg/Getty Images)*

Radiofrequency energy and cancer risk

Definition

Radiofrequency (RF) energy is radiation in the radio wave region at the low end of the electromagnetic spectrum. It is low-energy, low-frequency, long-wavelength, nonionizing radiation emitted by communication devices such as radios and cell phones. Unlike higher-energy ionizing radiation—such as some ultraviolet (UV) light, **x-rays**, and gamma rays—RF energy cannot cause **cancer** by damaging DNA. However, there has been some concern that it may increase cancer risk by other means.

Description

The electromagnetic spectrum is the radiation of energy, ranging from very high-energy, high-frequency gamma rays and x-rays to UV and visible light and low-energy, low-frequency infrared microwaves, RF energy, electromagnetic fields (EMF) emitted from power lines, and even heat radiated by the human body. RF energy is at the low end of the electromagnetic spectrum, with higher energy than extremely low-frequency electromagnetic radiation but lower energy than nonionizing radiation such as infrared and visible light. High-energy radiation—such as gamma rays, x-rays, and higher-energy UV—is called ionizing radiation because it has sufficient energy to ionize or remove an electron from an atom or molecule.

Ionizing radiation can damage DNA, which increases the risk of cancer. Nonionizing radiation, such as visible light and RF energy, has only enough energy to vibrate atoms, and RF energy has even less energy than visible light. If enough RF energy is absorbed by water-containing materials, such as food or body tissues, it can produce heat, as occurs in a microwave oven. A large number of studies have examined the effects of nonionizing radiation from sources such as microwave ovens, radar, and cell phones. There is no consistent evidence that non-ionizing radiation increases cancer risk.

RF energy sources

Sources of RF energy include:

- the earth, sky, lightning strikes, sun, and outer space
- radio and television signals
- signals from cell phones, cordless phones, cell phone towers, satellite phones, WiFi, and Bluetooth
- microwave ovens
- radar
- medical procedures that destroy body tissues with heat
- millimeter-wave full-body scanners used for security screening in airports

Although some people have significant workplace exposure to RF energy, most people have much lower levels of exposure from their phones, WiFi, televisions, and radios. Although microwave ovens use very high levels of RF energy to heat food, the radiation is contained within the oven. Damaged or modified ovens that leak energy could potentially cause burns.

CELL PHONES. Cell phones and cell phone towers transmit and receive signals using RF energy, and there have been concerns that this energy use may increase the risk of cancer or other health problems. Depending on the country and the network, cell phones operate in a frequency range of 800–2,600 megahertz (MHz); in the United States, their frequency range is approximately 1,800–2,200 MHz. Cordless phones often operate at radiofrequencies similar to cell phones, but because they have a limited range—from the phone to its base—their signals are usually much less powerful than those of cell phones. Radios and televisions operate at lower radiofrequencies than cell phones, whereas RF sources such as radar, microwave ovens, industrial equipment, and **magnetic resonance imaging** (MRI) equipment operate at somewhat higher frequencies.

Body tissues nearest to a cell phone can absorb RF energy that could theoretically cause heating; however, cell phones do not cause a measurable increase in body temperature. Current exposure guidelines for RF radiation are designed to protect against heat-induced injury

since, as of 2014, there is no convincing evidence that cell phones increase cancer risk. However, given the ubiquity of cell phones—with their total number approaching that of the entire global population—and the increasing amount of time that people spend on their phones, if cell phones do increase cancer risk, the result would be a global pandemic. Because cell phones have not been in use for enough time to reveal potential long-term risks, large prospective epidemiologic studies of cell phone use and cancer risk are ongoing.

Despite their increased use, RF energy exposure from cell phones is probably decreasing. Since the early 2000s, cell phones in the United States have been digital rather than analog. Digital phones operate at a different frequency and lower power than the analog phones that were commonly used in some earlier studies of cell phones and cancer risk. Texting and wired and wireless cell phone headsets have also reduced the exposure of the head to RF energy.

FULL-BODY SECURITY SCANNERS. Full-body scanners are now used in airports around the world to screen passengers for concealed security threats. In the United States, full-body airport x-ray scanners have been replaced with millimeter-wave scanners that do not use x-rays. Passive millimeter-wave scanners detect the very low levels of natural radiation emitted from the body. Active scanners emit low-energy RF radiation that passes through clothing, bounces off the skin and anything concealed under clothing, and is detected by receivers that project an image of a generic body showing the location of any concealed object. The amount of RF radiation exposure from a full-body active millimeter-wave scan is much less than that from a cell phone and has no known health effects.

Full-body x-ray scanners emit low-energy or higher-energy x-rays that bounce off or pass through the body, respectively. Although ionizing radiation doses from these types of scanners are very low, they do add to an individual's total lifetime radiation dose, which could increase cancer risk.

Precautions

The only known potential risks from RF energy are heat and burns. RF energy focused on a particular area of the body can cause burns and tissue damage. RF energy focused on the eye can cause the formation of cataracts. It is not clear whether RF energy at levels below those that cause heating have any physiological effects.

If RF energy were to increase cancer risk, children would theoretically be at greater risk than adults because their developing nervous systems are more vulnerable. Their smaller heads have greater proportional exposure to

KEY TERMS

Electromagnetic spectrum—The entire range of wavelengths or frequencies of radiation, extending from high-energy gamma rays to extremely low-frequency radio waves, including visible light and radiofrequency energy.

Ionizing radiation—Electromagnetic radiation with enough energy to remove electrons from atoms, causing those atoms to become ionized or charged; high-frequency radiation including x-rays and gamma rays.

Microwaves—Relatively low-frequency electromagnetic radiation of wavelengths ranging from about 1 millimeter to 1 meter.

Millimeter-wave scanners—The technology used in full-body security scanners, such as in airports, that directs millimeter-length radiofrequency energy that penetrates clothing and bounces off the skin and concealed objects.

Nonionizing radiation—Low-frequency electromagnetic radiation with insufficient energy to ionize atoms, including radio waves, microwaves, and radiofrequency energy from cell phones.

RF energy from cell phones, and their lifetime exposure will be greater than that of adults. However, as of 2014, data from studies of children with brain cancer have not found an association with cell phone use. International studies of childhood cancer risk from communications technologies, including cell phones, are ongoing.

Research and general acceptance

Research

It is generally accepted that DNA damage is necessary for the development of cancer, and nonionizing radiation, such as RF energy, does not damage DNA in cells. Most animal and other laboratory studies have found no increased cancer risk from RF energy, although a few studies have reported biological effects that could be linked to cancer. Studies exposing laboratory animals to RF energy enable scientists to carefully control for other factors that may increase cancer risk, but it is not always clear how applicable such studies are to human exposure and risk.

The primary concern about the health effects of cell phone use has been the potential for an increased risk of brain cancer, since most RF exposure from cell phones is to the head. Most epidemiologic studies have found no association between cell phone use and **brain tumors**, although there have been a few findings of statistically significant associations in certain subgroups of people. Studies comparing cancer risk in groups of people with and without exposure to RF energy from cell phones can be difficult to interpret because of uncontrolled factors. First of all, it is impossible to avoid exposure to RF energy from a variety of sources other than cell phones. Furthermore, epidemiologic studies generally use participant recall questionnaires to determine exposure. These are notoriously unreliable, especially among people diagnosed with brain cancer. Most analyses of the international Interphone Study—the largest case-controlled study of cell phone use and head and neck tumors—have reported no associations. One analysis reported a small but significant increase in gliomas among participants who spent the most total time using cell phones; however, the total times reported appeared unlikely, and people who reported lower total times appeared to have less risk of glioma than participants who did not use cell phones. Another study found no relationships between the location of brain tumors and exposures of the head to RF energy from cell phones. The **National Cancer Institute**, which tracks cancer incidence in the United States, found no increase in brain or other central nervous system cancers between 1987 and 2007, despite the dramatic increase in cell phone use. Similar results have been reported from other countries. Studies of workers exposed to high levels of RF energy for long periods of time have found no increased risk of brain tumors. Other studies of people with workplace RF energy exposure—such as radio operators and people who work with radar or communications antennas—have found no clear increased cancer risk.

There are several ongoing studies of cell phone use and cancer risk. The results of a case-control study called Mobi-Kids are expected in 2016. This study is comparing 2,000 young people with newly diagnosed brain tumors with 4,000 healthy young people. COSMOS, a European study launched in 2010, will be examining possible long-term health effects of cell phone use in some 290,000 adults over the next 20–30 years.

Expert opinion

Concerns about cancer risk from cell phone RF energy increased when the International Agency for Research on Cancer (IARC) classified RF radiation as "possibly carcinogenic to humans." Although the IARC admitted that the research findings were conflicting and the studies were generally of low quality, they based their classification primarily on the one study showing a possible link between cell phone use and one type of brain tumor.

QUESTIONS TO ASK YOUR DOCTOR

- Am I at increased cancer risk because of my cell phone use?
- Do microwave ovens increase cancer risk?
- Should I avoid full-body airport scanners?
- What types of environmental radiation increase my cancer risk?
- How can I reduce my exposure to radio-frequency energy?

Among U.S. organizations as of 2014:

- The U.S. Environmental Protection Agency (EPA) and the National Toxicology Program (NTP) of the National Institute of Environmental Health Sciences have not formally ruled on the cancer-causing potential of RF energy. The NTP has been carrying out further studies.

- The American Cancer Society has stated that further studies are needed and that people who are concerned about RF exposure should use an earpiece and limit cell phone use, especially their children's use.

- The U.S. Food and Drug Administration (FDA), which regulates the safety of devices that emit radiation (including cell phones), has stated that most human epidemiologic studies have failed to show an association between cell phone RF energy exposure and health problems and that studies that have indicated biological effects have not been replicated.

- The U.S. Centers for Disease Control and Prevention (CDC) has stated that studies have raised concerns, but that research as a whole does not support an association between cell phone use and health effects.

- The Federal Communications Commission (FCC) has concluded that there is no scientific evidence that wireless phone use can cause cancer or other health effects.

Prevention

Because RF energy is ubiquitous in the environment, there is no way to completely avoid exposure. People who are concerned about RF energy can reduce their exposure by avoiding appliances and equipment that emit RF energy and using devices that prevent cell phone antennas—the source of RF energy—from being placed against the ear. People can also limit their use of cell phones. People who are concerned about RF exposure

from full-body security scanners can request to be screened in a different manner.

Resources

BOOKS

Kempson, Cynthia, and Eugene Rahm, eds. *Cell Phone Use and Health Risks: Assessments and State of Research.* Hauppauge, NY: Nova, 2013.

Naff, Clay Farris, ed. *Do Cell Phones Cause Cancer?* Detroit: Greenhaven, 2013.

PERIODICALS

Yaros, Ronald A., Elia Powers, and Soo-Kwang Oh. "Incorrect Terms Used to Portray Possible Cell Phone Risk." *Newspaper Research Journal* 35, no. 1 (Winter 2014): 96–107.

OTHER

"Cell Phone Radiofrequency Radiation Studies." National Toxicology Program. February 2014. http://www.niehs.nih.gov/health/assets/docs_a_e/cell_phone_radiofrequency_radiation_studies_508.pdf#search=radiofrequency%20energy%20AND%20cancer%20risk (accessed October 24, 2014).

WEBSITES

"Cell Phones and Cancer Risk." National Cancer Institute. June 24, 2013. http://www.cancer.gov/cancertopics/factsheet/Risk/cellphones (accessed October 24, 2014).

Institute of Physics. "Could Your Phone Harm Your Health?" physics.org. http://www.physics.org/article-questions.asp?id=84 (accessed October 24, 2014).

"Microwaves, Radio Waves, and Other Types of Radiofrequency Radiation." American Cancer Society. October 16, 2013. http://www.cancer.org/cancer/cancercauses/radiationexposureandcancer/radiofrequency-radiation (accessed October 24, 2014).

ORGANIZATIONS

American Cancer Society, 250 Williams Street NW, Atlanta, GA 30303, (800) 227-2345, http://www.cancer.org.

International Agency for Research on Cancer, 150 Cours Albert Thomas, Lyon, FranceCEDEX 0869372, 33 (0)4 72 73 84 85, Fax: 33 (0)4 72 73 85 75, http://www.iarc.fr.

National Cancer Institute, 6116 Executive Boulevard, Suite 300, Bethesda, MD 20892-8322, (800) 4-CANCER (422-6237), http://www.cancer.gov.

National Institute of Environmental Health Sciences, PO Box 12233, MD K3-16, Research Triangle Park, NC 27709, (919) 541-3345, Fax: (919) 541-4395, webcenter@niehs.nih.gov, http://www.niehs.nih.gov.

Margaret Alic, PhD

Radionuclide bone scan *see* **Nuclear medicine scans**

Radionuclide imaging *see* **Nuclear medicine scans**

Radiopharmaceuticals

Definition

Radiopharmaceuticals are drugs that contain radioactive substances called radioisotopes. They are prepared by pharmaceutical companies for use in diagnosing and treating disease, particularly **cancer**.

Purpose

Radioactive pharmaceuticals are made in nuclear reactors by several pharmaceutical suppliers in different parts of the world. The radiopharmaceutical drugs are obtained locally from radiopharmaceutical pharmacies. All radiopharmaceuticals are produced based on different ways of combining radionuclides, called radioactive isotopes or radioisotopes, with other biological substances for use in nuclear medicine, a branch of radiology. The two main purposes of radiopharmaceuticals are diagnosing and treating various diseases, especially cancer. For diagnostic purposes, radiopharmaceuticals are applied as tracers that emit gamma rays inside the body. The use of radioactive tracers allows the functions of different organ systems in the body to be evaluated in **imaging studies** such as **positron emission tomography** (PET). For the purpose of cancer treatment, therapeutic radiopharmaceuticals are prepared in different forms for delivery by injection, by mouth, or placed into a body cavity. The radioisotopes are used in smaller doses for diagnostic imaging and larger doses to deliver radiation to the part of the body being treated. The focus here is the use of radiopharmaceuticals in the treatment of cancer, a form of radiotherapy called radionuclide therapy (RNT).

About 10,000 hospitals around the world use radiopharmaceuticals. Diagnostic procedures represent 90% of their use and treatments about 10%, but their role in treating cancer is increasing. The most common radioisotope used for diagnostic procedures is technetium-99, which is used in over 30 different preparations for 40 million procedures each year (16.7 million in the United States in 2012). Fluorine-18 is the radioactive tracer used in PET for cancer diagnosis.

The most common radiopharmaceuticals used in cancer treatment include:

- phosphorus-32 (chromic phosphate or sodium phosphate with radioactive phosphorus), mainly for the treatment of brain cancer

- iodine-131 (sodium iodide with radioactive iodine) for treating different types of thyroid cancer and other thyroid diseases

---

KEY TERMS

Half-life—Length of time for the decay of one half of the radiation in a sample of a given radioactive isotope.

Isotopes—Forms of a chemical element that have the same number of protons (atomic number) but different numbers of neutrons and different atomic weights.

Lymph nodes—Small bean-shaped glands found throughout the body that produce lymphatic fluid, cells, and proteins to fight infection. They also clean and filter foreign and toxic cells, such as bacteria or cancer cells, out of the lymph fluid.

Metastasis—Spread of cancer from its point of origin to other parts of the body, such as nearby tissue, distant organs, and bone.

Millicurie—Unit for measuring radioactivity.

Platelets—Tiny blood cells that are an essential component of the body's coagulation system.

Thyroid glands—Small glands on each side of the trachea (windpipe) that secrete hormones to regulate metabolism and growth.

- strontium-89, samarium-153, and radium-223 for treating metastatic bone cancer

- lutetium-177 and ytterbium-90 as radiolabeled monoclonal antibodies for treating non-Hodgkin lymphoma and liver cancer

Description

The principle behind the use of therapeutic radiopharmaceuticals is that rapidly dividing cells are particularly sensitive to radiation, and irradiation of certain types of cancerous growths can control the growth of cancer cells and even stop their growth in some cases. Internal radiopharmaceutical use requires the administration of a small source of radiation in the target cancer site. When the target area is within short range, internal use is known as brachytherapy, a technique that is becoming widely used for certain types of cancer, such as **thyroid cancer**, **endometrial cancer**, and **prostate cancer**.

Radiopharmaceuticals used in cancer treatment are small, simple substances that contain a radioactive isotope of an element with an atomic weight less than that of bismuth. Treatment using radiopharmaceuticals, called radionuclide therapy (RNT), is targeted to specific areas of the body where cancer is present so that radiation emitted from the radioisotope will kill cancer cells. These isotopes have short half-lives, meaning that most of the radiation is gone within a few days or weeks. A study of thousands of radiopharmaceutical administrations, both for PET and for cancer treatment, found that no hospitalizations or deaths occurred following treatment, suggesting that the incidence of adverse events associated with radiopharmaceuticals has remained stable for two decades.

Phosphorus-32

Phosphorus-32 is a salt of chromium and phosphoric acid (chromic phosphate), containing a radioactive form of the element phosphorus. Another preparation of phosphorus-32 uses sodium phosphate, a salt of sodium and phosphoric acid, containing a radioactive form of the element phosphorus. Phosphorus-32 is used primarily for brain cancer, but also for breast and prostate cancers that have metastasized to the bone, and for some other cancers. In addition, it is used to treat fluid accumulations (**ascites**) that can result from lung, ovarian, or uterine cancers. It is 50% to 80% effective in stopping fluid leakage from these organs; the fluid sometimes can fill the abdominal cavity and lower extremities, resulting in complications. Phosphorus-32 is also used to kill cancer cells that may remain after surgery for uterine cancer. It may be used to treat ovarian or prostate cancers directly without being combined with external beam radiation, and is sometimes used in conjunction with **chemotherapy**.

Radiopharmaceuticals for treating thyroid cancer

Iodine-131 (sodium iodide), also called radioactive iodine or radioiodine, is a salt of sodium and a radioactive form of the element iodine. Iodine-131 is taken up by the thyroid gland, which absorbs most of the iodine in the body. Radioiodine can destroy the thyroid gland while having only minor effects on other parts of the body. Therefore, it is used following surgery for thyroid cancer to destroy any remaining cancer cells in thyroid tissue, or to destroy thyroid cancer that has spread (metastasized) to lymph nodes or other tissues. Iodine-131 is standard treatment for differentiated thyroid cancer that has spread to the neck and other parts of the body. Its use improves the survival rate for such patients. Radioiodine may be beneficial for treating small cancers of the thyroid that have not metastasized to other tissues. It is also used to treat noncancerous thyroid tumors.

Radiopharmaceuticals for treating metastatic bone cancer

Several radiopharmaceuticals are used to treat bone cancer, particularly metastatic bone cancer originating from invasive prostate cancer or **breast cancer**. When radiopharmaceuticals are injected into a vein, they accumulate in the cancerous bone tissue and emit radiation. This treatment has been shown to kill cancer cells and relieve pain in a majority of patients. Sometimes the radiopharmaceuticals are used in conjunction with external beam radiation directed at the most painful areas. The most common radiopharmaceutical for treating bone cancer or metastatic prostate cancer is strontium-89 (Metastron). Men with advanced prostate cancer who are responding to chemotherapy appear to have a better chance of survival if bone metastases are treated with strontium-89 every six weeks in conjunction with a chemotherapy drug.

Samarium-153 (Quadramet) and radium-223 (Xofigo) are also used primarily to treat prostate cancer that has metastasized to the bone. In addition, two other radioactive isotopes, rhenium-186 and rhenium-188, are sometimes used to treat metastatic bone cancer originating from prostate cancer.

Other radiopharmaceuticals

Lutetium-177 is a strong emitter of beta radiation used to destroy cancer cells. It is derived from ytterbium-176. Both lutetium-177 and ytterbium-90, another ytterbium compound, are used as radiolabeled **monoclonal antibodies** in the treatment of **non-Hodgkin lymphoma** and **liver cancer**.

Recommended dosage

Dosages of radiopharmaceuticals vary with the individual, considering age, weight, the type of cancer, and the type of treatment. Red and white blood cell counts are also considered. Dosages of radioactive materials are expressed in units called millicuries. Dosage is determined by the oncologist. The drug may be delivered by injection, placement into a body cavity, inhalation, or orally.

Phosphorus-32 is provided in a suspension that is delivered through a catheter, or tube, inserted into the sac surrounding the lungs, or into the abdominal or pelvic cavities. The usual dosage is 15–20 millicuries for abdominal administration and 10 millicuries for administration to the lung sac. Phosphorus-32 also may be injected into the ovaries or prostate.

Iodine-131 is taken by mouth as a capsule or a solution. The dose range for treating thyroid cancer is 30–200 millicuries, depending on age and body size. Doses may be repeated. Treatment usually requires two to three days of hospitalization. For this therapy to be effective there must be high levels of thyroid-stimulating hormone (TSH, or thyrotropin) in the blood. This hormone can be injected prior to treatment.

Strontium-89 is injected into a vein. The usual dosage is four millicuries, depending on age, body size, and blood cell counts. Repeat doses may be required.

The usual dosage of samarium-153 is one millicurie per kg (0.45 millicurie per lb.) of body weight, injected slowly into a vein. Repeat doses may be necessary.

The dosage of phosphorus-32 depends on the patient's age, body size, blood cell counts, the type of cancer, and the type of treatment. The usual dosages range from 1–5 millicuries. Repeat doses may be required.

Precautions

Some individuals may have an allergic reaction to strontium-89, samarium-153, phosphorus-32, or other radiopharmaceuticals. Such allergic reactions are treated on an individual basis.

Because radiopharmaceuticals collect in the urine for elimination, they will also accumulate in the bladder. Consequently, patients are advised to drink plenty of liquid prior to treatment and to urinate as often as possible after treatment. This precaution reduces the irradiation of the bladder and helps avoid urinary tract problems after treatment.

Radiopharmaceuticals are not usually recommended for use during pregnancy. It is recommended that women do not become pregnant for a year after treatment with sodium iodide-131. Breastfeeding is not possible during treatment with radiopharmaceuticals.

Precautions before treatment with iodine-131

The patient is advised to avoid foods containing iodine, such as iodized salt, seafood, cabbage, kale, or turnips, for several weeks prior to treatment with iodine-131. The iodine in these foods will be taken up by the thyroid, thereby reducing the amount of radioiodine that can be taken up. Radiopaque agents containing iodine sometimes are used to improve imaging on an x-ray. A recent x-ray exam that included such an agent may interfere with the ability of the thyroid to take up radioiodine.

Diarrhea or vomiting may cause iodine-131 to be lost from the body, resulting in less effective treatment and the risk of outside contamination. Kidney disease may prevent the excretion of radioiodines, increasing the risk of side effects from the drug.

Precautions after radiopharmaceutical treatment

Strontium-89, samarium-153, and large doses of iodine-131 may temporarily lower the number of circulating white blood cells, which are necessary for fighting infections. The number of blood platelets (important for blood clotting) also may be lowered. Precautions for reducing the risk of infection and bleeding include:

- avoiding people with infections
- seeking medical help at the first sign of infection or unusual bleeding
- using care when cleaning teeth
- avoiding touching the eyes or inside of the nose
- avoiding cuts and injuries

Patients are advised to drink plenty of clear liquids and to urinate often after treatment with iodine-131. This helps to flush the radioiodine from the body. To reduce the risk of contaminating the environment or other people, patients are advised to adhere to the following procedures for 48–96 hours after treatment with iodine-131:

- avoid kissing and sex
- avoid food preparation and handling other people's eating utensils
- avoid close contact with others, especially pregnant women
- wash the tub and sink after each use
- wash hands after using or cleaning the toilet
- use separate washcloths and towels
- wash clothes, bed linens, and dishes separately
- flush the toilet twice after each use

Strontium-89 and samarium-153 also are excreted in the urine. To prevent radioactive contamination, special measures should be followed for one week after receiving strontium-89 and for 12 hours after receiving samarium-153:

- use a toilet rather than a urinal
- flush the toilet several times after each use
- wipe up and flush any spilled urine or blood
- wash hands after using or cleaning a toilet
- wash soiled clothes and bed linens separately from other laundry.

Individuals with bladder control problems are advised to follow special measures after treatment to prevent contamination by radioactive urine.

Side effects

Some side effects of the different radiopharmaceuticals may be rare and temporary, since the drugs are eliminated fairly quickly. However, certain milder side effects are common with these drugs, but will typically be of short duration. More serious side effects are usually related to the type and location of the cancer being treated and may require treatment with specific medications.

Each radiopharmaceutical may have certain characteristic side effects; not all of those shown are applicable.

The more common side effects of radiopharmaceuticals include:

- loss of appetite (anorexia)
- abdominal cramps
- diarrhea
- nausea and vomiting
- weakness or fatigue
- dry cough
- sore throat
- tenderness in the salivary glands or neck
- painful or difficult urination

More serious side effects may include:

- decreased red blood cell (anemia) and white blood cell (neutropenia) counts
- severe abdominal pain
- severe nausea and vomiting
- fever
- chills
- chest pain
- difficulty breathing
- irregular heartbeat
- temporary increase in bone pain
- bleeding or bruising

Signs of a low platelet count after treatment with strontium-89, samarium-153, or iodine-131 may include tiny red spots on the skin, bruising, bleeding, and black, tar-like stools.

Large total doses of radioiodine may cause infertility in men, especially those being treated for prostate cancer.

Flushing and transient increased **bone pain** are among the more common side effects of strontium-89.

Signs of infection due to low white blood cell counts may occur after treatment with strontium-89, samarium-153, or iodine-131, including:

- fever or chills
- cough or hoarseness
- lower back or side pain

A long-term effect of thyroid treatment with iodine-131 may be an increased risk of developing another type of cancer, including possibly leukemia.

Because children and older adults are particularly sensitive to radiation, they may experience more side effects during and after treatment with radiopharmaceuticals.

Interactions

Radiation therapy or **anticancer drugs** may increase the harmful effects of strontium-89, samarium-153, or other drugs used in treating bone cancer. Medicines containing calcium may prevent strontium-89 from being taken up by bone tissue. Etidronate (Didronel), one of several **bisphosphonates** that are sometimes used to prevent or treat osteoporosis, may prevent samarium-153 or other radiopharmaceuticals from working effectively.

Research

Therapeutic radiopharmaceuticals are the focus of intensive medical research worldwide. Radionuclides are being attached to highly specific biological compounds such as monoclonal antibodies. Boron-10, for example, is an experimental radiopharmaceutical that concentrates in the tumor itself. Then the patient is given radiotherapy with neutrons that attach to the boron and the resulting high-energy alpha particles kill cancer cells. Radiopharmaceuticals are gaining widespread recognition as an effective targeted cancer treatment and many are being researched for effectiveness in diagnosing and treating different types of cancer.

Resources

BOOKS
Haller, D. G., L. D. Wagman, K. A. Camphausen, and W. J. Hoskins, eds. *Cancer Management: A Multidisciplinary Approach.* 14th ed. Philadelphia: Karger, 2012.

PERIODICALS
Repetto-Llamazares, A., N. Abbas, O. S. Bruland, J. Dahle, and R. H. Larsen. "Advantage of Lutetium-177 Versus Radioiodine Immunoconjugate in Targeted Radionuclide Therapy of B-cell Tumors." *Anticancer Research* 34 (July 2014): 424–30.
Silberstein, E. B. "Prevalence of Adverse Events to Radiopharmaceuticals from 2007 to 2011." *Journal of Nuclear Medicine* 55 (May 2014): 1308–10.
Wieder, H. A., M. Lassmann, and M. S. Allen-Auerbach, et al. "Clinical Use of Bone-targeting Radiopharmaceuticals with Focus on Alpha-emitters." *World Journal of Radiology* 6 (July 2014): 480–85.

WEBSITES
American Cancer Society "Radiopharmaceuticals" http://cancer.org/treatment/treatmentsandsideeffects/treatmenttypes/radiation/radiationtherapyprinciples/radiation-therapy-principles-how-is-radiotherapy-given-radiopharmaceuticals (accessed September 23, 2014).

ORGANIZATIONS
American Cancer Society, 1599 Clifton Rd. NE, Atlanta, GA 30329-4251, (800) ACS-2345 http://www.cancer.org.

International Radiosurgery Support Association (IRSA), 3005 Hoffman Street, Harrisburg, PA 17110, (717) 260-9808 http://www.irsa.org.

Margaret Alic, PhD

REVISED BY L. LEE CULVERT

REVIEWED BY KEVIN GLAZA, RPH

Raloxifene

Definition

Raloxifene (Evista) is an oral medication classified as a selective estrogen receptor modulator or SERM. This classification means that its action on the estrogen receptor is different in various tissues, allowing it to selectively inhibit or stimulate estrogen-like action in different tissues of the body. It stimulates the action of estrogen on the bones, but blocks the effects of estrogen on breast and uterine tissues.

Purpose

Raloxifene is a hormone therapy drug that protects against bone loss (osteoporosis) in postmenopausal women. It was approved by the Food and Drug Administration (FDA) for the prevention of osteoporosis in postmenopausal women in 1997 and for the treatment of osteoporosis in postmenopausal women in 1999. In 2007, the FDA approved raloxifene as a treatment to reduce the risk of invasive **breast cancer** in postmenopausal women diagnosed with osteoporosis. As of 2014, however, raloxifene was *not* indicated for the treatment of invasive breast **cancer**. It cannot be used to prevent the recurrence of breast cancer in women who have already been treated for it, and it cannot be used to reduce the risk of noninvasive breast cancer.

Description

Raloxifene belongs to a family of compounds called selective estrogen receptor modulators or SERMs. It acts on estrogen receptors in different ways in various tissues, allowing it to selectively inhibit or stimulate estrogen-like action in different tissues of the body. Its antiestrogen activity can used in cancer therapy to inhibit the effects of estrogen on target tissues. Estrogen is a steroid hormone secreted by the granulosa cells of a maturing follicle within the female ovary. Depending on the target tissue, estrogen can stimulate the growth of female reproductive organs and breast tissue, play a role in the female menstrual cycle, and protect against bone loss by

---

KEY TERMS

Anticoagulant—An agent preventing the coagulation (clotting) of blood.

Estrogen receptors—A group of proteins found inside cells that are activated by the sex hormone estrogen.

Granulosa cells—Cells that form the wall of the ovarian follicle and produce various steroid hormones.

Indication—A valid reason for prescribing a certain medication.

Ovarian follicle—Several layers of cells that surround a maturing egg in the ovary.

Selective estrogen receptor modulator (SERM)—A drug that has estrogenic effects in some body tissues and antiestrogenic effects in other tissues.

Thromboembolism—A blood clot that blocks a blood vessel in the cardiovascular system.

---

binding to estrogen receptors on the outside of cells within the target tissue.

Raloxifene selectively inhibits the effects of estrogen on breast tissue and uterine tissue, while selectively mimicking the effects of estrogen on bone (by increasing bone mineral density). Its effects on breast and uterine tissue are thought to make raloxifene an excellent therapeutic agent against the risk of breast cancer and uterine cancer by depriving potential tumors of the estrogen they need to grow.

In its pure form, raloxifenc hydrochloride is a whitish or pale yellow solid that is only slightly soluble in water. It is presently available only in tablet form.

Recommended dosage

The standard dose of raloxifene for any of its indications is one 60 mg tablet by mouth daily, without regard to mealtimes or time of day, although patients should take it at the same time each day. Postmenopausal women prescribed raloxifene to reduce the risk of invasive breast cancer should take the drug at this 60 mg daily dosage for five years. If a dose is missed, patients should not double the next dose. Instead, they should go back to their regular schedule and contact their doctor.

Raloxifene should be kept at room temperature, tightly capped, away from children, and away from excess heat and moisture (thus it should not be stored in the bathroom).

Precautions

Women taking raloxifene should eat foods that are rich in calcium and vitamin D, or take calcium and vitamin supplements.

Although raloxifene is approved for use only by women past the childbearing years, researchers emphasize that it is not recommended for women who are pregnant or breastfeeding. In test animals, raloxifene caused birth defects and miscarriages. Although it is not known whether raloxifene is present in breast milk, it is possible that its presence may be toxic to infants. Further, this drug is not recommended for use in children. The effects of its use (if any) in men are unknown.

Patients at risk for the formation of deep venous thrombosis or pulmonary thromboembolisms should use raloxifene with caution. Those with past episodes of venous thrombosis should not use the drug at all. Women with coronary heart disease (CHD) are at increased risk of stroke if they take raloxifene, and others not presently diagnosed with CHD are at increased risk of developing it. Raloxifene can cause a higher risk of developing blood clots. In addition, women with kidney or liver disease should use raloxifene with caution. Patients should tell their doctor if they have ever smoked, have ever been treated for high blood pressure, have ever had a stroke or mini-stroke, or have ever been diagnosed with an irregular heartbeat.

Patients taking raloxifene should stop taking the drug and call their doctor *at once* if they notice any of the following symptoms: swelling of the hands, feet, ankles, or lower legs; sudden chest pain; shortness of breath; coughing up blood; loss of vision or blurred vision; sensations of warmth in the lower legs; or pain in the legs.

Side effects

Although raloxifene is usually well tolerated by patients, it also has side effects. Commonly reported side effects include mild nausea, vomiting, hot flashes, weight gain, **bone pain**, and hair thinning, which are not severe enough to stop therapy. Other side effects include leg cramps, flu-like symptoms, insomnia, joint pain, and heavy sweating.

Interactions

The usefulness of raloxifene can be diminished if patients also are on hormone replacement therapy (HRT) or such cholesterol-lowering cholestyramines as Questran. Cholestyramines decrease the absorption of raloxifene into the blood, while estrogen supplements increase the amount of estrogen competing with raloxifene for binding sites on target cells' estrogen receptors. Raloxifene also interacts with **diazepam** (Valium), lidocaine, colestipol, and diazoxide (Proglycem, used to treat low blood sugar). Patients should tell their doctor if they are taking any of these medications, or if they are likely to require local anesthesia for dental work or minor surgery.

Raloxifene interferes with the anticoagulant effect of **warfarin** with severe consequences and even death. Patients using warfarin should make sure their physician is aware prior to commencing treatment with raloxifene.

See also Toremifene.

Resources

BOOKS

Huang, Xianhai, and Robert G. Aslanian, eds. *Case Studies in Modern Drug Discovery and Development.* Hoboken, NJ: John Wiley and Sons, 2012.

Jordan, V. Craig, ed. *Estrogen Action, Selective Estrogen Receptor Modulators, and Women's Health: Progress and Promise.* Hackensack, NJ: World Scientific Publishing Co., 2013.

PERIODICALS

Gizzo, S., et al. "Update on Raloxifene: Mechanism of Action, Clinical Efficacy, Adverse Effects, and Contraindications." *Obstetrical and Gynecological Survey* 68 (June 2013): 467–481.

Komm, B. S., and S. Mirkin. "An Overview of Current and Emerging SERMs." *Journal of Steroid Biochemistry and Molecular Biology* 143C (September 2014): 207–222.

Moyer, C. A., and the USPSTF. "Medications to Decrease the Risk for Breast Cancer in Women: Recommendations from the U.S. Preventive Services Task Force Recommendation Statement." *Annals of Internal Medicine* 159 (November 19, 2013): 698–708.

Pinkerton, J. V., and S. Thomas. "Use of SERMs for Treatment in Postmenopausal Women." *Journal of Steroid Biochemistry and Molecular Biology* 142 (July 2014): 142–154.

Reimers, L., and K. D. Crew. "Tamoxifen vs Raloxifene vs Exemestane for Chemoprevention." *Current Breast Cancer Reports* 4 (September 1, 2012): 207–215.

Visvanathan, K., et al. "Use of Pharmacologic Interventions for Breast Cancer Risk Reduction: American Society of Clinical Oncology Clinical Practice Guideline." *Journal of Clinical Oncology* 31 (August 10, 2013): 2942–2962.

WEBSITES

Drugs.com. "Raloxifene Hydrochloride." http://www.drugs.com/monograph/raloxifene-hydrochloride.html (accessed September 23, 2014).

Food and Drug Administration (FDA) news release. "FDA Approves New Uses for Evista." http://www.fda.gov/

newevents/newsroom/pressannouncements/2007/ucm108981.htm (accessed September 23, 2014).

MedlinePlus. "Raloxifene." http://www.nlm.nih.gov/medlineplus/druginfo/meds/a698007.html (accessed September 23, 2014).

WebMD. "Raloxifene." http://www.webmd.com/osteoporosis/raloxifene-for-osteoporosis (accessed September 23, 2014).

ORGANIZATIONS

Food and Drug Administration (FDA), 10903 New Hampshire Avenue, Silver Spring, MD 20993, (888) INFO-FDA (463-6332), http://www.fda.gov/AboutFDA/ContactFDA/default.htm, http://www.fda.gov/default.htm.

Sally C. McFarlane-Parrott
Teresa G. Odle
REVISED BY REBECCA J. FREY, PhD

Ramucirumab

Definition

Ramucirumab (Cyramza) is a drug for treating stomach cancers, including gastroesophageal junction cancers—cancers at the junction of the stomach and esophagus—that are advanced or have spread to other parts of the body (metastasized). Ramucirumab is a type of targeted-therapy drug called a monoclonal antibody. It may also be referred to as an antiangiogenic agent, meaning that it helps prevent the tumor from forming its own blood vessels.

Purpose

The U.S. Food and Drug Administration (FDA) approved ramucirumab injection in 2014 to treat advanced or metastatic stomach and gastroesophageal junction adenocarinomas that have progressed during or following **chemotherapy** with fluoropyrimidine- or platinum-containing drugs. The approval was based on improved overall survival in a multinational clinical trial of 355 patients receiving either ramucirumab and "best supportive care" or a placebo and best supportive care. Median overall survival in the ramucirumab group was 5.2 months compared with 3.8 months for the placebo group. Median progression-free survival (PFS)—the period of survival without the **cancer** progressing—was also longer in the group receiving ramucirumab.

Ramucirumab is being studied in the treatment of other cancers. In 2014, it was shown in a large phase 3

clinical trial to significantly improve overall survival and PFS of metastatic **non-small cell lung cancer**.

Description

Ramucirumab is a monoclonal antibody produced in the laboratory. The antibody is fully "humanized," which means that the patient's immune system will not recognize and destroy it as foreign. Ramucirumab binds specifically to a receptor called vascular endothelial growth factor receptor-2 (VEGFR-2). By binding to VEGFR-2, ramucirumab prevents vascular endothelial growth factors (VEGFs) from binding to VEGFR-2 and activating the receptor to initiate angiogenesis—the formation of blood vessels that the tumor needs to grow and metastasize. VEGFR-2 is a receptor on the surface of endothelial cells (cells lining internal body cavities) that is required for the formation of new blood vessels. Inhibition of this receptor by ramucirumab results in a decrease in the tumor's nutrient supply and may slow or stop cancer growth.

U.S. brand names

Ramucirumab is made by Eli Lilly and Company and is marketed as Cyramza. It is also known as anti-VEGFR-2 fully humanized monoclonal antibody IMC-1121B.

Recommended dosage

Ramucirumab is administered by infusion into a vein (IV) over a period of about an hour. It is infused by a doctor or nurse in a hospital or medical facility, usually once every two weeks. The dosage is 8 milligrams (mg) per kg (2.2 lb.) of body weight. Before each infusion, patients are given an IV antihistamine such as **diphenhydramine** (Benadryl) to reduce the risk of an allergic reaction. Patients may also be given acetaminophen (Tylenol) and a corticosteroid such as **dexamethasone**, especially if they previously had a reaction to ramucirumab. The length of treatment depends on the patient's response to the drug and side effects.

Precautions

Ramucirumab injection has a boxed warning explaining that it may cause severe or life-threatening bleeding. Symptoms that require immediate medical attention include:

- any unusual bleeding or bruising
- coughing up or vomiting blood or material that looks like coffee grounds
- pink, red, or dark-brown urine
- red or tarry-black bowel movements

KEY TERMS

Adenocarcinomas—Cancers originating in glandular cells that line certain internal organs and release substances.

Angiogenesis—Blood vessel formation.

Antiangiogenic agent—A drug that inhibits angiogenesis.

Gastroesophageal junction—The connection between the esophagus (the muscular tube extending from the pharynx) and the stomach.

Humanizing—The process of replacing the animal portions of a protein, such as an antibody produced in an animal, with human portions so that the human immune system does not recognize the drug as foreign.

Metastasis—Cancer that has spread from its site of origin to other parts of the body.

Monoclonal antibody—Monospecific antibodies that recognize and bind to a specific protein; often used as targeted drugs.

Placebo—An inactive substance or preparation given to a control group in a clinical trial to test the effectiveness of the real medication or treatment; usually study participants do not know if they are receiving the drug or the placebo.

Progression-free survival (PFS)—The length of time patients survive without their cancer progressing; used in clinical trials to measure the effectiveness of a drug.

Receptor—A molecule, usually a protein, inside or on the surface of a cell that binds with a specific chemical group or molecule, such as a hormone or growth factor, to initiate a sequence of events.

Targeted therapy—A drug that interferes with a specific molecule involved in cancer cell growth and/or survival.

Vascular endothelial growth factors (VEGFs)—Factors that stimulate angiogenesis by binding to receptors on endothelial cells.

Vascular endothelial growth factor receptor-2; VEGFR-2—The receptor that binds vascular endothelial growth factors to initiate angiogenesis; the target of ramucirumab.

- nosebleeds
- unusual vaginal bleeding
- bleeding gums during tooth brushing

- lightheadedness

Ramucirumab can cause allergic infusion reactions in some people during or shortly after administration, especially with the first two treatments. Mild reactions are usually **fever** and chills. More serious reactions are less common but may be dangerous. Symptoms of a more serious reaction include:

- dizziness or lightheadedness from low blood pressure
- fainting
- headache
- feeling warm or flushed
- itching
- hives
- shortness of breath
- wheezing
- increased heart rate
- back or chest pain
- swelling of the face, tongue, or throat

Ramucirumab may also:

- affect fertility
- cause bleeding in the brain—a type of stroke
- cause or worsen high blood pressure (blood pressure is checked before and during treatment and may require medication to control it)
- increase the risk of problems from blood clots, including heart attack, stroke, mini-stroke (transient ischemic attack), blood clots in leg veins (deep venous thrombosis), and blood clots in the lungs (pulmonary embolism), even in patients taking blood thinners
- inhibit wound healing, so it should not be administered before surgery or until after a surgical wound has healed
- cause kidney damage (urine is checked for high protein levels before and during treatment)
- rarely, cause a hole (perforation) in the stomach or intestines
- rarely, cause a serious brain condition called reversible posterior leukoencephalopathy syndrome

Pediatric

The safety and effectiveness of ramucirumab in pediatric patients has not been established. Animal studies suggest that it would be harmful.

Geriatric

Clinical trials of ramucirumab did not include enough patients aged 65 and over to determine whether they respond differently than younger patients.

Pregnant or breastfeeding

Ramucirumab may affect the fetus if administered during pregnancy. Women who could become pregnant should use effective birth control during treatment and for at least three months after treatment is ended. Women should not breastfeed while receiving ramucirumab.

Other conditions and allergies

Patients should inform their doctors if they:

- are allergic to anything, including drugs, dyes, additives, or foods
- have ever had heart disease or a heart attack, stroke, transient ischemic attack, or blood clots in the legs or lungs
- have ever coughed up blood or had serious bleeding
- have ever had high blood pressure
- have any type of liver problem or disease, including hepatitis or cirrhosis, since ramucirumab can worsen liver function, leading to brain swelling or fluid buildup in the abdomen
- have any other medical conditions, such as kidney disease, congestive heart failure, diabetes, gout, or infections
- had any recent surgery or are planning surgery or any type of dental procedure

Side effects

Ramucirumab has no common side effects. Less common side effects are:

- high blood pressure
- diarrhea
- headache
- excess protein in the urine
- low blood sodium levels

    Rare side effects are:

- infusion reaction
- low white blood cell count with increased risk of infection
- low red blood cell count (anemia)
- nosebleeds
- skin rash
- intestinal blockage
- stroke, transient ischemic attack, or heart attack
- hole in the intestines (bowel perforation)
- bleeding in the lungs, brain, intestines, or other parts of the body
- death due to perforations or bleeding in the intestines, bleeding in the lungs or brain, stroke, heart attack, or other causes

Other conditions and allergies

Rarely, ramucirumab can slow the healing of a wound or surgical incision, or cause the reopening of a

---

QUESTIONS TO ASK YOUR DOCTOR

- Will any of my prescription or over-the-counter drugs interact with ramucirumab?
- What types of over-the-counter remedies should I avoid while on ramucirumab?
- May I drink alcohol while on ramucirumab?
- What side effects can I expect from ramucirumab?
- What symptoms require immediate medical attention?

---

healing wound. It can also worsen liver damage in patients with cirrhosis, although this is rare as well.

Interactions

As of 2014, ramucirumab was not known to directly interact with any drugs or foods. However, patients should tell their doctors about all prescription and over-the-counter medications, supplements, **vitamins**, and herbs that they are taking. Ramucirumab interferes with blood clotting and can increase the risk of bleeding. Therefore, it is very important that doctors are aware of any other drugs a patient may be taking that increase bleeding risk, including:

- nonsteroidal anti-inflammatory drugs (NSAIDs), such as aspirin, ibuprofen (Advil, Motrin), naproxen (Aleve, Naprosyn), and many others, including many cold, flu, fever, and headache remedies that contain aspirin or ibuprofen
- warfarin (Coumadin), dabigatran (Pradaxa), rivaroxaban (Xarelto), apixaban (Eliquis), or other blood thinners, and any type of heparin injections
- anti-platelet drugs, such as clopidogrel (Plavix) or prasugrel (Effient)
- vitamin E

Resources

OTHER

"Ramucirumab." American Cancer Society. April 23, 2014. http://www.cancer.org/acs/groups/cid/documents/webcontent/acspc-042589-pdf.pdf (accessed October 17, 2014).

WEBSITES

Berkrot, Bill. "Eli Lilly Drug Prolongs Survival in Large Lung Cancer Trial." Reuters. May 31, 2014. http://www.reuters.com/article/2014/05/31/us-health-cancer-lung-eli-lilly-idUSKBN0EB0CR20140531 (accessed October 17, 2014).

Pazdur, Richard. "FDA Approval for Ramucirumab." National Cancer Institute. April 30, 2014. http://www.cancer.gov/cancertopics/druginfo/fda-ramucirumab (accessed October 17, 2014).

"Ramucirumab Injection." MedlinePlus. June 15, 2014. http://www.nlm.nih.gov/medlineplus/druginfo/meds/a614026.html (accessed October 17, 2014).

ORGANIZATIONS

American Cancer Society, 250 Williams Street NW, Atlanta, GA 30303, (800) 227-2345, http://www.cancer.org.

National Cancer Institute, 6116 Executive Boulevard, Suite 300, Bethesda, MD 20892-8322, (800) 4-CANCER (422-6237), http://www.cancer.gov.

U.S. Food and Drug Administration, 10903 New Hampshire Avenue, Silver Spring, MD 20993-0002, (888) INFO-FDA (463-6332), http://www.fda.gov.

Margaret Alic, PhD

Ranitidine *see* **Histamine 2 antagonists**

Receptor analysis

Definition

Receptor analysis is a diagnostic test that determines an important biological characteristic of the cells in a tumor—their response to normal growth factors.

Purpose

The goal of receptor analysis is to reveal whether the **cancer** cells in a tumor have specific molecules, termed receptors, on the cell surface. A receptor is an area of the cell's membrane that is triggered to respond to the presence of a specific chemical (such as a hormone, growth factor, or neurotransmitter). Activation of a receptor by an appropriate chemical can prompt cellular growth, division, invasion of local tissue, or other cellular activities. Evaluating the presence of a receptor can give information about appropriate therapies to treat a particular cancer and can aid in tailoring treatment to a specific individual, as well as helping to predict prognosis. This test is routinely performed for **breast cancer** as well as other tumors.

Description

Cancer cells have unique characteristics that often vary from the corresponding normal cells in tissue and blood. In some respects, cancer treatment depends upon the differences in behavior between malignant (cancerous) cells and normal cells. For example, tumor cells

KEY TERMS

Antiestrogen—A drug, for example tamoxifen, that prevents the hormone estrogen from influencing the behavior of specific types of cells.

Biopsy—A piece of tissue removed for diagnostic examination.

HER2—Human epidermal growth factor receptor 2; a protein involved in cell growth that is found in some types of cancer cells. Patients with excess amounts of HER2 are believed to have worse prognoses.

Receptors—Molecules, usually found on the surface of a cell, that are required for cells to be influenced by hormones and other growth factors.

often grow faster than normal (noncancerous) cells. The changes that occur as normal cells become cancerous are progressive. As a tumor develops, the cells generally become less similar to normal cells and behave in a biologically different way. Some cancer treatments make use of the ways that cancer cells in a tumor can be like cells in the normal surrounding tissue.

One of the most fundamental ways in which the early stages of some cancers resemble healthy tissue is that the growth of the cells in the tumor responds to some of the same factors that control the growth of normal tissues. The most common example of this is the response of breast cancer cells to estrogen. During the normal menstrual cycle, the mammary glands respond to changes in the levels of two hormones, estrogen and progesterone. In many cases, the growth of breast cancer tumor cells also responds to the presence or absence of estrogen. The response of both normal and tumor cells to these hormones depends upon the presence of molecules termed estrogen and progesterone receptors. If cells in a breast tumor have these receptors, it is possible to inhibit the growth of the cancer cells by preventing estrogen from stimulating their growth. This prevention is generally accomplished through the use of antiestrogen drugs such as **tamoxifen**.

Receptor analysis usually involves a special technique called immunocytochemistry to examine a small piece of the tumor tissue. A tissue section (a slice of the tumor) is placed on a glass microscope slide. These tissue sections, which are very similar to those used in the initial diagnosis of the patient's breast cancer, are incubated with antibody preparations that will react with estrogen and progesterone receptors. Special reagents lead to a chemical reaction that produces a visible color in cells that have hormone receptors. A pathologist then looks at the section with a microscope to determine the percentage of tumor cells that are receptor-positive.

The information from the analysis can be used to decide whether a woman with breast cancer should be treated with antiestrogens. In addition, the presence of estrogen receptors helps doctors determine a patient's prognosis, or outlook. Tumors that have high levels of estrogen receptors are generally less aggressive. Taken together with information such as the patient's age, the size and grade of the tumor, and whether there is lymph node involvement, it is possible for a doctor to have some idea of the likelihood that the patient will remain disease-free after initial treatment.

For some time now, estrogen receptor analysis has been an important and generally accepted part of managing breast cancer. More recently, assays for other cell surface receptors have been explored and introduced for the management of breast and other cancers. Examples of these include androgen receptors in **prostate cancer** and epidermal growth factor receptor (EGFR) in a variety of cancers, including **non-small cell lung cancer**. Testing has also begun for a cell surface molecule designated HER2. Patients whose tumors express higher-than-normal amounts of HER2 are believed to have worse prognoses. However, these patients may be treated with a specific reagent, a monoclonal antibody, which is targeted toward the HER2 protein. Analysis for HER2 can be performed in a similar way to estrogen receptor immunocytochemical assays or by using a different type of test that directly examines the gene for HER2. Treatment with the monoclonal antibody to HER2 can improve the survival of patients who express higher-than-normal levels of HER2 in their tumor cells.

Precautions

Because this test is performed on a piece of tissue that has already been removed during a surgical or diagnostic procedure, it does not require any precautionary measures on behalf of the patient.

Risks

This test is performed on a piece of tissue that has been removed during the initial surgery or diagnostic procedure used to establish the nature of the tumor. It does not require any new surgery on the patient and does not entail any risk to the patient.

Results

Receptor assays measure molecules that play normal and essential roles in the natural function of various tissues. Abnormal results depend upon the particular tissue and the type of cancer involved. The presence of the appropriate

---

QUESTIONS TO ASK YOUR DOCTOR

- What fraction of the cells in my tumor have normal receptors?
- Do the results of the receptor assay on the biopsy of my tumor make me a candidate for antiestrogen treatment?
- How do the results of the receptor assays of my tumor influence your decision as to my treatment and prognosis?

---

receptor (for example, estrogen receptors in breast tumors) may be indicative that the cancer can be treated with compounds that can inhibit the growth of the cells that make up the tumor. In other cases, receptor assays may enable a doctor to know the origin of a tumor. That is, sometimes it is not possible for a pathologist to examine a **biopsy** and be certain what type of cancer a tumor represents. Knowing the identity of the receptors found on the tumor cells may then provide important information for establishing the diagnosis and best course of treatment for such patients. Certain proteins may trigger growth of a cancer or help to halt cancer cell growth, so finding receptors for these proteins also can improve cancer treatment. As doctors learn more, they can better target treatments specifically to these receptors, sparing normal cells.

Resources

BOOKS

Abeloff, M. D., et al. *Clinical Oncology*, 5th ed. New York: Churchill Livingstone, 2013.

Niederhuber, J. E., et al. *Clinical Oncology*, 5th ed. Philadelphia: Elsevier, 2014.

PERIODICALS

Nishimura, R., et al. "Usefulness of Liquid-Based Cytology in Hormone Receptor Analysis of Breast Cancer Specimens." *Virchows Archiv: An International Journal of Pathology* 458, no. 2 (2011): 153–58.

WEBSITES

Breastcancer.org. "How to Read Hormone Receptor Test Results." http://www.breastcancer.org/symptoms/diagnosis/hormone_status/read_results (accessed November 10, 2014).

Pruthi, Sandhya. "HER2-Positive Breast Cancer: What Is It?" Mayo Clinic. http://www.mayoclinic.org/breast-cancer/expert-answers/FAQ-20058066 (accessed November 10, 2014).

Warren Maltzman, PhD

REVISED BY TERESA G. ODLE
REVIEWED BY ROSALYN CARSON-DEWITT, MD

Reconstructive surgery

Definition

Reconstructive surgery is a type of plastic surgery performed to reshape abnormal structures of the body to improve function and appearance. Reconstructive surgery is different from cosmetic surgery, which is performed to reshape normal structures of the body to improve a patient's appearance and self-esteem.

Purpose

The goals of reconstructive surgery are to reshape abnormal structures of the body, to improve function, and/or to allow a person to have a more normal appearance. Abnormal structures of the body that are corrected during reconstructive surgery may be the result of birth defects, developmental abnormalities, trauma or injury, infection, tumors, or disease. The three most commonly performed reconstructive surgeries in the United States are tumor ablation (removal) and reconstruction; hand surgery; and **breast reconstruction**.

Description

The most commonly performed reconstructive surgeries of cancer patients are breast reconstruction, laceration repair, scar revision, and tumor removal.

Breast reconstruction

Breast reconstruction surgeries can be performed as part of the procedure to remove the breast (immediate **mastectomy**). They may also be performed as a separate procedure after recuperation from a mastectomy (delayed). There are two major types of breast reconstruction: autogenous free flap reconstruction and breast implants. Women may also choose to forgo breast reconstruction if they are concerned about the possibility of muscle weakness or have health problems that increase the difficulty of reconstructive procedures. As of 2014, about 20% of women who have had mastectomies choose not to undergo breast reconstruction.

An autologous free flap reconstruction uses tissue from another part of the patient's own body to form the reconstructed breast. This category of breast reconstruction includes the techniques called TRAM (transverse rectus abdominis myocutaneous); LD (latissimus dorsi); VRAM (vertical rectus abdominis myocutaneous); and DIEP (deep inferior epigastric perforator) flaps. These names refer to the location from which the tissue for reconstruction is taken. TRAM, in which tissue is taken from the abdominal region, is the most common breast reconstruction procedure in the United States, but DIEP

KEY TERMS

Autologous—Referring to tissue transplanted from one part of the body to another within the same person.

Cosmetic surgery—A form of plastic surgery performed to alter normal tissue to improve the appearance of that tissue.

Flap surgery—A procedure in which a portion of living tissue is moved from one part of a patient's body to another to restore shape and/or function to the targeted location.

Mohs surgery—A form of microscopically controlled surgery that allows for the precise removal of cancerous tissue. It is commonly used to treat various types of skin cancer, particularly in areas of the body where preserving as much tissue as possible is essential. Mohs surgery is also known as micrographic surgery.

Plastic surgery—A type of surgery that is performed to alter the physical characteristics of a patient. This medical discipline is subdivided into cosmetic surgery and reconstructive surgery.

Reconstructive surgery—A form of plastic surgery that is performed to repair or reshape abnormally formed tissue to improve the form and/or function of that tissue.

Scar revision—A surgical procedure that attempts to diminish the physical appearance of a scar. This procedure is also used to add flexibility and range of motion to joints and muscles that were previously restricted by a particular scar.

Z-plasty—A technique used in plastic surgery to elongate a scar as part of scar revision surgery. The name comes from the Z shape of the incision made by the surgeon.

---

is preferred when the reconstruction involves both breasts. Newer options for flap reconstructions include the GAP (gluteal artery perforator) flap, in which tissue is taken from the buttocks area; and the TUG (transverse upper gracilis) flap, in which the graft tissue is removed from the upper portion of the inner thigh. As of 2014, however, the GAP and TUG flap procedures are not available everywhere in North America.

The surgeon may use one of several techniques to create a nipple and areola (the pinkish or dark area around the nipple) on the reconstructed breast. One option is to harvest portions of the nipple and areola from the healthy breast and graft it to the reconstructed breast. A second option is to create a flap in the reconstructed breast to produce a raised area of skin, create an areola with a circular incision that is then resutured, and then tattoo the new nipple and areola to match the patient's other breast.

Breast implants involve the placement of an artificial object in the body to simulate the shape and size of the natural breast. The implant is most commonly a saline (salt water) or silicone-filled bag. Because of the health problems reported by many women after silicone breast implants, this technique is no longer as widespread as it once was, particularly for reconstructive surgeries. A newer type of breast implant, called a form-stable implant, contains a thicker gel known as cohesive gel. Unlike the older silicone implants, form-stable implants will not lose their shape or leak if accidentally cut. The U.S. Food and Drug Administration (FDA) approved these implants for use in the United States in 2013. Other alternative types of breast implants are in **clinical trials** as of 2014.

A technique that is still in the experimental stage is fat grafting, which seeks to use a relatively small amount of the patient's own adipose (fatty) tissue taken from the thighs, abdomen, or buttocks by liposuction to create a larger volume of material that can be used to reconstruct the breast. As of 2014 one of the limitations on fat grafting is the need to use fairly large amounts of adipose tissue from the patient's body. In addition, no large-scale studies of the technique have been done to date, and one of the risks of the procedure is that the grafted fat may be reabsorbed by the body, and the reconstructed breast may lose some of its volume.

Breast reconstruction usually involves more than one operation; in fact the average number of secondary procedures required is four for reconstruction of one breast and more than five for reconstruction of both breasts. The factors that complicate breast reconstruction include delaying the reconstruction after the mastectomy; the need for **radiation therapy**; and the presence of other risk factors affecting the patient's health.

Laceration repair

Laceration repair includes the repair of large wounds caused by the removal of large tumors or tumors associated with the skin. It also includes the surgical repair of wounds that fail to heal or heal improperly. Laceration repair can be subdivided into four general categories: direct closure, skin grafts, tissue expansion, and flap surgery.

Direct closure (stitches) is usually only performed on wounds that are not very deep beneath the surface of the skin and that have straight edges of skin on either side of the wound. The primary goal in direct closure is to provide a permanent closure of the wound with a minimum of scarring.

Skin grafts are used for wounds that are wide and difficult or impossible to close directly. This technique involves removing healthy skin from a location on the patient (the donor site) and using it to cover the wound site. The skin will grow back at the donor site but often leaves a color mismatch. The donor site is chosen to best match the color of the skin needed in the graft area.

Tissue expansion is used to grow extra skin by stretching skin near the site that will require the skin. A small inflatable balloon is placed under the skin next to the area where the skin will be removed. Over time, this balloon is slowly filled with salt water until the skin has grown to the required size. The surgical procedure that involves the loss of skin is then performed and closed with the extra skin that was formed during the tissue expansion process. The major advantage associated with tissue expansion is that skin grown in this way remains connected to its original blood and nerve supply, so the risk of loss of sensation in the area of the wound is greatly diminished. Also, the scars that result from tissue expansion are generally less noticeable than those from skin grafts or skin flaps. A final advantage of this method is the near-perfect match in color provided by this skin.

Flap surgery involves taking a section of living tissue, with its blood supply, from one part of the patient and moving it to the area where it is needed. In most flap surgeries, one end of the flap remains attached to its original blood supply so that it continues to be nourished as it grows to heal the wound. In cases where the flap is completely removed and transplanted to another part of the body, the surgery involves the reconnection of all the tiny blood vessels of the flap tissue to the blood vessels of the new location (microsurgery). Flap surgery has the advantage of being able to restore both form and function to areas of the body that have lost skin, fat, muscle, and/or skeletal support. The most commonly performed flap surgeries are the autologous breast reconstructions discussed above. This procedure is used elsewhere on the body with considerable success.

Scar revisions

Many cancer patients have scarring that results from their particular form of cancer or from the number or severity of surgical procedures or radiation that they have undergone. In some of these cases, surgeries to minimize or reshape the scar(s) may be undertaken. Most physicians will recommend that a scar be allowed to heal for at least one year prior to a recommendation of scar revision. This timetable may be shortened in extreme cases of loss of mobility, increased sensitivity, or inflamed and irritable scars that do not respond to topical steroid creams.

Scar revision surgery is considered by most insurance companies to be a cosmetic surgery that is not covered as an insurance benefit. The most common reason for scar revision to be classified as a reconstructive rather than a cosmetic procedure is a loss of mobility of muscles or joints caused by the scar.

The most common procedure for scar revision is called Z-plasty. In this procedure, the old scar is removed and the two sides of the wound are cut into a z-shape that is designed to follow the natural lines and contours of the surrounding skin. This z-shaped wound is then closed with stitches. Other scar revision procedures include skin grafts and flap surgeries.

Tumor removal

The surgical procedure used to remove a tumor will be chosen by the surgeon based on the type and size of the tumor. Other factors influencing the surgical technique chosen for tumor removal include: the location of the tumor within the body; the potential for recurrence of the tumor at this, or another, location in the body; and, the stage of development of both the tumor itself and the underlying cancer.

Skin cancers are generally removed by excision of the cancerous portion of skin, with the wound closed by stitches or left to heal on its own. In cases of large or spreading skin cancers, major surgery involving skin grafts or flap surgeries may be required. For skin cancers in the facial area, **Mohs surgery** with primary or flap closure may be performed.

Precautions

Reconstructive surgery should not be performed on patients who are not healthy enough to withstand a surgical procedure performed under general anesthetic. People with severe diabetes, an autoimmune disorder such as AIDS, or a suppressed immune system should not undergo reconstructive surgery. This type of surgery is also contraindicated in patients with a history of excessive smoking, obesity, poor wound healing, abnormal scarring, and/or a bleeding disorder. Women who are pregnant should not undergo reconstructive surgeries.

Patients who have received recent radiation treatments for **cancer** (generally within the last three to six months) should not undergo surgical procedures involving these tissues. Recently irradiated tissue is highly prone to infection and has poorer wound healing.

In some cases, it is necessary after **tumor removal** to monitor the affected tissue for redevelopment of the tumor. Patients requiring this type of postoperative surveillance should not undergo further reconstructive surgeries because these procedures could obscure the results of imaging techniques (x-ray, **computed tomography**, or **magnetic resonance imaging**) used to monitor tumor recurrence.

Patients with an allergy to collagen, beef, or beef products should not receive collagen injections.

Preparation

The preparation for a reconstructive surgery depends on the type of surgery that is to be performed. Some reconstructive surgeries can be performed on an outpatient basis. These procedures require only a local anesthetic and very little patient preparation other than counseling about the risks, possible achievable outcomes, and alternatives to the surgery. Other reconstructive surgeries are considered major operations. These require hospitalization, a general anesthetic, and much more extensive counseling and discussion of possible alternatives.

Prescription medications that may interfere with the performance of reconstructive surgery should be discontinued approximately two weeks prior to surgery, unless the surgeon advises otherwise. These medications include any medicines that may interfere with the anesthetic or that may increase bleeding. Such over-the-counter medications as aspirin and **nonsteroidal anti-inflammatory drugs** (NSAIDs) should not be taken for at least one week prior to surgery unless approved by the doctor who will be performing the surgery. Patients undergoing surgeries that require a general anesthetic will be asked not to eat after midnight prior to the surgery and not to drink at least eight hours prior to surgery. The purpose of this precaution is to ensure that the stomach is empty while the patient is unconscious. Otherwise, the stomach contents could be inhaled into the lungs, causing complications with the surgery or the recovery.

For procedures involving skin flaps, the patient may be asked to donate blood for possible use in a later transfusion.

In the case of tissue expansion procedures, the amount of time that will be required for the expansion of the tissue depends on the amount of tissue that must be grown to ensure an adequate closure of the wound. This process may take a matter of days or several weeks.

Psychological and emotional preparation is important in reconstructive surgery to manage patient expectations. The patient should not expect cosmetically perfect results. Complete understanding of the limitations, as well as the benefits, of this surgery is necessary for a successful outcome.

Aftercare

The aftercare of a patient who has undergone a reconstructive surgery depends on the surgery, the overall health of the patient, and the wound care process. Some outpatient procedures require little aftercare other than a follow-up examination to determine the success of the procedure. Other procedures may require an extended hospitalization followed by extensive **physical therapy**. Smoking should be avoided, as it can cause delayed wound healing and higher risk of complications, including infection.

Women who have had breast reconstruction surgery should avoid overhead lifting, strenuous athletic activity, and some types of sexual activity for four to six weeks after surgery. Women who have had breast implants are recommended to have periodic MRIs every two to three years after surgery to make sure the implant is not leaking, and they will also need to inform the doctor and technician whenever they have a mammogram.

Procedures involving skin flaps or grafts require careful monitoring in the first days after surgery to ensure that proper blood circulation is taking place. Bandages and drainage tubes will remain in place for at least a day.

Scars may remain reddened and raised for a month or longer and may cause **itching**. Many people find that inflammation or severe itching from postsurgical scars is lessened or completely eliminated by topical treatments with vitamin E or steroidal creams.

After tumor removal, many patients require follow-up treatments and medical imaging to ensure that the tumor has not recurred.

Risks

The risks associated with all reconstructive surgeries are infection, bleeding, an unsightly scar, improper wound closure, and adverse reactions to anesthesia. Complications associated with flap reconstruction of the breasts include tissue necrosis (death of the transplanted tissue), unusual firmness of the fatty tissue (fat necrosis), partial flap loss, fluid collection beneath the flap site, and muscle weakness (including abdominal hernias) at the donor site. For breast implants, complications include the formation of fibrous tissue around an implant, rupture or leakage of the implant, or movement of the implant from its intended location.

Results

The normal result of a reconstructive surgery is an improved ability to function and/or an improved **body image** as a result of the surgery. A normal result also depends on the patient's realistic goals and expectations. The patient should understand that the feeling and appearance of the reconstructed area will be improved but not fully restored to its unaffected state.

QUESTIONS TO ASK YOUR DOCTOR

- What are the alternatives to this surgical procedure?
- What will the scars look like, and can I expect them to decrease over time?
- How many reconstructions have you performed previously?
- Will this procedure be covered by my insurance?
- How long will the preoperative waiting period, the hospital stay, and the recovery period take?

Abnormal results

An abnormal result of reconstructive surgery is a major infection or other long-lasting health complication as a result of the surgery. Another abnormal result is a degradation in the ability to function and/or a loss of self-confidence caused by the loss of sensation or scarring that may accompany such procedures.

See also Breast cancer.

Resources

BOOKS

Bristow, Robert E., and Dennis S. Chi, eds. *Radical and Reconstructive Gynecologic Cancer Surgery.* New York: McGraw-Hill Education Medical, 2015.

Genden, Eric M., ed. *Head and Neck Surgery: Reconstructive Surgery.* Philadelphia, PA: Wolters Kluwer Health, 2014.

Serletti, Joseph M., ed. *Current Reconstructive Surgery.* New York: McGraw-Hill Medical, 2013.

Steligo, Kathy. *The Breast Reconstruction Guidebook: Issues and Answers from Research to Recovery*, 3rd ed. Baltimore, MD: Johns Hopkins University Press, 2012.

PERIODICALS

Albornoz, C.R., et al. "Diminishing Relative Contraindications for Immediate Breast Reconstruction: A Multicenter Study." *Journal of the American College of Surgeons* 219, no. 4 (2014): 788–95.

Berbers, J., et al. "'Reconstruction: Before or After Postmastectomy Radiotherapy?' A Systematic Review of the Literature." *European Journal of Cancer* 50, no. 6 (2014): 2752–62.

Buchel, E.W., K.R. Dalke, and T.E. Hayakawa. "The Transverse Upper Gracilis Flap: Efficiencies and Design Tips." *Canadian Journal of Plastic Surgery* 21 (Fall 2013): 162–166.

Fischer, J.P., et al. "Mastectomy with or without Immediate Implant Reconstruction Has Similar 30-Day Perioperative Outcomes." *Journal of Plastic, Reconstructive & Aesthetic Surgery* 67, no. 11 (2014): 1515–22.

Grosfeld, E.C., et al. "Facial Reconstruction Following Mohs Micrographic Surgery: A Report of 622 Cases." *Journal of Cutaneous Medicine and Surgery* 18 (July–August 2014): 265–270.

Largo, R.D., et al. "Efficacy, Safety and Complications of Autologous Fat Grafting to Healthy Breast Tissue: A Systematic Review." *Journal of Plastic, Reconstructive, and Aesthetic Surgery* 67 (April 2014): 437–448.

Sbitany, H., et al. "Immediate Implant-Based Breast Reconstruction Following Total Skin-Sparing Mastectomy: Defining the Risk of Preoperative and Postoperative Radiation Therapy for Surgical Outcomes." *Plastic and Reconstructive Surgery* 134 (September 2014): 396–404.

Tsoi, B., et al. "Safety of Tissue Expander/Implant Versus Autologous Abdominal Tissue Breast Reconstruction in Postmastectomy Breast Cancer Patients: A Systematic Review and Meta-analysis." *Plastic and Reconstructive Surgery* 133 (February 2014): 234–249.

OTHER

American Cancer Society (ACS). "Breast Reconstruction After Mastectomy." http://www.cancer.org/acs/groups/cid/documents/webcontent/002992-pdf.pdf (accessed September 6, 2014).

WEBSITES

American Society of Plastic Surgeons (ASPS). "Reconstructive Procedures." http://www.plasticsurgery.org/reconstructive-procedures.html (accessed September 7, 2014).

BreastCancer.org. "Breast Reconstruction." http://www.breastcancer.org/treatment/surgery/reconstruction (accessed September 6, 2014).

BreastCancer.org. "Reconstruction Options: A Comparison Chart." http://www.breastcancer.org/treatment/surgery/reconstruction/types/comparison-chart (accessed September 6, 2014).

WebMD. "Reconstructive Surgery." http://www.webmd.com/a-to-z-guides/reconstructive-surgery (accessed September 6, 2014).

ORGANIZATIONS

American Academy of Facial Plastic and Reconstructive Surgery (AAFPRS), 310 South Henry Street, Alexandria, VA 22314, (703) 299-9291, Fax: (703) 299-8898, info@aafprs.org, http://www.aafprs.org/.

American Cancer Society (ACS), 250 Williams Street NW, Atlanta, GA 30303, (800) 227-2345, http://www.cancer.org.

American Society of Plastic Surgeons, 444 E. Algonquin Rd., Arlington Heights, IL 60005, (847) 228-9900, (800) 514-5058, memserv@plasticsurgery.org, http://www.plastic-surgery.org.

Paul A. Johnson, EdM
Rebecca J. Frey, PhD

Rectal cancer

Definition

The rectum is the portion of the large bowel that lies in the pelvis and terminates at the anus. **Cancer** of the rectum is the disease characterized by the development of malignant cells in the lining or epithelium of the rectum. Malignant cells have changed such that they lose normal control mechanisms governing growth. These cells may invade surrounding local tissue or they may spread throughout the body and invade other organ systems.

Description

The rectum is the continuation of the colon (part of the large bowel) after it leaves the abdomen and descends into the pelvis. It is about 4.7 inches long in adult humans and is divided into equal thirds: the upper, middle, and lower rectum.

The pelvis and other organs in the pelvis form boundaries to the rectum. Behind, or posterior to, the rectum is the sacrum (the lowest portion of the spine, closest to the pelvis). Laterally, on the sides, the rectum is bounded by soft tissue and bone. In front, the rectum is bounded by different organs in the male and female. In the male, the bladder and prostate are present; in the female, the vagina, uterus, and ovaries are present.

The upper rectum receives its blood supply from branches of the inferior mesenteric artery from the abdomen. The lower rectum has blood vessels entering from the sides of the pelvis. Lymph, a protein-rich fluid that bathes the cells of the body, is transported in small channels known as lymphatics. These channels run alongside the blood supply of the rectum. Lymph nodes are small filters through which the lymph flows on its way back to the bloodstream. Cancer spreads elsewhere in the body by invading the lymph and vascular systems.

When a cell or cells lining the rectum become malignant, they first grow locally and may invade partially or totally through the wall of the rectum. The tumor here may invade surrounding tissue or the organs nearby, a process known as local invasion. In this process, the tumor penetrates and may invade the lymphatics or the capillaries locally and gain access to the circulation in this way. As the malignant cells work their way to other areas of the body, they again become locally invasive in the new area to which they have spread. These tumor deposits, originating from the primary tumor in the rectum, are then known as metastases. If metastases are found in the regional lymph nodes, they are known as regional metastases. If they are distant from the primary tumor, they are known as distant

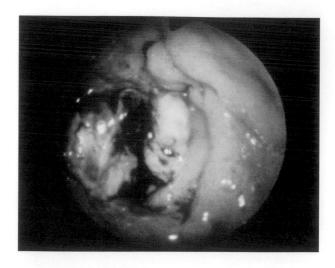

Rectal cancer seen through an endoscope. *(Benjamin/ Custom Medical Stock Photo)*

metastases. The patient with distant metastases may have widespread disease, also referred to as systemic disease. The cancer originating in the rectum begins locally but, given time, may become systemic.

By the time the primary tumor is originally detected, it is usually larger than one centimeter (about 3/8 inch) in size and has over one million cells. This amount of growth is estimated to take about three to seven years. Each time the cells double in number, the size of the tumor quadruples. Thus, like most cancers, the part that is identified clinically is later in the progression than would be desired. Screening becomes a very important step in earlier detection of this disease.

Passage of red blood with the stool (noticeable bleeding with defecation) is much more common in rectal cancer than that originating in the colon because the tumor is much closer to the anus. Other symptoms (constipation and/or **diarrhea**) are caused by obstruction and, less often, by local invasion of the tumor into pelvic organs or the sacrum. When the tumor has spread to distant sites, these metastases may cause dysfunction of the organ they have invaded. Distant **metastasis** usually occurs in the liver, less often in the lung(s), and rarely in the brain.

Demographics

The **National Cancer Institute** (NCI) projected that about 40,000 cases of rectal cancer would be diagnosed in the United States in 2014. Worldwide, about 1.2 million cases are diagnosed each year, with 608,000 deaths. Together, colon and rectal cancers account for 10% of cancers in men and 11% of cancers in women in developed countries. It is the second most common site-specific cancer affecting both men and women.

Approximately 50,300 people died from colon and rectal cancer in the United States in 2014. In recent years the incidence of this disease has decreased very slightly, and the mortality rate has also dropped, partly as a result of more effective screening and partly as a result of more effective treatments. As of 2014, African Americans have higher rates of rectal cancer than members of other ethnic and racial groups; the reason for this difference is not yet completely understood.

Cancer of the rectum is thought to arise sporadically in about 80% of those who develop the disease. About 20% of cases probably arise from genetic predisposition; some people have a family history of rectal cancer occurring in a first-degree relative. Development of rectal cancer at an early age suggests a genetically transmitted form of the disease as opposed to the sporadic form.

Causes and symptoms

Causes of rectal cancer are probably environmental in sporadic cases (80%), and genetic in the heredity-predisposed (20%) cases. Since malignant cells have a changed genetic makeup, this means that in 80% of cases, the environment spontaneously induces change. Those born with a genetic predisposition are either destined to develop the cancer, or it will take less environmental exposure to induce the cancer. Exposure to agents in the environment that may induce mutation is the process of **carcinogenesis** and is caused by agents known as **carcinogens**. Specific carcinogens have been difficult to identify; however, dietary factors seem to be involved.

Rectal cancer is more common in industrialized nations. Dietary factors may be the reason. Diets high in fat, red meat or processed meat (hot dogs, luncheon meat), total calories, and alcohol seem to increase the risk. Diets high in fiber are associated with a decreased risk. High-fiber diets may be related to less exposure of the rectal epithelium to carcinogens from the environment, as the transit time through the bowel is faster with a high-fiber diet than with a low-fiber diet.

Age plays a definite role in rectal cancer risk. Rectal cancer is rare before age 40. This incidence increases substantially after age 50 and doubles with each succeeding decade; 90% of people diagnosed with rectal cancer are above age 50. There is also a slight increase of risk for rectal cancer in smokers.

Patients who suffer from an inflammatory disease of the colon known as ulcerative colitis are also at increased risk, as are people with type 2 diabetes and women with a personal history of breast, ovarian, or **endometrial cancer**.

KEY TERMS

Adenocarcinoma—Cancer beginning in epithelial cells that line certain organs and have secretory properties.

Adjuvant therapy—Treatment involving radiation, chemotherapy (drug treatment), hormone therapy, or a combination of all three given after the primary treatment for the possibility of residual microscopic disease.

Anastomosis—Surgical reconnection of the ends of the bowel after removal of a portion of the bowel.

Anemia—Condition caused by too few circulating red blood cells, often manifested in part by fatigue.

Carcinogens—Substances in the environment that cause cancer with prolonged exposure, presumably by inducing mutations.

Defecation—The act of having a bowel movement.

Epithelium—A type of tissue that forms the surface or the lining of body structures.

Lymph nodes—Cellular filters through which lymph flows.

Lymphatics—Channels that are conduits for lymph.

Malignant—Cancerous; referring to cells that have been altered such that they have lost normal control

mechanisms and are capable of local invasion and spreading to other areas of the body.

Metastasis (plural, metastases)—Site of invasive tumor growth that originated from a malignancy elsewhere in the body.

Mutation—A change in the genetic makeup of a cell that may occur spontaneously or be environmentally induced.

Occult blood—Presence of blood that cannot be detected visually.

Polyps—Localized growths of the epithelium that can be benign, precancerous, or malignant.

Resect—To remove surgically.

Sacrum—The posterior bony wall of the pelvis.

Systemic—Referring to a disease that spreads throughout the body.

Targeted therapy—In cancer treatment, a type of drug therapy that blocks tumors by interfering with specific molecules that the cancer cells need for growth. Also called biologic therapy, targeted therapy is less harmful to normal cells than traditional chemotherapy.

Genes that have been linked to rectal cancer include the *APC, PTEN, BRAF, KRAS, MSH2*, and *MLH1* genes. On chromosome 5 is the *APC* gene, associated with familial adenomatous polyposis (FAP) syndrome. There are multiple mutations that occur at this site, yet they all cause a defect in tumor suppression that results in early and frequent development of **colon cancer**. This gene is transmitted to 50% of offspring and each of those affected will develop colon or rectal cancer, usually at an early age. Persons of Ashkenazi Jewish heritage are at increased risk of rectal cancer due to mutations in the *APC* gene.

Another syndrome, hereditary nonpolyposis colon cancer (HNPCC), is related to mutations in any of four genes responsible for DNA mismatch repair. In patients with colon or rectal cancer, the *TP53* gene is mutated 70% of the time. When the *TP53* gene is mutated and ineffective, cells with damaged DNA escape repair or destruction, allowing the damaged cells to multiply. Continued replication of the damaged DNA may lead to tumor development. Though these syndromes (FAP and HNPCC) have a very high incidence of colon or rectal cancer, family history without the syndromes is also a

substantial risk factor. When considering first-degree relatives, a history of one close relative with colon or rectal cancer raises the baseline risk from 2% to 6%, and the presence of a second close relative raises the risk to 17%.

The development of polyps of the colon or rectum commonly precedes the development of rectal cancer. Polyps are growths of the rectal lining. They can be unrelated to cancer, precancerous, or malignant. Polyps, when identified, are removed for diagnosis. If the polyp or polyps are benign, the patient should undergo careful surveillance for the development of more polyps or the development of colon or rectal cancer.

Symptoms of rectal cancer most often result from the local presence of the tumor and its capacity to invade surrounding pelvic structures:

- bright red blood present with stool
- abdominal distention (stretching from internal pressure), bloating, inability to have a bowel movement
- narrowing of the stool, so-called ribbon stools
- pelvic pain

- unexplained weight loss
- persistent chronic fatigue
- rarely, urinary infection or passage of air in urine in males (late symptom)
- rarely, passage of feces through the vagina in females (late symptom)

If the tumor is large and obstructing the rectum, the patient will not be evacuating stool normally and will feel bloated and have abdominal discomfort. The tumor itself may bleed, and, because it is near the anus, the patient may see bright red blood on the surface of the stool. Blood alone (without stool) may also be passed. Thus hemorrhoids are often incorrectly blamed for bleeding, delaying the diagnosis. If **anemia** develops, which is rare, the patient will experience chronic **fatigue**. If the tumor invades the bladder in the male or the vagina in the female, stool will accumulate where it doesn't belong and cause infection or discharge. (This condition is also rare.) Patients with widespread disease lose weight secondary to the chronic illness.

Diagnosis

Screening evaluation of the colon and rectum are accomplished together. Screening involves a physical exam, simple laboratory tests, and the visualization of the lining of the rectum and colon. **X-rays** (indirect visualization) and endoscopy (direct visualization) are used to visualize the organs' lining.

The physical examination involves the performance of a digital rectal exam (DRE). At the time of this exam, the physician checks the stool on the examining glove with a chemical to see whether any occult (invisible) blood is present. At home, after having a bowel movement, the patient is asked to swipe a sample of stool obtained with a small stick on a card. After three such specimens are placed on the card, the card is then chemically tested for occult blood. These exams are accomplished as an easy part of a routine yearly physical exam.

Proteins are sometimes produced by cancers and these may be elevated in the patient's blood. When this elevation occurs, the protein produced is known as a tumor marker. There is a tumor marker for cancer of the colon and rectum known as carcinoembryonic antigen (CEA). Unfortunately, this marker may be produced by other adenocarcinomas, or it may not be produced by a particular colon or rectal cancer. Therefore, screening by chemical analysis for CEA has not been helpful. CEA has been helpful in patients treated for colon or rectal cancer if their tumor makes the protein. It is used in a follow-up rather than a screening role. Another tumor marker sometimes found in patients with rectal cancer is CA-19.

Direct visualization of the lining of the rectum is accomplished using a scope or endoscope. The physician introduces the instrument into the rectum and is able to see the epithelium of the rectum directly. A simple rigid tubular scope may be used to see the rectal epithelium; however, screening of the colon is done at the same time. The lower colon may be visualized using a fiberoptic flexible scope in a procedure known as flexible **sigmoidoscopy**. When the entire colon is visualized, the procedure is known as total **colonoscopy**. Each type of endoscopy requires pre-procedure preparation (evacuation) of the rectum and colon.

The American Cancer Society has recommended the following screening protocol for colon and rectal cancers for people over age 50:

- yearly fecal occult blood test
- flexible sigmoidoscopy at age 50
- flexible sigmoidoscopy repeated every 5 years
- double-contrast barium enema every five years
- colonoscopy every 10 years

If the patient has such predisposing factors as a positive family history, history of polyps, or a familial syndrome, screening evaluations should start sooner—at age 40 or 10 years before the youngest case in the immediate family, whichever is earlier. African Americans should start having screening evaluations at age 45.

Evaluation of patients with symptoms

When patients visit their physician because they are experiencing symptoms that could possibly be related to colon or rectal cancer, the entire colon and rectum must be visualized. Even if a rectal lesion is identified, the entire colon must be screened to rule out a syndromic polyp or cancer of the colon. The combination of a flexible sigmoidoscopy and double-contrast **barium enema** may be performed, but the much-preferred evaluation of the entire colon and rectum is that of complete colonoscopy. Colonoscopy allows direct visualization, photography, as well as the opportunity to obtain a **biopsy** (a sample of tissue) of any abnormality visualized. If, for technical reasons, the entire colon is not visualized endoscopically, a double-contrast barium enema should complement the colonoscopy. A patient who is identified as having a problem in one area of the colon or rectum is at greater risk of having a similar problem in another area of the colon or rectum. Therefore, the entire colon and rectum need to be visualized during the evaluation.

Colorectal cancer screening guidelines for adults over 50

Type of exam*	Occurrence
Fecal immunochemical test	Annually
Fecal occult blood test	Annually
Flexible sigmoidoscopy	Every 5 years
Double-contrast barium enema	Every 5 years
Virtual colonoscopy	Every 5 years
Colonoscopy	Every 10 years

*Not all of these tests are needed. Patients should talk to their physicians about which tests are right for them.

SOURCE: American Cancer Society, "American Cancer Society Guidelines for the Early Detection of Cancer." http://www.cancer.org/healthy/findcancerearly/cancerscreeningguidelines/american-cancer-society-guidelines-for-the-early-detection-of-cancer.

Table listing colorectal cancer screening guidelines for adults over 50. *(Illustration by PreMediaGlobal. © Cengage Learning®.)*

The diagnosis of rectal cancer is actually made by the performance of a biopsy of any abnormal lesion in the rectum. In some cases the tissue sample may be tested for mutations in the *BRAF* or *KRAS* genes, as patients with mutations in either of these genes do not benefit from targeted therapy (described below). Many rectal cancers are within reach of the examiner's finger. Identifying how close to the anus the cancer has developed is important in planning the treatment. Another characteristic ascertained by exam is whether the tumor is mobile or fixed to any surrounding structure. Again, this feature will have implications related to primary treatment. As a general rule, it is easier to identify and adequately obtain tissue for evaluation in the rectum as opposed to the colon. This is because the lesion is closer to the anus.

If the patient has advanced disease, areas where the tumor has spread, such as the liver, may require biopsy. Such biopsies are usually obtained using a special needle under local anesthesia.

Once a diagnosis of rectal cancer has been established by biopsy, in addition to the physical exam, an **endorectal ultrasound** will be performed to assess the extent of the disease. For rectal cancer, endorectal ultrasound is the preferred method for staging both depth of tumor penetration and local lymph node status. An endorectal ultrasound:

- differentiates areas of invasion within large rectal adenomas that may appear benign
- determines the depth of tumor penetration into the rectal wall
- determines the extent of regional lymph node invasion, thereby determining the metastatic status

- can be combined with other tests (chest x-rays and computed tomography scans, or CT scans) to determine the extent of cancer spread to such distant organs as the liver and/or the lungs

The resulting rectal cancer staging allows physicians to determine the need for— and order of— radiation, surgery, and **chemotherapy**. An MRI may help physicians determine whether a tumor can be resected (removed surgically) and the risk of cancer recurrence.

Treatment team

Surgery, radiation treatment, and chemotherapy are used in the therapy of cancer of the rectum. The extent of the primary tumor dictates whether surgery or radiation will be utilized first. When surgery is the primary local therapy, radiation often has an adjunctive role in helping to prevent local recurrence. Chemotherapy may also be used as an adjunct to decrease recurrence and improve overall survival. Thus, teamwork is required utilizing the skills of the surgeon and the radiation and medical oncologists.

Clinical staging

Once the diagnosis has been confirmed by biopsy and the endorectal ultrasound has been performed, the clinical stage of the cancer is assigned. The treating physicians use staging to plan the specific treatment protocol for the patient. In addition, the stage of the cancer at the time of presentation gives a statistical likelihood of the treatment outcome (prognosis).

Rectal cancer first invades locally and then progresses to regional lymph nodes or to other organs. The stage is derived from: the characteristics of the primary tumor; its depth of penetration through the rectum; local invasion into pelvic structures; and the presence or absence of regional or distant metastases. A CT scan of the pelvis is helpful in staging because tumor invasion into the sacrum or pelvic sidewalls may mean surgical therapy is not initially possible. On this basis, clinical staging is used to begin treatment. The pathologic stage is defined when the results of analyzing the surgical specimen are available (typically stage I and II).

Rectal cancer is assigned stages 0 through IV, based on the following general criteria:

- Stage 0: the tumor is confined to the epithelium (layer of cells covering the surface) or has not penetrated through the first layer of muscle in the rectal wall. A tumor in this stage is sometimes referred to as a carcinoma in situ.

- Stage I: the tumor has grown into one of the intermediate layers in the wall of the rectum, but has not spread to nearby lymph nodes or distant sites.

- Stage II: the tumor has penetrated through to the outer wall of the colon or has gone through it, possibly invading other local tissues or organs.

- Stage III: any depth or size of tumor associated with regional lymph node involvement. The tumor has not yet spread to distant sites, however.

- Stage IV: any of the previous criteria associated with distant metastases in one or more organs, most often the lungs or liver. It may also have spread to the lining of the abdominal cavity.

Treatment

Surgery

Surgical resection remains the mainstay of therapy in the treatment of rectal cancer. Stage I, II, and even suspected stage III disease are treated by surgical removal of the involved section of the rectum (resection) along with the complete vascular and lymphatic supply. In some cases, robotic surgery may be used, and this approach was being intensively studied as of 2014. Because of the improvement in staging methods (principally endorectal ultrasound), many rectal cancers are now selected for presurgical treatment with radiation and, often, chemotherapy. The use of chemotherapy prior to surgery is known as neoadjuvant chemotherapy, and it is used for Stage II and Stage III rectal cancers. Following neoadjuvant treatment, the remaining tumor (often only a scar) is resected. In some cases, such neoadjuvant treatment avoids the need for permanent **colostomy** by major tumor shrinkage prior to surgery. Following surgery, chemotherapy is completed.

For patients with stage I tumors, transanal endoscopic microsurgery (TEM) may be used. This technique is less invasive than abdominal surgery and has been linked to fewer side effects and shorter recovery periods. Some patients with small Stage I lesions may receive surgical therapy followed by additional radiation and chemotherapy (as opposed to before). In a small group of patients with small Stage I lesions, endoluminal radiation alone is performed as a curative treatment.

When determining primary treatment for rectal cancer, the surgeon's ability to reconnect the ends of the rectum must be considered. The pelvis is a confined space that makes surgical reconnection more difficult to do safely when the tumor is in the lower rectum. The upper rectum does not usually present a substantial problem to the surgeon restoring bowel continuity after the cancer has been removed. Mid-rectal tumors,

especially in males where the pelvis is usually smaller than a woman's, may present technical difficulties in attaching the proximal bowel to the remaining rectum. Technical advances in stapling instrumentation have largely overcome these difficulties. If the anastomosis (surgical connection) leaks postoperatively, infection can occur. In the past, infection was a major cause of complications in resection of rectal cancers. Today, utilizing the stapling instrumentation, an anastomosis at the time of the original surgery is much safer. If the surgeon feels that the connection is compromised or may leak, a colostomy may be performed. A colostomy is performed by bringing the colon through the abdominal wall and sewing its end to the skin. In these cases the stool is diverted away from the anastomosis, allowing it to heal and preventing the infectious complications associated with leakage. Later, when the connection has completely healed, the colostomy can be reversed and bowel continuity restored.

Stapling devices have allowed the surgeon to get closer to the anus and still allow the technical performance of an anastomosis, but there are limits. It is generally felt that there should be at least three centimeters of normal rectum below the tumor or the risk of recurrence locally will be excessive. In addition, if there is no residual native rectum, the patient will not have normal sensation or control and will have problems with loss of bowel control (incontinence). For these reasons, patients with low rectal tumors may undergo total removal of the rectum and anus. This procedure is known as an abdominal-perineal resection. A permanent colostomy is performed in the lower left abdomen.

Radiation

Radiation therapy may help shrink the size of stage II and III tumors prior to surgery. The other roles for radiation therapy are as an aid to surgical therapy in locally advanced cancer that has been removed, and in the treatment of certain distant metastases. Radiation administered postoperatively and in combination with chemotherapy has been shown to reduce the risk of local recurrence in the pelvis by 46% and death rates by 29%. The **National Comprehensive Cancer Network** advises undergoing such treatment for at least six months. Such combined therapy is recommended in patients with locally advanced primary tumors that have been removed surgically. Radiation has been helpful in treating the effects of distant metastases, particularly in the brain. In very few cases, radiation alone may be the curative treatment for rectal cancer.

Chemotherapy

Adjuvant chemotherapy (treating the patient who has no evidence of residual disease but who is at high risk of recurrence) is considered in patients whose tumors deeply penetrate or locally invade (late stage II and stage III). If the tumor is not locally advanced, this form of chemotherapeutic adjuvant therapy may be recommended without radiation. This therapy is identical to that of colon cancer and leads to similar results. Standard postoperative therapy drug combinations include the FOLFOX6 protocol (**fluorouracil** (5-FU), **leucovorin**, and oxaliplatin), weekly or biweekly infusions of 5-FU and leucovorin, **capecitabine**, and CapeOx (capecitabine and oxaliplatin). The drug **levamisole**, which seems to stimulate the immune system, may be substituted for leucovorin. These protocols reduce the rate of recurrence by about 15% and reduce mortality by about 10%. The regimens have some toxicity, but usually are tolerated fairly well; FOLFOX and CapeOx have been associated with more severe side effects.

For stage IV disease or if a cancer progresses and metastasis develops, the following drug combinations may be used:

- FOLFOX
- FOLFOX with bevacizumab
- FOLFOX with panitumumab (only used for cancer linked to specific genetic mutations)
- CapeOx
- CapeOx with bevacizumab

The chemotherapy may produce a temporary regression of the cancer, but unfortunately, these patients eventually succumb to the disease. In **clinical trials**, the agent **irinotecan** has improved response rates from 20% to 39%, added two to three months to disease-free survival, and prolonged overall survival by a little more than two months. The National Comprehensive Cancer Network provides additional information on the various chemotherapy regimens and drug combinations.

Targeted therapy

Targeted therapy is a newer form of pharmacotherapy that treats cancers with drugs that target the changes in genes or proteins that cause cancer cells to grow and spread. It is most often used to treat advanced or metastatic rectal cancer. The drugs most often used to treat rectal cancer are **cetuximab** and **panitumumab**, which attack the epidermal growth factor receptor (EGFR), a molecule found on the surface of cancer cells that helps them grow. Other drugs used include **bevacizumab** and **regorafenib**. These targeted drugs will not work, however, in patients with mutations in the *BRAF* or *KRAS* gene, which is why patients diagnosed with rectal cancer are often now tested for these mutations. Side effects of targeted therapy may include

an acne-like rash on the face and chest, headache, tiredness, **fever**, and diarrhea.

Palliative treatment

Palliative treatment refers to any form of treatment given to control symptoms and relieve pain rather than bring about a cure. In cases of advanced-stage or metastatic rectal cancer, radiation therapy might be used to relieve the symptoms of cancer that has spread to the bones. Chemotherapy may be given to shrink a tumor that is starting to block the bowels. Patients with late-stage rectal cancer nearing the end of life may wish to consider **hospice care**.

Alternative and complementary therapies

Most alternative therapies have not been studied in clinical trials. Large doses of **vitamins**, fiber, and green tea are among the various therapies tried. Before initiating any alternative therapies, patients should consult with their physician to be sure that these therapies do not complicate or interfere with the recommended therapy.

Patients may find such complementary therapies as meditation, prayer, guided imagery, massage therapy, music therapy, or relaxation techniques helpful in coping with the stress of cancer diagnosis and the side effects of treatment for rectal cancer.

Prognosis

Prognosis is the long-term outlook or survival after therapy. Overall, about 50% of patients treated for colon and rectal cancer survive the disease. As expected, the survival rates are dependent upon the stage of the cancer at the time of diagnosis, making early detection crucial.

According to the NCI, about 15% of patients present with stage I disease, or are diagnosed with stage I disease when they initially visit a doctor, and about 75% survive 5 years later. Stage II represents 20–30% of cases and 65% survive; 30–40% comprise the stage III presentation, of which 55% survive. The remaining 20–25% present with stage IV disease and have a 5-year survival rate of about 6%. It is important to keep in mind, however, that most patients with rectal cancer are older than the general population and may have other serious health conditions that affect their mortality during the first five years after treatment; the number of people who survive rectal cancer by itself may actually be somewhat higher than the NCI's figures indicate.

Coping with cancer treatment

For those with familial syndromes causing colon cancer, genetic counseling may be appropriate. Psychological counseling may help anyone having trouble coping with a potentially fatal disease. Local cancer support groups are often identified by contacting local hospitals or the American Cancer Society. Another good source of information and support is the Colon Cancer Alliance.

Clinical trials

Clinical trials are scientific studies in which new therapies are compared to current standards in an effort to identify therapies that offer better results. In 2014, there were 313 open clinical trials in the United States for rectal cancer, ranging from comparisons of robotic to standard surgery and comparisons of different chemotherapeutic agents to studies of patients' quality of life and studies of the effect of genetic mutations on patients' response to treatment.

Prevention

There is no absolute method for preventing colon or rectal cancer as of 2014. However, an individual can lessen risk or identify the precursors of colon and rectal cancer. The patient with a familial history can enter screening and surveillance programs earlier than the general population. High-fiber diets and vitamins, avoiding obesity, and staying active lessen the risk. Avoiding **cigarettes** and alcohol may be helpful. By controlling these environmental factors, an individual can lessen risk and to this degree potentially prevent the disease.

By undergoing appropriate screening when uncontrollable genetic risk factors have been identified, an individual may be rewarded by the identification of benign polyps that can be treated, as opposed to having these growths degenerate into a malignancy.

Special concerns

Polyps are growths of the epithelium of the colon. They may be completely benign, premalignant, or cancerous. The association of colon and rectal cancers in patients with certain types of polyps is that many polyps begin as a benign growth and later acquire malignant characteristics. There are two types of polyps: pedunculated and sessile. This terminology comes from their appearance. Those that are pedunculated are on a stalk like a mushroom and the sessile polyps are broad-based and have no stalk. Unless a pedunculated polyp gets large, its malignant potential is very small. This type may also be easily removed during endoscopy. The sessile polyp is also known as a villous **adenoma**, and as many as one-third of these harbor a malignancy. Therefore, the villous adenoma is considered premalignant. Sessile polyps may or may not be easily managed with the colonoscope and may need surgical removal because of their premalignant nature.

Polyps commonly present with occult blood in the stool. Since they are associated with the development of cancer, patients who have developed polyps need to enter a program of careful surveillance.

Elderly or debilitated patients with rectal cancers that seem localized may be treated by local destruction of the tumor through the anus. If the tumor is amenable to local resection or destruction by laser or cautery through the anus, the patient may be treated this way. This select group of patients may not be able to tolerate the standard therapy. Local control becomes the main issue while avoiding high-risk surgery and its inherent complications.

Resources

BOOKS

Abeloff, Martin D., et al. *Clinical Oncology*. 4th ed. New York: Churchill Livingstone/Elsevier, 2008.

Ahuja, Nita, and Brenda S. Nettles. *Johns Hopkins Patients' Guide to Colon and Rectal Cancer*. Burlington, MA: Jones and Bartlett Learning, 2014.

Ruggieri, Paul, and Addison R. Tolentino. *Colon and Rectal Cancer: From Diagnosis to Treatment*, 2nd ed. Omaha, NE: Addicus Books, 2012.

Scholefield, John H., and Cathy Eng, eds. *Colorectal Cancer: Diagnosis and Clinical Management*. Chichester, UK: John Wiley and Sons, 2014.

Valentini, Vincenzo. *Multidisciplinary Management of Rectal Cancer*. New York: Springer, 2012.

PERIODICALS

Fornaro, L., et al. "Bevacizumab in the Pre-operative Treatment of Locally Advanced Rectal Cancer: A Systematic Review." *World Journal of Gastroenterology* 20 (May 28, 2014): 6081–6091.

Kasagi, Y., et al. "A Case of Panitumumab-responsive Metastatic Rectal Cancer Initially Refractory to Cetuximab." *Case Reports in Oncology* 6 (July 20, 2013): 382–386.

Mak, T. W., et al. "Robotic Surgery for Rectal Cancer: A Systematic Review of Current Practice." *World Journal of Gastrointestinal Oncology* 6 (June 15, 2014): 184–193.

Park, K. K., et al. "Laparoscopic Resection for Middle and Low Rectal Cancer." *Journal of Minimal Access Surgery* 10 (April 2014): 68–71.

Sermeus, A., et al. "Advances in Radiotherapy and Targeted Therapies for Rectal Cancer." *World Journal of Gastroenterology* 20 (January 7, 2014): 1–5.

Turgeon, D. K., and M. T. Ruffin IV. "Screening Strategies for Colorectal Cancer in Asymptomatic Adults." *Primary Care* 41 (June 2014): 331–353.

Ung, L., T. Chua, and A. F. Engel. "A Systematic Review of Local Excision Combined with Chemoradiotherapy for Early Rectal Cancer." *Colorectal Disease* 16 (July 2014): 502–515.

Walker, A. S., et al. "Future Directions for the Early Detection of Colorectal Cancer Recurrence." *Journal of Cancer* 5 (March 16, 2014): 272–280.

OTHER

American Cancer Society (ACS). "Colorectal Cancer." http://www.cancer.org/acs/groups/cid/documents/webcontent/003096-pdf.pdf (accessed September 3, 2014).

WEBSITES

American College of Gastroenterology (ACG). "Colorectal Cancer." http://patients.gi.org/topics/colorectal-cancer/ (accessed September 3, 2014).

eMedicineHealth. "Rectal Cancer." http://www.emedicine-health.com/rectal_cancer/article_em.htm (accessed September 3, 2014).

National Cancer Institute (NCI). "Rectal Cancer Treatment (PDQ)." http://www.cancer.gov/cancertopics/pdq/treatment/rectal/HealthProfessional/page1/AllPages (accessed September 3, 2014).

National Comprehensive Cancer Network. "NCCN Chemotherapy Order Templates: Rectal Cancer." http://www.nccn.org/ordertemplates/default.asp?did=4 (accessed September 3, 2014).

ORGANIZATIONS

American Cancer Society (ACS), 250 Williams Street NW, Atlanta, GA 30303, (800) 227-2345, http://www.cancer.org/aboutus/howwehelpyou/app/contact-us.aspx, http://www.cancer.org/index.

American College of Gastroenterology (ACG), 6400 Goldsboro Road, Suite 200, Bethesda, MD 20817, (301) 263-9000, info@acg.gi.org, http://gi.org//.

American Society of Clinical Oncology (ASCO), 2318 Mill Road, Suite 800, Alexandria, VA 22314, (571) 483-1300, (888) 651-3038, contactus@cancer.net, http://www.asco.org.

Colon Cancer Alliance, 1025 Vermont Avenue NW, Suite 1066, Washington, DC 20005, (202) 628-1023, (877) 422-2030, Fax: (866) 304-9075, http://ccalliance.org/.

National Cancer Institute (NCI), BG 9609 MSC 9760, 9609 Medical Center Drive, Bethesda, MD 20892-9760, (800) 4-CANCER (422-6237), http://www.cancer.gov/global/contact/email-us, http://www.cancer.gov/.

National Comprehensive Cancer Network, 275 Commerce Dr., Ste. 300, Fort Washington, PA 19034, (215) 690-0300, Fax: (215) 690-0280, http://www.nccn.org.

Office of Cancer Complementary and Alternative Medicine (OCCAM), 9609 Medical Center Dr., Room 5-W-136, Rockville, MD 20850, (240) 276-6595, Fax: (240) 276-7888, ncioccam1-r@mail.nih.gov, http://cam.cancer.gov/.

Richard A. McCartney, MD
Teresa G. Odle
REVISED BY REBECCA J. FREY, PhD

Rectal resection

Definition

A rectal resection is the surgical removal of a portion of the rectum.

Purpose

Rectal resections repair damage to the rectum caused by diseases of the lower digestive tract, such as **cancer**, diverticulitis, and inflammatory bowel disease (ulcerative colitis and Crohn's disease). Injury, obstruction, and ischemia (compromised blood supply) may require rectal resection. Masses and scar tissue can grow within the rectum, causing blockages that prevent normal elimination of feces. Other diseases, such as diverticulitis and ulcerative colitis, can cause perforations in the rectum. Surgical removal of the damaged area can return normal rectal function.

Description

During a rectal resection, the surgeon removes the diseased or perforated portion of the rectum. If the diseased or damaged section is not very large, the separated ends are reattached. Such a procedure is called rectal anastomosis.

Demographics

The American Cancer Society estimated 142,820 new colorectal cancer diagnoses in the United States for 2013, with 50,830 deaths. **Rectal cancer** incidence is approximately 28% of the total colorectal incidence rate. Surgery is the optimal treatment for rectal cancer, resulting in cure for 45% of patients. Recurrence due to surgical failure is low, from 4%–8%, when the procedure is meticulously performed.

Crohn's disease and ulcerative colitis, both chronic inflammatory diseases of the colon, each affect approximately 500,000 young adults. Surgery is recommended when medication fails patients with ulcerative colitis. Nearly three-fourths of all Crohn's patients will require surgery to remove a diseased section of the intestine or rectum.

Diagnosis

A number of tests identify masses and perforations within the intestinal tract:

- A lower GI (gastrointestinal) series is a series of x-rays of the colon and rectum that can help identify ulcers, cysts, polyps, diverticuli (pouches in the intestine), and cancer. The patient is given a barium enema to coat the intestinal tract, making disease easier to see on the x-rays.

- Flexible sigmoidoscopy involves insertion of a sigmoidoscope, a flexible tube with a miniature camera, into the rectum to examine the lining of the rectum and the sigmoid colon, the last third of the intestinal tract. The sigmoidoscope can also remove polyps or tissue for biopsy.

- A colonoscopy is similar to the flexible sigmoidoscopy, except the flexible tube examines the entire intestinal tract.

- Magnetic resonance imaging (MRI), used both prior to and during surgery, allows physicians to determine the precise margins for the resection so that all of the diseased tissue can be removed. This imaging also identifies patients who could most benefit from adjuvant therapy such as chemotherapy or radiation.

Preparation

To cleanse the bowel, the patient may be placed on a restricted diet for several days before surgery, then placed on a liquid diet the day before, with nothing by mouth after midnight. A series of enemas and/or oral preparations (GoLytely, Colyte, or senna) may be ordered to empty the bowel. Oral anti-infectives (neomycin, erythromycin, or kanamycin sulfate) may be ordered to decrease bacteria in the intestine and help prevent postoperative infection. The operation can be done with an abdominal incision (laparotomy) or using minimally invasive techniques with small tubes to allow insertion of the operating instruments (**laparoscopy**).

Aftercare

Postoperative care involves monitoring blood pressure, pulse, respiration, and temperature. Breathing tends to be shallow because of the effect of the anesthesia and the patient's reluctance to breathe deeply due to discomfort around the surgical incision. The patient is taught how to support the incision during deep breathing and coughing, and given pain medication as necessary. Fluid intake and output is measured, and the wound is observed for color and drainage.

Fluids and electrolytes are given intravenously until the patient's diet can be resumed, starting with liquids, then adding solids. The patient is helped out of bed the evening of the surgery and allowed to sit in a chair. Most patients are discharged in two to four days.

Risks

Rectal resection has potential risks similar those of other major surgeries. Complications usually occur while the patient is in the hospital, and the patient's general health prior to surgery will be an indication of the risk potential. Patients with heart problems and stressed immune systems are of special concern. Both during and following the procedure, the physician and nursing staff will monitor the patient for:

- excessive bleeding
- wound infection
- thrombophlebitis (inflammation and blood clot in the veins in the legs
- pneumonia
- pulmonary embolism (blood clot or air bubble in the lungs' blood supply)
- cardiac stress due to allergic reaction to the general anaesthetic

Symptoms that the patient should report, especially after discharge, include:

- increased pain, swelling, redness, drainage, or bleeding in the surgical area
- flu-like symptoms such as headache, muscle aches, dizziness, or fever

---

• increased abdominal pain or swelling, constipation, nausea or vomiting, or black, tarry stools

Results

Complete healing is expected without complications. The recovery rate varies, depending on the patient's overall health prior to surgery. Typically, full recovery takes six to eight weeks.

Morbidity and mortality rates

Mortality has decreased from nearly 28% to under 6%, through the use of prophylactic **antibiotics** before and after surgery.

Alternatives

If the section of the rectum to be removed is very large, the rectum may not be able to be reattached. Under those circumstances, a **colostomy** would be performed. The distal end of the rectum would be closed and left to atrophy. The proximal end would be brought through an opening in the abdomen to create an opening (a stoma) for feces to be removed from the body.

Health care team roles

Rectal resections are performed by general surgeons and colorectal surgeons as inpatient surgeries under general anesthesia.

Resources

BOOKS

American Cancer Society. *QuickFACTS Colorectal Cancer.* Chicago: American Cancer Society, 2012.

Johnston, Lorraine. *Colon & Rectal Cancer: A Comprehensive Guide for Patients and Families.* Sebastopol, CA: O'Reilly, 2000.

Levin, Bernard, et al. *American Cancer Society's Complete Guide to Colorectal Cancer.* Atlanta: American Cancer Society, 2006.

PERIODICALS

Fernandez, Ramiro, et al. "Laparoscopic versus Robotic Rectal Resection for Rectal Cancer in a Veteran Population." *American Journal of Surgery* 206, no. 4 (2013): 509–17. http://dx.doi.org/10.1016/j.amjsurg.2013.01.036 (accessed October 3, 2014).

Turina, Matthias, et al. "Quantification of Risk for Early Unplanned Readmission after Rectal Resection: A Single-Center Study." *Journal of the American College of Surgeons* 217, no. 2 (2013): 200–208. http://dx.doi.org/10.1016/j.jamcollsurg.2013.05.016 (accessed October 3, 2014).

WEBSITES

American Cancer Society. "Surgery for Colorectal Cancer." http://www.cancer.org/cancer/colonandrectumcancer/overviewguide/colorectal-cancer-overview-treating-surgery (accessed February 5, 2015).

Society of American Gastrointestinal Endoscopic Surgeons. "Guidelines for Laparoscopic Resection of Curable Colon and Rectal Cancer." http://www.sages.org/publications/guidelines/guidelines-for-laparoscopic-resection-of-curable-colon-and-rectal-cancer (accessed October 3, 2014).

ORGANIZATIONS

American Board of Colon and Rectal Surgery, 20600 Eureka Rd., Ste. 600, Taylor, MI 48180, (734) 282-9400, Fax: (734) 282-9402, admin@abcrs.org, http://www.abcrs.org.

Society of American Gastrointestinal Endoscopic Surgeons (SAGES), 11300 W. Olympic Blvd., Ste. 600, Los Angeles, CA 90064, (310) 437-0544, Fax: (310) 437-0585, webmaster@sages.org, http://www.sages.org.

Janie Franz

Reglan *see* **Metoclopramide**

Regorafenib

Definition

Regorafenib (Stivarga) is used to treat colon and rectal cancers that have spread to other parts of the body (metastasized) and that have not responded to treatment with certain other drugs. Regorafenib is also used to treat gastrointestinal stromal tumor (GIST). Regorafenib is a type of targeted therapy called a kinase inhibitor.

Purpose

Regorafenib was first approved in 2012 by the U.S. Food and Drug Administration (FDA) for treating metastatic colorectal **cancer** in patients who had been treated previously with fluoropyrimidine-, oxaliplatin-, and irinotecan-based **chemotherapy**, and with a therapy targeting vascular endothelial growth factor (VEGF). Patients whose cancers do not have mutations in the *KRAS* gene must also have been treated previously with therapy targeting the epidermal growth factor receptor (EGFR). FDA approval was based on the significant prolonging of overall survival and a median survival time of 6.4 months for patients receiving regorafenib compared with 5.0 months for patients administered a placebo. The median progression-free survival (PFS) time was 2.0 months in the regorafenib group compared with 1.7 months in the placebo group.

In 2013, the FDA expanded regorafenib approval to the treatment of GIST that was locally advanced (spread from its origin to nearby tissue or lymph nodes); could not be surgically removed; or had metastasized in patients whose cancers were resistant to or no longer responding to treatment with **imatinib mesylate** and **sunitinib** malate, the two other FDA-approved drugs for GIST. Regorafenib was given an expedited review under the FDA priority review program because there were no other satisfactory therapies for GIST. Regorafenib was also granted orphan product designation because GIST is considered a rare disease—there are 3,300–6,000 new cases in the United States each year, primarily in older adults. In the clinical trial, the median PFS was 4.8 months for patients receiving regorafenib, compared with 0.9 months for patients treated with a placebo, although 85% of placebo patients switched to regorafenib when their cancers progressed. Regorafenib is being studied in the treatment of other types of cancer.

Description

Regorafenib is a small molecule that binds to and inhibits abnormal growth factor receptors on the surfaces or inside of cancer cells. These receptors are proteins called kinases. When growth factors bind to these kinases, they activate signaling pathways that tell cancer cells either to grow and multiply (proliferate) or to form new blood vessels (**angiogenesis**) that enable the tumor to grow and metastasize. By binding to these receptors, regorafenib prevents growth factors from binding and inhibits the activities of the receptors, which helps to slow or halt the spread of cancer cells. Because regorafenib or its active metabolites bind to and inhibit several different receptors and other kinases, it inhibits several different cell-signaling pathways that are involved in both normal and cancerous cellular processes, including cell proliferation and angiogenesis. Regorafenib has only one atom that differs from the cancer drug **sorafenib**. This change enables it to also block angiogenesis by a second mechanism.

KEY TERMS

Angiogenesis—Blood vessel formation that is necessary for tumor growth and metastasis.

Epidermal growth factor receptor (EGFR)—A protein on the cell surface that can initiate cell growth and proliferation.

Gastrointestinal stromal tumor (GIST)—A type of tumor that usually starts in cells of the gastrointestinal tract wall.

Kinase inhibitor—A drug such as regorafenib that inhibits kinase enzymatic activity in a cell-signaling pathway.

Kinases—Proteins that add phosphates to other proteins in cell-signaling pathways.

KRAS—A gene that is mutated in 30–40% of colorectal tumors.

Metastasis—Cancer that has spread from its site of origin to other parts of the body.

Placebo—An inactive substance or preparation given to a control group in a clinical trial to test the effectiveness of the real medication or treatment; usually study participants do not know if they are receiving the drug or the placebo.

Progression-free survival (PFS)—The length of time patients survive without their cancer progressing; used in clinical trials to measure the effectiveness of a drug.

Receptor—A molecule, usually a protein, inside or on the surface of a cell that binds a specific chemical group or molecule, such as a hormone or growth factor, to initiate a sequence of events.

Sorafenib—A drug used to treat several types of cancer that differs in only one atom from regorafenib.

Targeted therapy—A drug that interferes with specific molecules involved in cancer cell growth and/or survival.

Vascular endothelial growth factor (VEGF)—A factor that stimulates angiogenesis by binding to receptors on endothelial cells.

Brand names

Regorafenib is marketed as Stivarga tablets in the United States, Canada, and internationally. It is manufactured by Bayer HealthCare Pharmaceuticals, Inc. Regorafenib is approved for GIST in Canada, Chile, Ecuador, Japan, Uruguay, and Venezuela. As of 2014, European approval was pending. Stivarga was formerly known as BAY 73-4506 and fluoro-sorafenib.

Recommended dosage

Regorafenib is supplied as 40 milligram (mg) tablets taken by mouth. The usual starting dose is 160 mg (four tablets) taken once per day for 21 days, followed by seven days off. This 28-day cycle is then repeated. The tablets are swallowed whole at the same time each day along with a low-fat breakfast. The breakfast must have less than 30% of its calories from fat—such as two slices of white toast with one tablespoon (tbsp.) low-fat margarine and 1 tbsp. jelly and 8 oz. (237 mL) skim milk or one cup of cereal, 8 oz. skim milk, one slice of toast with jelly, apple juice, and one cup (237 mL) of coffee or tea. The tablets should not be chewed, split, or crushed. The tablets should be kept in the container they came in along with the packet of desiccant. Regorafenib must be taken exactly as prescribed—no more or less. If a dose is missed, it should be taken as soon as possible on the same day, but two doses should not be taken in the same day. Any unused tablets should be discarded 28 days after opening the container. Patients may be instructed to lower the dose or delay or stop treatment depending on side effects and how the drug is working. Regorafenib is not available from retail pharmacies—it is mailed to the patient or doctor from a specialty pharmacy.

Precautions

Regorafenib comes with a boxed warning of possible severe or life-threatening liver damage. It cannot be used to treat patients with severe liver problems. Patients are examined and given blood tests before and during treatment to check liver function. Symptoms of liver damage include:

- yellowing of the skin or eyes
- nausea
- vomiting
- loss of appetite
- flu-like symptoms
- dark-colored urine
- pain in the upper right belly
- fatigue
- lack of energy
- unusual bleeding or bruising
- changing sleep habits

Regorafenib may affect fertility. It may also cause:

- bleeding from the stomach, intestines, lungs, or other areas, which in some cases could be fatal
- high blood pressure, which in rare cases may be life-threatening, so blood pressure is checked before and regularly during treatment (patients whose high blood pressure is controlled with medication can take regorafenib)
- skin rash
- hand-foot syndrome—pain, numbness, tingling, redness, or swelling in the hands or feet, or peeling, blistering, or open sores in severe cases
- decreased blood flow to the heart and increased risk of heart attacks
- problems with wound healing—the drug should be stopped at least two weeks before planned surgery
- rarely, holes (perforations) or abnormal connections (fistulas) in the digestive tract, which can be life-threatening
- rarely, a brain condition called reversible posterior leukoencephalopathy syndrome

Symptoms of regorafenib overdose can include:

- rash or other skin changes
- hoarseness or voice changes
- diarrhea
- swelling inside the nose or mouth
- dry mouth
- decreased appetite
- fatigue

Pediatric

The safety and effectiveness of regorafenib has not been established in patients under 18. Animal studies suggest that the drug is not safe for pediatric patients.

Geriatric

In **clinical trials**, 37% of patients were 65 or older, and 8% were 75 or older. No overall differences in safety and effectiveness were observed between older and younger patients.

Pregnant or breastfeeding

Regorafenib can harm a fetus if taken at the time of conception or during pregnancy, so pregnancy must be avoided. Couples who could become pregnant must use effective birth control during and for at least two months after treatment. The drug may pass into breast milk, so breastfeeding is not recommended while taking regorafenib.

Other conditions and allergies

Patients should tell their doctors if they have:

- a history of any type of liver disease, including hepatitis

- any allergies, including allergies to medicines, dyes, additives, foods, or any ingredients in regorafenib
- a history of high blood pressure
- a history of chest pain, heart attack, or other heart problems
- a history of any bleeding problems
- an unhealed wound, had recent surgery, or are planning to have surgery—patients must stop taking regorafenib at least two weeks before surgery
- any other medical conditions, such as kidney disease, diabetes, gout, or infections

Side effects

In clinical trials, 98% of patients receiving regorafenib reported drug-related adverse events, as did 68% of patients receiving the placebo. Less than 1% of patients had serious side effects that included liver damage, severe bleeding, blistering and peeling skin, very high blood pressure requiring emergency treatment, heart attacks, and perforations in the intestines. The most common events, occurring in at least 30% of patients receiving regorafenib, were:

- weakness/fatigue
- decreased appetite and food intake
- weight loss
- infection
- voice changes or hoarseness
- high blood pressure
- mouth or throat sores
- hand-foot skin reactions
- diarrhea

Other common side effects of regorafenib are:

- fever
- rash
- low blood cell counts
- low blood mineral levels
- abnormal blood tests suggesting effects on the liver
- protein in the urine suggesting possible kidney damage

Less common side effects are:

- headache
- hair loss
- taste changes
- muscle or joint stiffness

Rare side effects are:

- dry mouth
- hypothyroidism

QUESTIONS TO ASK YOUR DOCTOR

- How will I get regorafenib?
- Can you give me a copy of the information sheet for regorafenib and a list of ingredients?
- How should I take this medication?
- What over-the-counter remedies can I take with regorafenib?
- How do I dispose of unused regorafenib?

- tremor
- heartburn
- severe liver damage
- heart attack
- vision loss
- perforation or fistula in the stomach or intestines
- brain changes causing headache, confusion, seizures, or blindness
- death from liver damage, bleeding, or other problems

Interactions

Regorafenib can interact with many drugs and supplements. Patients should tell their doctors about any prescription or over-the-counter drugs and supplements—including **vitamins** and herbs—that they are taking or are planning to take. Grapefruit, grapefruit juice, or grapefruit extract may affect the amount of regorafenib in the body and should be avoided. The cancer drug **irinotecan** may interact with regorafenib. Drugs and supplements that may interfere with blood clotting and increase the risk of bleeding with regorafenib include:

- vitamin E
- nonsteroidal anti-inflammatory drugs (NSAIDs), such as aspirin, ibuprofen (Advil, Motrin), naproxen (Aleve, Naprosyn), and many others, including many cold, flu, fever, and headache remedies that contain aspirin or ibuprofen
- warfarin (Coumadin)
- ticlopidine (Ticlid)
- clopidogrel (Plavix)

Drugs and supplements that can lower the levels of regorafenib in the blood, possibly making it less effective, include:

- antiseizure drugs, such as carbamazepine, phenobarbital, and phenytoin

- tuberculosis drugs, such as rifampin, rifabutin, and rifapentine
- the steroid dexamethasone
- St. John's wort, an herbal supplement

Drugs that may cause regorafenib to build up in the blood, possibly worsening side effects or causing other problems, include:

- some antibiotics, such as erythromycin, clarithromycin, telithromycin, and similar drugs
- some antifungal medicines, such as ketoconazole, itraconazole, posaconazole, and voriconazole
- some antidepressants, such as nefazodone
- some HIV drugs, such as indinavir, ritonavir, nelfinavir, atazanavir, saquinavir, and others

Resources

PERIODICALS

Songdej, Natthapol, and Margaret von Mehren. "GIST Treatment Options after Tyrosine Kinase Inhibitors." *Current Treatment Options in Oncology* 15, no. 3 (September 2014): 493–506.

WEBSITES

Pazdur, Richard. "FDA Approval for Regorafenib." National Cancer Institute. July 3, 2013. http://www.cancer.gov/cancertopics/druginfo/fda-regorafenib (accessed October 19, 2014).

"Regorafenib." American Cancer Society. February 26, 2013. http://www.cancer.org/treatment/treatmentsandsideeffects/guidetocancerdrugs/regorafenib (accessed October 19, 2014).

"Regorafenib." MedlinePlus. February 15, 2013. http://www.nlm.nih.gov/medlineplus/druginfo/meds/a613004.html (accessed October 19, 2014).

"Stivarga (Regorafenib)." GIST Support International. October 18, 2013. http://www.gistsupport.org/treatments-for-gist/stivarga.php (accessed October 19, 2014).

ORGANIZATIONS

American Cancer Society, 250 Williams Street NW, Atlanta, GA 30303, (800) 227-2345, http://www.cancer.org.

GIST Support International, 12 Bomaca Drive, Doylestown, PA 18901, (215) 340-9374, gsi@gistsupport.org, http://www.gistsupport.org.

National Cancer Institute, 6116 Executive Boulevard, Suite 300, Bethesda, MD 20892-8322, (800) 4-CANCER (422-6237), http://www.cancer.gov.

U.S. Food and Drug Administration, 10903 New Hampshire Avenue, Silver Spring, MD 20993-0002, (888) INFO-FDA (463-6332), http://www.fda.gov.

Margaret Alic, PhD

Renal cell carcinoma *see* **Kidney cancer**

Renal pelvis tumors

Definition

Renal pelvis tumors are rare kidney cancers appearing in a specific part of the kidney known as the pelvis (or collecting system) of the kidney.

Description

The word *renal* means having to do with the kidneys. A part of each kidney in the human body is called the renal pelvis. The renal pelvis in each kidney is the portion of the collecting system that empties into the ureters (tubes that carry urine from the kidneys to the bladder).

Renal pelvis tumors usually appear after an earlier condition called renal papillary necrosis has already developed. The tumors may be composed of any one of several different types of cells. Most commonly, these tumors are of a type of cell known as a **transitional cell carcinoma**.

A transitional cell is intermediate between the flat squamous cell and the tall columnar cell. It is restricted to the epithelium (cellular lining) of the urinary bladder, ureters, and the renal pelvis. Transitional cell carcinomas have a wide range of appearance depending on their locations. Some of these carcinomas are flat in appearance, some are papillary (small elevation), and others are in the shape of a node. Under the microscope, however, most of these carcinomas have a papillary-like look. There are three generally recognized grades of transitional cell **carcinoma**. The grade of the carcinoma is determined by particular characteristics found in the cells

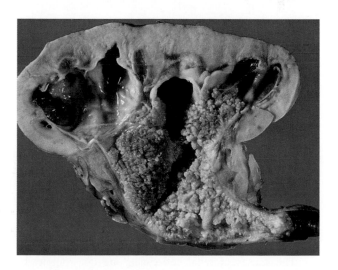

Transitional cell carcinoma of the renal pelvis. *(BIOPHOTO ASSOC/Science Source)*

KEY TERMS

Cystoscopy—A medical procedure involving the use of a medical instrument that permits the physician to look directly at portions of the urinary tract.

Pyelography—A type of x-ray procedure applied to a portion of the urinary tract, of which the kidneys form part.

Renal—Having to do with the kidneys.

Renal papillary necrosis—A medical condition affecting the kidney that increases a person's risk of developing a tumor of the renal pelvis.

Renal pelvis—That portion of the collecting system of the kidney that empties into the ureter.

Ureteroscopy—A diagnostic procedure that increases the diagnostic accuracy of the examination of possible renal pelvis tumors. Ureteroscopy may cause damage to some portion of the urinary tract. Therefore, ureteroscopy is usually reserved for those patients for whom unanswered questions remain after conventional diagnostic approaches have been completed.

Urography—A type of x-ray procedure applied to a portion of the urinary tract, of which the kidneys form part.

of the tumor. Transitional cell carcinoma typically affects the mucosa (the moist tissue layer that lines hollow organs or the cavity of the body) in the areas where it originates—in this case, the kidney.

Demographics

Because statistics on these tumors are gathered with statistics on other kidney tumors, little information specific to tumors of the pelvic area of the kidney is available. These tumors are relatively uncommon, and account for no more than 7% of cancers of the kidney and upper urinary tract. This percentage would indicate that about 4,400 Americans (2,700 men and 1,700 women) were diagnosed with **cancer** of the renal pelvis in 2014 and 950 patients died of the disease. Renal pelvis cancers are more common in men than in women, as the statistics indicate, and appear most often in people over the age of 65.

Causes and symptoms

The causes of renal cell cancer are not completely understood as of 2014, but are thought to be a combination of genetic (inherited) mutations and the excretion of irritating substances in the urine. The appearance of renal pelvis tumors is often associated with a history of cigarette smoking and the overuse of certain pain medicines, as well as with a history of either kidney stones or **bladder cancer**. People who have worked in the rubber, paint, dye, printing, textile, and plastic industries and have been exposed to certain chemicals are also at increased risk of this type of cancer.

Approximately four out of five patients have symptoms of blood in the urine at the time of diagnosis. Approximately one out of three patients experiences pain in the side or lower back. Other frequent symptoms include urinary frequency or urgency, unintentional **weight loss**, brown or rusty-colored urine, and **fatigue**. Some patients may have no symptoms, while others may feel generally ill, visit the doctor for this general complaint, and have the cancer diagnosed at that time.

Diagnosis

The doctor may have the urine examined to measure amounts of its contents and may order urine **cytology**, which examines cells in the urine for the possible presence of cancer cells shed from the kidney. Ultrasound uses high-energy sound waves and echoes to create images of the ureters and kidneys. Either urography or pyelography may be used to diagnose renal pelvis tumors. Both urography and pyelography are types of x-ray procedures that may be used to visualize portions of the urinary tract. The kidneys are part of the urinary tract.

A technique called ureteroscopy increases the diagnostic accuracy doctors are able to attain. Doctors insert a thin scope through the urethra. A light and lens on the end of the scope help the doctor look for abnormal areas inside the bladder, ureter, or renal pelvis.

The doctor may also order an x-ray of the chest, a bone scan, and liver function tests to see whether the cancer has spread.

Clinical staging

Tumor stage and grade provide important information on how an individual patient's renal pelvis tumor(s) will be treated and on the patient's prognosis. The primary tumor is staged on the basis of whether it remains superficial or has settled into the kidney. Patients with more superficial tumors have the best prognosis. However, even these patients may develop new tumors later. Staging also relies on whether the tumor has spread to distant organs and tissues, which is called **metastasis**.

Another factor important in determining treatment and prognosis is to determine the type and character of the individual cells that make up the tumor. Cells with a well-differentiated structure are associated with longer patient survival than cells with poorly differentiated structure.

Treatment

Surgery constitutes the standard treatment for renal pelvis tumors. One surgical procedure is called a radical nephroureterectomy, and involves the removal of the ureter and a portion of the bladder as well. A segmental resection of the ureter is removal of the part of the ureter containing cancer, along with some of the healthy tissue around the cancer cells. The surgeon reattaches the remaining portions of the ureter.

New treatments are often tested in **clinical trials**, and these include:

- segmental resection of the renal pelvis, which removes only the cancer cells and some healthy tissue around it when some of the kidney needs to be spared

- fulguration, which burns away tissue with an electric current applied with a needle-shaped electrode

- laser surgery, which uses a laser beam to cut away tissue

- regional chemotherapy and regional immunotherapy, which combines chemotherapy drugs aimed at the area where the cancer is located and immunotherapy (also called biologic therapy) to boost the patient's immune system to better fight cancer

Of course, patients with a single tumor comprised of well-differentiated cells are likely to have a better long-term outcome following a limited surgical procedure than are patients with several tumors comprised of poorly differentiated cells. It should be understood, however, that more limited procedures may involve a greater likelihood that the cancer will return.

Patients who have advanced, metastatic, and recurrent renal pelvic cancer may receive **chemotherapy**, often as part of a clinical trial. Some **kidney cancer** patients with advanced cancer have benefited from a bone marrow or blood stem cell transplant. In this procedure, the patient is treated with high doses of chemotherapy, and immature cells called stem cells are donated by a volunteer and transplanted into the patient's body to replace damaged ones. As researchers continue to learn more about the genetics of cancer, they will likely begin to better understand the reasons why renal pelvic tumors form and to develop targeted therapies that destroy the specific cancer cells responsible. In 2014, researchers identified a number of biomarkers responsible for a similar cancer called urothelial carcinoma.

Prognosis

In terms of patient survival, almost all patients with superficial tumors composed of relatively well-differentiated cells live more than five years. In contrast, patients with poorly differentiated (abnormal in maturity and function) tumors that have invaded deep into the kidney and transplanted cells to other parts of the body may live only one year or less.

Approximately two out of five patients given limited surgical treatment for renal pelvis tumors will have new tumors develop. Therefore, it is important that these patients receive careful and regular follow-up. Some authorities recommend examinations for new tumors of and near the renal pelvis at 3, 6, 9, 12, 18, and 24 months following surgery, and then annually afterward.

Coping with cancer treatment

Cancer patients need supportive care to help them through the treatment period with physical and emotional strength intact. Many patients experience feelings of **depression**, anxiety, and fatigue, and many experience nausea, vomiting, and other side effects during treatment. Studies have shown that these can be managed effectively if the patient discusses these issues with the treating physician.

Prevention

Smoking cessation is the most important step. In addition, persons working in the rubber, paint, dye, printing, textile, and plastic industries might speak with their doctor about whether they are at elevated risk of developing this cancer.

Resources

BOOKS

Abeloff, M. D., et al. *Clinical Oncology.* 5th ed. New York: Churchill Livingstone, 2013.

WEBSITES

American Cancer Society (ACS). "What's New in Kidney Cancer Research and Treatment?" http://www.cancer.org/cancer/kidneycancer/detailedguide/kidney-cancer-adult-new-research (accessed November 1, 2014).

National Cancer Institute. "General Information About Transitional Cell Cancer of the Renal Pelvis and Ureter." http://www.cancer.gov/cancertopics/pdq/treatment/transitional-cell/Patient/page1 (accessed November 1, 2014).

ORGANIZATIONS

American Urological Association, 1000 Corporate Boulevard, Linthicum, MD 21090, (410) 689-3700, (866) 746-4282, http://www.auanet.org.

Urology Care Foundation, 1000 Corporate Blvd., Linthicum, MD 21090, (410) 689-3700, (800) 828-7866, Fax: (410) 689-3998, info@urologycarefoundation.org, http://www.urologyhealth.org.

Bob Kirsch
Rebecca J. Frey, PhD
REVISED BY TERESA G. ODLE
REVIEWED BY ROSALYN CARSON-DEWITT, MD

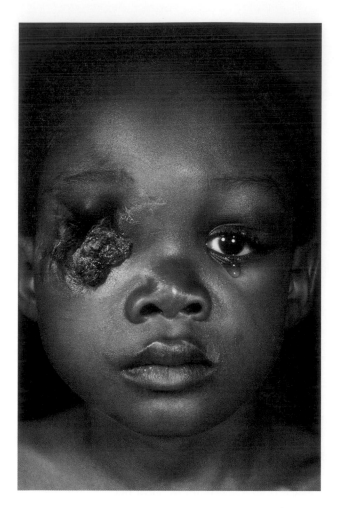

Child with retinoblastoma. *(M.A. Ansary/Science Source)*

Retinoblastoma

Definition

Retinoblastoma is a malignant tumor originating in the retina of one or both eyes that usually affects children under age five. Although rare, it is the most common eye **cancer** in children and the seventh most common childhood cancer in the United States.

Description

The retina is the innermost of the three layers of the eye. The sclera is the outer protective white layer. The choroid is the middle layer with blood vessels that nourish the eye. The front portion of the choroid is the colored iris. The pupil is the opening in the iris that allows light to enter and that usually appears black. The pupil contracts (closes) in bright light and dilates (opens) in low light so that the appropriate amount of light enters the eye. Light entering through the pupil passes through the lens, which focuses it onto the retina. The retina transforms the light into information transmitted by the optic nerve to the brain.

Retinoblastoma is a malignant tumor that can metastasize (spread) from the retina to other parts of the eye and eventually to other parts of the body. In most cases, however, retinoblastoma is diagnosed before it spreads past the eye (intraocular); it has a very good prognosis. The prognosis is poorer if the cancer has spread beyond the eye (extraocular).

The majority (60–75%) of retinoblastomas are unilateral—developing in only one eye. The remainder are bilateral—developing independently in both eyes. Occasionally retinoblastomas are multifocal—multiple tumors in one or both eyes. Trilateral retinoblastoma affects both eyes, along with an independent brain tumor, often in the pineal gland, in children with inherited retinoblastoma. Trilateral retinoblastoma has a poor prognosis.

Although 90% of patients have no family history of retinoblastoma, approximately 40% are caused by an inherited (germline) gene mutation. The other 60% are the result of sporadic or spontaneous (somatic) gene mutations that are not inherited. Bilateral, multifocal, and trilateral retinoblastomas are much more likely to be inherited.

Demographics

The incidence of retinoblastoma varies by country, from 3.4 per million live births to 42.6 per million. Among children under five in the United States, the incidence is 11.8 per million live births, or 6.1% of all cancers in this age group. There are about 350 new cases diagnosed in the United States each year. Retinoblastoma typically occurs in children under age four but occasionally affects older children and adults. It affects males and females equally. The incidence of bilateral retinoblastoma is believed to be slightly higher among African American children than among Caucasian or Asian American children. In the United States and other developed countries, the survival rate for retinoblastoma is above 95%; however, the fatality rate is very high in the developing world.

Causes and symptoms

Causes

Retinoblastoma is caused by changes (mutations) in or the absence (deletion) of a gene called *RB1*, which was identified in 1986. *RB1* is located on chromosome 13q14.2. Cells of the body, or somatic cells, contain 23 pairs of chromosomes. Because somatic cells contain two of each chromosome, they have two copies of the *RB1* gene. Each egg and sperm cell contains only one chromosome 13; therefore only one copy of the *RB1* gene is found in an egg or sperm cell.

The *RB1* gene produces a tumor-suppressor protein that normally limits the growth or cell cycle of retinal cells. Without this control, cells can become cancerous—rapidly undergoing many cell divisions without dying. Adjacent cancer cells can form a mass called a tumor, and malignant tumors can spread to other parts of the body. Retinoblastoma can result from just one retinal cell replicating out of control. The tumor suppressor produced by the *RB1* gene prevents retinal cells from becoming cancerous. A single functioning *RB1* gene in a retinal cell is sufficient for preventing the cell from becoming cancerous. If both *RB1* genes are nonfunctional, a retinal cell can become cancerous, leading to retinoblastoma.

Approximately 40% of patients with retinoblastoma inherited a nonfunctional or deleted *RB1* gene from either their mother or father. Therefore, every cell in their body has a dysfunctional *RB1* gene. If the second normal *RB1* gene in a retinal cell is mutated, patients have a 90% risk of developing retinoblastoma. Environmental triggers such as chemicals and radiation can cause such a

mutation, although in most cases, the trigger or mutagen is unknown.

The average age of onset for inherited retinoblastoma is one year—earlier than for the sporadic form. Children with inherited retinoblastoma are also more likely to have tumors in both eyes and/or multifocal retinoblastoma in one or both eyes. They are also at increased risk of trilateral retinoblastoma, especially **neuroendocrine tumors** in the brain. Only about 15% of inherited retinoblastomas are unilateral.

People who have inherited a deleted or nonfunctional *RB1* gene have a 50% chance of passing on the defect to each of their offspring. The risk of inheriting the mutated/deleted gene and actually developing retinoblastoma is approximately 45% for each child. However, the majority of children with inherited retinoblastoma have no family history of the disease, usually because the affected parent retained a functioning *RB1* gene. It is also possible that the affected parent developed a retinal tumor that was destroyed by the immune system. In some cases, a parent has two normal *RB1* genes in every somatic cell, but some of their egg or sperm cells contain a mutated/deleted *RB1* gene—a condition called gonadal mosaicism.

Approximately 60% of retinoblastoma patients have the sporadic form, in which both *RB1* genes spontaneously mutated in a retinal cell, while remaining normal in all other cells of the body. Such people are not at increased risk of having a child with retinoblastoma. Sporadic retinoblastoma is usually unifocal and has an average age of onset of approximately two years.

There are at least three other genes that appear to be involved in retinoblastoma. An oncogene called *SYK* is overactive in retinoblastoma cells. The gene *MDM4* also seems to be involved in the development of the cancer. Finally, a very small number of retinoblastomas develop in people who appear to have normal *RB1* genes but have too many copies of a gene called *MYCN*.

Symptoms

The most common symptom of retinoblastoma is a white pupil reflex or leukocoria, in which the pupil reflects white instead of black or red on a flash photograph. Parents are often the first to notice this abnormal "cat's eye" reflex. Other symptoms may include:

- a crossed eye or strabismus
- poor vision
- a red, painful, or irritated eye
- inflamed tissue around the eye
- an enlarged or dilated pupil
- different-colored irises (heterochromia)

- extra fingers or toes
- malformed ears
- developmental delays
- failure to thrive

Diagnosis

Children with symptoms of retinoblastoma are usually first evaluated by their pediatrician. A red reflex test is used to diagnose or confirm leukocoria: medicated eye drops keep the pupils dilated when exposed to bright light, and the eyes are examined with an ophthalmoscope. Leukocoria can also be diagnosed by taking a flash Polaroid photograph of a patient who has been in a dark room for three to five minutes.

Suspected cases are usually referred to an ophthalmologist (eye doctor) who has experience with retinoblastoma. The ophthalmologist examines the eyes using an indirect ophthalmoscope to visualize the retina. This test is usually performed with anesthetic eye drops or under general anesthesia. Eye drops are used to dilate the pupils, and a metal clip holds the eyes open. A cotton swab or metal instrument with a flattened tip is pressed on the outer lens of the eye to visualize the front of the retina. Sketches or photographs of the tumor are obtained.

Ultrasound is used to confirm the presence of the tumor and evaluate its size. **Computed tomography** (CT) scans are used to determine whether the tumor has spread beyond the eye or to the brain. **Magnetic resonance imaging** (MRI) may also be used to examine the eyes, eye sockets, and brain for **metastasis**. If the cancer appears to have spread beyond the eye, other assessments, such as blood tests, spinal tap (**lumbar puncture**), and/or **bone marrow biopsy** may be necessary.

Genetic testing

It is important to determine whether retinoblastoma is inherited or somatic. Inherited retinoblastoma increases the risk of unilateral retinoblastoma progressing to bilateral involvement, as well as recurrent tumors or other types of cancer, especially if treated with radiation. Furthermore, the inherited form increases the risk of retinoblastoma in other family members. Families of a child diagnosed with inherited retinoblastoma usually consult with a genetic specialist and may undergo **genetic testing**. A family history of retinoblastoma, as well as bilateral, trilateral, or multifocal retinoblastoma, usually indicates the inherited form. Free testing for retinoblastoma patients to determine the status of the *RB1* gene in their germline is available through the eyeGENE program of the National Eye Institute.

Approximately 5–8% of patients with retinoblastoma have a chromosomal abnormality involving the *RB1* gene that can be detected by microscopic examination of chromosomes obtained from a blood sample. If a chromosomal abnormality is detected in a child, the parents' chromosomes are analyzed for an abnormality that puts them at risk of having other children with retinoblastoma. Chromosome analysis may be recommended for other family members as well.

In most cases, specialized DNA tests on a tumor sample and blood cells are required to look for mutations in the *RB1* gene. If an *RB1* gene is deleted or changed in all of the tested blood cells, patients are assumed to have the inherited form, with a 50% chance of passing the mutated/deleted *RB1* gene to each of their children. Both parents will undergo testing for the same *RB1* gene change/deletion. If the mutation is identified in one of the parents, their other children have a 50% chance of inheriting the altered gene. Blood relatives of that parent may also be at risk for developing retinoblastoma. If the *RB1* gene change/deletion is not identified in either parent, there is a 90–94% likelihood that the retinoblastoma was not inherited. If the mutated *RB1* gene change/deletion is detected in only some of the patient's blood cells, it is assumed that the retinoblastoma is the somatic form, and siblings and other relatives are not at increased risk. Patients' offspring could be at increased risk, however, since some of their egg or sperm cells might contain the changed/deleted *RB1* gene. The risk to offspring is probably less than 50%.

PRENATAL TESTING. If chromosome or DNA testing identifies an inherited *RB1* gene mutation/deletion in a parent, prenatal testing can be performed. Amniocentesis or chorionic villus sampling is used to obtain fetal cells that can then be analyzed for the *RB1* gene mutation or chromosomal abnormality.

Prenatal detection of tumors by ultrasound may be performed for at-risk fetuses. During ultrasound, a handheld instrument is placed on the mother's abdomen or inserted vaginally. It produces sound waves that are reflected back from the fetal structures, producing a picture on a video screen. If a tumor is detected, the baby may be delivered a few weeks early to allow intervention and treatment to begin immediately.

Treatment team

If possible, retinoblastoma should be treated at a medical center with a team of cancer specialists. The team may include a primary-care pediatrician, an ophthalmologist experienced in treating retinoblastoma, pediatric medical oncologists, pediatric surgeons, radiation oncologists, rehabilitation specialists, pediatric nurse specialists, genetic specialists, and social workers.

KEY TERMS

Amniocentesis—Prenatal testing performed at 16–20 weeks of gestation by inserting a needle through the mother's abdomen and obtaining a small sample of amniotic fluid containing fetal cells for biochemical and/or DNA testing.

Bilateral retinoblastoma—A form of retinoblastoma in which tumors affect both eyes.

Brachytherapy—Cancer treatment that involves radioactive material administered directly to the site of a tumor.

Chorionic villus sampling (CVS)—Prenatal testing performed at 10–12 weeks of gestation for biochemical and/or DNA testing of fetal cells.

Chromosomes—The structures within each cell that contain the genes; human somatic cells have 23 pairs of chromosomes.

Cryotherapy—Cancer treatment that destroys a tumor by freezing.

DNA (deoxyribonucleic acid)—The hereditary material that makes up genes that control development and function.

DNA testing—Genetic testing for gene mutations.

Enucleation—Surgical removal of an eye.

Extraocular retinoblastoma—Cancer that has spread beyond the eye.

Gene—A building block of inheritance, made up of DNA and containing instructions for the production of a particular protein; each gene has a specific location on a chromosome.

Germline—A genetic trait such as a mutation that is carried in the egg or sperm and transmitted to offspring.

Intraocular retinoblastoma—Cancer that is confined to the eye and has not spread to other parts of the body.

Leukocoria—An abnormal red reflex; a pupil that reflects white instead of black or red on a flash photograph; indicative of retinoblastoma.

Malignant tumor—Cancer; an abnormal proliferation of cells that can spread to other sites.

Multifocal—Referring to more than one independent tumor.

Mutation—An inherited or spontaneous change in the DNA sequence of a gene.

Oncogene—A gene that has the potential to turn a cell cancerous.

Oncologist—A physician who specializes in the diagnosis and treatment of cancer.

Ophthalmologist—A physician who specializes in diseases of the eye.

Optic nerve—The nerve fibers that transmit signals from the eye to the brain.

Photocoagulation—Cancer treatment that destroys a tumor with an intense beam of laser light.

Prenatal testing—Testing for a disease, such as a genetic condition, in an unborn baby.

RB1—A cell-cycle control and tumor-suppressor gene; deletion or mutation of RB1 can lead to retinoblastoma.

Retina—The light-sensitive layer of the eye that receives images and sends them to the brain.

Scotoma—An area of lost or depressed vision within the visual field that is surrounded by an area of normal vision.

Somatic—Referring to all the cells of the body except egg and sperm cells; a noninheritable mutation that occurs spontaneously or sporadically in a cell other than an egg or sperm.

Trilateral retinoblastoma—Retinoblastomas in both eyes and an independent brain tumor.

Tumor—Tissue growth that results from the uncontrolled proliferation of cells.

Tumor suppressor gene—A gene that controls normal cell growth and prevents cancer.

Unifocal retinoblastoma—A single tumor in one eye.

Unilateral retinoblastoma—Cancer that affects only one eye.

Clinical staging

There are several different staging (classification) systems to establish the severity of retinoblastoma and aid in choosing an appropriate treatment plan. During the 1990s, preferred treatment shifted from radiation to **chemotherapy** due to the risk of secondary tumors following radiation, and new staging systems were developed to reflect this change. The International Retinoblastoma Staging System (IRSS) is based on cancer remaining after surgical removal of the tumor and whether the cancer has spread:

• stage 0—the tumor is treated without surgery and the eye is not removed

- stage I—no cancer cells are detected after removal of the eye (enucleation)
- stage II—cancer cells are detectable only microscopically after enucleation
- stage IIIa—cancer has spread to tissues around the eye socket
- stage IIIb—cancer has spread to lymph nodes near the ear or in the neck
- stage IVa—cancer has spread to the blood, but not to the brain or spinal cord, and there are one or more tumors
- stage IVb—cancer has spread to the brain or spinal cord and possibly other parts of the body

Intraocular retinoblastoma may involve only the retina or other parts of the eye. Extraocular disease may involve only tissues surrounding the eye or metastasis to the brain or other body parts. It is also important to establish whether the cancer is unilateral, bilateral, trilateral, unifocal, or multifocal. Multifocal retinoblastoma involves tumors that have arisen independently rather than from metastasis.

Treatment

Treatment is based on the stage of the cancer. The goal is to cure the cancer and preserve as much vision as possible. Since the late 1990s, chemotherapy and focal therapies have replaced enucleation and external-beam **radiation therapy** whenever possible. Improved methods of chemoreduction (tumor shrinkage) have greatly increased preservation of affected eyes, often with some visual function.

Chemotherapy

Intraocular retinoblastoma is treated with mild intravenous chemotherapy with one or more drugs to shrink tumors prior to laser treatment, **cryotherapy**, or plaque brachytherapy. Occasionally, chemotherapy is used alone to treat very small tumors. Periocular chemotherapy involves the application of high doses of **carboplatin** directly to the eye, with fewer effects on the rest of the body. It may be administered multiple times. Intra-arterial chemotherapy is a new treatment for advanced disease, in which the drug is injected directly into the artery leading to the eye. Systemic (whole-body) chemotherapy almost never cures intraocular retinoblastoma.

Enucleation

Enucleation remains the most common treatment, because by the time unilateral retinoblastoma is diagnosed, the tumor is often so large that useful vision cannot be preserved. The eye is surgically removed under general anesthesia. The procedure usually takes less than an hour, and most children can leave the hospital the same day. A temporary ball is placed in the eye socket. Approximately three weeks following the operation, a plastic artificial eye (prosthesis) that looks like the normal eye is inserted into the eye socket. When both eyes are affected, the more involved eye may be enucleated, while the second eye is treated with vision-preserving therapy.

Radiation

External-beam radiation therapy is often used to treat large tumors when sight preservation is possible. If the tumor has not spread extensively, the radiation beam can be focused on the cancerous retinal cells. If the cancer is extensive, radiation treatment of the entire eye may be necessary. External-beam radiation is performed on an outpatient basis, usually over a period of three to four weeks. Newer forms of therapy, such as intensity-modulated radiation, stereotactic radiation therapy, and proton-beam therapies, target the tumor while sparing nearby tissues. Some patients may need sedatives prior to the treatment.

Radiation therapy sometimes results in temporary loss of a patch of hair on the back of the head and a small area of "sunburned" skin. Long-term side effects may include cataracts, vision problems, bleeding from the retina, and decreased growth of the bones on the side of the head. People with inherited retinoblastoma are at increased risk of developing other cancers as a result of this therapy.

Other treatments

Laser therapy includes photocoagulation, in which intense light is focused through the pupil to destroy the cancer, and laser **hyperthermia**, which kills cancer cells with high temperature. These therapies are very effective in destroying smaller tumors. A new laser delivery system called a DioPexy probe aims the light through the wall of the eye rather than the pupil. Laser therapy is performed under local or general anesthesia and does not usually cause postprocedural pain.

Cryotherapy freezes smaller tumors. It is performed under local or general anesthesia. A pen-like probe is placed on the sclera adjacent to the tumor. Cryotherapy often must be repeated multiple times to successfully destroy all of the cancer cells.

Plaque brachytherapy is the application of radioactive material to the outer surface of the eye at the base of the tumor. It is generally used for medium-sized tumors and requires a surgical procedure to attach the material and a second surgery to remove it. The plaques, containing the radioactive isotope iodine-125, are custom-made for each child. The patient is usually hospitalized for three to seven days during the procedure. Long-term side effects can include cataracts and damage to the retina, which can impair vision.

Alternative and complementary therapies

There are no alternative or complementary therapies specific to retinoblastoma. Most drug-based alternative therapies for general cancer are not appropriate for young children. However, a well-balanced diet, including certain fruits, vegetables, and vitamin supplements, helps ensure that the body is strengthened in its fight against cancer. Some practitioners advocate the use of visualization, in which patients visualize their body's immune cells attacking and destroying the cancer cells.

Prognosis

In the United States, more than 95% of children treated for retinoblastoma are cured; more than 90% retain at least one eye; and more than 80% retain 20/20 vision. The majority of children with bilateral retinoblastoma recover with good vision in at least one eye and often retain vision in both eyes. Visual-field defects are common after treatment, especially scotomas—areas of lost or depressed vision within an area of normal vision. The size and type of these visual defects are determined by the size and type of the original tumor and the type of therapy used to treat it. However, bilateral retinoblastoma and the 15% of unilateral retinoblastomas that are inherited put children at significantly increased lifelong risk of other cancers, especially if they were treated with radiation. Furthermore, inherited unilateral retinoblastoma has a 70% risk of developing in the other eye, compared to a 5% risk in patients with somatic unilateral retinoblastoma. Retinoblastoma only rarely metastasizes to the brain, spinal cord, and bones. Children with inherited retinoblastoma are more likely to die of second tumors than of metastasized retinoblastoma. Trilateral retinoblastoma has a very poor prognosis. Children with any form of retinoblastoma in developing countries may have a poor prognosis due to lack of access to treatment.

Coping with cancer treatment

Side effects of chemotherapy can include nausea, vomiting, and hair loss. There are a number of drugs that can decrease or even eliminate **nausea and vomiting**. Hair loss can be very traumatic for older children, but a wig may be helpful until the hair grows back. Chemotherapy also can temporarily decrease the levels of:

• white blood cells, thereby increasing susceptibility to infection and requiring early recognition and treatment

with antibiotics—high fevers should be reported immediately and may require hospitalization

• red blood cells, which can result in fatigue or shortness of breath

• platelets, which can increase the risk of bruising or prolonged bleeding after an injury and which sometimes require platelet transfusions

Retinoblastoma and its treatments, such as enucleation and radiation, can result in vision impairment and some mild disfigurement around the eye. Children can often be helped by programs for the visually impaired. It is recommended that children who have undergone enucleation wear glasses to protect the remaining eye. Special glasses may be recommended for contact sports. If necessary, **reconstructive surgery** following enucleation or radiation treatment can improve the appearance of the area around the eye. Eye drops and ointments are used to counteract side effects, such as swelling and inflammation, that are associated with cancer treatments such as brachytherapy and cryotherapy.

Clinical trials

As of 2014, there were 27 open trials listed for retinoblastoma. Information is available at http://clinicaltrials.gov/search/open/condition=%22Retinoblastoma%22.

Prevention

Retinoblastoma cannot be prevented, but appropriate screening and surveillance of all at-risk children can ensure that the tumor(s) are diagnosed at an early stage. Early diagnosis increases the likelihood of retaining the affected eye and preserving vision. Several professional academies have jointly recommended red-reflex screening for all newborns prior to discharge from the neonatal nursery and for all infants and children on subsequent health checkups.

Post-treatment screening

Children treated for retinoblastoma require periodic dilated retinal examinations until the age of five and periodic eye exams thereafter. Those with bilateral or inherited retinoblastoma may require periodic screening for **brain tumors**. All lumps and complaints of **bone pain** should be thoroughly evaluated.

Screening of relatives

Parents and siblings of a child diagnosed with inherited retinoblastoma should have a dilated retinal examination by an ophthalmologist experienced with the disease. Siblings should undergo periodic retinal examinations under anesthesia until age three and periodic eye examinations until age seven. Children of anyone diagnosed with

QUESTIONS TO ASK YOUR DOCTOR

- Which form and stage of retinoblastoma does my child have? Has the cancer spread beyond the eye?
- Is this an inherited disease? Should other family members be tested?
- What treatment options are appropriate?
- What are the chances of preserving my child's vision?
- Are there support groups in the area to help my family cope with this diagnosis?

retinoblastoma should also undergo periodic retinal exams. Retinal examinations are unnecessary if DNA testing indicates that the patient has a non-inherited form or if the sibling or other family member has not inherited the *RB1* mutation. Any relatives who are found through genetic testing to have inherited an *RB1* gene mutation/deletion should undergo surveillance procedures.

Special concerns

Since retinoblastoma primarily affects young children, parents have the difficult task of helping the doctor explain the condition and prognosis to their child. A diagnosis of retinoblastoma can be very frightening for children. It is very important for parents to be open and honest about the disease. Some parents have found it helpful to read their child a story about another child facing the same condition. Talking to other children with the same diagnosis can also be helpful. Talking to a counselor or using relaxation therapies may help children deal with their emotions and fears.

Children with retinoblastoma may experience difficulties with self-image due to the temporary loss of hair or the loss of one or both eyes. It is important to remind children about their many positive qualities. It is also important to teach them strategies for coping with questioning or teasing by other children.

A diagnosis of retinoblastoma affects the entire family. For some, therapy may be necessary to ensure that the family can cope with stresses associated with this diagnosis. Talking with other families who have children with retinoblastoma may be helpful.

In general, most children and families cope very well with diagnosis and treatment for retinoblastoma. The prognosis is usually very good, so it is important that parents strive to maintain a positive outlook.

Resources

BOOKS

Edelman, Emily, et al. "Genetics of Retinoblastoma." In *Genetic Diseases of the Eye,* edited by Elias I. Traboulsi. 2nd ed. New York: Oxford University, 2012.

Judd, Sandra J. *Eye Sourcebook.* 4th ed. Detroit: Omnigraphics, 2012.

Judd, Sandra J. *Genetic Disorders Sourcebook.* 5th ed. Detroit: Omnigraphics, 2014.

PERIODICALS

Abramson, David H. "Retinoblastoma: Saving Life With Vision." *Annual Review of Medicine* 65 (2014): 171.

Wong, Jeannette R., et al. "Retinoblastoma Incidence Patterns in the US Surveillance, Epidemiology, and End Results Program." *Archives of Ophthalmology* 132, no. 4 (April 2014): 478.

WEBSITES

American Academy of Ophthalmology. "What Is Retinoblastoma?" eyeSmart. http://www.geteyesmart.org/eyesmart/diseases/retinoblastoma.cfm (accessed June 19, 2014).

Choe, Christina, and Joan M. O'Brien. "Retinoblastoma." EyeWiki. January 22, 2013. http://eyewiki.aao.org/Retinoblastoma (accessed June 19, 2014).

"Eye Cancer." MedlinePlus. June 16, 2014. http://www.nlm.nih.gov/medlineplus/eyecancer.html (accessed June 19, 2014).

"Retinoblastoma." American Cancer Society. http://www.cancer.org/cancer/retinoblastoma/index (accessed June 19, 2014).

"Retinoblastoma." National Cancer Institute. http://www.cancer.gov/cancertopics/types/retinoblastoma (accessed June 19, 2014).

"Retinoblastoma." Pediatric Cancer Care. Memorial Sloan Kettering Cancer Center. http://www.mskcc.org/pediatrics/childhood/retinoblastoma (accessed June 19, 2014).

ORGANIZATIONS

American Academy of Ophthalmology, PO Box 7424, San Francisco, CA 94120-7424, (415) 561-8500, Fax: (415) 561-8533, aaoe@aao.org, http://www.aao.org.

American Cancer Society, 250 Williams Street NW, Atlanta, GA 30303, (800) 227-2345, http://www.cancer.org.

National Cancer Institute, 6116 Executive Boulevard, Suite 300, Bethesda, MD 20892-8322, (800) 4-CANCER (422-6237), http://www.cancer.gov.

National Eye Institute Information Office, 31 Center Drive, MSC 2510, Bethesda, MD 20992-3655, (301) 496-5248, 2020@nei.nih.gov, http://www.nei.nih.gov.

Retinoblastoma International, 18030 Brookhurst Street, Box 408, Fountain Valley, CA 92708.info@retinoblastoma.net, http://www.retinoblastoma.net.

Lisa Andres, M.S., C.G.C.
Rebecca J. Frey, PhD
Margaret Alic, PhD

Rhabdomyosarcoma

Definition

Rhabdomyosarcoma is a childhood **cancer**. It begins in cells that will become skeletal muscle cells. Skeletal muscle is attached to bones and is different from the smooth muscle that lines the intestinal tract (esophagus, stomach, small and large intestines). With rhabdomyosarcoma, these muscle cells grow uncontrollably and form masses or lumps called tumors. They can start almost anywhere in the body where there is skeletal muscle.

Description

Rhabdomyosarcomas can start in any organ that contains skeletal muscle cells, but most commonly tumors are found in the head and neck and in the prostate, bladder, and vagina. From 5%–8% of all cancers diagnosed in children are rhabdomyosarcomas.

Demographics

Rhabdomyosarcoma occurs most frequently in children ages 2 to 6 and 15 to 19 years old. More males than females develop rhabdomyosarcomas. Among younger children, the tumor is usually in the head and neck and may involve the area surrounding the eye. Less often, young children develop rhabdomyosarcomas of the genitourinary tract (bladder, prostate, vagina).

In the older age group, the most likely site is the male genitourinary tract, especially the testes and surrounding area. Other body parts where rhabdomyosarcoma may begin are on the arms, legs, trunk, or deep inside the abdomen (retroperitoneum).

Some cases of rhabdomyosarcoma run in families and are linked to genetic syndromes. Immediate family members of children with rhabdomyosarcoma are at increased risk of developing certain cancers that are not rhabdomyosarcomas, such as breast and **brain tumors**.

Causes and symptoms

The causes of rhabdomyosarcoma are not known. Certain inherited conditions that run in families increase the risk of developing this cancer. Rhabdomyosarcoma has been linked to medical conditions such as fetal alcohol syndrome, neurofibromatosis, Gorlin's syndrome, and **Li-Fraumeni syndrome**.

The symptoms of rhabdomyosarcoma depend on the site of the tumor and whether it has spread. When rhabdomyosarcoma begins in the head, it may involve the area surrounding the eye, the nasal passages, or the ear and throat. Tumors in these areas may cause swelling, especially around the eye; blocked nasal passages or sinuses; ear pain and bleeding; and difficulties swallowing. Rhabdomyosarcomas in the head and neck may also put pressure on the brain or nerves.

When rhabdomyosarcoma affects an arm, leg or other body part, the swelling may be mistaken for a bruise or other injury. When the genitals or urinary tract are involved, there may be symptoms such as recurring urinary tract infections, blood in the urine, incontinence, or blockage of the urinary tract or rectum.

Rhabdomyosarcoma affecting the testes may cause swelling of the scrotum. When the uterus or vagina is affected, there may be a mass or small tumor pushing into the vaginal canal.

Diagnosis

Some patients who have rhabdomyosarcomas go to the doctor because they have discovered a lump or mass or swelling on a body part. Others have symptoms related to the part of the body affected by the tumor. The patient's doctor will take a detailed medical history to investigate the symptoms. The history is followed by a complete physical examination with special attention to the suspicious symptom or body part.

Depending on the location of the tumor (mass or lump), the doctor will order **imaging studies** such as x-ray, ultrasound, **computed tomography** (CT) scans, and **magnetic resonance imaging** (MRI) to help determine the size, shape, and exact location of the tumor. The doctor may also order bone scans to determine whether the tumor has spread to bones. Blood tests will be done and an examination of the bone marrow also may be performed.

A **biopsy** of the tumor is necessary to make the diagnosis of rhabdomyosarcoma. During a biopsy, some tissue from the tumor is removed. The tissue sample is

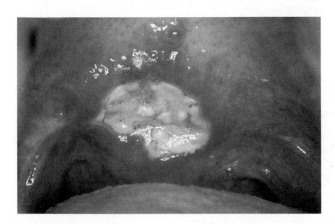

Rhabdomyosarcoma, a malignant tumor affecting the inside of the mouth. *(SPL/Custom Medical Stock Photography)*

KEY TERMS

Biopsy—The surgical removal and microscopic examination of living tissue for diagnostic purposes.

Chemotherapy—Treatment of cancer with synthetic drugs that destroy the tumor either by inhibiting the growth of cancerous cells or by killing them.

Metastasis—The spread of cancer cells from a primary site to distant parts of the body.

Oncologist—A doctor who specializes in cancer medicine.

Pathologist—A doctor who specializes in the diagnosis of disease by studying cells and tissues under a microscope.

Radiation therapy—Treatment using high-energy radiation from x-ray machines, cobalt, radium, or other sources.

Stage—A term used to describe the size and extent of spread of cancer.

examined by a pathologist, a doctor who specializes in the study of diseased tissue.

Types of biopsy

The type of biopsy done depends on the location of the tumor. For some small tumors, such as those on the arm or leg, the doctor may perform an excisional biopsy, removing the entire tumor and a margin of surrounding normal tissue. Most often, the doctor will perform an incisional biopsy, a procedure that involves cutting out only a piece of the tumor. This biopsy provides a core of tissue from the tumor that is used to determine its type and grade.

Treatment team

Patients with rhabdomyosarcoma are usually cared for by a multidisciplinary team of health professionals. The patient's pediatrician or primary care doctor may refer the patient to other physician specialists, such as surgeons and oncologists (doctors who specialize in cancer medicine). Radiologic technicians perform x-ray, CT, and MRI scans, and nurses and laboratory technicians may obtain samples of blood, urine, and other laboratory tests.

Before and after any surgical procedures, specially trained nurses may explain the procedures and help to prepare patients and families. Depending on the tumor location and treatment plan, patients may also benefit from rehabilitation therapy with physical therapists and nutritional counseling from dieticians.

Clinical staging

The purpose of staging a tumor is to determine how far it has advanced. This step is important because treatment varies depending on the stage. Stage is determined by the size of the tumor, whether the tumor has spread to nearby lymph nodes, and whether the tumor has spread elsewhere in the body.

Tumors are staged using numbers to designate stages I through IV. The higher the number, the further the tumor has advanced. Stage I rhabdomyosarcomas have not extended beyond the site where they began; they are limited to a single muscle or organ. Stage II tumors show signs of spread beyond the muscle or organ where they began. Stage III rhabdomyosarcomas are tumors that could not be removed in their entirety by surgery. As a result, some tumor remains at the site where it began. Stage IV rhabdomyosarcomas have involved either lymph nodes or have spread to distant parts of the body.

Treatment

Treatment for rhabdomyosarcoma varies depending on the location of the tumor, its size and grade, and the extent of its spread. By the time most cases of rhabdomyosarcoma are diagnosed, there has already been some spread of the disease. For these patients, the goals of treatment are to remove or control the tumor and combat the spread of the cancer.

Generally, when completely removing the tumor will not sharply reduce function, rhabdomyosarcoma tumors are surgically removed. The site, size, and extent of the tumor determine the type of surgery performed. The goal of removing as much tumor as possible is to reduce the amount of radiation needed after surgery. The part of the body where the tumor was removed is treated with radiation to destroy remaining tumor cells. Many patients also receive **chemotherapy**.

When the disease has spread throughout the body, there may be no benefit from surgical removal of the tumor. These cases, usually patients with stage IV tumors, are treated with chemotherapy.

Side effects

The surgical treatment of rhabdomyosarcoma carries risks related to the surgical site, such as loss of function resulting from head and neck surgeries. Head and neck surgeries may also result in deformities that may be cosmetically unsatisfactory. There are also the medical risks associated with any surgical procedure, such as reactions to general anesthesia or infection after surgery.

The side effects of **radiation therapy** depend on the site being irradiated. Radiation therapy can produce side effects such as **fatigue**, skin rashes, nausea, **diarrhea**, and secondary cancers. Most of the side effects lessen or disappear completely after the radiation therapy has been completed.

The side effects of chemotherapy vary depending on the medication, or combination of **anticancer drugs**, used. Nausea, vomiting, **anemia**, lowered resistance to infection, and hair loss are common side effects. Medication may be given to reduce the unpleasant side effects of chemotherapy.

Alternative and complementary therapies

Many patients explore alternative and complementary therapies to help to reduce the stress associated with illness, improve immune function, and feel better. While there is no evidence that these therapies specifically combat disease, activities such as biofeedback, relaxation, therapeutic touch, massage therapy, and guided imagery have been reported to enhance well-being.

Prognosis

The outlook for patients with rhabdomyosarcoma varies. It depends on the site of the tumor, how the cancer cells look under the microscope, and the extent of spread. For example, patients with tumors affecting the area around the eye and the bladder are more likely to do well than patients with tumors that begin deep within the chest or abdomen.

Rhabdomyosarcoma may spread to areas near the tumor and to nearby lymph glands. To spread to distant parts of the body, the cells travel in the blood or through the lymph glands. The most common sites for **metastasis** (spread) are the lymph glands near the tumor, the lung, liver, bone marrow, and brain. In general, tumors that have spread widely throughout the body are not associated with favorable survival rates.

Patients with stage I tumors that are completely removed surgically have excellent prognoses; eight-year survival is nearly 75%. Sixty-five percent of patients with stage II tumors are disease free after 8 years. Stage I and II rhabdomyosarcomas account for about 40% of all cases.

About 40% of patients with stage III and 15% of those with stage IV rhabdomyosarcomas are disease free after 8 years. Patients with tumors that do not respond to treatment and those who suffer recurrences have poor outlooks for long-term survival.

Coping with cancer treatment

Toddlers, children, and teens undergoing cancer treatment have special needs. The diagnosis of a life-threatening illness, surgery, and radiation or chemotherapy may cause fear, anxiety, **depression**, and loss of self-esteem. Toddlers may be especially fearful when they are separated from their parents for medical tests and hospital stays. Disruption of their normal routines and discomfort from diagnostic tests and treatment may also cause anxiety. Older children face additional social problems, including making up missed schoolwork, explaining the illness and treatment to friends, and coping with physical limitations or disability.

Teens with serious illnesses and disabilities face special conflicts and challenges. One conflict is between the teen's growing desire for independence and the reality of dependence on others for the activities of daily living. It is important for teens to be fully informed about their disease and treatment plan and involved in treatment decision making. Many teens benefit from continuing contact with friends, classmates, teachers, and family during hospital stays and recovery at home.

Depression, emotional distress, and anxiety associated with the disease and its treatment may respond to counseling from a mental health professional. Play therapy often helps toddlers and young children to reveal and express their feelings about illness and treatment. Many cancer patients and their families find that participation in mutual aid and group support programs helps to relieve feelings of isolation and loneliness. By sharing problems with others who have lived through similar difficulties patients and families can exchange ideas and coping strategies.

Clinical trials

About 25 clinical studies were under way during 2014. Several studies were examining the proteins in people with rhabdomyosarcoma to find changes in DNA and other **tumor markers** in order to help improve diagnosis and treatment methods.

To learn more about clinical trials, visit the **National Cancer Institute** (NCI) website at http://www.cancer.gov/clinicaltrials/search.

Prevention

Since the causes of rhabdomyosarcoma are not known, there are no recommendations about ways to prevent its development. Among families with an inherited

QUESTIONS TO ASK YOUR DOCTOR

- What stage is the rhabdomyosarcoma?
- What are the recommended treatments?
- What are the side effects of the recommended treatments?
- Is treatment expected to cure the disease or only to prolong life?

tendency to develop soft tissue sarcomas, careful monitoring may help to ensure early diagnosis and treatment of the disease.

Special concerns

Rhabdomyosarcoma, like other cancer diagnoses, may produce a range of emotional reactions in patients and families. Education, counseling, and participation in group support programs can help to reduce feelings of guilt, fear, anxiety, and hopelessness. For many parents suffering from spiritual distress, visits with clergy members and participation in organized prayer may offer comfort.

Resources

PERIODICALS

Chauhan, K., Jain, M., Shukla, P., Grover, R.K. "Rhabdomyosarcoma Infiltrating Bone Marrow." *International Journal of Hematology* (October 28, 2014): e-pub ahead of print. http://dx.doi.org/10.1007/s12185-014-1692-x (accessed November 14, 2014).

WEBSITES

A.D.A.M. Medical Encyclopedia. "Rhabdomyosarcoma." Medline Plus. http://www.nlm.nih.gov/medlineplus/ency/article/001429.htm (accessed November 14, 2014).
American Cancer Society. "What is Rhabdomyosarcoma?" http://www.cancer.org/cancer/rhabdomyosarcoma/detailedguide/rhabdomyosarcoma-what-is-rhabdomyosarcoma (accessed November 14, 2014).

ORGANIZATIONS

American Cancer Society, 250 Williams St. NW, Atlanta, GA 30303, (800) 227-2345, http://www.cancer.org.
National Cancer Institute, 9609 Medical Center Dr., BG 9609 MSC 9760, Bethesda, MD 20892-9760, (800) 4-CANCER (422-6237), http://www.cancer.gov.
National Children's Cancer Society (NCCS), 500 N. Broadway, Ste. 800, St. Louis, MO 63102, (314) 241-1600, http://www.thenccs.org.

Barbara Wexler, M.P.H.

Richter syndrome

Definition

Richter syndrome is a rare and aggressive type of acute adult leukemia that results from a transformation of **chronic lymphocytic leukemia** into diffuse large-cell **lymphoma**.

Description

Leukemia is a group of cancers of the white blood cells. In adults, white blood cells are made in the bone marrow of the flat bones (skull, shoulder blades, ribs, hip bones). There are three main types of white blood cells: granulocytes, monocytes, and lymphocytes. Richter syndrome concerns only the lymphocytes.

Lymphocytic leukemia develops from lymphocytes in the bone marrow. Unlike many other cancers in which a tumor starts growing in one particular location, lymphocytic leukemia is a disease of blood cells that travel throughout the body. In chronic (long-term) lymphocytic leukemia (CLL), lymphocytes do not follow a normal life cycle; eventually, too many will exist in the blood. These cells are abnormal and do not fight infections well.

In a small percentage of people, CLL, even when it is treated, transforms into a new kind of aggressive blood **cancer** called diffuse large-cell lymphoma. When this transformation occurs, it is called Richter syndrome. The disease is named for the American pathologist Maurice Nathaniel Richter, who practiced medicine early in the twentieth century.

Demographics

Richter syndrome is a disease of older adults. It is an extremely rare disease. The American Cancer Society estimated that in 2014, there were 15,720 new cases of chronic lymphocytic leukemia. Of these, only a handful (about 500 per year in the United States) will develop into Richter syndrome. In general, people who are more likely to get CLL are those who smoke, have been exposed to high doses of radiation, or have had long-term exposure to herbicides and **pesticides**. People who have close relatives (parent, siblings, or children) with CLL are also more likely to develop the disease. However, none of these risk factors predict whether CLL will develop into Richter syndrome.

Causes and symptoms

Scientists have yet to understand why some people develop Richter syndrome and others do not. So far, no firm genetic or environmental links have been found.

KEY TERMS

Lymph nodes—Small, bean-shaped collections of tissue found in lymph vessels. They produce cells and proteins that fight infection and filter lymph. Nodes are sometimes called lymph glands.

Lymphatic system—Primary defense against infection in the body. The tissues, organs, and channels (similar to veins) that produce, store, and transport lymph and white blood cells to fight infection.

Lymphoma—A cancer of the lymphatic system.

When the transformation from CLL to Richter syndrome occurs, a change occurs in the way the lymphocytes look under the microscope. In addition, lymph nodes swell; tumors grow rapidly in the lymphatic system; and the patient may experience **fever**, **night sweats**, and **weight loss**. The patient's health deteriorates rapidly and severely.

Diagnosis

Diagnosis is made by examining blood cells under microscope and by a **bone marrow biopsy**. This is the same test used to diagnose CLL. A small amount of bone marrow from one of the flat bones is drawn out with a needle for laboratory examination. In some cases, lymph nodes are also removed and examined in the laboratory.

Treatment team

Because a person who develops Richter syndrome is already a cancer patient, a treatment team is already in place. This team usually includes an oncologist (cancer specialist), a hematologist (blood specialist), and possibly a radiation oncologist (specialist in **radiation therapy**), radiation or **chemotherapy** technicians, and nurses with special training in cancer care. With the development of Richter syndrome, a social worker or counselor may be added to the team.

Treatment

Chemotherapy is used to treat Richter syndrome, but treatments are often unsuccessful. In addition, allogeneic **bone marrow transplantation** is currently being tried in some patients. This treatment is not common and is not done at many cancer centers. For Richter syndrome, the median survival rate (the time to which half the patients survive) is less than one year.

Alternative and complementary therapies

Alternative and complementary therapies range from herbal remedies, vitamin supplements, and special diets to spiritual practices, acupuncture, massage, and similar treatments. When these therapies are used in addition to conventional medicine, they are called complementary therapies. When they are used instead of conventional medicine, they are called alternative therapies.

There are no specific alternative therapies directed toward Richter syndrome. However, good nutrition and activities that reduce stress and promote a positive view of life have no unwanted side effects and may help improve the patient's quality of life.

Unlike traditional pharmaceuticals, complementary and alternative therapies are not evaluated by the United States Food and Drug Administration (FDA) for either safety or effectiveness. Patients should be wary of "miracle cures." In order to avoid any harmful side effects or interference with regular cancer treatment, patients should notify their doctors if they are using any herbal remedies, vitamin supplements, or other unprescribed treatments. Alternative and experimental treatments normally are not covered by insurance.

Coping with cancer treatment

Richter syndrome is usually fatal within a short time. Coming to grips with this is tremendously stressful for both the patient and family members. In addition, chemotherapy treatments can cause **fatigue**, nausea, vomiting, and other uncomfortable side effects. Some patients decide to end treatment rather than undergo this discomfort when their chance of recovery is almost non-existent. Others wish to continue full treatment.

This and many other personal decisions are issues to discuss with loved ones. It is often helpful for loved ones to have the support of a therapist, religious leader, or other counselor at this time when emotions are intense and often conflicting. Hospice staff members or hospital social workers or chaplains can direct patients and family members to resources that address their individual needs.

Clinical trials

Many ongoing **clinical trials** related to chronic lymphocytic lymphoma may be appropriate for people with Richter syndrome. Participation is always voluntary. The selection of clinical trials under way changes frequently. Current information on what clinical trials are available and where they are being held is available by entering the search term "chronic lymphocytic lymphoma" at http://www.cancer.gov/clinicaltrials or http://clinicaltrials.gov/.

Prevention

There is no known way to prevent the transformation of CLL into Richter syndrome.

Resources

PERIODICALS

Hillmen, P. "Richter's Syndrome: CLL Taking a Turn for the Worse." *Oncology* 26, no. 12 (2012): 1155–6. http://www.cancernetwork.com/oncology-journal/richters-syndrome-cll-taking-turn-worse (accessed November 14, 2014).

WEBSITES

Cancer Research UK. "Richter's Syndrome." http://www.cancerresearchuk.org/about-cancer/cancers-in-general/cancer-questions/what-is-richters-syndrome (accessed November 14, 2014).

National Cancer Institute. "Richter Syndrome." http://www.cancer.gov/dictionary?cdrid=489396 (accessed November 14, 2014).

ORGANIZATIONS

American Cancer Society, 250 Williams St. NW, Atlanta, GA 30303, (800) 227-2345, http://www.cancer.org.

Leukemia & Lymphoma Society, 1311 Mamaroneck Ave., Ste. 310, White Plains, NY 10605, (914) 949-5213, Fax: (914) 949-6691, infocenter@lls.org, http://www.lls.org.

National Cancer Institute, 9609 Medical Center Dr., BG 9609 MSC 9760, Bethesda, MD 20892-9760, (800) 4-CANCER (422-6237), http://www.cancer.gov.

Tish Davidson, A.M.

Ritalin *see* **Methylphenidate**

Rituxan *see* **Rituximab**

Rituximab

Definition

Rituximab is a monoclonal antibody that selectively binds to CD20, a protein found on the surface of normal and malignant B cells. A monoclonal antibody is a type of protein produced in a laboratory. Rituximab is used to reduce the numbers of circulating B cells, a type of immune system cell, in patients who have B-cell **non-Hodgkin lymphoma** (NHL). Rituximab is sold as Rituxan in the United States.

Purpose

Rituximab is a type of biological therapy, also called **immunotherapy**. The monoclonal antibody is used to treat NHL, which is characterized by overgrowth of B cells, the cell involved in about 85% of NHL malignancies. Of all the B-cell cancers, more than 90% express a protein called CD20 on the cell surface. By binding the CD20 protein on the B cell, the antibody in rituximab targets it for removal from the circulation. Based on data gathered in the laboratory, developers believe that rituximab triggers two kinds of activity to attack the B cells in NHL. First, the antibody attaches to the CD20 protein receptor and programs it with a signal to die. Second, the monoclonal antibody can bring other immune cells into the circulation to help destroy the B cells.

Rituximab has been most effective against low-grade (indolent) or follicular B-cell NHL. Low-grade (slow progression) NHL often responds well to initial treatment but frequently relapses, making rituximab a welcome addition to the treatment options. Additionally, rituximab has been used for a second course of treatments after relapse with some success. As most patients with NHL are in stage III or IV by the time of diagnosis and treatment, rituximab treatment is primarily used in those stages of the disease.

As of 2014, rituximab had also been approved for use in patients with **chronic lymphocytic leukemia**, a slow-growing blood and bone marrow **cancer**. **Clinical trials** were testing the ability of this drug to work against several other types of cancers, including newly diagnosed acute lymphoblastic leukemia (ALL) and newly diagnosed mature B-cell ALL, treatment of NHL or B-cell ALL in younger patients, use of the drug for **mantle cell lymphoma**, and several trials comparing the use of rituximab with other drugs and therapy approaches.

Description

Rituximab is produced in the laboratory using genetically engineered single clones of B cells. Like all

KEY TERMS

Antibody—A protective protein made by the immune system in response to an antigen, also called an immunoglobulin.

Apoptosis—Internal system for cell death, also called programmed cell death.

CD20—A protein found on the surface of normal and malignant B cells.

Humanization—Fusing the constant and variable framework region of one or more human immunoglobulins with the binding region of an animal immunoglobulin, done to reduce human reaction against the fusion antibody.

Monoclonal—Referring to genetically engineered antibodies specific for one antigen.

antibodies, it is a Y-shaped molecule that can bind to one particular substance, the antigen for that monoclonal antibody. For rituximab, that antigen is CD20, a protein found on the surface of B cells. Rituximab is a humanized antibody, meaning that the regions that bind CD20, located on the tips of the Y branches, are derived from mouse antibodies, but the rest of the antibody is a human sequence. The presence of the human sequences helps to reduce the **immune response** by the patient against the antibody itself—a problem seen when complete mouse antibodies were used for cancer therapies. The human sequences also help to ensure that the various cell-destroying mechanisms of the human immune system are properly triggered with binding of the antibody.

In 1997, rituximab was the first unconjugated (not linked to a radioactive isotope or toxin) antibody approved for use by the FDA to treat cancer. It was specifically approved for treatment of low-grade or follicular B-cell NHL. Administration of the antibody resulted in either complete or partial responses in a little less than half of those patients.

Rituximab can be used alone or in combination with other chemotherapeutic drugs. Specifically, very good results have been seen when rituximab is used in combination with the CHOP **chemotherapy** regimen (**cyclophosphamide**, **doxorubicin**, **vincristine**, and prednisone). When used in combination, dosages of the antibody given before beginning chemotherapy, alternating with the other drugs, then after the chemotherapy as a "mop-up" therapy have proven effective.

There are a number of clinical trials in progress testing the ability of rituximab to work in combination with other chemotherapy drugs, treatments, and cytokines. Some substances and treatments being tested include interleukins 2 and 11, **stem cell transplantation**, radioimmunotherapy, vaccination, and a wide variety of other chemotherapy combinations.

Recommended dosage

The recommended dosage for patients with low-grade or follicular NHL is 375 mg/m^2 infused intravenously. The infusion is given at weekly intervals for four total dosages. Acetaminophen and **diphenhydramine** hydrochloride are given 30–60 minutes before the infusion to help reduce side effects. If given as a retreatment, the dosage is the same. Generally, a decrease in symptoms occurs at an average of 55 days after the last administration of the antibody.

Precautions

Serious (even fatal) infusion reactions, especially with the first infusion, have been known with this drug. There are a number of patient conditions that can make taking this drug more dangerous. Specifically, heart problems such as arrhythmias and high blood pressure, and the medications taken to treat those conditions, can lead to problems with this treatment.

Side effects

Most side effects occur after or during the first infusion of the drug. Some common side effects include dizziness, swelling in the tongue or throat, **fever** and chills, flushing of the face, headache, **itching**, **nausea and vomiting**, runny nose, shortness of breath, skin rash, and unusual **fatigue**.

Less common side effects include: black tarry stools; blood in urine or stools; fever or chills with cough or hoarseness; lower back or side pain, or painful or difficult urination; pain at place of injection; pinpoint red spots on skin; red, itchy lining of eye; swelling of feet or lower legs; unusual bleeding or bruising; and unusual weakness.

Although severe side effects are very rare, this drug does have potentially serious side effects, such as chest pain and irregular heartbeat, particularly in patients with heart conditions. It can also cause serious effects on the blood cells, such as low red blood cell count (**anemia**) and low white blood cell count (**neutropenia**). Additionally, this drug has caused low blood pressure (hypotension).

In patients with high tumor burden (a large number of circulating malignant B cells), this drug can cause a side effect called **tumor lysis syndrome**. Thought to be due to the release of the lysed cells' contents into the

QUESTIONS TO ASK YOUR DOCTOR

- What are the potential risks of using this drug?
- May I take my other drugs and vitamins while receiving rituximab?
- Will this treatment cure my disease?
- Can I do anything to lessen the side effects of this treatment?

bloodstream, it can cause an imbalance of urea, uric acid, phosphate, and calcium in the urine and blood. Patients at risk of this side effect must keep hydrated and can be given **allopurinol** (an antigout medication) before infusion.

Interactions

Rituximab can interact with the chemotherapy drug **cisplatin**, resulting in kidney damage. Doctors will advise patients to stop taking blood pressure medicines on the day of treatment because of rituximab's effect of lowering blood pressure. Likewise, because the drug can lower the number of platelets in the blood, patients should talk to doctors about any drugs or supplements they take related to blood clotting.

See also Monoclonal antibodies.

Resources

WEBSITES

AHFS Consumer Medication Information. "Rituximab Injection." American Society of Health-System Pharmacists. Available from: http://www.nlm.nih.gov/medlineplus/druginfo/meds/a607038.html (accessed October 12, 2014).

American Cancer Society. "Rituximab." http://www.cancer.org/treatment/treatmentsandsideeffects/guidetocancerdrugs/rituximab (accessed October 12, 2014).

National Cancer Institute. "Rituximab." http://www.cancer.gov/cancertopics/druginfo/rituximab (accessed October 12, 2014).

"Rituxan (Rituximab)." Genentech USA. http://www.rituxan.com (accessed October 12, 2014).

ORGANIZATIONS

U.S. Food and Drug Administration, 10903 New Hampshire Ave., Silver Spring, MD 20993, (888) INFO-FDA (463-6332), http://www.fda.gov.

Michelle Johnson, MS, JD
REVISED BY TERESA G. ODLE

Rofecoxib *see* **Cyclooxygenase 2 inhibitors**

S

Salagen *see* **Pilocarpine**

Salivary gland tumors

Definition

A salivary gland tumor is an uncontrolled growth of cells that begins in one of the many saliva-producing glands in the mouth.

Description

The tongue, cheeks, and palate (the hard and soft areas on the roof of the mouth) contain many glands that produce saliva. Saliva contains enzymes, or catalysts, that begin the breakdown (digestion) of food while it is still in the mouth. The glands are called salivary glands because of their function.

There are three pairs of larger salivary glands in addition to many smaller ones. The parotid glands, submandibular glands, and sublingual glands are the large paired salivary glands. The parotids are located inside the cheeks, one below each ear. The submandibular glands are located on the floor of the mouth, with one on the inner side of each part of the lower jaw, or mandible. The sublingual glands are also on the floor of the mouth, but they are under the tongue.

The parotids are the salivary glands most often affected by tumors. Yet most of the tumors that grow in the parotid glands are benign, or not cancerous. Approximately 8 out of 10 salivary tumors diagnosed are in a parotid gland. One in 10 diagnosed is in a submandibular gland. The remaining 10% are diagnosed in other salivary glands.

In general, glands more likely to show tumor growth are also glands least likely to show malignant tumor growth. Thus, although tumors of the sublingual glands are rare, almost all of them are malignant. In contrast, about one in four tumors of the parotid glands is malignant.

Cancers of the salivary glands begin to grow in epithelial cells, or the flat cells that cover body surfaces. Thus, they are called carcinomas.

Demographics

Salivary gland cancers are rare. Cancers in the mouth account for fewer than 2% of all cases of **cancer** and about 1.5% of cancer deaths. About 7% of all cancers diagnosed in the head and neck region are diagnosed in a salivary gland. Men and women are at equal risk, and the risk increases as people reach their 60s.

Mortality from salivary gland tumors in the United States is higher among male African Americans below the age of 50 than among older people of any race or either sex; the reasons for this difference are not yet known.

Causes and symptoms

Age, male sex, and having a close relative who has had salivary gland cancer are risk factors for the cancer. When survivors of the 1945 atomic bombings of Nagasaki and Hiroshima began to develop salivary gland tumors at a high rate, radiation was suspected as a cause. Ionizing radiation, particularly gamma radiation, is a factor that contributes to tumor development. So is **radiation therapy**. Adults who received radiation therapy for enlarged adenoids or tonsils when they were children are at greater risk of salivary gland tumors.

Another reported risk factor is an association between wood dust inhalation and **adenocarcinoma** of the minor salivary glands of the nose and paranasal sinuses. Occupational exposure to dust from certain metals and minerals likely increases risk.

Researchers are beginning to understand how changes in certain chromosomes and genes can lead to some types of salivary gland cancers. A genetic process called translocation, which is the switching of some DNA

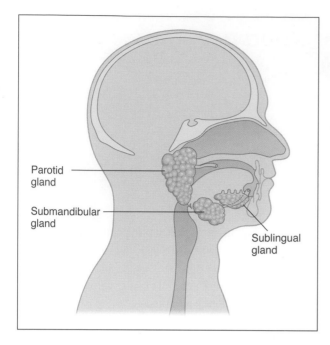

Illustration of the head and neck showing the location of the three main salivary glands: parotid, submandibular, and sublingual. *(Illustration by Electronic Illustrators Group. © Cengage Learning®.)*

on chromosomes, can sometimes cause cancerous cells to grow and may increase the risk of salivary gland cancer. Learning more about these causes could help doctors develop new targeted treatments that would be more effective and cause fewer side effects.

Symptoms are often absent until the tumor is large or has metastasized (spread to other sites). In many cases, the tumor is first discovered by the patient's dentist. During regular dental examinations, the dentist looks for masses on the palate or under the tongue or in the cheeks, and such checkups are a good way to detect tumors early. Some symptoms are:

- lump or mass in the mouth
- swelling in the face
- pain in the jaw or the side of the face
- difficulty swallowing
- difficulty breathing
- difficulty speaking

Diagnosis

A physical examination and medical history are the first steps toward diagnosing salivary gland tumors. A tissue sample will be taken for study via a **biopsy**. Usually an incision is necessary to take the tissue sample. Sometimes it is possible to take a tissue sample with a needle.

Magnetic resonance imaging (MRI) and **computed tomography** (CT) scans are also used to evaluate the tumor. They help determine whether the cancer has spread to sites adjacent to the salivary gland where it is found. MRI offers a good way to examine the tonsils and the back of the tongue, which are soft tissues. CT is used as a way of studying the jaw, which is bone.

Treatment team

Generally, physicians with special training in surgery of the ears, nose, and throat take responsibility for the care of a patient with a salivary gland cancer. They are called otolaryngologists or otorhinolaryngologists.

Otolaryngologists are usually labeled ENT (for Ear, Nose and Throat) specialists. An ENT specializing in cancer will probably lead the team. An oncologist or radiation therapist might be involved, and nurses, as well as a nutritionist, speech therapist, and social worker, will also be part of the team. Depending on the extent of the cancer when diagnosed, some surgery and other treatments result in extensive changes in the throat, neck, and jaw. The social worker, speech therapist, and nutritionist are important in helping the patient cope with the changes caused by surgery and radiation treatment. If there is great alteration to the neck because of surgery, rehabilitation will also be part of the recovery process, and a rehabilitation therapist will become a member of the team.

Clinical staging

To assess the stage of growth of a salivary gland tumor, many features are examined, including its size and the type of abnormal cell growth. Analysis of the types of abnormal cell growth in tissue is so specific that many salivary gland tumors are given unique names.

Salivary gland cancer is staged according to the **American Joint Committee on Cancer** TNM system for cancer staging. The T stands for tumor, and generally indicates tumor size and invasion of nearby tissues. N refers to whether the cancer has spread to nearby lymph nodes, and M refers to the cancer's **metastasis**, or spread to distant areas of the body. The most common organ for metastasis of salivary gland cancer is the lungs. Doctors cannot complete staging information until biopsy results are obtained, and often not until after surgery to remove the tumor.

Treatment

A promising form of treatment for patients at high risk of tumor recurrence in the salivary glands near the base of the skull is gamma knife surgery. Used as a booster treatment following standard neutron radiotherapy, gamma knife surgery appears to be well tolerated by the patients and to have minimal side effects. Doctors also are learning new techniques for surgery to reach tumors that have spread to tissues at the base of the skull. Called skull-base surgery, the technique involves operating through a small incision in the patient's nose and inserting a thin tube called an endoscope to perform the operation. Skull-base surgery is less invasive than traditional head and neck surgery.

Tumors in small salivary glands that are localized can usually be removed without much difficulty. The outlook for survival once the tumor is removed is very good if it has not metastasized.

Alternative and complementary therapies

Techniques such as yoga, meditation, or biofeedback can help a patient cope with anxiety over the condition. Some alternative and complementary therapies also can relieve discomfort from treatment side effects. Patients should discuss alternative and complementary therapies with their oncologist or otolaryngologist.

Prognosis

Most early-stage salivary gland tumors are removed and do not return. Those that do return, or recur, are the most troublesome and reduce the chance that an individual will remain cancer-free. Five-year survival rates for salivary

gland cancers range from 91% for early-stage tumors to 39% for patients whose cancers are diagnosed in late stages, after the cancer has begun to spread to surrounding tissues or distant organs.

Coping with cancer treatment

Many patients are encouraged to join a support group during the course of treatment and follow-up. They should also be encouraged to take an active role in following the recommendations and decisions made by the treatment team.

Clinical trials

There are a number of **clinical trials** in progress. Two trials involve the study of eribulin, a synthetic medication similar to a natural substance produced by marine sponges that inhibits cell division, as a treatment for salivary gland cancer. Participation in clinical trials can provide better treatment options for some patients. Participation is voluntary.

Information on clinical trials can be found online at http://clinicaltrials.gov.

Prevention

Minimizing intake of alcoholic beverages may decrease the risk of developing salivary gland cancer, as may avoiding unnecessary exposure of the head to radiation. The use of condoms may also lower the risk of salivary gland cancer, because some of these cancers have been linked to the sexually transmitted **human papillomavirus** (HPV).

Special concerns

Salivary gland tumors are considered rare. Because there are so many salivary glands, and so many types of salivary tumors, most physicians (even those who specialize in diseases of the ears, nose and throat) are challenged when they must interpret biopsies of salivary gland tissue. For treatment of a salivary gland tumor, it is best to find a medical facility that specializes in diseases of the head and neck. Such a facility will be better able to match treatment to the specific characteristics of the tumor.

See also Oral cancer; Oropharyngeal cancer.

Resources

BOOKS

Beers, Mark H., MD, and Robert Berkow, MD, editors. "Disorders of the Oral Region: Neoplasms." Section 9, Chapter 105. In *The Merck Manual of Diagnosis and Therapy.* Whitehouse Station, NJ: Merck Research Laboratories, 2002.

Woo, Sook-bin. *Oral Pathology: A Comprehensive Atlas and Text.* Philadelphia: Elsevier/Saunders, 2012.

PERIODICALS

Day, T. A., J. Deveikis, M. B. Gillespie, et al. "Salivary Gland Neoplasms." *Current Treatment Options in Oncology* 5 (February 2004): 11–26.

Douglas, J. G., D. L. Silbergeld, and G. E. Laramore. "Gamma Knife Stereotactic Radiosurgical Boost for Patients Treated Primarily with Neutron Radiotherapy for Salivary Gland Neoplasms." *Stereotactic and Functional Neurosurgery* 82 (March 2004): 84–89.

Lawler, B., A. Pierce, P. J. Sambrook, et al. "The Diagnosis and Surgical Management of Major Salivary Gland Pathology." *Australian Dental Journal* 49 (March 2004): 9–15.

Wilson, R. T., L. E. Moore, and M. Dosemeci. "Occupational Exposures and Salivary Gland Cancer Mortality among African American and White Workers in the United States." *Journal of Occupational and Environmental Medicine* 46 (March 2004): 287–297.

Zheng, R., L. E. Wang, M. L. Bondy, et al. "Gamma Radiation Sensitivity and Risk of Malignant and Benign Salivary Gland Tumors: A Pilot Case-Control Analysis." *Cancer* 100 (February 1, 2004): 561–567.

OTHER

American Cancer Society. "Salivary Gland Cancer." http://www.cancer.org/acs/groups/cid/documents/webcontent/003137-pdf.pdf (accessed August 28, 2014).

WEBSITES

American Society of Clinical Oncology. "Salivary Gland Cancer: Overview." Cancer.Net. http://www.cancer.net/cancer-types/salivary-gland-cancer/overview (accessed August 28, 2014).

Johns Hopkins Medicine. "Skull Base Surgery." http://www.hopkinsmedicine.org/healthlibrary/test_procedures/neurological/skull_base_surgery_135,43/ (accessed August 28, 2014).

National Cancer Institute. "General Information About Salivary Gland Cancer." http://www.cancer.gov/cancertopics/pdq/treatment/salivarygland/Patient (accessed August 28, 2014).

ORGANIZATIONS

American Cancer Society, 250 Williams Street NW, Atlanta, GA 30303, (800) 227-2345, http://www.cancer.org.

National Cancer Institute, 9609 Medical Center Drive, Bethesda, MD 20892, (800) 422-6237, http://www.cancer.gov.

Support for People With Head and Neck Cancer, PO Box 53, Locust Valley, NY 11560, (800) 377-0928, Fax: (516) 671-8794, info@spohnc.org, http://www.spohnc.org/.

Diane M. Calabrese
Rebecca J. Frey, PhD
REVISED BY TERESA G. ODLE

Samarium SM 153 Lexidronam *see* **Radiopharmaceuticals**

Sandimmune *see* **Cyclosporine**

Sarcoma

Definition

A general term for any **cancer** of the bone, cartilage, fat, muscle, blood vessels, or other connective or supportive tissues. Sarcomas can be divided into soft tissue and bone (osteogenic) sarcomas. Liposarcomas (cancerous tumors of fat tissue) are an example of soft tissue sarcomas, while **Ewing sarcoma** is considered an osteogenic sarcoma.

Resources

BOOKS

Brennan, Murray F., Cristina R. Antonescu, and Robert G. Maki. *Management of Soft-tissue Sarcoma.* New York: Springer, 2013.

WEBSITES

American Cancer Society. "Sarcoma - Adult Soft Tissue Cancer." http://www.cancer.org/cancer/sarcoma-adultsoft-tissuecancer/ (accessed November 14, 2014).

National Cancer Institute. "General Information About Adult Soft Tissue Sarcoma." http://www.cancer.gov/cancertopics/pdq/treatment/adult-soft-tissue-sarcoma/Patient/page1 (accessed November 14, 2014).

Kate Kretschmann

Sargramostim

Definition

Sargramostim is a medicine used to increase the blood cell counts after bone marrow transplants and **chemotherapy**. Sargramostim may be referred to as GM-CSF or granulocyte-macrophage colony stimulating factor.

Purpose

Sargramostim is a drug approved by the U.S. Food and Drug Administration (FDA) to decrease the time it takes for the bone marrow blood counts to recover after a bone marrow transplant. This therapy decreases the risk of infection, the amount of time patients are treated with **antibiotics**, and the amount of time patients are in the hospital.

Sargramostim is approved for use after chemotherapy to increase the recovery of the white cell counts and decrease the length of time a patient may have a **fever** and infection due to a low white cell count.

Sargramostim can be used after **bone marrow transplantation**. Once the new healthy bone marrow has been given back to a patient, sargramostim can be administered to help increase the blood cell counts and decrease the risk of fever and infection. Sargramostim can be used in patients when bone marrow is not recovering after a bone marrow transplant.

Sargramostim can be used for patients who will undergo a peripheral blood stem cell transplant. Patients will receive the sargramostim before the transplant. The sargramostim in these patients causes young undeveloped blood cells, known as stem or progenitor cells, to move from the bone marrow to the blood where they will then be removed from a patient by the process of apheresis. These blood cells are stored until after the patient receives large doses of chemotherapy that destroy the bone marrow and the **cancer**. The patient then receives these stored cells back by an intravenous infusion. The stored cells repopulate the bone marrow and develop into the many types of functioning blood cells.

Description

Sargramostim is known under the brand name Leukine. It has been available for use in bone marrow transplant patients for almost a decade. In cancer patients, chemotherapy destroys white blood cells temporarily. These white blood cells will be produced again, but during the time that the levels are low, patients are at an increased risk of developing fevers and infection. Sargramostim acts to stimulate the bone marrow to make more white blood cells, which can either prevent the white count from dropping below normal or shorten the time that the level is low. This activity helps patients avoid fevers and infections and allows them to receive their next doses of chemotherapy without delay.

Recommended dosage

Sargramostim is a clear colorless liquid that is dosed based on a mathematical calculation that measures a person's body surface area (BSA). This number is dependent on a patient's height and weight. The larger the

person, the greater the body surface area. Body surface area is measured in units known as square meters (m^2). The body surface area is calculated and then multiplied by the drug dosage in milligrams per square meter (mg/m^2). This formula calculates the actual dose a patient is to receive.

Sargramostim is kept refrigerated until ready to use and it is administered to patients as an injection directly underneath the skin, subcutaneously. Subcutaneous is the preferred way to give the drug; it can be given in the back of the arms, upper legs, or stomach area. Sargramostim can also be administered to patients as a short intravenous infusion into a vein over 15 to 30 minutes.

To treat chemotherapy-related neutropenia in AML patients

The starting dose for AML patients who have just finished induction chemotherapy is 250 micrograms per square meter per day. This dose is given beginning four days after the chemotherapy has ended or approximately day number eleven of therapy. The dose is administered as an intravenous infusion over a period of four hours. The doctor will inform the patient when it is time to stop the sargramostim based on blood count monitoring.

For patients receiving bone marrow transplant

The recommended dose is 250 micrograms per square meter per day administered as a two-hour infusion intravenously. This medication should begin within 2 to 4 hours of the patient receiving the bone marrow infusion.

If the patient's counts are not returning after the bone marrow has been received, sargramostim can be administered at a dose of 250 micrograms per square meter per day intravenously over a two hour time period for 14 consecutive days. This dose can be repeated after a seven-day rest for two more cycles. The doctor may increase the dose to 500 micrograms per square meter per day if the white blood cell count does not rise.

For patients prior to receiving a peripheral blood stem cell transplant

The recommended dose is 250 micrograms per square meter per day. This dose can be given either as a once daily dose administered under the skin, or intravenously as a continuous infusion over 24 hours. This dosage should continue until the last day of collection.

For patients after receiving a peripheral blood stem cell transplant

The recommended dose is 250 micrograms per square meter per day. This dose can be given either as a once daily dose administered under the skin, or intravenously as a continuous infusion over 24 hours. This dosage should begin right after the patient receives the stem cell infusion and continue until the white blood cell count rises to acceptable levels.

Precautions

Sargramostim should not be received by a patient in the 24-hour time frame before or after receiving chemotherapy.

Blood counts will be monitored frequently while on sargramostim. This precaution allows the doctor to determine whether the drug is working and when to stop treatment.

Sargramostim can affect patients who have kidney or liver problems before beginning treatment. These patients will be monitored by the doctor for any changes in kidney or liver function.

It is not recommended to give sargramostim to patients who have certain types of leukemias.

Sargramostim should be used with caution in patients who have fluid problems, including heart and lung problems.

Patients with a known previous allergic reaction to sargramostim or yeast-derived substances should tell their doctor before receiving this drug.

Patients who may be pregnant or trying to become pregnant should tell their doctor before receiving sargramostim.

Side effects

One of the most common side effects of sargramostim is **bone pain**. The drug causes bone marrow to produce more white blood cells, and the process causes the patient to experience pain in their bones.

Other common side effects due to sargramostim administration are fever, muscle aches, chills, and weakness.

An uncommon but serious side effect of sargramostim is increased fluid retention in patients. This swelling with fluid can occur in the body as a whole, legs, arms, around the heart, and in the lungs.

Patients who have received sargramostim treatment have reported: **nausea and vomiting**, muscle pain, abdominal pain, rash, **diarrhea**, hair loss (**alopecia**), mouth sores, **fatigue**, allergic reactions and **itching**, shortness of breath, weakness, dizziness, heart problems, pain at the injection site, blood clots, headache, cough, rash, constipation, and change in kidney and/or liver function. These side effects may be due to chemotherapy received prior to the administration of sargramostim.

Interactions

Sargramostim should not be given at the same time as chemotherapy or **radiation therapy**. Dosing should begin at least 24 hours after the last dose of treatment.

Patients on lithium or steroids should tell their doctor before starting sargramostim therapy, as these drugs can affect the white blood cell count.

Resources

BOOKS

Chu, Edward, and Vincent T. DeVita Jr. *Physicians' Cancer Chemotherapy Drug Manual 2014*. Burlington, MA: Jones & Bartlett Learning, 2014.

WEBSITES

National Cancer Institute. "Sargramostim." http://www.cancer. gov/drugdictionary?cdrid=40566 (accessed November 14, 2014).

The Scott Hamilton CARES Initiative. "Sargramostim." Chemocare.com http://chemocare.com/chemotherapy/ drug-info/Sargramostim.aspx (accessed November 14, 2104).

Nancy J. Beaulieu, RPh, BCOP

Saw palmetto

Definition

Saw palmetto is a natural plant remedy used to treat men who are experiencing difficulty when urinating. According to the Academy of Nutrition and Dietetics, saw palmetto is one of the most commonly used dietary supplements among Americans between the ages of 50 and 76.

Purpose

Saw palmetto is not used to treat **cancer**. It is used to treat nonmalignant enlargement of the prostate gland, also called benign prostatic hyperplasia (BPH).

Although saw palmetto has also been used to treat prostatitis and chronic pelvic pain syndrome (CPPS) in men, it does not appear to be useful for these conditions. A group of researchers at Columbia University reported in early 2004 that men given saw palmetto for CP/CPPS showed no appreciable improvement at the end of a year-long trial.

Description

The prostate gland is found only in men. It is located where the bladder drains into the urethra. The urethra is the tube that takes urine out of the body. The prostate gland contributes to the fluid in which sperm are ejaculated (semen).

It is common for the prostate to enlarge in men over age 50. This enlargement often is not malignant. It is thought to occur because of the action of **testosterone**, a male hormone, on the cells of the prostate. As the prostate grows, it can press on the urethra and narrow it. This causes men to have problems with urination that include the frequent urge to urinate (especially at night) and a weak, dribbling, interrupted urine stream.

Saw palmetto (*Serenoa repens*) is a bushy palm that grows to a height of about 18 feet (6 m) along the coast of the United States from South Carolina to Florida, and in Southern California. It is also found in Europe along the Mediterranean coastline. Other names for this plant are American dwarf palm, cabbage palm, serenoa, or sable. The medicinal part of the saw palmetto is an extract derived from the dark, olive-sized berries.

Saw palmetto has a long history of use by Native Americans in treating bladder inflammation, urinary difficulties, sexual difficulties, and respiratory tract infections. Of these uses, the only scientifically substantiated claim is that saw palmetto eases urinary difficulties and increases urine output. Although the exact mechanism of action of saw palmetto has not been determined, it is believed to interfere with the action of testosterone on the prostate gland. Finasteride (Proscar) is a prescription drug used to treat BPH that works in the same way. It is important to remember that BPH is not cancer, and saw palmetto is not a treatment for cancer.

Recommended dosage

Extract of saw palmetto is available in health food stores in capsules, liquid concentrate, tablets, and as dried, ground berries. An average daily dose of the drug is 1–2 grams, of which 320 mg are the active ingredients. Dosage may vary from manufacturer to manufacturer.

Saw palmetto is classified as a dietary supplement. The United States Food and Drug Administration does not test or certify it. Unlike traditional pharmaceuticals, its manufacture is largely unregulated. Dietary supplements such as saw palmetto are not required to meet standards of purity or effectiveness in controlled **clinical trials**. Men interested in using saw palmetto should look for a reputable manufacturer of supplements who provides adequate testing and label information. The cost of dietary supplements is not covered by insurance.

Precautions

Men who are having trouble urinating should see a doctor before taking any remedies on their own. **Prostate cancer** is a serious, sometimes life-threatening disease, and its symptoms can be similar to those of BPH. A blood test and physical examination are used to diagnose prostate cancer. It is believed that saw palmetto may interfere with this blood test (called a prostate-specific antigen or PSA test). Men should have this blood test done before they begin taking saw palmetto to make sure they get accurate results.

Side effects

Saw palmetto has few side effects, and is generally regarded as safe. Medical authorities in Germany, France, and Italy all officially recognize it as a safe and generally effective treatment for symptoms of BPH. Side effects that have been reported are uncommon but include headache, upset stomach, and **diarrhea**.

Interactions

Because saw palmetto is a natural remedy, few controlled studies have been done on how it interacts with other herbal remedies or traditional pharmaceuticals. Saw palmetto extract should be used with caution with blood thinners or with such over-the-counter drugs as aspirin or NSAIDs because it increases the risk of bleeding. Persons taking birth control pills, estrogen replacement therapy, or testosterone replacement therapy should consult their doctor before taking saw palmetto. Patients taking any supplements such as **vitamins** or herbs should tell their doctor.

Resources

BOOKS

Bagetta, Giacinto, et al., eds. *Herbal Medicines: Development and Validation of Plant-Derived Medicines for Human Health*. Boca Raton, FL: CRC Press, 2012.

WEBSITES

American Cancer Society. "Saw Palmetto." http://www.cancer.org/treatment/treatmentsandsideeffects/complementaryandalternativemedicine/herbsvitaminsandminerals/saw-palmetto (accessed November 14, 2014).

Micromedex. "Saw Palmetto (*Serenoa Repens, Serenoa Serrulata*)." Mayo Clinic. http://www.mayoclinic.org/drugs-supplements/saw-palmetto/background/hrb-20059958 (accessed November 14, 2014).

ORGANIZATIONS

National Center for Complementary and Alternative Medicine, 9000 Rockville Pike, Bethesda, MD 20892, (888) 644-6226, TTY: (866) 464-3615, http://nccam.nih.gov.

Office of Cancer Complementary and Alternative Medicine (OCCAM), 9609 Medical Center Dr., Rockville, MD 20850, (240) 276-6595, nccioccam1-r@mail.nih.gov, http://cam.cancer.gov.

Tish Davidson, AM
Rebecca J. Frey, PhD

Scintigraphy *see* **Nuclear medicine scans**

Scopolamine

Definition

Scopolamine, also called hyoscine hydrobromide, is used in **cancer** treatment to prevent **nausea and vomiting** that results from movement of the head.

Purpose

Chemotherapy causes nausea and vomiting in many people. These conditions can occur for several different reasons. Scopolamine is used to treat nausea and vomiting that result from movement of the head. In many ways, this type of nausea is similar to motion sickness.

Other uses of scopolamine include preanesthesia sedation. In combination with morphine, scopolamine may be given to women in childbirth to induce "twilight sleep." Last, scopolamine is used in an ophthalmic solution to dilate the pupil of the eye before an eye examination.

Description

Scopolamine is a natural product and is familiar to many people as a motion sickness medicine. In its most common form, it comes as a patch that a person with motion sickness wears behind the ear. It is also known by the brand names Scopace, Transderm-Scop, and Transderm-V.

As a motion sickness drug, scopolamine has been used for many years with few side effects. It is approved by the United States Food and Drug Administration (FDA), and its cost is usually covered by insurance. In cancer treatment, scopolamine is used to treat a particular type of nausea and vomiting that occur as a result of chemotherapy.

Scopolamine is classified as an anticholinergic drug. It works by blocking the nerve impulses that send information from the part of the inner ear that controls the sense of balance. In motion sickness, a person vomits because conflicting information arrives in the brain from

Narrow-angle glaucoma—A subtype of glaucoma in which the drainage angle in the eye is unusually small, allowing for a sudden buildup of fluid pressure inside the eye, acute pain, and potential damage to the optic nerve and blindness.

the inner ear and the eye. Some chemotherapy drugs also cause the brain to receive conflicting information, so that when patients move their head, they feel nauseated. People vary in their sensitivity to this condition. This drug is effective in helping most people control nausea and vomiting that arises from this source.

Recommended dosage

Scopolamine comes in a patch that the patient applies behind the ear. The patch stays in place for three days and releases a continuous supply of the drug. To be effective, the patch must be applied at least four hours before chemotherapy is begun. After three days, the patch is removed. Unused patches should be stored at room temperature.

Precautions

People applying or removing a scopolamine patch should wash their hands well immediately after handling the patch so that they do not accidentally transfer any of the drug to other parts of their body (for example, by rubbing their eyes). Scopolamine should not be used in children, should be kept away from pets, and should be used with caution in the elderly.

The patch should be used with caution in patients with a history of either seizures or psychosis, because scopolamine may make either of these disorders worse.

Side effects

About 65% of the people who use scopolamine get a dry mouth. About 17% of people report feeling drowsy from the drug. Other less common side effects include blurred vision, disorientation, restlessness, confusion, dizziness, difficulty urinating, constipation, skin rash, dry red itchy eyes, extreme sensitivity to light, and narrow-angle glaucoma.

Interactions

Many drugs interact with nonprescription (over-the-counter) drugs and herbal remedies. Patients should always tell their health care providers about these remedies, as well as prescription drugs they are taking.

Patients should also mention if they are on a special diet such as low salt or high protein.

Scopolamine interferes with the absorption of ketoconazole (Nizoral), an antifungal drug, sometimes used to treat **prostate cancer**. It may also interact with other anticholinergic drugs (drugs that block nerve impulses), antidepressants, and antihistamines. Scopolamine decreases the absorption of phenothiazines (antipsychotic drugs), and interferes with the effectiveness of levodopa, a drug given to treat Parkinson's disease.

Resources

PERIODICALS

LeGrand, S.B., Walsh, D. "Scopolamine for Cancer-Related Nausea and Vomiting." *Journal of Pain and Symptom Management* 40, no. 1 (2010): 136–41. http://www.jpsmjournal.com/article/S0885-3924(10)00304-0/abstract (accessed November 14, 2014).

WEBSITES

American Cancer Society. "Scopolamine." http://www.cancer.org/treatment/treatmentsandsideeffects/guidetocancerdrugs/scopolamine (accessed November 14, 2014).

Healthwise. "Scopolamine." Norris Cotton Cancer Center, Dartmouth. http://cancer.dartmouth.edu/pf/health_encyclopedia/d00986a1 (accessed November 14, 2014).

ORGANIZATIONS

U.S. Food and Drug Administration, 10903 New Hampshire Ave., Silver Spring, MD 20993, (888) INFO-FDA (463-6332), http://www.fda.gov.

Tish Davidson, A.M.
Rebecca J. Frey, PhD

Screening test

Definition

A screening test is a procedure that is performed to detect the presence of a specific disease. The individual or group of individuals (as in mass screenings) does not present any symptoms of the disease.

Purpose

The purpose of a **cancer** screening test is to identify the presence of a specific cancer in an individual that does not demonstrate any symptoms. Screening allows for early detection of cancer and can save the life of the person who might have died if the cancer had not been detected by screening. If cancers are detected early, the

KEY TERMS

BRCA-1 and BRCA-2—Tumor suppressor genes whose inherited mutations have been associated with hereditary forms of breast cancer.

Digital rectal exam—A manual examination in which the physician will feel the prostate for irregular symmetry by inserting a gloved finger into the rectum.

Genetic test—A test for the presence of specific genes or the presence of mutations on specific genes.

Prostate-specific antigen test—A test that measures the level of prostate antigen in the blood to identify the presence of prostate cancer.

Transrectal ultrasonography—A test that uses a small rectal probe to create an image of the prostate gland.

treatment can be more effective and often less costly than if the cancer had progressed and needed drastic treatment.

Precautions

Most screening tests have been developed to be non-invasive or mildly invasive. For example, breast self-exams, mammograms, and pelvic exams may be uncomfortable but are noninvasive. Therefore, most screening tests will not be affected by medications that a patient may be taking or other unrelated conditions a patient may be experiencing.

Description

Before developing or administering a screening test, the effectiveness of the test needs to be evaluated. There are several criteria to consider when deciding whether to screen. First, is the cancer highly fatal and common? If yes, then it is suitable for screening. Second, in order to screen a cancer, there must be detectable pre-symptomatic indicators. Finally, the reliability of results needs to be evaluated. A test can have one of four following outcomes: true positive, false positive, true negative, and false negative. Randomized controlled trials also help to identify effective screening.

Screening tests exist for many of the more common cancers such as **prostate cancer**, **breast cancer**, **colon cancer**, lung cancer, and **cervical cancer**. Each screening test has an advisable age to begin screening and a recommended frequency at which the test should be performed. As people age, cancer becomes more prevalent; therefore, more screening tests are recommended.

Prostate cancer screening

Prostate cancer affects many men each year. Screening includes a digital rectal exam, tests for prostate-specific antigen (PSA), and transrectal **ultrasonography** (TRUS). Each of these tests takes less than half an hour to perform. The PSA test is an excellent tool as it is highly sensitive, reasonably priced, and well tolerated by patients. Men should be counseled about the benefits and risks of detecting and treating an indolent tumor (this cancer may not have caused symptoms). The treatment may cause urinary and sexual problems.

Breast cancer screening

After **skin cancer**, breast cancer is the most common malignancy diagnosed in women. There are several screening methods that can be performed, including **breast self-exam** (performed by the patient), clinical breast exam, **mammography**, and *BRCA-1* and *BRCA-2* **genetic testing**. Genetic testing is offered to patients who have a familial history of breast cancer. All of these tests can be performed in the doctor's office and take less than half an hour. Genetic testing requires a blood sample, and it takes a few days to receive the results. Counseling is strongly advised prior to genetic testing.

Colon cancer

Colon cancer (colorectal cancer) is the third leading cause of cancer death in the United States and is the third most diagnosed cancer among both men and women. Screening tests include **fecal occult blood test**, flexible **sigmoidoscopy**, **barium enema**, and **colonoscopy**. High-risk patients (significant familial history) should begin screening at puberty or 10 years prior to the age at which a family member's tumor occurred. Sigmoidoscopy and colonoscopy are slightly invasive, completed under mild sedative in the hospital on an outpatient basis, and take about 15 and 30 minutes respectively. Screening with colonoscopy is considered reliable because it allows visualization of the entire colon.

Preparation

Most screening procedures are noninvasive in order to make them convenient for patients and cost-effective. Screening such as breast exams, mammography, pelvic exams, digital rectal exams, and tests that require blood samples require no preparation by the patient. However, barium enema, sigmoidoscopy, and colonoscopy all require prior preparation of the bowel. Patients will be

QUESTIONS TO ASK YOUR DOCTOR

- Which medications may interfere with the results of this test?
- Which tests can be performed to confirm that the results of this screening test are accurate?
- What is the most accurate and cost-effective screening test for the type of cancer in question?
- Who will have access to the test results? Can the results be kept private?
- Will my insurance company pay for this test?

asked to consume a clear liquid diet 24 hours prior to the exams, followed by liquid laxative about 2 hours prior to the exam. An enema or two may be required until the bowel is clear.

Aftercare

Because most screening exams are noninvasive, there is no required aftercare. However, patients are encouraged to monitor themselves for any related symptoms of the cancer in question.

Risks

Since no medical tests are perfect, there are several negative consequences associated with screening. First, if a patient's prognosis would be the same with or without the screening, then the patient experiences a longer time of being sick. Second, if the results of the tests are a false negative, then the patient may be negligent in identifying symptoms and warning signals. Conversely, if the results of the test are a false positive, then the patient may be subjected to unnecessary diagnostic procedures and psychological trauma.

Results

Normal results vary for each test and need to be analyzed for false negative results.

Abnormal results

Doctors schedule more diagnostic testing if abnormal results arise. Normally, a **biopsy** is administered on the tissue in question in order to view the cells for typical cancer traits.

See also Pap smear; Tumor grading; Tumor staging.

Resources

WEBSITES

American Cancer Society. "Cancer Screening Guidelines." http://www.cancer.org/healthy/findcancerearly/cancer-screeningguidelines/ (accessed November 14, 2014).

Cancer Research UK. "Screening for Cancer." http://www.cancerresearchuk.org/about-cancer/cancers-in-general/causes-symptoms/screening-for-cancer (accessed November 14, 2014).

National Cancer Institute. "Screening and Testing to Detect Cancer: Types of Screening Tests." http://www.cancer.gov/cancertopics/screening/types (accessed November 14, 2014).

Sally C. McFarlane-Parrott

Second cancers

Definition

Second cancers are new primary cancers that develop at least two months—but often many years—after the end of treatment for a different primary **cancer**. Second cancers may be associated with treatment for the first cancer or with genetic or other factors, such as smoking, that contributed to the first cancer. Survivors of childhood cancer in particular are at increased risk of a second cancer later in life.

Description

Second cancers are referred to as late effects or second primary neoplasms. They are among the most serious of potential late complications of cancer and its treatments. The type of second cancer depends, at least in part, on the type of original cancer and its treatment. **Radiation therapy** and **chemotherapy** can eventually result in second cancers, regardless of the type of primary cancer. Many second cancers occur near the site of the original tumor or affect parts of the body that were exposed to radiation.

Because second cancers can take a very long time to develop, they have been best characterized in patients who have survived for a long time after primary cancer treatment. These include survivors of **childhood cancers** and of other cancers that were among the first with treatments resulting in long-term survival.

- Blood-based malignancies, such as leukemias, usually occur within a few years of the original cancer treatment. Myelodysplastic syndrome (MDS) and acute myelogenous leukemia (AML) may develop within less

KEY TERMS

Acute lymphoblastic leukemia (ALL)—Childhood leukemia with rapid onset and progression.

Acute myelogenous leukemia (AML)—The most common second cancer caused by chemotherapy.

Alkylating agent—A mutagenic chemotherapy drug that inhibits cell division and growth.

Childhood Cancer Survivor Study (CCSS)—The National Cancer Institute's long-term study of the health of many thousands of survivors of childhood cancer.

Cisplatin—A platinum-containing chemotherapy drug that acts as an alkylating agent and increases the risk of developing difficult-to-treat leukemia.

Complete blood count (CBC) with differential—Counts of red blood cells and platelets, the types and numbers of white blood cells, the amount of hemoglobin in red blood cells, and a hematocrit (the proportion of red cells in the blood); used to screen for second cancers.

Hodgkin lymphoma—Also called Hodgkin disease (HD); a malignant cancer of the lymphatic system.

Human papillomavirus (HPV)—A large family of viruses, some of which cause cervical and other cancers.

Late effect—A consequence of illness or therapy that becomes evident only after long-term patient monitoring.

Leukemia—Acute or chronic cancers characterized by overproduction of white blood cells.

Melanoma—A benign or malignant skin tumor that originates in melanocytes (pigmented cells) of normal skin or moles.

Myelodysplastic syndrome (MDS)—A group of bone marrow disorders that are late effects of cancer treatment and that may progress to acute myelogenous leukemia.

Neoplasm—An abnormal tissue growth that may be benign or malignant.

Non-Hodgkin lymphoma (NHL)—Various malignant lymphomas that are distinct from Hodgkin lymphoma.

Sarcoma—A malignant tumor originating in mesodermal tissue, such as connective tissue, bone, cartilage, or muscle.

Solid tumor—A cancer that originates in an organ or tissue rather than in bone marrow or the lymphatic system.

Topoisomerase II inhibitors—Chemotherapy drugs that may cause second cancers.

---

than ten years of diagnosis of a primary cancer—such as Hodgkin lymphoma, acute lymphoblastic leukemia (ALL), or sarcoma—that was treated with chemotherapy.

- There exists a more than 20% risk of a second cancer in the first two decades after successful treatment for Hodgkin lymphoma.

- The risk of MDS and acute leukemia is linked to chemotherapy with alkylating agents, with the MOPP combination (mechlorethamine, vincristine/oncovin, prednisone, and procarbazine), or chemotherapy preceding a stem-cell transplant. The highest risk is to people aged 35 or older at the time of treatment.

- Radiation for Hodgkin lymphoma also increases the risk of solid tumors, with breast cancer the most common second cancer in female survivors. Lung and thyroid cancer risks are also higher.

- Non-Hodgkin lymphoma (NHL) survivors have about a 15% increased risk of second cancers.

- Breast cancer survivors have a three- to four-fold increased risk of a new primary cancer in the unaffected breast. They are also at increased risk of ovarian, uterine, lung, colon, rectum, connective-tissue cancers, melanoma, and leukemia. Some of these second cancers have the same genetic or hormonal causes as the first cancer.

- Cervical cancer is caused by the human papillomavirus (HPV), and survivors are at increased risk of other HPV-associated cancers, including throat, anus, vulvar, and vaginal cancers. Smoking is linked to cervical cancer, and survivors are at increased risk of smoking-linked cancers including lung, bladder, and pancreatic cancers.

- Ovarian cancer survivors are at increased risk of colon, rectum, small intestine, renal pelvis, breast, bladder, and bile duct cancers, melanoma of the eye, and leukemia. Second cancers may result from radiation therapy, chemotherapy, or genetic factors that contributed to the original ovarian cancer.

- Men treated with radiation for prostate cancer have a higher risk of bladder, colon, and rectal cancers than men who had their prostates removed.

- Cancer in one testicle leaves men at a 2–5% risk of developing cancer in the other testicle, although this is not related to treatment, and the risk is actually lower for men treated with chemotherapy. However, testicular cancer survivors are at twice the risk of a second cancer outside the testicle, especially cancers of the bladder, colon, pancreas, and stomach. They are also at increased risk of leukemia.

Solid tumors may not become evident until 10 to 20 years after primary cancer diagnosis and treatment. These include:

- thyroid cancer following neck radiation for Hodgkin lymphoma, brain tumors, or ALL
- thyroid cancer after radioactive iodine treatment for neuroblastoma
- thyroid cancer after total-body irradiation for a stem-cell transplant
- brain tumors following radiation to the head, especially in combination with intrathecal methotrexate chemotherapy for a primary brain tumor, ALL, or NHL
- bone tumors following radiation for retinoblastomas, Ewing sarcoma, or other bone cancers
- bone tumors after treatment with an alkylating agent
- sarcomas after radiation, with the risk increasing with the dosage
- sarcomas after chemotherapy with anthracyclines
- stomach, liver, or colorectal cancers after abdominal irradiation (with the risk increasing with the dosage), after chemotherapy alone, or after chemotherapy combined with radiation
- non-melanoma skin cancer following radiation therapy, usually developing in the irradiated area
- malignant melanoma after radiation therapy or combination chemotherapy with alkylating agents and antimitotic drugs, especially for Hodgkin lymphoma, hereditary retinoblastoma, soft-tissue sarcoma, or gonadal tumors
- oral cavity cancers after chemotherapy followed by a stem-cell transplant or chronic graft-versus-host disease
- kidney cancer following neuroblastoma treatment, radiation to the mid-back, or chemotherapy with cisplatin or carboplatin

Demographics

Patients with a cancer diagnosis have almost double the risk of a second cancer in the future. As of 2014, there were more than 14.5 million cancer survivors living in the United States, and this number is expected to grow to 19 million over the next decade. The rate of second cancers is expected to rise along with the population of long-term cancer survivors. However, many cancer treatments have improved dramatically in recent years. Safer chemotherapy

drugs have been developed, and radiation therapy is often much more focused than previously. Thus, the risk of second cancers may be lower in the future.

Some 80% of children remain alive five years after a cancer diagnosis, and many are ultimately considered cured. A child who develops cancer before the age of 15 is eight times more likely to develop a new primary cancer than a child of the same age who has not had cancer. Children treated for **Hodgkin lymphoma** are most at risk of developing a second cancer within 20 years. People who survive for at least five years after treatment for NHL are at the lowest risk of a second cancer.

Causes and symptoms

Causes

Some second cancers result from factors responsible for the original cancer. Some childhood cancer survivors may be at increased risk because of a family history or an inherited genetic syndrome such as Li-Fraumeni syndrome. Certain inherited gene changes can increase a woman's risk of both breast and **ovarian cancer**. Exposure to certain cancer-causing substances increases the risk of second cancers. Many second cancers are caused by radiation or chemotherapy that damages normal cells or suppresses the immune system.

RADIATION. Radiation has long been recognized as a risk factor for cancer. The risk of a second cancer from radiation treatment is influenced by:

- the type and amount of radiation
- the patient's age at treatment
- the patient's personal and family medical history

Chronic and acute myelogenous leukemias, ALL, and MDS—a bone-marrow disorder that can lead to acute leukemia—are associated with radiation. Risk depends on the total amount of radiation, the extent of exposed bone marrow, and the radiation dose rate—the amount, length, and frequency of each dose. Patient age does not appear to be a factor. Peak development of second cancers occurs five to seven years after exposure, after which the risk slowly declines.

Solid tumors do not usually develop until at least 10–15 years after radiation exposure. Risk depends on the radiation dose, the area treated, and the patient's age at treatment. Second cancers tend to develop in or near the irradiated area. Certain organs, such as the breast and thyroid, appear to be more susceptible to second cancers from radiation. **Breast cancer** risk appears to be highest in women who were treated as children, and risk decreases with increasing age at treatment.

Radiation treatment in women over age 40 presents little or no increased risk of breast cancer. Early menopause lowers the breast cancer risk. Risk for other solid cancers, such as lung and thyroid cancers, bone **sarcoma**, and **gastrointestinal cancers**, also decreases with increasing age at radiation treatment. However, smoking significantly increases the risk of lung cancer after radiation treatment. The risk of some second cancers is increased if radiation therapy is combined with chemotherapy.

CHEMOTHERAPY. Chemotherapy is a stronger risk factor for leukemia than radiation. AML is the second cancer most often linked to chemotherapy, and MDS often precedes the development of AML. ALL and some solid tumors, such as **testicular cancer**, are also linked to chemotherapy. The risk of leukemia from alkylating agents increases with drug dose, longer treatment times, and higher dose intensity—higher doses over a shorter time. Leukemias peak at five to ten years after treatment, and incidence then declines. MDS and leukemia after treatment with alkylating agents can be hard to treat and may have poor prognoses. Alkylating agents that can cause MDS and leukemias include:

- mechlorethamine
- chlorambucil
- cyclophosphamide
- melphalan
- lomustine
- carmustine
- prednimustine
- busulfan
- dihydroxybusulfan
- ifosfamide
- dacarbazine

Other chemotherapy agents also increase the risk of leukemias:

- Cisplatin attacks cancer cells in a similar manner to alkylating agents and appears to increase the risk of leukemias that are hard to treat and have a poor prognosis. The risk of leukemia rises with the cisplatin dose or accompanying radiation treatment.
- Topoisomerase II inhibitors—such as etoposide and teniposide—also cause leukemia, primarily AML. Leukemia usually develops within two to three years, faster than with alkylating agents, but tends to respond better to treatment and has a better prognosis.
- Anthracyclines—such as doxorubicin, daunorubicin, epirubicin, and mitoxantrone—are also topoisomerase

II inhibitors that may cause AML, although the risk is lower.

Symptoms

Symptoms are specific to the type of second cancer.

Research

With so many more patients surviving cancer, increased research is being focused on second cancers and other **late effects of cancer treatment**. The **National Cancer Institute** initiated the Childhood Cancer Survivor Study (CCSS) in 1994 to study late effects. It has followed more than 14,000 childhood cancer survivors in the United States and Canada who were diagnosed between 1970 and 1986, along with about 4,000 of their healthy siblings. All of the survivors had one or more primary treatments—surgery, radiation, and/or chemotherapy. A second group of 14,000 adults treated for cancer as children between 1987 and 1999 and 4,000 of their siblings were recruited beginning in 2007. Results from the CCSS have begun to significantly increase knowledge of second cancers and the treatments that increase risk, with the goals of reducing the incidence of second cancers and improving early detection. Researchers are also investigating the processes that transform cancer treatments into sources of new tumors and are studying ways to maintain or improve survival rates with gentler types of chemotherapy or radiation doses too low to inflict the cellular damage that causes second cancers.

Prevention

To help prevent second cancers, cancer survivors should:

- follow a healthy lifestyle
- avoid known causes of cancer, such as smoking or prolonged sun exposure
- follow all recommendations for cancer screenings and other forms of medical surveillance
- have a physical exam and medical history at least once a year
- get immediate medical attention for any changes or new symptoms

Children who were treated with an alkylating agent or topoisomerase II inhibitor for leukemia should have a complete blood count (CBC) with differential every year for ten years after treatment ends. Leukemia patients treated with radiation may require:

- annual exams for signs of skin cancer, especially in the treated area
- monthly breast self-exams

Journal of Clinical Oncology 18, no. 6 (December 2013): 1078–84.

QUESTIONS TO ASK YOUR DOCTOR

- What is my risk of developing a second cancer?
- What second cancers am I at risk of developing?
- How can I reduce my risk of developing a second cancer?
- Which screenings should I have for second cancers?
- What is my prognosis if I develop a second cancer?

- clinical breast exams every six months from puberty until age 25 if treated with radiation to the chest
- annual mammograms or magnetic resonance imaging (MRI) beginning eight years after treatment or at age 25 if treated with radiation to the chest
- a colonoscopy every five years, beginning ten years after treatment or at age 35 if treated with radiation to the abdomen, pelvis, or spine

The Institute of Medicine recommends that all cancer survivors receive individualized **survivorship care plans** to monitor their long-term health. The American College of Surgeons (ACS) Commission on Cancer has pushed to require all ACS-accredited facilities, where the majority of cancer patients are treated, to provide these plans. However, there is some debate regarding whether oncologists or primary care physicians should provide the follow-up care.

Special concerns

Improved long-term cancer survival has increased concerns about the physical and psychological effects of the disease and its treatments. Radiation and chemotherapy doses are continually being fine-tuned to eradicate all of the cancer while minimizing risks of late effects, including second cancers. Cancer patients should be aware of the risks of second cancers, although the benefits of cancer treatment far outweigh the risks.

Resources

BOOKS

Keene, Nancy, Wendy Hobbie, and Kathy Ruccione. *Childhood Cancer Survivors: A Practical Guide to Your Future*. 3rd ed. Bellingham, WA: Childhood Cancer Guides, 2012.

PERIODICALS

Okajima, Kaoru, et al. "Multiple Primary Malignancies in Patients with Prostate Cancer: Increased Risk of Secondary Malignancies After Radiotherapy." *International*

Rosenthal, Eric T. "Deadline for Survivorship Care Plan Compliance Being Rethought." *Oncology Times* 36, no. 13 (2014): 1, 14–16. http://dx.doi.org/10.1097/01.COT.0000452080.35411.d6 (accessed August 14, 2014).

Smith-Gagen, Julie, George A. Goodwin, and Jonathan Tay. "Multiple Primary Tumors Following Stage II and III Rectal Cancer in Patients Receiving Radiotherapy, 1998–2010." *Journal of Cancer Research & Clinical Oncology* 140, no. 6 (June 2014): 949–55.

WEBSITES

American Cancer Society. "Second Cancers Caused by Cancer Treatment." http://www.cancer.org/cancer/cancercauses/othercarcinogens/medicaltreatments/secondcancerscausedbycancertreatment/second-cancers-caused-by-cancer-treatment-intro (accessed June 21, 2014).

American Cancer Society. "Survivorship Care Plans." http://www.cancer.org/treatment/survivorshipduringandaftertreatment/survivorshipcareplans/index (accessed August 14, 2014).

National Cancer Institute. "The Childhood Cancer Survivor Study: An Overview." http://www.cancer.gov/cancertopics/coping/survivorship/ccss (accessed June 21, 2014).

National Cancer Institute. "Second Cancers." Late Effects of Treatment for Childhood Cancer (PDQ). May 17, 2014. http://www.cancer.gov/cancertopics/pdq/treatment/lateeffects/Patient/page2 (accessed June 21, 2014).

ORGANIZATIONS

American Cancer Society, 250 Williams Street NW, Atlanta, GA 30303, (800) 227-2345, http://www.cancer.org.

National Cancer Institute, 6116 Executive Boulevard, Suite 300, Bethesda, MD 20892-8322, (800) 4-CANCER (422-6237), http://www.cancer.gov.

Maureen Haggerty
Margaret Alic, PhD

Secondary liver cancer *see* **Liver cancer**

Secondhand smoke

Definition

Secondhand smoke is tobacco smoke that is inhaled involuntarily or passively by a person who is not smoking. That person may inhale smoke that is either exhaled by a person who is smoking a cigarette, cigar, or pipe (exhaled smoke is known as mainstream smoke), or generated from smoldering tobacco (known as sidestream smoke). Secondhand smoke contains at least 69 chemicals that are known to cause lung **cancer**, even in nonsmokers. Secondhand smoke increases the likelihood of heart disease, including heart attacks, and various breathing problems.

Description

Secondhand smoke, also known as passive smoking or environmental tobacco smoke, can cause disease and premature death in nonsmoking adults and children, because tobacco smoke contains toxic chemicals that increase health risks. The amount of smoke created by a tobacco product is related to the amount of tobacco in that product. According to the **National Cancer Institute**, secondhand smoke emitted from one large cigar is similar to that of an entire pack of **cigarettes**. Because of tobacco's effects on both smokers and nonsmokers, smoking constitutes a universal public health risk.

Babies and young children are especially susceptible to the effects of secondhand smoke. According to the Tobacco Control Research Branch of the National Cancer Institute:

- Babies who are exposed to secondhand smoke after birth, or whose mothers smoked while pregnant, are more likely to die from sudden infant death syndrome than babies who do not breathe secondhand smoke.
- Mothers who breathe secondhand smoke while pregnant are more likely to have a baby weighing 5.5 pounds or less. Underweight babies often experience serious health problems.
- Bronchitis, pneumonia, and other lung problems, as well as middle-ear infections, are more common among children who have smoking parents.

Demographics

Secondhand smoke can affect anyone. Approximately 126 million people in the United States are exposed to secondhand smoke at home and at work. Studies show that secondhand smoke exposure has, however, declined. Secondhand smoke results in nearly 50,000 deaths in adult nonsmokers annually, including about 3,400 due to lung disease and 46,000 due to heart disease. Nonsmokers who are exposed to secondhand smoke at home or at work have a 25%–30% higher risk of heart disease and a 20%–30% higher risk of lung cancer.

Infants and children are more susceptible to the effects of secondhand smoke, yet among those aged six or younger, almost three million (11%) are exposed to secondhand smoke at least four days per week. As many as 300,000 children and infants experience **pneumonia**, bronchitis, and other respiratory infections as a result, and up to 15,000 are hospitalized each year. Secondhand

smoke also can cause severe attacks among children who already have asthma. More than 40% of all children who are rushed to an emergency room for severe asthma attacks live in homes with smokers. In addition, according to the U.S. Environmental Protection Agency (EPA), secondhand smoke can cause new cases of asthma in children who have not previously shown symptoms.

Causes and symptoms

Causes

Secondhand smoke contains dozens of cancer-causing chemicals. These include arsenic, **benzene**, nickel, and vinyl chloride. It also contains about 7,000 other chemicals, hundreds of which are known to be toxic. Some of these include formaldehyde and toluene.

Symptoms

Many patients experiencing effects of secondhand smoke report coughing, increased phlegm production, and breathing problems. Those who have other conditions associated with secondhand smoke, such as heart disease, bronchitis, or cancer, have various symptoms indicative of those illnesses.

Diagnosis

Secondhand smoke exposure may be measured by checking the indoor air for nicotine or other chemicals that are found in tobacco smoke. To determine exposure in a nonsmoker, scientists measure the level of a substance called cotinine in bodily fluids. Cotinine is a byproduct produced as the body breaks down nicotine inhaled from tobacco smoke. During 1988–91, about 87.9% of nonsmokers had measurable levels of cotinine. The proportion dropped to 52.5% in 1999–2000, and to 40.1% in 2007–8, according to a report from the Centers for Disease Control and Prevention (CDC). Those declines are correlated with the increasing number of smoking restrictions (bans) in the workplace and in public places, such as restaurants; the decline in smoking rates overall; and the rise in the number of private citizens who restrict smoking in their own homes.

Prevention

The most effective way to prevent the dangers of secondhand smoke is to avoid those places where smoking occurs, but this can be difficult. Although restrictions are now in place to prohibit smoking in many public places, secondhand smoke is still common in the everyday environment, and neither air-cleaning systems

KEY TERMS

Mainstream smoke—The tobacco smoke exhaled by a smoker.

Nicotine—A substance found in tobacco and other plants of the nightshade family (Solanaceae) that acts as a stimulant. Nicotine is highly addictive.

Sidestream smoke—The smoke emitted from burning tobacco (not exhaled by a smoker).

nor ventilation can fully eliminate secondhand smoke exposure, according to the CDC.

Smoking bans

In the United States, each state has jurisdiction to enact smoking bans. From 2000 to 2014, the number of states (including the District of Columbia and U.S. territories) that had enacted laws to prohibit smoking in indoor areas of worksites, restaurants, and bars increased from 0 to 26, according to the CDC and Americans for Nonsmokers' Rights.

Other

Besides public smoking bans, additional efforts may contribute to reducing secondhand smoke. These include taxation, media campaigns, increasing law enforcement for underage users, advertisement restrictions, youth education, cessation services, and other programs, laws, and policies that focus on prevention and helping current smokers to quit.

Resources

BOOKS

Committee on Secondhand Smoke Exposure and Acute Coronary Events. *Secondhand Smoke Exposure and Cardiovascular Effects: Making Sense of the Evidence.* Washington, DC: National Academies Press, 2010.

U.S. Department of Health and Human Services. *How Tobacco Smoke Causes Disease: The Biology and Behavioral Basis for Smoking-Attributable Disease: A Report of the Surgeon General.* Atlanta: U.S. Department of Health and Human Services, Centers for Disease Control and Prevention, National Center for Chronic Disease Prevention and Health Promotion, Office on Smoking and Health, 2010.

PERIODICALS

Centers for Disease Control and Prevention. "State Smoke-Free Laws for Worksites, Restaurants, and Bars—United States, 2000–2010." *Morbidity and Mortality Weekly Report* 60, no. 15 (2011): 1472–75. http://www.cdc.gov/mmwr/ preview/mmwrhtml/mm6015a2.htm (accessed October 10, 2014).

Centers for Disease Control and Prevention. "Vital Signs: Nonsmokers' Exposure to Secondhand Smoke—United States, 1999–2008." *Morbidity and Mortality Weekly Report* 59, no. 35 (2010): 1141–46.

OTHER

American Cancer Society Cancer Action Network. *Saving Lives, Saving Money: A State by State Report on the Health and Economic Impact of Comprehensive Smoke-Free Laws.* 2011. http://www.acscan.org/pdf/tobacco/ reports/acscan-smoke-free-laws-report.pdf (accessed October 10, 2014).

American Nonsmokers' Rights Foundation. "U.S. 100% Smokefree Laws in Non-Hospitality Workplaces AND Restaurants AND Bars." October 2014. http://www.no-smoke. org/pdf/WRBLawsMap.pdf (accessed October 10, 2014).

Environmental Protection Agency. "Fact Sheet: National Survey on Environmental Management of Asthma and Children's Exposure to Environmental Tobacco Smoke." http://www.epa.gov/smokefre/pdfs/survey_fact_sheet.pdf (accessed October 10, 2014).

U.S. Department of Health and Human Services. *The Health Consequences of Smoking—50 Years of Progress. A Report of the Surgeon General.* Atlanta: U.S. Department of Health and Human Services, Centers for Disease Control and Prevention, National Center for Chronic Disease Prevention and Health Promotion, Office on Smoking and Health, 2014. http://www.surgeongeneral. gov/library/reports/50-years-of-progress/full-report.pdf (accessed October 10, 2014).

WEBSITES

Environmental Protection Agency. "Health Effects of Exposure to Secondhand Smoke." http://www.epa.gov/smokefre/ healtheffects.html (accessed October 10, 2014).

National Cancer Institute. "Secondhand Smoke and Cancer." http://www.cancer.gov/cancertopics/factsheet/Tobacco/ ETS (accessed October 10, 2014).

Tobacco Control Research Branch of the National Cancer Institute. "Secondhand Smoke." Smoke-Free.gov. http:// smokefree.gov/topic-secondhand_smoke.aspx (accessed October 10, 2014).

ORGANIZATIONS

Americans for Nonsmokers' Rights, 2530 San Pablo Ave., Ste. J, Berkeley, CA 94702, (510) 841-3032, http://www. no-smoke.org.

Centers for Disease Control and Prevention, 1600 Clifton Rd., Atlanta, GA 30333, (800) CDC-INFO (232-4636), http:// www.cdc.gov.

U.S. Environmental Protection Agency, 1200 Pennsylvania Ave. NW, Washington, DC 20460, http://www2.epa.gov.

National Cancer Institute, 9609 Medical Center Dr., BG 9609 MSC 9760, Bethesda, MD 20892-9760, (800) 4-CANCER (422-6237), http://www.cancer.gov.

Leslie Mertz, PhD

Second-look surgery

Definition

Second-look surgery is performed after a procedure or course of treatment to determine whether the patient is free of disease. If disease is found, additional procedures may or may not be performed at the time of second-look surgery.

Purpose

Second-look surgery may be performed under numerous circumstances on patients with various medical conditions.

Cancer

A second-look procedure is sometimes performed to determine whether a **cancer** patient has responded successfully to a particular treatment. Examples of cancers that are assessed during second-look surgery are **ovarian cancer** and colorectal cancer. In many cases, before a round of **chemotherapy** and/or **radiation therapy** is started, a patient will undergo a surgical procedure called cytoreduction to reduce the size of a tumor. This debulking increases the sensitivity of the tumor and decreases the number of necessary treatment cycles. Following cytoreduction and chemotherapy, a second-look procedure may be necessary to determine whether the area is cancer-free.

An advantage to second-look surgery following cancer treatment is that if cancer is found, it may be removed during the procedure in some patients. In other cases, if a tumor cannot be entirely removed, the surgeon can debulk the tumor and improve the patient's chances of responding to another cycle of chemotherapy. However, second-look surgery cannot definitively prove that a patient is free of cancer; some microscopic cancer cells can persist and begin to grow in other areas of the body. Even if no cancer is found during second-look surgery, the rate of cancer relapse is approximately 25%.

Pelvic disease

Second-look surgery may benefit patients suffering from a number of different conditions that affect the pelvic organs. Endometriosis is a condition in which the tissue that lines the uterus grows elsewhere in the body, usually in the abdominal cavity, leading to pain and scarring. Endometrial growths may be surgically removed or treated with medications. A second-look procedure may be performed following the initial surgery or course of medication to determine if treatment was successful in reducing the number of growths. Additional growths may be removed at this time.

Second-look surgery may also be performed following the surgical removal of adhesions (bands of scar tissue that form in the abdomen following surgery or injury) or uterine fibroids (noncancerous growths of the uterus). If the results are positive, an additional procedure may be performed to remove the adhesions or growths. Patients undergoing treatment for infertility may benefit from a second-look procedure to determine whether the cause of infertility has been cured before ceasing therapy.

Abdominal disease

In patients suffering from bleeding from the gastrointestinal (GI) tract, recurrence of bleeding after attempted treatment remains a significant risk; approximately 10%–25% of cases do not respond to initial treatment. Second-look surgery following treatment for GI bleeding may be beneficial in determining whether bleeding has recurred and, if necessary, in treating the cause of the bleeding before it becomes more extensive.

Patients suffering from a partial or complete blockage of the intestine are at risk of developing bowel ischemia (death of intestinal tissue due to a lack of oxygen). Initial surgery is most often done to remove the diseased segment of bowel; a second-look procedure is commonly performed to ensure that only healthy tissue remains and that the new intestinal connection (called an anastomosis) is healing properly.

Other conditions

A variety of other conditions can be assessed with second-look surgery. Patients who have undergone surgical repair of torn muscles in the knee might undergo a procedure called second-look arthroscopy to assess whether the repair is healing. A physician may use second-look mastoidoscopy to visualize the middle ear after removal of a cholesteatoma (a benign but destructive growth in the middle ear). A second endoscopic procedure may be performed on a patient who underwent endoscopic treatment for sinusitis (chronic infection of the sinuses) to evaluate the surgical site and remove debris.

Description

Second-look surgery may be performed within hours, days, weeks, or months of the initial procedure or treatment. The time interval depends on the patient's condition and the type of procedure.

Laparotomy

A laparotomy is a large incision through the abdominal wall to visualize and explore the structures inside the abdominal cavity. After placing the patient under general anesthesia, the surgeon first makes a large incision through the skin, then through each layer under the skin in the region that the surgeon wishes to explore. The incision may include the muscle, fascia, and subcutaneous layers. The area will then be assessed for evidence of remaining disease. For example, in the case of second-look laparotomy following treatment for endometriosis, the abdominal organs will be examined for evidence of endometrial growths. In the case of cancer, a washing of the abdominal cavity may be performed; sterile fluid is instilled into the abdominal cavity and washed around the organs, then extracted with a syringe. The fluid is then analyzed for the presence of cancerous cells. Biopsies may also be taken of various abdominal tissues and analyzed.

If the surgeon discovers evidence of disease or a failed surgical repair, additional procedures may be performed to remove the disease or repair the dysfunction. For example, if adhesions are encountered during a second-look procedure on an infertile female patient, the surgeon may remove the adhesions at that time. Upon completion of the procedure, the incision is closed.

Laparoscopy

Laparoscopy is a surgical technique that permits a view of the internal abdominal organs without an extensive surgical incision. During laparoscopy, a thin lighted tube called a laparoscope is inserted into the abdominal cavity through a tiny incision. Images taken by the laparoscope are seen on a video monitor connected to the scope. The surgeon may then examine the abdominal cavity, albeit with a more limited operative view than with laparotomy. Procedures such as the removal of growths or repair of deformities can be performed by instruments inserted through other small incisions or trocars in the abdominal wall. After the procedure is completed, any incisions are closed with stitches or surgical glue products. Surgical glues are also known as wound adhesives or sealants.

Other procedures

Depending on the area of the body in question, other procedures may be used to perform second-look surgery:

- Arthroscopy uses a thin endoscope to visualize the inner space of a joint such as the knee or elbow. Second-look arthroscopy may be used to determine whether previous surgery on the joint is healing properly.

- Percutaneous nephrolithotomy (PNL) is a minimally invasive procedure used to remove kidney stones. Second-look PNL may be used to remove fragments of stones that could not be removed during the initial procedure.

- A hysteroscope is an instrument used to visualize and perform procedures on the inner cavity of the uterus. Second-look hysteroscopy may be used after surgery or medical treatment to treat adhesions or benign growths in the uterus to determine whether they have been effectively removed.

- Mastoidectomy is a surgical procedure used to treat cholesteatoma; a second-look procedure is generally performed to ensure that the entire cholesteatoma was removed during the initial procedure.

Resources

BOOKS

Hatch, Kenneth D. *Laparoscopy for Gynecology and Oncology.* Philadelphia: Wolters Kluwer/Lippincott Williams & Wilkins Health, 2008.

Karakousis, Constantine P. *Atlas of Operative Procedures in Surgical Oncology.* New York: Springer, 2014.

Sabel, Michael S., Vernon K. Sondak, and Jeffrey J. Sussman, eds. *Surgical Foundations: Essentials of Surgical Oncology.* Philadelphia: Mosby/Elsevier, 2007.

PERIODICALS

Ahn, J. H., et al. "Second-Look Arthroscopic Findings of 208 Patients after ACL Reconstruction." *Knee Surgery, Sports Traumatology, Arthroscopy* 15 (March 2007): 242–48.

Dell Anna, T., et al. "Systematic Lymphadenectomy in Ovarian Cancer at Second-Look Surgery: A Randomised Clinical Trial." *British Journal of Cancer* 107 (August 21, 2012): 785–92. http://dx.doi.org/10.1038/bjc.2012.336 (accessed September 12, 2013).

Marmo, Riccardo, et al. "Outcome of Endoscopic Treatment for Peptic Ulcer Bleeding: Is a Second Look Necessary?" *Gastrointestinal Endoscopy* 57, no. 1 (January 2003): 62–67.

Shenoy, Ashok M., et al. "The Utility of Second Look Microlaryngoscopy after Trans Oral Laser Resection of Laryngeal Cancer." *Indian Journal of Otolaryngology and Head & Neck Surgery* 64, no. 2 (2012): 137–41. http://dx.doi.org/10.1007/s12070-012-0496-7 (accessed October 3, 2014).

Sood, A. K. "Second-Look Laparotomy for Ovarian Germ Cell Tumors: To Do or Not to Do?" *Journal of Postgraduate Medicine* 52 (October–December 2006): 246–47.

Yanar, H., et al. "Planned Second-Look Laparoscopy in the Management of Acute Mesenteric Ischemia." *World Journal of Gastroenterology* 13 (June 28, 2007): 3350–353.

WEBSITES

Horlbeck, Drew. "Middle Ear Endoscopy." Medscape Reference. http://emedicine.medscape.com/article/860570-overview (accessed October 3, 2014).

Murphy, Kate. "Second Look Surgery for Peritoneal Carcinomatosis." FightColorectalCancer.org. http://fightcolorectalcancer.org/uncategorized/2011/05/second_look_surgery_for_peritoneal_carcinomatosis (accessed October 3, 2014).

ORGANIZATIONS

American College of Surgeons, 633 N. Saint Clair St., Chicago, IL 60611-3211, (312) 202-5000, (800) 621-4111, Fax: (312) 202-5001, postmaster@facs.org, http://www.facs.org.

Society of Surgical Oncology, 9525 W. Bryn Mawr Ave., Ste. 870, Rosemont, IL 60018, (847) 427-1400, info@surgonc.org, http://surgonc.org.

Stephanie Dionne Sherk
REVISED BY REBECCA FREY, PhD

Segmentectomy

Definition

Segmentectomy is the excision (removal) of a portion of any organ or gland. The procedure has several variations and many names, including wide excision, **lumpectomy**, tumorectomy, **quadrantectomy**, and partial **mastectomy**.

Purpose

The purpose of this procedure is to surgically remove a portion of an organ or gland that contains a cancerous tumor.

Description

Common organs that have segments are the breasts, lungs, and liver. When **cancer** is confined to a segment, removal of that portion may offer cancer-control results equivalent to larger operations. This is especially true for breast and liver cancers. In cases of lung cancer, **lobectomy** (surgical removal of all or part of the lung) is preferable, but if the patient does not have sufficient pulmonary function to tolerate this larger operation, then a segmentectomy may be necessary. For breast and lung cancers, this procedure is often combined with removal of some or all regional lymph nodes.

Precautions

Because of the need for radiotherapy after segmentectomy, some patients, such as pregnant women and those with syndromes not compatible with radiation treatment, may not be candidates for this procedure. As with any surgery, patients should alert their physician about all allergies and any medications they are taking.

Preparation

Routine preoperative preparations, such as having nothing to eat or drink the night before surgery, are typically ordered for a segmentectomy. Information about expected outcomes and potential complications is also part of the preparation for this surgery.

Aftercare

After a segmentectomy, patients are usually cautioned against any moderate lifting for several days.

Other activities may be restricted (especially if lymph nodes were removed) according to individual needs. Pain is often enough to limit inappropriate motion. Women who undergo segmentectomy of the breast are often instructed to wear a well-fitting support bra both day and night for approximately one week after surgery. Pain is usually well controlled with prescribed medication. If it is not, the patient should contact the surgeon, as severe pain may be a sign of a complication that needs medical attention.

Radiation therapy is usually started four to six weeks after surgery and will continue for four to five weeks. The timing of additional therapy is specific to each individual patient.

Risks

Risk of infection in the area affecting a segmentectomy occurs in 3% to 4% of patients.

Results

Successful removal of the tumor.

Abnormal results

Major bleeding and/or infection at the wound after surgery.

Clinical trials

Using a segmentectomy to remove breast cancers (as a technique that conserves the aesthetic appearance of a breast) is being investigated for large tumors after several cycles of preoperative **chemotherapy**. Segmentectomy is also being investigated for treating small-cell lung cancers. Information about clinical trial options is available from the **National Cancer Institute** at http://www.nci.nih.gov.

Resources

BOOKS

Hiroaki, Nomori. *Illustrated Anatomical Segmentectomy for Lung Cancer.* New York, NY: Springer Science+Business Media, LLC, 2012.

PERIODICALS

Ohtaki, Y., Shimizu, K. "Anatomical Thoracoscopic Segmentectomy for Lung Cancer." *General Thoracic and Cardiovascular Surgery* 62, no. 10 (2014): 586–93. http://www.ncbi.nlm.nih.gov/pubmed/24791926 (accessed November 14, 2014).

WEBSITES

Cancer Research UK. "Types of Surgery for Lung Cancer." http://www.cancerresearchuk.org/about-cancer/type/lung-cancer/treatment/surgery/types-of-surgery-for-lung-cancer (accessed November 14, 2014).

Laura Ruth, PhD

Self image *see* **Body image/self image**

Semustine

Definition

Semustine, also known as methyl-CCNU, is one of a group of antineoplastic (antitumor) drugs known as alkylating agents. It is an investigational drug.

Purpose

Semustine has been used in the treatment of **brain tumors**, lymphomas, colorectal **cancer**, and **stomach cancer**. It is not clearly superior to other treatments for these diseases. It has also been associated with an increased risk of secondary (that is, treatment-related) leukemia. Thus, semustine is not used in the United States.

Description

Like many antineoplastic (antitumor) therapies, semustine acts by killing quickly growing cells. Since cancerous cells are generally growing faster than normal cells, drugs that kill quickly growing cells generally affect tumors more than normal cells. However, some normal cells, such as white blood cells and platelets, also grow quickly, and can be severely affected by antineoplastic drugs. Antitumor therapies create a situation in which the drug is racing to kill the tumor before it causes irreparable damage to normal tissues. The ideal situation is one in which the growth of the tumor is severely affected, but the growth of normal cells is unaffected.

However, not every situation is ideal. Some patients taking antitumor drugs may have to discontinue treatment or decrease the dose because of side effects.

Semustine is included in the group of **anticancer drugs** known as alkylating agents.

Semustine is an investigational drug in the United States, which means that the FDA has not approved this drug for marketing. Generally, **investigational drugs** are made available through participation in research studies.

Many drugs have toxic side effects, some of which are difficult to detect. **Clinical trials** are used to determine the side effects, drug interactions, and precautions for medicines, as well as their efficacy. Successful completion of multi-step clinical trials results in FDA approval of a drug. Many drugs that are used in clinical trials never gain FDA approval, however, possibly because of severe side effects that outweigh the benefits of the medication, or because the medication does not perform the function for which it was tested. Final approval of a drug is also expensive. Some drugs may not receive the financial support necessary to achieve final approval. Because of semustine's carcinogenic (cancer-causing) effects, it is no longer used in trials in the United States.

Recommended dosage

Because semustine is investigational, there is no recommended dosage. Different dosing schedules have been reported in the literature for different cancers.

Side effects

In the published reports of semustine use, a common side effect is **myelosuppression**, the damage to white blood cells and platelets. Such damage may result in infection and bleeding, respectively. The myelosuppression from semustine is prolonged, meaning that it takes longer for blood cells to recover than is seen with many other anticancer drugs. Therefore, the interval between courses of semustine is longer than with other agents. Semustine also causes **nausea and vomiting**. Sometimes **anorexia**, or loss of appetite, persists after nausea and vomiting. As noted above, semustine has also been associated with the development of secondary leukemia.

Interactions

Semustine has been linked with other alkylating agents that can cause leukemia.

Resources

BOOKS
Chu, Edward, and Vincent T. DeVita Jr. *Physicians' Cancer Chemotherapy Drug Manual 2014.* Burlington, MA: Jones & Bartlett Learning, 2014.

WEBSITES
National Cancer Institute. "Semustine." http://www.cancer.gov/drugdictionary?cdrid=43727 (accessed November 14, 2014).
U.S. National Library of Medicine. "Semustine." PubMed Health. http://pubchem.ncbi.nlm.nih.gov/compound/semustine (accessed November 14, 2014).

Michael Zuck, PhD

Senna *see* **Laxatives**
Senokot *see* **Laxatives**

Sentinel lymph node biopsy

Definition

Sentinel **lymph node biopsy** (SLNB) is a minimally invasive procedure in which a lymph node near the site of a cancerous tumor is first identified as a sentinel node and then removed for microscopic analysis. A lymph node is

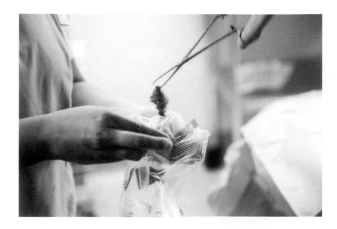

Surgeon removing the sentinel lymph node—the first node affected by the spread of a cancer—for biopsy. *(Garo/ Phanie/Alamy)*

called "sentinel" when it serves as a sentry; that is, the first or nearest lymph node to which **cancer** cells would likely spread from a primary tumor. Sometimes more than one sentinel node can be present. SLNB removes a sample of the sentinel lymph node, and histologic examination by a pathologist helps determine the extent or stage of cancer.

The ability to map the lymph nodes throughout the body using blue dye led to the development of SLNB. SLNB is used primarily for staging **breast cancer** and **melanoma**, but is also used in the diagnosis and treatment of colorectal cancer, **esophageal cancer**, head and neck cancer, **thyroid cancer**, and non-small cell lung cancer.

Purpose

Sentinel lymph node **biopsy** has several purposes, including:

- Catch the spread of cancer to nearby lymph nodes as early as possible.
- Improve the accuracy of staging the cancer (cancer staging) by measuring the extent of the spread of cancer cells in the body; cancer staging helps to guide treatment decisions.
- Define homogeneous patient populations for clinical trials of new cancer treatments.

Description

A sentinel lymph node biopsy is most often performed during surgery to remove the primary tumor, although it may also be performed before or after surgery to remove the tumor. SLNB is accomplished in two stages. The first stage takes place in the nuclear medicine department of the hospital. It involves a two-hour imaging study called lymphoscintigraphy, in which images of the tumor are taken for analysis before the SLNB and before the tumor surgery if the procedures are combined. A physician who specializes in nuclear medicine first numbs the area around the tumor with a local anesthetic and then injects a radioactive colloid along with a blue dye. A gamma camera then takes images of the lymph nodes before surgery.

After the lymphoscintigraphy, the patient must wait several hours for the dye and the radioactive material to travel from the tissues around the tumor to the sentinel lymph node. Then the patient will be taken to the operating room and put under general anesthesia. Next, the surgeon injects more blue dye into the area around the tumor and uses a handheld probe connected to a gamma ray counter to scan the area for the sentinel node, which is highlighted by the blue dye. The sentinel lymph node is pinpointed by the sound made by the gamma ray counter as it recognizes the radioactive material that was injected. When the node has been identified, the surgeon

either makes a small incision to remove it (lymph node resection), or removes it when the primary tumor is resected. The sample of lymph node tissue is then sent to the pathology laboratory for staining and histologic examination. The pathologist examines the stained tissue microscopically to determine whether cancer cells are present. If cancer cells are present, the biopsy is said to be positive. If the patient is undergoing surgery to remove the primary tumor, additional lymph nodes may be removed while the patient is still under anesthesia. If only SLNB is performed, additional nodes will be removed in a follow-up surgery.

SLNB is often combined with diagnostic imaging during surgery. For example, intraoperative 3D imaging using freehand single-photon emission **computed tomography** (fhSPECT) is used to improve the accuracy of identification of SLNB during surgery for treating oral cancer. In treating patients with melanoma, ultrasound-guided fine needle aspiration performed along with SLNB allows more accurate staging of the cancer. SLNB is also used along with preoperative computed tomography lymphography (CTLG). Methods such as these are used during surgery to more accurately identify sentinel nodes, help avoid the use of radioactive materials, and eliminate the need for second surgeries to remove axillary lymph nodes when the SLNB is positive.

Precautions

As with all surgical procedures, SNLB may produce short-term effects such as mild discomfort after the procedure, pain and swelling at the surgical site, and skin or allergic reactions to the blue dye. These are usually treated effectively with medications. Lymph node surgery sometimes has adverse effects related to the removal of multiple lymph nodes. These may include tissue swelling (lymphedema) due to disruption of the normal flow of lymphatic fluid throughout the body, buildup of lymph fluid (seroma) at the site of the surgery, numbness or tingling at the surgical site, and difficulty moving the affected body part. A patient may experience pain or swelling of an arm or leg or other effects when extensive lymph node surgery is performed in the underarm area or groin.

Preparation

No specific preparation is necessary for performing SLNB before or after surgery to remove the primary tumor. However, the patient must be evaluated for fitness to undergo the procedure, as SLNB is not appropriate for all patients. Patients who might be excluded are: women with cancer in more than one part of the breast; women who have had previous breast surgery of any kind, including plastic surgery; women with breast cancer in advanced stages; and women who have had **radiation therapy**. Melanoma patients who have undergone wide excision (removal of surrounding skin as well as the tumor) of the original **skin cancer** are also not candidates for SLNB.

Aftercare

A sentinel lymph node biopsy alone does not require extensive aftercare. In most cases, the patient will go home after the procedure or after an overnight stay in the hospital.

The surgeon or the patient's oncologist will discuss the laboratory findings with the patient. If the sentinel node was found to contain cancer cells, the surgeon will usually recommend a full axillary **lymph node dissection** (ALND) in a follow-up surgery. This is a more invasive surgical procedure in which a larger number of lymph nodes—usually 12–15—is surgically removed. A drainage tube is placed for two to three weeks after the surgery, and the patient must undergo **physical therapy** to regain muscle strength at the surgical site area.

Risks

Risks associated with SLNB include those associated with any surgery, such as reaction to anesthesia, bleeding or bruising at the surgical site, and risk of infection. The possibility of obtaining a false negative biopsy report is also a risk. A false negative means that cancer actually exists in other lymph nodes in spite of the absence of cancer in the sentinel node. False negatives sometimes result from poor timing of the dye injection, the way in which the tissue was prepared for examination, or the existence of previously undiscovered sentinel nodes. In rare instances, when multiple lymph nodes have been removed surgically, postoperative lymphedema becomes chronic and can lead to cancer of the lymphatic vessels (lymphangiosarcoma).

Results

Sentinel lymph node biopsies are highly accurate and have relatively few false negatives. A negative histology report means that chances are greater than 95% that other nearby lymph nodes are also free of cancer.

Morbidity and mortality rates

Compared to axillary lymph node dissection, sentinel lymph node biopsy has a significantly lower rate of complications, including a lower rate of postoperative pain and infection, as well as a lower long-term risk of lymphedema.

Alternatives

Breast cancer patients who are not candidates for SNLB usually undergo axillary lymph node dissection to

---

QUESTIONS TO ASK YOUR DOCTOR

- Am I a candidate for sentinel lymph node biopsy?
- How many SLNB procedures have you performed?
- Do you perform this procedure on a regular basis?
- What is your false negative rate?
- What can I expect in the way of pain or discomfort after having an SNLB?
- What are the adverse effects or risks of having this procedure?

---

determine whether their cancer has spread. Melanoma patients who have already had a wide excision of the original melanoma may have nearby lymph nodes removed to prevent the cancer from spreading; this procedure is called a prophylactic lymph node dissection.

Health care team roles

SLNB is usually performed in the department of nuclear medicine in a hospital, although it is sometimes performed as an outpatient procedure. The procedure involves close cooperation between nuclear medicine physicians, surgeons, and pathologists. The radioactive material and/or dye is injected by a physician who specializes in nuclear medicine. The sentinel lymph node is removed by a surgeon with experience in the technique. It is then analyzed in the hospital laboratory by a pathologist, who is a doctor specializing in the causes and effects of disease through the laboratory examination of body fluids and tissues.

The accuracy of a sentinel lymph node biopsy depends greatly on the skill of the surgeon who removes the node. Most doctors need to perform 20–30 SLNBs before they achieve an 85% success rate in identifying the sentinel node(s) and 5% or fewer false negatives. Training for this procedure is accomplished through special residency programs, fellowships, or training protocols. It is vital for patients to ask their surgeon how many SLNB procedures he or she has performed, as those who do these biopsies on a regular basis generally have a higher degree of accuracy.

Resources

BOOKS

Niederhuber, J. E., et al. "Sentinel Lymph Node Biopsy." In *Abeloff's Clinical Oncology*, edited by Martin D. Abeloff. 5th ed. New York: W.B. Saunders, 2013.

PERIODICALS

Amersi, F., and Hansen, N. M. "The Benefits and Limitations of Sentinel Lymph Node Biopsy." *Current Treatment Options in Oncology* 7 (March 2006) 141–51.

Bluemel, C., et al. "Intraoperative 3-D Imaging Improves Sentinel Lymph Node Biopsy in Oral Cancer." *European Journal of Nucear Medicine and Molecular Imaging* (July 2014): PMID: 25077931.

Jaffer, Shabnam, and Ira Bleiweiss. "Evolution of Sentinel Lymph Node Biopsy in Breast Cancer, In and Out of Vogue?" *Advances in Anatomic Pathology* 21, no. 6 (November 2014) 433–42. http://dx.doi.org/10.1097/PAP.0000000000000041 (accessed October 30, 2014).

WEBSITES

National Cancer Institute. "Fact Sheet: Sentinel Lymph Node Biopsy." http://www.cancer.gov/cancertopics/factsheet/detection/sentinel-node-biopsy (accessed October 27, 2014).

ORGANIZATIONS

American Cancer Society, 250 Williams St. NW, Atlanta, GA 30303, (800) 227 2345, http://www.cancer.org.

National Cancer Institute, 9609 Medical Center Dr., BG 9609 MSC 9760, Bethesda, MD 20892-9760, (800) 4-CANCER (422-6237), http://www.cancer.gov.

Society of Nuclear Medicine and Molecular Imaging, 1850 Samuel Morse Dr., Reston, VA 20190, (703) 708-9000, Fax: (703) 708-9015, http://www.snmmi.org.

Rebecca Frey, PhD

REVISED BY L. LEE CULVERT

REVIEWED BY MELINDA GRANGER OBERLEITNER, RN, DNS, APRN, CNS

Sentinel lymph node mapping

Definition

Sentinel lymph node mapping is a method of determining whether **cancer** has metastasized (spread) beyond the primary tumor and into the lymphatic system. The mapping procedure is used in conjunction with **sentinel lymph node biopsy** or dissection.

Purpose

The lymphatic system is the body's primary defense against infection. Lymph vessels carry clear, slightly yellow fluid called lymph that contains proteins to help rid the body of infection. Lymph nodes are small, bean-shaped collections of tissue found along the lymphatic vessels. Cancer cells can break off from the original tumor and spread through the lymphatic system to distant parts of the body where secondary tumors are formed.

One job of the lymph nodes is to clean the lymph by trapping foreign cells, such as bacteria or cancer cells, and identifying foreign proteins for antibody response.

The sentinel lymph node is the first lymph node that filters the fluid draining away from the primary tumor. If cancer cells are breaking off and entering the lymphatic system, the first filtering node (not necessarily the closest to the tumor) will be most likely to contain the breakaway cancer cells.

There are about 600 lymph nodes in the body. About 200 are in the head and neck and another 30–50 are in the armpit. Others are located in the groin. The sentinel node, or first filtering lymph node, will be different for each tumor and for each individual. Sentinel lymph node mapping is a technique for pinpointing which node is the most likely to receive the primary drainage from the tumor and therefore the most likely to contain cancer, so that it can be surgically removed and examined under the microscope for cancer.

If the sentinel node is cancer-free, there is a very high probability that cancer has not spread to any other node. If cancer cells are present in the sentinel node, it is likely that other nodes in the lymphatic system also contain cancer cells. This information is important in staging the cancer and individualizing cancer treatment for maximum benefit.

Sentinel lymph node mapping is a relatively new technique. It was first used in 1977 by researchers studying cancer of the penis. Later it was used successfully in staging **melanoma** (a type of **skin cancer**). In 1993, researchers first used the technique in **breast cancer** patients. Since then, **clinical trials** in breast cancer patients have demonstrated the accuracy and effectiveness of sentinel lymph node mapping and dissection in the staging of breast cancer. Researchers hope to be able to apply the sentinel node technique to other cancers in the future.

Advantages of sentinel lymph node mapping

Before sentinel node mapping was developed, there was no way of knowing whether and how far cancer had spread without removing and examining samples from many lymph nodes under the microscope. For example, in breast cancer patients, after a **lumpectomy** or **mastectomy** it was conventional treatment to remove most of the axillary nodes. These are the lymph nodes in the armpit. Removing axillary nodes causes frequent complications in as many as 80% of women. These complications include swelling (lymphedema), numbness, burning sensation in the armpit, reduction in arm and shoulder movement, and increased risk of infection.

Sentinel **lymph node dissection** limits the extent of surgery. It provides the following advantages:

- Less surgical trauma because only one lymph node or a small cluster of nodes is removed. For example, in breast cancers, two or three nodes are generally removed.

- Fewer side effects from surgery.

- The lymphatic system is left intact and is better able to transport fluid and fight infection.

- Fewer risks of impairment of arm and shoulder movements.

- With only a small amount of tissue being removed, it can be studied much more exhaustively in the laboratory for the presence of cancer.

- Significant reduction in post-mastectomy pain.

How accurate are sentinel lymph node mapping and dissection?

Sentinel lymph node mapping is used primarily in cases of melanoma and breast cancer. The technique is relatively new, and several breast cancer clinical trials are underway. One purpose is to determine the most accurate methods of finding the sentinel node. Another is to compare the control of cancer and survival rates of sentinel node **biopsy** with conventional axillary lymph node dissection in women whose sentinel nodes are both positive and negative for cancer. Up-to-date information about these clinical trials can be obtained from the **National Cancer Institute** at http://www.cancer.gov/clinicaltrials or (800) 4-CANCER.

Since sentinel lymph node mapping and dissection are relatively new, they are not done at every hospital. Doctors need special training in order to perform these procedures. Studies consistently have shown that the ability to locate the sentinel node increases the more experience doctors have with the procedure. Experienced physicians can pinpoint the sentinel node with about 95% to 98% accuracy. Similarly, studies have shown that there is a learning curve for surgeons and pathologists (doctors who examine the nodes in the laboratory) in sentinel lymph node dissection. The more experience they have, the more accurate they are.

Overall, accurate diagnoses from sentinel lymph node dissection are very high (92% or more). However, it is important that the patient find out how much training and experience the treatment team has with this procedure, and if necessary ask for a referral to another facility with more experienced staff. Some insurers may also consider the procedure experimental. Patients should check with their insurers about coverage, as the acceptance of this procedure is evolving.

Precautions

Women with breast cancer who are the best candidates for sentinel node dissection are those with early-stage breast cancer with low-to-moderate risk of lymph node involvement. Women who are not good candidates for sentinel node dissection are those who:

- Are believed to have cancer in the lymph nodes.

- Have had prior surgery (such as breast reduction surgery) that would change the normal pattern of lymph flow near the primary tumor.

- Have already received chemotherapy, because chemotherapy can create tissue changes that alter normal lymph flow.

- Are older, because lymph flow alters with age and the sentinel node may not be accurately detected.

To get valid results, people with melanoma must have sentinel **lymph node biopsy** performed before wide excision of the original melanoma.

Description

Sentinel lymph node mapping and dissection is done in a hospital under general anesthesia. There are two methods of detecting the sentinel node. In the dye method, a vital blue tracer dye is injected near the tumor. The dye enters the lymphatic system and then collects in the sentinel or first filtering node. The surgeon looks for the accumulation of dye and removes the blue node.

In the radioactive technique, a low-level radioactive tracer is injected near the tumor. It is absorbed into the lymph system and travels to the sentinel node. A hand-held Geiger counter (a device that measures radioactivity) is passed over the area near the tumor until the spot with the most radioactivity is located. The radioactive ("hot") node is then removed. Because accuracy in locating the sentinel node is increased by 10% to 15% if both radioactive and dye tracers are used together, this method is generally done.

Once the sentinel nodes are removed, they are sent to the laboratory to be examined for cancer. If no cancer cells are present, there is rarely a need to remove more lymph nodes. If cancer cells are present, it is likely that more lymph nodes will be removed. In any event, information from the sentinel node biopsy will be used to determine the best way to treat the cancer.

Preparation

Standard preoperative blood and liver function tests are performed before sentinel node mapping and dissection. The patient will also meet with an anesthesiologist before the operation and should tell the anesthesiologist about all medication (prescription, nonprescription, or herbal) that he or she is taking and about all drug allergies.

Aftercare

Because only a small amount of tissue is removed, patients generally recover quickly from sentinel node mapping and dissection. They may feel tired from the anesthesia and may experience minor burning, pain, and slight swelling at the site of the incision. If tracer dye is used, the dye stays in the body for up to nine months and may be visible under the skin.

Risks

The greatest risk associated with sentinel lymph node mapping is that the sentinel node cannot be identified and conventional removal of many lymph nodes will be necessary. Failure to locate the sentinel node happens in less than 5% of patients.

The second greatest risk is of a false-negative reading (approximately 5% to 8% for breast cancer), finding no cancer in the tissue sample when it is actually present. As discussed above, this test is extremely accurate when performed by an experienced treatment team.

Other risks associated with sentinel lymph node mapping are allergic reaction to the dye, infection at the incision site, and allergic reaction to anesthesia.

QUESTIONS TO ASK YOUR DOCTOR

- Am I a good candidate for sentinel lymph node mapping and biopsy?
- How much experience do you have with this procedure?
- If you have limited experience, can you refer me to a center where this operation is frequently performed?
- Where can I find out about clinical trials involving sentinel node mapping and biopsy?
- If I am not a good candidate for sentinel lymph node biopsy, what are my options?

Results

If no cancer cells are found in the sentinel node, other lymph nodes do not need to be removed.

Abnormal results

If cancer cells are found in the sentinel lymph node the treatment team may recommend an operation to remove more lymph nodes and/or radiation or **chemotherapy** to control the cancer.

Resources

PERIODICALS

Abu-Rustum, N.R. "Sentinel Lymph Node Mapping For Endometrial Cancer: A Modern Approach To Surgical Staging." *Journal of the National Comprehensive Cancer Network* 12, no. 2 (2014): 288–97. http://www.ncbi.nlm.nih.gov/pubmed/24586087 (accessed November 14, 2014).

Brucker, S.Y., Taran, F.A., and Wallwiener, D. "Sentinel Lymph Node Mapping in Endometrial Cancer: A Concept Ready For Clinical Routine?" *Archives of Gynecology and Obstetrics* 290, no. 1 (2014): 9–11.

Giammarile, F., Vidal-Sicart S., and Valdés Olmos, R.A. "Uncommon Applications of Sentinel Lymph Node Mapping: Urogenital Cancers." *Quarterly Journal of Nuclear Medicine and Molecular Imaging* 58, no. 2 (2014): 161–79. http://www.minervamedica.it/en/journals/nuclear-med-molecular-imaging/article.php?cod=R39Y2014N02A0161 (accessed November 14, 2014).

WEBSITES

National Cancer Institute. "Sentinel Lymph Node Biopsy." http://www.cancer.gov/cancertopics/factsheet/detection/sentinel-node-biopsy (accessed November 14, 2014).

ORGANIZATIONS

American Cancer Society, 250 Williams St. NW, Atlanta, GA 30303, (800) 227-2345, http://www.cancer.org.

National Cancer Institute, 9609 Medical Center Dr., BG 9609
    MSC 9760, Bethesda, MD 20892-9760, (800) 4-CANCER
    (422-6237), http://www.cancer.gov.

Radiological Society of North America, 820 Jorie Blvd., Oak
    Brook, IL 60523-2251, (800) 381-6660, Fax: (630) 571-
    7837, http://www.rsna.org.

Tish Davidson, A.M.

Septic shock *see* **Infection and sepsis**

Sexual issues for cancer patients

Definition

Sexuality issues can arise following diagnosis and
during and after treatment for **cancer**. They can include
sexual dysfunction, pain, necessary modifications in
sexual activities, early menopause, loss of sexual desire,
psychological and emotional changes, negative **body
image**, anxiety, **depression**, and/or infertility.

Description

Many types of cancer and their treatments can result in
temporary or permanent sexuality issues; however, these
issues are most common with prostate, breast, and
gynecological cancers. The most common problems are loss
of sexual desire, erectile dysfunction (ED) in men, and
painful intercourse in women. Less commonly, men may be
unable to ejaculate, have ejaculation that reverses into the
bladder, be unable to reach orgasm, or have weaker or shorter
orgasms. Although weaker orgasms are a normal part of
aging, severe orgasmic weakening often accompanies ED
and may not improve with ED treatment. Men who
experience dry orgasms after cancer treatment sometimes
report reduced sensation. Pain during vaginal intercourse in
women is often due to treatment-related dryness or changes
in vaginal tissue or vaginal size. Cancer treatments may cause
sudden premature menopause and a tight, dry vagina. This
condition can lead to vaginismus—a tensing of the muscles
around the opening to the vagina that makes penetration
difficult and painful. Female cancer patients may also
experience pain or numbness in the genitals or some other
part of the body, such as a sore arm following a **mastectomy**
(removal of part or all of a breast), or tingling or numbness in
the hands or feet from **chemotherapy**. Less commonly,
women have trouble reaching orgasm.

Other common sexuality issues in men and women
include:

• concerns about intimacy following treatment

• inability to have satisfactory sexual experiences

• anxiety over sexual performance

• genital or urinary tract bleeding from some types of
cancer—such as cervical or bladder cancer—that can
interfere with sexual activity

• negative body image and feelings of unattractiveness

• fear of rejection

• infertility

Sexuality issues are linked to needs for intimacy,
love and caring, and physical contact. Sexuality issues in
cancer patients can affect self-esteem, relationships, and
quality of life. Unfortunately, many patients are uncomfortable discussing sexuality issues with their partners
and their physicians.

Sexuality during treatment

Sexual activity is usually safe during cancer
treatment. Small amounts of a few chemotherapy drugs
may be present in vaginal fluids or semen, so it may be
necessary to use a condom when having sex during the
period when chemotherapy is being administered and
for about two weeks after treatment ends. An implanted
chemotherapy infusion catheter must be protected
during sexual activity. Pregnancy should be avoided
during chemotherapy and for some time afterward to
prevent birth defects. Some types of radiation treatment
require temporary precautions such as condom use.
Women who are not bleeding heavily can have sex
during pelvic **radiation therapy**, although waiting
about four weeks may reduce the risk of tearing
damaged tissue. Intercourse may not be possible with
radioactive implants (brachytherapy). Both chemotherapy and radiation can damage the immune system and
increase the risk of sexually transmitted infections
(STIs). Sexual activity following surgery may cause
bleeding or strain on an incision, or increase the risk of
infection. Abstinence may be necessary until healing is
complete.

Risk factors

Risk factors for sexuality issues in cancer patients
include:

• prostate cancer

• testicular or penile cancers

• breast cancer

• cancers of the ovaries, uterus, cervix, or vagina

• anal cancer

• radiation therapy—especially for ovarian or prostate
cancer—that destroys tissue

• ED before diagnosis and treatment

KEY TERMS

Abdominoperineal (AP) resection—Surgical removal of the lower colon and rectum and possibly other organs to treat colon cancer.

Brachytherapy—Cancer treatment that administers radioactive material directly to the site of a tumor.

Cystectomy—Surgical removal of part or all of the bladder and possibly other organs to treat bladder cancer.

Erectile dysfunction (ED)—The consistent inability to achieve or maintain a penile erection.

Hormone replacement therapy (HRT)—Treatment of menopausal symptoms with the female hormones estrogen and/or progesterone.

Hormone therapy—Cancer treatment that affects the hormone balance of the body, such as by blocking estrogen receptors or preventing estrogen production.

Hysterectomy—Surgical removal of the uterus and possibly adjacent tissues.

Kegel exercises—Repetitive contractions of the muscles used to halt urinary flow, in order to enhance sexual responsiveness and control incontinence.

Mastectomy—Surgical removal of part or all of the breast and possibly associated lymph nodes and muscle to treat breast cancer.

Menopause—The female developmental stage at which menstruation ceases.

Penile rehabilitation—Frequent use of erectile dysfunction drugs, penile injections, or a vacuum constriction device to achieve erections to keep the tissue healthy and low-dose ED drugs to improve blood flow to healing nerves following cancer surgery.

Prostatectomy—Surgical removal of the prostate gland to treat prostate cancer.

Sexually transmitted infection (STI)—An infection transmitted through sexual activity.

Vacuum constriction device (VCD)—A cylinder placed over the penis that creates a vacuum to achieve and maintain an erection.

Vaginal dilator—A rubber or plastic tube used to stretch the vagina following radiation or surgery to treat cancer.

Vaginismus—Painful spasmodic contractions of the vagina.

- negative sexual feelings or sexuality issues that were present before diagnosis and treatment
- older age, which is often associated with decreased sexual desire and performance

Demographics

Sexuality issues are very common in both male and female cancer patients, regardless of sexual orientation. More than half of all survivors of prostate, breast, gynecological, and colorectal cancers have post-treatment sexuality issues. The **National Cancer Institute** (NCI) estimates that between 40% and 100% of patients experience some degree of sexual dysfunction following various cancer treatments. Erectile dysfunction (ED) affects 60–90% of men treated with radical **prostatectomy** (removal of the entire prostate gland and some of the surrounding tissue, including seminal vesicles) for **prostate cancer**, and 67–85% of men treated with external-beam radiation for prostate cancer. About half of all women treated for breast and gynecological cancers—including ovarian, uterine, and vaginal cancers—experience long-term sexual dysfunction. About 25% of patients treated for **testicular cancer** and **Hodgkin lymphoma** experience sexual dysfunction.

Causes and symptoms

Chemotherapy

Chemotherapy is associated with a temporary loss of sexual desire in both men and women. Chemotherapy side effects—including nausea, vomiting, **diarrhea**, constipation, mouth sores, hair loss, smell and taste changes, and weight changes—or catheters that remain in place can interfere with attraction and desire.

Chemotherapy can reduce **testosterone** in men and estrogen in women. Decreased estrogen may cause vaginal dryness, shrinking, inelasticity, hot flashes, urinary tract infections, irritability, **fatigue**, or mood swings. Chemotherapy can cause painful intercourse and difficulty reaching orgasm in women. Yeast infections or a flare-up of genital herpes or genital warts can occur because chemotherapy weakens the immune system.

Radiation

Radiation side effects—including fatigue, nausea, vomiting, and diarrhea—may decrease sexual desire. Pelvic radiation therapy in men may cause ED, weaker orgasms, changes in penis length, or urinary incontinence. Brachytherapy for prostate cancer has less effect on erectile function and ejaculation. Pelvic radiation in women can cause sudden menopause or scarring and thickening of the vaginal walls and shortening or narrowing of the vagina, leading to painful intercourse. It can also cause the vaginal lining to become thin and fragile.

Surgery in men

Cancer surgeries that can cause ED—usually from damage to nerves or blood vessels—include:

- radical prostatectomy
- radical cystectomy—removal of the bladder, upper urethra, prostate, and seminal vesicles for bladder cancer
- abdominoperineal (AP) resection—removal of the lower colon and rectum for colon cancer
- total pelvic exenteration—removal of the bladder, prostate, seminal vesicles, and rectum, usually for a large colon tumor

Many men experience problems with orgasm, changes in penis length, or urinary incontinence after radical prostatectomy, or problems with ejaculation or orgasm after surgery for **rectal cancer**. However, newer nerve-sparing techniques for radical prostatectomy and bladder, colon, and/or rectum removal usually lead to a faster return of erectile function.

Testicular cancer and its treatment, including removal of a testicle, usually affects sexual function only temporarily. Removal of both testicles is more likely to interfere with sexual desire and function.

Surgery in women

Mastectomy for **breast cancer** is associated with loss of sexual interest. Feeling less attractive is the most common sexual side effect of breast surgery. The breasts and nipples are also a source of sexual pleasure. **Breast reconstruction** following a mastectomy restores appearance but not the same degree of sensation. However, breast-preserving surgery or breast reconstruction following mastectomy appears to lead to far fewer sexuality issues. For most such women, frequency of sex, ability to reach orgasm, and overall sexual satisfaction are similar to their experiences before diagnosis and treatment.

Surgery to remove the uterus, ovaries, bladder, or other pelvic or abdominal organs can reduce vaginal size and moisture, and may cause sexual pain and dysfunction. However, most women regain normal vaginal and genital sensations and can have pain-free intercourse and achieve orgasm.

- Hysterectomy (removal of the uterus) does not usually affect sexual pleasure—the vagina is shortened, but the vagina and clitoris usually remain sensitive. If cancer was causing bleeding or pain during intercourse, a

hysterectomy may improve sexual relations. Most reported sexual issues following radical hysterectomy (removal of the uterus, cervix, and adjacent tissues and lymph nodes) disappear within six months.

- Radical cystectomy for bladder cancer removes the bladder, uterus, ovaries, fallopian tubes, cervix, front wall of the vagina, and urethra, and may cause pain during intercourse and difficulty reaching orgasm. Vaginal reconstruction during the surgery often eliminates these problems.
- AP resection for colon cancer removes the lower colon and rectum and sometimes the uterus, ovaries, and rear wall of the vagina, requiring vaginal reconstruction. It does not damage the nerves that supply genital sensation.
- Vulvectomy (removal of the vulva) may cause painful intercourse, genital numbness, or difficulty reaching orgasm. Orgasm may be impossible if the clitoris must be removed.

Other surgical procedures

UROSTOMY OR COLOSTOMY. Urostomy and **colostomy** are surgical procedures that reroute urine and other excrement to an opening in the abdomen (stoma). Before sexual activity, the partners should ensure that the urostomy fits correctly, and the bag should be emptied to reduce the chance of a leak. A patterned pouch may be worn over it to cover it. Sexual activity with a colostomy can be performed with the same precautions. Partners may wish to plan sexual activity at a time when the colostomy is not active and avoid gas-producing foods that day. Direct communication and reassurances from a loving partner can be extremely helpful.

LIMB AMPUTATION. Treatment mainly of primary tumors of bone may include amputating a limb. The partners may wish to decide whether the prosthesis needs to be worn during sex. A prosthesis can help with movement and balance but the straps that attach it can get in the way. If the prosthesis is not used, pillows could be used instead for balance.

TREATMENT OF FACIAL CANCER. Some cancers of the head and neck may be treated by partial removal of the facial bony structure. The resulting scars can be psychologically damaging for some patients. Following such surgery, speech may also be affected. Recent advances in facial prosthesis and plastic surgery may help regain a more natural appearance and speech.

Hormone therapy

Hormone therapy for prostate cancer often causes decreased sexual desire, ED, or difficulty reaching orgasm. **Tamoxifen** for breast cancer in women over

45 may cause menopausal symptoms, decreased sexual desire, vaginal discharge and pain, and trouble reaching orgasm.

Other drugs

Some cancer drug therapies affect nerves, blood vessels, and hormones that control sexual feelings and function. Drugs known as **aromatase inhibitors** used to treat breast cancer in postmenopausal women can affect sexual desire and function. **Opioids** for pain and antidepressants can also affect sexuality.

Psychological and emotional issues

Depression is common in cancer patients, and decreased sexual desire and pleasure are common symptoms of depression. Hair loss, weight gain, or body changes from surgery may negatively affect self-image and decrease the desire for sex. Concern over a partner's reaction to the cancer or bodily changes can also affect sexual desire. Stress from a cancer diagnosis and treatment can negatively affect sexual relationships. Anxiety and mental distraction can overwhelm sexual feelings and cause a woman's vagina to remain tight and dry, making intercourse uncomfortable or painful.

Diagnosis

Examination

A gynecological examination during or following cancer treatment may reveal potential problems with sexual functioning, such as vaginal dryness. Physical examinations are generally not useful in men.

Tests

There are no tests that measure sexual function in women. The primary test for sexual function in men is the ability to obtain and maintain an erection sufficient for penetration. Erections during sleep indicate that there is probably not a physical cause for ED. Nighttime erections are measured with a snap gauge or electronic monitor. Blood tests may indicate abnormal hormone levels that can affect sexuality.

Procedures

Sexuality issues are usually self-diagnosed by cancer patients, since they depend on a patient's age, sex, personal attitudes, and religious and cultural values. Physicians should bring up sexuality issues associated with the specific type of cancer and treatment, and patients should talk to their doctors about issues that come up at diagnosis and during and after treatment. Discussions may include the patient's partner.

Assessment of sexuality issues can include:

- sexual desire, arousal, and enjoyment
- energy for sexual activity
- ability of male patients to obtain and maintain erections
- expansion and lubrication of the female vagina
- ability to reach orgasm and types of orgasmic stimulation, such as self-touching, use of a vibrator, caressing, oral stimulation, or intercourse
- pain during sex
- whether issues existed before diagnosis or treatment
- medications and their dosages
- relationships with partners
- lifestyle issues, such as smoking and alcohol consumption
- specific problems and concerns

Treatment

The goal of treatment is to help cancer patients, survivors, and their partners discover or rediscover their sense of sexual pleasure and sensuality. Lubricants, drugs, and devices are of little use if sexual desire is impaired. Counseling by a mental health professional or sex therapist can be useful for approaching sex from a new perspective or dealing with fear, anxiety, depression, or misbeliefs about sexuality and cancer. Specialized cancer centers may have staff experts for assessing and treating sexuality issues.

ED that does not respond to medications may be treated with a vacuum constriction device (VCD) placed over the penis or with an implanted penile prosthesis.

Treatments for women include vaginal lubricants and dilators that can ease pain. The lubricant should be a water-based gel without perfumes, colorings, spermicides, flavors, or herbal extracts that could irritate delicate tissues. Vaginal moisturizers are over-the-counter, non hormonal products that are used several times a week to keep the vagina moist and at a normal acidic balance. Vitamin E gel caps can be used as a vaginal moisturizer by making a small hole in the cap with a clean needle.

Drugs

ED is usually treated with sildenafil (Viagra), vardenafil (Levitra), or tadalafil (Cialis). These drugs may not be effective for the first year or two after surgical nerve damage; however, if the penile tissues weaken during this time, a natural erection will become impossible. Since it is thought that any type of erection will help keep the tissues healthy while the nerves heal, penile rehabilitation is begun within weeks or months after surgery. An ED drug, VCD, or penile injections are used two to three times per week to achieve an erection hard enough for penetration. Urethral pellets are drugs inserted in the urethra (opening of the penis) with an applicator to cause an erection. In addition, a low dose (about one-quarter tablet) of an ED drug is taken on days without an erection to increase blood flow around the nerves to encourage healing.

Vaginal atrophy—dry, thin, inelastic vaginal walls—can be treated with topical or systemic estrogen therapy (HRT) in postmenopausal women. Hormones applied to the genital area or vagina as gels, creams, tablets, or rings are safer than HRT supplied in a pill or a patch, which can increase the risk of breast and uterine cancers.

Alternative

Alternative and complementary treatments include meditation, biofeedback, acupuncture, yoga, creative imagery, and hypnosis. Medical marijuana may be helpful in states where it is legal. **Vitamins**, minerals such as zinc, special diets, or herbs and supplements such as **saw palmetto** or yohimbe may also be helpful. However, many herbs and supplements for ED may be ineffective, may not contain the listed ingredients, or may contain potentially dangerous ingredients that are not listed on the label. For example, yohimbe can cause priapism (a painful and long-lasting erection), and chronic marijuana use has been studied as a potential cause of sexual dysfunction.

Home remedies

The most effective treatments for sexuality issues in cancer patients may be open, honest communication between partners and adaptation—discovering new ways of giving and receiving sexual pleasure and reaching orgasm. Cancer patients often find that sexual touching alone is satisfying. Sexual fantasizing and self-stimulation can be helpful. Women can experiment with different leg positions, rhythmically tightening and relaxing vaginal muscles, or use a vibrator for extra stimulation. Other recommendations include:

- planning sexual activity for times when pain is minimal, such as an hour after taking pain medication
- finding positions and activities and using support pillows to avoid putting pressure on sore areas
- focusing on pleasurable feelings and excitement
- changing negative thoughts
- staying active and sociable
- dealing with grief and loss
- rebuilding self-esteem

To strengthen their climax, men can repeatedly slow down when approaching orgasm and then rebuild excitement. This technique can be practiced during self-stimulation. Fantasizing and extended foreplay can also help.

Female genital pain may be avoided or minimized by:

- using Kegel exercises and vaginal dilators to relax the vaginal muscles
- using large amounts of lubricating gel
- ensuring full arousal before penetration
- showing a partner the types of touching and positions that are not painful
- using positions that enable the woman to control movement

Couples usually adjust to a shortened post-surgical vagina. Extended caressing and foreplay can adequately lengthen a well-lubricated vagina. Different sexual positions can limit the depth of penetration. There are also methods for increasing the perception of greater vaginal depth.

Women who are uncomfortable with changes in their body after cancer treatment may try touching and looking at their genitals, using whole-body stroking, and finding new places that are pleasurable to the touch. Wearing a wig, hat, or scarf to cover hair loss or a breast form prosthesis is helpful for some women.

Prognosis

The ability of cancer patients to resolve sexuality issues varies, depending on the individual and the type and severity of the cancer. Many patients resume the same type and degree of sexual activity as before their cancer or adapt to changes in their sexual functioning. Many patients discover that their sexuality was lacking before cancer and that the changes are improvements. Most women who had orgasms before cancer treatment can have them afterward, although it may take practice. However, unlike many other side effects of cancer and its treatment, sexual problems can worsen over time, so learning to adapt is very important.

Radical prostatectomy that spares nerves on both sides of the prostate is less likely to cause sexual problems than radiation therapy for prostate cancer. However, it may take up to two years for the nerves and blood vessels to heal enough to regain erections. Recovery following radiation occurs over two to three years. Younger men with good erections before surgery are more likely to regain full erections than older men who may have had some degree of ED before treatment. Peyronie's disease, a painful curve in the erect penis usually resulting from scar tissue, has been linked to

QUESTIONS TO ASK YOUR DOCTOR

- How will my cancer treatment affect my sexuality?
- What can I do before my cancer treatment to minimize my risk of sexuality issues after treatment?
- May I be sexually active during my cancer treatment?
- How can my partner help with my sexuality issues?
- Would a sex counselor or therapist be helpful?

some cancer surgeries, including prostatectomy. It can be treated with drug injections or surgery.

Prevention

Learning about possible effects of cancer treatment on sexuality—and realizing that regardless of the type of treatment, sexual pleasure is still possible—are important for preventing sexuality issues.

Women can often prevent tight scar tissue from forming by stretching the vaginal walls with vagina-penetrating sex or a vaginal dilator three to four times per week, beginning about four weeks after radiation treatment. Since scarring can develop over many years following radiation, ongoing dilator use may be necessary. Following surgery that rebuilds the vagina with skin grafts, a specially designed dilator may be worn continuously for a time.

Using a condom for vaginal, oral, and anal sex can prevent STIs. It is very important to avoid touching the vagina or urethra after contact with the anal area to prevent infections. Urinating after sex can wash away bacteria and help prevent urinary tract infections.

Resources

OTHER

American Cancer Society. *Sexuality for the Man with Cancer.* http://www.cancer.org/acs/groups/cid/documents/ webcontent/002910-pdf.pdf (accessed November 17, 2014).

American Cancer Society. *Sexuality for the Woman with Cancer.* http://www.cancer.org/acs/groups/cid/documents/webcon tent/002912-pdf.pdf (accessed November 17, 2014).

WEBSITES

American Cancer Society. "Sexuality After Breast Cancer." http://www.cancer.org/cancer/breastcancer/detailedguide/breast-cancer-after-sexuality (accessed November 14, 2014).

National Cancer Institute. "Sexuality and Reproductive Issues." http://www.cancer.gov/cancertopics/pdq/supportivecare/ sexuality/HealthProfessional/page1 (accessed November 14, 2014).

ORGANIZATIONS

American Cancer Society, 250 Williams Street NW, Atlanta, GA 30303, (800) 227-2345, http://www.cancer.org.

American Psychosocial Oncology Society, 154 Hansen Road, Suite 201, Charlottesville, VA 22991, (434) 293-5350, Fax: (434) 977-1856, (866) APOS-4-HELP (276-7443), info@apos-society.org, http://www.apos-society.org.

National Cancer Institute, 6116 Executive Boulevard, Suite 300, Bethesda, MD 20892-8322, (800) 4-CANCER (422-6237), http://www.cancer.gov.

Margaret Alic, PhD

Sézary syndrome

Definition

Sézary syndrome is a type of **cutaneous T-cell lymphoma**, characterized by skin abnormalities, extreme **itching**, enlarged lymph glands, and abnormal blood cells.

Description

Sézary syndrome is a type of **lymphoma**, which is a disease in which lymphocytes (a type of white blood cell) increase to very large numbers in a person's blood. Sézary syndrome is a specific type of lymphoma known as a cutaneous T-cell lymphoma, meaning that it is a disease in which the white blood cells known as T-lymphocytes increase to large numbers.

Sézary syndrome can affect many organs. In early-stage disease, the skin is the only organ affected; however, later-stage disease can affect other organ systems.

Demographics

Sézary syndrome is relatively rare, affecting about one in one million people. The incidence of the syndrome increases with age, with most cases appearing in people in their 50s or 60s. Men appear to be affected more often than women, and black males appear to be at higher risk of developing the syndrome than white males.

Causes and symptoms

There are no known causes of Sézary syndrome. Early in the course of study of the syndrome, it was thought that exposure to certain chemicals could trigger the disease. However, later studies have not shown any relation between industrial chemical exposure and Sézary syndrome.

The symptoms of Sézary syndrome can be very subtle; because of this, it is often not diagnosed for many years. Early symptoms include skin lesions that can look like eczema and psoriasis. Later symptoms can include skin tumors, especially in body folds. Enlarged lymph glands in the neck, armpits, and groin can accompany the skin tumors. Later in the course of Sézary syndrome, its symptoms may relate to other areas of disease involvement.

Diagnosis

The diagnosis of Sézary syndrome is made by careful clinical evaluation. Generally, a patient with Sézary syndrome seeks treatment for skin lesions that are not responsive to ordinary medications. If the doctor suspects a cutaneous T-cell lymphoma, a blood test is ordered to see if there are any abnormalities, such as an increase or decrease in lymphocytes and the presence or absence of Sézary cells, which are white blood cells with a distinctive shape when viewed under a microscope. Finally, a sample (**biopsy**) of one the skin lesions is done to see whether the lesion is part of Sézary syndrome or caused by some other disease.

Clinical staging, treatment, prognosis

Staging for cutaneous T-cell lymphoma, including Sézary syndrome, is based on the extent of skin involvement and the presence or absence of other manifestations of the syndrome. Stage I is characterized by mild skin involvement. In stage II there is extensive skin involvement, including skin tumors. Patients in stages III and IV have extensive skin involvement, blood abnormalities including Sézary cells, and swollen lymph nodes.

There are multiple therapies for Sézary syndrome. However, unless the disease is in an early stage, the chances for a complete cure are small. Nonspecific treatment includes skin lubricants and moisturizers to help treat the skin irritation and dryness that is common with the syndrome. Low-potency steroid creams or ointments may be used to help treat itching and skin inflammation.

The first therapy used with some success against Sézary syndrome is **mechlorethamine**, or nitrogen mustard. It is applied daily to the entire skin surface (except for sensitive areas such as eyelids and genitalia) for six to twelve months, then three times a week for one to two years more. Several studies have investigated the effectiveness of nitrogen mustard therapy, and have found that in stage I or II disease, the therapy causes complete remission in 60–80% of patients. Side effects are minimal, but dry skin, irritation, and change in skin pigmentation can occur.

Another treatment that has been used for many years, especially for stage II and III disease, is electron beam **radiation therapy**. Treatment with electron beam radiation therapy has been used since 1953, with good response rates seen in 50–70% of patients. Side effects can include excessive skin dryness, skin blistering, loss of hair on treated areas, and increased risk of **skin cancer**.

ECP, or photopheresis, has been approved by the FDA as a treatment for Sézary syndrome. In this mode of treatment, phototherapy with ultraviolet light is combined with leukapheresis. In leukapheresis, a person's blood is taken out and passed through special filters that remove circulating Sézary cells; the cells are treated with ultraviolet radiation, then reinfused into the patient. Response rates range from 55% to 75%, with some reports showing a 15–25% cure rate. Side effects can include nausea and **fever**.

Systemic **chemotherapy** is often used in patients who are in later stages of the disease. Using standard **cancer** chemotherapeutic agents such as **cyclophosphamide**, **vincristine**, and **doxorubicin**, response rates up to 19 months have been seen. No studies have shown an increased survival rate in patients getting aggressive, high-dose chemotherapy versus those getting more standard doses.

The prognosis for patients with Sézary syndrome is based on placing the patient in one of three categories: good, intermediate, or poor. Patients with good prognosis have the condition limited to their skin. Their general survival time is more than 10 years. Patients in the intermediate category have skin lesions including tumors and plaques, but no blood involvement. Their survival time is five years. Patients in the poor risk category have extensive skin lesions along with blood abnormalities, including high levels of Sézary cells. Patients in this category, even with extensive treatment, generally have survival times of only one year or less.

Coping with cancer treatment

There are multiple ways to help patients cope with side effects brought about by the treatment of Sézary syndrome. Lubricants can be used to help dryness, scaling, and itching of the skin caused by the use of topical treatments such as nitrogen mustard and electron beam therapy. Symptoms such as **nausea and vomiting**, caused by ECP and systemic chemotherapy, can be treated with standard anti-nausea and vomiting medication (antiemetics).

Clinical trials

In 2014, many **clinical trials** were under way to investigate several forms of innovative treatment for Sézary syndrome. Interferon has been used with some success in both early- and late-stage disease. Common side effects include a decrease in white blood cells and chronic **fatigue**. The use of **monoclonal antibodies** in treating late-stage disease (III and IV) has also been studied. Early studies have shown response rates of around 30%. Side effects include allergies to the monoclonal antibodies, fever, and fatigue.

Prevention

There are no known ways to prevent Sézary syndrome.

Resources

BOOKS

Zackheim, Herschel S., ed. *Cutaneous T-cell Lymphoma: Mycosis Fungoides and Sézary Syndrome.* Boca Raton, FL: CRC Press, 2005.

WEBSITES

National Cancer Institute. "Mycosis Fungoides and the Sézary Syndrome Treatment." http://www.cancer.gov/cancer topics/pdq/treatment/mycosisfungoides/Patient/page1/All Pages (accessed November 14, 2014).

Edward R. Rosick, D.O., M.P.H., M.S.

Shingles *see* **Herpes zoster**

Shunt *see* **Peritoneovenous shunt**

SIADH *see* **Syndrome of inappropriate antidiuretic hormone**

Sigmoidoscopy

Definition

Sigmoidoscopy is a diagnostic and screening procedure in which a rigid or flexible tube with a camera on the end (a sigmoidoscope) is inserted into the anus to examine the rectum and lower colon (bowel) for bowel disease, **cancer**, precancerous conditions, or causes of bleeding or pain.

Purpose

Sigmoidoscopy is used most often in screening for colorectal cancer or to determine the cause of rectal bleeding. It is also used in diagnosis of inflammatory bowel disease, microscopic and ulcerative colitis, and Crohn's disease.

Cancer of the rectum and colon is the second most common cancer in the United States. About 148,300 new cases are diagnosed annually. Between 55,000 and 60,000 Americans die each year of cancer in the colon or rectum.

After reviewing a number of studies, experts recommend that people over 50 be screened for colorectal cancer using sigmoidoscopy every three to five years. Individuals with inflammatory bowel conditions such as Crohn's disease or ulcerative colitis, and thus at increased risk for colorectal cancer, may begin their screenings at a younger age, depending on when their disease was diagnosed. Many physicians screen such persons more often than every three to five years. Screening should also be performed in people who have a family history of colon or **rectal cancer**, or small growths in the colon (polyps).

Some physicians do this screening with a colonoscope, which allows them to see the entire colon. Most physicians prefer sigmoidoscopy, which is less time-consuming, less uncomfortable, and less costly.

Studies have shown that one-quarter to one-third of all precancerous or small cancerous growths can be seen with a sigmoidoscope. About one-half are found with a 1 ft. (30 cm) scope, and two-thirds to three-quarters can be seen using a 2 ft. (60 cm) scope.

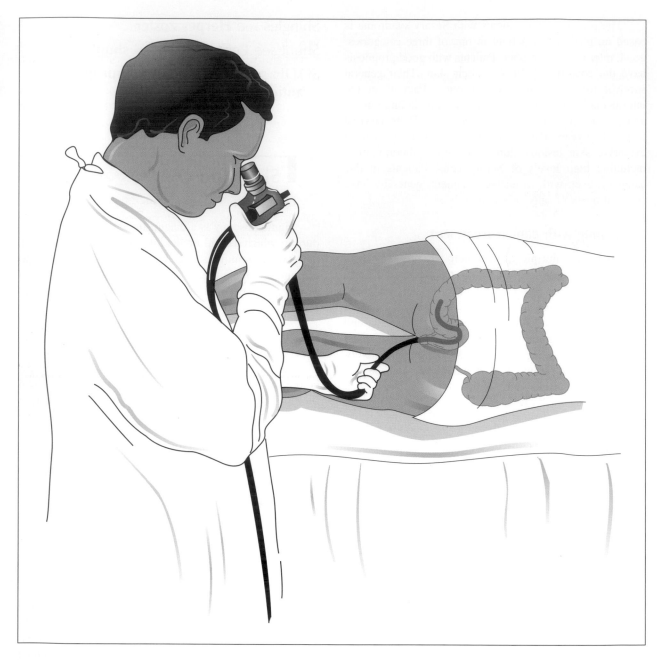

Sigmoidoscopy is a procedure used to screen for colorectal cancer. The physician views the rectum and colon through a sigmoidoscope, a flexible fiberoptic tube that contains a light source and a camera lens. *(Illustration by Electronic Illustrators Group. © Cengage Learning®.)*

In some cases, the sigmoidoscope can be used therapeutically in conjunction with other equipment such as electrosurgical devices to remove polyps and other lesions found during the sigmoidoscopy.

Description

Sigmoidoscopy may be performed using either a rigid or flexible sigmoidoscope. A sigmoidoscope is a thin tube with fiberoptics, electronics, a light source, and camera. A physician inserts the sigmoidoscope into the anus to examine the rectum (the first 1 ft [30 cm] of the colon) and its interior walls. If a 2 ft (60 cm) scope is used, the next portion of the colon can also be examined for any irregularities. The camera of the sigmoidoscope is connected to a viewing monitor, allowing the interior of the rectum and colon to be enlarged and viewed on the monitor. Images can then be recorded as still pictures, or the entire procedure can be videotaped. The still pictures are useful for comparison purposes with the results of future sigmoidoscopic examinations.

KEY TERMS

Biopsy—The removal of a small portion of tissue during sigmoidoscopy to perform laboratory tests to determine whether the tissue is cancerous.

Colonoscopy—A diagnostic endoscopic procedure that uses a long flexible tube called a colonoscope to examine the inner lining of the entire colon; it may be used for colorectal cancer screening or for a more thorough examination of the colon.

Colorectal cancer—Cancer of the large intestine, or colon, including the rectum.

Electrosurgical device—A medical device that uses electrical current to cauterize or coagulate tissue during surgical procedures; often used in conjunction with laparoscopy, colonoscopy, or sigmoidoscopy.

Inflammatory bowel diseases—Ulcerative colitis or Crohn's disease: chronic conditions characterized by periods of diarrhea, bloating, abdominal cramps, and pain, sometimes accompanied by weight loss and malnutrition because of the inability to absorb nutrients.

Pathologist—A doctor who specializes in the diagnosis of disease by studying cells and tissues under a microscope.

Polyp—A small growth, usually not cancerous, but often precancerous when it appears in the colon.

If polyps, lesions, or other suspicious areas are found, the physician biopsies them for analysis. During the sigmoidoscopy, the physician may also use forceps, graspers, snares, or electrosurgical devices to remove polyps, lesions, or tumors.

A typical sigmoidoscopy procedure requires 15 to 20 minutes to perform. Preparation begins one day before the procedure. There is some discomfort when the scope is inserted and throughout the procedure, similar to that experienced when a physician performs a rectal exam using a finger to test for occult blood in the stool (another important **screening test** for colorectal cancer). Individuals may also feel some minor cramping pain. There is rarely severe pain, except for persons with active inflammatory bowel disease.

Private insurance plans almost always cover the cost of sigmoidoscopy examinations for screening in healthy individuals over 50, or for diagnostic purposes. Medicare covers the cost for diagnostic exams, and may cover the costs of screening exams. Medicaid benefits vary by state, but sigmoidoscopy is not a covered procedure in many states. Some community health clinics offer the procedure at reduced cost, but it can only be done if a local gastroenterologist (a physician who specializes in treating stomach and intestinal disorders) is willing to donate personal time to perform the procedure.

Precautions

Individuals need to be careful about medications before having sigmoidoscopy. They should not take aspirin, products containing aspirin, or products containing ibuprofen for one week prior to the exam, because these medications can exacerbate bleeding during the procedure. They should not take any iron or **vitamins** with iron for one week prior to the exam, since iron can cause color changes in the bowel lining that interfere with the examination. They should take any routine prescription medications, but may need to stop certain medications. Prescribing physicians should be consulted regarding routine prescriptions and their possible effect(s) on sigmoidoscopy.

Individuals with renal insufficiency or congestive heart failure need to be prepared in an alternative way, and must be carefully monitored during the procedure.

Preparation

The purpose of preparation for sigmoidoscopy is to cleanse the lower bowel of fecal material or stool so the physician can see the lining. Preparation begins 24 hours before the procedure, when an individual must begin a clear liquid diet. Preparation kits are available in drug stores. In normal preparation, about 20 hours before the exam, a person begins taking a series of **laxatives**, which may be oral tablets or liquid. The individual must stop drinking any liquid four hours before the exam. An hour or two prior to the examination, the person uses an enema or laxative suppository to finish cleansing the lower bowel.

Aftercare

There is no specific aftercare necessary following sigmoidoscopy. If a **biopsy** was taken, a small amount of blood may appear in the next stool. Persons should be encouraged to pass gas following the procedure to relieve any bloating or cramping that may occur after the procedure. In addition, an infection may develop following sigmoidoscopy. Persons should be instructed to call their physician if a **fever** or pain in the abdomen develops over the few days after the procedure.

Risks

There is a slight risk of bleeding from the procedure. This risk is heightened in individuals whose blood does not clot well either due to disease or medication, and in those with active inflammatory bowel disease. Rarely, trauma to the bowel or other organs can occur, resulting in an injury (perforation) that must be repaired, or peritonitis, which must be treated with medication.

Sigmoidoscopy may be contraindicated in persons with severe active colitis or toxic megacolon (an extremely dilated colon). In general, people experiencing continuous ambulatory peritoneal dialysis are not candidates due to a high risk of developing intraperitoneal bleeding.

Results

The results of a normal examination reveal a smooth colon wall, with sufficient blood vessels for good blood flow. An abnormal result is one or more noncancerous or precancerous polyps or clearly cancerous polyps. People with polyps have an increased risk of developing colorectal cancer in the future and may be required to undergo additional procedures such as **colonoscopy** or more frequent sigmoidoscopic examinations.

Small polyps can be completely removed. Larger polyps may require the physician to remove a portion of the growth for laboratory biopsy. Depending on the laboratory results, a person is then scheduled to have the polyp removed surgically, either as an urgent matter if it is cancerous, or as an elective procedure within a few months if it is noncancerous.

In a diagnostic sigmoidoscopy, an abnormal result shows signs of active inflammatory bowel disease, either a thickening of the intestinal lining consistent with ulcerative colitis, or ulcerations or fissures consistent with Crohn's disease.

Alternatives

A screening examination for colorectal cancer is a test for fecal occult blood. A dab of fecal material from toilet tissue is smeared onto a card. The card is treated in a laboratory to reveal the presence of bleeding. This test is normally performed prior to a sigmoidoscopic examination.

A less invasive alternative to a sigmoidoscopic examination is an x-ray of the colon and rectum. Barium is used to coat the inner walls of the colon. This lower GI (gastrointestinal) x-ray may reveal the outlines of suspicious or abnormal structures. It has the disadvantage of not allowing direct visualization of the colon. It is less costly than a sigmoidoscopic examination.

QUESTIONS TO ASK YOUR DOCTOR

- Is the supervising physician appropriately certified to conduct a sigmoidoscopy?
- How many sigmoidoscopy procedures has the doctor performed?
- What other steps will be taken as a result of my test findings?

A more invasive procedure is direct visualization of the colon during surgery. This procedure is rarely performed in the United States.

Health care team roles

A colonoscopy procedure is usually performed by a gastroenterologist, a physician with specialized training in diseases of the colon. Alternatively, general surgeons or experienced family physicians perform sigmoidoscopic examinations. In the United States, the procedure is usually performed in an outpatient facility of a hospital or in a physician's professional office.

Persons with rectal bleeding may need full colonoscopy in a hospital setting. Individuals whose blood does not clot well (possibly as a result of blood-thinning medications) may require the procedure to be performed in a hospital setting.

Resources

BOOKS

Balakrishnan, V., ed. *Practical Gastroenterology*. 3rd ed. Tunbridge Wells, Kent, UK: Anshan Ltd., 2007.

Gillison, W., and H. Buchwald. *Pioneers in Surgical Gastroenterology*. Shrewsbury, Shropshire, UK: TFM Publishing, 2006.

PERIODICALS

Carter, Xiaolu Wu, et al. "Role of Anxiety in the Comfort of Nonsedated Average-Risk Screening Sigmoidoscopy." *Southern Medical Journal* 106, no. 4 (2013): 280–84. http://dx.doi.org/10.1097/SMJ.0b013e31828de613 (accessed October 3, 2014).

Holme, Ø., et al. "Flexible Sigmoidoscopy versus Faecal Occult Blood Testing for Colorectal Cancer Screening in Asymptomatic Individuals." *Cochrane Database of Systematic Reviews* 9, art. no. CD009259 (September 30, 2013). http://dx.doi.org/10.1002/14651858.CD009259. pub2 (accessed October 3, 2014).

van Dam, L., et al. "What Influences the Decision to Participate in Colorectal Cancer Screening with Faecal Occult Blood Testing and Sigmoidoscopy?" *European Journal of*

Cancer 49, no. 10 (2013): 2321–30. http://dx.doi.org/ 10.1016/j.ejca.2013.03.007 (accessed October 3, 2014).

WEBSITES

American Cancer Society. "Frequently Asked Questions about Colonoscopy and Sigmoidoscopy." http://www.cancer. org/healthy/findcancerearly/examandtestdescriptions/faq-colonoscopy-and-sigmoidoscopy (accessed October 3, 2014).

American Society for Gastrointestinal Endoscopy. "Six Questions That Could Save Your Life (Or the Life of Someone You Love): What Women Need to Know about Colon Cancer Screening." http://www.asge.org/patients/patients. aspx?id=374 (accessed October 3, 2014).

National Cancer Institute. "Colorectal Cancer Screening (PDQ®)." http://www.cancer.gov/cancertopics/pdq/ screening/colorectal/Patient (accessed October 3, 2014).

National Digestive Diseases Information Clearinghouse. "Flexible Sigmoidoscopy." National Institute of Diabetes and Digestive and Kidney Diseases. http://digestive.niddk. nih.gov/ddiseases/pubs/sigmoidoscopy (accessed October 3, 2014).

ORGANIZATIONS

American Academy of Family Physicians (AAFP), 11400 Tomahawk Creek Pkwy., Leawood, KS 66211-2680, (913) 906-6000, (800) 274-2237, Fax: (913) 906-6075, http://www.aafp.org.

American Society for Gastrointestinal Endoscopy, 1520 Kensington Rd., Ste. 202, Oak Brook, IL 60523, (630) 573-0600, (866) 353-ASGE (2743), Fax: (630) 573-0691, info@asge.org, http://www.asge.org.

National Digestive Diseases Information Clearinghouse (NDDIC), 2 Information Way, Bethesda, MD 20892-3570, (800) 891-5389, TTY: (866) 569–1162, Fax: (703) 738–4929, nddic@info.niddk.nih.gov, http://www.digestive. niddk.nih.gov.

Society of American Gastrointestinal Endoscopic Surgeons (SAGES), 11300 West Olympic Blvd., Ste. 600, Los Angeles, CA 90064, (310) 437-0544, Fax: (310) 437-0585, webmaster@sages.org, http://www.sages.org.

L. Fleming Fallon, Jr., MD, DrPH

Simple mastectomy

Definition

Simple **mastectomy** is the surgical removal of one or both breasts. The adjacent lymph nodes and chest muscles are left intact. If a few lymph nodes are removed, the procedure is called an extended simple mastectomy. Breast-sparing techniques may be used to preserve the patient's breast skin and nipple, which is helpful in cosmetic **breast reconstruction**.

Purpose

Removal of a patient's breast is usually recommended when **cancer** is present in the breast or as a prophylactic measure when the patient has severe fibrocystic disease and a family history of **breast cancer**. The choice of a simple mastectomy may be determined by evaluating the size of the breast, the size of the cancerous mass, where the cancer is located, and whether any cancer cells have spread to adjacent lymph nodes or other parts of the body. If the cancer has not been contained within the breast, it calls for a **modified radical mastectomy**, which removes the entire breast and all of the adjacent lymph nodes. Only in extreme circumstances is a radical mastectomy, which also removes part of the chest wall, indicated.

A larger tumor usually is an indication of more advanced disease and will require more extensive surgery such as a simple mastectomy. In addition, if a woman has small breasts, the tumor may occupy more area within the contours of the breast, necessitating a simple mastectomy in order to remove all of the cancer.

Very rapidly growing tumors usually require the removal of all breast tissue. Cancers that have spread to adjacent tissues such as the chest wall or skin make simple mastectomy a good choice. Similarly, multiple sites of cancer within a breast require that the entire breast be removed. In addition, simple mastectomy is also recommended when cancer recurs in a breast that has already undergone a **lumpectomy**, which is a less invasive procedure that removes just the tumor and some surrounding tissue without removing the entire breast.

Sometimes, surgeons recommend simple mastectomy for women who are unable to undergo the adjuvant **radiation therapy** required after a lumpectomy. Radiation treatment is not indicated for pregnant women, those who have had previous therapeutic radiation in the chest area, and patients with collagen vascular diseases such as scleroderma or lupus. In these cases, simple mastectomy is the treatment of choice.

Some women with family histories of breast cancer and who test positive for a cancer-causing gene choose to have one or both of their breasts removed as a preventive for future breast cancer. This procedure is highly controversial. Though prophylactic mastectomy reduces the occurrence of breast cancer by 90% in high-risk patients, it is not a foolproof method. There has been some incidence of cancer occurring after both breasts were removed.

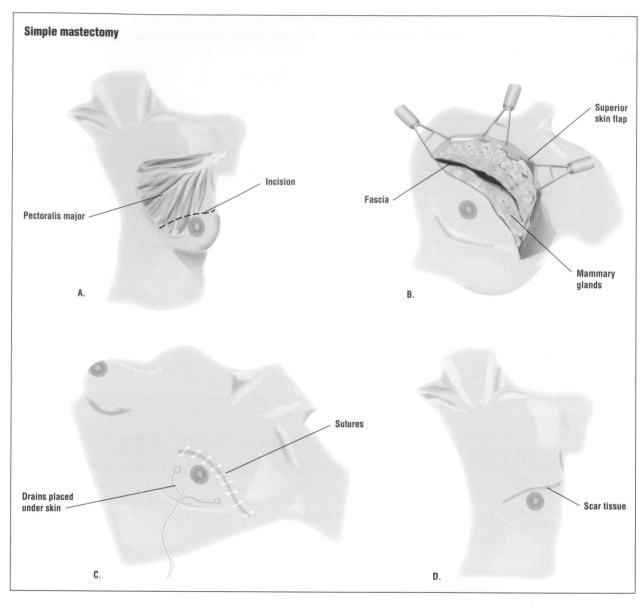

Simple mastectomy

A.
- Pectoralis major
- Incision

B.
- Superior skin flap
- Fascia
- Mammary glands

C.
- Drains placed under skin
- Sutures

D.
- Scar tissue

In a simple mastectomy, the skin over the tumor is cut open (A). The tumor and tissue surrounding it is removed (B), and the wound is closed (C). *(Illustration by GGS Information Services. © Cengage Learning®.)*

Description

Simple mastectomy is one of several types of surgical treatments for breast cancer. Some techniques are rarely used; others are quite common. These common surgical procedures include:

- Radical mastectomy. Radical mastectomy is rarely used, and then only in cases where cancer cells have invaded the chest wall and the tumor is very large. The breast, muscles under the breast, and all of the lymph nodes are removed. This procedure produces a large scar and severe disability to the arm nearest the removed breast.

- Modified radical mastectomy. Modified radical mastectomy was the most common form of mastectomy until the 1980s. The breast is removed along with the lining over the chest muscle and all of the lymph nodes.

- Simple mastectomy. Simple, sometimes called total, mastectomy has been the treatment of choice in the late 1980s and 1990s. Generally, only the breast is removed; sometimes one or two lymph nodes may be removed as well.

- Partial mastectomy. Partial mastectomy is used to remove the tumor, the lining over the chest muscle underneath the tumor, and a good portion of breast

KEY TERMS

Lumpectomy—A less invasive procedure that removes the tumor and some surrounding tissue without removing the entire breast.

Lymphedema—Swelling, usually of the arm after a mastectomy, caused by the accumulation of fluid from faulty drainage in the lymph system.

Mammogram—A special x-ray image of the breast that looks for anomalies in breast tissue.

tissue, but not the entire breast. This is a good treatment choice for early-stage cancers.

• Lumpectomy. Lumpectomy or breast-conserving surgery removes the tumor and a small amount of tissue surrounding it. Some lymph nodes may be removed as well. This is the most commonly used surgical procedure for the treatment of breast cancer in the early twenty-first century.

Two other surgical procedures are variations on the simple mastectomy. The skin-sparing mastectomy is a surgical procedure in which the surgeon makes an incision, sometimes called a keyhole incision, around the areola. The tumor and all breast tissue are removed, but the incision is smaller and scarring is minimal. About 90% of the skin is preserved and allows a cosmetic surgeon to perform breast reconstruction at the same time as the mastectomy. The subcutaneous mastectomy, or nipple-sparing mastectomy, preserves the skin and the nipple over the breast.

During a simple mastectomy, the surgeon makes a curved incision along one side of the breast and removes the tumor and all of the breast tissue. A few lymph nodes may be removed. The tumor, breast tissue, and any lymph nodes will be sent to the pathology lab for analysis. If the skin is cancer-free, it is sutured in place or used immediately for breast reconstruction. One or two drains will be put in place to remove fluid from the surgical area. Surgery takes from two to five hours; it is longer with breast reconstruction.

Breast reconstruction

Breast reconstruction, especially if it is begun at the same time as the simple mastectomy, can minimize the sense of loss that women feel when having a breast removed. Although there may be other smaller surgeries later to complete the breast reconstruction, there will not be a second major operation nor an additional scar.

If there is not enough skin left after the mastectomy, a balloon-type expander is put in place. In subsequent weeks, the expander is filled with larger amounts of saline (salt water) solution. When it has reached the appropriate size, the expander is removed and a permanent breast implant is installed.

If there is enough skin, an implant is installed immediately. In other instances, skin, fat, and muscle are removed from the patient's back or abdomen and repositioned on the chest wall to form a breast.

None of these reconstructions have nipples at first. Nipples are later reconstructed in a separate surgery. Finally, the areola is tattooed in to make the reconstructed breast look natural.

Breast reconstruction does not prevent a potential recurrence of breast cancer.

Demographics

According to the American Cancer Society, 232,340 new cases of invasive breast cancer in women were diagnosed in 2013. New cases of breast cancer in men were expected to reach 2,240.

For approximately 80% of women, the first indication of cancer is the discovery of a lump in the breast, found either by themselves in a monthly self-exam; by a partner; or by a mammogram, a special x-ray of the breast that looks for anomalies. Early detection of breast cancer means that smaller tumors are found, which require less intensive surgery and have better treatment outcomes. Simple mastectomy has been the standard treatment of choice for breast cancer for the past 60 years. Newer breast-conserving surgery techniques have gained acceptance since the mid-1980s. For larger hospitals, facilities in urban areas, and health care institutions with a cancer center or high cancer patient volume, these newer techniques are being utilized at a more rapid rate, especially on the East Coast.

In 2003, the **National Cancer Institute** found that American women were 21% more likely to have a mastectomy than their counterparts in the United Kingdom. Though breast-conserving procedures are available and have proven to be viable options, some physicians and women still think breast removal will also remove all their risk of cancer recurrence. It is clear that treatment options for cancer are highly individual and often emotionally charged.

Preparation

If a mammogram has not been performed, it is usually ordered to verify the size of the lump the patient has reported. A **biopsy** of the suspicious lump and/or lymph nodes is usually ordered and sent to the pathology lab before surgery is discussed.

When a simple mastectomy has been determined, preoperative tests such as blood work, a chest x-ray, and an electrocardiogram may be ordered. Blood-thinning medications such as aspirin should be stopped several days before the surgery date. The patient is also asked to refrain from eating or drinking the night before the operation.

At the hospital, the patient will sign a consent form, verifying that the surgeon has explained what the surgery is and what it is for. The patient will also meet with the anesthesiologist to discuss the patient's medical history and determine the choice of anesthesia.

Aftercare

If the procedure is performed as an outpatient surgery, the patient may go home the same day of the surgery. The length of the hospital stay for inpatient mastectomies ranges from one to two days. If breast reconstruction has taken place, the hospital stay may be longer.

The surgical drains will remain in place for five to seven days. Sponge baths will be necessary until the stitches are removed, usually in a week to 10 days. It is important to avoid overhead lifting, strenuous sports, and sexual intercourse for three to six weeks. After the surgical drains are removed, stretching exercises may be begun, though some physical therapists may start a patient on shoulder and arm mobility exercises while in the hospital.

Since breast removal is often emotionally traumatic for women, seeking out a support group is often helpful. Women in these groups offer practical advice about matters such as finding well-fitting bras and swimwear, and emotional support because they have been through the same experience.

For women who chose not to have breast reconstruction, it may be necessary to find the proper fitting breast prosthesis. Some are made of cloth, and others are made of silicone, which are created from a mold from the patient's other breast.

In some case, the patient may be required to undergo additional treatments such as radiation, **chemotherapy**, or hormone therapy.

Risks

The risks involved with simple mastectomy are the same for any major surgery; however, there may be a need for more extensive surgery once the surgeon examines the tumor, the tissues surrounding it, and the

lymph nodes nearby. A biopsy of the lymph nodes is usually performed during surgery and a determination is made whether to remove them. Simple mastectomy usually has limited impact on range of motion of the arm nearest the breast that is removed, but **physical therapy** may still be necessary to restore complete movement.

There is also the risk of infection around the incision. When the lymph nodes are removed, lymphedema may also occur. This condition is a result of damage to the lymphatic system. The arm on the side nearest the affected breast may become swollen. It can either resolve itself or worsen.

As in any surgery, the risk of developing a blood clot after a mastectomy is a serious matter. All hospitals use a variety of techniques to prevent blood clots from forming. It is important for the patient to walk daily when at home.

Finally, there is the risk that not all cancer cells were removed. Further treatment may be necessary.

Results

The breast area will fully heal in three to four weeks. If the patient had breast reconstruction, it may take up to six weeks to recover fully. The patient should be able to participate in all of the activities she has engaged in before surgery. If breast reconstruction is done, the patient should realize that the new breast will not have the sensitivity of a normal breast. In addition, dealing with cancer emotionally may take time, especially if additional treatment is necessary.

Morbidity and mortality rates

Deaths due to breast cancer have declined by 1.4% each year between 1989 and 1995, and by 3.2% each year thereafter. The largest decreases have been among younger women as a result of cancer education campaigns and early screening, which encourage more women to go to their physicians to be checked.

Research performed between 2000 and 2004 demonstrated that the five-year survival rate for cancers confined to the breast is 98%. For cancers that had spread to areas within the chest region, the rate was 83.5%, and it was only 26.7% for cancers occurring in other parts of the body after breast cancer treatment. The best survival rates were for early-stage tumors.

Two 20-year longitudinal studies concluded in 2002 indicated that the survival rate for patients with modified radical mastectomy (the removal of the entire breast and all lymph nodes) was no different from that of breast-conserving lumpectomy (the removal of the tumor alone). These studies suggest that the removal of the entire breast may not afford greater protection against future cancer than breast-conserving techniques; however, the majority of cancer recurrences happen within the first five years for both those with mastectomies and those with lumpectomies.

Alternatives

Skin-sparing mastectomy, also called nipple-sparing mastectomy, is becoming a treatment of choice for women undergoing simple mastectomy. In this procedure, the skin of the breast, the areola, and the nipple are peeled back to remove the breast and its inherent tumor. Biopsies of the skin and nipple areas are performed immediately to ensure that they do not have cancer cells in them. Then, a cosmetic surgeon performs a breast reconstruction at the same time as the mastectomy. The breast regains its normal contours once prostheses are inserted. Unfortunately, the nipple will lose its sensitivity and its function, since all underlying tissue has been removed. If cancer is found near the nipple, this procedure cannot be done.

Health care team roles

Simple mastectomy is performed by a general surgeon or a gynecological surgeon. If reconstructive breast surgery is to be done, a cosmetic surgeon performs it. Patients undergo simple mastectomies under general anesthesia as inpatients in a hospital. There is a growing trend, due to reductions in insurance coverage and patient preference, to perform simple mastectomies without reconstructive breast surgery as outpatient procedures.

Resources

BOOKS

Khatri, V. P., and J. A. Asensio. *Operative Surgery Manual.* Philadelphia: Saunders, 2003.

Lentz, Gretchen, et al. *Comprehensive Gynecology.* 5th ed. St. Louis: Mosby/Elsevier, 2012.

Niederhuber, John E., et al. *Abeloff's Clinical Oncology.* 5th ed. Philadelphia: Saunders/Elsevier, 2013.

Townsend, Courtney M., et al. *Sabiston Textbook of Surgery.* 19th ed. Philadelphia: Saunders/Elsevier, 2012.

PERIODICALS

Bugelli, George J., Walid A. Samra, and Karen Stuart Smith. "Simple Mastectomy and Axillary Lymph Node Biopsy Performed under Paravertebral Block and Light Sedation in a Patient with Severe Cardiorespiratory Comorbidities: Proposed Management of Choice in High-Risk Breast Surgery Patients." *Clinical Breast Cancer* 13, no. 2 (2013): 153–55. http://dx.doi.org/10.1016/j.clbc.2012.12.003 (accessed October 3, 2014).

Johansen, Helge, et al. "Extended Radical Mastectomy Versus Simple Mastectomy followed by Radiotherapy in Primary Breast Cancer. A Fifty-Year Follow-Up to the Copenhagen Breast Cancer Randomised Study." *Acta Oncologica* 47, no. 4 (2008): 633–38. http://dx.doi.org/10.1080/02841860801989753 (accessed October 3, 2014).

WEBSITES

American Cancer Society. "Surgery for Breast Cancer." http://www.cancer.org/cancer/breastcancer/detailedguide/breast-cancer-treating-surgery (accessed October 3, 2014).

American Cancer Society. "What Are the Key Statistics about Breast Cancer?" http://www.cancer.org/cancer/breastcancer/detailedguide/breast-cancer-key-statistics (accessed October 3, 2014).

American Cancer Society. "What Are the Key Statistics about Breast Cancer in Men?" http://www.cancer.org/cancer/breastcancerinmen/detailedguide/breast-cancer-in-men-key-statistics (accessed October 3, 2014).

Breastcancer.org. "Skin-Sparing Mastectomy." http://www.breastcancer.org/treatment/surgery/mastectomy/skinsparing (accessed October 3, 2014).

Susan G. Komen for the Cure. "Mastectomy." http://ww5.komen.org/BreastCancer/Mastectomy.html (accessed October 3, 2014).

ORGANIZATIONS

American Cancer Society, 250 Williams St. NW, Atlanta, GA 30303, (800) 227-2345, http://www.cancer.org.

American Society of Plastic Surgeons, 444 E. Algonquin Rd., Arlington Heights, IL 60005, (847) 228-9900, (800) 514-5058, memserv@plasticsurgery.org, http://www.plasticsurgery.org.

National Cancer Institute, 6116 Executive Blvd., Ste. 300, Bethesda, MD 20892-8322, (800) 4-CANCER (422-6237), http://cancer.gov.

Janie Franz

Sipuleucel-T

Definition

Sipuleucel-T, sold under the brand name Provenge, is the first drug to be developed and approved in a new class of drugs called autologous cellular immunotherapies.

Purpose

Sipuleucel-T was approved by the U.S. Food and Drug Administration (FDA) in 2010 for the treatment of advanced **prostate cancer** in men whose **cancer** is not yet causing symptoms and for men whose prostate cancer has metastasized and is causing minimal symptoms but has been resistant to treatment with hormonal therapies designed to treat prostate cancer.

Description

The exact mechanism of action of sipuleucel-T is not yet known. Sipuleucel-T works by harnessing the actions of the patient's own immune cells to target and treat that patient's biologically unique prostate cancer. Each dose of the drug is designed specifically for an individual patient using the process of leukapheresis, which is scheduled three days prior to a scheduled treatment with Provenge. In leukapheresis, a cell collection process, some of the patient's own immune cells are collected. The collected cells are then packaged, labeled, and shipped to a drug manufacturing facility. Once at the facility, the patient's cells are placed in a culture with a human recombinant protein. This protein works to activate the patient's immune cells to function specifically as a prostate-associated antigen whose purpose is to trigger the patient's own immune system to recognize and kill prostate cancer cells. Another purpose of the end product is to stimulate the immune system. Once the process is completed at the drug manufacturing facility, the activated cells are shipped back to a treatment center and are reinfused into the patient from whom they were originally collected. The patient's immune system is then activated to destroy prostate cancer cells.

Biologically active components of Provenge include autologous-presenting cells (APCs) and remnants of a recombinant human protein designated as PAP-GM-CSF. PAP-GM-CSF consists of prostatic acid phosphatase (PAP), an antigen expressed by prostate cancer tissue, which is then combined with granulocyte-macrophage colony-stimulating factor (GM-CSF). GM-CSF stimulates immune cells to activate. In addition to the components derived from the recombinant human protein, the precise cellular composition of Provenge varies depending on the exact composition of the cells

obtained from the patient during leukapheresis. The resulting product will likely contain immune cells such as T cells, B cells, natural killer cells, and other cells, in addition to the autologous APCs.

Each dose of the drug is placed in suspension in 250 milliliters of Ringer's Lactate solution in a sealed infusion bag that is to be administered intravenously to one specific patient. No additives or preservatives are added to the solution during the manufacturing process.

The completed product cannot be administered to any patient other than the original patient whose immune cells were collected during the leukapheresis process.

Recommended dosage

According to the manufacturer, each dose of Provenge contains a minimum of 50 million CD54+ cells that have been activated by human recombinant protein technology. The exact number of cells present in each dose varies. CD54 is a molecule on the surface of cells and is considered to be a marker of immune cell activity.

Administration of Provenge occurs in a three-dose schedule at intervals spaced about every two weeks. The drug is administered intravenously over a period of about an hour. No further treatment with Provenge is required after the initial three doses.

Precautions

This drug is not to be administered to patients other than the patient from whom immune cells were collected during leukapheresis. The identity of the patient receiving Provenge must match the patient identifying information on the infusion bag.

A cell filter must not be used during infusion of Provenge.

Prior to infusion, the patient should be premedicated with oral acetaminophen and an antihistamine such as **diphenhydramine**. The infusion time may have to be slowed or stopped if severe infusion reactions occur during administration of this product.

The product has not been tested for infectious diseases that can be transmitted to others. Therefore, any infectious diseases that are present may be transmitted to healthcare workers during product handling or administration. Universal precautions should be adhered to by health care workers when handling this product.

If a patient is unable to receive a scheduled dose of Provenge, the patient will be required to undergo an additional leukapheresis procedure if treatment is to be continued. Patients should be informed of this possibility prior to the beginning of the treatment process.

Side effects

In **clinical trials**, the most common adverse reactions associated with Provenge administration included chills, **fever**, **fatigue**, back pain, nausea, pain in the joints, and headache. Some patients may experience acute and severe infusion reactions during administration of Provenge. Should these occur, the infusion may be slowed or stopped depending on the severity of the reaction. Severe reactions may occur after the administration is complete and typically occur within one day of drug administration.

Interactions

The concurrent use of Provenge with **chemotherapy** or other medications that have the potential to suppress the immune system has not been studied. The use of immunosuppressive drugs concurrently with the use of Provenge may result in decreased effectiveness of Provenge. Patients on immunosuppressive drugs such as **corticosteroids** may be required to reduce or discontinue the use of these drugs during therapy with Provenge.

Resources

PERIODICALS

Dawson, Nancy A., and Erin E Roesch. "Sipuleucel-T and Immunotherapy in the Treatment of Prostate Cancer." *Expert Opinion on Biological Therapy* 14, no. 5 (2014): 709–19. http://dx.doi.org/10.1517/14712598.2014.896897 (accessed October 9, 2014).

Higano, C. S., et al. "Integrated Data from 2 Randomized, Double-Blind, Placebo-Controlled, Phase 3 Trials of Active Cellular Immunotherapy with Sipuleucel-T in Advanced Prostate Cancer." *Cancer* 115 (2009): 3670–79.

Kantoff, P. W., et al. "Sipuleucel-T Immunotherapy for Castration-Resistant Prostate Cancer." *New England Journal of Medicine* 363, no. 5 (July 29, 2010): 411–12.

WEBSITES

American Cancer Society. "Sipuleucel-T." http://www.cancer.org/treatment/treatmentsandsideeffects/guidetocancerdrugs/sipuleucel-t (accessed October 9, 2014).

National Cancer Institute. "FDA Approval for Sipuleucel-T." http://www.cancer.gov/cancertopics/druginfo/fda-sipuleucel-T (accessed October 9, 2014).

ORGANIZATIONS

U.S. Food and Drug Administration, 10903 New Hampshire Ave., Silver Spring, MD 20993, (888) INFO-FDA (463-6332), http://www.fda.gov.

Melinda Granger Oberleitner, RN, DNS, APRN, CNS

Sirolimus

Definition

Sirolimus is a macrolide drug indicated by the Food and Drug Administration (FDA) to be used after a kidney transplant to prevent the body from rejecting the new kidney. Sirolimus may also have a role in prevention of organ rejection in heart or lung transplantation, and prevention of **graft-versus-host disease** in patients undergoing **bone marrow transplantation**. Sirolimus (formerly known as rapamycin) became available at the end of 1999 and is marketed under the brand name Rapamune by Wyeth-Ayerst Laboratories.

Description

Sirolimus belongs to a class of macrolide **antibiotics** and is isolated from an organism named *Streptomyces hygroscopicus*.

Sirolimus prevents the immune system from attacking the transplanted organ by decreasing the growth of certain chemicals in the body responsible for immune function (B and T lymphocytes). Sirolimus works differently from other immunosuppressants used to prevent organ rejection after transplantation (**azathioprine**, **mycophenolate mofetil**, **tacrolimus**, **cyclosporine**, and steroids). It should be given in combination with cyclosporine and steroids to prevent acute rejection of a

KEY TERMS

Immune system—The body's mechanism to fight infections, toxic substances, and to recognize and neutralize or eliminate foreign material (for example, a body organ transplanted from another person).

Immunosuppressant—An agent that decreases the activity of the immune system (for example, radiation or drugs).

Lymphocele—A mass surrounded by an abnormal sac that contains lymph (fluid collected from tissues throughout the body) from diseased or injured lymphatic channels.

Lymphoma—Any malignant (cancerous) disorder of lymphoid tissue.

Steroids—Drugs such as prednisone or dexamethasone, which resemble the body's natural hormones and are often used to decrease inflammation or to suppress the activity of the immune system.

Transplant—Tissue transferred from one part of the body to another or from one person to another.

transplanted kidney. This drug is available as a tablet and a liquid and can be used in children and adults.

Recommended dosage

Adults

KIDNEY TRANSPLANTATION. The first dose of 3 tablets (2 mg each) or 6 milliliters of oral solution should be given as soon as possible after a kidney is transplanted. A maintenance dose of 2 mg should then be given once a day.

Children over 13 years of age and adults less than 40 kg (88 lb.)

KIDNEY TRANSPLANTATION. 3 mg of sirolimus per square meter of body surface area on day one after transplantation, followed by a maintenance dose of 1 mg per square meter per day.

Children less than 13 years of age

Check with a specialist physician.

Administration

Sirolimus should be administered in combination with cyclosporine and steroids. To decrease the risk of side effects, sirolimus should be given four hours after cyclosporine. To avoid variations in blood levels, sirolimus should be taken consistently—either always with food or always without food. Sirolimus oral solution should be mixed with water or orange juice and consumed immediately. Juices or liquids other than water or orange juice should not be used to mix sirolimus. Bottled sirolimus solution should be stored in the refrigerator but not frozen. Refrigerated sirolimus solution may develop a slight haze. If haze is noticed, the drug should be left at room temperature and gently shaken until the haze disappears. If a dose is missed, it should taken as soon as possible unless it is almost time for the next dose. Two doses should not be taken at the same time.

Precautions

Sirolimus may increase the risk of the following conditions:

- infections caused by viruses and bacteria
- lymphoma or skin cancer
- elevated blood lipids (cholesterol and triglycerides)
- decreased kidney function
- lymphocele formation after a kidney transplantation

Patients with the following conditions should use sirolimus with caution:

- An allergic reaction to tacrolimus (has a similar structure to sirolimus).
- Liver disease (dose of sirolimus may need to be decreased).
- Treatment with medications that are broken down in the liver and that may interact with sirolimus.
- Pregnancy. These patients should use an effective method of birth control started before therapy with sirolimus and continued for 12 weeks after stopping this medication.

Patients should immediately alert their doctor if any of these symptoms develop:

- fever, chills, sore throat
- fast heartbeat
- trouble breathing
- unusual bleeding or bruising

Sirolimus should be taken consistently with regard to meals (either always taken with food or always taken on an empty stomach) and at least four hours after cyclosporine to decrease variability of blood sirolimus levels. Patients should avoid grapefruit or grapefruit juice because it may increase sirolimus levels in the blood. Those taking sirolimus will need to see a physician regularly to check blood and urine.

Side effects

The most common side effects include mild dose-related risk of bleeding, elevated blood cholesterol and triglyceride values, decreased kidney function, high blood pressure, **diarrhea** or constipation, rash, acne, joint pain, nausea, vomiting, stomachache, and decreased blood potassium and phosphate values. Sirolimus can decrease the number of red blood cells, which can cause a patient to look pale, feel tired, short of breath, and drowsy, and experience heart palpitations. People who are allergic to tacrolimus may develop an allergy when taking sirolimus.

Interactions

Sirolimus is broken down in the liver by the same enzyme system that also breaks down cyclosporine and tacrolimus. Because cyclosporine can increase sirolimus blood levels, sirolimus should be given four hours after the morning cyclosporine dose to decrease the risk of side effects. Diltiazem (Cardizem, Tiazac, Dilacor) and ketoconazole (Nizoral) can increase sirolimus blood levels. The use of ketoconazole should be avoided in patients taking sirolimus. Other drugs that are likely to increase sirolimus blood levels and increase its side effects include calcium channel blockers (used to treat high blood pressure), drugs that treat fungal infections (ketoconazole, itraconazole, fluconazole), macrolide antibiotics (erythromycin, clarithromycin), and anti-HIV drugs (ritonavir, nelfinavir, indinavir). Rifampin can greatly decrease sirolimus blood levels, potentially making it less effective. Other drugs that may decrease effectiveness of sirolimus include phenobarbital, **carbamazepine**, rifabutin, and **phenytoin**. Anyone who is taking these drugs should ask their physician if they can safely take sirolimus.

Resources

BOOKS

Chu, Edward, and Vincent T. DeVita Jr. *Physicians' Cancer Chemotherapy Drug Manual 2014.* Burlington, MA: Jones & Bartlett Learning, 2014.

WEBSITES

National Cancer Institute. "Sirolimus." http://www.cancer.gov/drugdictionary?cdrid=42555 (accessed November 14, 2014).

U.S. Food and Drug Administration. "Rapamune (sirolimus): Drug Monitoring Recommendations." http://www.fda.gov/safety/medwatch/safetyinformation/safetyalertsforhumanmedicalproducts/ucm197059.htm (accessed November 14, 2014).

Olga Bessmertny, Pharm.D.

6-Mercaptopurine *see* **Mercaptopurine**

6-Thioguanine *see* **Thioguanine**

Skin biopsy

Definition

A skin **biopsy** is a procedure in which a small piece of living skin is removed from the body for examination, usually under a microscope. Skin biopsies are usually brief, straightforward procedures performed by a skin specialist (dermatologist) or family physician. They are performed to help the physician make a diagnosis when a skin disorder is suspected. Information from the biopsy also helps the doctor choose the best treatment for the patient.

Purpose

Doctors perform skin biopsies to:

- make a diagnosis

- confirm a diagnosis made from the patient's medical history and a physical examination

- check whether a treatment prescribed for a previously diagnosed condition is working

- check the edges of tissue removed with a tumor to make certain it contains all of the diseased tissue

Skin biopsies also serve a therapeutic purpose. Many skin abnormalities (lesions) can be removed completely during a biopsy procedure, even if they are not negatively affecting a patient's health.

Skin biopsy

Certain features of skin lesions might be indicative of a need for a skin biopsy. Stay alert for changes in moles over time, especially related to:

Asymmetrical shape
Border
Color
Diameter

SOURCE: Melanoma Research Foundation, "ABCDE's of Melanoma." Available online at: http://www.melanoma.org/learn-more/melanoma-101/abcdes-melanoma.

Warnings for skin cancer include changes in mole shape, border, color, and size, particularly changes that take place over time (evolution). *(Illustration by PreMediaGlobal. © Cengage Learning®.)*

KEY TERMS

Benign—Noncancerous.

Dermatitis (plural, dermatitides)—Any skin disorder that causes inflammation; that is, redness, swelling, heat, and pain.

Dermatologist—A doctor who specializes in skin care and treatment.

Dermatosis (plural, dermatoses)—A noninflammatory skin disorder.

Lesion—An area of abnormal or injured skin.

Malignant—Cancerous.

Pathologist—A physician who specializes in studying diseases. In particular, this person examines the structural and functional changes in the tissues and organs of the body that are caused by disease or that cause disease themselves.

Description

The first step in a skin biopsy is obtaining a sample of tissue that best represents the lesion being evaluated. Many biopsy techniques are available. The choice of technique and precise location from which to take the biopsy material are determined by factors such as the type and shape of the lesion. Biopsies can be classified as excisional, when the lesion is completely removed, or incisional, when a portion of the lesion is removed.

There are four common biopsy techniques:

- In a shave biopsy, the doctor uses a scalpel or razor blade to shave off a thin layer of the lesion parallel to the skin surface.

- In a punch biopsy, a small cylindrical punch is screwed into the lesion through the full thickness of the skin and a plug of tissue is removed. A stitch or two may be needed to close the wound.

- In a scalpel biopsy, the doctor makes a standard surgical incision or excision to remove tissue. This technique is most often used for large or deep lesions. The wound is closed with stitches.

- In a scissors biopsy, surface (superficial) skin growths or lesions growing from a stem or column of tissue are snipped off with surgical scissors. Such growths are sometimes seen on the eyelids or neck.

After the biopsy tissue is removed, bleeding may be controlled by applying pressure or heat. **Antibiotics** are often applied to the wound to prevent infection. Depending on the type of biopsy performed, stitches may be placed in the wound, or the wound may be bandaged and allowed to heal on its own.

The tissue sample is placed immediately in an appropriate preservative, such as formaldehyde, to prevent drying and structural damage. It is then sent to the laboratory. A variety of laboratory techniques may be used to process the biopsy tissue, including tissue stains and examination with any of several different kinds of microscopes. There are many skin disorders (broadly called dermatoses and dermatitides), so the pathologist studying the sample has had extensive training in their accurate identification. Cases of **melanoma**, the most malignant kind of **skin cancer**, have almost tripled in the past 30 years. Because melanoma grows very rapidly in the skin, quick and accurate diagnosis is important.

Precautions

A patient taking aspirin or another blood thinner (anticoagulant) may be asked to stop taking it a week or more before the skin biopsy. This adjustment in medication will prevent excessive bleeding during the procedure and allow for normal blood clotting.

Some patients are allergic to lidocaine, the numbing agent most frequently used during a skin biopsy. The doctor can usually substitute another anesthetic agent.

Preparation

The area of the biopsy is cleansed thoroughly with alcohol or a disinfectant containing iodine. Sterile cloths (drapes) may be positioned, and a local anesthetic, usually lidocaine, is injected into the skin near the lesion. Sometimes the anesthetic contains epinephrine, a drug that helps reduce bleeding during the biopsy. Sterile gloves and surgical instruments are used in excision procedures to reduce the risk of infection. They are not required for shave or punch biopsies.

Aftercare

If stitches have been placed, they should be kept clean until removed. Sometimes the patient is instructed to put protective ointment on the stitches before or after showering; the doctor should provide specific instructions on how to care for the wound. Stitches are usually removed five to ten days after the biopsy. Wounds that have not been stitched should be cleaned with soap and water daily until they heal. Any adhesive strips should be left in place for two to three weeks. Pain medications usually are not necessary.

Risks

Infection and bleeding rarely occur after skin biopsy. If the skin biopsy may leave a scar, the patient usually is asked to give informed consent before the test.

Results

If the biopsy reveals a lesion, it is classified as either benign (noncancerous) or malignant (cancerous). Some benign lesions may require treatment, but all malignant lesions require treatment.

Resources

BOOKS

Schwartz, Robert A., ed. *Skin Cancer: Recognition and Management.* Malden, MA: Wiley-Blackwell, 2008.

WEBSITES

A.D.A.M. Medical Encyclopedia. "Skin Lesion Biopsy." MedlinePlus. http://www.nlm.nih.gov/medlineplus/ency/article/003840.htm (accessed October 10, 2014).

MedlinePlus. "Skin Cancer." U.S. National Library of Medicine, National Institutes of Health. http://www.nlm.nih.gov/medlineplus/skincancer.html (accessed October 10, 2014).

UW Health. "Skin Biopsy." University of Wisconsin-Madison. http://www.uwhealth.org/health/topic/medicaltest/skin-biopsy/hw234496.html (accessed October 10, 2014).

ORGANIZATIONS

American Academy of Dermatology, PO Box 4014, Schaumburg, IL 60168-4014, Fax: (847) 240-1859, (866) 503-SKIN (7546), http://www.aad.org.

Collette L. Placek

Skin cancer

Definition

Skin **cancer** refers to abnormal cells of the skin that grow uncontrollably. If untreated, these cells can grow deeper into the skin and invade other tissues. There are three main types of skin cancer: **basal cell carcinoma**, squamous cell **carcinoma**, and **melanoma**. All three types are related to excessive sun exposure.

Description

Cancer is a group of diseases in which abnormal cells continuously grow out of control. These cells can spread to other organs and if not controlled can result in death. Skin cancer is the most common type of cancer but certainly not the most fatal. Although skin cancer most often occurs on areas of the skin that are exposed to sunlight, this is not always the case.

There are three main types of skin cancer; melanoma, basal cell carcinoma, and squamous cell carcinoma. Each develops from a different cell type of the skin's epidermal layer. Basal cell carcinoma and squamous cell carcinoma are the most common and most treatable if they are found early. Melanoma is a more serious form of skin cancer affecting deeper layers of the skin and has a higher potential to spread to other parts of the body.

Basal cell carcinoma (BCC) is the most common type of skin cancer, accounting for about 80% of all skin cancers. It develops from cells of the lowest layer of the epidermis, the basal cells or basal keratinocytes. These are the cells that produce new skin cells. BCC occurs primarily on the parts of the skin exposed to the sun and is most common in people living in areas near the equator, at high altitudes, or in areas of severe ozone depletion. Light-skinned people are at greater risk of developing basal cell carcinoma than dark-skinned people. Basal cell carcinoma grows very slowly; however, if it is not treated, it can invade deeper skin layers causing extensive damage and can be fatal. This type of cancer can appear as a shiny translucent nodule on the skin or as a red, wrinkled and scaly area.

Squamous cell carcinoma (SCC) is the second most frequent type of skin cancer overall but the most common type in dark-skinned people. It arises from the outer keratinizing layer of skin just below the surface. Squamous cell carcinoma grows faster than basal cell carcinoma and is more likely to metastasize to the lymph nodes as well as to distant sites. Squamous cell carcinoma most often appears on the arms, head, and neck. Fair-skinned people of Celtic descent are at high risk of developing squamous cell carcinoma. This type of cancer is rarely life-threatening but can cause serious problems if it spreads; it can also cause disfigurement. Squamous cell carcinoma usually appears as a scaly, slightly elevated area of damaged skin. It can also appear in an area of chronic inflammation on the skin.

Malignant melanoma is the most serious type of skin cancer. It develops from the melanocytes or pigment-producing cells of the skin. These cells are found in the lowest layer of the epidermis. Melanocytes are stimulated

KEY TERMS

Actinic keratosis—A precancerous skin condition in which skin exposed to the sun forms thick, scaly, or crusty patches. Untreated actinic keratosis has a 20% chance of progressing to skin cancer.

Basal cell—A keratinocyte in the basal layer, the deepest of the five layers of cells in the epidermis.

Biopsy—Removal of a small sample of tissue for examination under a microscope; used for the diagnosis and treatment of cancer and precancerous conditions.

Dermis—The layer of skin just below the epidermis.

Epidermis—The outer covering of skin in mammals. In humans, it consists of five layers of cells.

Epithelial tissue—The collection of cells that cover the exterior and line the interior surfaces of the body.

Immunity—Ability to resist the effects of agents, such as bacteria and viruses, that cause disease.

Keratinocyte—The basic type of cell in the epidermis (uppermost layer) of the skin, comprising about 90% of its cells.

Lymph node—A concentration of lymphatic tissue and part of the lymphatic system that collects fluid from around the cells and returns it to the blood vessels, and helps with the immune response.

Melanocyte—A specialized skin cell that makes pigment. Tanning of the skin results from an increase in the number and activity level of melanocytes.

Mohs surgery—A form of microscopically controlled surgery that allows for the precise removal of cancerous tissue. It is commonly used to treat various types of skin cancer, particularly in areas of the body where preserving as much tissue as possible is essential. Mohs surgery is also known as micrographic surgery.

Nevus (plural, nevi)—The medical term for a common skin mole. Atypical moles are called dysplastic nevi.

Squamous cells—Flat epithelial cells, which usually make up the outer layer of epithelial tissue, the layer farthest from the surface the epithelium covers.

Targeted therapy—In cancer treatment, a type of drug therapy that blocks tumors by interfering with signaling pathways or specific molecules that the cancer cells need for growth. Also called biologic therapy, targeted therapy is less harmful to normal cells than traditional chemotherapy.

Topical—Referring to a medication applied directly to the skin or other outer surfaces of the body.

---

by the sun to produce more melanin or pigment. It is this pigment that protects skin cells from sun damage and explains why darker-skinned persons have a lower risk of melanoma. Although melanoma is the least common skin cancer, it is the most aggressive. It spreads (metastasizes) to other parts of the body—especially the lungs and liver—as well as invading surrounding tissues. Melanomas in their early stages resemble moles. In Caucasians, melanomas appear most often on the trunk, head, and neck in men and on the arms and legs in women. Melanomas in African Americans, however, occur primarily on the palms of the hand, soles of the feet, and under the nails. Melanomas appear only rarely in the eyes, mouth, vagina, or digestive tract. Although melanomas are associated with exposure to the sun, the greatest risk factor for developing melanoma may be genetic. People who have a first-degree relative with melanoma have an increased risk up to eight times greater of developing the disease.

Besides the three major types of skin cancer, there are a few other less common forms of skin cancer as well as some precancerous skin lesions.

• Kaposi sarcoma (KS) occurs primarily in people whose immune system is depressed, such as AIDS patients, or those who have had organ transplants. When KS occurs with AIDS, it is usually more aggressive.

• Merkel cell carcinoma is a rare skin cancer usually found on sun-exposed areas. Merkel cell carcinoma grows more rapidly than basal and squamous cell carcinoma and can spread.

• Sebaceous gland carcinoma is an aggressive cancer that begins in the oil glands of the skin. These are hard, painless nodules that can develop anywhere, but most often on the eyelid.

Precancerous skin lesions include:

• Actinic keratosis (AK) is also known as solar keratosis. It appears as rough, scaly patches that are red, pink, or brown. The patches appear most often on the face, ears, lower arms, and hands. This condition is not cancer but may develop into squamous cell carcinoma. Actinic keratosis is the most common precancerous skin disorder in the United States, affecting about 58 million Americans.

- Dysplastic nevi are common moles on the surface of the skin. A dysplastic nevus is a type of mole that looks different from common moles; it may be larger than a common mole or have a different color, border, or surface texture. Dysplastic nevi are not cancerous by themselves but may develop into melanoma.

- Leukoplakia occurs inside the mouth as white patches. It is related to constant irritation that might be caused by smoking, rough edges on teeth, dentures, or fillings.

- Actinic cheilitis is a type of actinic keratosis or leukoplakia that occurs on the lips.

- Bowen disease is a type of skin inflammation (dermatitis) that sometimes looks like squamous cell carcinoma. This may be a superficial type of squamous cell carcinoma that appears as a persistent, scaly patch. It can resemble eczema or psoriasis.

- Keratoacanthoma is a dome-shaped tumor that can grow quickly and appear like squamous cell carcinoma. Although it is usually benign, it should be removed to ensure that it is not a carcinoma.

Risk factors

Risk factors for skin cancer include the following:

- Excessive exposure to ultraviolet light or a history of sunburns. Severe sunburns in childhood increase the risk of skin cancer in later life.

- Having fair skin or less pigmentation in the skin.

- A family history of skin cancer or a personal history of previously having skin cancer.

- Exposure to certain environmental chemicals, including arsenic, pitch, creosote, radium or coal tar.

- Having large areas of scar tissue, burns, skin ulcers, or other types of skin inflammation.

- Human papillomavirus (HPV) infection. Certain types of HPV can infect the skin and may increase the risk of squamous cell skin cancer. These are not, however, the same types of HPV associated with cervical cancer.

- Age. Most types of skin cancer take years to develop and are more common in people over 50. The exception is melanoma, which is the most common form of cancer for young adults 25–29 years old and the second most common form of cancer for young people between the ages of 15 and 29.

- A weakened immune system due to HIV/AIDS, leukemia, or drugs that suppress the immune system.

- Having a high number (more than 50) of moles on the body.

Frequent use of **tanning** beds and tanning booths has been linked to the development of skin cancer. Women who use tanning beds or booths more frequently than once per month are at greatest risk and are 55% more likely to develop malignant melanoma. The risk is greatest for individuals who are fair-skinned; those who have blonde or red hair; or those have blue, green, or gray-colored eyes. People who burn easily after sun exposure, those who have previously been treated for skin cancer and individuals with a family member diagnosed with skin cancer are at greater risk for the development of skin cancer after using tanning beds or booths.

Exposure to toxic chemicals such as arsenic, tar, coal, paraffin, and certain types of oil can increase the risk of **non-melanoma skin cancer**. **Radiation therapy** used for cancer as well as drugs used to treat psoriasis can also increase the risk of non-melanoma skin cancer. Skin cancer most often develops on areas of the skin that are exposed to the sun. The most common locations are the scalp, face, lips, ears, neck, chest, arms, and hands. Skin cancer can, however, also occur on areas of the body that do not see much light, such as the palms, the skin between the toes, and the genital area.

Demographics

Cancer of the skin is the most common type of cancer in the United States, with 2.8 million Americans estimated to be diagnosed with skin cancer each year. The exact number is difficult to determine because unlike other cancers, skin cancers are not reported to cancer registries. The average American has a one in five chance of being diagnosed with skin cancer over the course of his or her lifetime. Skin cancers account for as much as 50% of all cases of cancer, more than the combined incidence of cancers of the breast, prostate, lung and colon.

It is estimated that there will be 76,100 new cases of melanoma diagnosed and 9,710 deaths will occur in the United States in 2014. Melanoma accounts for less than 2% of skin cancer cases, but the great majority of skin cancer deaths.

The incidence of skin cancers continues to rise. This increase is attributed to better detection practices, increased exposure to the ultraviolet radiation in sunlight, and the increasing age of the general population. Deaths from non-melanoma-type skin cancers are relatively uncommon, with about 2,000 deaths occurring each year. Despite increasing incidence rates of skin cancer, deaths from skin cancers have continued to decline over the last three decades.

Causes and symptoms

All three main types of skin cancer are related to excessive sun exposure. Ultraviolet light from the sun damages the DNA found in the cells. This damage to the DNA causes changes in the cell that can lead to increased and uncontrolled growth. Although it was once thought that only UVB rays were responsible for the DNA damage that leads to cancer, we now know it is both UVA and UVB rays. Since tanning beds deliver high levels of UVA, they can put people at significant risk of the development of skin cancer.

Basal cell carcinoma appears as a pearly or waxy bump or a flat flesh-colored or brown mark. It is difficult to distinguish this type of mark from a normal mole without performing a **biopsy**. A basal cell carcinoma can take months or years before it becomes sizable. Squamous cell carcinoma can appear as a firm red nodule or a flat mark with a scaly crusted surface.

Melanoma, the most serious of the skin cancers, appears as a large brownish spot. This spot can change in color or size or have an irregular border. It can also appear as a shiny, firm, dome-shaped bump. Melanomas can vary greatly in their appearance, but often the first sign is a change in the appearance of a mole. Early detection of melanoma is important for successful treatment.

Kaposi sarcoma appears as red or purple patches on the skin or mucous membranes. This type of cancer tends to be more common in people with immune suppression such as those with AIDS or those who have undergone organ transplants.

The American Cancer Society (ACS) has introduced an ABCDE system that provides an easy way to remember the important characteristics of moles when one is examining the skin:

• Asymmetry: A normal mole is round, whereas a suspicious mole is unevenly shaped.

• Border: A normal mole has a clear-cut border with the surrounding skin, whereas the edges of a suspect mole are often irregular or scalloped.

• Color: Normal moles are uniformly tan or brown, but cancerous moles may appear as mixtures of red, white, blue, brown, purple, or black.

• Diameter: Normal moles are usually less than 5 millimeters in diameter. A skin lesion greater than 0.25 inches across (6.5 mm, or about the size of a pencil eraser) may be suspected as cancerous.

• Evolving: A mole that changes over time in color or shape or develops itchiness or bleeding can be suspect.

Diagnosis

Examination

A person who finds a suspicious-looking mole, a change in the appearance or texture of a mole, new areas of skin growth, or a bothersome area of skin should consult a physician. As with many cancers, early detection and treatment are important in increasing the chances of treating the cancer successfully. A physician can do a thorough inspection of the skin, noting any suspicious-looking areas. If any suspect areas are found, the patient's primary care physician will most likely refer him or her to a dermatologist, a physician who specializes in diagnosing and treating skin diseases.

Procedures

The dermatologist may first inspect the suspicious area of skin with a dermatoscope, which is an instrument with a special magnifying lens and an attached light source. In some cases this inspection is enough to determine that the skin lesion is not cancerous. The next step in diagnosis is a **skin biopsy**, during which a small sample of skin is taken by the doctor and analyzed by a lab. The skin biopsy is often done in the physician's office under local anesthesia. A shave biopsy removes a tiny bit of superficial tissue; a punch biopsy removes a slightly larger, deeper sample. If the tumor has grown into deeper layers of the skin, the doctor may perform either an incisional biopsy, which removes part of the tumor, or an excisional biopsy, which removes the entire growth.

If cancer is present, the stage of the cancer is then determined. This is a rating of how advanced the cancer is and will help determine the appropriate treatment for the cancer. Stages include stage 0, stage I, stage II, stage III, and stage IV, often with substages as well. Each stage represents a progressively larger and more invasive tumor. Stage 0 refers to a precancerous lesion of suspicious cells and stage IV refers to a severe tumor that has spread to other parts of the body.

Treatment

Treatment depends on the type of cancer and the severity. Basal cell carcinoma is fairly easy to treat when detected early, as is squamous cell carcinoma. There are four main types of treatment for skin cancer. They include surgery, radiation therapy, **chemotherapy**, and **photodynamic therapy**. There are always new types of treatment being tested in **clinical trials**. One new type is targeted therapy, used to treat advanced cases of cancer. Targeted therapy is a type of drug therapy that blocks the growth of skin cancers by interfering with signaling pathways or specific molecules that the cancer cells need for growth.

Surgery is often the best choice if the tumor is localized and easily removable. There are several different surgical procedures used. Excision surgery involves using a scalpel to cut around the tumor and remove it from the skin. This surgery can also be done by shaving the tumor off the surface of the skin. Mohs micrographic surgery involves removing the skin lesion in small layers and immediately examining each layer under a microscope to see when the surgery has gone deep enough to remove the cancerous cells. Mohs micrographic surgery has the highest cure rates of all surgical treatments for basal skin carcinomas, with a 96% cure rate. It is a more time-consuming surgery, though, and not always available. Cryosurgery freezes and destroys the tumor cells. Laser surgery uses a laser beam to cut the skin to remove the tumor. Dermabrasion removes the upper layer of skin and can be used for very small superficial tumors.

Radiation therapy uses high-energy **x-rays** directed towards the tumor to kill cancer cells. It is often used for cancers that occur on the face or ears, where **reconstructive surgery** would be difficult.

Chemotherapy refers to drugs taken internally either by injection or orally that travel through the bloodstream. Chemotherapy is intended to either stop the growth of cancer cells or to kill the cancer cells. Chemotherapy often has rather serious side effects as it affects other cells in the body besides the cancer cells. Occasionally, for non-melanoma skin cancers, the chemotherapy drug 5-fluorouracil (5-FU) can be delivered in a cream form to use topically. Imiquimod is another drug used in topical form to treat early-stage basal cell carcinomas.

Photodynamic therapy uses both a drug and a laser to kill cancer cells. The drug is a photosensitizer which becomes active only after light of a specific wavelength from the laser contacts it. This method allows more control over preventing damage to healthy tissue. Photodynamic therapy is a relatively new therapy, however, and not always available.

A newer method of treatment for advanced skin cancer is targeted therapy, in which drugs that target genetic changes in cancer cells are used to prevent the abnormal cells from reproducing. The targeted therapy used to treat advanced basal cell carcinoma is a drug called vismodegib (Erivedge), which targets genes in a cell signaling pathway known as hedgehog. Vismodegib comes in pill form and is taken once a day. It cannot be used by pregnant women, however, because the hedgehog pathway is also involved in fetal development.

Special concerns

Because many skin cancers are found on the face and neck, cosmetic concerns are a priority for many patients. If there is a risk of noticeable scarring or disfigurement, a patient may wish to ask about alternative types of removal or inquire about the services of a plastic surgeon.

Prognosis

Prognosis depends upon the type of cancer and its severity. Skin cancer is the most common type of cancer in the United States but accounts for less than 1% of cancer deaths. Basal cell carcinoma is fairly easy to treat when caught early. Squamous cell carcinoma also is not usually serious and has a very high treatment rate when caught early. If not detected and diagnosed in early stages, skin cancer can be more difficult to treat and treatment for the cancer can result in some disfigurement. A small number of squamous cell carcinomas can spread to other organs.

Melanoma is a more serious type of skin cancer; however, if it is caught early it is still curable. Melanoma is the most likely skin cancer to spread to other parts of the body, which worsens the prognosis. According to the American Cancer Society, as of 2014, for stage I melanoma, the five-year survival rates range from 92% to 97%. The five-year survival rates for stage II melanomas range from 53% to 81%. The five-year survival rate for stage III melanoma decreases to 40% to 78%, and for stage IV melanoma, five-year survival drops to 15%. Patients over the age of 70 typically have five-year survival rates on the lower side, as do African Americans and persons with weakened immune systems.

Prevention

There are many interventions to decrease the risk of skin cancer:

- Wear protective clothing (long sleeves, sunglasses, and hat) while in the sun. Some companies now make clothing that is more tightly woven and coated with special products to block out UV radiation.

- Use sunscreen of at least 15 SPF when outside. Sunscreens as high as 100 SPF are now available, but study results vary on the effectiveness of sunscreens higher than SPF 30. SPF 15 sunscreens filter out about 93% of UVB rays, while SPF 30 sunscreens filter out about 97%. Always check the expiration date on sunscreen products; most are good for two to three years.

- Avoid being outside when the sun is brightest, between 10 A.M. and 4 P.M.

- Avoid the use of sunlamps and tanning beds and booths. Legislation has been proposed in several states as of 2014 to prohibit minors from visiting tanning salons. On May 29, 2014, the U.S. Food and Drug Administration (FDA) issued a formal warning about

QUESTIONS TO ASK YOUR DOCTOR

- What type of skin cancer do I have?
- What are my various treatment options?
- Are there any clinical trials that would be relevant for my type of cancer?
- What is your experience in treating this type of cancer?
- How advanced is my cancer?
- What is the goal of treatment, to eradicate the cancer or to alleviate symptoms?
- Should I go to a specialized cancer center for treatment?

the use of sunlamps and similar indoor tanning devices, stating that they must carry warning labels regarding the increased risk of skin cancer associated with their use, and that they should not be used by persons under the age of 18.

- Children need special protection against the sun as their skin burns more easily, they spend more time outdoors than most adults, and they are less knowledgeable about the dangers of too much sun. Babies younger than six months should be kept out of direct sunlight.

- Keep in mind that UV rays can be reflected from the surface of the ocean, sandy beaches, or snow-covered ski slopes. It is a good idea to check the local weather forecast for the UV index for the day before heading outdoors.

- Check your skin periodically for abnormal moles. The American Academy of Dermatology recommends doing this on your birthday: "Check your birthday suit on your birthday." Although self-examination will not prevent skin cancer, early detection improves prognosis.

These precautions are just as important for African Americans, Native Americans, and others with darker skin tones as they are for Caucasians; dermatologists are now working to warn members of these groups about the dangers of excessive sun exposure. It is thought that one reason that ethnic and racial minorities with darker skin are more likely to have advanced skin cancers at the time of diagnosis is that they mistakenly believe they are at little risk of skin cancer.

See also Merkel cell carcinoma; Skin cancer, non-melanoma; Squamous cell carcinoma of the skin.

Resources

BOOKS

Baldi, Alfonso, Paola Pasquali, and Enrico P. Spugnini, eds. *Skin Cancer: A Practical Approach.* New York: Humana Press, 2014.

Cognetta, Armand B., Jr., and William M. Mendenhall, eds. *Radiation Therapy for Skin Cancer.* New York: Springer, 2013.

Nouri, Keyvan, ed. *Mohs Micrographic Surgery.* New York: Springer, 2012.

Oro, Anthony E., and Fiona M. Watt, eds. *Skin and Its Diseases: A Subject from the Cold Spring Harbor Perspectives in Medicine.* Cold Spring Harbor, NY: Cold Spring Harbor Laboratory Press, 2014.

PERIODICALS

Abello-Poblete, M.V., et al. "Histologic Outcomes of Excised Moderate and Severe Dysplastic Nevi." *Dermatologic Surgery* 40 (January 2014): 40–45.

Agbai, O.N., et al. "Skin Cancer and Photoprotection in People of Color: A Review and Recommendations for Physicians and the Public." *Journal of the American Academy of Dermatology* 70 (April 2014): 748–762.

Clark, C.M., et al. "Basal Cell Carcinoma: An Evidence-Based Treatment Update." *American Journal of Clinical Dermatology* 15, no. 3 (2014): 197–216.

Dreier, J., et al. "Basal Cell Carcinoma: A Paradigm for Targeted Therapies." *Expert Opinion on Pharmacotherapy* 14 (July 2013): 1307–1318.

Hawryluk, E.B., and M.G. Liang. "Pediatric Melanoma, Moles, and Sun Safety." *Pediatric Clinics of North America* 61 (April 2014): 279–291.

Holman, D.M., et al. "Strategies to Reduce Indoor Tanning: Current Research Gaps and Future Opportunities for Prevention." *American Journal of Preventive Medicine* 44 (June 2013): 672–681.

Kolk, A., et al. "Melanotic and Non-melanotic Malignancies of the Face and External Ear—A Review of Current Treatment Concepts and Future Options." *Cancer Treatment Reviews* 40 (August 2014): 819–837.

Mancebo, S.E., J.Y. Hu, and S.Q. Wang. "Sunscreens: A Review of Health Benefits, Regulations, and Controversies." *Dermatologic Clinics* 32 (July 2014): 427–438.

Maru, G.B., et al. "The Role of Inflammation in Skin Cancer." *Advances in Experimental Medicine and Biology* 816 (2014): 437–469.

Micali, G., et al. "Topical Pharmacotherapy for Skin Cancer: Part I. Pharmacology." *Journal of the American Academy of Dermatology* 70 (June 2014): 965.e1–965.e12.

OTHER

American Cancer Society (ACS). "Skin Cancer: Basal and Squamous Cell." http://www.cancer.org/acs/groups/cid/documents/webcontent/003139-pdf.pdf (accessed June 17, 2014).

American Cancer Society (ACS). "Skin Cancer Prevention and Early Detection." http://www.cancer.org/acs/groups/cid/documents/webcontent/003184-pdf.pdf (accessed June 23, 2014).

WEBSITES

American Academy of Dermatology (AAD). "Basal Cell Carcinoma." http://www.aad.org/dermatology-a-to-z/diseases-and-treatments/a—d/basal-cell-carcinoma (accessed June 17, 2014).

eMedicine Health. "Skin Cancer." http://www.emedicinehealth.com/skin_cancer/article_em.htm (accessed June22, 2014).

National Cancer Institute (NCI). "What Does a Mole Look Like?" http://www.cancer.gov/cancertopics/prevention/skin/molephotos (accessed June 23, 2014).

National Cancer Institute (NCI). "What You Need to Know about Melanoma and Other Skin Cancers." http://www.cancer.gov/cancertopics/wyntk/skin/page1/AllPages (acccssed June 23, 2014).

Skin Cancer Foundation. "Skin Cancer Facts." http://www.skincancer.org/skin-cancer-information/skin-cancer-facts (accessed June 23, 2014).

ORGANIZATIONS

American Academy of Dermatology (AAD), P.O. Box 4014, Schaumburg, IL 60168, (847) 240-1280, (866) 503-SKIN (7546), Fax: (847) 240-1859, http://www.aad.org/Forms/ContactUs/Default.aspx, http://www.aad.org/.

American Cancer Society (ACS), 250 Williams Street NW, Atlanta, GA 30303, (800) 227-2345, http://www.cancer.org/aboutus/howwehelpyou/app/contact-us.aspx, http://www.cancer.org/index.

American Society of Clinical Oncology (ASCO), 2318 Mill Road, Suite 800, Alexandria, VA 22314 , (571) 483-1300, (888) 651-3038, contactus@cancer.net, http://www.asco.org/.

National Cancer Institute (NCI), BG 9609 MSC 9760, 9609 Medical Center Drive, Bethesda, MD 20892-9760, (800) 4-CANCER (422-6237), http://www.cancer.gov/global/contact/email-us, http://www.cancer.gov/.

Office of Cancer Complementary and Alternative Medicine (OCCAM), 9609 Medical Center Dr., Room 5-W-136, Rockville, MD 20850, (240) 276-6595, Fax: (240) 276-7888, ncioccam1-r@mail.nih.gov, http://cam.cancer.gov/.

Skin Cancer Foundation, 149 Madison Avenue, Suite 901, New York, NY 10016, (212) 725-5176, http://www.skincancer.org/contact-us, http://www.skincancer.org/.

Cindy L. Jones, PhD
Melinda Granger Oberleitner, R.N., D.N.S.,
A.P.R.N., C.N.S.
REVISED BY REBECCA J. FREY, PhD

▌Skin cancer, non-melanoma

Definition

Non-melanoma **skin cancer** is a malignant growth of the external surface or epithelial layer of the skin. The main types of non-melanoma skin **cancer** are basal cell carcinomas (BCCs) and squamous cell carcinomas (SCCs).

Description

Skin cancer is the growth of abnormal cells capable of invading and destroying other associated skin cells. Skin cancer is often subdivided into either **melanoma** or non-melanoma. Melanoma is a dark-pigmented, usually malignant tumor arising from a skin cell capable of making the pigment melanin (a melanocyte). Non-melanoma skin cancer most often originates from the external skin surface as a squamous cell **carcinoma** or a **basal cell carcinoma**.

The cells of a cancerous growth originate from a single cell that reproduces uncontrollably, resulting in the formation of a tumor. Exposure to sunlight is documented as the main cause of more than one million cases of non-melanoma skin cancer diagnosed each year in the United States. The incidence increases for those living where direct sunshine is plentiful, such as near the equator.

Basal cell carcinoma (BCC) is the most common type of skin cancer, accounting for about 80% of all skin cancers. It develops from cells of the lowest layer of the epidermis, the basal cells or basal keratinocytes. These are the cells that produce new skin cells. BCC occurs primarily on the parts of the skin exposed to the sun and is most common in people living in areas near the equator, at high altitudes, or in areas of high ozone depletion. Light-skinned people are at greater risk of developing basal cell carcinoma than dark-skinned people. Basal cell carcinoma grows very slowly; however, if it is not treated it can invade deeper skin layers causing extensive damage and can be fatal. This type of cancer can appear as a shiny, translucent nodule on the skin or as a red, wrinkled and scaly area.

Squamous cell carcinoma (SCC) is the second most frequent type of skin cancer overall but the most common type in dark-skinned people. It arises from the outer keratinizing layer of skin just below the surface. Squamous cell carcinoma grows faster than basal cell carcinoma and is more likely to metastasize to the lymph nodes as well as to distant sites. Squamous cell carcinoma most often appears on the arms, head, and neck. Fair-skinned people of Celtic descent are at high risk of developing squamous cell carcinoma. This type of cancer is rarely life threatening but can cause serious problems if it spreads and can also cause disfigurement. Squamous cell carcinoma usually appears as a scaly, slightly elevated area of damaged skin. It can also appear in an area of chronic inflammation on the skin.

KEY TERMS

Actinic keratosis—A precancerous skin condition in which skin exposed to the sun forms thick, scaly, or crusty patches. Untreated actinic keratosis has a 20% chance of progressing to skin cancer.

Basal cell—A keratinocyte in the basal layer, the deepest of the five layers of cells in the epidermis.

Biopsy—Removal of a small sample of tissue for examination under a microscope; used for the diagnosis and treatment of cancer and precancerous conditions.

Dermis—The layer of skin just below the epidermis.

Epidermis—The outer covering of skin in mammals. In humans, it consists of five layers of cells.

Epithelial tissue—The collection of cells that cover the exterior and line the interior surfaces of the body.

Immunity—Ability to resist the effects of agents, such as bacteria and viruses, that cause disease.

Keratinocyte—The basic type of cell in the epidermis (uppermost layer) of the skin, comprising about 90% of its cells.

Lymph node—A concentration of lymphatic tissue and part of the lymphatic system that collects fluid from around the cells and returns it to the blood vessels, and helps with the immune response.

Melanocyte—A specialized skin cell that makes pigment. Tanning of the skin results from an increase in the number and activity level of melanocytes.

Mohs surgery—A form of microscopically controlled surgery that allows for the precise removal of cancerous tissue. It is commonly used to treat various types of skin cancer, particularly in areas of the body where preserving as much tissue as possible is essential. Mohs surgery is also known as micrographic surgery.

Squamous cells—Flat epithelial cells, which usually make up the outer layer of epithelial tissue, the layer farthest away from the surface the epithelium covers.

Targeted therapy—In cancer treatment, a type of drug therapy that blocks tumors by interfering with signaling pathways or specific molecules that the cancer cells need for growth. Also called biologic therapy, targeted therapy is less harmful to normal cells than traditional chemotherapy.

Topical—Referring to a medication applied directly to the skin or other outer surfaces of the body.

Risk factors

Risk factors for skin cancer include the following:

- Excessive exposure to ultraviolet light or a history of sunburns. Severe sunburns in childhood increase the risk of skin cancer in later life.

- Having fair skin or less pigmentation in the skin.

- A family history of skin cancer or a personal history of previously having skin cancer.

- Exposure to certain environmental chemicals, including arsenic, pitch, creosote, radium or coal tar.

- Frequent use of tanning beds or sunlamps.

- Having large areas of scar tissue, burns, skin ulcers, or other types of skin inflammation.

- Human papillomavirus (HPV) infection. Certain types of HPV can infect the skin and may increase the risk of squamous cell carcinoma. These are not, however, the same types of HPV associated with cervical cancer.

- Age. Skin cancer often takes years to develop and is more common with age. The sunburn you get as a teen can increase your risk of skin cancer when you are 40.

- A weakened immune system due to HIV/AIDS, leukemia, or drugs that suppress the immune system.

Exposure to such toxic chemicals as arsenic, tar, coal, paraffin, and certain types of oil can increase the risk of non-melanoma skin cancer. **Radiation therapy** used for cancer as well as drugs used to treat psoriasis can also increase the risk of non-melanoma skin cancer. Skin cancer most often develops on areas of the skin that are exposed to the sun. The most common locations are the scalp, face, lips, ears, neck, chest, arms and hands. It can, however, also occur on areas that do not see much light such as the palms, between the toes and the genital area.

Demographics

Cancer of the skin is the most common type of cancer in the United States; about 3.5 million basal and squamous cell skin carcinomas are diagnosed each year, occurring in about 2.2 million Americans. The exact number is difficult to determine, however, because unlike most cancers, skin cancers are not reported to cancer registries. About 80% of these skin cancers are BCCs; SCCs are less common. The average American has a one in five chance of being diagnosed with skin cancer over the course of his or her lifetime. Skin cancers account for as much as 50% of all cases of cancer, more than the combined incidence of cancers of the breast, prostate, lung, and colon.

The incidence of skin cancers continues to rise. This increase is attributed to better detection practices, increased exposure to the ultraviolet radiation in sunlight, and to the increasing age of the general population.

Deaths from non-melanoma skin cancers are relatively uncommon, with about 2,000 deaths occurring from these skin cancers each year. Despite increasing incidence rates of skin cancer, deaths from skin cancers have continued to decline over the last three decades.

Causes and symptoms

Cumulative sun exposure is considered a significant risk factor for non-melanoma skin cancer. There is evidence suggesting that early, intense exposure causing blistering sunburn in childhood may also play an important role in the cause of non-melanoma skin cancer. Basal cell carcinoma most frequently affects the skin of the face, with the next most common sites being the ears, the backs of the hands, the shoulders, and the arms. It is prevalent in both sexes and most commonly occurs in people over 40.

About 1–2% of all skin cancers develop within burn scars; squamous cell carcinomas account for about 95% of these cancers, with 3% being basal cell carcinomas and the remainder malignant melanomas.

Basal cell carcinomas usually appear as small skin lesions that persist for at least three weeks. This form of non-melanomatous skin cancer looks flat and waxy, with the edges of the lesion translucent and rounded. The edges also contain small fresh blood vessels. An ulcer in the center of the lesion gives it a dimpled appearance. Basal cell carcinoma lesions vary from 4–6 mm in size, but can slowly grow larger if untreated.

Squamous cell carcinoma also involves skin exposed to the sun, such as the face, ears, hands, or arms. This form of non-melanoma is also most common among people over 40. Squamous cell carcinoma presents itself as a small scaly raised bump on the skin with a crusting ulcer in the center, but without pain and **itching**. It may be preceded by a skin condition called actinic keratosis or AK. Also known as solar keratosis, AK appears as rough, scaly patches that are red, pink, or brown. They appear most often on the face, ears, lower arms, and hands. AK is not cancer but may develop into squamous cell carcinoma. Actinic keratosis is the most common precancerous skin disorder in the United States, affecting about 58 million Americans.

Basal cell and squamous cell carcinomas can grow more easily when people have a suppressed immune system because they are taking immunosuppressive drugs or are exposed to radiation. Some people must take immunosuppressive drugs to prevent the rejection of a transplanted organ or because they have a disease in which the immune system attacks the body's own tissues (autoimmune illnesses); others may need radiation therapy to treat another form of cancer. Because of this increased risk of skin cancer, everyone taking these immunosuppressive drugs or receiving radiation treatments should undergo complete skin examination at regular intervals. If proper treatment is delayed and the tumor continues to grow, the tumor cells can spread (metastasize) to muscle, bone, nerves, and possibly the brain.

Diagnosis

Examination

To diagnose skin cancer, doctors must carefully examine the lesion and ask the patient about how long it has been there, whether it itches or bleeds, and other questions about the patient's medical history. If any suspect areas are found, the patient's primary care physician will most likely refer him or her to a dermatologist, a physician who specializes in diagnosing and treating skin diseases.

Procedures

The dermatologist may first inspect the suspicious area of skin with a dermatoscope, which is an instrument with a special magnifying lens and an attached light source. In some cases this inspection is enough to determine that the skin lesion is not cancerous. If skin cancer cannot be ruled out, however, a sample of the tissue is removed and examined under a microscope (a **biopsy**). A definitive diagnosis of squamous or basal cell carcinoma can be made only with microscopic examination of the tumor cells. Once skin cancer has been diagnosed, the stage of the disease's development is determined. The information from the biopsy and staging allows the physician and patient to plan for treatment and possible surgical intervention.

Treatment

A variety of treatment options are available for those diagnosed with non-melanoma skin cancer. Some carcinomas can be removed by cryosurgery, the process of freezing with liquid nitrogen. Uncomplicated and previously untreated basal cell carcinoma of the trunk and arms is often treated with curettage and electrodesiccation, which is the scraping of the lesion and the destruction of any remaining malignant cells with an electrical current. Removal of a lesion layer by layer down to normal margins (**Mohs surgery**) is an effective treatment for both basal and squamous cell carcinoma. Mohs micrographic surgery has the highest cure rate of all surgical treatments for basal skin carcinomas, with a 96% cure rate.

Radiation therapy is best reserved for older, debilitated patients or for those in whom the tumor is considered inoperable. Laser therapy in combination with a photosensitizing drug, a treatment known as **photodynamic therapy**, can be used to treat some non-melanoma skin cancers. The topical application of the **chemotherapy** drug 5-fluorouracil (5-FU), may be used as a treatment option for non-melanoma skin cancers. Imiquimod is another drug used in topical form to treat early-stage basal cell carcinomas.

A newer type of treatment option is targeted therapy, used to treat advanced cases of skin cancer. Targeted therapy is a type of drug therapy that blocks the growth of skin cancers by interfering with signaling pathways or specific molecules that the cancer cells need for growth.

Alternative treatment

Alternative medicine aims to prevent rather than treat skin cancer. **Vitamins** have been shown to prevent sunburn and possibly skin cancer. Some dermatologists have suggested that taking vitamins E and C may help prevent sunburn. Other antioxidant nutrients, including beta carotene, selenium, zinc, and the bioflavonoid quercetin have been suggested as possibly preventing skin cancer. Such antioxidant herbs as bilberry (*Vaccinium myrtillus*), hawthorn (*Crataegus laevigata*), turmeric (*Curcuma longa*), and ginkgo (*Ginkgo biloba*) also have been presented as helpful in preventing skin cancers.

Researchers are also looking at botanical compounds that could be added to skin care products applied externally to lower the risk of skin cancer. Several botanical compounds had been tested on animals and found to be effective in preventing skin cancer, but further research needs to be done on human subjects. In any case, people at increased risk of skin cancer should first use standard methods of reducing sun exposure before relying on alternative methods of prevention.

Prognosis

Both squamous and basal cell carcinomas are curable with appropriate treatment, although basal cell carcinomas have about a 5% rate of recurrence. Skin cancer is the most common type of cancer in the United States, but non-melanoma skin cancers account for less than 1% of cancer deaths. Early detection remains critical for a positive prognosis. Although it is rare for basal cell carcinomas to metastasize, their metastases can rapidly lead to death if they invade the eyes, ears, mouth, or the membranes covering the brain.

Prevention

There are many interventions to decrease the risk of non-melanoma skin cancer:

- Wear protective clothing (long sleeves, sunglasses, and hat) while in the sun. Some companies now make clothing that is more tightly woven and coated with special products to block out UV radiation.

- Use sunscreen of at least 15 SPF when outside. Sunscreens as high as 100 SPF are now available. SPF 15 sunscreens filter out about 93% of UVB rays; SPF 30 sunscreens filter out about 97%; SPF 50 sunscreens about 98%; and SPF 100 sunscreens about 99%. Always check the expiration date on sunscreen products; most are good for 2–3 years.

- Avoid being outside when the sun is brightest, between 10 A.M. and 4 P.M.

- Avoid the use of sunlamps and tanning beds and booths. Legislation has been proposed in several states as of 2014 to prohibit minors from visiting tanning salons. On May 29, 2014, the Food and Drug Administration (FDA) issued a formal warning about the use of sunlamps and similar indoor tanning devices, stating that they must carry warning labels regarding the increased risk of skin cancer associated with their use, and that they should not be used by persons under the age of 18.

- Children need special protection against the sun, as their skin burns more easily, they spend more time outdoors than most adults, and they are less knowledgeable about the dangers of too much sun. Babies younger than six months should be kept out of direct sunlight.

- Keep in mind that UV rays can be reflected from the surface of the ocean, sandy beaches, or snow-covered ski slopes. It is a good idea to check the local weather forecast for the UV index for the day before heading outdoors.

These precautions are just as important for African Americans, Native Americans, and others with darker skin tones as they are for Caucasians; dermatologists are now working to warn members of these groups about the dangers of excessive sun exposure. It is thought that one reason ethnic and racial minorities with darker skin are more likely to have advanced skin cancers at the time of

QUESTIONS TO ASK YOUR DOCTOR

- What type of skin cancer do I have?
- What are the recommended treatment options for my type of skin cancer?
- How long will treatment last?
- Are the recommended treatments available in my community?
- How long will I need follow-up after treatment?
- What can I do to prevent a recurrence of my skin cancer after treatment?

diagnosis is that they mistakenly believe they are at little risk of skin cancer.

Resources

BOOKS

Baldi, Alfonso, Paola Pasquali, and Enrico P. Spugnini, eds. *Skin Cancer: A Practical Approach*. New York: Humana Press, 2014.

Cognetta, Armand B., Jr., and William M. Mendenhall, eds. *Radiation Therapy for Skin Cancer*. New York: Springer, 2013.

Nouri, Keyvan, ed. *Mohs Micrographic Surgery*. New York: Springer, 2012.

Oro, Anthony E., and Fiona M. Watt, eds. *Skin and Its Diseases: A Subject from the Cold Spring Harbor Perspectives in Medicine*. Cold Spring Harbor, NY: Cold Spring Harbor Laboratory Press, 2014.

PERIODICALS

Agbai, O.N., et al. "Skin Cancer and Photoprotection in People of Color: A Review and Recommendations for Physicians and the Public." *Journal of the American Academy of Dermatology* 70 (April 2014): 748–762.

Clark, C.M., et al. "Basal Cell Carcinoma: An Evidence-Based Treatment Update." *American Journal of Clinical Dermatology* 15, no. 3 (2014): 197–216.

Cleavenger, J., and S.M. Johnson. "Non-Melanoma Skin Cancer Review." *Journal of the Arkansas Medical Society* 110 (April 2014): 230–234.

Dreier, J., et al. "Basal Cell Carcinoma: A Paradigm for Targeted Therapies." *Expert Opinion on Pharmacotherapy* 14 (July 2013): 1307–1318.

Holman, D.M., et al. "Strategies to Reduce Indoor Tanning: Current Research Gaps and Future Opportunities for Prevention." *American Journal of Preventive Medicine* 44 (June 2013): 672–681.

Mancebo, S.E., J.Y. Hu, and S.Q. Wang. "Sunscreens: A Review of Health Benefits, Regulations, and Controversies." *Dermatologic Clinics* 32 (July 2014): 427–438.

Maru, G.B., et al. "The Role of Inflammation in Skin Cancer." *Advances in Experimental Medicine and Biology* 816 (2014): 437–469.

Micali, G., et al. "Topical Pharmacotherapy for Skin Cancer: Part I. Pharmacology." *Journal of the American Academy of Dermatology* 70 (June 2014): 965.e1–965.e12.

Wang, J., et al. "Role of Human Papillomavirus in Cutaneous Squamous Cell Carcinoma: A Meta-analysis." *Journal of the American Academy of Dermatology* 70 (April 2014): 621–629.

OTHER

American Cancer Society (ACS). "Skin Cancer: Basal and Squamous Cell." http://www.canccr.org/acs/groups/cid/documents/webcontent/003139-pdf.pdf (accessed June 17, 2014).

American Cancer Society (ACS). "Skin Cancer Prevention and Early Detection." http://www.cancer.org/acs/groups/cid/documents/webcontent/003184-pdf.pdf (accessed June 23, 2014).

WEBSITES

American Academy of Dermatology (AAD) "Basal Cell Carcinoma." http://www.aad.org/dermatology-a-to-z/diseases-and-treatments/a—d/basal-cell-carcinoma (accessed June 17, 2014).

eMedicine Health. "Skin Cancer." http://www.emedicinehealth.com/skin_cancer/article_em.htm (accessed June22, 2014).

National Cancer Institute (NCI). "What You Need to Know about Melanoma and Other Skin Cancers." http://www.cancer.gov/cancertopics/wyntk/skin/page1/AllPages (accessed June 23, 2014).

Skin Cancer Foundation. "Skin Cancer Facts." http://www.skincancer.org/skin-cancer-information/skin-cancer-facts (accessed June 23, 2014).

ORGANIZATIONS

American Academy of Dermatology (AAD), P.O. Box 4014, Schaumburg, IL 60168, (847) 240-1280, (866) 503-SKIN (7546), Fax: (847) 240-1859, http://www.aad.org/Forms/ContactUs/Default.aspx, http://www.aad.org/.

American Cancer Society (ACS), 250 Williams Strcct NW, Atlanta, GA 30303, (800) 227-2345, http://www.cancer.org/aboutus/howwehelpyou/app/contact-us.aspx, http://www.cancer.org/index.

American Society of Clinical Oncology (ASCO), 2318 Mill Road, Suite 800, Alexandria, VA 22314 , (571) 483-1300, (888) 651-3038, contactus@cancer.net, http://www.asco.org/.

National Cancer Institute (NCI), BG 9609 MSC 9760, 9609 Medical Center Drive, Bethesda, MD 20892-9760, (800) 4-CANCER (422-6237), http://www.cancer.gov/global/contact/email-us, http://www.cancer.gov/.

Office of Cancer Complementary and Alternative Medicine (OCCAM), 9609 Medical Center Dr., Room 5-W-136, Rockville, MD 20850, (240) 276-6595, Fax: (240) 276-7888, ncioccam1-r@mail.nih.gov, http://cam.cancer.gov/.

Skin Cancer Foundation, 149 Madison Avenue, Suite 901, New York, NY 10016, (212) 725-5176, http://www.skincancer.org/contact-us, http://www.skincancer.org/.

Jeffrey P. Larson, RPT
Melinda Granger Oberleitner, R.N., D.N.S., A.P.R.N., C.N.S.
REVISED BY REBECCA J. FREY, PhD

Skin cancer, squamous cell *see* **Squamous cell carcinoma of the skin**

Skin check

Definition

A skin check is a self-examination or an examination by a physician that checks the entire skin for signs of possible **skin cancer**.

Purpose

The purpose of skin checks is to detect skin **cancer** at the earliest possible stage when it is easier to cure. Skin cancer is the most common type of cancer, and skin cancers have been increasing in recent decades. One in five Americans will be diagnosed with skin cancer during their lifetime. There are more than 3.5 million diagnoses of skin cancer in the United States each year—more than all other cancer diagnoses combined.

The two main types of skin cancer are squamous cell **carcinoma** (SCC) and **basal cell carcinoma** (BCC). SCC and BCC originate in keratinocytes, the most common type of skin cell. Although much less likely than other types of skin cancer to spread to other parts of the body (metastasize) and become life-threatening, untreated BCC—and especially SCC—can grow and spread to nearby tissues and organs, potentially causing scarring, deformity, and possible loss of function; in some cases, they may even be fatal. Melanomas are skin cancers that originate in melanocytes, the cells that produce the brown pigment of skin color and moles. Although much less common than SCC and BCC, melanomas are much more serious. Like SCC and BCC, melanomas are almost always curable at early stages; however, untreated **melanoma** often metastasizes and can become very difficult to treat. The other types of skin cancers together account for less than 1% of all skin cancers. These include **Merkel cell carcinoma**, **Kaposi sarcoma**, cutaneous (skin) **lymphoma**, skin adnexal tumors that originate in hair follicles or glands in the skin, and various types of sarcomas.

With regular self-exams and periodic skin checks by a physician, most skin cancers can be found early. Careful skin checks are part of routine cancer-related checkups. Skin checks are especially important for people at high risk of skin cancer, including those who have had previous skin cancers, have reduced immune-system function, or have a strong family history of skin cancer. People at average skin cancer risk should have a professional skin check by a primary care physician or dermatologist every one to two years, especially if they tend to develop moles. People with previous skin cancer or a strong family history of the disease may need more frequent skin checks.

Description

Skin checks consist of examining all of the skin for new spots or skin areas that are changing in appearance, **itching**, or bleeding. BCC and SCC are strongly associated with exposure to the sun, and they usually develop on exposed body parts, such as the head and neck; however, they can occur anywhere on the body. Melanomas can also occur anywhere on the body, but they are most common on the chest and back of men and the legs of women. The neck and face are also common sites of melanomas.

KEY TERMS

ABCDE—A simple way to remember suspicious signs on the skin that could suggest melanoma—Asymmetry, Borders, Color, Diameter, Evolution.

Actinic keratoses—Solar keratoses; dry, scaly lesions or patches on the skin from long-term sun exposure that are considered the earliest stage in the development of squamous cell carcinoma.

Basal cell carcinoma (BCC)—Cancer originating in basal cells of the skin.

Keratinocytes—The most common type of skin cell; keratinocytes produce the protein keratin that provides strength for skin, hair, and nails.

Melanocytes—Skin cells that produce the pigment melanin.

Melanoma—A malignant skin tumor that originates in melanocytes (pigmented cells) of normal skin or moles.

Metastasis—The spreading of cancer from its site of origin to other parts of the body.

Mole—A pigmented spot, mark, or permanent protrusion on the skin.

Squamous cell carcinoma (SCC)—Cancer that originates in the squamous cells of the skin or linings of various organs.

Self-exams

Regular self-exams help people learn the normal appearance of their skin so that changes over time are evident. People learn the locations, appearance, and feel of their moles. When a person performs a self-exam for the first time, he or she should go over the entire surface of the skin carefully to learn the patterns of moles, freckles, birthmarks, blemishes, and other marks so that any changes will be noticeable. To assist with self-exams, the American Academy of Dermatology has a downloadable body mole map available at https://www.aad. org/File%20Library/Global%20navigation/For%20the%20public/aad-body-mole-map.pdf.

The steps of a skin check are as follows:

• Facing a mirror, the person first examines the face, neck, ears, and scalp. A comb or blow dryer can be used to move hair aside for a better view of the scalp. It can be difficult to check one's own scalp, so it may be preferable to ask a family member or friend to check through the hair.

• The chest and belly are examined next. Women should lift their breasts to examine the area under the breasts.

• The tops of the arms, the underarms, and both sides of the arms are checked with the arms straight and bent.

• The tops of the hands, the palms, between the fingers, and the fingernails are checked.

• The sides of the body are examined with the arms raised.

• Sitting down, the person checks the front of the thighs, shins, tops of the feet, between the toes, and the toenails.

• A hand mirror is used to check the soles of the feet, calves, and backs of the thighs, examining first one leg and then the other.

• A hand mirror is also used to check the genital area, buttocks, upper and lower back, and the backs of the neck and ears. The back can be examined in a wall mirror using a hand mirror. Alternatively, a family member or close friend can examine the back, buttocks, backs of the thighs, and back of the ears, along with the scalp.

• People with darker skin should carefully check for changes in less-pigmented areas of the body, such as the palms, soles of the feet, and nail beds.

The date of the skin check and anything of note should be recorded. Some people find it useful to take photos of certain skin areas.

What to look for

Skin changes to note include:

• new growths, spots, or bumps

• a new firm, flesh-colored bump

• a new red or darker-colored flaky patch that may be slightly raised

• a sore that does not heal, including shaving cuts that fail to heal in a few days and may bleed readily

• a new mole that appears different from one's other moles

BCC and SCC can both develop as flat areas that appear only very slightly different than normal skin. BCCs are often flat, firm, and pale or small, raised, and pink or red. They can also be clear, shiny, pearly bumps that may bleed easily. BCCs may also have one or more abnormal blood vessels, be lower at the center, and have blue, brown, or black areas. Large BCCs can have crusty or oozing areas. SCCs are growing lumps and often have a rough, scaly, or crusted surface. They can also be slow-growing, flat, reddish patches.

Actinic or solar keratoses are spots caused by sun exposure that are sometimes precancerous. They are usually small—less than 0.25 in. (6 mm) in diameter—rough or scaly, and flesh-colored or pink-red. They most often occur on the face, ears, arms, or backs of the hands, but they can also occur on other areas exposed to the sun. People who develop one actinic keratosis usually develop many more. They are often benign (noncancerous) and may disappear on their own, but some of them can develop into SCC.

Melanoma

Harmless skin changes are not unusual as people age, but some spots appear very similar to melanoma, so regular professional examinations are necessary. Almost all moles are harmless. Most people have moles that are present at birth or develop during childhood or young adulthood. They are evenly colored tan, brown, or black; flat or raised; and round or oval, usually less than 0.25 in. (6 mm). Most moles do not change, although sometimes they fade away with age. New moles later in adulthood or changes in the size, color, or shape of a mole or a spot that looks different from all other spots on the skin should be checked by a doctor, as such changes could indicate an early melanoma.

The ABCDE rule is a guide to moles or other spots that could be signs of melanoma:

• Asymmetry: The two halves of a mole or birthmark do not match.

• Border: The mole has irregular, ragged, notched, or blurred edges.

• Color: The mole is irregularly colored with different shades of brown or black or with pink, red, white, or blue patches.

• Diameter: The mole is new or larger than 0.25 in. (6 mm), although possibly smaller.

• Evolving: The mole is changing in size, shape, or color or is starting to itch, hurt, or bleed.

Other signs of possible melanoma include:

• a non-healing sore

• spread of pigment to the surrounding skin

• redness or swelling beyond the border of a spot

• a change in sensation, such as itchiness, tenderness, or pain

• changes to the surface of a mole, such as scaliness, oozing, bleeding, or the development of a bump or nodule

Mole mapping

If a person has a lot of moles or is concerned about developing skin cancer, he or she may wish to undergo mole mapping. Mole mapping is a more in-depth type of skin check in which all the patient's moles are individually photographed and recorded; this process is known as total body photography. The photographs are analyzed and serve as a record. During future visits, the patient's moles are checked against the photographs for changes.

Preparation

Skin checks should be performed monthly, preferably after a bath or shower. They should be performed in a well-lit room with a full-length mirror. A hand mirror or a family member or close friend is needed to check areas that cannot be seen with the wall mirror.

Aftercare

When a self-exam reveals skin spots that are changing, itching, or bleeding, they should be shown to a doctor. Actinic keratoses should also be seen by a doctor, who can help decide whether they require treatment. The doctor will take a medical history; a family history of any skin cancer; and a history of the patient's sun exposure, including sunburns and **tanning** practices. The doctor will ask when the spot appeared or changed and about any other symptoms. In addition to the suspicious spot, the physician will do a body skin check. The lymph nodes under the skin near the area may be felt for enlargement or firmness, as some skin cancers spread to nearby lymph nodes. A primary care doctor may refer the patient to a dermatologist.

QUESTIONS TO ASK YOUR DOCTOR

• How often should I perform skin checks?

• What should I look for when performing a skin check?

• Are there any areas on my skin that I should watch especially closely?

• What should I do if I find a suspicious area or spot?

• How often should I have a professional skin check?

Results

A skin cancer or precancer may be further tested or treated. A small localized spot may be removed with a **biopsy** or surgery. More widespread cancers, especially melanoma, may require more extensive treatment.

Resources

BOOKS

Schwartz, Robert A. *Skin Cancer: Recognition and Management.* 2nd ed. Malden, MA: Blackwell Publishing, 2008.

OTHER

American Cancer Society. "Skin Cancer Prevention and Early Detection." http://www.cancer.org/acs/groups/cid/documents/webcontent/003184-pdf.pdf (accessed October 13, 2014).

WEBSITES

American Academy of Dermatology. "How to Perform a Self-Exam." https://www.aad.org/spot-skin-cancer/understanding-skin-cancer/how-do-i-check-my-skin/how-to-perform-a-self-exam (accessed October 13, 2014).

American Academy of Dermatology. "What to Look For: The ABCDEs of Melanoma." https://www.aad.org/spot-skin-cancer/understanding-skin-cancer/how-do-i-check-my-skin/what-to-look-for (accessed October 13, 2014).

American Cancer Society. "Skin Self-Exam Gallery." http://www.cancer.org/cancer/skincancer/galleries/skin-self-exam-images (accessed October 13, 2014).

National Cancer Institute. "How to Check Your Skin for Skin Cancer." http://www.cancer.gov/cancertopics/prevention/skin/selfexam (accessed October 13, 2014).

Skin Cancer Foundation. "Early Detection and Self Exams." http://www.skincancer.org/skin-cancer-information/early-detection (accessed October 13, 2014).

Skin Foundation of South Africa. "Mole Mapping." http://skincancerfoundation.org.za/patient-information/mole-mapping/ (accessed November 6, 2014).

ORGANIZATIONS

American Academy of Dermatology, PO Box 4014, Schaumburg, IL 60168, (847) 240-1280, Fax: (847) 240-1859, (866) 503-SKIN (7546), http://www.aad.org.

American Cancer Society, 250 Williams Street NW, Atlanta, GA 30303, (800) 227-2345, http://www.cancer.org.

National Cancer Institute, 6116 Executive Boulevard, Suite 300, Bethesda, MD 20892-8322, (800) 4-CANCER (422-6237), http://www.cancer.gov.

Skin Cancer Foundation, 149 Madison Avenue, Suite 901, New York, NY 10016, (212) 725-5176, http://www.skincancer.org.

Margaret Alic, PhD

Small cell lung cancer *see* **Lung cancer, small cell**

Small intestine cancer

Definition

Cancer of the small intestine is a rare disease that occurs when abnormal, malignant cells divide out of control in the part of the body's digestive system called the small intestine. The small intestine connects the stomach and the large intestine.

Description

The small intestine is a long tube inside the abdomen divided into three sections: the duodenum, jejunum, and ileum. The function of the small intestine is to break

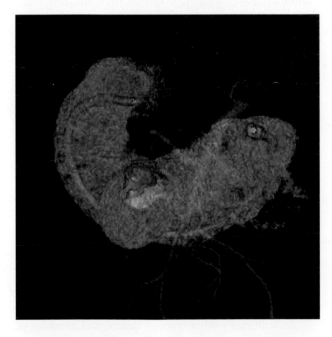

Computed tomography (CT) scan showing an intestinal tumor (in red). *(Barrau-CCN/Phanie/Alamy)*

down food and to remove proteins, carbohydrates, fats, **vitamins**, and minerals for the body to use. Obstruction of the small intestine by cancer may impair normal passage and digestion of food and nutrients. Cancers in this location consist primarily of **adenocarcinoma**, **lymphoma**, **sarcoma**, and carcinoid tumors.

Adenocarcinoma

These malignancies most often start in the lining of the small intestine, usually occurring in the duodenum and jejunum, the sections closest to the stomach. These tumors may obstruct the bowel, causing digestive problems. Adenocarcinoma is the most common cancer of the small intestine, but accounts for only 2% of all tumors in the gastrointestinal tract and 1% of all deaths related to cancer of the gastrointestinal tract. Carcinomas of the small intestine may appear at multiple sites.

Lymphoma

This fairly uncommon cancer is typically a non-Hodgkin type that starts in the lymph tissue of the small intestine. (The body's immune system is made up of lymph tissue, which assists in fighting infections.) Malignant lymphoma is not often found as a solitary tumor.

Sarcoma

Sarcoma malignancies of the small intestine are usually **leiomyosarcoma**. They most often occur in the smooth muscle lining of the ileum, the last section of the small intestine. Liposarcoma and angiosarcoma occur more rarely in the small intestine.

Carcinoid tumors

Carcinoid tumors are most often found in the ileum. In approximately 50% of cases, they appear as multiple tumors.

Demographics

Slightly more than 9,000 people in the United States are diagnosed with small intestine cancer each year. Approximately 30% of small intestine cancers are adenocarcinomas. Still, these cancers make up only 1% to 2% of all **gastrointestinal cancers**.

Causes and symptoms

Doctors know little about the causes of small intestine cancers, but as researchers learn more about the biology of cancer cells, more is revealed. There are some DNA changes in small intestine adenocarcinoma cells that probably cause the cancer cells to grow out of control. Mutations in genes can trigger certain proteins that signal cancer cells to grow or cause other signals that stop uncontrolled growth to malfunction and fail to work as they should. Scientists still need to learn what causes these mutations, some of which might occur as cells age along with an individual.

Factors that may contribute to the development of small intestine cancer include exposure to **carcinogens** such as chemicals, radiation, cigarette smoke, and alcohol. Eating a high-fat diet likely increases risk, but eating a diet high in fiber could lower risk. Some association has been shown between eating smoked and cured foods and the development of small intestine cancer. Some GI diseases may contribute to the incidence of small intestine cancer, including celiac disease and Crohn's disease. **Colon cancer** survivors have an increased risk of developing cancer in the small intestine. Familial adenomatous polyposis, a genetic disorder characterized by intestinal polyps, is also associated with an increased risk of small intestine cancer.

Often cancer of the small intestine does not initially produce any symptoms. Gastrointestinal bleeding, which shows up in the stool, is perhaps the most common symptom. A doctor should be consulted if any of these symptoms are present:

- unexplained weight loss
- a lump in the abdominal region
- blood in the stool
- pain or cramping in the abdominal region

Diagnosis

Evaluation begins by taking a patient's medical history and conducting a physical examination. Stool may be examined for the presence of blood that is not visible to the eye (occult blood). If a patient experiences symptoms, a doctor may suggest the following tests:

- Upper gastrointestinal x-ray/upper GI series: To allow the stomach to be seen more easily on an x-ray, the patient drinks a liquid called barium. This test can be conducted in either a doctor's office or a radiology department in a hospital.
- CT scan (computed tomography): A computerized x-ray that takes a picture of the abdomen.
- MRI scan (magnetic resonance imaging): An imaging technique that uses special magnets and radiofrequency waves with a computer to take a picture of the abdomen.
- Ultrasound: An imaging technique that uses sound waves to locate tumors.
- Endoscopy: An endoscope is a thin, lighted tube that is placed down the throat to reach the first section of the small intestine (duodenum). During this procedure, the doctor may take a biopsy, in which a small piece of

---

KEY TERMS

Adenocarcinoma—A cancer that starts in glandular tissue.

Angiosarcoma—A malignant tumor that develops either from blood vessels or from lymphatic vessels.

Carcinogen—Any substance that causes cancer.

Carcinoid—A tumor that develops from neuroendocrine cells.

Leiomyosarcoma—A cancerous tumor of smooth (involuntary) muscle tissue.

Liposarcoma—A cancerous tumor of fat tissue.

Lymphoma—A cancer of the lymphatic tissue.

Malignant—Cancerous; a tumor or growth that often destroys surrounding tissue and spreads to other parts of the body.

Metastasis—The spread of cancer from the original site to other body parts.

Polyp—An abnormal growth of tissue projecting from a mucous membrane.

Radiation therapy—Also called radiotherapy, it uses high-energy rays to kill cancer cells.

Sarcoma—A malignant tumor of soft tissue, including fat, muscle, nerve, joint, blood vessel, and deep skin tissues.

Staging—Performing exams and tests to learn the extent of the cancer within the body, especially whether the disease has spread from the original site to other parts of the body.

---

tissue is removed for the examination of potentially cancerous cells under a microscope.

If small intestine cancer is evident, more tests will be conducted to determine if cancer has spread to other parts of the body.

Treatment team

Cancer treatment often requires a team of specialists and may include a surgeon, medical oncologist, radiation oncologist, nurse, physical therapist, occupational therapist, dietitian, and a social worker.

Clinical staging

As with many other types of cancer, malignancies of the small intestine can be classified as localized, regional spread, or distant spread.

- Localized: The cancer has not spread beyond the wall of the organ in which it developed.
- Regional spread: The cancer has spread from the organ it started in to other tissues, such as muscle, fat, ligaments, or lymph nodes.
- Distant spread: The cancer has spread to tissues or organs beyond its original location, such as the liver, bones, or lungs.

Treatment

Treatment options for small intestine cancer most often include surgery, and possibly **radiation therapy**, **chemotherapy**, and/or biologic therapy. Cancer of the small intestine is treatable and sometimes curable depending on its histology. Removing the cancer through surgery is the most common treatment. If the tumor is large, a small portion may be removed if resection of the small intestine is possible. For larger tumors, surgery requires removing a greater amount of the surrounding normal intestinal tissue, in addition to some surrounding blood vessels and lymph nodes. Sometimes a patient requires bypass surgery, which allows food to go around a tumor that is blocking the small intestine and cannot be removed.

Radiation therapy kills cancer cells and reduces the size of tumors through the use of high-energy **x-rays**. Radiation therapy may come from an external source using a machine or an internal source. Internal-based therapy involves the use of radioisotopes to administer radiation through thin plastic tubes to the area of the body where cancer cells are found. Side effects of radiation therapy include:

- fatigue
- loss of appetite
- nausea and vomiting
- diarrhea
- gas
- bloating
- mild temporary sunburn-like skin changes
- difficulty tolerating milk products

Chemotherapy kills cancer cells with drugs taken orally or by injection in a vein or muscle. It is referred to as a systemic treatment due to the fact that it travels through the bloodstream and kills cancer cells outside the small intestine. **Adjuvant chemotherapy** may be given following surgery to ensure all cancer cells are killed. Some side effects of chemotherapy are:

- nausea and vomiting
- loss of appetite (anorexia)
- temporary hair loss (alopecia)

- mouth sores
- fatigue as a result of a low red blood cell count
- higher likelihood of infection or bleeding due to low white blood cell counts and low blood platelets, respectively

Radiation and chemotherapy are seldom beneficial in small intestinal cancers. As of 2014, research was studying the use of **bevacizumab** in treating small intestine cancer. The drug has been approved for treatment of colon cancer. New targeted therapies show more promise. Targeted therapies are treatments that identify and attack only cancer cells, sparing normal cells near a tumor or throughout the body. Many of these are in development for a number of cancers, or are being tested in **clinical trials**. An example is imatinib, which has been used with success in gastrointestinal stromal tumors. These tumors are found in the stomach and small intestine. In 2013, the U.S. Food and Drug Administration approved the use of **sunitinib** as a targeted therapy for patients in whom imatinib failed to work.

Utilizing the body's immune system, biological therapy stimulates the body to combat cancer. Natural materials from the body or other laboratory-produced agents are designed to boost, guide, or restore the body's ability to fight disease. Another name for biologic therapy is **immunotherapy**.

Treatment options for small intestine cancers are based on the type of cells found—adenocarcinoma, lymphoma, sarcoma, or carcinoid tumor—rather than the clinical staging system.

Treatment of adenocarcinoma of the small intestine may consist of:

- Surgical removal of the tumor.
- Surgery to bypass the cancer to allow food to travel through the intestine.
- Symptom relief with radiation therapy.
- Chemotherapy or biological therapy in a clinical trial setting.
- A clinical trial involving radiation and drug therapy (with or without chemotherapy) to elicit greater sensitivity to radiation using radiosensitizers.

Treatment of lymphoma of the small intestine may consist of:

- Surgical removal of the cancer and lymph nodes in close proximity to it.
- Surgery accompanied by radiation therapy or adjuvant chemotherapy. If the disease is localized to the bowel wall, then surgical resection alone or combined chemotherapy should be considered. If the disease has extended to the regional lymph nodes, then surgical

resection and combination chemotherapy is suggested at the time of diagnosis.

- For extensive lymphoma or lymphoma that cannot be removed surgically, chemotherapy with or without additional radiation therapy is frequently used to reduce the risk of recurrence.

Treatment of leiomyosarcoma of the small intestine may consist of:

- Surgical removal of the cancer.
- When cancer cannot be removed by resection, surgical bypass of the tumor is recommended to allow food to pass.
- Radiation therapy.
- For unresectable metastatic disease, surgery, radiation therapy, or chemotherapy is suggested in order to alleviate symptoms.
- For unresectable primary or metastatic disease, a clinical trial evaluating the benefits of new anticancer drugs (chemotherapy) and biological therapy is recommended.

For recurrent small intestine cancer, treatment may consist of the following measures, if the cancer has returned to one area of the body only:

- Surgical removal of the cancer.
- Symptom relief using chemotherapy or radiation therapy.
- A clinical trial using radiation and drug therapy (with or without chemotherapy) to elicit greater sensitivity to radiation using radiosensitizers.

For recurrent metastatic adenocarcinoma or leiomyosarcoma, there is no standard effective chemotherapy treatment. Patients should be regarded as candidates for clinical studies assessing new **anticancer drugs** or biological agents.

For carcinoid tumors less than 1 cm in size, surgical removal of the tumor and surrounding tissue is possible. Carcinoid tumors often grow and spread slowly; therefore, approximately half are found at an early or localized stage. By the time of surgery, 80% of the tumors over 2 cm in diameter have metastasized locally or to the liver.

Alternative and complementary therapies

Some popular herbs that are purported to have therapeutic effects in cancer treatment include echinacea, garlic, ginseng, and ginger. Laboratory studies have shown that echinacea has the potential to control the growth of cancerous cells, but more studies are needed to confirm its use in humans. In addition, dosage and toxicity levels still need to be established. Some studies suggest that diets high in garlic reduce the risk of stomach, esophageal, and colon cancers. There is still debate regarding the best form of garlic to take—whole raw garlic or garlic in tablet form; aged or fresh garlic; garlic with odor or "deodorized" garlic. Ginger is often recommended for its beneficial effects on the digestive system, but evidence has not confirmed any efficacy in cancer treatment. Ginseng in excessive amounts can be very toxic, causing vomiting, bleeding, and death. Patients should not take herbal remedies without consulting their physicians, particularly if they intend to combine the herbs with prescription drugs. Herb and drug combinations can sometimes result in toxic interactions.

Prognosis

The prognosis or likelihood of recovery depends on the type of cancer, the overall health of the patient, and whether the cancer has spread to other regions or is localized in the small intestine. A cure depends on the ability to remove the cancer completely with surgery. Adenocarcinoma is most common in the duodenum; however, patient survival is less likely for individuals with cancer in this area compared with those patients with tumors in the jejunum or ileum due to reduced rates of surgery to remove cancer. Surgery is the preferred treatment for smooth muscle tumors. Little benefit was found for irradiation or chemotherapy, or for these therapies combined. Patients over 75 years of age have a significantly poorer survival rate than younger people. In addition, patients with poorly differentiated tumors have a poorer prognosis than those with moderately or well-differentiated tumors. The five-year survival rate decreases with progression of disease by stage: localized, 47.6%; regional, 31%; distant, 5.2%.

Coping with cancer treatment

Pain is a common problem for people with some types of cancer, especially when the cancer grows and presses against other organs and nerves. Pain may also be a side effect of treatment. However, pain can generally be relieved or reduced with prescription medicines or over-the-counter drugs as recommended by the doctor. Other ways to reduce pain, such as relaxation exercises, may also be useful. It is important for patients to report pain to their doctors, so that steps can be taken to help relieve it.

Depression may affect approximately 15–25% of cancer patients, particularly if the prognosis for recovery is poor. A number of antidepressant medications are available from physicians to alleviate feelings of depression. Counseling with a psychologist or psychiatrist also may help patients deal with depression.

Clinical trials

There are fewer clinical trials conducted regularly for small intestine cancer than for some other types because so few people have this type of cancer. However, clinical trials continue to investigate new treatments for

QUESTIONS TO ASK YOUR DOCTOR

- What is my diagnosis?
- Is there any evidence the cancer has spread?
- What is the stage of the disease?
- What are my treatment choices?
- What new treatments are being studied?
- Would a clinical trial be appropriate for me?
- What are the expected benefits of each kind of treatment?
- What are the risks and possible side effects of each treatment?
- How often will I have treatments?
- How long will treatment last?
- Will I have to change my normal activities?
- What is the treatment likely to cost?
- Is infertility a side effect of cancer treatment? Can anything be done about it?
- What is my prognosis?

the cancer. In 2014, active trials included the testing of new chemotherapy or targeted therapy drugs, and one trial was investigating the use of **hyperthermia** (heat therapy) with chemotherapy to treat metastatic tumors that could not be treated with surgery, including those of the small intestine area.

Clinical trials may be suitable for patients who have small intestine cancer. The principal investigator should be contacted regarding participation in appropriate trials. Participation in trials is voluntary. For information about cancer trials, patients can visit the **National Cancer Institute** website at http://www.cancer.gov/clinicaltrials/search.

Prevention

Most people who develop cancer do not have inherited genetic abnormalities. Their genes have been damaged after birth by substances in their environment. By stopping smoking and improving dietary habits, people can help prevent their risk of small intestine cancer. For prevention of cancer, it is important to avoid carcinogens (smoking, chemicals) and known risk factors, and to pursue a healthy lifestyle that includes moderate alcohol intake, regular exercise, a low-fat diet, and a diet rich in fruits and vegetables. Modifying genetic predispositions through risk factor reduction can also assist in prevention.

Special concerns

Due to the side effects of radiation and chemotherapy, individuals must make a deliberate effort to eat as nutritiously as possible. Those who experience pain, nausea, or **diarrhea** may want to discuss treatment options with their doctor to ease these side effects.

Eating well during cancer treatment means getting enough calories and protein to help prevent **weight loss** and maintain strength. Eating nutritiously may also help an individual feel better.

Resources

BOOKS

Abeloff, M. D., et al. *Clinical Oncology*, 5th ed. New York: Churchill Livingstone, 2013.

Niederhuber, J. E., et al. *Clinical Oncology*, 5th ed. Philadelphia: Elsevier, 2014.

OTHER

American Cancer Society. "Small Intestine Cancer." http://www.cancer.org/acs/groups/cid/documents/webcontent/003140-pdf.pdf (accessed October 25, 2014).

WEBSITES

MD Anderson Cancer Center. "Carcinoid Tumor Treatment." http://www.mdanderson.org/patient-and-cancer-information/cancer-information/cancer-types/carcinoid-tumors/treatment/index.html (accessed October 25, 2014).

National Cancer Institute. "General Information About Small Intestine Cancer." http://www.cancer.gov/cancertopics/pdq/treatment/smallintestine/HealthProfessional (accessed October 25, 2014).

ORGANIZATIONS

American Cancer Society, 250 Williams Street NW, Atlanta, GA 30303, (800) 227-2345, http://www.cancer.org.

National Cancer Institute, 9609 Medical Center Drive, Bethesda, MD 20892, (800) 422-6237, http://www.cancer.gov.

Crystal Heather Kaczkowski, MSc
REVISED BY TERESA G. ODLE

Smoking cessation

Definition

Smoking cessation is the process of quitting tobacco smoking. Giving up smoking is considered a vital part of **cancer prevention**, since smoking is known as the single most preventable cause of death from **cancer**. Tobacco smoking is at epidemic levels worldwide. It is accountable for 100 million deaths globally in the twentieth century and is estimated to cause one billion deaths in the twenty-first century. Over 20% of all deaths in the United States are related to tobacco use. Although smoking is most often thought of in connection with lung cancer, it is also associated with cancers of the mouth, throat, voice box (larynx), esophagus, pancreas, kidney, and bladder. Women who smoke increase their risk of cancer of the cervix. The number of years someone has smoked and the type of tobacco used may influence cancer development. Quitting smoking, however, greatly reduces the risk of developing cancer and other smoking-related diseases such as heart and lung diseases; 15 years after quitting, a former smoker's risk of cancer is almost as low as that of someone who has never smoked.

Description

Methods for smoking cessation include several different approaches, ranging from medications and individual or group counseling to special classes and programs. The smoking habit is difficult to break because it involves many different aspects of an individual's emotions and social life as well as physical addiction to nicotine. Most people who quit smoking successfully use a combination of treatments or techniques to help them quit.

Demographics

About 70% of smokers in the United States say they want to quit and many have already tried. People who are trying to quit smoking are often concerned about:

- Withdrawal symptoms: Nicotine, the substance in tobacco that gives smokers a pleasurable feeling, is as addictive as heroin or cocaine. Withdrawal from nicotine may produce depression, anger, fatigue, headaches, problems with sleep or concentration, or increased appetite for food. These symptoms usually start several

hours after the last cigarette. They may last for several days or several weeks.

- Weight gain: Many people, particularly women, gain between 2 and 10 pounds after giving up smoking. This mild weight gain, however, is not nearly as great a danger to health as continuing to smoke. Getting more exercise can help.

- Stress: Many smokers say they smoke as a way to cope with stress and tension. Finding other methods—exercise, meditation, biofeedback, massage, and others—can help reduce the temptation to smoke when stress arises.

- Side effects of nicotine replacement products: Smokers who use these products to help them quit may experience headaches, nausea, sore throat, or long-term dependence. Side effects can often be reduced or eliminated by using a lower dosage of the product or switching to another form of nicotine replacement.

Treatment

Nicotine replacement therapy

Nicotine replacement therapy gives the smoker a measured supply of nicotine without the more than 4,000 other harmful chemicals in tobacco. Drugs that replace nicotine help reduce the physical craving for **cigarettes** so that the smoker can handle the emotional and psychological aspects of quitting more effectively. Using nicotine replacement therapy combined with counseling is more effective than using either one alone.

Four forms of nicotine replacement therapy have been FDA approved:

- Transdermal patches: Patches, which are nonprescription items, supply measured doses of nicotine through the skin. The doses are lowered over a period of weeks, thus helping the smoker reduce the need for nicotine gradually.

- Nicotine gum: Nicotine gum provides a fast-acting nicotine replacement that is absorbed through the mouth tissues. The smoker chews the gum slowly and then keeps it against the inside of the cheek for 20 to 30 minutes. The gum is also available without prescription.

- Nasal spray: Nicotine nasal spray provides nicotine through the tissues that line the nose. It acts much more rapidly than the patches or gum, but requires a doctor's prescription.

- Inhalers: Nicotine inhalers are plastic tubes containing nicotine plugs. The plug gives off nicotine vapor when the smoker puffs on the tube. Some smokers prefer inhalers because they look more like cigarettes than other types of nicotine replacement. They also require a doctor's prescription.

QUESTIONS TO ASK YOUR DOCTOR

- What methods would you recommend to help me quit smoking?
- How can I cope with withdrawal symptoms and other side effects of quitting?
- Are there any smoking cessation programs in my local area that you would recommend?

Non-nicotine products are also available by prescription to help reduce the symptoms of withdrawal while smokers are in the process of quitting. Bupropion (Zyban) is an antidepressant medication given to lower the symptoms of withdrawal from nicotine. Bupropion by itself can help people quit smoking, but its success rate is even higher when it is used together with nicotine replacement therapy. Other drugs that are given for nicotine withdrawal include buspirone (BuSpar), an antianxiety medication, and varenicline tartrate, an antidepressant (Chantix).

Stop-smoking programs and groups

Stop-smoking programs help by reinforcing a smoker's decision to give up tobacco. These programs teach smokers to recognize common problems that occur during quitting and offer emotional support and encouragement. The most successful methods of smoking cessation combine both stop-smoking programs and medications or nicotine replacement therapy; each method is less successful when used on its own. The most effective programs include either individual or group psychological counseling. Many state Medicaid plans now cover the costs of smoking cessation programs.

The Great American Smokeout has been held annually since 1977 on the third Thursday in November to call attention to the high human costs of smoking. Smokers are asked to quit for the day and donate the money saved on cigarettes to high school scholarship funds.

Nicotine Anonymous is an organization that applies the Twelve Step program of Alcoholics Anonymous (AA) to tobacco addiction. Local group meetings are free of charge.

Alternative and complementary therapies

Hypnosis is reported to help some smokers to quit. Acupuncture has also been used, but there are no large-scale studies comparing it to other stop-smoking treatments. A list of physicians who are also licensed acupuncturists is available from the American Academy of Medical Acupuncture at (800) 521-2262.

Other complementary approaches that have been shown to be useful in quitting smoking include movement therapies such as yoga, t'ai chi, and dance. Prayer and meditation have also helped many smokers learn to handle stress without using tobacco.

Some sources recommend the use of electronic cigarettes as a smoking cessation aid, but studies have found conflicting results. E-cigarettes still contain nicotine, and the long-term effects of e-cigarettes on health are not yet known.

See also Esophageal cancer; Laryngeal cancer; Lung cancer, non-small cell; Lung cancer, small cell; Oral cancers.

Resources

BOOKS

"Smoking Cessation." In *The Merck Manual of Diagnosis and Therapy*, edited by Robert S. Porter and Justin L. Kaplan. 19th ed. Whitehouse Station, NJ: Merck Research Laboratories, 2011.

PERIODICALS

Buczkowski, K., et al. "Motivations toward Smoking Cessation, Reasons for Relapse, and Modes of Quitting: Results from a Qualitative Study among Former and Current Smokers." *Patient Preference and Adherence* 8 (October 1, 2014): 1353–63. http://dx.doi.org/10.2147/PPA.S67767 (accessed October 24, 2014).

Bullen, Christopher, et al. "Electronic Cigarettes for Smoking Cessation: A Randomised Controlled Trial." *Lancet* 382, no. 9905 (2013): 1629–37. http://dx.doi.org/10.1016/S0140-6736(13)61842-5 (accessed August 14, 2014).

OTHER

Office of the Surgeon General. *The Health Consequences of Smoking—50 Years of Progress: A Report of the Surgeon General.* U.S. Department of Health and Human Services, 2014. http://www.surgeongeneral.gov/library/reports/50-years-of-progress/full-report.pdf (accessed October 24, 2014).

WEBSITES

American Cancer Society. "Guide to Quitting Smoking." http://www.cancer.org/healthy/stayawayfromtobacco/guidetoquittingsmoking/index (accessed October 24, 2014).

American Association for Respiratory Care. YourLungHealth.org. http://www.yourlunghealth.org (accessed November 17, 2014).

ORGANIZATIONS

American Association for Respiratory Care, 9425 N. MacArthur Blvd., Suite 100, Irving, TX 75063-4706,

(972) 243-2272, Fax: (972) 484-2720, info@aarc.org, http://www.aarc.org.

American Lung Association, 55 W. Wacker Dr., Ste. 1150, Chicago, IL 60601, (800) LUNG-USA (586-4872), Fax: (202) 452-1805, http://www.lung.org.

National Heart, Lung, and Blood Institute, 31 Center Dr. MSC 2486, Bldg. 31, Rm. 5A52, Bethesda, MD 20892, (301) 592-8573, nhlbiinfo@nhlbi.nih.gov, http://www.nhlbi.nih.gov.

Nicotine Anonymous, 6333 E. Mockingbird #147-817, Dallas, TX 75214.info@nicotine-anonymous.org, http://www.nicotine-anonymous.org.

L. Lee Culvert

Rebecca J. Frey, PhD

Smooth muscle cancer *see* **Leiomyosarcoma**

Sodium iodide I 131 *see* **Radiopharmaceuticals**

Sodium phosphate P 32 *see* **Radiopharmaceuticals**

Soft tissue sarcoma

Definition

Soft tissue sarcomas are rare cancerous (malignant) tumors that develop in mesodermal tissues. Mesodermal tissues are tissues that surround, support, and connect the structures and organs of the body, which include muscle, fat, fibrous tissue, and blood vessels. There are more than 50 types of soft tissue sarcomas, of which **rhabdomyosarcoma** and soft-tissue Ewing tumors are the most common.

Description

Soft tissues include muscles and tendons, fat, fibrous (connective) tissues, synovial tissues surrounding the joints, peripheral nerve tissues, blood and lymph vessels, and deep-skin tissues. About one-half of all soft tissue sarcomas develop in the arms, legs, hands, or feet. About 40% occur in the trunk, internal organs, or the retroperitoneum—the back of the abdominal cavity; the remaining 10% occur in the head and neck. Soft tissue sarcomas may invade surrounding tissue or spread (metastasize) to distant sites in the body. Together, soft tissue sarcomas account for less than 1% of all newly diagnosed cancers.

The appearance of the cells of each type of soft tissue **sarcoma** differ according to the tissue in which

they originate. However, analysis is not always simple, because the cells of different types often appear similar to each other. Therefore, many sarcomas are of uncertain type. For example, new methods of analysis have demonstrated that most cancers previously classified as **malignant fibrous histiocytoma** (MFH) are actually high-grade liposarcomas, rhabdomyosarcomas, leiomyosarcomas, other sarcomas, carcinomas, lymphomas, or unclassified sarcomas now referred to as pleomorphic undifferentiated sarcomas.

Muscle tissue sarcomas

Rhabdomyosarcoma (RMS)—a skeletal muscle tumor—is the most common soft tissue sarcoma in children. Embryonal rhabdomyosarcoma (ERMS) is more common than alveolar rhabdomyosarcoma (ARMS). ERMS commonly develops in the head, neck, or reproductive or urinary tract organs. ARMS develops in the large muscles of the arms, legs, or trunk. All other soft tissue sarcomas in children are classified as non-rhabdomyosarcoma or non-RMS.

Leiomyosarcomas are smooth muscle tumors that occur most often in the retroperitoneum or internal organs but can also occur in the deep soft tissues of the arms or legs. **Leiomyosarcoma** is linked to **Epstein-Barr virus** in children with HIV/AIDS and inherited **retinoblastoma** (eye **cancer**).

Fat tissue sarcomas

Liposarcomas account for 25% of all soft tissue sarcomas. They can develop in fat tissue anywhere in the body but occur most often in the thigh or retroperitoneum. Most liposarcomas in children and teens are low-grade myxoid liposarcomas that grow and spread slowly and respond well to treatment. Pleomorphic liposarcoma is usually high grade, grows and spreads rapidly, and is more difficult to treat.

Fibrous tissue sarcomas

Fibrous tissue sarcomas occur in connective tissue:

- Fibrosarcoma is a cancer of the tendons and ligaments. Infantile or congenital fibrosarcoma is usually due to a chromosomal translocation and may be seen with prenatal ultrasound.
- Desmoid tumors may be low-grade fibrosarcomas or a unique type of fibrous tissue tumor.
- Fibrohistiocytic tumors include plexiform fibrohistiocytic tumors affecting children and young adults and originating as a painless growth on or under the skin of the hand, wrist, or arm, and undifferentiated pleomorphic sarcoma—a second cancer following radiation therapy or treatment for retinoblastoma.

KEY TERMS

Alveolar rhabdomyosarcoma (ARMS)—A soft tissue sarcoma in the large muscles of the arms, legs, or trunk that primarily affects older children.

Brachytherapy—Radiation administered by direct contact with a cancer.

Dermatofibrosarcoma protuberans (DFSP)—A low-grade cancer of fibrous tissue under the skin, usually in the limbs or trunk.

Desmoid tumors—Fibrous tumors that can develop anywhere in the body and may or may not be cancerous.

Embryonal rhabdomyosarcoma (ERMS)—The most common type of RMS in children; it usually occurs in the head, neck, or genitourinary tract and resembles fetal skeletal-muscle tissue.

Epithelioid hemangioendothelioma (EHE)—Hemangioendothelioma in adults.

Ewing sarcoma—A cancerous bone tumor.

Extraosseous Ewing tumor (EOE)—Extraskeletal Ewing tumor; a soft tissue tumor outside bone tissue with some characteristics of embryonic nerve tissue.

Fine-needle aspiration (FNA)—A biopsy using a very thin needle to remove small pieces of a superficial suspected sarcoma.

Hemangioendothelioma—A low-grade sarcoma of the blood vessels of soft tissues or internal organs such as the lungs or liver.

Leiomyosarcoma—A cancer of smooth-muscle cells.

Liposarcoma—A cancer arising from immature fat cells of the bone marrow.

Lymph nodes—The filtering system for lymphatic vessels that carry immune-system white blood cells throughout the body.

Malignant fibrous histiocytoma (MFH)—A former designation for 40% of all soft tissue sarcomas.

Mesoderm—The middle layer of embryonic cells that gives rise to skin, connective tissue, blood and lymph vessels, the urogenital system, and most muscles.

Non-RMS—All soft tissue sarcomas in children that are not rhabdomyosarcoma.

Primitive neuroectodermal tumor (PNET)—A type of Ewing tumor in soft tissue with some characteristics of embryonic nerve tissue.

Retroperitoneum—The space between peritoneum and the back abdominal wall that contains the kidneys and pancreas.

Rhabdomyosarcoma (RMS)—A cancerous tumor of skeletal muscle; the most common soft tissue sarcoma in children.

TNM—A cancer staging system, in which T indicates the size and location of the primary tumor, N signifies lymph node involvement, and M is metastasis to distant parts of the body.

• Dermatofibrosarcoma protuberans (DFSP) is a rare, low-grade cancer of fibrous tissue under the skin, usually in the limbs or trunk.

Synovial sarcoma

Synovial sarcomas are tumors of the synovium—the tough tissue that surrounds joints. They occur most often in leg and arm joints, especially the knee. They are the most common non-RMS in children and teens.

Peripheral nerve sarcomas

Malignant peripheral nerve sheath tumors—also called malignant schwannomas, neurofibrosarcomas, or neurogenic sarcomas—are tumors in cells surrounding the peripheral nerves that run throughout the body. Ewing sarcomas are a group of related cancers that share characteristics with nerve tissue of developing embryos. Ewing tumors that occur in soft tissue are extraosseous or extraskeletal (outside the bones) Ewing (EOE) tumors and primitive neuroectodermal tumors (PNETs).

Blood and lymph vessel sarcomas

• Angiosarcomas include hemangiosarcomas in blood vessels and lymphangiosarcomas in lymph vessels. They are usually slow growing.

• Epithelioid hemangioendothelioma (EHE) in adults is a low-grade cancer in the blood vessels of soft tissue or internal organs such as the lungs or liver. In infants, these tumors are usually benign and may disappear without treatment.

• Hemangiopericytoma is a sarcoma of the perivascular tissues around blood vessels that help control blood flow. It most often develops in the legs, pelvis, or retroperitoneum.

• Kaposi sarcoma is a tumor formed by cells similar to those that line blood and lymph vessels.

Other soft tissue sarcomas

Some soft tissue sarcomas are of uncertain origin:

• Mesenchymoma is a combination of tissue types that resemble fibrosarcomas and others.

• Alveolar soft-part sarcoma most commonly develops in the legs.

• Epithelioid sarcoma usually develops deep under the skin of the hands, forearms, lower legs, or feet.

• Clear cell sarcoma of soft tissue originates in a tendon and may spread to nearby lymph nodes.

• Desmoplastic small round cell tumors usually occur in the abdomen, pelvis, or tissues around the testes.

• Extrarenal rhabdoid tumors are rare, fast-growing sarcomas that originate in soft tissues such as those of the liver or peritoneum. They usually occur in newborns or young children.

• Extraskeletal myxoid chondrosarcoma is a rare mix of bone and cartilage cells in children and teens that often spreads to the lymph nodes and lungs.

Demographics

The American Cancer Society estimates 12,020 new diagnoses of soft tissue sarcomas in the United States in 2014—6,550 in males and 5,470 in females—and 4,740 deaths. About 900 children are diagnosed with soft tissue sarcomas each year, most frequently during infancy or after age ten.

• More than 85% of RMS occur in infants, children, and teenagers. RMS accounts for almost 60% of soft tissue sarcomas in children up to age four, but only 23% in 16–19-year-olds. ERMS accounts for 75% of RMS in children aged 1–14. ARMS can affect children in all age groups but is more prevalent among older children.

• Adolescents are more likely to develop leiomyosarcoma in the trunk, whereas in adults it is more common in the uterus or digestive tract.

• Liposarcoma is most common in people aged 60–65.

• Synovial sarcomas usually occur in young adults.

• Soft tissue Ewing tumors are relatively common in children and very rare in adults.

• Teenagers and adults can develop malignant peripheral nerve sheath tumors in the arms, legs, or trunk.

• Hemangiopericytoma is more common in adults, although infantile hemangiopericytoma occurs in children up to age four.

• Mesenchymoma is a rare sarcoma in children.

• Aveolar soft-part sarcoma is rare, usually affecting young adults.

• Alveolar soft-part sarcoma of the muscular nerves of the arms or legs can affect children in all age groups but is more prevalent in older children.

• Epithelioid sarcoma usually affects adolescents and young adults.

• Desmoplastic small cell tumors are rare and primarily affect adolescent and young adult males.

Causes & symptoms

Causes

Most soft tissue sarcomas have no known cause, although in children they are often associated with changes or translocations in chromosomes. Other soft tissue sarcomas are caused by changes (mutations) in DNA sequences carried on chromosomes. Some of these mutations are inherited, but most are acquired, sometimes from exposure to radiation during previous cancer treatment or cancer-causing chemicals. Most soft tissue sarcomas develop in people with no known risk factors; however:

• Long-term swelling (lymphedema) in the arms or legs is a risk factor for soft tissue sarcoma.

• Leiomyosarcoma and some other soft tissue sarcomas have been linked to the Epstein-Barr virus in people with HIV/AIDS.

• A high percentage of patients with angiosarcoma of the liver have been exposed to vinyl chloride.

• Angiosarcomas sometimes develop in an area that has been exposed to radiation.

• Kaposi sarcoma appears to be related to infection with human herpesvirus-8.

• Lymphangiosarcomas can develop where lymph nodes have been surgically removed or damaged by radiation.

• Some hormones, especially estrogen, cause desmoid tumors to grow.

The only known risk factors in children are congenital (present at birth) abnormalities and genetic (inherited) conditions:

• Li-Fraumeni syndrome increases the risk of soft tissue sarcomas and other cancers, and there is a high risk of developing soft tissue sarcoma in an area that was irradiated to treat another cancer.

• Children with inherited retinoblastoma are at increased risk of soft tissue sarcoma.

- Tuberous sclerosis (Bourneville disease), Wermer syndrome (adult progeria), and nevoid basal cell carcinoma syndrome (Gorlin syndrome) are risk factors.
- Children with Beckwith-Wiedemann syndrome are at risk of RMS.
- Familial adenomatous polyposis (Gardner syndrome) is a risk factor for desmoid tumors in the abdomen.
- Neurofibromatosis type 1 (von Recklinghausen disease) is characterized by benign neurofibromas that develop into malignant peripheral nerve sheath tumors in about 5% of cases.

Symptoms

Symptoms are not usually evident in the early stages of soft tissue sarcomas. A new or growing lump anywhere in the body or a painless swelling or lump in an arm or leg that grows over weeks or months may be a symptom of soft tissue sarcoma. As a tumor grows, it can press against normal tissue, causing soreness, pain, or difficult breathing. Synovial sarcoma causes tenderness, pain, or swelling in a joint.

RMS often develops in easily detectable regions, such as a lump just under the skin or around the testes. RMS in:

- an eye muscle can cause the eye to bulge
- the nasal cavity may cause nosebleeds
- the bladder or genitourinary tract can cause difficult urination or blood in the urine
- the abdomen or pelvis may cause vomiting, abdominal pain, or constipation

About one-third of abdominal sarcomas cause increasing pain. Although symptoms may be nonspecific, abdominal tumors can grow large enough to be felt or cause blockage or bleeding in the stomach or bowels, leading to blood in vomit or stool or very black and tarry stools.

Diagnosis

Only about 50% of soft tissue sarcomas are diagnosed at early stages before the cancer has spread. Soft tissue sarcomas in children may be particularly difficult to diagnose.

Diagnosis may include:

- medical history of risk factors
- physical examination
- complete blood cell count
- blood chemistries to measure substances in the blood released by tissues and organs
- ultrasound for visualizing internal organs and masses

- computed tomography (CT) scans to help determine whether a sarcoma has spread to the liver or other organs
- magnetic resonance imaging (MRI) for detailed images of organs or masses
- chest x-rays to determine whether a sarcoma has spread to the lungs
- positron emission tomography (PET) to scan the entire body for metastasized cancer

Biopsies

The size of a soft tissue sarcoma may be less important than the appearance of the cancer cells. Cells that appear similar to normal cells of the same tissue are referred to as well-differentiated or moderately differentiated. Sarcoma cells that appear very different from normal tissue are referred to as poorly differentiated or undifferentiated. For example, ERMS cells resemble developing skeletal muscle cells in a 6–8-week-old fetus, and ARMS cells resemble normal muscle cells of a 10-week-old fetus. Therefore, microscopic examination of sarcoma cells obtained by a biopsy—the removal of sarcoma tissue—is very important for determining the clinical stage, probable growth rate, likelihood of **metastasis**, and prognosis.

A fine-needle aspiration (FNA) **biopsy** uses a very thin needle and syringe to remove small fragments of a superficial (near the surface), easily accessed sarcoma. The needle may be guided by feel for a mass near the surface or by CT scanning. Although FNA biopsy is less invasive than other types of biopsies, FNA may not provide enough tissue to identify a sarcoma, determine its type, and grade it. FNA is most useful for identifying benign tumors, other types of cancer, infection, or some other disease. FNA also is used to determine whether tumors in other organs are metastases of the sarcoma.

If FNA indicates a sarcoma, a second biopsy is used to confirm the diagnosis:

- A core needle biopsy removes a cylindrical piece of tissue about one-sixteenth in. (0.15 cm) in diameter and 0.5 in. (1.3 cm) long. Although a core biopsy avoids an incision and may not require general anesthesia, the small sample size may cause a cancer to be missed or misdiagnosed.
- If the sarcoma is small, near the surface, and away from vital tissues, an excisional biopsy may be used to remove the entire mass and surrounding normal tissue. This type of biopsy combines diagnosis with surgical treatment.
- An incisional biopsy removes a small portion of a large sarcoma.

• An open surgical biopsy under general anesthesia is used to diagnose RMS in children. In addition to the tumor sample, nearby lymph nodes may be removed for testing.

Testing

In addition to analysis of the cells under a microscope, biopsy samples may undergo special testing to type and grade a sarcoma. The grade depends on the appearance of the cells and how fast they are dividing. High-grade tumors usually grow and spread faster than low-grade tumors:

• An immunohistochemical test treats the sample with antibodies that recognize cell proteins typical of some types of sarcomas. When an antibody binds such a cell protein, a color change is detected.

• For cytogenetic techniques, biopsied cells are grown in the laboratory for about a week and examined microscopically for chromosomal abnormalities.

• Fluorescent *in situ* hybridization (FISH) may be used to detect chromosome or gene abnormalities without first growing the cells.

• Flow cytometry analyzes the number of live cells in a sample and their characteristics, such as size, shape, and the presence of tumor markers on the cell surface.

Treatment team

Soft tissue sarcomas are treated by a multidisciplinary team of specialists, including:

• pathologists
• hematologists
• oncologists
• surgeons
• radiation oncologists

Children and adolescents are treated at medical centers specializing in **childhood cancers**, with treatment teams that include:

• a primary care physician
• pediatric hematologists/oncologists
• pediatric surgeons
• radiation oncologists
• pediatric oncology nurses
• nurse practitioners
• rehabilitation and physical therapists
• psychologists
• child-life specialists
• nutritionists
• social workers
• educators

Clinical staging

Cancer staging, treatment choices, and prognosis are based on the examinations and tests used in diagnosis and biopsy results. Biopsy of the sentinel lymph node—the first lymph node to receive drainage from the tumor—is used to determine whether the cancer has spread to the lymphatic system. Sometimes a patient is treated initially with **radiation therapy** or **chemotherapy**, and the sarcoma is then restaged.

Grading

Soft tissue sarcomas are graded according to the microscopic appearance of the cells, where G is the histological grade:

• GX—cannot be assessed
• G1 or low grade—cells appear normal, well-differentiated, slow-growing; these rarely metastasize
• G2 or intermediate—cells are moderately differentiated and fast growing
• G3 or high grade—cells are poorly differentiated and faster growing
• G4—cells are abnormal, poorly differentiated or undifferentiated, and very fast growing

TNM

Soft tissue sarcomas often are staged according to the TNM system, in which T is the primary tumor size and location, N represents involvement of neighboring lymph nodes, and M is metastasis to distant organs. Although RMS and synovial and epithelioid sarcomas commonly spread to lymph nodes, lymph node involvement occurs in less than 3% of adult soft tissue sarcomas.

• TX—cannot be assessed
• T0—no evidence of a primary tumor
• T1—sarcoma is 2 in. (5 cm) or less
• T2—sarcoma is more than 2 in. (5 cm)
• T2a—tumor is superficial
• T2b—tumor is deep in a limb or the abdomen
• NX—cannot be assessed
• N0—lymph nodes free of sarcoma cells
• N1—regional lymph nodes with sarcoma cells
• MX—cannot be assessed
• M0—sarcoma has not spread
• M1—distant metastases

Clinical staging

Stage I sarcomas are low-grade cancers, stage II sarcomas are mid-grade or high-grade cancers, and stages III and IV are any grade or high-grade:

- stage IA—G1–2, T1a or b, N0, M0
- stage IB—G1–2, T2a, N0, M0
- stage IIA—G1–2, T2b, N0, M0
- stage IIB—G3–4, T1a–b, N0, M0
- stage IIC—G3–4, T2a, N0, M0
- stage III—G3–4, T2b, N0, M0
- stage IVA—any G, any T, N1, M0
- stage IVB—any G, any T, any N, M1.

Childhood cancers

There is no standard grading system for childhood soft tissue sarcomas. Staging is commonly based on:

- grade and size of the tumor
- amount of tumor left after surgical removal
- spread to the lymph nodes or elsewhere in the body

In one staging method:

- group I—cancer completely removed by surgery
- group II—microscopic cancer remaining at the edge of tissue removal and/or in nearby lymph nodes
- group III—tumor visible after surgery or biopsy but has not spread
- group IV—metastatic cancer

Treatment

Treatment options and prognosis depend on:

- type and location of the sarcoma
- size, grade, and stage of the tumor
- how fast the cancer cells are growing and dividing
- whether surgery removed all of the tumor
- the patient's age and health
- whether the cancer has recurred after previous treatment

Treatment of non-RMS childhood sarcomas is generally the same as in adults. However, soft tissue sarcomas in children may respond differently to treatment. In general, children who are diagnosed with a sarcoma have a better prognosis than do adults, but children are much more susceptible to radiation, and the long-term effects of treatment are of greater concern.

Surgery

Most stages I, II, and III soft tissue sarcomas are treated surgically, with the goal of complete removal (resectioning) the tumor, as well as at least 0.8–1.2 in. (2–3 cm) of surrounding tissue. Many soft tissue sarcomas in infants and young children are treated successfully by surgery alone. Only about 5% of arm or leg sarcomas require **amputation** of the limb. Most patients have limb-sparing surgery followed by radiation therapy. Amputation may be necessary when invading sarcoma cells surround essential nerves, arteries, or muscles, or when limb-sparing surgery would result in a dysfunctional limb or chronic pain. Amputation is not recommended if the sarcoma has metastasized to the lungs or other organs. Abdominal sarcomas are difficult to remove because they can be quite large and adjacent to vital organs.

Stage IVA sarcomas and nearby lymph nodes are surgically removed. Sometimes the removal of stage IVB sarcomas and all of their metastases is attempted. Surgery may be preceded by high-dose radiation and/or chemotherapy to shrink the tumor or treat high-grade sarcomas that are at risk of metastasizing. If the only metastasis is in the lungs, sometimes the lung tumor can be removed.

Radiation therapy

Radiation therapy uses high-energy rays such as x-rays to kill cancer cells. External-beam radiation—delivered from outside the body—is aimed directly into the sarcoma. This is the most common radiation treatment for soft tissue sarcomas. Internal radiation therapy (brachytherapy) delivers small pellets of radioactive material directly into the sarcoma through thin plastic tubes. It may be used alone or in combination with external-beam radiation. Tumors of the retroperitoneum, trunk, head, or neck may be treated with fast-neutron therapy.

Radiation may be used:

- before and/or after surgery for all sarcoma stages
- for inoperable stage I and II sarcomas
- as the primary treatment for patients with health conditions that preclude surgery
- to kill small clusters of cancer cells
- to relieve symptoms of stage IVB sarcoma
- as an adjuvant treatment 6–9 weeks after chemotherapy
- for recurrent sarcomas that were not treated previously with radiation
- to treat pain accompanying recurrences

Short-term side effects of radiation therapy may include:

- fatigue
- mild skin conditions
- infections
- nausea, vomiting, and diarrhea after irradiation of the abdomen
- mouth sores and loss of appetite after head or neck irradiation

• swelling, weakness, or pain following irradiation of large portions of a limb

Longer-term radiation effects can include:

• worsening of chemotherapy side effects

• breathing difficulties and lung damage from chest irradiation

• bone fractures, sometimes occurring years later

• headaches and mental problems one or two years after radiation therapy for metastatic sarcoma in the brain

Chemotherapy

Most types of soft tissue sarcoma do not respond especially well to chemotherapy, although synovial sarcomas respond more readily. Chemotherapy usually does not prevent metastasis, and the benefits of postoperative chemotherapy in children have been questioned. However, chemotherapy may be used:

• as primary therapy for some sarcomas

• to shrink a stage II tumor prior to surgery

• as postoperative treatment for stage II sarcomas

• before or after surgery for stage III sarcomas to reduce the risk of recurrence

• to treat metastasized sarcomas

• to reduce pain with stage IV sarcomas

• for recurrence at a distant site

When used alone, only **doxorubicin** and **ifosfamide** have response rates above 20%. Doxorubicin alone or in combination with **dacarbazine** is the most frequently used chemotherapy for advanced sarcomas. High-dose ifosfamide is used to relieve symptoms of inoperable sarcomas. Other drugs include:

• trabectedin

• methotrexate

• vincristine

• cisplatin

• paclitaxel

• mesna for protecting the bladder from severe irritation caused by ifosfamide

Postoperative chemotherapy for ERMS is usually **vincristine** and **dactinomycin** (actinomycin-D). For groups II and III RMS, **cyclophosphamide** is added for a three-drug combination called VAC. **Topotecan** also may be included.

Temporary side effects of chemotherapy may include:

• nausea and vomiting

• loss of appetite

• hair loss

• mouth sores

Most side effects disappear when chemotherapy ends, although some drugs damage blood-producing bone marrow cells, increasing the risk of **fatigue**, bruising or bleeding, and infection. Some drugs also cause infertility. Doxorubicin can weaken the heart, and ifosfamide and cyclophosphamide can cause permanent kidney or bladder damage.

Other drugs

• Sunitinib is a targeted drug—a drug that does not harm normal cells—that appears to slow the growth of many sarcomas.

• Pazopanib is a tyrosine kinase inhibitor for treating progressive or recurrent soft tissue sarcomas.

• Antiangiogenesis drugs that starve sarcomas by preventing new blood vessel formation are used to treat alveolar soft part sarcomas and blood vessel tumors.

• Hormone therapy may be used if the cancer cells have receptors for specific hormones. Antiestrogens—drugs that block estrogen—may be used for childhood soft tissue sarcoma.

• A nonsteroidal anti-inflammatory drug (NSAID) called sulindac may be used to block cancer cell growth.

Watchful waiting

Sometimes soft tissue sarcoma is monitored closely without treatment until signs or symptoms develop or change. Watchful waiting may be used when:

• complete tumor removal is not possible

• no treatments are available

• the tumor does not threaten vital organs

Recurrences

Treatment of recurrent soft tissue sarcomas depends on the initial type and treatment. If the initial treatment was minimal, a local recurrence may be treated with surgery and radiation. If the original treatment was aggressive, limb amputation may be necessary. The lungs are the most common distant site of sarcoma recurrences—usually within two to three years after the initial diagnosis—and are treated as stage IV disease. In older patients, symptoms of recurrence may be treated by the sequential use of single chemotherapy drugs. Synovial sarcomas tend to recur locally and involve regional lymph nodes; however, distant metastasis occurs in about 50% of cases, sometimes many years later.

Prognosis

Stage I and II soft tissue sarcomas rarely metastasize, although they may recur locally if inadequately treated:

- Stage I sarcomas have a five-year survival rate of 99% and only a 20% risk of recurrence within five years.
- Stage II sarcomas have an 82% five-year survival rate and a five-year-recurrence risk of 35%.
- Stage III sarcomas have a five-year survival rate of 50% and a five-year-recurrence risk of about 65%.
- Stage IV sarcomas are usually incurable, with a five-year survival rate of 10–15%.
- Surgery to remove metastatic lung sarcomas has a five-year survival rate of 20–30%, but occasionally there is a complete cure.
- Patients over age 60 have a poorer prognosis than younger adults.

In children:

- stage I—90% do not recur
- stage II—long-term survival of about 89% with about 50% of recurrences cured in the second round of treatment
- stage III—about 70% long-term survival
- stage IV—five-year survival rate of less than 30%, but with a 50% survival rate for children under age ten with metastatic embryonal tumors

Younger children with RMS have higher survival rates than older children and adolescents. ERMS has a more favorable prognosis than ARMS. More than 70% of children survive ERMS, and second malignancies arise in less than 25% of survivors, usually in children with more advanced disease.

Children with non-RMS generally have a better prognosis than adults, although if the sarcoma is not completely removed, metastasizes, or recurs, the prognosis is poor.

- Leiomyosarcoma has a good prognosis unless it is within the gastrointestinal tract.
- Liposarcomas have a good prognosis if completely removed.
- Desmoid tumors rarely metastasize and have an excellent prognosis.
- Infantile fibrosarcoma—which occurs in children under five—has an excellent prognosis when treated with surgery alone.
- Adult-type fibrosarcomas have a survival rate of about 60% in both children and adults.
- Synovial sarcoma has a survival rate of 80%.

QUESTIONS TO ASK YOUR DOCTOR

- What type of sarcoma do I have?
- What stage is the cancer? Has it spread?
- What are my treatment options?
- Which treatment do you recommend and why?
- What are the risks and side effects of each treatment?
- What are the risks of recurrence after each treatment?
- How should I prepare for treatment?
- How much work or school will I miss?
- What is the recovery time after treatment?
- What is my estimated length of survival?

- Neurofibrosarcoma has a very good prognosis with complete removal; otherwise the prognosis is poor.
- The prognoses for angiosarcomas and hemangioendotheliomas depend on their removal, the extent of the disease, and the grade of the malignancy.
- Hemangiopericytoma has an excellent prognosis in young children and an overall survival rate of 30–70%.
- Alveolar and clear cell soft-part sarcomas have a 50% survival rate, and late relapses are common.

High-grade retroperitoneal sarcoma has a less favorable prognosis because of the difficulty of completely removing the tumor and the limitations on high-dose radiation therapy. Local recurrence is the most common cause of death.

Clinical trials

As of 2014, the **National Cancer Institute** listed 41 active **clinical trials** for adult soft tissue sarcoma. One trial was studying regional **hyperthermia** therapy, in which high temperature is used to damage or kill cancer cells or make them more susceptible to chemotherapy. A trial of isolated limb perfusion administers chemotherapy directly to an affected arm or leg.

Prevention

People with a family history of sarcomas or other cancers occurring at a young age may have **genetic testing** to assess their risk of certain soft tissue sarcomas. Since early detection is very important, a healthcare professional should be consulted about any unexplained lumps, growths, or other symptoms.

Special concerns

Since advanced soft tissue sarcoma has a high risk of metastasis and recurrence, patients must be closely monitored following treatment. They will require frequent physical examinations and possibly chest x-rays, ultrasound, or CT or MRI scans.

See also AIDS-related cancers; Osteosarcoma.

Resources

BOOKS

Brennan, Murray F., Cristina R. Antonescu, and Robert G. Maki. *Management of Soft Tissue Sarcoma*. New York: Springer, 2013.

Newman, Michael E. *Soft Tissue Sarcomas: Current and Emerging Trends in Detection and Treatment*. New York: Rosen, 2012.

PERIODICALS

Gronchi, Alessandro, and Paolo G. Casali. "Adjuvant Therapy for High-Risk Soft Tissue Sarcoma in the Adult." *Current Treatment Options in Oncology* 14, no. 3 (September 2013): 415–24.

Johannesmeyer, David, et al. "The Impact of Lymph Node Disease in Extremity Soft-Tissue Sarcomas: A Population-Based Analysis." *American Journal of Surgery* 206, no. 3 (September 2013): 289.

Tejani, Mohamedtaki A., et al. "Head and Neck Sarcomas: A Comprehensive Cancer Center Experience." *Cancers* 5, no. 3 (2013): 890–900.

WEBSITES

American Cancer Society. "Sarcoma—Adult Soft Tissue." Learn About Cancer. http://cancer.org/cancer/sarcoma-adultsofttissuecancer/index (accessed June 23, 2014).

"Soft Tissue Sarcoma." MedlinePlus. June 17, 2014. http://www.nlm.nih.gov/medlineplus/softtissuesarcoma.html (accessed June 23, 2014).

"Soft Tissue Sarcoma." National Cancer Institute. http://www.cancer.gov/cancertopics/types/soft-tissue-sarcoma (accessed June 22, 2014).

"Soft Tissue Sarcoma in Children." CureSearch for Children's Cancer. http://www.curesearch.org/Articleview2.aspx?id=9614 (accessed June 23, 2014).

ORGANIZATIONS

American Cancer Society, 250 Williams Street NW, Atlanta, GA 30303, (800) 227-2345, http://www.cancer.org.

CureSearch for Children's Cancer, 4600 East-West Highway, Suite 600, Bethesda, MD 20814, Fax: (301) 718-0047, (800) 458-6223, info@curesearch.org, http://www.curesearch.org.

National Cancer Institute, 6116 Executive Boulevard, Suite 300, Bethesda, MD 20892-8322, (800) 4-CANCER (422-6237), http://www.cancer.gov.

Margaret Alic, PhD

REVIEWED BY MARIANNE VAHEY, MD

▌Sorafenib

Definition

Sorafenib (Nexavar) is an anticancer drug used to treat some types of **kidney cancer** and **liver cancer**.

Purpose

Sorafenib is used to treat a type of kidney **cancer** known as renal cell **carcinoma**. Sorafenib is used for advanced renal cell carcinoma, often when the cancer cannot be treated well with surgery and when the cancer is metastatic or has spread to other parts of the body. Sorafenib is also used for a type of liver cancer known as hepatocellular carcinoma. In 2013, the U.S. Food and Drug Administration (FDA) approved use of the drug in treatment of late-stage differentiated **thyroid cancer**. In late stages of thyroid cancer, the cancer cells have metastasized to other areas of the body.

Description

Sorafenib is manufactured in pill or tablet form and taken orally. Sorafenib is an anticancer drug that acts on receptor tyrosine kinases to inhibit the growth of tumors. Receptor tyrosine kinases are receptors for growth factors that are a natural part of cell development and necessary for normal cell growth. When tyrosine kinase receptors are activated, they trigger chemical signals that tell the cell how to grow and develop. Normal tyrosine kinase receptors turn on and off as needed for usual amounts of growth. However, when cells have constantly activated tyrosine kinase receptors, the abnormal growth of cancer can occur. Drugs in the sorafenib class inhibit these overly active tyrosine kinase receptors, thereby slowing or stopping the rapid growth of tumor cells.

Sorafenib acts on other drug targets that affect tumor growth called serine/threonine kinases. By acting on these additional kinases, sorafenib increases the range of tumor cell surface targets and the effectiveness of **chemotherapy**.

Once they reach a certain size, solid tumor cells need to form their own blood supply to grow and remain alive. This process is known as **angiogenesis**. Angiogenesis is a part of tumor progression and one of the processes critical to tumor growth and survival. Sorafenib is thought to act on signals to inhibit the angiogenesis process.

Studies have shown that the use of sorafenib increases progression-free survival compared to a placebo. The term *progression-free survival* describes the length of time during and after treatment in which a patient is living with a disease that does not get worse. In a clinical trial designed to test a cancer drug in humans,

KEY TERMS

Angiogenesis—Physiological process involving the growth of new blood vessels from pre-existing blood vessels, process used by some cancers to create their own blood supply.

Blood electrolytes—Ions present in the blood that are necessary for health such as sodium and potassium.

Blood platelets—Blood components responsible for normal blood clotting to seal wounds.

Cytochrome P450—Enzymes present in the liver that metabolize drugs.

Erectile dysfunction—Sexual disorder involving the inability to develop or maintain a penile erection.

Hemorrhage—Extensive bleeding that may be life threatening.

Hepatocellular carcinoma—Malignant cancer of the liver that may arise in the liver or metastasize to the liver from elsewhere in the body.

Metastasis—The process by which cancer spreads from its original site to other parts of the body.

Receptor tyrosine kinases—Cell surface receptors that interact with growth factors and hormones to affect the normal life cycle of a cell.

Renal cell carcinoma—Cancer of the kidney that originates in the very small tubes in the kidney that filter the blood and remove waste products.

Serine/threonine kinases—Cell surface receptors that interact with growth factors and hormones to affect the normal life cycle of a cell.

progression-free survival is a way to measure the effectiveness of a treatment.

Recommended dosage

Sorafenib is taken orally in pill form. The usual adult dose for either renal cell carcinoma or hepatocellular carcinoma is 400 mg (200 mg taken twice a day). The presence of fat in food decreases the amount of sorafenib available to fight cancer in the body. Sorafenib needs to be taken either one hour before or two hours after meals, and should be swallowed with water. Therapy with sorafenib is continued as long as there is clinical benefit, or until the development of intolerable side effects or toxicity. In patients who develop severe side effects, the dose may be adjusted to 400 mg taken once daily, or discontinued altogether if toxicity occurs.

Studies done in Japanese patients suggest that less of the drug may be present in the body after the usual dose when compared with Caucasian patients. The clinical significance of this finding and its implications for dosing are unknown. Patients should never take higher doses of sorafenib than those set by their physician. If a dose of sorafenib is missed and remembered near the time of the next dose, that dose is skipped. Patients should never double the dose to catch up on missed doses.

Precautions

Sorafenib is a pregnancy category D drug. Pregnancy category D drugs are drugs for which there is evidence of human fetal risk based on data from marketing experience or studies done in humans, but for which the potential medical benefit is great enough that it may warrant use of the drug in pregnant women despite the risks. Sorafenib use during pregnancy may result in death to the fetus. Sorafenib is used in pregnancy only if medically necessary for survival of the mother, and is not recommended for use during breastfeeding. Both male and female patients undergoing sorafenib treatment should avoid a pregnancy. At least two forms of reliable birth control methods need to be used during treatment and for two weeks after the last dose.

Sorafenib has not been approved for use in individuals less than 18 years of age. Patients should not have any vaccinations while taking sorafenib without the consent of their treating physician, and live vaccines should not be given. Patients taking sorafenib should also avoid being around people who have recently had the oral polio vaccine or the inhaled flu vaccine, as these are both live vaccines.

Sorafenib may not be appropriate for use in patients with pre-existing heart disease or disorders, a recent heart attack, excessive bleeding or bleeding disorders, inflammation of the pancreas, depressed immune system, decreased blood platelets, impaired kidneys or kidney disease, impaired liver or liver disease, or damage to the gastrointestinal tract. In addition, sorafenib may not be appropriate for use in patients who have recently had surgical procedures. Sorafenib increases the risk of causing high blood pressure or exacerbation of existing high blood pressure, especially within the first six weeks of treatment. Blood pressure is monitored regularly while in treatment with sorafenib.

Side effects

Sorafenib is used when the medical benefit is judged to be greater than the risk of side effects. Many patients

QUESTIONS TO ASK YOUR DOCTOR

- How long must I take this drug before you can tell whether it helps me?
- Must I have blood work and other laboratory tests done to check the effect the drug is having?
- Is this drug safe to take with the other drugs that I am currently taking?
- What side effects should I watch for? When should I call the doctor about them?
- Are there any clinical trials of this drug combined with other therapies that might benefit me?

undergoing sorafenib treatment do not develop medically serious side effects. The most commonly seen side effects associated with sorafenib treatment are abdominal pain and cramping, nausea, vomiting, **diarrhea**, constipation, bone and joint pain, muscle pain, weakness, **fatigue**, flu-like symptoms, **fever**, flushed skin, rash, peeling inflamed skin, hair loss, acne, headache, loss of appetite, **weight loss**, difficulty breathing, cough, hoarseness, **anemia**, high blood pressure, inflammation of the inner lining of the mouth, **depression**, erectile dysfunction, hemorrhage (severe bleeding) of the gastrointestinal and respiratory tracts, blood electrolyte imbalances, depressed immune system, nervous system damage in the arms and legs, and blood disorders such as decreased blood platelets.

Sorafenib also commonly causes severe hand-foot syndrome, caused by leakage of sorafenib out of small blood vessels in the hands and feet. During some types of chemotherapy, small amounts of medication in the bloodstream leak out of capillaries in the palms of the hands and the soles of the feet. Drug leakage is increased by heat exposure or friction. The result is redness, tenderness, and sometimes peeling of the skin of the palms and soles. The appearance of sunburn, numbness, and tingling may develop, and may interfere with the activity level of the patient.

Rarely, sorafenib treatment is associated with chronic heart failure, heart attacks, and other cardiac disorders, severe inflammation of the pancreas, inflammation of the gastrointestinal tract, heartburn, abnormal breast development in males, extreme high blood pressure, ringing in the ears, and short periods of decreased oxygen flow to the brain.

Interactions

Patients should make their doctor aware of any and all medications or supplements they are taking before using sorafenib. Sorafenib interacts with many other drugs. Some drug interactions may make sorafenib unsuitable for use, while others may be monitored and attempted. Use of sorafenib with the agent **docetaxel** may cause docetaxel toxicity, so caution is advised. Multiple agents may have toxic effects when used in the same time period as sorafenib. Sorafenib may have dangerous additive effects with other drugs that also cause bleeding disorders. Drugs that interact with sorafenib in this way include **warfarin** and **heparin**.

Sorafenib is metabolized by a set of liver enzymes known as cytochrome P450 (CYP-450) subtype 3A4. Drugs that induce, or activate, these enzymes increase the metabolism of sorafenib. This activation results in lower levels of therapeutic sorafenib, thereby negatively affecting treatment of cancer. For this reason drugs that induce CYP-450 subtype 3A4 may not be used with sorafenib. These include some antiepileptic drugs such as **carbamazepine**, some anti-inflammatory drugs such as **dexamethasone**, antituberculosis drugs such as rifampin, and the herb St. John's wort.

Drugs that act to inhibit the action of CYP-450 subtype 3A4 may cause undesired increased levels of sorafenib in the body. This interaction could lead to toxic doses. Some examples are **antibiotics** such as clarithromycin, antifungal drugs such as ketoconazole, antiviral drugs such as indinavir, antidepressants such as fluoxetine, and some cardiac agents such as verapamil. Grapefruit juice may also increase the amount of sorafenib in the body. Patients should avoid drinking grapefruit juice or eating grapefruit while taking sorafenib.

Resources

BOOKS

Brunton, Laurence, Bruce Chabner, and Bjorn Knollman. *Goodman and Gilman's The Pharmacological Basis of Therapeutics.* 12th ed. New York: McGraw-Hill Medical Publishing, 2012.

Tarascon Pharmacopoeia Library Edition. Jones and Bartlett Publishers, 2009.

WEBSITES

American Cancer Society. "Sorafenib." http://www.cancer.org/treatment/treatmentsandsideeffects/guidetocancerdrugs/sorafenib (accessed November 3, 2014).

"Sorafenib." MedlinePlus. http://www.nlm.nih.gov/medlineplus/druginfo/meds/a607051.html (accessed November 3, 2014).

U.S. Food and Drug Administration. "FDA Approves Nexavar to Treat Type f Thyroid Cancer."

http://www.fda.gov/NewsEvents/Newsroom/Press Announcements/ucm376443.htm (accessed November 3, 2014).

ORGANIZATIONS

National Cancer Institute, 9609 Medical Center Dr., BG 9609 MSC 9760, Bethesda, MD 20892-9760, (800) 4-CANCER (422-6237), http://www.cancer.gov.

U.S. Food and Drug Administration, 10903 New Hampshire Ave., Silver Spring, MD 20993, (888) INFO-FDA (463-6332), http://www.fda.gov.

Maria Basile, PhD
REVISED BY TERESA G. ODLE
REVIEWED BY KEVIN GLAZA, RPH

Sperm banking *see* **Fertility issues**

Spinal axis tumors

Definition

Spinal axis tumors are tumors that affect the spinal cord—the bundle of nerves that lies inside the backbone. Another term for spinal axis tumors is spinal cord tumors.

Description

Spinal axis tumors form on or near the spinal cord and produce pressure on the nerves and blood vessels of the spinal cord. There are three types of spinal axis tumors: extradural, extramedullary intradural, and intramedullary.

Extradural spinal axis tumors

Extradural tumors are found outside the dura mater, the outermost of the three membranes that encase the spinal cord. Extradural tumors are wedged between the dura mater and the bone of the spine. Types of extradural tumors include chordomas, osteoblastomas, osteomas, and hemangiomas.

Extramedullary intradural spinal axis tumors

Extramedullary intradural tumors are found inside the dura mater but outside the nerves of the spinal cord itself. Types of extramedullary tumors include meningiomas and neurofibromas.

Intramedullary spinal axis tumors

Intramedullary tumors are found inside the nerves of the spinal cord. Types of intramedullary tumors include astrocytomas, ependymomas, and hemangioblastomas.

KEY TERMS

Astrocytoma—A tumor that begins in the brain or spinal cord in cells called astrocytes.

Chordoma—A type of bone cancer.

Dura mater—The outermost tough membrane that encases the nerves of the spinal cord.

Ependymoma—A tumor that begins in the tissue that lines the central canal of the spinal cord and the ventricles of the brain. About 85% of these tumors are benign.

Hemangioblastoma—A tumor composed of capillaries and disorganized clumps of capillary cells or angioblasts.

Hemangioma—A benign tumor consisting of a mass of blood vessels.

Meningioma—A tumor that occurs in the meninges, the membranes that cover the brain and spinal cord. Meningiomas usually grow slowly and primarily affect adults.

Metastatic tumor—A tumor that results from the spreading of one type of cancer to other parts of the body.

Neurofibroma—A fibrous tumor of nerve tissue.

Osteoblastoma—A benign tumor that most frequently occurs in the vertebrae, leg bones, or arm bones of children and young adults.

Osteoma—A usually benign tumor of bone tissue.

Spinal cord—The bundle of nerves that runs inside the backbone.

Benign vs. malignant

Spinal axis tumors are classified as either benign (noncancerous) or malignant (cancerous). The cells of malignant tumors are very different from normal cells; they grow quickly and usually spread easily to other parts of the body. Benign tumors have cells that are similar to normal cells, grow slowly, and tend to be localized. However, even benign tumors can cause significant problems when they grow within the confined space inside the backbone.

Demographics

Primary spinal axis tumors, or tumors that originate in the spinal axis itself, are extremely rare and represent only 0.5% of all diagnosed tumors. Malignant primary spinal axis tumors constitute about 65% of all spinal axis tumors. However, most spinal axis tumors result from **metastasis**, or spreading, of other types of **cancer** to the spinal axis. Other cancers that can spread to the spinal axis include head and neck cancer, **thyroid cancer**, **skin cancer**, **prostate cancer**, lung cancer, **breast cancer**, and others. The American Cancer Society estimates that brain and spinal cord cancers (primary only) represent approximately 1.4% of all cancers and 2.4% of all cancer-related deaths among adults. In 2014, the Central Brain Tumor Registry reported that tumors of the cranial nerves and spinal cord accounted for 9.6% of all **brain and central nervous system tumors**.

Half of all spinal axis tumors occur in the thoracic, or chest, region as opposed to the neck (cervical) or lower back (lumbar) region.

Spinal axis tumors occur with equal frequency in members of all races and ethnic groups. There does not appear to be any relationship between spinal axis tumors and any geographic region. Males and females are affected in equal numbers by spinal axis tumors.

Causes and symptoms

The cause, or causes, of primary spinal axis tumors is not known. The cause of metastatic spinal axis tumors is cancer that begins in another part of the body and then spreads to the spine.

The symptoms of spinal axis tumors are the result of increased pressure on the nerves of the spine. These symptoms include:

- constant and severe burning or aching pain
- numbness of the skin or decreased temperature sensation
- muscle weakness, wasting, or even paralysis
- problems with bladder and bowel control
- muscle spasticity or problems in walking normally

The location of the tumor determines where the symptoms are most noticeable. A tumor in the cervical region can cause symptoms in the neck or arms, while a tumor in the thoracic region may cause chest pain. A tumor in the lumbar region can result in observable symptoms in the back, bladder and bowel, and legs.

Diagnosis

The diagnosis of spinal axis tumors begins with a medical history and physical examination when the patient brings his or her symptoms to the doctor's attention. The diagnosis may be difficult to make due to the similarity of tumor symptoms to those caused by disc herniation or other spinal cord injuries.

If the doctor suspects a spinal axis tumor, further diagnostic tests are ordered. These tests are performed by a neurological specialist. Imaging tests that may be ordered include:

- magnetic resonance imaging (MRI)
- computed tomography (CT)
- bone scan
- spinal tap and myelogram (a specialized x-ray technique)

Treatment team

Treatment of any primary central nervous system tumor, including spinal axis tumors, is different from treating tumors in other parts of the body. Spinal cord surgery carries serious risks and requires a high level of precision. Also, the thoracic area, where most spinal axis tumors are located, is highly sensitive to radiation. The most up-to-date treatment opportunities are available from experienced, multidisciplinary medical professional teams made up of doctors, nurses, and technologists who specialize in cancer (oncology), neurosurgery, medical imaging, drug or radiation oncology, and anesthesiology.

Standard treatment may include surgery from a team of specialists in spinal cord tumors; **chemotherapy**, often regional chemotherapy directed at the area where the tumor is located; and internal or external **radiation therapy**. New types of treatment are continuously tested in **clinical trials**, in which patients may choose to participate before, during, or after having standard treatment. Some patients with advanced spinal axial cancer may receive high-dose chemotherapy with a stem-cell transplant. In this treatment, immature blood or bone marrow cells are destroyed by high doses of chemotherapy and new ones after the patient's healthy cells are stored. The healthy cells are then returned to the patient or new cells from a matched donor are transfused into the patient.

The treatment of spinal axis tumors depends on the location of the tumor and the severity of the symptoms. Many spinal axis tumors can be treated by surgical removal of the tumor. Medical advances in surgical techniques, such as microsurgery and laser surgery, have greatly improved the success rate of spinal cord surgeries.

Other treatments may include the use of steroids to reduce swelling and pressure on the spinal cord, surgical decompression and fusion of the spine, and chemotherapy in selected cases. These may be the only treatments used if the spinal axis tumor is due to the metastasis of another primary cancer.

QUESTIONS TO ASK YOUR DOCTOR

- Which type of spinal axis tumor do I have?
- Is my tumor operable?
- Is there a clinical trial that offers a new treatment option for this type of tumor?

Prognosis

Malignant tumors of the spinal axis may spread (metastasize) to other parts of the central nervous system, but almost never spread to other parts of the body. As of mid-2014, there was no formal staging system for spinal axis tumors. The most important factors in determining prognosis for individuals with these tumors are the type of cell involved (e.g., astrocyte, ependyma, etc.), the overall health of the patient, and the grade of the tumor (an indicator of the aggressiveness of the tumor cells). Grade I tumors have cells that are not malignant and are nearly normal in appearance. Grade II tumors have cells that appear to be slightly abnormal. Grade III tumors have cells that are malignant and clearly abnormal. Grade IV tumors contain fast-spreading abnormal cells. In general, the survival rate for some types of spinal cord tumors, such as extradural tumors and low-grade astrocytomas, is better than for other types, such as ependymomas. For childhood spinal cord tumors, doctors may base treatment and prognosis on the child's age and whether the tumor can be removed with surgery.

Prevention

Because the causes of spinal axis tumors are not known, there are no known preventive measures.

Special concerns

If left untreated, spinal axis tumors can cause loss of muscle function up to and including paralysis. This characteristic makes the proper diagnosis and management of spinal axis tumors important.

See also Astrocytoma; Brain and central nervous system tumors; Chordoma; Ependymoma.

Resources

PERIODICALS

Oh, M. C., et al. "Prognosis by Tumor Location in Adults with Spinal Ependymomas." *Journal of Neurosurgery: Spine* 18, no. 3 (2013): 226–35.

Ostrum, Quinn T., et al. "CBTRUS Statistical Report: Primary Brain and Central Nervous System Tumors Diagnosed in the United States 2007–2011." *Neuro-Oncology* 16, suppl 4 (2014): iv1–iv63.

WEBSITES

American Association of Neurological Surgeons. "Spinal Tumors." http://www.aans.org/Patient%20Information/Conditions%20and%20Treatments/Spinal%20Tumors.aspx (accessed November 6, 2014).

National Cancer Institute. "General Information About Childhood Brain and Spinal Cord Tumors." http://www.cancer.gov/cancertopics/pdq/treatment/childbrain/Patient (accessed October 19, 2014).

National Institute of Neurological Disorders and Stroke. "NINDS Brain and Spinal Tumors Information Page." http://www.ninds.nih.gov/disorders/brainandspinaltumors/brainandspinaltumors.htm (accessed November 6, 2014).

ORGANIZATIONS

American Association of Neurological Surgeons, 5550 Meadowbrook Dr., Rolling Meadows, IL 60008-3852, (847) 378-0500, (888) 566-AANS (2267), info@aans.org, http://www.aans.org.

National Institute of Neurological Disorders and Stroke (NINDS), NIH Neurological Institute, PO Box 5801, Bethesda, MD 20824, (301) 496-5751, (800) 352-9424, http://www.ninds.nih.gov.

Paul A. Johnson, EdM
REVISED BY TERESA G. ODLE

Spinal cord compression

Definition

Spinal cord compression occurs when something presses down with sufficient force on the nerves within the spinal cord so that they lose their ability to function properly. Although trauma, degenerative back disease, and genetic disorders can cause pressure on the spinal cord, the term *spinal cord compression* is usually reserved for cases in which the presence of a tumor results in pressure on the spinal cord. The tumor may originate in a number of areas and either directly or indirectly put pressure on the cord.

Description

In order to understand spinal cord compression, it is useful to understand the structure of the spinal cord and to understand the difference between the spinal cord and the vertebral column. The vertebral column includes the bony structure surrounding the spinal cord and the spinal cord itself. Also an important part of the vertebral column, the intervertebral disks are found between vertebrae. They act as shock absorbers. The spinal cord, however, is the series of nerves that run down the hollow part of the vertebrae. Thus, the bony vertebrae and shock-absorbing disks protect the spinal cord from physical damage and compression.

The spinal cord is responsible for most functions of the body, including but not limited to the "fight or flight" response, the movement of arms and legs, and feeling below the neck. Each nerve is responsible for different functions, such as movement, and each has a different position within the structure of the spinal cord. Thus, depending on the angle from which the spinal cord is compressed, a person could experience numbness versus a loss of ability to control muscles (often seen as an odd limp), depending on which area is compressed.

Not only do the different nerve clusters of the spinal cord have different functions, but each has nerves branching off from the spinal cord at many levels. Each of these branches controls different parts of the body. For example, nerves branching off the spinal cord in the lower back control movement of the legs, and nerves branching off the spinal cord at the level of the neck are responsible for most of the movements of the arm. Thus, compression of the spinal cord at different levels can result in very different symptoms.

Vertebrae are, in order, divided into cervical, thoracic, lumbar, and sacral sections. The cervical vertebrae correspond to the neck, the thoracic vertebrae correspond to most of the torso, the lumbar vertebrae are found in the lower back, and the sacral vertebrae correspond to the area of the buttocks. There are seven cervical, twelve thoracic, five lumbar, and five sacral vertebrae (although the sacrum is one bony structure and contains no intervertebral disks). The level of compression is indicated by using the first letter of the type of vertebra and then the number of the vertebra within the group. The topmost vertebrae are numbered lowest, so the first cervical vertebra is the vertebra closest to the head, and is known as C1. C7 is the cervical vertebra furthest down the spine. Compression of the spinal cord in this region would be known as compression at C7. The closer the compression is to the head, the more symptoms the patient is likely to have, since compression of the spinal cord affects all levels of nerves below the area of compression that are part of the same nerve branch. For example, if movement were affected at C2 and below, a person would have difficulty using both arms and legs, whereas compression at T12 might result in difficulty using just the legs.

Causes and symptoms

Causes

The most common cause of cancerous spinal cord compression is a vertebral **metastasis**. A metastasis is a cancerous lesion that arises from another tumor somewhere else in the body. Vertebral metastases account for 85% of cases of spinal cord compression, and 70% of those metastases occur in the thoracic vertebrae. About 5% to 10% of patients with **cancer** will develop metastases to the spinal cord. Tumors may also grow from the nerves themselves; from the connective tissue surrounding the nerves; or, rarely, from the bony vertebrae themselves. Tumors that grow from outside the vertebral column may cause pressure by either growing into the hollow space in the vertebral column or by pressing the vertebrae into an abnormal conformation. More rarely, tumors in the vertebrae may cause compression indirectly by causing the vertebrae to collapse. Tumors that originate in the spinal cord or in the connective tissue overlying the spinal cord cause direct pressure because there is a limited space in which they can grow before impinging on the cord directly.

Symptoms

The first symptom patients usually display prior to actual spinal cord compression is pain, especially pain that is not relieved by lying down and that has lasted one month or more. This kind of pain should be sufficient to suspect imminent spinal cord compression due to cancerous causes. Also, there may be damage to nerve roots at the level of compression that can lead to symptoms in other parts of the body. For example, if the cord compression is in the lower part of the spine, then parts of the legs may be affected with numbness, tingling, and loss of power and movement. Similarly, if the problem lies in the upper part of the spinal column, there may be a loss of power and sensation in parts of the arms or hands. If the cord compression becomes more severe, it can affect lower muscle functions such as bowel and bladder control.

Diagnosis

If symptoms develop, prompt diagnosis and rapid treatment are crucial in order to avoid any permanent damage to the sensitive nerve tissue of the spinal cord. Usually, **magnetic resonance imaging** (MRI) or **computed tomography** (CT) scans will be performed to confirm cord compression and fully define the level and extent of the lesion. High-dose **corticosteroids** (oral or IV **dexamethasone**) may be promptly administered in order to reduce inflammation and pressure.

Treatment

The goal of therapy for spinal cord compression includes pain control, avoidance of complications, preserving or improving neurologic functions, or reversing impaired neurologic functions. Treatment usually involves treatment of the underlying tumor. For most patients with cancer-induced compression, **radiation therapy** is the treatment of choice. However, if radiation therapy is unavailable or if neurologic signs worsen despite medical therapy, surgical decompression should be performed. Surgery is also indicated when a **biopsy** is needed, when the spine is unstable, when tumors have recurred after radiation therapy, or when any abscess is present. Finally, in some tumors known to be highly chemoresponsive, **chemotherapy** alone or in combination with other modalities may be used.

Resources

PERIODICALS

Robson, P. "Metastatic Spinal Cord Compression: A Rare But Important Complication of Cancer." *Clinical Medicine* 14, no. 5 (2014): 542–5. http://www.clinmed.rcpjournal.org/content/14/5/542.long (accessed November 14, 2014).

WEBSITES

Canadian Cancer Society. "Spinal Cord Compression." http://www.cancer.ca/en/cancer-information/diagnosis-and-treatment/managing-side-effects/spinal-cord-compression/?region=on (accessed November 14, 2014).

Cancer Reasearch UK. "What Spinal Cord Compression Is." http://www.cancerresearchuk.org/about-cancer/coping-with-cancer/coping-physically/spinal/what-spinal-cord-compression-is (accessed November 14, 2014).

Michael Zuck, PhD

Spinal tap *see* **Lumbar puncture**

Spiritual and ethical concerns

Definition

Spiritual and ethical concerns refer to a set of issues affecting **cancer** patients that relate to questions about the ultimate meaning and purpose of life and the moral principles that guide one's actions during illness and at the end of life. While *ethics*, or moral philosophy, is a longstanding intellectual discipline, *spirituality* is much more difficult to define. In the twenty-first century, it is generally used to distinguish an interest in subjective experiences of transcendence or connection with the universe from the objective practices (prayer and worship) and formal theological systems of organized *religion*. There is, however, no universally accepted definition of spirituality, and certainly most active members of religious communities would describe themselves as spiritual. The important point to note is that spirituality, religious faith, and concerns about right conduct are genuine issues to cancer patients, particularly those confronting terminal illness. Ethical concerns about the role of medical professionals at the end of a cancer patient's life are also important to patients and their families and friends.

Description

Spirituality, religion, and ethical concerns influence cancer patients' sense of well-being and response to treatment at all points along the course of illness, not just at the end of life.

Spirituality and well-being

The NCI has compiled data that indicate that cancer patients—and their caregivers—draw on their spirituality and religious practices to cope with the anxiety and other stressors of cancer diagnosis and therapy. It is difficult, however, to compile precise data on the relationship between spiritual or religious practices and patient health. Investigators use a variety of different criteria (attendance at church or synagogue, frequency of private prayers, etc.) to measure people's degree of religious involvement or the extent of their beliefs; in particular, the difficulty of defining spirituality complicates comparisons of the findings reported in various studies. In addition, while many cancer patients who consider themselves religious or spiritual have less fear of death, cope better with pain, and are less likely to withdraw from others socially, some patients undergo intense spiritual distress during cancer treatment and may lose the religious faith they once claimed.

An instrument that has been used to measure spiritual well-being or distress in cancer patients is the Functional Assessment of Chronic Illness Therapy–Spiritual Well-Being (FACIT-Sp). A recent Yale study indicated that spiritual well-being is more closely related to improved quality of life in patients diagnosed with advanced cancer than either physical or emotional well-being. Other physicians have found the FACIT-Sp helpful in identifying which patients are at increased risk of **depression**. Although the FACIT-Sp was developed as a research tool, some clinicians find it a useful way for opening a conversation with cancer patients regarding their spirituality, their need or desire for further exploration of religious or spiritual issues, and the presence of spiritual distress. The FACIT-Sp has an advantage in that its questions do not assume that the patient believes in God; it can be administered to anyone, regardless of belief.

Spirituality and CAM

One unexpected finding of research conducted by the NCI in the area of spirituality is that while relatively few cancer patients identify "spiritual needs" as such with complementary and alternative medicine (CAM), about 20% of health care providers do. This result may be due to

KEY TERMS

Advance directive—A legal document in which a person states the type of care that he or she wishes or does not wish to receive in the event of losing his or her ability to make decisions or express them. "Do not resuscitate" (DNR) orders and living wills are types of advance directives.

Distress—A condition marked by emotional, social, spiritual, or physical pain or suffering that may affect caregivers as well as cancer patients.

Ethics—The branch of philosophy that discusses and analyzes what is the best way for humans to live, and which actions may be right or wrong in specific circumstances. The English word is derived from the Greek word for habit or custom.

Euthanasia—The practice of intentionally ending life to relieve prolonged pain or suffering.

Health care proxy—A document in which a person appoints someone else (known as an agent) to make health care decisions in the event of the loss of the ability to do so.

Hospice—A program that provides specialized medical and spiritual care for patients at the end of life. Hospice care may be provided in the patient's home, in hospitals, or in separate facilities.

Informed consent—A process for obtaining a patient's permission before a medical intervention, or obtaining a research subject's permission prior to enrollment in a clinical trial.

Palliative care—Care intended to relieve the symptoms of a disease rather than cure the disease.

Spirituality—In general, a subjective experience of or interest in the transcendent, connection with the universe, or a search for ultimate meaning. There is, however, no universally agreed-upon definition of spirituality.

Supportive care—In regard to cancer, the prevention or management of the adverse effects of cancer and cancer treatment.

the fact that prayer and meditation are often grouped under the general heading of mind/body CAM approaches, and that such movement therapies as yoga and t'ai chi entered the West from Eastern spiritual traditions. While mainstream medical professionals are often reluctant to ask patients about their use of CAM therapies, a conversation about CAM may be helpful in encouraging patients to discuss their spiritual needs as well, as patients who consider themselves spiritual or religious are more likely to have used CAM therapies or are interested in doing so.

A growing number of health care professionals are open to incorporating CAM approaches within the patient's conventional cancer therapy. This coordination of standard mainstream cancer therapies with complementary approaches is known as integrative medicine or IM. IM is particularly appealing to cancer patients who desire full partnership with their physicians in the treatment process; want all dimensions of their being taken into account, spirit as well as body; and prefer a highly personalized approach to their care. Several major cancer centers have added IM programs to their therapy programs, including at-home care; two such programs are noted in the Resources.

Ethical issues

Issues of medical ethics arise as soon as a cancer patient is diagnosed and continue through treatment to survivorship and ultimately to the end of the patient's life. The core principles that guide health care professionals in Canada and the United States can be outlined as follows:

- First, do no harm. Sometimes seen in its Latin form—*primum non nocere*—this principle has guided physicians since the days of Hippocrates. It includes acting in the patient's best interests as well as avoiding harm to the patient.

- Respect the patient's autonomy. This principle refers to allowing the patient to choose or refuse a treatment and have an equal voice in medical decision making. Although at one time doctors expected patients to accept their treatments unquestioned, the patients' rights movement of the 1970s (sometimes called the patient empowerment movement) led to a greater acceptance of patients as full participants in their care.

- Be honest and truthful. This principle requires health care professionals to tell patients the truth, not only about their diagnosis and prognosis, but also about the nature and side effects of their cancer treatments. The informed consent that patients must provide before a medical intervention is one aspect of this principle.

- Consider justice and fairness. This principle applies to the use of scarce health care resources and decisions about which patients should receive specific therapies.

In regard to end-of-life care, this principle is often invoked in decisions to halt heroic measures that extend a patient's life.These principles can, however, conflict with one another, and resolving the conflict may involve spiritually as well as emotionally agonizing decisions or painful disagreements between the patient and his or her caregivers and physicians.

End-of-life care is associated with several specific ethical issues:

- Decisions regarding do-not-resuscitate (DNR) orders or other specific wishes regarding end-of-life care. Cancer patients are encouraged to make advance directives, which are legal documents specifying the care the patient wishes (or does not want) to receive in the event of being unable to make or state decisions for him- or herself. Living wills and appointing health care proxies are two specific forms of advance directives.

- Depression. The NCI notes that cancer patients— particularly males—are at increased risk of suicide, often shortly after being diagnosed with cancer. Physicians and nurses who treat cancer patients are increasingly trained to assess patients for depression and to encourage them to discuss any suicidal thoughts. It is a myth that talking about suicide increases the patient's risk of taking his or her life; in many cases, the simple opportunity to discuss suicidal feelings helps the patient to move past them.

- Physician-assisted suicide (PAS). Sometimes called assisted dying, physician-assisted suicide is defined by the Canadian Medical Association (CMA) as "knowingly and intentionally providing a person with the knowledge or means or both required to commit suicide, including counselling about lethal doses of drugs, prescribing such lethal doses or supplying the drugs." Cancer patients with terminal illness sometimes request PAS; however, it is illegal in all but four states of the United States (Washington, Oregon, Vermont, and New Mexico, with Montana taking no public stand against PAS). In Canada, it is illegal in all provinces except for Quebec, which legalized it in June 2014. Most hospice physicians recommend pain control and other palliative and supportive measures that relieve the patient's distress without an irreversible action like PAS.

- Euthanasia. Euthanasia, which comes from two Greek words meaning "good death," refers to the intentional ending of the life of a person with an incurable or painful disease. Sometimes called mercy killing, it is a controversial issue. Health care professionals usually distinguish between passive euthanasia, which is the withholding of treatments that might prolong life in a terminally ill patient; and active euthanasia, which is the deliberate causation or hastening of the patient's death. They also distinguish between voluntary euthanasia, in which the patient knowingly requests death and is competent to make that decision; and involuntary euthanasia, in which the patient is killed or is allowed to die without his or her consent. Health care professionals as well as ethicists express concern about the possibility that widened acceptance of euthanasia could put family or social pressure on vulnerable patients to allow themselves to be euthanized. According to the NCI, most cancer patients who favor euthanasia are male, not religious or spiritual, and likely to hold strong beliefs about the extreme suffering of cancer patients.

Demographics

The **National Cancer Institute** (NCI) notes that the general population of the United States still considers religion and spirituality important in their lives. One survey reported that 90% of adults expressed a belief in God, and 70% stated that religion is "one of the most important influences in their lives." On the other hand, the specific content of people's beliefs varies widely depending on religious background (if any), ethnicity, and level of education. Some studies indicate that Hispanics, African Americans, and persons self-identified as Christians are more likely to feel a sense of being comforted by God during illness than are members of other groups.

What is common, however, across different ethnic groups and faith traditions is patients' desire for medical professionals to pay more attention to their spiritual and religious needs. A survey of hospital inpatients found that 77% wished that hospital staff would take spiritual needs more seriously, and that 37% wanted physicians to acknowledge the significance of religious beliefs more often. (The reader should note that these patients were not asking health care professionals to pray with them or discuss specific beliefs, only to inquire about whether their beliefs were important to them.) The inpatients who stated that their spiritual or religious needs were not met scored quality of care lower and were more likely to express dissatisfaction with that care. A study at a cancer center in Boston in 2013 reported that the center's doctors and nurses consider some provision of spiritual care as part of their role, while patients reported receiving such care infrequently.

Health care team roles

The roles of various members of the health care team have changed in recent years. In particular, medical professionals are encouraged to become partners with cancer patients, caregivers, and hospital chaplains in attending to the patients' spiritual needs. This development is an outgrowth of patients' increased desire for greater autonomy in decision making; for fuller participation in their cancer treatment; and for closer attention to their spirituality.

Chaplains

Most large hospitals, nursing homes, assisted living facilities, and hospices in the United States have one or more chaplains to minister to the spiritual needs of patients or residents, although chaplains are not always available in outpatient facilities or smaller hospitals. While the majority of chaplains are ordained clergy of one faith tradition or another, women who belong to traditions that do not ordain women can serve as hospital chaplains provided they are commissioned by their faith group and meet all other educational and certification requirements. As of 2014, American hospital chaplains must hold the M.Div. degree (three years of post-college theological study); be endorsed by their church or faith group; and have completed 1600 hours of clinical pastoral education in a hospital or other health care setting for board certification. There are four organizations that presently offer board certification for hospital chaplains in the United States: the American Association of Pastoral Counselors, the Association for Clinical Pastoral Education, the Healthcare Chaplains Ministry Association, and the College of Pastoral Supervision and Psychotherapy.

In addition to ministering to the spiritual needs of cancer patients, hospital chaplains also meet with the patient's caregivers and health care staff when needed. They arrange visits for patients who wish to pray with or receive Christian sacraments from an ordained pastor or priest of their own tradition; this practice is often comforting for patients who are being treated in a cancer center far from home.

Physicians and nurses

As noted above, health care professionals have begun to devote more attention to the spiritual needs to cancer patients. Several studies have indicated, however, that doctors and nurses tend to underestimate the degree to which patients want health care professionals to acknowledge their spiritual needs. Interventions related to spiritual care that are considered appropriate for doctors and nurses to provide include: exploration of spiritual concerns within the general context of medical care; encouraging the patient to have his or her own clergy (if local) visit in the hospital; referring the patient to a hospital chaplain; referring the patient to a support group that focuses on spirituality; or referring the patient to a faith-based therapist.

QUESTIONS TO ASK YOUR DOCTOR

- What is your opinion of the role of spirituality or religion in coping with cancer diagnosis or treatment?
- Have you ever conducted a spiritual assessment of a cancer patient?
- Do you feel comfortable discussing spiritual or ethical issues with patients?
- What is your opinion of physician-assisted suicide and euthanasia?
- Have you ever worked closely with hospital chaplains as part of a health care team?
- Have you ever treated a depressed patient who was considering suicide? If so, what was helpful for the patient?

According to the NCI, gentle and respectful inquiries on the part of doctors and nurses about religious or spiritual concerns are greatly appreciated by the majority of cancer patients without regard to their diagnosis or prognosis. In addition to the FACIT-Sp described earlier, other tools that are recommended by physicians and nurses in conducting spiritual assessments are the FICA Spiritual History Tool, the HOPE questions for spiritual assessment, and the Open Invite, which is an open-ended approach that allows the doctor or nurse to begin a conversation with the patient about his or her religious or spiritual beliefs and practices. The FICA tool and the HOPE questions may be found on the websites listed below.

Resources

BOOKS

Adams, Spencer B., ed. *Comfort and Care at the End of Life.* New York: Nova Science Publishers, 2011.

Angelos, Peter, Ed. *Ethical Issues in Cancer Patient Care*, 2nd ed. New York: Springer, 2008.

Cohen, Lorenzo, and Maurie Markman, eds. *Integrative Oncology: Incorporating Complementary Medicine into Conventional Cancer Care.* Totowa, NJ: Humana, 2008.

Lazenby, Mark, Ruth McCorkle, and Daniel P. Sulmasy, eds. *Safe Passage: A Global Spiritual Sourcebook for Care at the End of Life.* New York: Oxford University Press, 2014.

Lee, Colleen O., and Georgia M. Decker. *Cancer and Complementary Medicine: Your Guide to Smart Choices in Symptom Management.* Pittsburgh, PA: Hygeia Media, 2012.

Wills, Margaret A., ed. *Communicating Spirituality in Health Care.* Cresskill, NJ: Hampton Press, 2009.

PERIODICALS

Bai, M., et al. "Exploring the Relationship between Spiritual Well-being and Quality of Life among Patients Newly Diagnosed with Advanced Cancer." *Palliative and Supportive Care* (July 3, 2014): e-pub ahead of print. http://dx.doi.org/10.1017/S1478951514000820 (accessed November 19, 2014).

Best, M., P. Butow, and I. Olver. "Spiritual Support of Cancer Patients and the Role of the Doctor." *Supportive Care in Cancer* 22 (May 2014): 1333–1339.

Canada, A.L., et al. "Racial/Ethnic Differences in Spiritual Well-being among Cancer Survivors." *Journal of Behavioral Medicine* 36 (October 2013): 441–453.

Cooke, L., et al. "What Do I Say? Suicide Assessment and Management." *Clinical Journal of Oncology Nursing* 17 (February 2013): E1–E7.

Gonzalez, P., et al. "Spiritual Well-being and Depressive Symptoms among Cancer Survivors." *Supportive Care in Cancer* 22 (September 2014): 2393–2400.

Morrison, W., and T. Kang. "Judging the Quality of Mercy: Drawing a Line between Palliation and Euthanasia." *Pediatrics* 133 (February 2014): Suppl. 1: S31–S36.

Peteet, J.R., and M.J. Balboni. "Spirituality and Religion in Oncology." *CA: A Cancer Journal for Clinicians* 63 (July-August 2013): 280–289.

Piderman, K.M., et al. "Spiritual Quality of Life in Advanced Cancer Patients Receiving Radiation Therapy." *Psychooncology* 23 (February 2014): 216–221.

Rosenfeld, B., et al. "Does Desire for Hastened Death Change in Terminally Ill Cancer Patients?" *Social Science and Medicine* 111 (June 2014): 35–40.

Saguil, A., and K. Phelps. "The Spiritual Assessment." *American Family Physician* 86 (September 15, 2012): 546–550.

Trevino, K.M., et al. "Negative Religious Coping as a Correlate of Suicidal Ideation in Patients with Advanced Cancer." *Psycho-oncology* 23 (August 2014): 936–945.

WEBSITES

American Cancer Society (ACS). "Advance Directives: Frequently Asked Questions." This is a useful brief discussion about terminal illness and the options for end-of-life care as well as information about advance directives as such. http://www.cancer.org/treatment/findingandpayingfortreatment/understandingfinancialandlegalmatters/advancedirectives/advance-directives-faqs (accessed August 6, 2014).

American Cancer Society (ACS). "Spirituality and Prayer." http://www.cancer.org/treatment/treatmentsandsideeffects/complementaryandalternativemedicine/mindbodyandspirit/spirituality-and-prayer (accessed August 5, 2014).

Anandarajah, G., and E. Hight. "Spirituality and Medical Practice: Using the HOPE Questions as a Practical Tool for Spiritual Assessment." http://www.aafp.org/afp/2001/0101/p81.html (accessed August 5, 2014).

George Washington Institute for Spirituality and Health. "FICA Spiritual History Tool." FICA is an acronym for Faith and belief; Importance; Community; and Address in Care. http://smhs.gwu.edu/gwish/clinical/fica/spiritual-history-tool (accessed August 5, 2014).

M.D. Anderson Cancer Center. "Integrative Medicine Center." http://www.mdanderson.org/patient-and-cancer-information/care-centers-and-clinics/specialty-and-treatment-centers/integrative-medicine-center/index.html (accessed August 6, 2014).

Memorial Sloan Kettering Cancer Center. "Integrative Medicine." http://www.mskcc.org/cancer-care/integrative-medicine (accessed August 6, 2014).

National Cancer Institute (NCI). "Last Days of Life (PDQ)." http://www.cancer.gov/cancertopics/pdq/supportivecare/lasthours/healthprofessional/page1/AllPages (accessed August 5, 2014).

National Cancer Institute (NCI). "Spirituality in Cancer Care (PDQ)." http://www.cancer.gov/cancertopics/pdq/supportivecare/spirituality/HealthProfessional/page1/AllPages (accessed August 5. 2014).

Office of Cancer Complementary and Alternative Medicine (OCCAM). "Frequently Asked Questions about Cancer and CAM." Includes links to more detailed descriptions of specific CAM approaches. http://cam.cancer.gov/health_faq.html (accessed August 6, 2014).

ORGANIZATIONS

American Academy of Hospice and Palliative Medicine (AAHPM), 8735 West Higgins Road, Suite 300, Chicago, IL 60631, (847) 375-4712, Fax: (847) 375-6475, info@aahpm.org, http://aahpm.org/.

American Cancer Society (ACS), 250 Williams Street NW, Atlanta, GA 30303, (800) 227-2345, http://www.cancer.org/aboutus/howwehelpyou/app/contact-us.aspx, http://www.cancer.org/index.

Association for Clinical Pastoral Education (ACPE), One West Court Square, Suite 325, Decatur, GA 30030, (404) 320-1472, Fax: (404) 320-0849, acpe@acpe.edu, http://www.acpe.edu/.

HealthCare Chaplaincy Network, 65 Broadway, 12th Floor, New York, NY 10006-2503, (212) 644-1111, comm@healthcarechaplaincy.org, http://www.healthcarechaplaincy.org/.

National Cancer Institute (NCI), BG 9609 MSC 9760, 9609 Medical Center Drive, Bethesda, MD 20892-9760, (800) 4-CANCER (422-6237), http://www.cancer.gov/global/contact/email-us, http://www.cancer.gov/.

National Hospice and Palliative Care Organization (NHPCO), 1731 King Street, Alexandria, VA 22314, (703) 837-1500, Fax: (703) 837-1233, http://www.nhpco.org/.

Office of Cancer Complementary and Alternative Medicine (OCCAM), 9609 Medical Center Dr., Room 5-W-136, Rockville, MD 20850, (240) 276-6595, Fax: (240) 276-7888, ncioccam1-r@mail.nih.gov, http://cam.cancer.gov/.

Rebecca J. Frey, PhD

Splenectomy

Definition

A splenectomy is the total or partial surgical removal of the spleen, an organ that is part of the lymphatic system.

Purpose

The human spleen is a dark purple, bean-shaped organ located in the upper left side of the abdomen just behind the bottom of the rib cage. In adults, the spleen is about 4.8 × 2.8 × 1.6 in. (12 × 7 × 4 cm) in size, and weighs about 4–5 oz. (113–141 g). The spleen plays a role in the immune system of the body. It also filters foreign substances from the blood and removes wornout blood cells. The spleen regulates blood flow to the liver and sometimes stores blood cells—a function known as sequestration. In healthy adults, about 30% of blood platelets are sequestered in the spleen.

Splenectomies are performed for a variety of different reasons and with different degrees of urgency.

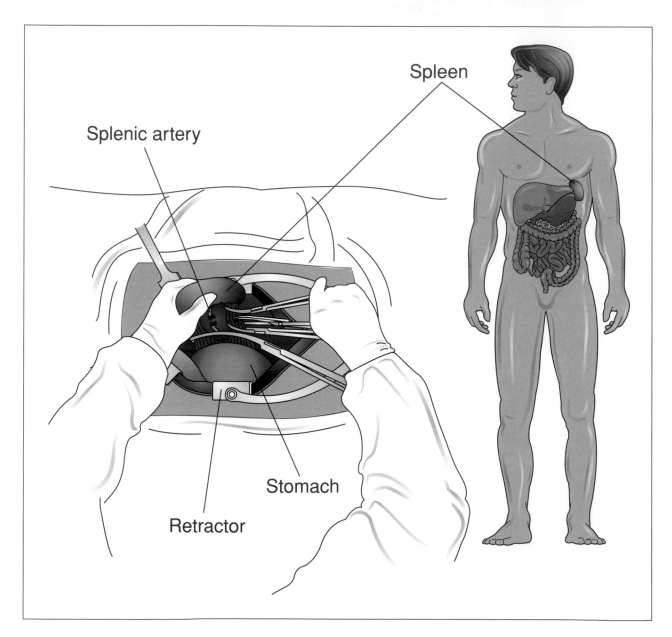

Splenectomy is the surgical removal of the spleen. This procedure is performed as a last resort in most diseases involving the spleen. In some cases, such as in many types of cancer, splenectomy does not cure the condition causing an enlarged spleen—it only relieves the symptoms. *(Illustration by Electronic Illustrators Group. © Cengage Learning®.)*

KEY TERMS

Computed tomography (CT) scan—An imaging technique that creates a series of pictures of areas inside the body taken from different angles. The pictures are created by a computer linked to an x-ray machine.

Embolization—A treatment in which foam, silicone, or another substance is injected into a blood vessel in order to close it off.

Endemic—Present in a specific population or geographical area at all times. Some diseases that may affect the spleen are endemic to certain parts of Africa or Asia.

Hereditary spherocytosis—A hereditary disorder that leads to a chronic form of anemia (too few red blood cells) due to an abnormality in the red blood cell membrane.

Idiopathic thrombocytopenia purpura (ITP)—A rare autoimmune disorder characterized by an acute shortage of platelets with resultant bruising and spontaneous bleeding.

Laparoscopy—A procedure in which a laparoscope (a thin, lighted tube) is inserted through an incision in the abdominal wall to evaluate the presence or spread of disease. Tissue samples may be removed for biopsy.

Lymphatic system—The tissues and organs that produce and store cells that fight infection, together with the network of vessels that carry lymph. The organs and tissues in the lymphatic system include the bone marrow, spleen, thymus gland, and lymph nodes.

Palpate—To examine by means of touch.

Platelet—A disk-shaped structure found in blood that binds to fibrinogen at the site of a wound to begin the clotting process.

Sequestration—A process in which the spleen withdraws blood cells from the circulation and stores them.

Spleen—An organ that produces lymphocytes, filters the blood, stores blood cells, and destroys those that are aging. It is located on the left side of the abdomen near the stomach.

Splenomegaly—Enlargement of the spleen.

Most splenectomies are done after a patient has been diagnosed with hypersplenism. Hypersplenism is not a specific disease but a syndrome (group or cluster of symptoms) that may be associated with different disorders. Hypersplenism is characterized by enlargement of the spleen (splenomegaly), defects in the blood cells, and an abnormally high turnover of blood cells. It is almost always associated with such specific disorders as cirrhosis of the liver or certain cancers. The decision to perform a splenectomy depends on the severity and prognosis of the disease that is causing the hypersplenism.

Splenectomy always required

There are two diseases for which a splenectomy is the only treatment—primary cancers of the spleen and a blood disorder called hereditary spherocytosis (HS). In HS, the absence of a specific protein in the red blood cell membrane leads to the formation of relatively fragile cells that are easily damaged when they pass through the spleen. The cell destruction does not occur elsewhere in the body and ends when the spleen is removed. HS can appear at any age, even in newborns, although doctors prefer to put off removing the spleen until the child is five to six years old.

Splenectomy usually required

There are some disorders for which a splenectomy is usually recommended. They include:

- Immune (idiopathic) thrombocytopenic purpura (ITP). ITP is a disease in which platelets are destroyed by antibodies in the body's immune system. A splenectomy is the definitive treatment for this disease and is effective in about 70% of cases of chronic ITP.

- Trauma. The spleen can be ruptured by blunt as well as penetrating injuries to the chest or abdomen. Car accidents are the most common cause of blunt traumatic injury to the spleen.

- Abscesses. Abscesses of the spleen are relatively uncommon but have a high mortality rate.

- Rupture of the splenic artery. This artery sometimes ruptures as a complication of pregnancy.

- Hereditary elliptocytosis. This is a relatively rare disorder. It is similar to HS in that it is characterized by red blood cells with defective membranes that are destroyed by the spleen.

Splenectomy sometimes required

Other disorders may or may not necessitate a splenectomy. These include:

• Hodgkin lymphoma, a serious form of cancer that causes the lymph nodes to enlarge. A splenectomy is often performed in order to find out how far the disease has progressed.

• Autoimmune hemolytic disorders. These disorders may appear in patients of any age but are most common in adults over 50. The red blood cells are destroyed by antibodies produced by the patient's own body (autoantibodies).

• Myelofibrosis. Myelofibrosis is a disorder in which bone marrow is replaced by fibrous tissue. It produces severe and painful splenomegaly. A splenectomy does not cure myelofibrosis but may be performed to relieve pain caused by the swelling of the spleen.

• Thalassemia. Thalassemia is a hereditary form of anemia that is most common in people of Mediterranean origin. A splenectomy is sometimes performed if the patient's spleen has become painfully enlarged.

Description

Complete splenectomy

REMOVAL OF ENLARGED SPLEEN. A splenectomy is performed under general anesthesia. The most common technique is used to remove greatly enlarged spleens. After the surgeon makes a cut (incision) in the abdomen, the artery to the spleen is tied to prevent blood loss and reduce the size of the spleen. Tying the splenic artery also keeps the spleen from further sequestration of blood cells. The surgeon detaches the ligaments holding the spleen in place and removes the organ. In many cases, tissue samples will be sent to a laboratory for analysis.

REMOVAL OF RUPTURED SPLEEN. When the spleen has been ruptured by trauma, the surgeon approaches the organ from its underside and ties the splenic artery before removing the ruptured organ.

Partial splenectomy

In some cases, the surgeon removes only part of the spleen. This procedure is considered by some to be a useful compromise that reduces pain caused by an enlarged spleen while leaving the patient less vulnerable to infection.

Laparoscopic splenectomy

Laparoscopic splenectomy, or removal of the spleen through several small incisions, has been performed more frequently in recent years. Laparoscopic surgery, which is sometimes called keyhole surgery, is done with smaller surgical instruments inserted through very short incisions, with the assistance of a tiny camera and video monitor. Laparoscopic procedures reduce the length of hospital stay, the level of postoperative pain, and the risk of infection. They also leave smaller scars. A laparoscopic procedure is contraindicated, however, if the patient's spleen is greatly enlarged. Most surgeons will not remove a spleen longer than 20 cm (as measured by a CT scan) by this method.

Diagnosis

The most important part of a medical assessment in disorders of the spleen is the measurement of splenomegaly. The normal spleen cannot be felt when the doctor palpates the patient's abdomen. A spleen that is large enough to be felt indicates splenomegaly. In some cases, the doctor will hear a dull sound when he or she thumps (percusses) the patient's abdomen near the ribs on the left side. **Imaging studies** that can be used to confirm splenomegaly include ultrasound tests, technetium-99m sulfur colloid imaging, and CT scans. The rate of platelet or red blood cell destruction by the spleen can also be measured by tagging blood cells with radioactive chromium or platelets with radioactive indium.

Preparation

Preoperative preparation for a splenectomy procedure usually includes:

• Correction of abnormalities of blood clotting and the number of red blood cells.

• Treatment of any infections.

• Control of immune reactions. Patients are usually given protective vaccinations about a month before surgery. The most common vaccines used are Pneumovax or Pnu-Imune 23 (against pneumococcal infections) and Meno-mune-A/C/Y/W-135 (against meningococcal infections).

Aftercare

Immediately following surgery, patients are given instructions for incision care and medications intended to prevent infection. Blood transfusions may be indicated for some patients to replace defective blood cells. The most important part of aftercare, however, is long-term caution regarding vulnerability to infection. Patients are asked to see their doctor at once if they have a **fever** or any other sign of infection, and to avoid travel to areas where exposure to malaria or similar diseases is likely. Children with splenectomies may be kept on antibiotic therapy until they are 16 years old. All patients can be given a booster dose of pneumococcal vaccine five to ten years after undergoing a splenectomy.

Risks

The main risk of a splenectomy procedure is overwhelming bacterial infection, or postsplenectomy sepsis. This condition results from the body's decreased ability to clear bacteria from the blood, and lowered levels of a protein in blood plasma that helps to fight viruses (immunoglobulin M). The risk of dying from infection after undergoing a splenectomy is highest in children, especially in the first two years after surgery. The risk of postsplenectomy sepsis can be reduced by vaccinations before the operation. Some doctors also recommend a two-year course of penicillin following splenectomy, or long-term treatment with ampicillin.

Other risks associated with the procedure include inflammation of the pancreas and collapse of the lungs. In some cases, a splenectomy does not address the underlying causes of splenomegaly or other conditions. Excessive bleeding after the operation is an additional possible complication, particularly for patients with ITP. Infection of the incision immediately following surgery may also occur.

Results

Results depend on the reason for the operation. In blood disorders, the splenectomy will remove the cause of the blood cell destruction. Normal results for patients with an enlarged spleen are relief of pain and the complications of splenomegaly. It is not always possible, however, to predict which patients will respond well or to what degree.

Recovery from the operation itself is fairly rapid. Hospitalization is usually less than a week (one to two days for laparoscopic splenectomy), and complete healing usually occurs within four to six weeks. Patients are encouraged to return to such normal activities as showering, driving, climbing stairs, light lifting, and work as soon as they feel comfortable. Some patients may return to work in a few days while others prefer to rest at home a little longer.

Alternatives

Splenic embolization is a surgical alternative to splenectomy that is used in some patients who are poor candidates for surgery. Embolization involves plugging or blocking the splenic artery with synthetic substances to shrink the size of the spleen. The substances that are injected during this procedure include polyvinyl alcohol foam, polystyrene, and silicone.

Health care team roles

A splenectomy is performed by a surgeon trained in gastroenterology, the branch of medicine that deals with the diseases of the digestive tract. An anesthesiologist is responsible for administering anesthesia, and the operation is performed in a hospital setting.

QUESTIONS TO ASK YOUR DOCTOR

- What happens on the day of surgery?
- What type of anesthesia will be used?
- How long will it take to recover from the surgery?
- When can I expect to return to work and resume normal activities?
- What are the risks associated with a splenectomy?
- How many splenectomies do you perform in a year?
- Will I have a large scar?

Resources

BOOKS

Gabrielson, Curt. *Surgical Diseases of the Spleen*. New York: Springer, 2012.

O'Malley, Dennis P. *Atlas of Spleen Pathology*. New York: Springer, 2013.

PERIODICALS

Jankulovski, N., et al. "Laparoscopic versus Open Splenectomy: A Single Center Eleven-Year Experience." *Acta Clinica Croatica* 52, no. 2 (2013): 229–34. http://dx.doi.org/10.1111/hepr.12234 (accessed October 3, 2014).

Nomura, Yoriko, et al. "Influence of Splenectomy in Patients with Liver Cirrhosis and Hypersplenism." *Hepatology Research* (September 3, 2013): e-pub ahead of print. http://dx.doi.org/10.1111/hepr.12234 (accessed October 3, 2014).

Wang, Xin, et al. "Laparoscopic Splenectomy: A Surgeon's Experience of 302 Patients with Analysis of Postoperative Complications." *Surgical Endoscopy* 27, no. 10 (2013): 3564–71. http://dx.doi.org/10.1007/s00464-013-2978-4 (accessed October 3, 2014).

WEBSITES

A.D.A.M. Medical Encyclopedia. "Spleen Removal." MedlinePlus. http://www.nlm.nih.gov/medlineplus/ency/article/002944.htm (accessed October 3, 2014).

American Academy of Family Physicians. "Splenectomy." FamilyDoctor.org. http://familydoctor.org/familydoctor/en/drugs-procedures-devices/procedures-devices/splenectomy.html (accessed October 3, 2014).

Platelet Disorder Support Association. "Splenectomy." http://www.pdsa.org/treatments/conventional/splenectomy.html (accessed October 3, 2014).

ORGANIZATIONS

American College of Gastroenterology, 6400 Goldsboro Rd., Ste. 200, Bethesda, MD 20817, (301) 263-9000, info@acg.gi.org, http://gi.org.

American Gastroenterological Association, 4930 Del Ray Ave., Bethesda, MD 20814, (301) 654-2055, Fax: (301) 654-5920, member@gastro.org, http://www.gastro.org.

National Cancer Institute, 6116 Executive Blvd., Ste. 300, Bethesda, MD 20892-8322, (800) 4-CANCER (422-6237), http://cancer.gov.

Teresa Norris, RN
Monique Laberge, PhD

Sprycel *see* **Dasatinib**

Squamous cell carcinoma of the skin

Definition

A squamous cell **carcinoma** is a **skin cancer** that originates from squamous keratinocytes in the epidermis, the top layer of the skin. *Squamous* is a term that indicates a surface with a scaly nature.

Description

The skin has three layers: the epidermis (or topmost layer), the dermis (or middle layer), and the subcutis (or lower layer). Squamous keratinocytes are flattened unpigmented skin cells in the middle of the epidermis. When they become cancerous, these cells invade the dermis and spread out into the normal skin. They become visible as a small growth or area of change in the skin's appearance.

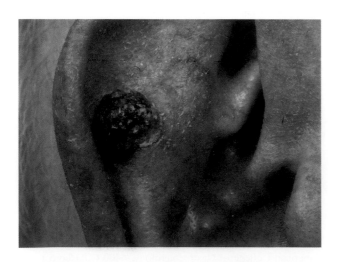

Squamous cell carcinoma on the ear. *(Girand/Science Source)*

Most squamous cell carcinomas appear on areas that have been exposed to the sun: the head and neck, forearms, backs of the hands, upper part of the torso, and lower legs. Many develop in precancerous patches called actinic keratoses. Actinic keratoses are rough, scaly patches on the skin that usually start to appear in middle age. They are associated with a lifetime's exposure to the sun. Estimates of the chance that an actinic keratosis will turn into a squamous cell carcinoma vary from 0.24% to 20%.

Squamous cell carcinomas can also originate in old scars and burns, long-standing sores, and other areas of chronic skin irritation. These tumors tend to be more dangerous than those that arise in actinic keratoses.

The least dangerous type of squamous cell carcinoma is called Bowen's disease, intraepithelial squamous cell carcinoma, or squamous cell carcinoma *in situ*. Bowen's disease can show up anywhere on the skin, but it is especially common on the head and neck. This **cancer** usually grows slowly, but it may evolve into a more serious spreading form if it is not removed.

Other types of squamous cell carcinomas grow fairly quickly and can develop within a few months. These tumors may spread in the skin along the blood vessels, nerves, and muscles. They can also metastasize, or spread to other areas. On the average, 2–6% of squamous cell carcinomas metastasize, but the rate varies with the tumor site. At least 95% of the tumors that originate in actinic keratoses remain in the skin, but up to 38% of the cancers from scars are metastatic. **Metastasis** is also more likely when the cancer originates on the ear, lip, or genitalia; is large or deep; or develops in someone with a severely suppressed immune system. Cancers that regrow after treatment and tumors that spread along the nerves are particularly dangerous.

Demographics

Skin cancer is the most common type of cancer, and squamous cell carcinoma is the second most common type of skin cancer in North America. The American Cancer Society estimates that about 440,000 cases are diagnosed each year in the United States, but because squamous and basal cell skin cancers are not required to be reported to cancer registries, the actual number is open to debate.

Squamous cell carcinomas are more common in the older adult population than in the young. The average age at diagnosis is about 70 years, although the cancer often appears earlier in individuals with compromised immune systems and certain other health problems. Overall, the chance of developing a squamous cell

KEY TERMS

Actinic keratosis (plural, actinic keratoses)—A rough, dry, scaly patch on the skin associated with sun exposure.

Antioxidant—A substance that can neutralize free radicals. Free radicals are damaging molecules formed by oxidation. Antioxidant vitamins include vitamin E, C, and beta-carotene, a form of vitamin A.

Biopsy—A sample of an organ or tissue taken to look for abnormalities.

Chronic—Long-standing or persistent.

Dermis—A layer of skin sandwiched between the epidermis and the fat under the skin. It contains the blood vessels, nerves, sweat glands, and hair follicles.

Epidermis—The thin layer of skin cells at the surface of the skin.

Fluorouracil—A prescription drug used to treat actinic keratoses, solar keratoses, and various forms of cancer.

Human papillomaviruses (HPV)—A family of viruses that cause common warts of the hands and feet, as well as lesions and warts in the genital and vaginal area. More than 50 types of HPV have been identified, some of which are linked to cancerous and precancerous conditions.

Local anesthetic—A liquid used to numb a small area of the skin.

Lymph node—A small organ full of immune cells, found in clusters throughout the body.

Nonmelanoma skin cancer—A squamous cell carcinoma or basal cell carcinoma.

Oncologist—A doctor who specializes in the treatment of cancer.

Pathologist—A doctor who specializes in examining samples of cells, tissues, or body fluids for abnormalities.

Precancerous—Abnormal and with a higher probability of turning into cancer, but not yet a cancer.

Squamous cells—Thin, flat cells on the surfaces of the skin and the linings of various organs.

carcinoma is about 7%–11%. The likelihood increases with exposure to the sun, and is greatest for fair-skinned individuals who tan poorly. Living near the equator, where ultraviolet light is more intense, also increases the risk. A weakened immune system, such as from an organ transplant or HIV infection, can also increase the risk of developing a squamous cell carcinoma by a factor of 5 to 250.

More people with fair skin develop squamous cell carcinomas, but this cancer tends to be most dangerous in individuals with dark skin, most likely because it is not diagnosed as early. The mortality rate for African Americans with squamous cell carcinomas is much higher than the death rate for Caucasian males with nonmelanoma skin cancer. One reason for this disparity is that the cancers that develop in dark skin are more likely to come from old scars and burns than from actinic keratoses.

Causes and symptoms

Squamous cell carcinoma is caused by genetic damage to a skin cell, usually by the ultraviolet rays in sunlight. Severe burns and infection with some human papillomaviruses are also risk factors.

Any of the following changes may be a warning sign that an actinic keratosis is developing into a squamous cell carcinoma:

- pain
- increased redness
- sores or bleeding
- hardening or thickening
- increased size

Most squamous cell carcinomas begin as a small red bump on the skin. Advanced squamous cell carcinomas have the following characteristics:

- a few millimeters to a few centimeters in diameter
- reddish-brown, flesh-colored, pink, or red
- bumpy or flat
- sharp, irregular edges in Bowen's disease; others may have no definite edge
- may be crusted or scaly
- may contain bleeding sores

Diagnosis

Squamous cell carcinomas are usually diagnosed with a **skin biopsy** taken in the doctor's office. This is generally a brief, simple procedure. After numbing the skin with an injection of local anesthetic, the doctor snips out the tumor or a piece of it. This skin sample is sent to a pathologist to be examined under a microscope. It can take up to a week for the **biopsy** results to come back. Squamous cell carcinomas are graded into categories of one through four. The grading is based on how deeply the tumor penetrates the skin and how abnormal its cells are. Higher grades are more serious.

Treatment team

Primary care physicians remove some squamous cell carcinomas. Other cancers, including larger or more complicated tumors, may be referred to a dermatologist. The services of a plastic surgeon are occasionally necessary. Metastatic tumors are often treated by an oncologist, surgeons, specially trained nurses, and specialists in radiation treatment.

Clinical staging

In stage 0 (Bowen's disease), the cancer is very small and has not yet spread from the epidermis to the dermis.

In stage I, the cancer is less than 0.8 in. (2 cm) in diameter. No cancer cells can be found in lymph nodes or other internal organs.

In stage II, the cancer is more than 0.8 in. (2 cm) in diameter. No cancer cells can be found in lymph nodes or other internal organs.

In stage III, cancer cells have been found in nearby lymph nodes or in the bone, muscle, or cartilage beneath the skin.

A stage IV cancer can be any size. In this stage, cancer cells have been discovered in internal organs that are distant from the skin. Squamous cell carcinomas tend to spread to nearby lymph nodes, the liver, and the lungs.

Treatment

The treatment options for a squamous cell carcinoma depend on the size of the tumor, its location, and the likelihood that it will spread aggressively or metastasize. All of the treatments described below generally have cure rates of approximately 90% to 99% for small, localized cancers. The five-year cure rates are highest with **Mohs surgery**, also called Mohs micrographic surgery.

One option is conventional surgery. The doctor numbs the area with an injection of local anesthetic, then cuts out the tumor and a small margin of normal skin around it. The wound is closed with a few stitches. One advantage of conventional surgery is that the wound usually heals quickly. Another benefit is that the complete cancer can be sent to a pathologist for evaluation. If cancer

cells are found in the skin around the tumor, additional treatments can be done.

Laser surgery may be an alternative. A disadvantage to laser surgery is that the wounds from some lasers heal more slowly than cuts from a scalpel. The advantage is that bleeding is minimal.

Another option is Mohs micrographic surgery. This technique is a variation of conventional surgery. In this procedure, the surgeon examines each layer of skin under the microscope as it is removed. If any cancer cells remain, another slice is taken from that area and checked. These steps are repeated until the edges of the wound are clear of tumor cells, then the wound is closed. The advantage to this technique is that all of the visible cancer cells are removed, but as much normal skin as possible is spared. Mohs surgery is often used for larger or higher-risk tumors and when cosmetic considerations are important. The main disadvantage is that it takes much longer than conventional surgery and requires a specially trained surgeon.

In cryosurgery, liquid nitrogen is used to freeze the tumor and destroy it. This treatment is another type of blind destruction; there is no skin sample to make sure the cancer cells have all been killed. Patients often report swelling and pain after cryosurgery, and a wound appears a few days later where the cells were destroyed. Healing takes about four to six weeks. When the site heals, it has usually lost its normal pigment. There is also a risk of nerve damage with this technique. Cryosurgery is generally used only for small cancers in stage 0 and stage I.

In electrodesiccation and curettage, the physician scoops out the cancer cells with a spoon-shaped instrument called a curette. After most of the tumor is gone, the rest is destroyed with heat from an electrical current. The wound is left open to heal like an abrasion. It leaks fluid, crusts over, and heals during the next two to six weeks. This method is generally used only for the smallest squamous cell carcinomas (stage 0 and stage I). One disadvantage is that there is no skin sample to confirm that the tumor is completely gone. Also, the electrical current used during this surgery can interfere with some artificial cardiac pacemakers.

Some cases of Bowen's disease can be treated by applying a lotion containing the **chemotherapy** drug 5-fluorouracil (**fluorouracil** or 5-FU) to the tumor for several weeks. This treatment usually gives good cosmetic results. The side effects from 5-fluorouracil include allergies to the ingredients, infections, redness, peeling, crusting, sensitivity to the sun, and changes in skin color. The main disadvantage to this treatment is that the drug cannot penetrate very far, and cancer cells in the deeper parts of the tumor may not be destroyed.

Radiation therapy is sometimes used for squamous cell carcinomas, especially when the tumor is at a site where surgery would be difficult or remove a sizeable amount of tissue. This treatment is sometimes combined with surgery for cancers that have metastasized or are likely to. One disadvantage is that tumors returning after radiation tend to grow more quickly than the original cancer. In addition, **x-rays** may promote new skin cancers. The cosmetic results are usually good. In some cases, the skin may lose a little pigment or develop spider veins. Some doctors reserve radiation treatment for those over age 60. One drawback of radiation therapy for squamous cell carcinomas in or near the mouth is that the radiation may cause the tissues inside the mouth to break down.

Chemotherapy is often added to surgery or radiation for stage IV cancers.

Alternative and complementary therapies

Alternative treatments for squamous cell carcinoma usually attempt to prevent rather than treat this cancer. Options being tested include antioxidant **vitamins**, minerals, and green tea extracts.

Prognosis

Because many squamous cell carcinomas are not staged, precise five-year survival rates for each stage are not available. In general, the prognosis is very good for small squamous cell carcinomas that originate in actinic keratoses. However, cancers that are not completely destroyed may regrow. Tumors can redevelop in the scar from the surgery, on the edges of the surgery site, or deep in the skin. Larger or higher-risk tumors, cancers that regrow after treatment, and tumors that have invaded local tissues or metastasized are more difficult to cure. Most metastases appear within the first two years after a skin tumor has been removed. The five-year survival rate for metastatic cancers is 34%.

Coping with cancer treatment

Most squamous cell carcinomas are removed with techniques that cause few, if any, lasting side effects. Patients who have cosmetic concerns may wish to discuss them with their doctors.

Clinical trials

Clinical trials are government-regulated studies of new treatments and techniques that may prove beneficial in diagnosing or treating a disease. Participation is always voluntary and at no cost to the participant. Clinical trials are conducted in three phases. Phase 1 tests the safety of the treatment and looks for harmful side effects. Phase 2 tests the effectiveness of the treatment.

QUESTIONS TO ASK YOUR DOCTOR

- What treatment(s) would you recommend for my tumor?
- How effective would you expect each treatment to be for a tumor of this size and in this location?
- How much cosmetic damage am I likely to see with each?
- Are there any alternatives?
- How should I prepare for the procedure?
- What is the risk that my tumor will grow again?

Phase 3 compares the treatment to other treatments available for the same condition.

The selection of clinical trials under way changes frequently. Patients and their families can search for open trials on the **National Cancer Institute** website at http://www.cancer.gov/clinicaltrials/search.

Prevention

The most important risk factor for squamous cell carcinoma is exposure to the sun or other sources of ultraviolet light (such as **tanning** beds), combined with a lighter complexion and inability to tan. Most people receive 80% of their lifetime exposure to the sun before they reach the age of 20. For this reason, prevention should start during childhood and adolescence. Some important steps to prevent squamous cell carcinoma as well as other skin cancers include:

- Wear protective clothing and a wide-brimmed hat in the sun.
- Stay out of the sun from 10 A.M. to 4 P.M.
- Use a sunscreen that has a high sun protection factor (SPF).
- Do not use tanning booths or tanning beds.

Special concerns

Because many squamous cell carcinomas are found on the face and neck, cosmetic concerns are a priority for many patients. If there is a risk of noticeable scarring or damage, a patient may wish to ask about alternative types of removal or inquire about the services of a plastic surgeon.

After treatment, it is important to return to the doctor periodically to check for regrowth or new skin cancers.

Approximately a third to a half of all patients with nonmelanoma skin cancers find a new skin cancer within the next five years.

See also Basal cell carcinoma; Chemoprevention; Reconstructive surgery.

Resources

BOOKS

Burnes, Samuel, and Graham Chamberlain. *Squamous Cell Carcinoma: Causes, Tests and Treatment Options.* CreateSpace, 2012.

WEBSITES

American Academy of Dermatologists. "Squamous Cell Carcinoma." http://www.cancer.org/cancer/skincancer-basalandsquamouscell/detailedguide/index (accessed August 26, 2014).

American Cancer Society. "Basal and Squamous Cell Skin Cancer." http://www.cancer.org/cancer/skincancer-basalandsquamouscell/index (accessed August 26, 2013).

"Skin Cancer." MedlinePlus, June 7, 2014. http://www.nlm.nih.gov/medlineplus/skincancer.html (accessed August 26, 2014).

ORGANIZATIONS

American Academy of Dermatology, PO Box 4014, Schaumburg, IL 60168-4014, (866) 503-7546, Fax: (847) 240-1859, MRC@aad.org, http://www.aad.org.

American Cancer Society, 1599 Clifton Rd., NE, Atlanta, GA 30329, (404) 320-3333, (800) ACS-2345, http://www.cancer.org.

National Cancer Institute, BG 9609 MSC 9760, 9609 Medical Center Drive, Bethesda, MD 20892-9760, (800) 4-CANCER, TTY: (800) 332-8615, http://www.cancer.gov.

Anna Rovid Spickler, DVM, PhD
Rebecca J. Frey, PhD
REVISED BY TISH DAVIDSON, AM

Staging *see* **Tumor staging**

▌Stem cell transplantation

Definition

Stem cells are cells that can continuously reproduce themselves and produce other, more specialized types of differentiated cells. A stem cell transplant is a procedure that replaces unhealthy stem cells with healthy ones. Stem cells can be harvested from bone marrow, from peripheral blood, and from umbilical cord blood.

Purpose

Physicians use stem cell transplants to treat many diseases that damage or destroy bone marrow, found in the soft fatty tissue inside the bones. Examples of these diseases are leukemia and **multiple myeloma**. Some patients develop bone marrow disorders because of aggressive **cancer** treatments or as result of diseases such as aplastic **anemia**, which causes abnormal blood cell production.

Recent advances in stem cell research have made it a treatment possibility for patients with certain types of lymphomas, genetic disorders, hereditary metabolic disorders, and autoimmune disorders. These stem cells are typically not bone marrow stem cells but other types of stem cells. Researchers are hoping eventually to harvest stem cells to treat diseases such as Parkinson's disease, type 1 diabetes, Alzheimer's disease, liver disease, arthritis, and spinal cord injuries.

Description

Stem cell transplants sometimes are called hematopoietic stem cell transplants, bone marrow transplants, or cord blood transplants. Nearly 100 years ago, physicians tried to give patients with leukemia and anemia bone marrow by mouth. These treatments were not successful, but led to experiments showing that healthy bone marrow transfused into the bloodstream could restore damaged bone marrow.

Today, two types of stem cell transplants are performed most often. When a patient's own stem cells are collected (harvested) and then returned to the same patient's body, it is called an autologous transplant. Using stem cells from another person, or a donor, is called an allogeneic transplant. A third type, which is rare, is called a syngeneic transplant, in which the donor is an identical twin. In many cases, donor cells come from a close relative, such as a brother or sister. However, the likelihood that a sibling will match the patient is 25%. Stem cells may need to come from a person not related to the recipient.

To find out whether a patient can receive stem cells from a donor, physicians developed human leukocyte antigen (HLA) testing to match tissue types. The next challenge became finding donors. Throughout the 1980s and 1990s, private individuals, hospitals, foundations, and states worked to set up a nationwide registry of bone marrow donors. The National Marrow Donor Program (NMDP) now has the largest stem cell donor registry in the world. As of 2014, there were more than 10.5 million donors registered through the NMDP. However, ethnic minorities represented only a small percentage of the donors to the NMDP, often making it more difficult to provide a donor to a member of an ethnic minority requiring a stem cell transplant.

Stem cell transplants normally take place at specialized centers. Procurement of stem cells from the donor can be accomplished in several ways: from the bone marrow; from the peripheral blood; and, less commonly, from umbilical cord blood.

Donor cells harvested directly from the bone marrow are taken in an operating room while the patient (or the donor) is under regional or general anesthesia. Bone marrow normally is harvested from the top of the hip bone. The marrow usually is filtered, treated, and either transplanted immediately or frozen for later use.

Stem cells can also be harvested from a donor's peripheral blood during apheresis once a process called stem cell mobilization has occurred. Hematopoietic stem cells are typically found in low concentrations in the circulating peripheral blood. Stem cells can be mobilized to enter the peripheral blood by administering the hematopoietic growth factor, granulocyte colony-stimulating factor (G-CSF) (**filgrastim** or lenograstim) to the donor. After about four days, enough stem cells are available in the circulating peripheral blood to be harvested. During a three- to four-hour apheresis collection process, more stem cells can typically be collected than during a bone marrow harvest, without the need for general anesthesia and an operating room setting.

Bone marrow transplantation is considered superior to peripheral blood stem cell transplant (PBSCT) for most nonmalignant conditions. Peripheral blood stem cell transplant is considered superior to bone marrow transplant when rapid engraftment of stem cells is needed. PBSCT is also associated with early hospital discharges, decreased relapse rates, and decreased mortality rates. However, PBSCT is associated with increased incidence of **graft-versus-host disease** (GVHD), a post-transplant complication.

Stem cells are transfused through an intravenous (IV) catheter that physicians insert in the patient's neck or chest. The procedure is usually done in the patient's hospital room. This part of the transplant process is referred to as the "rescue process." The stem cells replace malignant or defective cells. Transplanted donor cells travel to the bone cavities and begin replacing old bone marrow.

Demographics

The number of stem cell transplants performed continues to increase. It is estimated that between 30,000 to 40,000 transplantations are performed on an annual basis worldwide; this number is increasing by up to 20% yearly.

Precautions

The transplant team will weigh many factors when determining whether a patient is a candidate for stem cell transplantation, including overall health and function of many vital organ systems. Stem cell transplantation is an aggressive treatment and may not be recommended for some patients, including those with heart, kidney, or lung disorders. If the patient has an aggressive cancer that has spread throughout the body, he or she may not be considered a candidate for a stem cell transplant. It once was thought that stem cell transplants were not safe in patients over age 60, but research shows that some elderly patients can safely receive stem cells from donors.

Many ethical and legal factors are affecting the research and development into stem cell transplantation. Much debate surrounds scientific advances. For example, human embryos, fetal tissues and umbilical cords are sources of stem cells that may be transplanted or used for disease research. Some people have ethical problems with the use of embryos in fertility clinics for stem cell research or transplantation. Some link stem cell transplantation for disease with cloning and want to stop funding for stem cell research over fear of human cloning. A study released in 2005 stated that 63% of Americans back embryonic stem cell research and 70% support federal legislation to promote more research. Meanwhile, scientists continue to develop new and exciting possibilities for transplanting stem cells into the human body that may one day lead to new treatments for previously incurable diseases. Many do so with private funding. However, the most common type of stem cell transplant, with bone marrow, is not controversial.

Preparation

Standard preparation involves eliminating diseased and damaged cells. The exact process depends on the patient and the disease or condition being treated. In many cases when transplantation is done to treat cancer, the patient will receive **chemotherapy**, often in extremely high doses. Some also receive **radiation therapy**. Another goal of preparation is to suppress the immune system, which makes it less likely that the patient's body will reject the donated stem cells. This step is called the conditioning regimen and is considered a crucial element in stem cell transplantation. New advances have been made that allow some of the patient's diseased cells to remain and mix with the new cells. Immediately before transplantation, the treating physician and staff will give the patient special instructions and precautions, depending on his or her disease and exact procedure. Many serious side effects are associated with the preparative regimens, including nausea, vomiting, hair loss (**alopecia**), **diarrhea**, skin rashes, mouth sores, and ulcers, as well as lung, liver, and neurological toxicities. Another serious result of the conditioning regimen is infertility. Sperm banking may be an option for some men. Preservation of female fertility by banking of oocytes (eggs) has not been as successful.

Aftercare

Stem cells take up to three weeks or longer to begin producing new cells or bone marrow, a process called engraftment. Until engraftment is complete, patients may bleed easily and are at high risk for the development of life-threatening infections. To reduce the risk of infection, patients are hospitalized in high-efficiency particulate air (HEPA) filtered rooms that are sealed using positive air pressure. All individuals entering the room should practice strict hand hygiene to minimize the potential to spread infection. Patients may be required to stay in the hospital for at least one week following transplantation until blood cell counts reach a safe level. Patients who received autologous transplants can often be managed on an outpatient basis. Once home, patients must be closely monitored, must be careful not to risk infection, may be anemic, and may be extremely fatigued. Most patients will receive prophylactic antibiotic and **antifungal therapy** for 75–100 days after the transplant and will be monitored very closely for the occurrence of graft-versus-host disease and other transplant-related side effects.

Risks

In addition to the risk of a life-threatening infection following a stem cell transplant, patients receiving stem cells from donors risk serious complications from graft-versus-host disease (GVHD). GVHD is caused when the donor's cells react against the patient's (recipient's) tissue. Sometimes, the patient's body simply rejects the new cells. Researchers continue to explore ways to lessen risks of complications following stem cell transplants.

Resources

BOOKS

Rowley, S. D., and H. Benn. "Collection and Processing of Peripheral Blood Stem Cells and Bone Marrow." In *Blood Banking and Transfusion Medicine*, 2nd ed. Edited by C. D. Hillyer, L. E. Silberstein, and P. M. Ness. Philadelphia: Churchill Livingstone/Elsevier, 2007.

Wingard, John R., et al., eds. *Hematopoietic Stem Cell Transplantation: A Handbook for Clinicians.* 2nd ed. Bethesda, MD: AABB, 2015.

PERIODICALS

Copelan, E. A. "Hematopoietic Stem-Cell Transplantation." *New England Journal of Medicine* 354, no. 17 (2006): 1813–26.

Doubek, M., et al. "Autologous Hematopoietic Stem Cell Transplantation in Adult Acute Lymphoblastic Leukemia: Still Not Out of Fashion." *Annnals of Hematology* 88, no. 9 (2009): 881–7.

Lubin, B. H., and W. T. Shearer. "Cord Blood Banking for Potential Future Transplantation." *Pediatrics* 119, no. 1 (2007): 165–70.

WEBSITES

American Cancer Society. "Stem Cell Transplant (Peripheral Blood, Bone Marrow, and Cord Blood Transplants)." http://www.cancer.org/treatment/treatmentsandsideeffects/treatmenttypes/bonemarrowandperipheralbloodstemcelltransplant/bone-marrow-and-peripheral-blood-stem-cell-transplant-toc (accessed October 21, 2013).

Multiple Myeloma Research Foundation. "Treatment Options—Stem Cell Transplantation." http://www.themmrf.org/living-with-multiple-myeloma/patients-starting-treatment/treatment-options/stem-cell-transplantation.html (accessed October 21, 2013).

National Heart, Lung, and Blood Institute. "What Is a Blood and Marrow Stem Cell Transplant?" http://www.nhlbi.nih.gov/health/health-topics/topics/bmsct (accessed October 21, 2013).

National Institutes of Health. "Stem Cell Basics." http://stemcells.nih.gov/info/basics/Pages/Default.aspx (accessed October 21, 2013).

ORGANIZATIONS

International Myeloma Foundation (IMF), 12650 Riverside Dr., Ste. 206, North Hollywood, CA 91607–3421, (800) 452-CURE, http://www.myeloma.org.

National Marrow Donor Program (NMDP), 3001 Broadway St. NE, Ste. 100, Minneapolis, MN 55413–1753, (800) 627-7692, http://www.marrow.org.

Teresa G. Odle
Melinda Granger Oberleitner, RN, DNS, APRN, CNS

Stenting

Definition

Stenting is a procedure in which a cylindrical structure (stent) is placed into a hollow tubular organ to provide artificial support and maintain the patency of the opening. Although it is most often used for cardiovascular functioning, it is also utilized to manage obstructions in **cancer** patients.

Purpose

Stents are used in cancer patients to relieve obstructions due to:

- direct blockages within the tube (or lumen) due to cancer growth
- narrowing of the lumen from tumor growth outside pressing on the tube and narrowing the lumen
- occasionally from the buildup of scar tissue (fibrosis) from radiation therapy

Tumors most likely to cause obstruction requiring stent placement include **esophageal cancer**, **bronchogenic carcinoma**, **pancreatic cancer**, cancers of the bile duct, and occasionally colorectal carcinomas.

Description

Endoscopic retrograde cholangiopancreatography (ERCP) is the name of the procedure utilized to place most stents for pancreatic and biliary tumors. ERCP is performed with a flexible endoscope, which can be directed and moved around the many bends in the upper gastrointestinal tract. The newer video endoscopes have a tiny, optically sensitive computer chip at the end which transmits electronic signals through the scope to a computer that displays an image on a large video screen. The scope has an open channel that permits other instruments to be passed through it to perform biopsies,

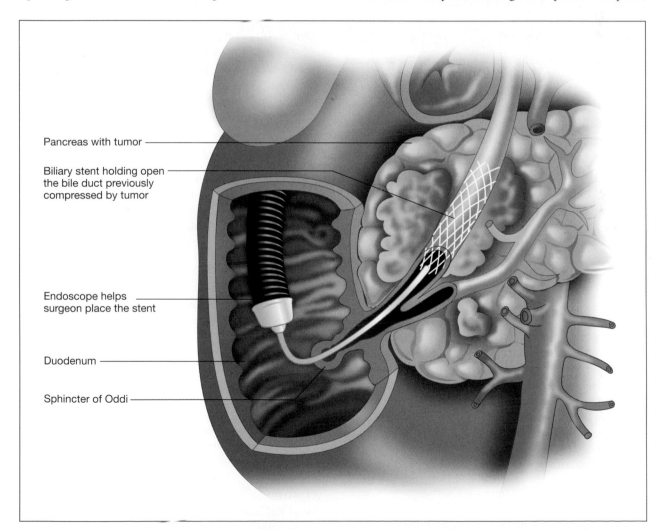

Pancreas with tumor

Biliary stent holding open the bile duct previously compressed by tumor

Endoscope helps surgeon place the stent

Duodenum

Sphincter of Oddi

Illustration showing the insertion of a biliary stent. (*Illustration by Electronic Illustrators Group. © Cengage Learning®.*)

inject solutions, or place stents. Since ERCP uses x-ray films, the procedure takes place in an x-ray area. Initially the throat is anesthetized with a spray solution and the patient is also usually mildly sedated. The endoscope is inserted into the upper esophagus and a thin tube is inserted through it to the main bile duct entering the intestinal area. Dye is injected into the bile duct and/or the pancreatic duct, and x-ray films are taken. The patient usually lies on the left side and then turns onto the stomach to allow complete visualization of the ducts. The patient is able to breathe easily throughout the exam and rarely gags. Any gallstones found may be removed, or if the duct has become narrowed, an incision can be made using electrocautery (electrical heat) to relieve the blockage. It is also possible to widen narrowed ducts by placing stents in these areas to keep them open. The patient is taken to recovery following the procedure, which takes 20–40 minutes.

Other endoscopes are used to place stents elsewhere in the body. For example, an esophagoscope is used to place stents in cases of esophageal cancer, a bronchoscope is used for procedures involving endobronchial obstructions, and a colonoscope is used in cases of colorectal obstructions.

Precautions

Every patient should be viewed individually, with special consideration given to the patient's present status. Generally, surgical procedures are for the correction of a problem; but in many cancer cases, relief of symptoms is the only therapeutic option. Since it is extremely difficult to remove or reposition these stents after they are placed, the degree of relief to be offered by stent insertion should be significant. The physician and the patient should discuss all alternatives and come to a mutual decision.

Preparation

The patient is instructed not to eat or drink anything for eight hours prior to the procedure. Some physicians may request that no aspirin be taken for a certain time period prior to the procedure to prevent excessive bleeding.

Aftercare

The patient may go home after the procedure or may spend one or two nights in the hospital. **Antibiotics** may be given, especially if there has been long-standing biliary obstruction. Dietary restrictions are common after esophageal and colorectal stenting.

Risks

The most serious risk associated with the placement of a stent is the risk of perforation. If a tear is made, leakage with life-threatening infection may occur. Migration or recurrent obstruction may necessitate repeat stenting if possible. Occasionally bleeding may occur.

Results

Relief of the obstruction with resumption of the ability to eat, breathe, normally clear fluids from the liver or pancreas, or allow normal passage of stool is the desired result of this procedure.

Abnormal results

A sudden change in the degree of pain and/or **fever** that persists, as well as any unusual changes, should be communicated immediately to a physician.

Resources

WEBSITES

Cancer Research UK. "Stents and Surgery for Advanced Gallbladder Cancer." http://www.cancerresearchuk.org/about-cancer/type/gallbladder-cancer/treatment/advanced/

stents-and-surgery-for-advanced-gallbladder-cancer (accessed November 14, 2014).

ORGANIZATIONS

American Cancer Society, 250 Williams St. NW, Atlanta, GA 30303, (800) 227-2345, http://www.cancer.org.

American Society of Clinical Oncology (ASCO), 2318 Mill Rd., Ste. 800, Alexandria, VA 22314, (571) 483-1300, (888) 651-3038, contactus@cancer.net, http://www.asco. org.

National Digestive Diseases Information Clearinghouse, 2 Information Way, Bethesda, MD 20892-3570, (800) 891-5389, TTY: (866) 569-1162, Fax: (703) 738-4929, nddic@info.niddk.nih.gov, http://www.digestive.niddk. nih.gov.

Linda K. Bennington, C.N.S., M.S.N.

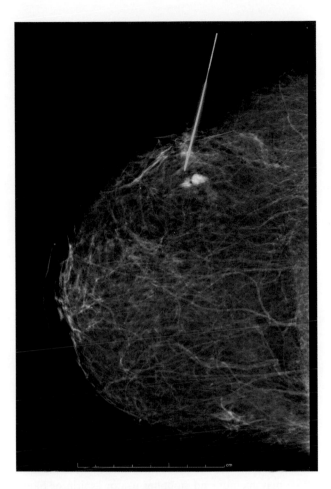

Stereotactic needle biopsy of the breast. *(Apogee/Science Source)*

Stereotactic needle biopsy

Definition

Needle **biopsy** is a way for doctors to collect a small sample of tissue from a tumor or other suspicious area, using imaging to guide the needle. Stereotactic needle biopsy uses a special imaging method with two angles to help a radiologist pinpoint a mass.

Purpose

Stereotactic needle biopsy is most often used to sample nonpalpable (unable to be felt) abnormalities of the breast found on a woman's mammogram. This biopsy procedure uses a large (core) or small (fine) needle that withdraws samples of the abnormal breast tissue. The doctor uses specially equipped **mammography** equipment to guide the needle to the site of the identified mass. The needle is used to remove tissue samples at the site for laboratory analysis. Doctors can take biopsies with needles using other types of imaging to guide them, such as ultrasound or **magnetic resonance imaging**. Stereotactic guidance is used often for breast biopsies because it is a mammography technique. With stereotactic guidance, radiologists can obtain a sample through the skin. This technique spares the patient from more invasive surgery.

Description

The patient is made comfortable with a local anesthesia injection before the procedure begins. First, the patient lies face down on a table with her breast suspended through an opening or sits with her breast placed on a mammography unit. The woman's breast is compressed, as it is for a screening mammogram. Then a certified mammographer, or radiologic technologist, takes mammograms of the suspicious area of the breast from several different angles. This technique creates a virtual three-dimensional (stereotactic) picture of the abnormal area. A computer is used to guide the needle to the site for sample removal. The samples are examined in the laboratory by a pathologist (a physician trained in identification of pathological or abnormal findings) to determine if **cancer** cells are present.

There are two different types of needles used for stereotactic needle biopsy. The procedures are similar, but the size of the needle varies. A fine-needle biopsy is most often used when a cyst is suspected. Fine-needle biopsy is often done with ultrasound guidance. The doctor is able to suction a sample of fluid or tissue through the needle and send it for analysis. The needle is smaller and so is the sample of fluid or tissue extracted. In a core needle biopsy, the needle is larger; has a cutting edge; and enables the physician to extract a larger tissue sample from the suspicious area, often with the assistance of a tiny vacuum to help pull the tissue sample into the collector. A larger tissue sample helps the pathologist more accurately identify the presence of cancer cells.

Usually the physician will use a local injectable anesthetic agent at the needle insertion site to numb the area. When the anesthetic is injected at the biopsy site, the patient will feel a stinging sensation. The physician will wait until the numbing agent takes effect and then proceed with the biopsy. The patient may feel a pressure sensation as the needle is guided to the biopsy site.

Preparation

A biopsy is used to confirm whether a finding on imaging or during a clinical breast examination is cancerous. Many biopsy results are negative, meaning that the lump, mass, or other abnormality does not indicate cancer. If a woman needs a breast biopsy, she should know that most biopsies result in negative findings. Pain and discomfort from image-guided breast biopsies is minimal for most patients, but studies have shown that if a woman is anxious or worried about pain, she is more likely to report pain after the procedure.

All patients should provide written informed consent before any biopsy. The consent document should explain the patient's treatment options, risks and benefits of the procedure, and potential complications. Patients do not need to prepare for the procedure, although the doctor's office may recommend stopping use of aspirin or blood thinners before the biopsy procedure. Women should avoid use of deodorant, talcum powder, lotion, perfume, or ointment under their arms and on their breasts the day of the procedure. Use of these products can affect the imaging results.

Precautions

Patients should discuss the reasons for undergoing a stereotactic needle biopsy with their doctor. The procedure has been studied extensively with positive outcomes for accuracy of results, but it might not be the best procedure for all patients. Some masses in the breast cannot be seen well using mammography. These women might be better candidates for ultrasound guidance or open biopsy.

Physicians decide to order a biopsy to diagnose **breast cancer** based on findings from mammograms and other imaging, clinical breast examination, and a woman's medical history. The American College of Radiology has developed a system used by radiologists to categorize findings that enable doctors to systematically determine and report whether a finding is suspicious enough to warrant a biopsy. For example, a category 5

QUESTIONS TO ASK YOUR DOCTOR

- What type of physician performs a stereotactic needle biopsy?
- How long will it take to interpret the biopsy results?
- What type of pain management will be used during the procedure?
- Can the biopsy give false negative results?
- Will I have a fine-needle biopsy or core biopsy? Why?

---

finding is highly suggestive of malignancy. The physician can use information from a stereotactic needle biopsy to confirm a breast cancer diagnosis and expedite treatment. Other categories with lower numbers suggest cancer but are not as certain. Doctors can determine whether a mass in the breast is a cancerous mass only by studying its cells.

Stereotactic needle biopsy is not indicated in all cases in which there is nonpalpable breast tissue abnormality. The size of the patient and size of the breast must be considered because a certain breast thickness is necessary for mammogram-guided biopsy. Areas of breast tissue microcalcification (tiny areas of thickened breast tissue that contain calcium) that are not closely clustered together can be difficult to visualize in a stereotactic system and therefore difficult to retrieve during biopsy. Finally, the patient must be able to remain still and lie face down for the duration of the biopsy procedure (20 minutes). Any movement by the patient can render the localization of the abnormal site invalid.

Aftercare

The patient might experience mild pain or discomfort at the biopsy site following the procedure. Mild bruising at the site also sometimes occurs. For these reasons, the physician might suggest that activities be limited for 24 to 48 hours after the procedure. The physician will suggest or prescribe a medication for discomfort relief. Often, a sport bra or other firm support garment will minimize breast movement and increase post-procedure comfort. Icing the area is often recommended. The physician will inform the patient of further follow-up care needed to monitor the patient's ongoing breast health and the subsequent intervals for follow-up imaging.

Risks

Patients who have a stereotactic needle biopsy procedure might need a repeat procedure. A repeat biopsy is necessary in the absence of concordance, or the presence of a discrepancy between the radiology reports and the pathologist's findings from laboratory analysis of the sample. Stereotactic imaging uses some radiation. To be well informed, patients should consult with their physician about the risks prior to undergoing stereotactic needle biopsy.

Results

Stereotactic needle biopsy is a diagnostic tool used to determine the presence of cancer cells. It is not a therapy used to remove or destroy area of abnormal tissue. The results of the biopsy help the physician to determine the best medical or surgical options available to the patient. The biopsy results are reviewed by the physician performing the biopsy and by the pathologist who analyzes the sample. Results are reviewed and discussed with the patient and options for further treatment or follow-up are presented. The patient, with the guidance and expertise of the physician, selects a course of therapy.

Resources

BOOKS

DeVita, Vincent T., Jr., Samuel Hellman, and Steven A. Rosenberg, editors. *Cancer: Principles and Practice of Oncology.* Philadelphia: Lippincott Williams & Wilkins, 2001.

PERIODICALS

Huang, M.L., et al. "Stereotactic Breast Biopsy: Pitfalls and Pearls." *Techniques in Vascular and Interventional Radiology* 17 (March 2014): 32–39.

WEBSITES

"Pain, Anxiety Linked in Image-Guided Core-Needle Breast Biopsies." DiagnosticImaging.com. http://www.diagnostic imaging.com/ultrasound/pain-anxiety-linked-image-guided-core-needle-breast biopsies (accessed August 1, 2014).
"Stereotactic Breast Biopsy." American College of Radiology and Radiological Society of North America. http://www. radiologyinfo.org/en/info.cfm?pg=breastbixr (accessed August 1, 2014).

OTHER

Bassett l., D. P. Winchester, R. B. Caplan, D. D. Dershaw, et al. "Stereotactic Core-Needle Biopsy of the Breast: A Report of the Joint Task Force of the American College of Radiology, American College of Surgeons, and College of American Pathologists."

Molly Metzler, R.N., B.S.N.
REVISED BY TERESA G. ODLE

Stereotactic surgery

Definition

Stereotactic surgery is a minimally invasive surgical technique that is performed to diagnose (**biopsy**) or treat a tumor. It is performed most often to diagnose and treat tumors in the brain and spinal cord but is also performed for other disorders related to damaged brain tissue, head injuries, or small tumors within the head. It has also been used for biopsy and surgery of the breast and certain small tumors in the lungs and liver.

The two most common stereotactic procedures are stereotactic neurosurgery and stereotactic radiosurgery. Stereotactic neurosurgery uses a conventional incision and drill to enter the patient's skull and remove tissue for biopsy or remove a cancerous (malignant) or noncancerous (benign) tumor. Stereotactic radiosurgery is a form of **radiation therapy** that focuses external beams of radiation precisely on the tumor to destroy cancerous tissue. It is not actually surgery and no incisions are made. The stereotactic

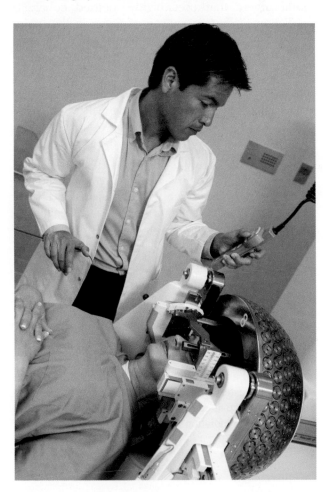

Patient preparing for stereotactic surgery. *(Monkey Business Images/Shutterstock.com)*

KEY TERMS

Atlas—In anatomy, a collection of medical illustrations of one specific subject, such as the brain or heart. Detailed atlases of the brain are important guides for surgeons performing stereotactic neurosurgery.

Biopsy—Removal of a small sample of tissue for examination under a microscope; used in the diagnosis of cancer.

Collimator—A metal tube designed to control the size and direction of a beam of radiation.

Cyclotron—A machine that accelerates charged atomic particles within a constant magnetic field.

Fractionated—In radiotherapy, treatment that is divided into several sessions of smaller doses of radiation rather than one large dose delivered in a single session.

Gamma knife—The name for a specific type of radiosurgery that uses highly focused cobalt-60 radiation to destroy cancerous tissue in the brain. It is not a knife in the conventional sense.

Hydrocephalus—A condition marked by the buildup of cerebrospinal fluid within the skull, causing increased pressure on the brain and a variety of neurologic symptoms. Stereotactic surgery can be used to place a catheter within the brain in order to drain the excess fluid.

Landmark—An anatomical structure that is easy to recognize and suitable as a reference point in locating other structures or making measurements.

Photon—A quantum of electromagnetic radiation with no mass and no charge.

Posterior commissure—A bundle of fibers that connects the two cerebral hemispheres near the third ventricle of the brain.

Radiosurgery—A form of radiation therapy in which tissue is destroyed by external beam radiation. In spite of its name, radiosurgery is not actually surgery and no incision is made.

Ventricles—Small cavities within the brain filled with cerebrospinal fluid.

---

procedures are often guided by **computed tomography** (CT) or **magnetic resonance imaging** (MRI).

Purpose

Stereotactic surgery is performed either to obtain a sample of tumor tissue for biopsy or to remove or destroy a tumor. A stereotactic biopsy is the preferred method of diagnosing a brain tumor because it is exceptionally precise and can obtain a tissue sample even when the tumor is located deep within the brain.

Stereotactic radiosurgery is most often used to treat movement disorders such as Parkinson disease, Huntington chorea, and essential tremor; however, it is sometimes used to treat malformations of blood vessels, malignant **brain tumors**, benign brain tumors (acoustic neuromas, pituitary adenomas, and meningiomas), and tumors of the spinal cord. It can also be used to treat cancers in the nose or other small and well-defined parts of the body, or as a follow-up booster treatment for patients with recurrent tumors who have already received the maximum safe dose of conventional radiation therapy.

Description

Stereotactic surgery

Stereotactic surgery is performed using a stereotactic frame, which consists of a plaster cap fitted to the patient with a head ring and an attached electrode carrier. The ring is attached to the patient's scalp as well as to the operating table to hold the patient's head steady. After taking CT or MRI scans, the surgeon is able to create a map or atlas of the patient's brain to guide the procedure. Specific coordinates are identified using these images to pinpoint the location of the drill entry site and of the tumor. These coordinates are entered into a computer that determines the final path of the surgeon's instruments. Another tool called an arc ring is then attached to the head ring to guide the surgeon's movements. The stereotactic system allows the surgeon to make only a tiny incision (less than one-quarter of an inch long) in the scalp and drill a hole smaller in diameter than a pencil in order to insert a biopsy needle or an electrode.

Some medical centers use a frameless method for stereotactic brain surgery. In this method, images of the patient's head from CT or MRI scans are uploaded into a computer for display on a monitor. Markers on the patient's skin are registered by a probe linked to the computer by a camera, which joins the position of the patient's head on the operating table to the images on the computer monitor. In addition, the surgeon's instruments contain light-emitting diodes (LEDs) that are tracked by the computer during the operation.

Stereotactic radiosurgery and radiotherapy

Stereotactic radiosurgery (SRS) is performed with three different types of computer-assisted medical devices that provide the radiation used to kill **cancer** cells. The gamma knife is a stationary unit that contains 201 sources of gamma rays derived from cobalt-60 that can be focused by a computer on a single small area of the brain. The radiation can be directed precisely to the tumor without destroying nearby healthy tissue. The patient lies on a couch with a large helmet attached to the head frame. The helmet contains holes that allow beams of radiation to enter. The couch then slides into a frame containing the cobalt-60. Treatment time varies from several minutes to over an hour, depending on the size, shape, and location of the tumor. Gamma knife radiosurgery is usually a single-dose treatment.

Radiosurgery can also be performed with a linear accelerator (also called a LINAC), a device that produces high-energy photons for treating larger tumors, metastatic tumors, or arteriovenous malformations (abnormal arteries or veins). Linear accelerators are preferred for multisession treatments using smaller doses of radiation. Radiosurgery performed with several smaller doses (as opposed to one large dose) is known as fractionated radiosurgery; some doctors prefer to call it fractionated stereotactic radiotherapy (FSR). The advantage of fractionated treatment is that it allows a higher total dose of radiation to be delivered to the tumor over time without harming nearby normal tissues. Unlike the gamma knife unit, the LINAC moves around the patient during treatment, delivering arcs of radiation matched by computer to the shape of the tumor.

The third type of device that can be used for radiosurgery is a cyclotron, which is a nuclear reactor used to accelerate charged particles (usually protons or ions) to high levels of energy that can be used for radiosurgery. Cyclotrons are available in only a few large medical centers specializing in cancer treatment. **Clinical trials** continue to compare radiosurgery performed with a cyclotron to radiosurgery using a gamma knife or LINAC.

Precautions

Stereotactic surgery or radiosurgery should be done only by qualified specialists who are experienced in these techniques and performed only in treatment centers with the necessary equipment.

Stereotactic radiosurgery with a gamma knife is most effective in treating relatively small tumors (an inch or less in diameter) with well-defined borders that have not invaded the brain; this procedure is usually reserved for patients with a life expectancy of six months or longer. Large brain tumors may require partial removal by conventional open surgery prior to treatment with stereotactic radiosurgery.

Preparation

Preparation for stereotactic surgery or radiosurgery can be invasive. No food or drink is allowed after midnight the night before the procedure, and the patient is given an intravenous sedative the morning of the procedure. A local anesthetic is applied at four points on the scalp without shaving the head. After the skin has been numbed, the surgeon fastens the base ring to the patient's skull with four pins, with the insertion points of the pins determined by the brain tumor location. CT or MRI scans are performed to provide images of the tumor and surrounding areas in three dimensions. The planning and procedure can take from 3 to 12 hours.

Some cancer centers use a less invasive form of patient preparation that consists of an individualized mouthpiece used to attach a headframe or "halo" to the patient's head, which prevents the head from moving during treatment.

Stereotactic radiosurgery is always preceded by a careful review of the patient's records to make sure that this type of treatment is appropriate for the tumor. The patient may be given steroid medications to control swelling of brain tissue or antiepileptic drugs to prevent seizures prior to radiosurgery.

Prior to receiving fractionated radiosurgery, a simulation scan will be performed to help the neurosurgeon plan the treatment. The simulation scan involves making a set of images that show the exact location of the tumor in relation to normal brain tissue. The first step of the procedure is to create a thermoplastic mask that allows the surgeon to precisely position the patient's head each time the patient receives a treatment. Next, the patient is placed in a scanner while wearing the mask. The simulation scan takes about two and a half hours. When the patient returns for additional treatment sessions, the molded thermoplastic mask is applied to reposition the patient's head in the exact location used for the simulation scan. Fractionated treatments usually take between 30 and 90 minutes each to complete.

A preparatory scan is not needed with newer lightweight linear accelerators that use robots to direct the radiation beam rather than a frame to hold the head in place. If the patient moves during treatment, the robot detects the movement and repositions the linear accelerator before the radiation beam is delivered.

Aftercare

Stereotactic surgery

When the procedure is finished, the surgeon closes the scalp incision with a single stitch and removes the base ring from its attachment points on the scalp by unscrewing the pins. These holes are small and require only a sterile cover rather than stitches. Antibiotic medication may be applied to prevent infection. The patient is taken to a recovery room and remains in the hospital overnight for observation. Patients are typically able to go home the next day but must arrange for transportation. A follow-up visit with the neurosurgeon is scheduled for 6 to 12 weeks after treatment.

Stereotactic radiosurgery

Patients receiving gamma knife treatment can be treated as outpatients, which means they are able to return home after the procedure. If pins were used to attach a head frame to the patient's scalp, the head will be wrapped with gauze for about two hours before the patient is discharged. Patients are sometimes hospitalized overnight for observation. Most patients resume normal activities within a day or two.

Side effects

Stereotactic neurosurgery and stereotactic radiosurgery have few side effects. The most common side effects are generally related to swelling of brain tissue and are of short duration; these may include nausea, vomiting, dizziness, and headaches. Patients may have hair loss in the area treated by stereotactic radiosurgery, but this condition will correct itself as the hair follicles heal. Delayed reactions can occur weeks and months after treatment, including cell death in the region of high-dose radiation, symptoms of tumor regrowth, or stroke.

Risks

Stereotactic surgery

The risks associated with stereotactic surgery are similar to those of other surgical procedures involving open incisions in the head or neck:

• infection

• scarring

• pain

• incomplete removal of the tumor

• swelling of brain tissue

• worsening of neurologic symptoms

• anesthesia reaction

Stereotactic radiosurgery

The risks associated with stereotactic radiosurgery are similar to those for other forms of radiation treatment of the brain or spinal cord:

• nausea and vomiting

• headaches

• dizziness

• fatigue

• hair loss

• radiation necrosis (a group or collection of dead brain cells)

• leukoencephalopathy (damage to the white matter of the brain)

• swelling of brain tissue

Results

Anticipated results of stereotactic surgery include obtaining an appropriate tissue sample for biopsy or removal of cancerous tissue. Anticipated results of stereotactic radiosurgery include destruction or death of cancer cells in the brain or spinal cord, drainage of excess cerebrospinal fluid, or improvement in tremor and other symptoms of Parkinson disease or Huntington chorea.

See also Brain and central nervous system tumors; Stereotactic needle biopsy.

Resources

BOOKS

Pazdur, Richard, et al, eds. *Cancer Management: A Multidisciplinary Approach.* 13th ed. Norwalk, CT: UBM Medica, 2010.

Porter, Robert S., Justin L. Kaplan, eds. "Neurologic Disorders." In *The Merck Manual of Diagnosis and Therapy*, sec. 13. Whitehouse Station, NJ: Merck Research Laboratories, 2011.

PERIODICALS

Ahmed, Z., Bet al. "Postoperative Stereotactic Radiosurgery for Resected Brain Metastases." *CNS Oncology* 3 (May 2014): 199–207.

Nieder, C., A. L. Grosu, and L. E. Gaspar. "Stereotactic Radiosurgery (SRS) for Brain Metastases: A Systematic Review." *Radiation Oncology* 9 (July 2014): 155.

Patil, C. G., et al. "Whole Brain Radiation Therapy (WBRT) Alone versus WBRT and Radiosurgery for the Treatment of Brain Metastases." *Cochrane Database System Review* 9 (Sept. 2012): CD006121.

Yen, C. P., et al. "Gamma Knife Surgery for Incidental Cerebral Arteriovenous Malformations." *Journal of Neurosurgery* 3 (Aug. 2014): 1–7.

Yen, C. P., and L. Steiner. "Gamma Knife Surgery for Brainstem Arteriovenous Malformations." *World Neurosurgery* 76 (Jul/Aug 2011): 87–95.

"The Use of Stereotactic Radiosurgery for the Treatment of Spinal Axis Tumors: A Review." *Clinical and Neurological Neurosurgery* 125C (August 2014): 166–72.

WEBSITES

American Brain Tumor Association (ABTA). "Stereotactic Radiosurgery." http://www.abta.org/brain-tumor-treatment/treatments/stereotactic-radiosurgery (accessed Sept. 5, 2014).

ORGANIZATIONS

American Brain Tumor Association, 8550 West Bryn Mawr Avenue, Chicago, IL 60631, (773) 577-8750, http://www.abta.org.

American Cancer Society, 1599 Clifton Rd. NE, Atlanta, GA 30329-4251, (800) ACS-2345 (227-2345), http://www.cancer.org.

International Radiosurgery Support Association (IRSA), 3005 Hoffman Street, Harrisburg, PA 17110, (717) 260-9808, http://www.irsa.org.

Rebecca Frey, PhD
REVISED BY L. LEE CULVERT
REVIEWED BY MARIANNE VAHEY, MD

STI-571 *see* **Imatinib mesylate**

Stilphostrol *see* **Diethylstilbestrol diphosphate**

Stivarga *see* **Regorafenib**

Stomach cancer

Definition

Stomach **cancer** (also known as gastric cancer) is a disease in which the cells forming the inner lining of the stomach become abnormal and start to divide uncontrollably, forming a mass called a tumor.

Description

The stomach is a J-shaped organ that lies in the left and central portion of the abdomen. The stomach produces many digestive juices and acids that mix with

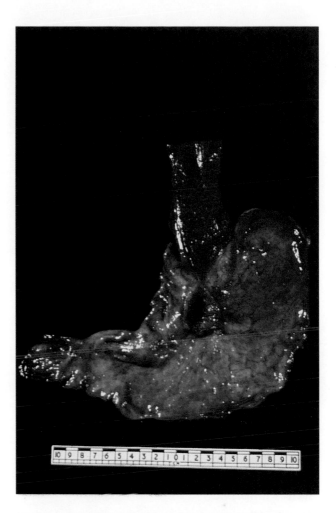

An excised section of a human stomach showing a cancerous tumor (center, triangular shape). *(SPL/Customer Medical Stock Photography)*

the food and aid in the process of digestion. There are five regions of the stomach that doctors refer to when determining the origin of stomach cancer. These are:

- the cardia, the area surrounding the cardiac sphincter that controls the movement of food from the esophagus into the stomach
- the fundus, the upper expanded area adjacent to the cardiac region
- the antrum, the lower region of the stomach where it begins to narrow
- the prepyloric region, just before or nearest the pylorus
- the pylorus, the terminal region where the stomach joins the small intestine

Cancer can develop in any of the five sections of the stomach; about 40% of cancers develop in the lower part; 40% in the middle part; and 15% in the upper part; 10% involve more than one part of the stomach. Symptoms and outcomes of the disease will vary depending on the location of the cancer. In the last twenty years a trend of decreasing incidence of gastric tumors diagnosed in the gastric body and distal stomach has been noted, while the incidence of cancers in the gastroesophageal junction and cardiac areas has increased dramatically. The reason for this change in incidence patterns is not yet fully understood.

Most gastric cancers are adenocarcinomas and begin in the gastric mucosa (the inner lining of the stomach). Adenocarcinomas comprise 90–95% of stomach tumors. Other less common types of stomach cancers are lymphomas, carcinoid tumors, and gastrointestinal stromal tumors (GISTs).

Risk factors

Risk factors associated with the development of stomach cancer include:

- Age: The risk of stomach cancer increases sharply after age 50.
- Sex: Men are more likely than women to develop stomach cancer.
- Race/ethnicity: Asian Americans/Pacific Islanders, Hispanic Americans, and African Americans have higher rates of stomach cancer than Caucasians. Native Americans have the lowest rates.
- Family history: People with a first-degree relative (parent, child, or sibling) with stomach cancer are at increased risk.
- Obesity: Obesity is associated with an increased risk of stomach cancer in men; it is not known as of 2014 whether it is a risk factor in women.
- Infection with the bacterium *Helicobacter pylori*: Chronic (long-term) infection of the stomach with these bacteria may lead to a particular type of cancer (lymphoma or mucosa-associated lymphoid tissue [MALT]) in the stomach.
- History of smoking: Smokers have twice the risk of stomach cancer as nonsmokers.
- Dietary habits: Increased consumption of foods containing nitrates or nitrites, commonly found in such foods as cured meats; increased consumption of smoked foods and foods high in salt; and consumption of a diet low in fresh fruits and vegetables have been linked to the development stomach cancer.
- Medical history: A personal history of prior gastric surgery, pernicious anemia, or atrophic gastritis (a precancerous condition), as well as having type A blood, may increase the risk of developing stomach cancer. Certain mutations in the E-cadherin (*CDH1*) gene are also associated with a hereditary form of gastric cancer.

Demographics

The American Cancer Society estimated that 22,220 Americans would be diagnosed with stomach cancer in 2014, 13,730 men and 8,490 women; and approximately 10,990 deaths would result from the disease, 6,720 men and 4,270 women. The risk for developing stomach cancer in the United States is about 1 in 100. The risk is higher for men than for women. The average age at time of diagnosis of stomach cancer is 70 years for men and 74 years for women. Two-thirds of stomach cancer cases are diagnosed in people older than age 65, but in families with a hereditary risk for stomach cancer, cases in younger individuals are more frequently seen. The average risk that a person will develop stomach cancer in his or her lifetime is about 1 in 111.

Although stomach cancer incidence has been decreasing, it is the fourth most commonly diagnosed cancer and the second leading cause of cancer deaths worldwide. It is the seventh leading cause of cancer deaths in the United States. Stomach cancer is one of the leading causes of cancer deaths in several areas of the world, most notably in Japan and China, and in countries in Eastern Europe and Latin America.

In Japan, gastric cancer is diagnosed almost ten times as frequently as in the United States. The number of new stomach cancer cases is decreasing in some areas, however, especially in developed countries. In the United States, the incidence of stomach cancer has declined since the 1960s. The use of refrigerated foods and increased consumption of fresh fruits and vegetables, instead of preserved foods with high salt content, may be a reason for the decline. Another reason for the decrease may be that **antibiotics** given to treat childhood illnesses can kill the bacterium *Helicobacter pylori*, which is a major cause of stomach cancer.

Causes and symptoms

Causes

Studies have shown that eating foods with high quantities of salt and nitrites increases the risk of stomach cancer. Making changes to the types of foods consumed has been shown to decrease likelihood of disease, even for individuals from countries at higher risk. The diet in a specific region can have a great impact on its residents. For example, Japanese people who move to the United States or Europe and change the types of foods they eat have a far lower chance of developing the disease than Japanese people who remain in Japan and do not change their dietary habits. Eating recommended amounts of fruit and vegetables may lower a person's chances of developing this cancer as well.

KEY TERMS

Acanthosis nigricans—A poorly defined brownish-black hyperpigmentation of the skin found in body folds (under the armpits, the groin, the folds of the neck, and similar areas).

Adenocarcinoma—A type of cancerous tumor that develops in the gland-like cells of epithelial tissue, which is the tissue that lines the inner and exterior surfaces of body organs.

Atrophic gastritis—A chronic inflammation of the gastric mucosa caused either by an autoimmune process or by infection with *Helicobacter pylori*. It is a risk factor for the development of gastric cancer.

Biopsy—The surgical removal and microscopic examination of living tissue for diagnostic purposes.

Computed tomography—A radiology test by which images of cross-sectional planes of the body are obtained.

Gastrectomy—Surgical removal of the stomach. A gastrectomy may be either partial or total.

Helicobacter pylori—A rod-shaped bacterium found in the stomach and associated with an increased risk of stomach cancer.

Lymph—An almost colorless fluid that bathes body tissues.

Lymph nodes—Cellular filters through which lymphatics flow.

Lymphatics—Channels that are conduits for lymph.

Malignant—A general term for cells and the tumors they form that can invade and destroy other tissues and organs.

Metastasis (plural, metastases)—The spread of tumor cells from one part of the body to another through blood vessels or lymphatic vessels.

Mucosa—The smooth moist inner lining of some body organs, including the stomach; also referred to as a mucous membrane.

Prophylactic—Referring to a drug given or procedure performed to prevent disease.

Resection—The surgical removal of a portion of an organ or body part.

Stent—A tube made of plastic or metal mesh inserted into a hollow structure (like a blood vessel or the digestive tract) to keep the structure open.

Targeted therapy—In cancer treatment, a type of drug therapy that blocks tumors by interfering with specific molecules that the cancer cells need for growth. Also called biologic therapy, targeted therapy is less harmful to normal cells than traditional chemotherapy.

Tumor—An abnormal growth resulting from a cell that loses its normal growth control restraints and starts multiplying uncontrollably.

Ultrasound—A radiology test utilizing high-frequency sound waves.

There are two hereditary syndromes that increase a person's risk of stomach cancer as well as of **colon cancer**. One is hereditary non-polyposis colorectal cancer (HNPCC) or Lynch syndrome; the other is familial adenomatous polyposis (FAP). HNPCC is related to mutations in any of four genes responsible for DNA mismatch repair (MMR). FAP is caused by a mutation in the *APC* gene on chromosome 5. In addition to these two syndromes, persons with either of the two genes associated with breast cancer—*BRCA1* and *BRCA2*—are also at increased risk of stomach cancer.

Symptoms

Stomach cancer is a slow-growing cancer. It may be years before a tumor grows very large and produces distinct symptoms. In the early stages of the disease, the patient may have mild discomfort, indigestion, heartburn, a bloated feeling after eating (also known as early satiety), and mild nausea. In the advanced stages, a patient has loss of appetite and resultant **weight loss**, stomach pains, vomiting, difficulty in swallowing, and blood in the stool. Stomach cancer often spreads (metastasizes) to such adjoining organs as the esophagus, adjacent lymph nodes, liver, or colon.

Diagnosis

Unfortunately, many patients diagnosed with stomach cancer experience pain or loss of appetite for two or three years before informing a doctor of their symptoms. When a doctor suspects stomach cancer from the symptoms described by the patient, a complete medical history (including a family history) is conducted to check for any related risk factors.

Examination

A thorough physical examination is conducted to assess all the symptoms. Advanced gastric cancer may be diagnosed by noting palpable nodes in the area above the left collarbone and in the left armpit, which are typically nodes affected by metastases from stomach cancer. Other areas that may harbor metastatic disease include ovarian or pelvic masses which may be palpable.

The physician may also note changes to the skin, including acanthosis nigricans (areas of dark, thick, velvety skin in such body folds as the armpits, groin, under the breasts or behind the neck) or the appearance of new areas of seborrheic keratoses (itchy, crusty, wart-like skin lesions).

Tests

Recommended laboratory tests include a complete blood count (CBC) and blood chemistry profile, including liver function tests. Laboratory tests may be ordered to check for blood in the stool (**fecal occult blood test**) and **anemia** (low red blood cell count), which often accompany gastric cancer.

The *H. pylori* test will also be ordered to determine whether the patient is infected with the bacterium. If the *H. pylori* test is positive, treatment will be initiated.

In some countries, such as Japan, it is appropriate for patients to undergo routine screening examinations for stomach cancer, as the risk of developing cancer in that society is very high. Such screening might be useful for all high-risk populations. Due to the low prevalence of stomach cancer in the United States, routine screening is usually not recommended unless a family history of the disease exists.

Imaging tests that may be ordered if a diagnosis of gastric cancer is suspected include **X-rays** of the chest, abdominal **computed tomography** (CT) scan with contrast, CT and ultrasound of the pelvis in females, and PET/CT or PET (**positron emission tomography**) scans.

During another test, known as **upper gastrointestinal endoscopy**, a thin, flexible, lighted tube (endoscope) is passed down the patient's throat and into the stomach. The doctor can view the lining of the esophagus and the stomach through the tube. Sometimes, a small ultrasound probe is attached at the end of the endoscope. This probe sends high-frequency sound waves that bounce off the stomach wall. A computer creates an image of the stomach wall by translating the pattern of echoes generated by the reflected sound waves. This procedure is known as an endoscopic ultrasound or EUS.

Endoscopy has several advantages because the physician is able to see any abnormalities directly. In addition, if any suspicious-looking patches are seen, **biopsy** forceps can be passed painlessly through the tube to collect some tissue for microscopic examination. This procedure is known as a biopsy. The tissue sample may be tested to see whether it contains a protein called HER2/neu. This protein is made by a gene called the *HER2/neu* gene. Tumors that are HER2-positive can be treated with targeted therapy, described below. Endoscopic ultrasound (EUS) is beneficial because it can provide valuable information on depth of tumor invasion.

After stomach cancer has been diagnosed and before treatment starts, another type of x-ray scan is taken. Computed tomography (CT) is an imaging procedure that produces a three-dimensional picture of organs or structures inside the body. CT scans are used to obtain additional information in regard to how large the tumor is and what parts of the stomach it borders; whether the cancer has spread to the lymph nodes; and whether it has spread to distant parts of the body (metastasized), such as the liver, lung, or bone. A CT scan of the chest, abdomen, and pelvis is taken. If the tumor has penetrated through the wall of the stomach and extends to the liver, pancreas, or spleen, the CT will often show it. Although a CT scan is an effective way of evaluating whether cancer has spread to some of the lymph nodes, it is less effective than EUS in evaluating whether the nodes closest to the stomach are free of cancer.

Clinical staging

More than 95% of stomach cancers are caused by adenocarcinomas, malignant cancers that originate in glandular tissues. The remaining 5% of stomach cancers include lymphomas and other types of cancers.

Staging of stomach cancer is based on how deeply the growth has penetrated the stomach lining; to what extent (if any) it has invaded surrounding lymph nodes; and to what extent (if any) it has spread to distant parts of the body (metastasized). In the United States, about 25% of stomach cancer patients are diagnosed with localized disease, 31% with regional disease, and 32% with distant metastatic disease. Staging of stomach cancers is as follows as of 2014:

- Stage 0: The cancer (called carcinoma in situ in this stage) is limited to the gastric mucosa.

- Stage I: The cancer has either spread to six nearby lymph nodes and the submucosa; or it has invaded the submucosa and the underlying muscle layer of the stomach but has not spread to nearby lymph nodes.

- Stage II: The tumor has invaded the submucosa and 7 to 15 nearby lymph nodes; or has invaded the muscular layer of the stomach and spread to 1 to 6 nearby lymph nodes; or has penetrated through the outer wall of the stomach but has not spread to nearby lymph nodes.

- Stage III: The cancer has invaded the muscular layer of the stomach and spread to 7 to 15 nearby lymph nodes; or has penetrated through the outer wall of the stomach and has spread to 1 to 15 nearby lymph nodes; or has spread to nearby organs (liver, spleen, or colon) but not to distant organs.
- Stage IV: The cancer has spread to more than 15 nearby lymph nodes; or has spread to distant organs.

Treatment

Because symptoms of stomach cancer are so mild, treatment often does not commence until the disease is well advanced. The three standard modes of treatment for stomach cancer are surgery, **radiation therapy**, and **chemotherapy**. When deciding on the patient's treatment plan, the doctor takes into account many factors. The location of the cancer and its stage are important considerations. In addition, the patient's age, general health status, and personal preferences are also taken into account.

It is important that gastric lymphomas be accurately diagnosed because these cancers have a much better prognosis than stomach adenocarcinomas. Approximately half of the people with gastric lymphomas survive five years after diagnosis. Treatment of gastric **lymphoma** involves surgery combined with chemotherapy and radiation therapy.

A hereditary form of gastric cancer that is more likely to develop in younger individuals has been linked to people with blood group A, a history of pernicious anemia, and with a genetic mutation in the *CDH1* gene. Prophylactic **gastrectomy** may be recommended for younger patients known to have this specific genetic mutation.

Surgery

In the early stages of stomach cancer, surgery may be used to remove the cancer. Surgical removal of an **adenocarcinoma** is the only treatment capable of eliminating the cancer. Prior to surgery, CT scans and endoscopic ultrasounds are performed to determine the extent of tumor involvement. If the cancer is widespread and cannot be removed with surgery, an attempt is made to remove blockage and control symptoms such as pain or bleeding. This type of surgery is known as palliative surgery.

Depending on the location of the cancer, a portion of the stomach may be removed, a procedure called a partial or subtotal gastrectomy. In a surgical procedure known as total gastrectomy, the entire stomach may be removed. However, doctors prefer to leave at least part of the stomach if possible.

Partial or total gastrectomy is often accompanied by other surgical procedures. Lymph nodes are frequently removed during gastric cancer surgery. The current recommendation in the United States is that a gastrectomy done to remove a gastric tumor should include the removal of at least 15 lymph nodes in the areas near the cancer to offer the best hope of survival for the patient. Because stomach cancer is a relatively rare cancer in the United States, it is recommended that surgery for stomach cancer be done by a surgeon experienced in this type of procedure and in a center with experience in treating large numbers of patients with gastric cancer. In addition to total or partial removal of the stomach along with adjacent lymph nodes, nearby organs, or parts of these organs, may be removed if the cancer has spread to them. Such organs may include the pancreas, colon, or spleen. Patients whose digestive tract is blocked by a late-stage tumor may be treated by radiation therapy to shrink the tumor; laser treatment to remove the tumor; or the placement of a stent to keep the digestive tract open.

Preliminary studies suggest that patients who have tumors that cannot be removed through surgery at the start of therapy may become candidates for surgery later. Combinations of chemotherapy and radiation therapy are sometimes able to reduce disease for which surgery is not initially appropriate.

Chemotherapy

Chemotherapy involves administering **anticancer drugs** either intravenously (through a vein in the arm) or orally (in the form of pills). This method can either be used as the primary mode of treatment or after surgery to destroy any cancerous cells that may have migrated to distant sites.

Although chemotherapy using a single medicine (the chemotherapy drug 5-FU) is sometimes used, the best response rates are often achieved with combinations of medicines. Some of the more commonly used chemotherapy drugs used to treat stomach cancer include 5-FU, **doxorubicin**, **capecitabine**, oxaliplatin, **irinotecan**, **methotrexate**, **epirubicin**, **etoposide**, and **cisplatin**. As of 2014, there is no standard combination of chemotherapy drugs used with all patients.

Radiation therapy

Radiation therapy is often used after surgery to destroy the cancer cells that may not have been completely removed during surgery. To treat stomach cancer, external beam radiation therapy is generally used. In this procedure, high-energy rays from a machine that is outside of the body are concentrated on the area of the tumor. In the advanced stages of stomach cancer, radiation therapy is used to ease symptoms such as pain and bleeding rather than to cure the cancer; this approach is called palliative therapy.

Targeted therapy

Targeted therapy is a newer form of pharmacotherapy that treats cancers with drugs that target the changes in genes or proteins that cause cancer cells to grow and spread. In April 2014, the Food and Drug Administration (FDA) approved **ramucirumab** (Cyramza), a drug that targets a protein in tumor cells that helps the cancer form new blood vessels to get nourishment, for the treatment of metastatic stomach cancer. The drug was shown in two **clinical trials** to extend patients' survival time. It can be given together with chemotherapy drugs or as a stand-alone treatment.

Stomach cancers that are HER2-positive (about 20% of adenocarcinomas) can be treated with **trastuzumab**, a monoclonal antibody that targets the HER2 protein. Trastuzumab is given together with chemotherapy.

Prognosis

As of 2014, the overall five-year survival rate for patients with stomach cancer is 28%. Patients with Stage I cancers have a five-year survival rate of 60–71%; those with Stage II cancers have a five-year survival rate of 30–40%, while patients with Stage III cancers have a survival rate of only 9–15%. The reason for the high mortality is that many people with stomach cancer are not diagnosed until their cancer has metastasized. Metastatic stomach cancer is presently considered incurable.

Prevention

Avoiding many of the risk factors associated with stomach cancer may prevent its development. Excessive amounts of salted, smoked, and pickled foods should be avoided, as should foods high in nitrates or nitrites. A diet that includes recommended amounts of fruits and vegetables is believed to lower the risk of several cancers, including stomach cancer. The American Cancer Society recommends eating at least five servings of fruits and vegetables daily and choosing six servings of food from other plant sources, such as grains, pasta, beans, cereals, and whole-grain bread. Following a healthy diet and balancing caloric intake with recommended amounts of physical activity may reduce obesity, which is itself a risk factor for stomach cancer, at least in men.

Quitting smoking and avoiding excessive amounts of alcohol reduces the risk of many cancers. In countries

---

QUESTIONS TO ASK YOUR DOCTOR

- Has the cancer spread to the lymph nodes?
- Has the cancer spread to the lungs, liver, or spleen?
- (If surgery is recommended) Do recent studies show that it might be a good idea to use chemotherapy or radiation therapy also?
- (If gastrectomy or partial gastrectomy was performed) How should I alter my diet and eating patterns?
- (Following surgery) What foods should I eat? Is there a registered dietitian I can speak with on a regular basis about what I should eat?

---

where stomach cancer is common, such as Japan, early detection is important for successful treatment.

Treatment for *H. pylori* infection, especially for those individuals with chronic infections, may reduce the risk of developing stomach cancer.

Resources

BOOKS

Bhullar, Jasneet Singh. *Gastric Cancer: Risk Factors, Treatment and Clinical Outcomes.* Hauppauge, New York: Nova Science Publishers, 2014.

Corso, Giovanni. *Spotlight on Familial and Hereditary Gastric Cancer.* New York: Springer, 2013.

Duncan, Marc D. *Johns Hopkins Patients' Guide to Cancer of the Stomach and Esophagus.* Sudbury, MA: Jones and Bartlett Learning, 2011.

Griffin, S. Michael, ed. *Oesophagogastric Surgery*, 5th ed. New York: Saunders/Elsevier, 2014.

Otto, Florian, and Manfred P. Lutz, eds. *Early Gastrointestinal Cancers.* New York: Springer, 2012.

PERIODICALS

Abreu, M.T., and R.M. Peek Jr. "Gastrointestinal Malignancy and the Microbiome." *Gastroenterology* 146 (May 2014): 1534–1546.

American Association for Cancer Research. "Ramucirumab Approved for Gastric Cancer." *Cancer Discovery* 4 (July 2014): 752–753.

Deng, J.Y., and H. Liang. "Clinical Significance of Lymph Node Metastasis in Gastric Cancer." *World Journal of Gastroenterology* 20 (April 14, 2014): 3967–3975.

Gomez-Martín, C., et al. "A Critical Review of HER2-positive Gastric Cancer Evaluation and Treatment: From Trastuzumab, and Beyond." *Cancer Letters* 351 (August 28, 2014): 30–40.

Kasper, S., and M. Schuler. "Targeted Therapies in Gastro-esophageal Cancer." *European Journal of Cancer* 50 (May 2014): 1247–1258.

Lasithiotakis, K., et al. "Gastrectomy for Stage IV Gastric Cancer. A Systematic Review and Meta-analysis." *Anticancer Research* 34 (May 2014): 2079–2085.

Lordick, F., et al. "Unmet Needs and Challenges in Gastric Cancer: The Way Forward." *Cancer Treatment Reviews* 40 (July 2014): 692–700.

Moyat, M., and D. Velin. "Immune Responses to *Helicobacter pylori* Infection." *World Journal of Gastroenterology* 20 (May 21, 2014): 5583–5593.

Pavlidis, T.E., and E.T. Pavlidis. "Role of Stenting in the Palliation of Gastroesophageal Junction Cancer: A Brief Review." *World Journal of Gastrointestinal Surgery* 6 (March 27, 2014): 38–41.

OTHER

American Cancer Society (ACS). "Stomach Cancer." http://www.cancer.org/acs/groups/cid/documents/webcontent/003141-pdf.pdf (accessed July 9, 2014).

WEBSITES

Cabebe, Elwyn C. "Gastric Cancer." Medscape Reference. http://emedicine.medscape.com/article/278744-overview (accessed July 9, 2014).

Cancer.Net. "Stomach Cancer." http://www.cancer.net/cancer-types/stomach-cancer (accessed July 9, 2014).

Food and Drug Administration (FDA). "FDA Approves Cyramza for Stomach Cancer." http://www.fda.gov/NewsEvents/Newsroom/PressAnnouncements/ucm394107.htm (accessed July 9, 2014).

National Cancer Institute (NCI). "What You Need to Know about Stomach Cancer." http://www.cancer.gov/cancertopics/wyntk/stomach/page1/AllPages (accessed July 9, 2014).

ORGANIZATIONS

American Cancer Society (ACS), 250 Williams Street NW, Atlanta, GA 30303, (800) 227-2345, http://www.cancer.org/aboutus/howwehelpyou/app/contact-us.aspx, http://www.cancer.org/index.

American College of Gastroenterology (ACG), 6400 Goldsboro Road, Suite 200, Bethesda, MD 20817, (301) 263-9000, info@acg.gi.org, http://gi.org//.

National Cancer Institute (NCI), BG 9609 MSC 9760, 9609 Medical Center Drive, Bethesda, MD 20892-9760, (800) 4-CANCER (422-6237), http://www.cancer.gov/global/contact/email-us, http://www.cancer.gov/.

Office of Cancer Complementary and Alternative Medicine (OCCAM), 9609 Medical Center Dr., Room 5-W-136, Rockville, MD 20850, (240) 276-6595, Fax: (240) 276-7888, ncioccam1-r@mail.nih.gov, http://cam.cancer.gov/.

Lata Cherath, PhD
Bob Kirsch
REVISED BY MELINDA OBERLEITNER, R.N., D.N.S.
REVISED BY REBECCA J. FREY, PhD

Stomatitis

Definition

Stomatitis is an inflammation of the mucous membranes and other tissues of the mouth, including the gums, tongue, inside of the cheeks and lips, and roof and floor of the mouth. Although "stomatitis" and "oral mucositis" are often used interchangeably, oral **mucositis** refers only to inflammation of the mouth mucous membranes. Stomatitis is a side effect of some types of **chemotherapy** and **radiation therapy** for **cancer**.

Description

The mouth includes several structures that together are referred to as the oral cavity: the lips, teeth, gums, tongue, pharynx, and salivary glands. Most of these structures are covered by mucous membranes—the shiny, pink, moist lining of the mouth. These are the membranes affected by stomatitis. Stomatitis is painful. Inflamed membranes in the mouth can become dry and irritated and may bleed. The membranes can also become infected by the many bacteria that normally live in the mouth. Although stomatitis is often a short-term problem, it is of major concern for cancer patients and their doctors because, in addition to causing discomfort and pain, it can interfere with adequate nutrition. Oral pain can cause **weight loss**, treatment delays, and reductions in chemotherapy doses, which can have adverse effects on the outcome of treatment.

Patients with blood cancers or those being treated with high-dose chemotherapy or a combination of chemotherapy and radiation for **head and neck cancers** are most susceptible to stomatitis. Children are particularly susceptible to stomatitis, although they often heal faster than older patients.

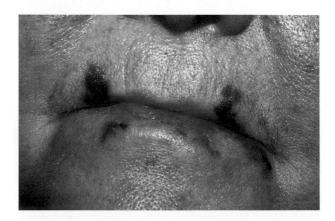

A close-up view of patient's mouth with gingivostomatitis cold sores. *(SPL/Custmer Medical Stock Photography)*

Causes and symptoms

Stomatitis is most often caused by cancer treatments such as chemotherapy and radiation therapy. Chemotherapy drugs work by killing rapidly dividing cancer cells. However, the drugs also kill healthy cells that normally divide rapidly. The outer layers of mucous membranes grow very rapidly and are susceptible to damage by chemotherapy and radiation therapy. When these cells are damaged, they slough off, leaving the lining of the mouth unprotected. This exposed lining can become inflamed, swollen, and dry and often develops ulcers or sores. 5-Fluorouracil, **methotrexate**, **doxorubicin**, and **bleomycin** are chemotherapy drugs that are most likely to cause stomatitis. Stomatitis resulting from these drugs is related to the dose and scheduling of the medication and can often be a dose-limiting toxic side effect of chemotherapy.

Stomatitis from cancer chemotherapy can cause pain, loss of taste, and reduced food intake. Reddened areas in the mouth may appear as early as three days after chemotherapy, but stomatitis usually develops in five to seven days. The first symptoms appear as reddened mucous membranes and sensitivity to spicy foods. The tongue may become dry or swollen. Inflammation can range from mild to severe. Patients can have difficulty swallowing and be unable to eat or drink. Ulceration sometimes occurs.

Stomatitis caused by radiation therapy normally develops in the area where the radiation is administered. It generally begins 7 to 14 days after the start of therapy. It will usually improve by about two to three weeks following treatment.

Stomatitis can also be an indirect result of cancer treatment or the cancer itself. Chemotherapy frequently causes a patient's infection-fighting white blood cells to drop below normal levels. When this occurs, the body can have difficulty maintaining the balance of normal organisms in the oral cavity; stomatitis, as well as infections such as **thrush** (oral candidiasis), may result. The severity of stomatitis is dependent upon various factors, including the type and stage of the cancer, the patient's age, the patient's oral health before cancer treatment, and the level of oral care during therapy. The duration and severity of a low white blood cell count is another factor. Dentures, braces, or other dental appliances that irritate mouth tissues can also cause or worsen stomatitis.

Treatment

If stomatitis is painful enough to interfere with eating and drinking; pain medications, including numbing medicines and non-narcotic or narcotic pain medicines, can be prescribed. Various measures may provide relief of symptoms:

• Warm or hot foods can further irritate the mouth and throat; serving foods cold or at room temperature is recommended.

• Choose soft and soothing foods including ice cream, custards, cottage cheese, milkshakes, soft fruits, mashed potatoes, baby foods, or cooked foods that are pureed in a blender.

• Rinsing the oral cavity after meals and before bedtime with a mild salt water or baking soda and water solution helps keep the mouth clean and free of debris.

• The mouth and teeth should be kept very clean with a soft-bristled toothbrush or soft foam tooth-cleaning device.

• Maintaining good nutritional intake and drinking adequate amounts of fluids help the body heal.

• Tobacco products and alcohol can irritate the lining of the mouth and should be avoided.

• Spicy, salty, and irritating and acidic foods (such as tomatoes and citrus fruits and juices) and rough, coarse, or dry foods, such as raw vegetables, granola, pretzels, or toast, should be avoided.

• Dentures should be removed at night and carefully cleansed with an antiseptic solution.

Alternative and complementary therapies

Some preliminary studies have indicated that the amino acid **glutamine** may be effective for shortening the duration of stomatitis. It has been suggested that topical vitamin E may also be effective. Small studies have suggested that sucking on ice chips or a chamomile mouthwash may decrease the severity of stomatitis. However, a randomized clinical study found that chamomile did not decrease stomatitis caused by 5-fluorouracil. Patients undergoing cancer treatment should always consult their physicians or other healthcare professionals before trying any alternative approaches.

Prognosis

Stomatitis is usually a short-term condition, lasting from just a few days to a few weeks. If complications, such as infection, are avoided, stomatitis usually heals completely within two to four weeks. However, patients should inform their doctors immediately if mouth sores develop, especially if they are painful or interfere with eating.

Prevention

Various measures can help prevent the occurrence or reduce the severity of stomatitis—especially good nutrition, good oral hygiene practices, and early detection of any oral lesions by the patient or healthcare provider. Practicing good oral hygiene before beginning cancer treatment can reduce the severity of stomatitis. Patients should have their teeth cleaned at least two weeks before beginning chemotherapy. They should have any dental work— such as treating cavities, abscesses, gum disease, or poorly fitting dentures— completed well before cancer treatment begins, to give the mouth sufficient time to heal. Patients should ask their dentists about the best ways to brush and floss their teeth during treatment. They should also ask about a daily decay-preventing fluoride gel or rinse, since chemotherapy can increase the risk of cavities.

Once cancer treatment has begun, patients should carefully examine their mouths daily and inform their healthcare professional about the appearance of any symptoms such as reddened areas, swelling, blisters, sores, white patches, or bleeding. It is important to brush the teeth and gums gently after every meal with an extra-soft bristle brush. Brushing too hard can further damage tissues. The toothbrush should be rinsed well after each use and stored in a dry place. Commercial mouthwashes should be avoided, since they often contain alcohol or other irritants.

Resources

BOOKS

Sonis, Stephen T. *Oral Mucositis*. London: Springer Healthcare, 2012.

WEBSITES

"Managing Oral Complications During and After Chemotherapy or Radiation Therapy." National Cancer Institute. April 24, 2014. http://www.cancer.gov/cancertopics/pdq/supportivecare/oralcomplications/Patient/page4 (accessed August 27, 2014).

"Mouth, Gum, Tongue, and Throat Problems During Chemo." American Cancer Society. August 24, 2014. http://www.cancer.org/treatment/treatmentsandsideeffects/treatment-types/chemotherapy/understandingchemotherapyaguide-forpatientsandfamilies/understanding-chemotherapy-more-side-effects-mouth-gum-throat-problems (accessed August 27, 2014).

ORGANIZATIONS

American Cancer Society, 250 Williams Street NW, Atlanta, GA 30303, (800) 227-2345, http://www.cancer.org.

National Cancer Institute, 6116 Executive Boulevard, Suite 300, Bethesda, MD 20892-8322, (800) 4-CANCER (422-6237), http://www.cancer.gov.

Deanna Swartout-Corbeil, R.N.
Rebecca J. Frey, PhD
REVISED BY MARGARET ALIC, PhD

Streptozocin

Definition

Streptozocin is one of the anticancer (antineoplastic) drugs called alkylating agents. It is available in the United States under the brand name Zanosar.

Purpose

Streptozocin is primarily used to treat **cancer** of the pancreas, specifically advanced islet-cell **carcinoma**.

Description

Streptozocin chemically interferes with the synthesis of the genetic material (DNA) of cancer cells, which prevents these cells from being able to reproduce.

Recommended dosage

Streptozocin is given by injection. The dosage prescribed varies widely depending on the patient, the cancer being treated, and whether or not other medications are also being taken.

Precautions

Streptozocin carries a risk of renal (kidney) toxicity. While receiving streptozocin, patients are encouraged to drink extra fluids, which can increase the amount of urine passed and help prevent kidney problems.

Streptozocin may cause an allergic reaction in some people. Patients with a prior allergic reaction to streptozocin should not take this medication.

Streptozocin also may cause serious birth defects if either the man or the woman is taking this drug at the time of conception or if the woman takes this drug during pregnancy. Streptozocin also may cause miscarriage.

It is not known whether streptozocin is passed from mother to child through breast milk. However, since many drugs are excreted in breast milk and since streptozocin has the potential to adversely affect an infant, breast feeding is not recommended while this medication is being taken.

Streptozocin suppresses the immune system (by damaging white blood cells) and interferes with the normal functioning of certain organs and tissues. For these reasons, it is important that the prescribing physician is aware of any of the following pre-existing medical conditions:

- a current case of or recent exposure to chicken pox
- diabetes mellitus
- herpes zoster (shingles)
- a current case or history of gout or kidney stones
- all current infections
- kidney disease
- liver disease

Also, because streptozocin damages white blood cells and platelets, patients taking this drug must exercise extreme caution to avoid contracting any new infections or sustaining any injuries that result in bruising or bleeding.

Side effects

The common side effects of streptozocin include:

- fatigue
- loss of appetite (anorexia)
- nausea and vomiting
- increased susceptibility to infection and bleeding
- swelling of the feet or lower legs
- unusual decrease in urination
- temporary hair loss (alopecia)

Diarrhea is a less common side effect that may also occur.

Because streptozocin can damage the kidneys, liver, white blood cells, and platelets, patients taking this medication should be closely monitored for evidence of these adverse side effects. Laboratory tests, including renal function, urinalysis, complete blood count, and liver function, should be done at frequent intervals (approximately weekly) during drug therapy. If evidence of these adverse side effects is found, treatment with streptozocin may be discontinued or the dose may be decreased.

Interactions

Streptozocin should not be taken in combination with any prescription drug, over-the-counter drug, or herbal remedy without prior consultation with a physician. It is particularly important that the prescribing physician be aware of the use of any of the following drugs:

- anti-infection drugs
- carmustine (an anticancer drug)
- cisplatin (an anticancer drug)
- cyclosporine (an immunosuppressive drug)
- deferoxamine (used to remove excess iron from the body)
- gold salts (used for arthritis)
- inflammation or pain medications other than narcotics
- narcotic pain medications containing acetaminophen (Tylenol) or aspirin
- lithium (used to treat bipolar disorder)
- methotrexate (an anticancer drug also used for rheumatoid arthritis and psoriasis)
- penicillamine (used to treat Wilson's disease and rheumatoid arthritis)
- phenytoin (an anticonvulsant)

- plicamycin (an anticancer drug)
- tiopronin (used to prevent kidney stones)

  See also Pancreatic cancer, endocrine.

Paul A. Johnson, EdM

Strontium-89 *see* **Radiopharmaceuticals**

Substance abuse

Definition

Substance abuse in the context of **cancer** treatment most often refers to the overuse and abuse of **pain management** drugs.

Description

The therapeutic use of drugs for palliative care in the cancer population requires careful management. This is particularly true of drugs given to relieve pain. Many of the most potent pain relievers are **opioids**, either derived directly from the opium poppy (*Papaver somniferum*) or synthesized in the laboratory. Although the use of opioids as analgesics goes back thousands of years, these compounds can also produce feelings of euphoria in some users, leading to their abuse as recreational drugs. Because of their high potential for abuse, most opioids prescribed in the United States are categorized as Schedule II drugs as defined by the Controlled Substances Act of 1970. The Schedule II classification means that while a drug on this schedule has accepted medical uses under strict supervision, abuse of the drug may lead to severe psychological or physical dependence.

One of the challenges in the use of opioids for pain management in cancer patients in recent years is the increasing popularity of painkillers as drugs of abuse. News articles, documentaries, and profiles of celebrity addicts in the mass media have made some cancer patients anxious about the use of opioid analgesics to manage cancer pain. Patients who have never abused drugs may fear becoming addicted to their pain medications, and those in recovery from drug abuse may fear that medications given to control their cancer pain will cause them to relapse into active drug abuse.

Diagnosis

Most recent discussions of drug misuse—defined as the use of a prescription medication for reasons other than that for which it was prescribed—and drug abuse in cancer patients begin by noting that the risk of addiction to or dependence on painkillers depends on the patient's previous history of medication use. A screening questionnaire that is frequently used to help identify patients at increased risk of opioid abuse is the Opioid Risk Tool (ORT). This survey gauges a patient's risk of substance abuse based on a family history of substance abuse, personal history of substance abuse, occurrence of preadolescent sexual abuse, history of **depression** or other mental health conditions, and age (patients aged 16–45 are at higher risk).

Recognizing specific signs of drug misuse

The following behaviors are clues that a cancer patient might be misusing pain medications:

- crushing drugs or breaking down capsules to feel an immediate "high"
- moving from opioid pain relievers to heroin or other drugs of abuse
- injecting medications intended to be taken by mouth
- forging prescriptions and/or stealing prescription pads
- stealing another patient's pain medications
- obtaining painkillers from nonmedical sources
- making frequent requests for higher doses of the drug
- hoarding drugs during periods of reduced pain symptoms

Treatment

One expert on drug dependence/abuse in cancer patients groups the patients into three categories: uncomplicated patients (those with no history of drug or alcohol abuse), patients with comorbid psychiatric disorders who use drugs to self-medicate, and addicted patients. Each type of patient requires a different approach to pain management for cancer pain.

Uncomplicated patients

Uncomplicated patients are those who have no history of substance abuse disorders. They are not likely to experience the euphoria or "high" sought by people addicted to opioids. While it is true that cancer patients taking opioid analgesics may develop tolerance—the need to take larger quantities of the drug to relieve their pain—or become physically dependent on the drug, neither tolerance nor physical dependence is the same thing as addiction, which involves psychological as well as physical dependence. When a patient without a history of substance abuse stops taking pain relievers given for cancer pain because the cancer has been effectively treated, he or she is usually able to discontinue the analgesic without difficulty. Cancer patients in this category usually do well with minimal structure, most often monthly checkups.

KEY TERMS

Addiction—The use of a drug or other substance in a manner that is out of control, compulsive, used in increasing amounts, and continued despite the risk of harm to the user.

Analgesic—Any drug that is given to relieve pain.

Dependence—A strong desire or a sense of compulsion to take a drug, combined with difficulty in controlling or stopping the use of the drug. Dependence may be physical, psychological, or both.

Drug misuse—The use of a drug for purposes other than those for which the drug is intended. The recreational use of prescription painkillers is an example of drug misuse.

Dual diagnosis—A term used to describe patients who suffer from a diagnosed mental disorder and comorbid substance abuse.

Euphoria—A state of intense pleasure, elation, or feelings of well-being that can be produced by normal human experiences but can also result from

taking opioids or other psychoactive drugs. Euphoria induced by drugs is often referred to as a "high."

Methadone—A synthetic opioid used as an anti-addictive treatment in patients who are dependent on or addicted to opioids.

Palliative care—Care that is given to relieve pain and other symptoms of a disease rather than cure the disease.

Tolerance—Decreased susceptibility to the effects of a drug as a result of its continued administration.

Withdrawal syndrome—A group of physical and psychological symptoms experienced by opioid addicts when the drug is abruptly discontinued. It lasts for two to seven days and includes chills, nausea, muscle pain, flu-like symptoms, restlessness, anxiety, panic attacks, depression, and mood swings. Withdrawal syndrome can also occur with sudden discontinuation of benzodiazepine tranquilizers.

The most serious risk in this group of patients is undertreatment for cancer pain. Because it was thought at one time that addiction arose from the use of opioids for pain, patients may be fearful of taking effective doses of pain relievers, and some health professionals may be reluctant to prescribe adequate dosages for pain management. The problem is compounded when **health insurance** companies or pharmacists question what they might regard as overly generous prescriptions for opioid analgesics. While this questioning is a response to the need to control opioid abuse and overdoses among the general population, it can cause feelings of guilt in cancer patients about the need for effective pain control.

Chemical copers

Chemical copers are people who use pain medications and other drugs as a way to cope with psychiatric problems. Sometimes called dual diagnosis patients, these patients are more likely to misuse opioids to relieve feelings of depression or anxiety rather than to do so for recreational purposes. These patients are treated with psychotherapy alongside their pain medication and are taught ways of coping with their psychological distress that do not involve drugs. The treating physicians often need to provide more structure for these patients and be judicious in the specific painkillers that are prescribed.

Chemically dependent patients

Cancer patients in this category include those who are currently addicted to drugs, who are in drug-free recovery, and who are on methadone maintenance. Patients at greatest risk of chemical dependence include the young, people with family histories of drug abuse, and people whose social and friendship networks include other drug users.

There can be complications with treating this patient group. Some patients might be reluctant to be truthful with the oncologist about their history of drug misuse or abuse, particularly if they are using multiple drugs. Lack of honesty in this area creates the risk that patients could develop withdrawal syndromes when they stop taking drugs other than opioids, particularly **benzodiazepines**, of which the physician is unaware. Also, patients with a history of substance abuse have often built up a tolerance to opioids and can require higher doses of these drugs for pain control than patients with no history of abuse.

Patients in this category require a great deal of structure in management of their cancer pain. General principles include giving the patient oral rather than injectable pain medications, prescribing long-acting analgesics with little or low street value, prescribing no more than a week's supply of pain medications at a time, placing the patient in a recovery program and psychotherapy, and taking periodic urine screens.

Setting realistic treatment goals

Some oncologists consider it unrealistic to expect cancer patients addicted to pain medications to achieve complete freedom from relapses, as there is not only a high rate of recurrence in general in drug addiction, but the diagnosis of cancer adds to the patient's stress level. Other stressors include the side effects of **radiation therapy** and **chemotherapy**, and the complexities of navigating the healthcare system. The patient's healthcare team can set limits and provide enough support to reduce the frequency and severity of the patient's relapses, even when complete abstinence from the drugs is not possible.

Alternative treatments

Educational interventions that help patients communicate better with their doctors can enhance the quality of their treatment. Relaxation techniques and such interventions as cognitive behavioral therapy (CBT) may help patients cope more effectively with feelings of anxiety or depression. A dietitian can help the patient plan a more nutritious diet, and a physical therapist can suggest appropriate forms of physical exercise tailored to the patient's age and general fitness level. Music and art therapy can be helpful, especially for patients who enjoy expressing themselves creatively. Some patients find it easier to deal with their pain by utilizing alternative or complementary (CAM) approaches such as yoga, acupuncture, and massage therapy.

Prevention

Cancer patients with a history of drug misuse or abuse often benefit from long-term structuring of their pain management. Forming a multidisciplinary team is appropriate for cancer patients in general and is critically important for patients with special needs, such as those who have substance abuse problems. The team should include healthcare practitioners best suited to meet the needs of the patient. Patients with substance abuse issues are likely to benefit from being under the care of a physician who specializes in pain medicine and palliative care, as well as a social worker and a psychologist who specializes in addiction. Physicians specializing in the treatment of pain come from a variety of medical specialties, such as anesthesiology, oncology, emergency medicine, psychiatry, and surgery. Ideally, a pain management team should be formed that works with the patient's primary care physician, oncologist, and radiation oncologist to provide comprehensive care to the patient.

Given the complex nature of pain management in cancer patients, much more research is needed regarding the best treatment options for patients with substance abuse problems coupled with cancer-related pain.

Resources

BOOKS

Abrahm, Janet L. *A Physician's Guide to Pain and Symptom Management in Cancer Patients*, 3rd ed. Baltimore, MD: Johns Hopkins University Press, 2014.

Sharma, Manohar, ed. *Practical Management of Complex Cancer Pain*. New York: Oxford University Press, 2014.

Smith, Howard S. *Opioid Therapy in the 21st Century*. New York: Oxford University Press, 2013.

PERIODICALS

Anghelescu, D.L., J.H. Ehrentraut, and L.G. Faughnan. "Opioid Misuse and Abuse: Risk Assessment and Management in Patients with Cancer Pain." *Journal of the National Comprehensive Cancer Network* 11 (August 2013): 1023–1031.

Barclay, J.S., J.E. Owens, and J.L. Blackhall. "Screening for Substance Abuse Risk in Cancer Patients Using the Opioid Risk Tool and Urine Drug Screen." *Supportive Care in Cancer* 22 (July 2014): 1883–1888.

Del Fabbro, E. "Assessment and Management of Chemical Coping in Patients with Cancer." *Journal of Clinical Oncology* 32 (June 1, 2014): 1734–1738.

Garland, E.L., et al. "The Downward Spiral of Chronic Pain, Prescription Opioid Misuse, and Addiction: Cognitive, Affective, and Neuropsychopharmacologic Pathways." *Neuroscience and Biobehavioral Reviews* 37 (December 2013): 2597–2607.

Granata, R., et al. "Rapid-onset Opioids for the Treatment of Breakthrough Cancer Pain: Two Cases of Drug Abuse." *Pain Medicine* 15 (May 2014): 758–761.

Ma, J.D., et al. "A Single-center, Retrospective Analysis Evaluating the Utilization of the Opioid Risk Tool in Opioid-treated Cancer Patients." *Journal of Pain and Palliative Care Pharmacotherapy* 28 (March 2014): 4–9.

Rauenzahn, S., and E. Del Fabbro. "Opioid Management of Pain: The Impact of the Prescription Opioid Abuse Epidemic." *Current Opinion in Supportive and Palliative Care* 8 (September 2014): 273–278.

OTHER

Webster, Lynn R. "Opioid Risk Tool (ORT)." Community Anti-Drug Coalitions of America. http://www.cadca.org/files/resources/5_opioid_risk_tool.pdf (accessed September 9, 2014).

WEBSITES

Cancer.Net. "Pain: Treating Pain with Medication." http://www.cancer.net/navigating-cancer-care/side-effects/pain-treating-pain-medication (accessed September 9, 2014).

DualDiagnosis.org. "Risk of Substance Abuse in Cancer Patients." http://www.dualdiagnosis.org/substance-abuse-cancer-patients/ (accessed September 8, 2014).

Memorial Sloan Kettering Cancer Center. "Will I Become Addicted to the Pain Medications I May Need During My Cancer Treatment?" http://www.mskcc.org/blog/will-i-become-addicted-pain-medications-i-may-need-during-my-treatment (accessed September 9, 2014).

National Cancer Institute (NCI). "Pain (PDQ)." http://www.cancer.gov/cancertopics/pdq/supportivecare/pain/Health-Professional/page1/AllPages (accessed September 9, 2014).

Neerkin, Jane, et al. "Guidelines for Cancer Pain Management in Substance Misusers." http://www.palliativedrugs.com/download/100615_Substance_misuse_pain_guidlines_final.pdf (accessed September 9, 2014).

SupportiveOncology.net. "Treating Cancer Pain in Patients Addicted to Drugs." http://www.oncologypractice.com/jso/journal/articles/0502063.pdf (accessed September 9, 2014).

U.S. Food and Drug Administration (FDA). "A Guide to Safe Use of Pain Medicine." http://www.fda.gov/downloads/ForConsumers/ConsumerUpdates/ucm095742.pdf (accessed September 9, 2014).

ORGANIZATIONS

American Academy of Pain Medicine (AAPM), 8735 West Higgins Road, Suite 300, Chicago, IL 60631, (847) 375-4731, Fax: (847) 375-6477, info@painmed.org, http://www.painmed.org/.

American Cancer Society (ACS), 250 Williams Street NW, Atlanta, GA 30303, (800) 227-2345, http://www.cancer.org/aboutus/howwehelpyou/app/contact-us.aspx, http://www.cancer.org/index.

Food and Drug Administration (FDA), 10903 New Hampshire Avenue, Silver Spring, MD 20993, (888) INFO-FDA (463-6332), http://www.fda.gov/AboutFDA/ContactFDA/default.htm, http://www.fda.gov/default.htm.

National Cancer Institute (NCI), BG 9609 MSC 9760, 9609 Medical Center Drive, Bethesda, MD 20892-9760, (800) 4-CANCER (422-6237), http://www.cancer.gov/global/contact/email-us, http://www.cancer.gov/.

National Hospice and Palliative Care Organization (NHPCO), 1731 King Street, Alexandria, VA 22314, (703) 837-1500, Fax: (703) 837-1233, http://www.nhpco.org/.

Lee Ann Paradise
REVISED BY REBECCA J. FREY, PHD

Sunitinib

Definition

Sunitinib is marketed by Pfizer under the trade name Sutent. It is a type of anticancer drug in a class called receptor tyrosine kinase inhibitors. It has been approved for use in treating a type of **kidney cancer** called renal cell **carcinoma**, gastrointestinal (GI) tumors called GISTs (gastrointestinal stromal tumors), and pancreatic **neuroendocrine tumors** (PNETs), which occur in certain cells of the pancreas.

Purpose

Sunitinib, or sunitinib malate, is a type of targeted **cancer** therapy. As of 2014, it was approved for use in patients with several types of cancer. Renal cell carcinoma occurs in small tubules in the kidney that help filter blood. It is a very common type of kidney cancer in adults. Sunitinib is also used for GISTs that are resistant to other agents or in patients who cannot tolerate the first regimen (imatinib) usually used to treat GISTs. GISTs are tumors that derive from connective tissue in the GI tract, and are generally benign when small to medium in size. When large enough, however, they may metastasize. Sunitinib was the first anticancer agent that was approved for use in treating two different types of cancer at the same time, and is part of the standard of care for these diseases. The drug was later approved for treatment of PNETs, or islet cell tumors. This type of cancer occurs in cells of the pancreas that make the hormones that control insulin. Sunitinib is being studied for use in treating other types of cancer.

Description

Sunitinib is an anticancer drug that acts on receptor tyrosine kinases to inhibit the growth of tumors. Receptor tyrosine kinases are receptors for growth factors that are a natural part of cell development and necessary for normal cell growth. When tyrosine kinase receptors are activated, they initiate chemical signals that tell the cell how to grow and develop. Normal tyrosine kinase receptors turn on and off as needed for usual amounts of growth. However, when cells have constantly activated tyrosine kinase receptors, they may undergo abnormal growth and lead to cancer. Drugs in the class of sunitinib inhibit these overly active tyrosine kinase receptors.

Once they reach a certain size, solid tumor cells need to form their own blood supply in order to grow and remain alive. New blood vessels need to be formed for the tumor to survive. This process is known as **angiogenesis**. Angiogenesis is a part of tumor progression, one of the processes critical to tumor growth and survival. Sunitinib is thought to act on many different receptor tyrosine kinases, which in addition to inhibiting individual tumor cell growth, inhibit the angiogenesis process as well.

Studies have shown that sunitinib affects both the time to tumor progression and progression-free survival. The term *time to tumor progression* describes a period of time from when disease is diagnosed (or treated) until the disease starts to get worse. *Progression-free survival* describes the length of time during and after treatment in which a patient is living with a disease that does not get worse. Both time to tumor progression and progression-free survival may be used in a clinical study or trial to

KEY TERMS

Angiogenesis—Physiological process involving the growth of new blood vessels from pre-existing blood vessels, used by some cancers to create their own blood supply.

Catheter—Tube inserted into a body cavity or blood vessel to allow drainage of fluids (as in a urinary catheter), injection of drugs, or insertion of a surgical instrument.

Cytochrome P450—Enzymes present in the liver that metabolize drugs.

Epilepsy—Neurological disorder characterized by recurrent seizures.

Gastrointestinal stromal tumor—Tumor of the gastrointestinal tract derived from connective tissue.

Hemolytic anemia—Type of anemia involving destruction of red blood cells.

Metastasis—The process by which cancer spreads from its original site to other parts of the body.

QT prolongation—Potentially dangerous heart condition that affects the rhythm of the heartbeat and alters the ECG reading of the heart.

Receptor tyrosine kinases—Cell surface receptors that interact with growth factors and hormones to affect the normal life cycle of a cell.

Renal cell carcinoma—Cancer of the kidney that originates in the very small tubes in the kidney that filter the blood and remove waste products.

Teratogen—Any drug or chemical agent that has the potential to cause birth defects in a developing fetus.

Tuberculosis—Potentially fatal infectious disease that commonly affects the lungs, is highly contagious, and is caused by an organism known as *Mycobacterium tuberculosis*.

help find out how well a new treatment works. In studies done on sunitinib, patients receiving sunitinib had a longer median time to tumor progression and a longer median progression-free survival than those receiving a placebo and other drugs tested.

Recommended dosage

Sunitinib is taken orally in capsule form. The drug is made in dosages of 12.5, 25, and 50 mg. The doses used to treat kidney cancer and GISTs are often 50 to 100 mg per day, and the dose for treating PNETs is about 37.5 mg per day, but doses may vary according to the patient's medical condition. A regimen of 100 mg a day would involve taking two 50 mg capsules once a day. Sunitinib is usually taken in four-week time periods with two weeks off in between.

For the treatment of GIST in adults, sunitinib may be given in six-week cycles at a dosage of 50 mg once daily for four consecutive weeks, followed by a two-week period without taking any drug. For the treatment of advanced renal cell carcinoma in adults, sunitinib is administered in six-week cycles at a recommended dosage of 50 mg once daily for four consecutive weeks, followed by a two-week period without the drug. For PNETs, sunitinib is given in 37.5 mg doses once daily without a scheduled off-period. In clinical studies done with sunitinib, these regimens were maintained for as long as the patient derived clinical benefit from sunitinib or until unacceptable toxicity occurred.

The dosage of sunitinib is adjusted in increasing or decreasing amounts of 12.5 mg daily (considered one dose level). Adjustments are made depending on the individual patient's health and ability to tolerate the treatment. Studies have shown that sunitinib does not act significantly differently in the body based on the adult age, ethnicity, or sex of a patient. However, sunitinib has not been evaluated in pediatric patients. Following an oral dose, peak blood concentrations of sunitinib are reached within 6 to 12 hours. It is administered with or without food. Taking food with sunitinib has no effect on the dose absorbed or the dose available to the body.

Precautions

Sunitinib can cause life-threatening damage to a patient's liver. The drug is not recommended for use in pregnant women. Birth control is recommended while using this drug. Sunitinib is a pregnancy Category D drug. Category D describes drugs in which there is evidence of potential human fetal risk based on adverse reaction data from investigational or marketing experience or studies in humans, but potential benefits may warrant use of the drug in pregnant women despite potential risks. For Category D drugs, medical necessity must be great enough to warrant risking harm to the fetus. Sunitinib is a teratogen (an agent that can cause birth defects) and has proven lethal to fetuses in animal studies. Sunitinib is not recommended for use in breastfeeding women.

Sunitinib is used only in adults, as the safety for use in patients less than 18 years of age has not been established. All patients taking sunitinib must remain well hydrated. Patients should not have any vaccinations

while taking sunitinib without the consent of their treating physician. Patients taking sunitinib should avoid contact with people who have recently had the oral polio vaccine or inhaled flu vaccine.

Sunitinib may not be suitable for patients with a history of liver failure, inflammation of the pancreas, bleeding disorders, heart failure, imbalances in body potassium or magnesium, very high blood pressure, seizure disorders, some heart rhythm abnormalities, or other heart conditions. Sunitinib may cause a heart condition that affects the rhythm of the heartbeat known as QT prolongation. Sometimes QT prolongation can cause a serious cardiac condition that includes a fast and irregular heartbeat, with severe dizziness and fainting. The risk of developing QT prolongation syndrome may be increased if the patient is taking other drugs that also affect the rhythm of the heart, or if the patient has cardiac problems. Low blood levels of potassium or magnesium may also increase the risk of QT prolongation. Sunitinib toxicity may cause other adverse side effects affecting heart function, and multiple other heart conditions may result from use of sunitinib.

Sunitinib may also negatively affect the function of the thyroid gland. A set of baseline thyroid function tests are done before patients receive sunitinib therapy. Patients are also monitored closely for evidence of thyroid dysfunction. Other precautionary tests such as blood pressure checks, heart function tests, pancreatic inflammation, and blood chemistry need to be monitored during sunitinib therapy.

Side effects

Sunitinib is used when the medical benefit is judged to be greater than the risk of side effects. Many patients who are prescribed sunitinib do not develop serious side effects. The most frequent side effects of sunitinib are abdominal pain and cramping, dizziness, changes in liver enzymes, loss of appetite, altered taste in the mouth, **nausea and vomiting**, joint pain, constipation or **diarrhea**, cough, dry skin, **fatigue**, **fever**, increased blood pressure, difficulty breathing, increased bleeding, hair loss, and rash. Less frequently seen side effects include eye tearing, muscle pain, thyroid dysfunction, increased infections such as **pneumonia** or catheter infections, nerve damage, black stool, vomit that looks like coffee grounds, changes in hair or skin color, and sore tongue. Sunitinib may decrease the ability of the body to fight off an infection, as it suppresses the immune system.

Interactions

Patients should make their doctor aware of any and all medications or supplements they are taking before using

sunitinib. Sunitinib interacts with many other drugs. Some drug interactions may make sunitinib unsuitable for use, while others may be monitored and attempted.

Sunitinib may have dangerous additive effects with other drugs that also cause QT prolongation. Drugs that interact with sunitinib in this way include amiodarone, dofetilide, pimozide, procainamide, quinidine, sotalol, and macrolide **antibiotics** such as erythromycin. Sunitinib has been combined with multiple other agents in **clinical trials** with no clinical problems. However, sunitinib is known to interact with one other **chemotherapy** agent called **bevacizumab**, causing a severe form of **anemia** known as **hemolytic anemia**.

Sunitinib is metabolized by a set of liver enzymes known as cytochrome P450 (CYP-450) subtype 3A4. Drugs that induce, or activate, these enzymes increase the metabolism of sunitinib. This activation results in lower levels of therapeutic sunitinib, thereby negatively affecting treatment of cancer. For this reason drugs that induce CYP-450 subtype 3A4 may not be used with sunitinib. This includes some antiepileptic drugs such as **carbamazepine**, some anti-inflammatory drugs such as **dexamethasone**, antituberculosis drugs such as rifampin, and the herb St. John's wort.

Drugs that act to inhibit the action of CYP-450 subtype 3A4 may cause undesired increased levels of sunitinib in the body. This interaction could lead to toxic doses. Some examples are antibiotics such as clarithromycin, antifungal drugs such as ketoconazole, antiviral drugs such as indinavir, antidepressants such as fluoxetine, and some cardiac agents such as verapamil. Grapefruit juice may also increase the amount of sunitinib in the body. Patients should avoid drinking grapefruit juice or eating grapefruit while taking sunitinib.

Resources

BOOKS

Brunton, Laurence, Bruce Chabner, and Bjorn Knollman. *Goodman and Gilman's The Pharmacological Basis of Therapeutics.* 12th ed. New York: McGraw-Hill Medical Publishing, 2012.

Hamilton, Richard J., ed. *Tarascon Pharmacopoeia 2014 Professional Desk Reference Edition.* Burlington, MA: Jones & Bartlett Learning, 2014.

WEBSITES

American Cancer Society. "Sunitinib." http://www.cancer.org/treatment/treatmentsandsideeffects/guidetocancerdrugs/sunitinib (accessed November 3, 2014).

"Sunitinib." MedlinePlus. http://www.nlm.nih.gov/medlineplus/druginfo/meds/a607052.html (accessed November 3, 2014).

ORGANIZATIONS

National Cancer Institute, 9609 Medical Center Dr., BG 9609 MSC 9760, Bethesda, MD 20892-9760, (800) 4-CANCER (422-6237), http://www.cancer.gov.

U.S. Food and Drug Administration, 10903 New Hampshire Ave., Silver Spring, MD 20993, (888) INFO-FDA (463-6332), http://www.fda.gov.

Maria Basile, PhD

REVISED BY TERESA G. ODLE
REVIEWED BY KEVIN GLAZA, RPH

Superior vena cava syndrome

Definition

The superior vena cava is a large vein in the chest that drains the blood from the upper body back to the heart. Compression or occlusion (blocking off) of this vein creates superior vena cava syndrome.

Description

When the superior vena cava (SVC) becomes compressed or occluded, the blood from the upper body cannot drain back to the heart properly. This blockage creates suffusion (the spreading of body fluids into surrounding tissue), which causes varying degrees of airway obstruction, swelling, and cyanosis (purple discoloration due to lack of oxygenation) of the face, neck, arms and chest area.

Causes and symptoms

Causes

Cancer is the most common cause of superior vena cava syndrome. Lung cancer, **lymphoma**, **breast cancer**, and **germ cell tumors** of the chest are commonly associated with SVC syndrome. Any cancer that invades or constricts the blood vessels in the chest can cause SVC syndrome. Other non-cancer causes of SVC syndrome are thyroid goiter, fungal infections, pericardial constriction, aortic aneurysm, and any other disease that creates swelling in the mediastinum (organs and vessels of the chest). Occasionally, SVC syndrome can be caused by a central vein catheter (an IV catheter that is placed into central circulation with its tip in the superior vena cava), which may cause a thrombosis (blockage) of the SVC.

Symptoms

Patients with superior vena cava syndrome (SVC syndrome) might experience facial swelling, causing the shirt collar to feel tight; shortness of breath; coughing; a change of voice; or confusion. A patient might also notice distention or enlargement of veins near the surface of the skin. The development of these signs and symptoms is usually a gradual process taking up to four weeks from onset of symptoms to diagnosis.

Diagnosis

The physician diagnoses SVC syndrome by starting with a complete patient history and physical examination. The physician will ask about onset of symptoms and the timeline of symptom development. The physician will recommend a chest x-ray and a **computed tomography** scan to visualize the chest area in order to confirm the presence of SVC syndrome. The physician may also order venous patency (flow of blood through the vein) studies using contrast dye and scanning techniques. The physician may order a scan done in a **magnetic resonance imaging** (MRI) lab, ultrasound lab, or in nuclear medicine to help assess the cause of the superior vena cava syndrome. These tests help the physician identify the site and nature of the obstruction. If cancer of the bronchi is suspected, the patient should also anticipate other testing such as sputum collection, **bronchoscopy**, and **biopsy** of the suspected cancer site. These tests are very important to the oncologist (a physician who specializes in the treatment of cancer), because they will help to identify the disease, determine its stage, and assign the appropriate course of treatment.

Risks

Many patients have the symptoms of superior vena cava syndrome for more than a week before seeing their doctor. Sometimes the diagnosis of SVC syndrome is the first sign that there is cancer present in the body (only 3–5% of patients with SVC syndrome do not have cancer). Most patients with SVC syndrome do not die from the syndrome itself, but from the underlying disease and the extent of the cancer invasion causing the syndrome. Physicians consider the presence of superior vena cava syndrome a life-threatening oncologic medical emergency when there is tracheal (airway) obstruction present. Further, if there is extensive suffusion causing swelling in the vessels in the brain, the patient's condition can rapidly deteriorate. Once the diagnosis of SVC syndrome is made, the physician will immediately commence determining the cause of the syndrome to avoid or minimize these risks.

Treatment

There are several treatment options to alleviate the symptoms of SVC syndrome. The feasibility of these options depends on the primary cause of the obstruction, the severity of the symptoms, the prognosis of the patient, and the patient's preferences and ultimate goals for therapy. The physician will need to determine the histology (cellular origin) of the obstructing cancer before proceeding with SVC syndrome treatment. Unless there is airway obstruction or swelling in the brain, treatment of SVC syndrome can be delayed to determine the stage of the underlying disease.

Medical management of SVC syndrome includes elevating the head, using steroids to minimize swelling, and diuretics to remove fluid from circulation. Some patients may develop collateral circulation (development of smaller vessel branches to assist with the excess fluid load on the SVC) and not need further treatment.

Chemotherapy is used on lymphomas or small cell lung cancers because they are sensitive to the drugs. Rapid initiation of chemotherapy in these situations can dramatically reduce the unpleasant symptoms of SVC syndrome in most patients. When chemotherapy is not the best choice for the cancer type, **radiation therapy** can provide some relief from symptoms.

Other treatment options include thrombolysis, in which a fibrinolytic agent (agent that breaks down a thrombus or clot) is injected into the obstructed SVC. This option is used when it is determined that the obstruction is inside the vein. Stent placement (placing a sterile mesh tube inside the SVC to keep the vessel open) has been used successfully in some patients, but may require ongoing anticoagulation therapy after placement. Finally, surgical bypass of the obstructed SVC is a possible option for some patients, but the procedure is extensive and the patient must have appropriately healthy veins to graft to the affected area.

QUESTIONS TO ASK YOUR DOCTOR

- What is the most likely cause of my SVC syndrome?
- What tests will be done to determine the cause of my SVC syndrome?
- What are my treatment options for SVC syndrome?
- Am I a candidate for a stent?
- If I am a candidate for thrombolytic therapy, will ongoing anticoagulation be used? Will it interfere with my cancer therapy?
- If I choose to do nothing (opt for no therapy), what may be the consequence?
- Is my SVC syndrome presenting an oncologic medical emergency?

Resources

PERIODICALS

Mehra, S., S. S. Atwal, and U. C. Garga. "Primary Pulmonary Ewing's Sarcoma: Rare Cause of Superior Vena Cava Syndrome in Children." *Journal of Clinical and Diagnostic Research* 8, no. 8 (2014): RD05–06.

WEBSITES

American Society of Clinical Oncology. "Superior Vena Cava Syndrome." Cancer.net http://www.cancer.net/navigating-cancer-care/side-effects/superior-vena-cava-syndrome (accessed November 14, 2014).

Molly Metzler, R.N., B.S.N.

Supratentorial primitive neuroectodermal tumors

Definition

Supratentorial primitive neuroectodermal tumors, or SPNETs, are primary **brain tumors** found mostly in children. The word *supratentorial* refers to the location of these tumors in the part of the brain called the cerebrum, above the tentorium (the tentlike membrane that covers the cerebellum). This term is used to differentiate these tumors from medulloblastomas, which are sometimes called infratentorial primitive neuroectodermal tumors (IPNETs) because they are located beneath the tentorium. *Primitive* refers to the fact that SPNETs arise from cells that have not yet separated into

KEY TERMS

Blastoma—An abnormal growth of embryonic cells. Supratentorial primitive neuroectodermal tumors are sometimes called cerebral neuroblastomas.

Calcification—A deposit of calcium within cells or tissues. Calcifications in the brain are often visible on imaging studies of SPNETs.

Cerebellum—The part of the brain that lies within the lower back portion of the skull behind the brain stem. The cerebellum helps to coordinate voluntary movements.

Cerebrum—The largest part of the brain in humans, occupying the upper part of the skull cavity. Supratentorial primitive neuroectodermal tumors are located in the cerebrum.

Medulloblastoma—A malignant tumor of the cerebellum that occurs mostly in children and is considered a type of primitive neuroectodermal tumor. Medulloblastomas are sometimes classified as infratentorial primitive neuroectodermal tumors because they develop underneath the tentorium.

Primary brain tumor—A tumor that starts in the brain, as distinct from a metastatic tumor that begins elsewhere in the body and spreads to the brain.

Primitive—Simple or undifferentiated. SPNETs are classified as primitive tumors because they arise from cells that have not yet separated into groups of more specialized cells.

Shunt—A tube inserted by a surgeon to relieve pressure on the brain from blocked cerebrospinal fluid. The tube allows the fluid to bypass the tumor that is blocking its flow.

Supratentorial—Located above the tentorium, which is the tentlike membrane that covers the cerebellum.

Ventricle—One of the small cavities located within the brain.

more specialized types of cells. The word *neuroectodermal* means that these tumors develop out of a layer of cells in the embryo that eventually gives rise to the baby's nervous system. Supratentorial primitive neuroectodermal tumors are also called cerebral neuroblastomas.

Description

SPNETs are rapidly growing tumors that are considered highly malignant. While they resemble medulloblastomas in

terms of the type of cells that give rise to them, they are far less common; the ratio of medulloblastomas to SPNETs is thought to be about 25:1.

The location of SPNETs in the cerebrum means that they occur in the largest part of the brain—the portion that governs speech, emotions, voluntary muscular movements, and the ability to think, reason, and solve problems. These tumors may metastasize, or spread, to other parts of the central nervous system (CNS) via the cerebrospinal fluid. A doctor looking at a CT scan of one of these tumors will usually see a large mass with clear margins that contains cysts, calcifications (deposits of calcium within the brain cells), and patches of dead tumor cells. In some cases the doctor will also see evidence of bleeding into nearby tissue.

Demographics

These tumors are extremely rare, accounting for only 0.5–2 percent of childhood tumors of the central nervous system (CNS). About 2,200 children below the age of 15 are diagnosed with malignant tumors of the brain and spinal cord each year in the United States; between 10 and 40 of these children will be diagnosed with SPNETs.

It is difficult to evaluate the statistical significance of racial or gender differences in such a small group; however, the available evidence from American cancer registries suggests that these cancers occur more frequently in Caucasian children than in African Americans, and more frequently in males than in females. The male:female ratio is thought to be about 1.8:1.

SPNETs occur almost exclusively in younger children, with very few cases reported in adolescents or adults. About 75% of these tumors occur in children below the age of 15, with 50% diagnosed in children below the age of 10. Most SPNETs diagnosed in adults occur in young adults between the ages of 21 and 40.

Causes and symptoms

The causes of SPNETs are not well understood. They do not run in families and are not known to be associated with carcinogens in the environment. It is thought that they result from sporadic (random) gene mutations, possibly associated with abnormalities in the short arm of chromosome 17.

The symptoms of a supratentorial primitive neuroectodermal tumor are often insidious, which means that they are gradual in onset. They are caused by the increased pressure of cerebrospinal fluid inside the skull. Depending on the size of the tumor and the child's age, symptoms may include the following:

• headache, usually worse in the morning, sometimes relieved by vomiting

• blurred vision

• nausea and intermittent vomiting

• weakness or loss of sensation on one side of the body

• difficulty with balance

• frequent crying (in children below the age of three)

• decreased interaction with other people

• lowered energy level or unusual need for sleep

• irritability and other personality changes

• unexplained changes in weight or appetite

Parents should note, however, that none of these symptoms are unique to SPNETs; they may be produced by other types of brain tumors, head trauma, meningitis, migraine headaches, or several other medical conditions. In any event, a child with these symptoms should be seen by a doctor at once.

Diagnosis

The diagnosis of a supratentorial primitive neuroectodermal tumor begins with a review of the child's medical history and a thorough physical examination. The child may be given several vision tests if he or she is seeing double or having other visual disturbances. The doctor may notice one or more of the following signs, although none of them are distinctive features of SPNETs:

• Papilledema. Papilledema refers to swelling of the optic disk, usually caused by increased fluid pressure behind the eye.

• Ataxia. This term refers to loss of muscular coordination.

• Nystagmus. This term refers to rapid involuntary movement of the eyeball. The doctor may be able to detect it by having the child look to the right or the left.

• Palsy of the lower cranial nerve.

• Dysmetria. This term refers to the loss of ability to estimate distance when using the muscles; an example would be overreaching when trying to pick up a small object.

The child's doctor will then order both laboratory tests and **imaging studies**. The laboratory tests are done to rule out such diseases as meningitis and to see whether the child's liver and other organs are functioning normally. The imaging studies are performed to determine the extent of the cancer and to assign the child to a risk group.

The diagnosis of SPNET cannot be confirmed, however, on the basis of a clinical examination. Instead, a neurosurgeon will perform what is known as an open **biopsy**. He or she will drill a small hole in the child's skull and remove a small piece of the tumor for examination by a pathologist.

Imaging tests

Imaging tests for SPNETs include the following:

• Magnetic resonance imaging (MRIs)

• Computed tomography (CT) scan

• Chest x-ray

• Bone scan (This test is necessary to determine whether the tumor has spread beyond the central nervous system.)

Laboratory tests

Standard laboratory tests for children with brain tumors include a complete blood count (CBC), electrolyte analysis, tests of kidney, liver, and thyroid function, and tests that determine whether the child has been recently exposed to certain viruses. In addition, a **lumbar puncture** will usually be performed to look for cancer cells in the child's spinal fluid.

Treatment team

Since the 1960s, most children diagnosed with brain tumors have been treated in specialized children's cancer centers. A child with a SPNET will usually have a pediatric oncologist as his or her primary doctor, along with one or more specialists. These specialists may include a neurosurgeon, pathologist, neuroradiologist, radiation oncologist, medical oncologist, endocrinologist, nutritionist, physical therapist or rehabilitation specialist, and psychologist or psychiatrist. The team will also include social workers, clergy, and other professionals to help the parents cope with the stresses of their child's illness and treatments.

Clinical staging

Supratentorial primitive neuroectodermal tumors are not staged in the same way as cancers elsewhere in the body. Instead, children with these tumors are divided into two risk groups, average risk and poor risk. Assignment to these groups is based on the following factors:

• child's age

• size and location of the tumor

• whether the tumor has spread to other parts of the central nervous system

• whether the tumor has spread beyond the CNS to other parts of the body

Average-risk children are those older than three years, with most or all of the tumor removed by surgery and no evidence that the cancer has spread beyond the cerebrum. Poor-risk children are those who are younger than three years, whose cancer was located near the center of the brain or could not be removed completely by surgery, and whose cancer has spread to or beyond other parts of the CNS. The risk of recurrence is higher for children in the poor-risk group.

Treatment

Treatments for SPNETs depend on the child's age and his or her risk group. Children younger than three years are not usually given **radiation therapy** because it can affect growth and normal brain development. They are usually treated with surgery first to remove as much of the tumor as possible, followed by **chemotherapy** if they are considered poor-risk patients. The drugs most commonly used to treat SPNETs include **lomustine**, **cisplatin**, **carboplatin**, and **vincristine**.

In addition to removing the tumor, the surgeon may also place a shunt to reduce pressure on the child's brain if the tumor is blocking the flow of cerebrospinal fluid. A shunt is a plastic tube with one end placed within the third ventricle of the brain. The rest of the shunt is routed under the skin of the head, neck, and chest with the other end placed in the abdomen or near the heart. About 30% of children treated for SPNETs require shunt placement.

Children three years and older are treated with surgery first, followed by radiation treatment of the entire brain and spinal cord. Those considered poor risks may also be given chemotherapy. Recurrent SPNETs are treated with further surgery and an additional course of chemotherapy.

Treatments being researched for supratentorial primitive neuroectodermal tumors include:

- gamma knife surgery (GKS)
- gene therapy
- high-dose chemotherapy—chemotherapy with topotecan has been reported to give promising results in treating SPNETS, as does high-dose chemotherapy combined with stem cell transplantation
- photodynamic therapy
- bone marrow transplantation
- newer drugs: irinotecan, tipifarnib, lapatinib, ixabepilone, cilengitide, and tariquidar

Alternative and complementary therapies

Some complementary therapies that are reported to help children with SPNETs include pet therapy, humor therapy, art therapy, and music therapy. All of these can be pleasurable for the child as well as relaxing. Ginger or peppermint may help to relieve the **nausea and vomiting** associated with chemotherapy.

Prognosis

The prognosis for children with SPNETs depends largely on their risk group. In general, however, these tumors have a poorer prognosis than other types of brain tumors in children, in part because of the difficulty of removing the complete tumor due to its large size, its extensive blood supply, and its location within the cerebrum. The overall five-year survival rate of children with supratentorial primitive neuroectodermal tumors is reported to be 50–60%, but is much lower in children younger than three years and in older children who do not respond to radiation therapy.

Recurrent tumors of this type are almost always fatal; there are no effective therapies for recurrent SPNETs.

Coping with cancer treatment

Children being treated for SPNETs can be given additional medications to treat nausea and other side effects of chemotherapy. With regard to homesickness and other emotional reactions to being away from home, children's cancer centers have social workers and child psychologists who can educate the child's family about the cancer as well as help the child deal with separation issues.

The side effects of radiation therapy in children with brain tumors may include the formation of dead tissue at the site of the tumor. This formation is known as radiation necrosis. It occurs in about 5% of children who receive radiation therapy and may require surgical removal. Radiation necrosis, however, is not as serious as recurrence of the tumor.

Children who have difficulty speaking after brain surgery, or who experience physical weakness, difficulty walking, visual impairment, or other sensory problems, are given **physical therapy** and/or speech therapy on either an inpatient or outpatient basis.

Clinical trials

Because SPNETs are so rare, the American Cancer Society recommends that children diagnosed with these tumors be enrolled in an appropriate clinical trial. As of 2014, there were about 149 **clinical trials** in the United States for children with various types of PNETs. Some of these trials involved gene testing to improve diagnosis of children with brain tumors, while others were exploring various combinations of chemotherapy (including new agents), **photodynamic therapy**, **stem cell transplantation**, and **bone marrow transplantation** as treatments for primitive neuroectodermal tumors.

Prevention

There is no way to prevent SPNETs because their cause is still unknown.

Special concerns

Children with SPNETs are like children with other long-term illnesses in that they may develop emotional problems in reaction to restrictions on their activities, uncomfortable treatments, or being treated in a cancer center away from home. These children may withdraw from others, become angry or bitter, or feel inappropriately guilty about their illness. It is important for parents to reassure the child that he or she did not cause the cancer or deserve it as a punishment for being "bad." Parents may benefit from consulting a child psychiatrist about these and other emotional problems.

Another special concern is the task of explaining the child's illness and treatments to other family members and friends in ways that they can understand. Members of the child's treatment team can be helpful in providing simplified descriptions for siblings or schoolmates.

A third area of concern with **childhood cancers** is the parents' relationships with their other children and with each other. Siblings may resent the amount of time and attention given to the child with cancer, or they may fear that they too will develop a brain tumor. Support groups for families of children with cancer can help by sharing strategies for coping with these problems as well

as allowing members to express anxiety and other painful feelings in a safe setting.

See also Medulloblastoma; Pineoblastoma.

Resources

BOOKS

Shiminski-Maher, Tania, Catherine Woodman, and Nancy Keene. *Childhood Brain and Spinal Cord Tumors: A Guide for Families, Friends and Caregivers.* 2nd ed. Bellingham, WA: Childhood Cancer Guides, 2014.

PERIODICALS

Perez-Martinez, A., A. Lassaletta, M. Gonzalez-Vincent, et al. "High-Dose Chemotherapy with Autologous Stem Cell Rescue for Children with High-Risk and Recurrent Medulloblastoma and Supratentorial Primitive Neuroectodermal Tumors." *Journal of Neurooncology* 71 (January 2005): 33–38.

OTHER

American Cancer Society. *Brain and Spinal Cord Tumors in Children.* http://documents.cancer.org/acs/groups/cid/documents/webcontent/003089-pdf.pdf (accessed November 17, 2014).

ORGANIZATIONS

American Academy of Child and Adolescent Psychiatry, 3615 Wisconsin Ave. NW, Washington, DC 20016-3007, (202) 966-7300, Fax: (202) 966-2891, http://www.aacap.org.

American Brain Tumor Association, 8550 W. Bryn Mawr Ave., Ste. 550, Chicago, IL 60631, (773) 577-8750, (800) 886-2282, Fax: (773) 577-8738, info@abta.org, http://www.abta.org.

CureSearch for Children's Cancer, 4600 East-West Highway, Suite 600, Bethesda, MD 20814, (800) 458-6223, Fax: (301) 718-0047, info@curesearch.org, http://www.curesearch.org.

Rebecca Frey, PhD

Suprefact *see* **Buserelin**

Suramin

Definition

Suramin (suramin hexasodium; CI-1003) is a polysulfonated naphthylurea. It is a growth factor antagonist that has been studied as a form of palliative treatment in hormone-refractory **prostate cancer** and hormone-responsive metastatic prostate **cancer**.

Purpose

Suramin has been used for years to combat African sleeping sickness and river blindness but it has also been

KEY TERMS

Antagonist—A drug that binds to a cellular receptor for a hormone, neurotransmitter, or another drug. Antagonists block the action of the substance without producing any physiologic effect itself.

Antineoplastic—Referring to a regimen of chemotherapy aimed at destroying malignant cells using a variety of agents that directly affect cellular growth and development.

Anthelmintic—An agent destructive to worms. Many anthelmintic drugs are toxic and should be given with care; the patient should be observed carefully for toxic effects after the drug is given.

Antiprotozoal—An agent destructive to protozoa.

Clinical trials—Highly regulated and carefully controlled patient studies, where either new drugs to treat cancer or novel methods of treatment are investigated.

DNA—Deoxyribonucleic acid; genetic information carried in chromosomes.

Growth factors—Compounds made by the body that function to regulate cell division and cell survival. Some growth factors are also produced in the laboratory by genetic engineering and are used in biological therapy.

Metastatic—The term used to describe a secondary cancer, or one that has spread from one area of the body to another.

Palliative—To alleviate disease without curing it.

Tumor—An abnormal mass of tissue that serves no purpose. Tumors may be either benign (noncancerous) or malignant (cancerous).

found beneficial in slowing the progression of prostate cancer. The drug is classified as an antiprotozoal or anthelmintic. In addition to combating prostate cancer, suramin has demonstrated antitumor activity against many types of tumors including endometrial, breast, ovarian, and lung cancer. It has a number of important biological functions for cancer treatment; it inhibits a number of growth factors and receptors needed for tumor growth including epidermal growth factor (EGF), platelet-derived growth factor (PDGF), fibroblast growth factor, and vascular endothelial growth factor. Suramin decreases blood plasma levels of insulin-like growth

factors 1 and 2. Suramin also inhibits tumor antigen, DNA synthesis, cell motility, and urokinase activity. It has also demonstrated significant improvements in pain response.

Description

While conducting research into suramin as a potential anti-HIV agent, the investigators found that tumors regressed in HIV-associated cancers. This discovery led investigators to evaluate the antineoplastic effects of suramin. Unfortunately, suramin did not prove effective as an anti-HIV agent.

Suramin has not been approved by the U.S. Food and Drug Administration (FDA) as a cancer treatment.

Recommended dosage

Since this drug is not FDA-approved for cancer treatment, dosing information is not obtainable.

Precautions

Due to a risk of adrenal insufficiency (which results from the inadequate production of adrenal hormones) and coagulopathy (a defect that interferes with the blood clotting mechanism), patients receiving suramin should be administered hydrocortisone and vitamin K.

Significant toxicities are associated the use of suramin. However, with careful monitoring of serum concentrations, these toxicities are manageable.

Side effects

Rash, edema, and asthenia are commonly reported, but are generally mild to moderate. Malaise and **fatigue** are the most common dose-limiting toxicities, affecting 41% of patients in **clinical trials** for prostate cancer. The majority of the side effects listed below are based on suramin's use as an antiprotozoal agent. Different doses used for cancer treatment may affect the side effect profile. Abdominal pain, **fever**, metallic taste, and a general feeling of discomfort may be bothersome but do not usually require medical attention. These effects may disappear during treatment as the body adjusts to the medicine. Other common side effects are cloudy urine; crawling or tingling sensation of the skin; **diarrhea**; faintness (particularly after missing meals); headache; increased skin color; irritability; **itching**; joint pain; loss of appetite (**anorexia**); **nausea and vomiting**; numbness or weakness in arms, hands, legs, or feet; stinging sensation on skin; swelling on skin; tenderness of the palms and the soles; and becoming easily tired.

Less common side effects may include extreme fatigue or weakness; increased sensitivity of eyes to light;

changes in or loss of vision; watery eyes; swelling around eyes; ulcers or sores in mouth; and painful and tender glands in the neck, armpits, or groin.

Interactions

Drug interaction information is not readily available for suramin. However, as with any treatment, patients should alert their doctor to any prescription, over-the-counter, or herbal remedies they are taking in order to avoid possible drug interactions.

Resources

PERIODICALS

Bhargava, S., et al. "Suramin Inhibits Not Only Tumor Growth and Metastasis but Also Angiogenesis in Experimental Pancreatic Cancer." *Journal of Gastrointestinal Surgery* 11, no. 2 (2007): 171–78.

Singla, A.K., A. Bondareva, and F.R. Jirik. "Combined Treatment with Paclitaxel and Suramin Prevents the Development of Metastasis by Inhibiting Metastatic Colonization of Circulating Tumor Cells." *Clinical and Experimental Metastasis* 31 (August 2014): 705–14.

WEBSITES

National Cancer Institute. "Suramin." NCI Drug Dictionary. http://www.cancer.gov/drugdictionary?cdrid=40052 (accessed October 9, 2014).

Crystal Heather Kaczkowski, MSc.

Surgical oncology

Definition

Surgical oncology is a specialized area of oncology that engages surgeons in the cure and management of **cancer**.

Purpose

Cancer has become a medical specialty warranting its own surgical area because of advances in the biology, pathophysiology, diagnostics, and staging of malignant tumors. Surgeons have traditionally been involved with the resection and radical surgeries of tumors, leaving the management of the cancer and the patient to other specialists. Advances in the early diagnosis of cancer, the staging of tumors, microscopic analyses of cells, and increased understanding of **cancer biology** have broadened the range of nonsurgical cancer treatments. These treatments include systematic **chemotherapy**, hormonal therapy, and radiotherapy as alternatives or adjunctive

therapy for patients with cancer. Specialists known as oncologists often work in conjunction with various specialized surgeons for treatment of patients with cancer.

Not all cancer tumors are manageable by surgery, nor does the removal of some tumors or metastases necessarily lead to a cure or longer life. The oncological surgeon looks for the relationship between tumor excision and the risk presented by the primary tumor. He or she is knowledgeable about patient management with more conservative procedures than the traditional excision or resection.

Description

Surgical oncology is guided by principles that govern the routine procedures related to the cancer patient's cure, palliative care, and quality of life. Surgical oncology performs its most efficacious work by local tumor excision; regional lymph node removal; the handling of cancer recurrence (local or widespread); and, in rare cases, with surgical resection of metastases from the primary tumor. Each of these areas plays a different role in cancer management.

Excision

Local excision has traditionally been the hallmark of surgical oncology. Excision refers to the removal of the cancer and its effects. Resection of a tumor in the colon can end the effects of obstruction, for instance, or removal of a breast **carcinoma** can stop the cancer. Resection of a primary tumor also stops the tumor from spreading throughout the body. The cancer's spread into other body systems, however, usually occurs before a local removal, giving resection little bearing upon cells that have already escaped the primary tumor. Advances in oncology through pathophysiology, staging, and **biopsy** offer a new diagnostic role to the surgeon using excision. These advances provide simple diagnostic information about size, grade, and extent of the tumor, as well as more sophisticated evaluations of the cancer's biochemical and hormonal features.

Regional lymph node removal

Lymph node involvement provides surgical oncologists with major diagnostic information. The sentinel node biopsy is superior to any biological test in terms of prediction of cancer mortality rates. Nodal biopsy offers very precise information about the extent and type of invasive effects of the primary tumor. The removal of nodes, however, may present pain and other morbid conditions for the patient.

KEY TERMS

Biopsy—The surgical excision of tissue to diagnose the size, type, and extent of a cancerous growth.

Cancer surgery—Surgery in which the goal is to excise a tumor and its surrounding tissue found to be malignant.

Resection—Cutting out and removing tissue to eliminate a cancerous tumor; usually refers to a section of the organ (e.g., colon, intestine, lung, stomach) that must be cut to remove the tumor and its surrounding tissue.

Tumor staging—The method used by oncologists to determine the risk from a cancerous tumor. A number—ranging from 1A to 4B—is assigned to predict the level of invasion by a tumor, and offer a prognosis for morbidity and mortality.

Local and regional recurrence

Radical procedures in surgical oncology for local and regional occurrences of a primary tumor provide crucial information on the spread of cancer and prognostic outcomes; however, they do not contribute substantially to the outcome of the cancer. According to most surgical oncology literature, the ability to remove a local recurrence must be balanced by the patient's goals related to aesthetic and pain control concerns. Historically, more radical procedures have not improved the chances of survival.

Surgery for distant metastases

In general, a cancer tumor that spreads further from its **primary site** is less likely to be controlled by surgery. According to research, except for a few instances where **metastasis** is confined, surgical removal of a distant metastasis is not warranted. Since the rapidity of discovering a distant metastasis has little bearing upon cancer survival, the usefulness of surgery is not time dependent. In the case of liver metastasis, for example, a cure is related to the pathophysiology of the original cancer and level of cancer antigen in the liver rather than the size or time of discovery. While surgery of metastatic cancer may not extend life, there may be indications for it such as pain relief, obstruction removal, control of bleeding, and resolution of infection.

Demographics

According to the American Cancer Society and the **National Cancer Institute**, about 580,350 people were expected to die of cancer in the year 2013. According to the American Cancer Society, about 1,660,290 new cancer cases were expected to be diagnosed in 2013—854,790 males and 805,500 females. Cancer is the second most common cause of death in the United States. The specific cases of newly diagnosed cancers estimated for 2013 in males in the United States were:

- prostate (28%)
- lung and bronchus (14%)
- colon and rectum (9%)
- urinary bladder (6%)
- melanoma of the skin (5%)
- kidney and renal pelvis (5%)
- non-Hodgkin lymphoma (4%)
- oral cavity and pharynx (3%)
- leukemia (3%)
- pancreas (3%)

The newly diagnosed cases of cancers estimated for females in the United States during 2013 were:

- breast (29%)
- lung and bronchus (14%)
- colon and rectum (9%)
- uterine corpus (6%)
- thyroid (6%)
- non-Hodgkin lymphoma (4%)
- melanoma of the skin (4%)
- kidney and renal pelvis (3%)
- pancreas (3%)
- ovary (3%)

Preparation

Surgery removes cancer cells and surrounding tissues. It is often combined with **radiation therapy** and chemotherapy. It is important for the patient to meet with the surgical oncologist to talk about the procedure and begin preparations for surgery. Oncological surgery may be performed to biopsy a suspicious site for malignant cells or tumor. It is also used for **tumor removal** from organs such as the tongue, throat, lung, stomach, intestines, colon, bladder, ovary, and prostate. Tumors of limbs, ligaments, and tendons may also be treated with surgery. In many cases, the biopsy and surgery to remove the cancer cells or tissues are done at the same time.

The impact of a surgical procedure depends upon the diagnosis and the area of the body that is to be treated by surgery. Many cancer surgeries involve major organs and require open abdominal surgery, which is the most extensive type of surgical procedure. This surgery requires a number of medical tests prior to surgery to assess the overall health of the patient and to make decisions about adjunctive procedures like radiation or chemotherapy. Preparation for cancer surgery requires psychological readiness for a hospital stay, postoperative pain, sometimes slow recovery, and anticipation of complications from tumor excision or resection. It also may require consultation with stomal therapists if a section of the urinary tract or bowel is to be removed and replaced with an outside reservoir or conduit, called an ostomy.

Aftercare

After surgery, the type and duration of side effects and the elements of recovery depend on where in the body the surgery was performed and the patient's general health. Some surgeries may alter basic functions in the urinary or gastrointestinal systems. Recovering full use of function takes time and patience. Surgeries that remove conduits such as the colon, intestines, or urinary tract require appliances for urine and fecal waste and the help of a stomal therapist. Breast or prostate surgeries yield concerns about cosmetic appearance and intimate activities. For most cancer surgeries, basic functions like tasting, eating, drinking, breathing, moving, urinating, defecating, or neurological ability may be changed in the short term. Resources to attend to deficits in daily activities need to be set up before surgery.

Risks

The type of risks that cancer surgery presents depends almost entirely upon the part of the body being biopsied or excised. Risks of surgery can be great when major organs are involved, such as the gastrointestinal system or the brain. These risks are usually discussed explicitly with the patient when making treatment decisions.

Results

Most cancers are categorized based upon their likelihood of being contained, of spreading, and of recurring. This assessment is referred to as **tumor grading** or **tumor staging**. The prognosis after surgery depends upon the stage of the disease and the type of cancer cell involved. General results of cancer surgery depend in large part on norms of success based upon the study of groups of patients with the same diagnosis. The results are often stated in percentages of the chance of cancer recurrence or its spread after surgery. After five disease-free years, patients are usually considered cured, because the recurrence rates decline drastically after five years. The benchmark is based upon the percentage of people known to reach the fifth year after surgery with no recurrence or spread of the primary tumor.

QUESTIONS TO ASK YOUR DOCTOR

- What are the alternatives to surgery for this cancer?
- What is the likelihood that this surgery will entirely eliminate the cancer?
- What are the risks involved?
- Is this a surgical procedure that is often performed in this hospital or surgical center?
- What type of treatments will be needed following the surgery?
- What are the costs involved?

Morbidity and mortality rates

Morbidity and mortality of oncological surgery are high if there is organ involvement or extensive excision of major parts of the body. Because there is an ongoing disease process and many patients may be very ill at the time of surgery, the complications of surgery may be quite complex. Each procedure is understood by the surgeon for its likely complications or risks, and these are discussed during the initial surgical consultations.

With any surgery, there are risks associated with the use of general anesthetic and the opening of body cavities. Open surgery has general risks associated with it that are not related to the type of procedure, such as the occurrence of blood clots or cardiac events.

There is an extensive body of literature about the complication and morbidity rates of surgery performed in high-volume treatment centers. Data show that in general, large volumes of surgery affect the quality outcomes of surgery, with smaller hospitals having lower rates of procedural success and higher operative and postoperative complications than larger facilities. It is not known whether the surgeon's experience or the advantages of institutional resources in operative or postoperative care contribute to these statistics.

Alternatives

Alternatives to cancer surgery exist for almost every cancer treated in the United States. Research into alternatives has been very successful for some—but not all—cancers. Most organizations dealing with cancer patients suggest alternative treatments. Physicians and surgeons expect to be asked about alternatives to surgery and are usually quite knowledgeable about their use as cancer treatments or as adjuncts to surgery.

Health care team roles

A surgeon who specializes in cancer surgery or oncology performs oncology surgery in a general hospital or **cancer research** center.

Resources

BOOKS

Casciatio, Dennis A. *Manual of Clinical Oncology.* 7th ed. Philadelphia: Lippincott Williams & Williams/Wolters Kluwer, 2012.

Lee, K. J. *Essential Otolaryngology: Head and Neck Surgery.* 10th ed. New York: McGraw-Hill, 2012.

Lentz, Gretchen, et al. *Comprehensive Gynecology.* 5th ed. St. Louis: Mosby/Elsevier, 2012.

Townsend, Courtney M., et al. *Sabiston Textbook of Surgery.* 19th ed. Philadelphia: Saunders/Elsevier, 2012.

Wein, Alan J., et al. *Campbell-Walsh Urology.* 10th ed. Philadelphia: Saunders/Elsevier, 2012.

PERIODICALS

Begue, Aaron, et al. "Retrospective Study of Multidisciplinary Rounding on a Thoracic Surgical Oncology Unit." *Clinical Journal of Oncology Nursing* 16, no. 6 (2012): E198–202. http://dx.doi.org/10.1188/12.CJON.E198-E202 (accessed October 3, 2014).

Macefield, R. C., K. N. L. Avery, and J. M. Blazeby. "Integration of Clinical and Patient-Reported Outcomes in Surgical Oncology." *British Journal of Surgery* 100, no. 1 (2013): 28–37. http://dx.doi.org/10.1002/bjs.8989 (accessed October 3, 2014).

Menezes, Amber S., et al. "Clinical Research in Surgical Oncology: An Analysis of ClinicalTrials.gov." *Annals of Surgical Oncology* (June 26, 2013): e-pub ahead of print. http://dx.doi.org/10.1245/s10434-013-3054-y (accessed October 3, 2014).

Povoski, Stephen P., and Nathan C. Hall. "Recognizing the Role of Surgical Oncology and Cancer Imaging in the Multidisciplinary Approach to Cancer: An Important Area of Future Scholarly Growth for BMC Cancer." *BMC Cancer* 13, no. 355 (July 23, 2013). http://dx.doi.org/10.1186/1471-2407-13-355 (accessed October 3, 2014).

Shuman, Andrew G., et al. "A New Care Paradigm in Geriatric Head and Neck Surgical Oncology." *Journal of Surgical Oncology* 108, no. 3 (2013): 187–91. http://dx.doi.org/10.1002/jso.23370 (accessed October 3, 2014).

Søreide, Kjetil, and Annbjørg H. Søreide. "Using Patient-Reported Outcome Measures for Improved Decision-Making in Patients with Gastrointestinal Cancer—The Last Clinical Frontier in Surgical Oncology?" *Frontiers in Clinical Oncology* 3, no. 157 (June 2013). http://dx.doi.org/10.3389/fonc.2013.00157 (accessed October 3, 2014).

Veronesi, Umberto, and Vaia Stafyla. "Grand Challenges in Surgical Oncology." *Frontiers in Surgical Oncology* 2, no. 127 (October 2012). http://dx.doi.org/10.3389/fonc.2012.00127 (accessed October 3, 2014).

OTHER

American Cancer Society. *Cancer Facts & Figures 2013.* Atlanta: American Cancer Society, 2013. http://www.cancer.org/Research/CancerFactsStatistics/CancerFactsFigures2013/2013-cancer-facts-and-figures.pdf (accessed October 3, 2014).

WEBSITES

American Cancer Society. "A Guide to Cancer Surgery." http://www.cancer.org/treatment/treatmentsandsideeffects/treatmenttypes/surgery/surgery-treatment-toc (accessed February 5, 2015).

Cancer Treatment Centers of America. "Surgical Oncology." http://www.cancercenter.com/treatments/surgical-oncology/ (accessed February 5, 2015).

National Cancer Institute. *Cancer Trends Progress Report—2011/2012 Update.* Online. Bethesda, MD: National Institutes of Health, August 2012. http://progressreport.cancer.gov (accessed October 3, 2014).

National Cancer Institute. "SEER (Surveillance Epidemiology and End Results) Stat Fact Sheets: All Sites." http://seer.cancer.gov/statfacts/html/all.html (accessed October 3, 2014).

ORGANIZATIONS

American Cancer Society, 250 Williams St. NW, Atlanta, GA 30303, (800) 227-2345, http://www.cancer.org.

Cancer Research Institute, One Exchange Plz., 55 Broadway, Ste. 1802, New York, NY 10006, (212) 688-7515, (800) 99-CANCER (992-2623), http://cancerresearch.org.

National Breast Cancer Coalition, 1101 17th St. NW, Ste. 1300, Washington, DC 20036, (202) 296-7477, (800) 622-2838, Fax: (202) 265-6854, http://www.breastcancerdeadline2020.org.

National Cancer Institute, 6116 Executive Blvd., Ste. 300, Bethesda, MD 20892-8322, (800) 4-CANCER (422-6237), http://cancer.gov.

Society of Surgical Oncology, 9525 W. Bryn Mawr Ave., Ste. 870, Rosemont, IL 60018, (847) 427-1400, info@surgonc.org, http://surgonc.org.

Nancy McKenzie, PhD
REVISED BY ROSALYN CARSON-DEWITT, MD
REVISED BY TAMMY ALLHOFF, CST/CSFA, AAS

Survivorship care plans

Definition

Survivorship care plans (SCPs) are records of patients' **cancer** histories and recommendations for follow-up care. An SCP details the responsibilities of all care providers, whether cancer-related, primary care, or psychosocial. The SCP is intended to help the survivor keep track of his or her follow-up appointments and treatments, improve coordination of the survivor's care among the various health care professionals involved, and avoid duplication of resources.

Description

Background

SCPs are a relatively recent development in the care of cancer survivors. They were first discussed and recommended during an Institute of Medicine (IOM) workshop held in the fall of 2006; sample SCPs were included in the IOM's follow-up report published in 2007. What prompted the IOM's concern is the remarkable increase in the number of long-term survivors of cancer. As recently as 1960, only 25% of cancer patients lived 5 years or longer post diagnosis, and the creation of survivorship care plans was not a priority of either clinicians or researchers. In the 1980s, however, the number of 5-year survivors of cancer approached 50%, and was close to 65% as of 2014.

In terms of numbers, the **National Cancer Institute** (NCI) reports that as of January 2014, there were 14.5 million cancer survivors in the United States—about 4% of the total population. Sixty percent of survivors were 65 years old or older, while only 5% were 40 or younger. Sixty-four percent survived five years or more after diagnosis, with 41% living 10 years or longer and 15% living 20 years or more. By 2024, the number of cancer survivors is expected to increase by 37% to 19.9 million persons. By any definition, this is a sizable group of people who need to plan for lifelong follow-up care after cancer. In the years following the IOM's workshop and follow-up reports, a number of different professional organizations and cancer centers have drawn up sample SCPs.

IOM and NCCS recommendations for a model SCP

The IOM's 2007 report recommended that a survivorship care plan should contain the following elements:

- the patient's cancer diagnosis
- descriptions of the treatments received
- descriptions of their potential long-term consequences
- specific information about the timing and content of recommended follow-up appointments
- recommendations about preventive measures and lifestyle changes to maintain health and well-being
- information about the patient's legal protections in regard to employment and health insurance
- information about the availability of psychosocial resources in the patient's community

---

KEY TERMS

Oncologist—A physician who specializes in the diagnosis, treatment, and follow-up care of cancer patients.

Survivorship—A term that refers to the life of a person with cancer after treatment is complete. It encompasses physical, emotional, and financial issues, such as late effects of cancer treatment, follow-up care, and family and caregiver relationships.

The National Coalition for Cancer Survivorship (NCCS) maintains that the following should be added to a comprehensive SCP:

- A complete list of surgery, chemotherapy, radiotherapy, transplantation, hormonal therapy, gene or other therapies provided, including agents used, treatment regimen, total dosage, identifying number and title of clinical trials (if any), indicators of treatment response, and toxicities experienced during treatment.
- A complete list of nutritional, psychosocial, and other supportive therapies provided.
- Full contact information for all treating institutions and the principal individual providers.
- Information about the possible late and long-term effects of treatment and symptoms of such effects, and the possible signs of recurrence or second cancers.
- Information about the possible effects of cancer on marital or partner relationships, sexual functioning, work, and parenting, and any potential future need for psychosocial support.
- When appropriate, recommendations to inform first-degree relatives about their increased risk and the need for cancer screening.
- As appropriate, information on genetic counseling and testing to identify high-risk individuals who could benefit from more comprehensive cancer surveillance, chemoprevention, or risk-reducing surgery.
- A list of referrals to specific follow-up care providers, support groups, and/or the patient's primary care provider.
- A list of cancer-related resources and sources of reliable information.

Present models

A number of different model SCPs have been published by the IOM or made available online since 2007. They include:

- Online SCPs that the patient can download, print, fill out, and share with the oncologist and primary care physician. The Journey Forward and the Minnesota Cancer Alliance (MCA) models are examples of this type. Some of these models consist of a series of separate sheets, while the MCA model is a complete booklet.

- Templates that the patient can download and have their oncologist and/or primary care doctor complete. The templates designed by ASCO are the most widely used, and were included in the IOM's 2007 report as model SCPs. They can be downloaded from the National Coalition for Cancer Survivorship (NCCS) website listed in the Resources section.

- An improvised record compiled by patients themselves about their cancer diagnosis; treatment dates; drug names and doses, including chemotherapy; surgeries performed; and, if radiation was received, the specific areas of the body that were irradiated; contact information for all physicians involved in the treatments; results of laboratory tests and other diagnostic studies; the facilities where these tests were performed; and the patient's blood type, current medication, and other relevant portions of his or her medical history. Once the record is compiled, the patient can photocopy any handwritten documents, scan them, and save them to a CD or flash drive. Printouts of the documents, the CD, or the flash drive can then be taken to the patient's medical appointments.

Survivors' feedback

The IOM included cancer survivors among the participants in its 2006 workshop. Only a few reported that they had received anything like a written document from either their oncologist or their primary care physician when treatment was ended. Most stated that they wished they had received an SCP, for the following reasons:

- An SCP would have been a comforting "vote of confidence" from the oncologist that they would survive.

- A written document would have helped them take in necessary information about follow-up care slowly, rather than feeling overwhelmed by a deluge of information given orally.

- A written document would have helped them explain their follow-up care to family members.

- Some survivors thought they would have had better clinical outcomes during follow-up care if they had an SCP.

The patients who attended the IOM workshop were also clear about their preferences regarding SCPs:

- Most wanted the plan to be given in both digital and paper formats.

- Most survivors felt strongly that the SCP should be written in language that the average person can understand rather than medical jargon.

- Many participants liked the idea of a Web-based personalized site that their doctors could update with new information, including new research findings.

- Most participants approved of the content and format of the IOM's draft template, but many commented that the more personalized and tailored to the individual patient, the better the SCP would be.

Several research studies were under way as of 2014 to evaluate both short-term and long-term effects of SCPs on survivors' health outcomes, health behaviors, and the coordination of their health care, but the results will take several years to evaluate and publish.

Problems and concerns

Although a number of cancer advocacy organizations—as well as the ACS, NCI, and IOM—have urged the widespread adoption of SCPs, there were a number of difficulties with their full implementation as of 2014. According to the American Cancer Society, only about 20% of oncologists consistently provide their patients with SCPs. The barriers to widespread adoption of survivorship care plans that were noted by the ACS include the following:

- Shortage of time in which to set up the SCP and discuss it with the patient. It will be seen that many of the models require substantial time to retrieve the relevant records or other information in order to complete an SCP template.

- Lack of compensation for the doctor's time and effort to complete the plan. One suggestion is payment reform that would reimburse cancer centers for the time required to draw up SCPs and review them with patients.

- Disagreement as to whether the patient's oncologist or the primary care physician should be primarily responsible for supervising and updating the SCP. According to the NCI, many oncologists maintain that they are better equipped to provide follow-up care, while many primary care physicians would prefer a shared management approach.

A report published in the journal *Cancer* in 2014 summarized the present situation of SCPs in the United States as sporadic in use, with only limited research on their implementation carried out to date, and only a limited amount of evidence of improved outcomes associated with their use. As the IOM predicted in its

QUESTIONS TO ASK YOUR DOCTOR

- Have you helped any other patients draw up survivorship care plans? How well do they work?

- Which model do you think works best for the majority of patients?

- What is your opinion of electronic SCPs? Are they more efficient than paper records?

- I am concerned about privacy. How safe are SCPs from data breaches? And who will have access to my SCP?

- Who will be responsible for entering and storing the data in the SCP?

- How and how often will the SCP be updated, and by whom?

2007 report, "Overall, a profound cultural shift will be required to change entrenched practice patterns."

Resources

BOOKS

Abeloff, M. D., et al. *Clinical Oncology.* 5th ed. New York: Churchill Livingstone, 2013.

Cassileth, Barrie, and Ian Yarett. *Survivorship: Living Well During and After Cancer.* Ann Arbor, MI: Spry Publishing, 2014.

Institute of Medicine (IOM). *Implementing Cancer Survivorship Care Planning: Workshop Summary.* Washington, DC: National Academies Press, 2007. http://books.nap.edu/openbook.php?record_id=11739 (accessed November 10, 2014).

LaTour, Kathy. *Understanding Cancer Survivorship Care Plans: A Nurse's Guide to Help Patients Plan for the Future.* Dallas, TX: Cure Media Group, 2014.

PERIODICALS

Barton, M. K. "Oncologists and Primary Care Physicians Infrequently Provide Survivorship Care Plans." *CA: A Cancer Journal for Clinicians* 64 (September 10, 2014): 291–92.

Blanch-Hartigan, D., et al. "Provision and Discussion of Survivorship Care Plans among Cancer Survivors: Results of a Nationally Representative Survey of Oncologists and Primary Care Physicians." *Journal of Clinical Oncology* 32 (May 2014): 1578–85.

Cheung, W. Y., et al. "Physician Preferences and Attitudes Regarding Different Models of Cancer Survivorship Care: A Comparison of Primary Care Providers and Oncologists." *Journal of Cancer Survivorship* 7 (September 2013): 343–54.

Daudt, H. M., et al. "Survivorship Care Plans: A Work in Progress." *Current Oncology* 21 (June 2014): e466–79.

Forsythe, L. P., et al. "Use of Survivorship Care Plans in the United States: Associations with Survivorship Care." *Journal of the National Cancer Institute* 105 (October 16, 2013): 1579–87.

Klabunde, C. M., et al. "Physician Roles in the Cancer-Related Follow-up Care of Cancer Survivors." *Family Medicine* 45 (July–August 2013): 463–74.

Mayer, D. K., et al. "Implementing Survivorship Care Plans for Colon Cancer Survivors." *Oncology Nursing Forum* 41 (May 2014): 266–73.

Mayer, D. K., et al. "Summing It Up: An Integrative Review of Studies of Cancer Survivorship Care Plans (2006–2013)." *Cancer* (September 23, 2014): e-pub ahead of print. http://dx.doi.org/10.1002/cncr.28884 (accessed November 10, 2014).

Phillips, Carmen. "A Tough Transition: Cancer Survivorship Plans Slow to Take Hold." *NCI Cancer Bulletin* 9 (June 26, 2012).

OTHER

American Cancer Society (ACS). "Cancer Treatment and Survivorship: Facts and Figures, 2014–2015." http://www.cancer.org/acs/groups/content/@research/documents/document/acspc-042801.pdf (accessed November 3, 2014).

Minnesota Cancer Alliance. "Cancer Survivor Care Plan." http://mncanceralliance.org/wp-content/uploads/2013/07/SurvivorCarePlan3202012_Final.pdf (accessed November 3, 2014).

National Coalition for Cancer Survivorship (NCCS). "Cancer Survival Toolbox Resource Booklet." http://www.canceradvocacy.org/wp-content/uploads/2013/02/Cancer-Survival-Toolbox-Resource-Booklet.pdf (accessed November 3, 2014).

WEBSITES

American Cancer Society (ACS). "Survivorship Care Plans." http://www.cancer.org/treatment/survivorshipduringandaftertreatment/survivorshipcareplans/index (accessed November 3, 2014).

American Society of Clinical Oncology (ASCO). "Medical Forms." Cancer.Net. http://www.cancer.net/navigating-cancer-care/managing-your-care/medical-forms (accessed November 3, 2014).

Journey Forward. "My Care Plan." http://www.journeyforward.org/sites/journeyforward/files/mycareplan.pdf (accessed November 3, 2014).

Memorial Sloan Kettering Cancer Center. "Survivorship Care Plan." http://www.mskcc.org/cancer-care/survivorship/survivorship-care-plan (accessed November 3, 2014).

National Coalition for Cancer Survivorship (NCCS). "Care Planning Templates." http://www.canceradvocacy.org/cancer-resources/examples-of-cancer-care-plans/ (accessed November 3, 2014).

National Comprehensive Cancer Network (NCCN). "Taking Charge of Follow-Up Care." http://www.nccn.org/patients/resources/life_after_cancer/survivorship.aspx (accessed November 3, 2014).

ORGANIZATIONS

American Cancer Society (ACS), 250 Williams Street NW, Atlanta, GA 30303, (800) 227-2345, http://www.cancer.org/aboutus/howwehelpyou/app/contact-us.aspx, http://www.cancer.org/index.

American Society of Clinical Oncology (ASCO), 2318 Mill Road, Suite 800, Alexandria, VA 22314, (571) 483-1300, (888) 651-3038, Fax: (571) 366-9537, contactus@cancer.net, http://www.asco.org/.

Children's Oncology Group (COG), 222 E. Huntington Drive, Suite 100, Monrovia, CA 91016, (626) 447-0064, Fax: (626) 445-4334, HelpDesk@childrensoncologygroup.org, http://www.childrensoncologygroup.org/.

National Cancer Institute (NCI) Office of Cancer Survivorship, BG 9609 MSC 9760, 9609 Medical Center Drive, Bethesda, MD 20892-9760, (240) 276-6690, http://www.cancer.gov/global/contact/email-us, http://cancercontrol.cancer.gov/ocs/index.html.

National Coalition for Cancer Survivorship (NCCS), 1010 Wayne Avenue, Suite 315, Silver Spring, MD 20910, (877) 622-7937, info@canceradvocacy.org, http://www.canceradvocacy.org.

National Comprehensive Cancer Network (NCCN), 275 Commerce Drive, Suite 300, Fort Washington, PA 19034, (215) 690-0300, Fax: (215) 690-0280, http://www.nccn.org.

Rebecca J. Frey, PhD
REVIEWED BY ROSALYN CARSON-DEWITT, MD

Sutent *see* **Sunitinib**

Symmetrel *see* **Amantadine**

Syndrome of inappropriate antidiuretic hormone

Description

The syndrome of inappropriate antidiuretic hormone production (SIADH) is a condition in which the body develops an excess amount of water and a decrease in sodium (salt) concentration as a result of improper chemical signals. Patients with SIADH may become severely ill, or may have no symptoms at all.

A syndrome is a collection of symptoms and physical signs that together follow a pattern. SIADH is one of the **paraneoplastic syndromes**, in which a **cancer** leads to widespread ill effects due to more than just the direct presence of a tumor.

Normal physiology

The body normally maintains very tight control over its total amount of water and its concentration of sodium.

Many organs, including the kidneys, heart, and the adrenal, thyroid, and pituitary glands participate in this regulation. One important contribution is the release of a chemical substance, or hormone, by the pituitary gland into the bloodstream. This chemical substance, called antidiuretic hormone (ADH), is also known as arginine vasopressin, or AVP.

The pituitary releases ADH into the bloodstream when receptors in various organs detect that the body has too little water or too high a concentration of salt. ADH then affects the way the kidneys control water and salt balance. ADH causes the kidneys to decrease their output of urine. The body thus saves water by undergoing antidiuresis, that is, not excreting urine.

Simultaneously, the concentration of sodium in the body serum decreases. This decrease results from a second effect of ADH on the kidneys. When the kidneys retain extra water, the existing concentration of sodium in the body decreases slightly as a result of dilution. These functions are all part of the body's extremely precise control over water and salt balance in health.

Abnormal physiology in SIADH

Certain disease states can upset the delicate balance of water and salt in the body. If there is too much ADH in the body, or if the kidneys overreact to the ADH they receive, the body retains excess water and the serum sodium concentration becomes diluted and falls to abnormal levels. The patient with SIADH develops symptoms based on the degree of abnormality in the serum sodium concentration and the speed with which this concentration falls.

Normal serum sodium concentration is 135–145 mEq/L (milliEquivalents of sodium per liter of body fluid). When the sodium concentration is 125–135 mEq/L the patient may have mild nausea, loss of appetite, **fatigue**, headache, or still remain free of symptoms. As the sodium level drops below 120 mEq/L, the patient experiences greater weakness, confusion, sleepiness, vomiting, and weight gain. As the sodium concentration approaches 110 mEq/L, the patient may suffer seizures, coma, and death.

Causes and symptoms

Causes

SIADH has many known causes, some of which particularly relate to cancer or its treatment. These causes include specific types of cancer, drugs used to treat cancer, drugs used to treat the effects of cancer, and conditions that arise as a consequence of cancer or its treatment.

About 14% of inpatients with SIADH and its attendant low sodium (hyponatremia) have underlying cancer.

SPECIFIC TYPES OF CANCER. SIADH results from numerous types of cancer. The malignancies known to cause SIADH include:

- Lung cancer, small cell type
- Gastrointestinal cancers (pancreatic cancer, exocrine; duodenal or stomach cancer)
- Genitourinary cancer (bladder cancer, prostate cancer, ovarian cancer)
- Lymphoma, including Hodgkin lymphoma
- Head and neck cancers (oral cancers, laryngeal cancer, nasopharyngeal cancer)
- Thymoma
- Brain and central nervous system tumors
- Breast cancer
- Melanoma

Certain cancers produce and secrete ADH. This production occurs without regard for the needs of the body. Thus, the kidneys receive repeated signals to save water, even when the body already has a marked excess of fluid. Of all the types of cancer that produce ADH, small-cell lung cancer is by far the most common. Small-cell cancer of the lung is the cause in 75% of the cases of SIADH caused directly by a tumor. In some cases, the appearance of SIADH may be the first indication that a cancer exists.

Also, primary or metastatic tumors in the brain may lead to SIADH. SIADH here results from an increase in intracranial pressure (pressure within the head), or from other effects of intracranial disease on the brain. Increased intracranial pressure commonly causes various parts of the brain to work improperly.

DRUGS USED TO TREAT CANCER. A variety of drugs used in cancer treatment may lead to SIADH. The mechanism of this effect may be that the drug causes the abnormal release of ADH, or that the drug makes existing ADH work in a stronger fashion than usual. **Chemotherapy** drugs that cause SIADH include:

- Vincristine, vinblastine, vinorelbine, and other vinca alkaloids (Oncovin, Velban, Navelbine)
- Cyclophosphamide, ifosfamide, melphalan, and other nitrogen mustards (Cytoxan, Ifex, Alkeran)
- Cisplatin (Platinol-AQ)
- Levamisole (Ergamisol)

DRUGS USED TO TREAT THE EFFECTS OF CANCER. SIADH may also result from general anesthesia or as a reaction to drugs used to treat side effects of cancer such as pain, **depression**, or seizures. These drugs include:

- narcotic pain medications (morphine, Oramorph SR, fentanyl, Duragesic)
- tricyclic antidepressants (amitriptyline, Elavil)
- carbamazepine (Tegretol)
- general anesthetics

CONDITIONS THAT ARISE AS A CONSEQUENCE OF CANCER. SIADH may result from some of the debilitating consequences of cancer. For example, people with cancer who are weak or unsteady have a higher risk of falling and hitting their head. Skull fractures and other types of head injury may damage the brain or increase the intracranial pressure, and thus lead to SIADH.

Also, cancer patients who are weak, malnourished, receiving chemotherapy, or spending excessive time in bed have an increased risk of **pneumonia** and other infections. Infections such as pneumonia, meningitis, and tuberculosis can cause SIADH.

Symptoms

The symptoms of SIADH vary widely from patient to patient. More severe symptoms include:

- depression
- mood swings
- memory changes
- nausea and vomiting
- cramps
- seizures
- coma

Treatment

The treatment of SIADH involves relief of the urgent symptoms and correction of the underlying problem. For immediate improvement, all patients with SIADH require sharp restriction of their daily water intake. As little as two cups of liquid (about 500 mL) may be the daily limit for some patients. In cases where the sodium concentration is already dangerously low, doctors may cautiously give an intravenous infusion of fluid with a high concentration of sodium (hypertonic saline solution). However, this treatment carries some risk of damaging the brain. Physicians may also use a medicine such as furosemide (Lasix) that promotes water excretion (diuresis). Another drug, **demeclocycline**, blocks the action of ADH in the kidney. Vasopressin-related drugs help limit the excretion of electrolytes in the urine. These include conivaptan and tolvaptan.

The most definitive way to relieve SIADH is to address the underlying problem. Thus, if a tumor produces abnormal ADH, then surgery, **radiation therapy**, or chemotherapy may help by removing the tumor or reducing its size. If SIADH results from the use of a drug, then the patient must discontinue the medicine. Finally, doctors try to identify and treat any other correctable cause, such as an infection.

Prognosis

The prognosis of SIADH depends largely on its cause. Until recently, many physicians believed that the appearance of SIADH indicated a poor prognosis for cancer. However, more recent reports contradict this belief. The patient's ability to observe severe restriction of fluid intake may determine the degree of ongoing symptoms. SIADH usually improves after stopping a drug or curing an infection when that is the cause. When cancer is the direct cause of SIADH, one hopes for similar improvement of SIADH from treatments that reduce the amount of cancer in the body.

Resources

BOOKS

Abeloff, M. D., et al. *Clinical Oncology*. 5th ed. New York: Churchill Livingstone, 2013.

Niederhuber, J. E., et al. *Clinical Oncology*. 5th ed. Philadelphia: Elsevier, 2014.

WEBSITES

Thomas, Christie P. "Syndrome of Inappropriate Antidiuretic Hormone Secretion." Medscape. http://emedicine.medscape.com/article/246650-overview (accessed November 3, 2014).

University of Rochester Medical Center. "Syndrome of Inappropriate Antidiuretic Hormone Secretion (SIADH)." Medscape. http://www.urmc.rochester.edu/encyclopedia/content.aspx?ContentTypeID=90&ContentID=P01974 (accessed November 14, 2014).

Kenneth J. Berniker, M.D.

REVISED BY TERESA G. ODLE

Tacrolimus

Definition

Tacrolimus belongs to a group of medicines known as immunosuppressive agents. It is used primarily to lower the body's natural immunity in order to prevent the rejection of organ transplants and to prevent **graft-versus-host disease**. Tacrolimus is also known as Prograf and FK506.

Purpose

Tacrolimus first saw use in transplant patients. By suppressing the activity of the immune system, tacrolimus makes it more likely that the recipient of a transplanted organ will accept that organ. It is especially used for kidney transplants.

In the fight against leukemia, grafts of stem cells from donors are sometimes given to the patient to encourage the blood of a recipient to begin production of normal cells. Tacrolimus may be given during the graft process because it seems to make the patient more receptive to the donated stem cells.

Description

Tacrolimus somehow suppresses—or prevents activity of—the cells in the lymphatic system, which are known as T cells. Under normal circumstances T cells mount an **immune response** to foreign materials in the body. However, during a transplant, T cells can cause the reaction that can lead to the rejection of a donor organ. The exact reason for the activity of tacrolimus is not understood.

Recommended dosage

Given by mouth, in a capsule, or by intravenous line, tacrolimus doses range from about 0.03 milligrams to 0.05 milligrams per kilogram (1 kilogram equals approximately 2.2 pounds) of body weight per day. Individuals with liver or kidney problems must be given a lower dose.

Precautions

Tacrolimus should be taken without food and long after a meal. If there is food in the stomach it will interfere with the way the drug makes its way into the body. Grapefruit juice can increase the activity of tacrolimus and should be avoided.

Side effects

Many serious side effects are associated with tacrolimus. Conditions affecting the brain brought on by the use of tacrolimus include coma (unconscious state) and delirium (uncontrolled and erratic conscious state). Most times the brain conditions are reversible. Headache, skin rashes, hair loss (**alopecia**), pain, sensitivity to light, and shock (anaphylaxis) are all side effects. Kidney damage, which cannot be reversed, is also a danger.

Use of tacrolimus greatly increases the likelihood a person will get **skin cancer** and **lymphoma**. Anyone using the drug should be monitored closely for changes in the skin, and all normal precautions for avoiding skin **cancer**, such as avoiding direct exposure to ultraviolet light, should be taken.

Interactions

This drug interacts with a long list of other drugs. It is important to tell the physician in charge of the care plan, each and every drug being taken, so that interactions can be avoided. Tacrolimus prevents effective vaccination, and vaccinations should not be given while the drug is in use.

KEY TERMS

Intravenous line—A tube that is inserted directly into a vein to carry medicine directly to the blood stream bypassing the stomach and other digestive organs that might alter the medicine.

Lymphatic system—The system that collects and returns fluid in tissues to the blood vessels and produces defensive agents for fighting infection and invasion by foreign bodies.

Stem cell—Cell that gives rise to a lineage of cells. Particularly used to describe the most primitive cells in the bone marrow from which all the various types of blood cell are derived.

Resources

BOOKS

Chu, Edward, and Vincent T. DeVita Jr. *Physicians' Cancer Chemotherapy Drug Manual 2014.* Burlington, MA: Jones & Bartlett Learning, 2014.

WEBSITES

AHFS Consumer Medication Information. "Tacrolimus." American Society of Health-System Pharmacists. Available from: http://www.nlm.nih.gov/medlineplus/druginfo/meds/a601117.html (accessed November 14, 2014).

Micromedex. "Tacrolimus (Oral Route)." Mayo Clinic. http://www.mayoclinic.org/drugs-supplements/tacrolimus-oral-route/description/drg-20068314 (accessed November 14, 2014).

Diane M. Calabrese

Tafinlar *see* **Dabrafenib**

Tamoxifen

Definition

Tamoxifen is a synthetic compound similar to estrogen. It mimics the action of estrogen on the bones and uterus, but blocks the effects of estrogen on breast tissue.

Purpose

Tamoxifen (Nolvadex) is used as adjuvant hormonal therapy immediately after surgery in early stages of **breast cancer** and to treat advanced metastatic breast **cancer** (stages III and IV) in women and men. Adjuvant therapy is treatment added to curative procedures (such as surgery) to prevent the recurrence of cancer. Tamoxifen may also be used to reduce the chance of breast cancer development in high-risk patients. Although tamoxifen is also used to treat malignant **melanoma**, **brain tumors**, and uterine cancer, these uses are not indicated on the product label.

Description

Tamoxifen belongs to a family of compounds called **antiestrogens**. Antiestrogens are used in cancer therapy to inhibit the effects of estrogen on target tissues. Estrogen is a steroid hormone secreted by the ovaries. Depending on the target tissue, estrogen can stimulate the growth of female reproductive organs and breast tissue, play a role in the female menstrual cycle, and protect against bone loss by binding to estrogen receptors on the outside of cells within the target tissue. Antiestrogens act selectively against the effects of estrogen on target cells in a variety of ways, thus they are called selective estrogen receptor modulators (SERMs).

Tamoxifen selectively inhibits the effects of estrogen on breast tissue, while selectively mimicking the effects of estrogen on bone (by increasing bone mineral density) and uterine tissues. These qualities make tamoxifen an excellent therapeutic agent against estrogen receptor-positive breast cancer. Tamoxifen competes with estrogen by binding to estrogen receptors on the membrane of target cells, which limits the effects of estrogen on breast tissue. Tamoxifen also may be involved in other anti-tumor activities affecting the expression of genes associated with cancer (oncogenes), promotion of cancer cell death (apoptosis), and growth factor secretion. Growth factors are hormones that influence cell division and proliferation, which may encourage the growth of cancer cells.

Tamoxifen has been used to reduce the risk of breast cancer since it was approved by the U.S. Food and Drug Administration (FDA) in 1990. Studies in thousands of women have shown that the use of tamoxifen over a five-year period effectively reduced the risk for breast cancer in high-risk, postmenopausal women. Some patients have received the drug for up to ten years, although this is still controversial. A study conducted by the **National Cancer Institute**, the Breast Cancer Prevention Trial, reported that women receiving tamoxifen had:

• 49% fewer diagnoses of invasive breast cancer

• 50% fewer diagnoses of noninvasive breast cancer (e.g., ductal carcinoma in situ)

• fewer fractures of the hip, wrist, and spine.

The study also revealed that the women receiving tamoxifen had more than twice the chance of developing **endometrial cancer** and an increased risk of developing blood clots, both in the lungs and in major veins, when compared to the women receiving a placebo (non-drug used for comparison).

Fertility preservation through ovarian stimulation is another important function of tamoxifen. Although originally developed in the 1960s as a contraceptive, tamoxifen was later found to stimulate ovarian follicle growth. After this discovery, it was used as an ovarian stimulant in Europe, but not the United States. Now, after extensive research, high-dose tamoxifen is used as an ovarian stimulant to preserve fertility in women who have been treated for breast cancer. A study of tamoxifen in breast cancer survivors found that it stimulated the ovaries and increased the number of embryos that could be retrieved. As a result, patients were able to freeze embryos for immediate or later attempts at in vitro fertilization and pregnancy. About 27,000 women each year are still in their child-bearing years when they are diagnosed with breast cancer. However, while advances in treating breast cancer have led to an increased number of survivors, ovarian failure remains a major long-term effect of cell-killing (cytotoxic) cancer treatments. Therefore, once patients have been successfully treated for breast cancer, the use of adjuvant tamoxifen reduces the chances of breast cancer recurrence, and at the same time can be used as an ovarian stimulant to preserve fertility.

A newer group of drugs called **aromatase inhibitors**, including anastrozole (Arimidex), letrozole (Femara), and exemestane (Aromasin), may be used after a course of tamoxifen. These drugs are forms of endocrine therapy that are considered alternatives to tamoxifen. When used as adjuvant therapy, aromatase inhibitors reduce the risk of recurrence and death from breast cancer in women who have hormone receptor-positive breast cancer. Although tamoxifen has been the standard therapy for preventing recurrence and increasing survival, which is still true for pre-menopausal women, these drugs are able to prevent recurrence as effectively as tamoxifen and with fewer side effects (although only letrozole has been shown to improve survival). Therefore, aromatase inhibitors may be prescribed after a course of tamoxifen to improve overall treatment results in post-menopausal women.

Recommended dosage

Tamoxifen is taken orally and is available in 10- and 20-milligram (mg) tablets. The standard dosage for metastatic breast cancer or ductal **carcinoma** in situ (DCIS) is 10 mg twice daily or 20 mg once daily for adult females and males. The response rate at this dosage is about 30%, and the response rate with complete

KEY TERMS

Anticoagulant—An agent preventing the coagulation (clotting) of blood.

Apoptosis—A type of cell death where cells are induced to commit suicide.

Double-blind study—A study where neither the participant nor the physician know who has received the drug in question.

Oncogene—A gene associated with cancer development, usually arising through mutation of a normal gene.

Thromboembolism—A blood clot that blocks a blood vessel in the cardiovascular system, most often in a lung.

remission occurs in 10% of patients. Patients aged 60 years and older have higher response rates. For patients using tamoxifen for adjuvant therapy after surgery, the typical dosage is 20 mg once daily for two to five years following surgery. Women at high risk for developing breast cancer usually take 20 mg daily for five years. If a scheduled dose is missed, patients are advised to take their next regularly scheduled dose, contact their doctor, and avoid doubling the dose. Tamoxifen can be taken with food.

The dosage of tamoxifen used for ovarian stimulation is 20 mg daily for five days.

Precautions

Women who are pregnant or nursing are advised not to use this drug since it has several side effects that, although rare, can be severe. It is known to cause miscarriages and birth defects. Women are encouraged to use birth control while taking tamoxifen; however, oral contraceptives can negatively alter the effects of tamoxifen and women are advised to explore nonhormonal birth control options. Tamoxifen is not recommended for use in children.

Tamoxifen is used with caution in patients taking the anticoagulant drug **warfarin** because tamoxifen can interfere with the effects of warfarin, and dose adjustments may be necessary. Patients who are predisposed to the formation of blood clots (thromboembolisms) are advised to use tamoxifen with caution. Smokers are at a higher risk for thromboembolism than nonsmokers.

Tamoxifen may not work effectively for every patient, because certain tumors tend to become resistant to tamoxifen therapy. The development of tamoxifen resistance is believed to be due to the pharmacologic structure of tamoxifen and its effect on the structure and function of the estrogen receptor in breast cancer. Genetic studies are being conducted to investigate what causes tamoxifen resistance and how it may influence the management of individual breast cancer patients.

Side effects

Although tamoxifen is usually well tolerated by patients, certain side effects may occur. About 25% of patients experience side effects such as mild nausea, vomiting, hot flashes, weight gain, **bone pain**, and hair thinning. These side effects are usually not severe enough to stop therapy and most are short-term effects. Patients using adjuvant tamoxifen for long periods of time may face unwanted effects years into therapy, which may warrant discontinuing the drug. Possible long-term effects include:

- increased risk of developing liver adenoma and uterine (endometrial) cancer
- eye problems such as retinal lesions, macular edema, and corneal changes (most resolve after tamoxifen is discontinued)
- neurological problems such as depression, dizziness, confusion, and fatigue
- gynecologic problems such as vaginal bleeding, vaginal discharge, and endometriosis
- increased risk of developing blood clots, both in the lungs and major blood vessels

Interactions

Tamoxifen can increase the anticoagulant action of the anticoagulant drug warfarin, and if these two drugs are used together, patients will be monitored very closely. It can also reduce blood levels of letrozole and anastrozole (aromatase inhibitors that may be used with tamoxifen). Phenobarbital and rifampin increase the breakdown of tamoxifen and may therefore reduce its level in the blood, decreasing its activity. Oral contraceptives also may interfere with the action of tamoxifen.

See also Alopecia; Nausea and vomiting; Toremifene.

Resources

BOOKS

Hirshaut, Yashar, and Peter I. Pressman. *Breast Cancer: The Complete Guide.* 5th ed. New York: Bantam, 2008.
Miller, Kenneth D. *Choices in Breast Cancer Treatment: Medical Specialists and Cancer Survivors Tell You What You Need to Know.* Baltimore: Johns Hopkins University Press, 2008.

PERIODICALS

Davies, C., H. Pan, and J. Godwin, et al. "Long-term Effects of Continuing Adjuvant Tamoxifen to 10 Years Versus Stopping at 5 Years After Diagnosis of Oestrogen Receptor-positive Breast Cancer: ATLAS, a Randomized Trial." *Lancet* 38 (Mar 2013): 805–816.
Oktay, K. "Fertility Preservation: We Are in This For a Long Haul." *American Journal of Obstetrics and Gynecology* 209 (Aug 2013): 77–79.
Salama, M., K. Winkler, and K. F. Murach, et al. "Female Fertility Loss and Preservation: Threats and Opportunities." *Annals of Oncology*: 24 (Mar 2013): 598–608.
Schiavon, G., and I. E. Smith. "Status of Adjuvant Endocrine Therapy for Breast Cancer." *Breast Cancer Research*: 16 (Feb 2014): 206–209.
Smith, G. L. "The Long and Short of Tamoxifen Therapy: A Review of the ATLAS Trial." *Journal of Advanced Practice Oncology* 5 (Jan 2014): 57–60.
van Agthoven, T., A. M. Sieuwerts, and D. Meijer, et al. "Selective Recruitment of Breast Cancer Anti-estrogen Resistance Genes and Relevance for Breast Cancer Progression and Tamoxifen Therapy Response." *Endocrine-Related Cancer*: 17 (Feb 2010): 215–230.

WEBSITES

American Cancer Society. "Tamoxifen." http://www.cancer.org/treatment/treatmentsandsideeffects/guidetocancer-drugs/tamoxifen (accessed October 12, 2014).

ORGANIZATIONS

American Cancer Society, 250 Williams St. NW, Atlanta, GA 30303, (800) 227-2345, http://www.cancer.org.
U.S. Food and Drug Administration, 10903 New Hampshire Ave., Silver Spring, MD 20993, (888) INFO-FDA (463-6332), http://www.fda.gov.

Sally C. McFarlane-Parrott
Teresa G. Odle
REVISED BY L. LEE CULVERT

Tanning

Definition

Tanning is the browning or darkening of skin from exposure to ultraviolet (UV) radiation, either from sunlight or from an artificial source.

Purpose

Many people consider tanning fashionable and pursue it for cosmetic purposes. Most Americans—including up to 80% of young people under age 25—believe that a tan improves their appearance. Tanning

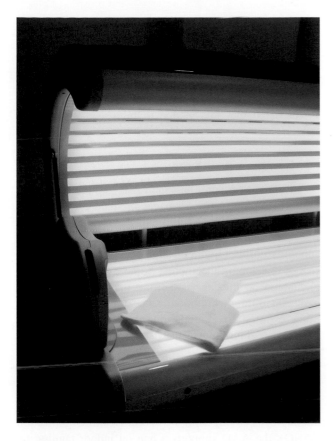

Tanning increases the risk of developing skin cancer.
(Pedro Miguel Sousa/Shutterstock.com)

beds or "sunbeds" that darken the skin using UV-radiating lights have become increasingly popular throughout the developed world, especially among young women. Many people also believe that tanning prevents sunburn.

Everyone needs some exposure to sunlight to produce vitamin D3 or cholecalciferol, which is synthesized in the skin after exposure to ultraviolet B (UV-B) light and converted into the active form of vitamin D. Vitamin D is required for calcium absorption for strong, healthy bones, as well as for a variety of other bodily functions. Light-colored skin absorbs more UV-B than darker skin. It has been proposed that lighter-colored skin evolved as humans migrated to northern climates with less year-round sunlight, which required maximizing absorbance of UV-B for synthesizing vitamin D. However, only 10 to 15 minutes of direct sunlight three times per week is adequate to meet the body's vitamin D requirement.

Description

Tanned skin is often associated with healthy outdoor activities and vacations in sunny climates. Unfortunately tanning is also an indication of damaged skin. Two types of UV radiation from the sun reach the skin. UV-B affects the upper layers of skin or epidermis and is responsible for sunburn; however most UV-B rays from the sun are absorbed by the ozone layer surrounding the earth. Therefore the majority of ultraviolet exposure is to ultraviolet A (UV-A), which passes through window glass. Tanning beds generally use UV-A, although full-spectrum tanning lights include UV-B. UV-A radiation penetrates to the lower layers of the epidermis, where it triggers cells called melanocytes to produce a brown pigment called melanin, which is responsible for tanning. Darker-skinned people tan more deeply than light-skinned people because their melanocytes produce more melanin.

Although melanin can protect skin from burning because the pigment absorbs UV radiation, it does not protect against skin cancer and other problems. UV-A radiation can turn melanocytes cancerous, causing melanoma. UV-A also causes skin aging and wrinkling. UV-A can penetrate through the epidermis to the dermis, which contains blood vessels and nerves, and there it can suppress the immune system, reducing its ability to protect against the development and spread of skin cancer. In addition to sunburn, UV-B rays can cause cataracts (clouding of the eye lens) and immune system damage, as well as contributing to skin cancer. Melanoma is thought to be associated with severe UV-B sunburns before the age of 20. UV radiation damages DNA in skin cells and, although the cells can repair this damage, excessive UV exposure eventually causes the damage to outpace the repair system. Therefore both types of UV radiation, whether from the sun or from artificial sources such as tanning beds and sunlamps, are classified as known **carcinogens**.

The U.S. Food and Drug Administration (FDA) and the American Academy of Dermatology (AAD) classify skin into six types based on susceptibility to tanning and burning:

- I—extremely sun-sensitive—always burns easily and never tans

- II—very sun-sensitive—usually burns easily and tans only minimally

- III—sun-sensitive—sometimes burns and gradually tans to light brown

- IV—minimally sun-sensitive—burns minimally and always tans to moderate brown

- V—sun-insensitive—rarely burns and tans well

- VI—sun-insensitive—never burns and is deeply pigmented

In 2014, the FDA required that tanning beds carry a warning stating that people younger than age 18 should not use them. The FDA warned that all indoor tanning beds, booths, and lamps expose skin to UV radiation that has been linked to increased risk of skin cancer, including melanoma.

Sunless tanning products, also called self-tanners, usually have dihydroxyacetone (DHA) as the active ingredient. DHA reacts with dead cells in the outermost layer of the skin to darken it. Although the color does not wash off, it fades as dead skin cells slough off, usually within a few days. These products are available as creams, gels, lotions, and sprays. Professional spray-on or airbrush tanning is also available. Although sunless tanning products are considered to be safe for applying to the skin, sunless tanning pills are unsafe. They usually contain the color additive canthaxanthin which, in large amounts, can turn the skin orange and cause hives, liver damage, and the formation of crystals in the retina of the eye.

Origins

Tanning has not always been considered desirable. In the past, tanning was often associated with outdoor manual labor and poverty. Then, in the 1920s, the designer Coco Chanel returned from a vacation on the Riviera with a deep tan. Tanning suddenly became fashionable and a symbol of wealth and leisure.

Demographics

Most people get 50%–80% of their lifetime sun exposure during childhood—before the age of 18. Teenage girls and young women account for much of the growth in the tanning bed industry. However, sun exposure, tanning, and especially sunburn, before the age of 15, are strongly associated with the development of **melanoma** and other forms of **skin cancer**. The incidence of skin **cancer** is reaching epidemic proportions in the United States, at a time when the incidence of many other types of cancer is leveling off or declining.

Skin cancers account for one-third of all cancers worldwide. Each year some 132,000 new cases of malignant melanoma—the deadliest form of skin cancer—and more than two million cases of other skin cancers are diagnosed around the world. More than 76,000 new cases of melanoma and more than two million new cases of other skin cancers are diagnosed each year in the United States. The incidence of melanoma is increasing faster than that of any other cancer. In the past, melanoma primarily affected people over age 50; however it has become the second most common cancer among 15–29–year–olds, especially

females. Other types of skin cancer are also being diagnosed more often in younger patients, including teens. Whereas older patients generally develop skin cancer on their heads and necks, young people more often develop skin cancer on their torsos. The torso is the most common location for melanoma in young women. It is suspected that this is due to high-risk outdoor and indoor tanning.

Common problems

Tanning can put a person at risk for sunburn, short-term or long-term eye damage, premature skin aging, immune system suppression, and the eventual development of skin cancer. Sunburns, especially blistering sunburns during childhood or adolescence, increase the risk of developing melanoma. Some experts believe that melanoma on the legs and trunk may result from sun exposure during childhood, since these areas are less often exposed to sunlight during adulthood. Tanning booths can contribute to the development of melanoma anywhere on the body.

Experts now agree that all tanning damages the skin and that no degree of tanning can be considered safe. There is particular agreement regarding the use of tanning beds. Along with the World Health Organization (WHO), the AAD supports a ban on indoor tanning by minors. The AAD also supports banning the manufacture and sale of indoor tanning equipment for non-medical purposes. Tanning salons are often unregulated and many fail to provide supervision or eye protection. In a National Cancer Institute–supported study published in 2009, female college students posed as fair-skinned, 15–year–olds who had never tanned. They telephoned more than 3,600 tanning facilities in all 50 states and inquired about their procedures. Fewer than 11% of the facilities followed the recommended schedule of no more than three sessions during the first week. Furthermore, 71% of the facilities promoted unlimited tanning packages and said that they would allow a teenager to tan every day during the first week.

The International Agency for Research on Cancer, a working group within the WHO that lists known carcinogens, or cancer-causing substances, added tanning beds and lamps to the official list of carcinogens and emphasized the particular danger of indoor tanning to young people.

Parental concerns

Parents should not promote tanning by their children and teens. It is particularly important to prevent sunburns in young children by limiting sun exposure and using sunscreen or sunblock. The AAD recommends that children and adults with all skin types use a water-resistant broad spectrum sun protection factor (SPF) of at least 30 SPF throughout the year, even on days when it is cool, windy, or cloudy. Sunscreen should be used even when very little time is spent outdoors, because up to 80% of sun exposure occurs during incidental day–to–day activities, rather than planned outside excursions. Unprotected skin can be damaged by as little as 15 minutes of sun exposure, although sunburn is sometimes not apparent until at least 12 hours later. Broad-spectrum sunscreen protects against both UV-A and UV-B rays. Titanium oxide, zinc oxide, and other products designed especially for infants and toddlers are especially made for the sensitive skin of children.

Babies have very thin, very sensitive skin and underdeveloped melanocytes. Therefore infants under six months should be kept in the shade, with their entire bodies covered. In general, babies under six months of age should not use sunscreen.

Sunscreen should be applied 15–30 minutes before going outdoors and reapplied every two hours and after swimming or sweating. Waterproof sunscreens may last up to 80 minutes in the water and some sunscreens are also sweat-and rub-proof. Studies have found that most people use only 25%–50% of the recommended amount of sunscreen. One ounce (28 grams) is considered the proper amount for covering exposed portions of the body.

UV rays reflect off snow, sand, and water, increasing the likelihood of sunburn. Other concerns include certain medications—especially some **antibiotics** and acne medications—that can cause any type of skin to burn very easily. Some cosmetics also can increase sensitivity to UV radiation.

Children should:

- Stay out of the sun between 10 a.m. and 4 p.m., when the sun is strongest, especially in the summer, at lower latitudes, and at high altitudes.
- Wear cool, lightweight, cotton clothing that covers the arms and legs.
- Wear sun-blocking shirts for swimming.
- Wear wide-brimmed hats that shade the face, scalp, ears, and neck.
- Wear sunglasses.
- Use a beach umbrella or pop-up tent for playing in the sun.

Children and teens should never use tanning beds or sunlamps. Many states restrict the use of tanning beds by minors or require parental consent; however these restrictions are often ignored by tanning facilities.

KEY TERMS

Dihydroxyacetone (DHA)—A chemical used for staining the skin to simulate a tan.

Melanin—Skin pigment that causes tanning.

Melanocyte—An epidermal skin cell that produces melanin.

Melanoma—A rapidly spreading and deadly form of cancer that usually occurs on the skin.

Ozone—A type of oxygen gas that occurs in a layer about 15 miles (24 kilometers) above Earth's surface and that helps protect living organisms from the damaging effects of the sun's ultraviolet rays.

SPF—Sun protection factor; a number assigned to sunscreens that indicates the amount of UV-B radiation that is required to produce sunburn in the presence of the sunscreen, relative to the amount of UV-B radiation required to burn unprotected skin.

Sunblock—A skin preparation containing an active ingredient, such as titanium oxide, that prevents sunburn by physically blocking out ultraviolet radiation.

Sunscreen—A skin preparation containing an active ingredient, such as benzophenone, that prevents sunburn by chemically absorbing ultraviolet radiation.

Ultraviolet radiation; UV—Invisible light rays with wavelengths shorter than those of visible light, but longer than those of x-rays.

Vitamin D—Any of several fat-soluble vitamins that are required for normal bone and teeth structure and various other physiological functions. Vitamin D is obtained from some foods and is produced in the body through the action of ultraviolet radiation.

Sunless options are available for teenagers who desire a tan, such as spray tans and bronzing lotions.

Resources
BOOKS
Brezina, Corona. *Skin Cancer.* Farmington Hills, MI: Greenhaven, 2010.

Fredericks, Carrie. *Frequently Asked Questions About Tanning and Skin Care.* New York: Rosen, 2010.

Redd, Nancy Amanda. *Body Drama.* New York: Gotham, 2008.

GALE ENCYCLOPEDIA OF CANCER, 4ᵀᴴ EDITION

1703

Wohlenhaus, Kim. *Skin Health Information for Teens*. 2nd ed. Detroit: Omnigraphics, 2009.

PERIODICALS

Fulmore, Jason S., et al. "Sun Protection Education for Healthy Children." *Childhood Education* 85, no. 5 (2009): 293–99.

Klingensmith, Dawn. "Cute, Cool and Covered; Kids' Swimwear Protects Against Sun's Harmful Rays." *Chicago Tribune* (May 21, 2008): 4.

WEBSITES

American Academy of Dermatology. "Sunscreen FAQs." http://www.aad.org/media/background/factsheets/fact_sunscreen.htm (accessed October 8, 2014).

American Cancer Society. "FDA Requires Warning on Tanning Beds." http://www.cancer.org/cancer/news/news/fda-requires-warning-on-tanning-beds (accessed September 25, 2014).

Centers for Disease Control and Prevention. "How Can I Protect My Children From The Sun?" http://www.cdc.gov/cancer/skin/basic_info/children.htm (accessed October 8, 2014).

MedlinePlus. "Sun Exposure." U.S. National Library of Medicine, National Institutes of Health. http://www.nlm.nih.gov/medlineplus/sunexposure.html (accessed September 28, 2014).

National Cancer Institute. "Skin Cancer Prevention." http://www.cancer.gov/cancertopics/pdq/prevention/skin/Patient/page3 (accessed September 28, 2014).

Skin Cancer Foundation. "Tanning Beds: WHO Issues Official Warning." http://www.skincancer.org/news/tanning/tanning-beds-who-issues-official-warning (accessed September 24, 2014).

U.S. Food and Drug Administration. "Indoor Tanning: The Risks of Ultraviolet Rays." For Consumers. (August 17, 2010). http://www.fda.gov/ForConsumers/ConsumerUpdates/ucm186687.htm#TanninginCh ildrenandTeens (accessed September 28, 2014).

ORGANIZATIONS

American Academy of Dermatology (AAD), PO Box 4014, Schaumburg, IL 60168, (866) 503-SKIN (7546), Fax: (847) 240-1859, http://www.aad.org.

American Academy of Pediatrics (AAP), 141 Northwest Point Blvd., Elk Grove Village, IL 60007-1098, (847) 434-4000, Fax: (847) 434-8000, http://www.aap.org.

National Cancer Institute, 9609 Medical Center Drive, Bethesda, MD 20892, (800) 422-6237, http://www.cancer.gov.

U.S. Food and Drug Administration (FDA), 10903 New Hampshire Ave., Silver Spring, MD 20993-0002, (888) 463-6332, http://www.fda.gov.

Margaret Alic, PhD
REVISED BY TERESA G. ODLE

Tarceva *see* **Erlotinib**

Targretin *see* **Bexarotene**

Tasigna *see* **Nilotinib**

▌Taste alteration

Definition

Taste alteration includes changes in how foods taste (dysgeusia), decreased taste (hypogeusia), the complete loss of the sense of taste (ageusia), or a metallic or medicine-like taste in the mouth. Taste alteration is one of the most common side effects of **cancer** treatments. It can also be caused by cancer itself or by an infection in the mouth.

Description

Taste alteration can have significant effects on the nutritional status of cancer patients. They may avoid certain foods, lose their appetite (**anorexia**), and lose weight. Problems associated with taste alteration can be compounded by dry mouth (**xerostomia**) or a mouth infection such as **thrush**, both of which can be side effects of cancer treatment.

Human taste buds distinguish five or six basic tastes: sweet, sour, bitter, salty, umami (a long-lasting savory or meaty taste), and possibly fat. Taste buds are located on the tongue, back portion of the roof of the mouth (soft palate), and the back of the throat. Each of the 10,000 or so taste buds is composed of clusters of 50–150 sensory receptors or taste cells that are replaced every one–two weeks. Hair-like structures (microvilli) projecting from the taste cells bind to food molecules dissolved in saliva to initiate the chain of events that results in taste perception. All taste buds are believed to be capable of detecting multiple combinations of basic tastes. Each receptor cell in a taste bud responds most strongly to one of the basic tastes and contributes to the specific taste sensation transmitted by the taste bud to the brain.

Causes and symptoms

Taste alteration can be caused by damage to taste buds from radiation or **chemotherapy** for cancer or by tumor invasion of the mouth by head or **neck cancers**, as well as xerostomia or infection. Between 88% and 93% of patients with head and neck tumors experience taste alteration. Cancer can also cause deficiencies in nutrients such as copper, niacin, nickel, vitamin A, and zinc, which can lead to taste alteration. Metallic or medicine-like tastes can be caused by zinc deficiency or increased levels of calcium or lactate. Cancer-related chemicals in the bloodstream may also affect taste.

The taste buds are very sensitive to radiation, and taste alteration can occur within the first two weeks of **radiation therapy** to the head, neck, or chest. Radiation therapy can decrease saliva production, which can alter the taste of salty and bitter foods. Surgery to the head or neck can also cause taste alteration.

Between 36% and 71% of patients undergoing chemotherapy experience taste alteration. Although the alterations vary, the most common complaints include a metallic taste, enhanced taste of bitter flavors (in foods such as beef, pork, coffee, and chocolate), and reduced taste of sweet flavors. Many other drugs used during cancer treatment, including **antibiotics**, pain relievers (analgesics), and antidepressants, can also affect taste. Chemotherapy drugs frequently associated with taste alteration include:

- 5-fluorouracil (5-FU)
- carboplatin
- cisplatin
- cyclophosphamide
- dacarbazine
- doxorubicin
- methotrexate
- nitrogen mustard
- vincristine

Taste alteration can cause food to be flavorless or taste too sweet or salty or metallic. Taste alteration is usually a temporary condition, although it may take a few months for taste to return to normal. However, surgery to the roof of the mouth (hard palate), tongue, or throat or high-dose radiation therapy can cause permanent taste alteration.

Treatment

There are no treatments for taste alteration, but there are various methods for overcoming the effects so that it does not interfere with caloric intake and nutritional requirements for proteins, **vitamins**, and minerals. Good oral hygiene and dental checkups are particularly important for cancer patients. The teeth should be brushed and flossed before eating to remove old tastes and refresh the mouth. Brushing and flossing should be performed carefully to prevent damage to weakened mouth tissues. Rinsing the mouth with saltwater, baking soda in water, tea, or ginger ale before eating may be helpful. Patients who have been following a special diet—such as a low-sodium, low-fat, or diabetes diet— may have to check with their doctor about temporarily lifting some restrictions, since increasing the variety of foods can help maintain adequate nutrition in the face of taste alterations. Sometimes medications can be adjusted to reduce or eliminate side effects such as taste alteration.

KEY TERMS

Ageusia—Impairment or absence of the sense of taste.

Anorexia—Prolonged loss of appetite.

Dysgeusia—Taste dysfunction.

Hypogeusia—Decreased taste sensitivity.

Thrush—An opportunistic infection with the fungus *Candida albicans* that causes white patches in the oral cavity.

Xerostomia—Dry mouth.

Measures to make food more flavorful or less offensive depend on the specific taste alteration, but may include:

- eating foods cold or at room temperature
- eating frozen fruits such as grapes, melons, or oranges
- eating fresh vegetables, which may taste better than frozen or canned vegetables
- flavoring foods with barbecue, soy, teriyaki or other sauces or marinades, wine, bits of meat, nuts, cheese (especially sharp cheese), or seasonings such as basil, catsup, chili powder, garlic, mint, mustard, onion, oregano, rosemary, or tarragon
- eating salty foods, such as cured meats and cheeses, for more flavor
- adding tart flavors such as lemon, citrus, or vinegar, unless the patient has mouth sores
- preparing appealing looking foods, which often makes them taste better
- selecting foods of various colors, textures, and temperatures
- using mints, gum, or lemon drops after eating to remove bad tastes
- if food tastes too salty, replacing salt, seasonings, and processed foods containing salt with bland or mild-flavored foods
- adding sugar or syrup to foods to reduce salty, acidic, or bitter tastes
- using brown sugar, maple syrup, honey, cinnamon, dates, or raisins on cereal in place of white sugar
- adding salt, lemon juice, plain yogurt, or milk to foods and nutritional beverages that taste too sweet; choosing less sweet beverages and desserts; using butter or margarine on cereal, toast, and pancakes in place of syrup, jam, or sugar

• if meat does not taste right, replacing it with other protein such as beans, peas, cheese, eggs, fish, nutritional beverages, nuts, peanut butter, poultry, tofu, tempeh, or yogurt; eating meat in stews, soups, chili, or pasta; seasoning meat with sauces, catsup, or other seasonings or marinades; choosing salty, spicy, or smoked meats

• using plastic utensils to reduce bitter or metallic tastes

Food safety is particularly important for patients undergoing cancer treatments that weaken the immune system. Foods should be kept at safe temperatures, and perishables should not sit out for more than one hour. Unpasteurized juice, cheese, or milk and raw or undercooked meat should be avoided.

Alternative and complementary therapies

Taste alteration related to zinc deficiency can be treated by the addition of zinc to the diet or taking zinc picolinate supplements. Foods that are rich sources of zinc include oysters, crab, beef, pork, eggs, nuts, yogurt, and whole grains. Although a small Italian study suggested that zinc supplements might help with loss of taste from radiation therapy for head or neck cancers, a large Mayo Clinic clinical trial found no effect. Zinc nasal sprays have been reported to permanently damage or destroy the senses of taste and smell.

Resources

WEBSITES

Mayo Clinic Staff. "Eating During Cancer Treatment: Tips to Make Food Tastier." Mayo Clinic. http://www.mayoclinic.org/diseases-conditions/cancer/in-depth/cancer/ART-20047536 (accessed October 12, 2014).

"Nutrition Cancer Care (PDQ)." National Cancer Institute. http://www.cancer.gov/cancertopics/pdq/supportivecare/nutrition/HealthProfessional (accessed October 12, 2014).

"Taste and Smell Changes." American Cancer Society. http://www.cancer.org/treatment/survivorshipduringandaftertreatment/nutritionforpeoplewithcancer/nutritionforthepersonwithcancer/nutrition-during-treatment-taste-smell-changes (accessed February 5, 2015).

ORGANIZATIONS

American Cancer Society, 250 Williams Street NW, Atlanta, GA 30303, (800) 227-2345, http://www.cancer.org.

National Cancer Institute, 6116 Executive Boulevard, Suite 300, Bethesda, MD 20892-8322, (800) 4-CANCER (422-6237), http://www.cancer.gov.

Belinda Rowland, PhD
REVISED BY MARGARET ALIC, PhD

Taxotere *see* **Docetaxel**

Tegretol *see* **Carbamazepine**

Temodar *see* **Temozolomide**

Temozolomide

Definition

A **chemotherapy** medicine used to reduce the size of a cancerous tumor and prevent the growth of new **cancer** cells. In the United States, temozolomide is known by the brand name Temodar and in the European Union as Temodal.

Purpose

Temozolomide is used as a treatment for a type of brain tumor called an anaplastic **astrocytoma**. Specifically, it is a treatment for patients who have experienced a relapse (or recurrence) of this disease while being treated with the drug **procarbazine**, one of a group of **anticancer drugs** known as nitrosoureas, which include **carmustine** and **lomustine**. It has also been investigated as a treatment for newly diagnosed and advanced stages of other brain/central nervous system tumors, such as oligodendrogliomas and ependymomas, and for an advanced malignant **melanoma** that has spread to the central nervous system.

Description

Temozolomide was first made in a British laboratory in the early 1980s and was approved for use in the United States in 1999.

It is included in the cancer drug category termed **antineoplastic agents**. These drugs slow or prevent the growth of cancerous tumors. Temozolomide is among a subset of antineoplastic agents that were designed to target rapidly dividing cells in the body, such as the cancerous cells that form tumors. These drugs work by altering the structure of the DNA in fast-growing cells, causing a cell to die or to fail to replicate itself.

the drug most frequently used for this cancer. If the cancer spreads to the central nervous system, temozolomide may be more effective than dacarbazine, because it, unlike dacarbazine, is able to move from the blood into the central nervous system.

A possible advantage to the use of temozolomide over other therapy options is that a patient may be able to continue the treatment over a longer period of time. Decreased bone marrow activity (**myelosuppression**) is a common reaction to many chemotherapy drugs, including temozolomide. But unlike other drugs, this condition is temporary in temozolomide patients; therefore, patients can physically tolerate a more extended treatment. Also, the side effects experienced with temozolomide are usually less severe compared to other drug treatment options, resulting in patients with a better quality of life.

Recommended dosage

Temozolomide is available in capsules and is taken orally. Dosage is determined based on a patient's body height and weight. The typical dose for the first treatment cycle is 150 mg per day taken for five consecutive days, with each treatment cycle lasting 28 days. The number of treatment cycles depends on how well a patient tolerates the treatment and its effectiveness in treating the cancer. The optimal number of treatment cycles is not known.

Because myelosuppression is a common reaction to this drug treatment, white blood cell and platelet counts are carefully monitored, particularly in the first few treatment cycles. A complete blood count is made on day 22 and day 29 of a treatment cycle. If blood counts are below a certain level, treatment is either postponed or the dosage is decreased in the next treatment cycle. The minimum recommended dosage is 100 mg. Blood counts within an acceptable range can result in an increased dosage for the next cycle.

Precautions

Food decreases the rate at which temozolomide is absorbed into the bloodstream. Although there are no foods that should be avoided while taking this drug, it should be taken on an empty stomach and swallowed whole with a glass of water.

Side effects

The most common side effects for patients treated with temozolomide are **nausea and vomiting**, headache, **fatigue**, and constipation. In a study of 158 brain tumor patients, 53% experienced nausea and 42% experienced vomiting, and most of these cases were moderate, with only about 10% of the patients experiencing severe forms of either condition. Avoiding food prior to taking temozolomide can decrease the occurrence of these effects, or they

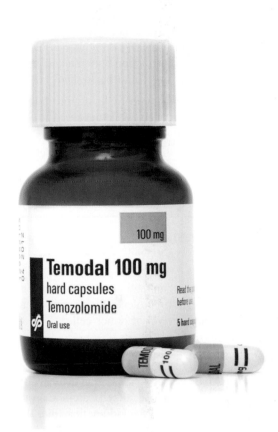

Bottle of temozolomide (Temodal). *(Leeds Teaching Hospitals NHS Trust/Science Source)*

The use of temozolomide as a treatment for cancers other than brain cancer and in combination with different cancer therapies is still experimental. Many ongoing **clinical trials** focus on the use of temozolomide as a cancer treatment not only for newly diagnosed and recurrent brain/central nervous system tumors, but also for advanced stages of **germ cell tumors**, lung cancer (non-small cell), **mycosis fungoides**, **Sézary syndrome**, and **gastrointestinal cancers**. Some clinical trials also involve experimental treatment of advanced brain cancer or malignant melanomas using a combination of temozolomide and other cancer drugs or therapies, such as **radiation therapy** and the drugs interleukin-12, **aldesleukin**, **thalidomide**, carmustine, **interferons**, and lomustine.

It is not yet known if temozolomide is more effective than other treatments, but it has been shown to stop or slow disease progression in patients with recurrent **brain tumors** who have not responded to other treatments, including other chemotherapy drugs, radiation therapy, or surgery. However, the duration of the response varies.

For the treatment of a malignant melanoma, temozolomide is as equally effective as **dacarbazine**,

can be controlled with medication. In the same study, 41% of the patients reported headaches, 34% reported feeling fatigued, and 33% experienced constipation.

Between 10% and 20% of the patients in the study experienced convulsions, partial paralysis, **diarrhea**, **fever**, feeling weak, a infection, dizziness, coordination problems, a **memory change**, or insomnia. Less than 10% of the 158 patients experienced **anorexia**, rash or **itching**, inflammation in the throat region, incontinence, back pain, an overactive adrenal gland, anxiety, comprehension problems, coughing, muscle pain, weight gain, **depression**, sinus problems, or abnormal vision.

Myelosuppression is experienced by 4% to 19% of patients. **Neutropenia** and **thrombocytopenia** are the most common forms, and the more severe cases of both are higher in women and in the elderly (patients older than age 70) than in men. When myelosuppression occurs, it usually appears late in the first few treatment cycles and does not worsen over time. On average, blood count levels return to normal 14 days after the lowest blood count is recorded.

Coping with side effects may require making some lifestyle changes or, in some cases, taking medication. For example, to treat constipation, patients may be told to increase the amount of fluid they drink, perform regular exercise, and eat more dietary fiber, while any infection will require medication. Treatment options for side effects should be discussed with a doctor.

Interactions

Valproic acid, a drug used to treat seizures, decreases the clearance of temozolomide from the body by about 5%. No other negative drug interaction has been reported, although its interaction with many conventional and alternative drugs has yet to be studied.

See also Cancer genetics; Chemoprevention; DNA cytometry; Drug resistance; Vaccines.

Monica McGee, M.S.

Temsirolimus

Definition

Temsirolimus is an anti-cancer drug designed to inhibit the synthesis of proteins that regulate proliferation, growth, and survival of tumor cells.

Purpose

Temsirolimus is used to treat renal cell **carcinoma**, a type of **kidney cancer**. Renal cell carcinoma originates in the very small tubes in the kidney that filter the blood and remove waste products.

Description

Temsirolimus was developed for the treatment of renal cell carcinoma by Wyeth Pharmaceuticals and approved for use by the U.S. Food and Drug Administration (FDA) in 2007. It is a derivative of the anti-cancer drug **sirolimus**. Temsirolimus is sold under the brand name Torisel. It is designed to inhibit an enzyme called mTOR in tumor cells that regulate their proliferation, growth, and survival. The enzyme mTOR is activated in the tumor cells of renal cell carcinoma. Activation of this enzyme leads to a series of chemical events called a signaling cascade. Renal cell carcinoma mTOR signaling causes an increase in two cellular signaling molecules called hypoxia-inducible factor 1a (HIF-1a) and vascular endothelial growth factor (VEGF). Both HIF-1a and VEGF are needed for tumor growth and survival. Hypoxia-inducible factor 1a affects cellular processes for tumor growth and survival and increases the amount of VEGF. Vascular endothelial growth factor is responsible for the formation of tumor blood vessels in the process of **angiogenesis**. Angiogenesis is the process of a tumor growing a new blood vessel system for tumor use. Once a solid tumor reaches a certain size, it needs blood vessels in order for its cells to remain alive,

KEY TERMS

Angiogenesis—Physiological process involving the growth of new blood vessels from pre-existing blood vessels; used by some cancers to create their own blood supply.

Cytochrome P450—Enzymes present in the liver that metabolize drugs.

Hemolytic anemia—Type of anemia involving destruction of red blood cells.

Humanized monoclonal antibody—Human-like antibodies usually genetically engineered in mice and used in a therapeutic manner.

Metastasize—The process by which cancer spreads from its original site to other parts of the body.

Renal cell carcinoma—Cancer of the kidney that originates in the very small tubes in the kidney that filter the blood and remove waste products.

Thrombophlebitis—Vein inflammation related to a blood clot.

Triglycerides—Blood component measured with cholesterol to make up the lipid profile, which helps determine the likelihood of an individual to develop heart disease.

VEGF—Vascular endothelial growth factor, chemical compound in the body that contributes to the growth of new blood vessels.

and to continue to grow. Blood vessels that grow in tumors also contribute to its **metastasis** to other parts of the body.

By inhibiting mTOR, temsirolimus inhibits tumor cell replication and growth, as well as inhibiting the process of angiogenesis. Studies done on renal cell carcinoma have shown that use of temsirolimus increases median survival time and progression-free survival compared to placebo or other agents tested. Median survival time is a term used to describe the time from either diagnosis or treatment at which half of the patients with a given disease are expected to still be alive. The term progression-free survival describes the length of time during and after treatment in which a patient is living with a disease that does not get worse. In a clinical trial designed to test out a **cancer** drug in humans, both median survival time and progression-free survival are ways to measure how effective a treatment is.

Recommended dosage

Temsirolimus is administered intravenously over 30 to 60 minute intervals. For adults with renal cell carcinoma, it is given at a dose of 25 mg once weekly. Therapy with temsirolimus is continued as long as clinical benefit to the patient is seen or until unacceptable levels of toxicity occur. The goal of temsirolimus administration is to use the dose that will be effective in the treatment of cancer while still avoiding toxicity. Once toxicity occurs either treatment is discontinued or the dose is adjusted. A dose of 20 mg per week may be attempted instead. In patients with diabetes, doses of anti-diabetes medication may need to be increased as temsirolimus may increase blood sugar levels. To minimize risk of hypersensitivity reactions, patients are intravenously pre-medicated with the antihistamine drug **diphenhydramine** hydrochloride at a dose of 25 to 50 mg about 30 minutes before beginning a temsirolimus infusion.

Precautions

Temsirolimus is a category D pregnancy drug. Category D pregnancy drugs are drugs in which there is evidence of risk to a human fetus based on clinical studies done in humans or marketing experience but that may be used during pregnancy if potential benefits to the patient are determined to outweigh potential risks to the fetus. Temsirolimus is contraindicated for use during pregnancy unless medically necessary, and may cause serious harm to a fetus. Birth control must be started prior to beginning treatment with temsirolimus and continued for at least 12 weeks after treatment. Both women and men receiving temsirolimus therapy need to use at least two reliable forms of contraception for this time period. Studies have shown fetal harm in animals. Temsirolimus should not be used during breast feeding. Temsirolimus has not been approved for use in individuals less than 18 years of age.

Patients should not have any vaccinations while taking temsirolimus without the consent of their treating physician. Patients taking temsirolimus should avoid being around people who have recently had the oral polio vaccine or the inhaled form of the flu vaccine, as these are live vaccines. If a physician determines that a patient taking temsirolimus requires a non-live vaccine during therapy, it should be administered during a treatment free period in the **chemotherapy** cycle of at least 14 days.

Treatment with temsirolimus increases risk for gastrointestinal perforations in susceptible individuals. There is also a possible increase in risk of adverse or toxic side effects in patients with history of stroke, diabetes mellitus, liver disease, high blood lipid levels, brain metastases, lung disease, kidney disease and those undergoing surgery. Fatal lung disease, bowel perforations, and kidney failure have occurred in treatment with temsirolimus.

Side effects

Temsirolimus is used when the medical benefit is judged to be greater than the risk of side effects. Potential side effects include abdominal pain and cramping, loss of appetite, nausea, vomiting, **anemia**, joint pain, muscle pain, back pain, chest pain, chills, **fever**, flushed skin, **diarrhea**, constipation, altered taste perception, headache, high blood sugar, difficulty breathing, **fatigue**, weakness, acne, high blood pressure, nose bleeds, increased blood lipids and triglycerides, insomnia, mouth and throat sores, inflamed throat, itchy skin, rash, **weight loss**, **depression**, impaired wound healing, compromised immune system, thrombophlebitis, and abnormal liver function tests. Temsirolimus also causes an increased risk of infections including urinary tract infections, **pneumonia**, and other upper respiratory tract infections.

Interactions

Patients should make their doctor aware of any and all medications or supplements they are taking before using temsirolimus. Temsirolimus interacts with many other drugs. Some drug interactions may make temsirolimus unsuitable for use, while others may be monitored and attempted. Medications such as ACE inhibitors have shown negative effects when used with temsirolimus. Use of anticoagulants with temsirolimus has resulted in bleeding reactions in the brain. Temsirolimus causes toxicity when used with another cancer drug called sirolimus. Oral contraceptive pills may cause toxic levels of temsirolimus during treatment. Use of the herb Echinacea may decrease the efficacy of temsirolimus if taken in the same time period.

Temsirolimus is metabolized by a set of liver enzymes known as CYP-450 subtype 3A4. Drugs that induce, or activate, these enzymes increase the metabolism of temsirolimus. This results in lower levels of therapeutic temsirolimus, thereby negatively affecting treatment of cancer. For this reason drugs that induce CYP-450 subtype 3A4 may not be used with temsirolimus. This includes some anti-epileptic drugs such as **carbamazepine**, some anti-inflammatory drugs such as **dexamethasone**, anti-tuberculosis drugs such as rifampin, and the herb St. John's Wort.

Drugs that act to inhibit the action of CYP-450 subtype 3A4 may cause undesired increased levels of

QUESTIONS TO ASK YOUR DOCTOR

- How long will I need to take this drug before you can tell if it helps for me?
- Is this drug safe to take with the other drugs that I am currently taking?
- What side effects should I watch for? When should I call the doctor about them?
- Are there any clinical trials of this drug combined with other therapies that might benefit me?

temsirolimus in the body. This could lead to toxic doses and be very dangerous. Some examples are **antibiotics** such as clarithromycin or erythromycin, antifungal drugs such as ketoconazole, antiviral drugs such as indinavir, antidepressants such as fluoxetine, and some cardiac agents such as amiodarone or verapamil. Grapefruit juice may also increase the amount of temsirolimus in the body. Eating grapefruit or drinking grapefruit juice is not advised while taking temsirolimus. If drugs that induce or inhibit CYP450 3A4 are medically necessary during treatment with temsirolimus, the dose of temsirolimus given may need to be adjusted.

Resources

BOOKS

Brunton, Laurence L., et al. *Goodman and Gilman's The Pharmacological Basis of Therapeutics, Eleventh Edition* McGraw Hill Medical Publishing Division, 2006.

Hamilton, Richard J., editor. *Tarascon Pharmacopoeia Library Edition.* Sudbury, MA: Jones and Bartlett Publishers, 2009.

WEBSITES

AHFS Consumer Medication Information. "Temsirolimus." American Society of Health-System Pharmacists. Available online at: http://www.nlm.nih.gov/medlineplus/druginfo/meds/a607071.html (accessed November 19, 2014).

ORGANIZATIONS

National Cancer Institute, 9609 Medical Center Dr., BG 9609 MSC 9760, Bethesda, MD 20892-9760, (800) 4-CANCER (422-6237), http://www.cancer.gov.

U.S. Food and Drug Administration, 10903 New Hampshire Ave., Silver Spring, MD 20993, (888) INFO-FDA (463-6332), http://www.fda.gov.

Maria Basile, PhD

Teniposide

Definition

Teniposide is a **chemotherapy** medicine used to treat **cancer** by destroying cancerous cells. Teniposide is also known as the brand name Vumon and may also be referred to as VM-26.

Purpose

Teniposide is approved by the Food and Drug Administration (FDA) as induction therapy (an initial, intensive course of chemotherapy) for refractory childhood acute lymphoblastic leukemia. Teniposide is used in combination with other chemotherapy drugs. It has also been used in some adult leukemias and lung cancers.

Description

Teniposide is a clear liquid for infusion into a vein. Teniposide is a semisynthetic derivative of podophyllotoxin found in extracts of the mandrake plant. It is a member of the group of chemotherapy drugs known as topoisomerase II inhibitors. Topoisomerase II is one of the enzymes involved in rearrangement of DNA structures, such as temporarily breaking DNA strands and resealing them. This process is necessary for cell replication, and topoisomerase II inhibitors interfere with this important process as it prevents the cells from further dividing and multiplying and the cells subsequently die.

Recommended dosage

A teniposide dose can be determined using a mathematical calculation that measures a person's body surface area (BSA). This number is dependent upon a patient's height and weight. The larger the person the greater the body surface area. Body surface area is measured in the units known as square meter (m^2). The body surface area is calculated and then multiplied by the drug dosage in milligrams per square meter (mg/m^2). This calculates the actual dose a patient is to receive.

To treat refractory childhood leukemia

Teniposide is dosed at 165 mg per square meter as an infusion into a vein over 30-60 minutes and is given with the chemotherapy drug **cytarabine** at a dose of 300 mg per square meter. This combination is given twice a week for eight to nine doses.

Other leukemia dosing includes teniposide 100 mg per square meter once or twice weekly, and teniposide 250 mg per square meter with the chemotherapy drug **vincristine** 1.5 mg per square meter given into a vein each week for four to eight weeks.

KEY TERMS

Anemia—Red blood cell count that is lower than normal.

Chemotherapy—Specific drugs used to treat cancer.

DNA—Deoxyribonucleic acid, the genetic material inside cells that allows cells to function, separate, into two cells, and make more cells.

Food and Drug Administration—A government agency that oversees public safety in relation to drugs and medical devices. The FDA gives the approval to pharmaceutical companies for commercial marketing of their products.

Induction therapy—Initial intensive course of chemotherapy designed to wipe out abnormal cells and allow regrowth of normal cells.

Intravenous—Administered into the body through a vein.

Neutropenia—White blood cell count that is lower than normal.

Refractory cancer—Cancer that is not responding to treatment.

Patients with significant kidney and liver problems may need to receive a smaller dose of teniposide than patients with normal kidney and liver function.

Patients with Down syndrome should receive a smaller dose with the initial treatment.

Precautions

Blood counts will be monitored regularly while on teniposide therapy. During a certain time period after receiving this drug, there is an increased risk of getting infections. Caution should be taken to avoid unnecessary exposure to germs. Patients with a known previous allergic reaction to chemotherapy drugs should tell their doctor before treatment. Patients who may be pregnant or trying to become pregnant should tell their doctor before receiving teniposide. Chemotherapy can cause men and women to be sterile (unable to have children). Patients should check with their doctors before receiving live virus vaccines while on chemotherapy.

Side effects

The most common side effect of teniposide is low blood counts, referred to as **myelosuppression**. When the white blood cell count is lower than normal, known as **neutropenia**, patients are at an increased risk of developing a **fever** and infections. Teniposide also causes the platelet count to fall. Platelets are blood cells in the body that allow for the formation of clots. When the platelet count is low patients are at an increased risk for bruising and bleeding. If the platelet count remains too low, a platelet blood transfusion is an option. Low red blood cell counts, referred to as **anemia**, may make patients feel tired, dizzy, and lacking energy. A drug known as erythropoietin may be given to increase a patient's red blood cell count.

Teniposide infusions given too quickly into the vein can cause a significant drop in blood pressure. This can usually be avoided by administering the drug over a time period of at least 30-60 minutes. Teniposide can also cause mild to moderate **nausea and vomiting**. Patients will be given medicines known as **antiemetics** before receiving teniposide to help prevent or decrease this side effect. **Diarrhea**, loss of appetite (**anorexia**), and mouth sores and inflammation are also common. Rarely, allergic or anaphylactic-type reactions that include fever, sweating, tongue swelling, chest tightness, **itching**, shortness of breath, low blood pressure, and increased heart rate have occurred.

Other less common side effects caused by teniposide include rash, itching, hair loss (**alopecia**), liver and kidney problems, **fatigue**, seizures, tingling, fever, development of another type of cancer or leukemia due to taking the drug, and redness and pain at the site of injection into the vein. All side effects a patient experiences should be reported to their doctor.

Interactions

There is an increase risk of worsening some of the side effects of teniposide when it is administered with the medicines sodium salicylate, tolbutamide (a drug to lower blood sugar levels), or sulfamethizole (an antibiotic).

Resources

BOOKS

Chu, Edward, and Vincent T. DeVita Jr. *Physicians' Cancer Chemotherapy Drug Manual 2014*. Burlington, MA: Jones & Bartlett Learning, 2014.

WEBSITES

AHFS Consumer Medication Information. "Teniposide Injection." American Society of Health-Systrem Pharmacists. Available from: http://www.nlm.nih.gov/medlineplus/druginfo/meds/a692045.html (accessed November 14, 2014).

National Cancer Institute. "Teniposide." http://www.cancer.gov/drugdictionary?cdrid=43671 (accessed November 14, 2014).

Nancy J. Beaulieu, R.Ph., B.C.O.P.

Teslac *see* **Testolactone**

Testicular cancer

Definition

Testicular **cancer** is the development of cancer cells in one or both testicles. The testicles—the testes or gonads and their enclosing structure—are located in a pouch (scrotum) beneath the penis.

Description

The testicles are an external part of the male reproductive system. They produce sperm and are the primary source of male hormones, especially **testosterone**.

There are several types of cells in the testicles, any of which can develop into one or more types of cancer. Over 95% of all testicular cancers begin in germ cells. Germ-cell tumors are classified into two types, seminomas and non-seminomas. Seminomas account for about 40% of all testicular germ-cell tumors. Non-seminomas include several different types of more aggressive cancers. Some testicular tumors contain elements of both seminoma and non-seminoma tumors. In such cases, the tumors are managed clinically as non-

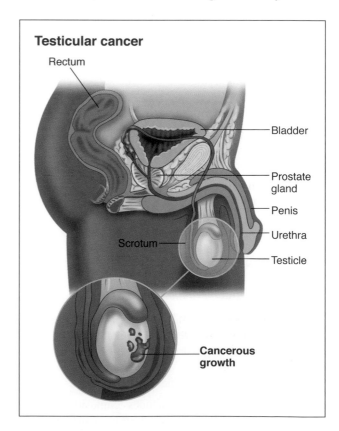

Testicular cancer

Rectum

Bladder

Prostate gland

Penis

Urethra

Scrotum

Testicle

Cancerous growth

Illustration of the male reproductive anatomy and surrounding organs, with a cancerous growth on the testicle. *(Illustration by Electronic Illustrators Group. © Cengage Learning®.)*

seminomas. Sertoli cell and Leydig cell tumors are rare testicular cancers that occur in non-germ cells.

Risk factors

The highest risk for testicular cancer occurs with a condition called cryptorchidism or undescended testicles, in which one or both testicles have not completely descended at birth and remain in the lower abdomen or have partially descended to the groin area but have not reached the scrotum. Cryptorchidism affects about 3% of all males at birth. In most cases, the testicles descend completely during the first year of life; if not, surgery called orchiopexy may be required to move them to the scrotum. The lifetime risk of testicular cancer is four times greater for boys with cryptorchidism than for the general male population. The risk of testicular cancer is somewhat greater if a testicle remains in the abdomen rather than partially descending. About 75% of testicular cancers occur in the undescended testicle and about 25% in a normally descended testicle. Orchiopexy performed on a younger child may reduce the risk of cancer; the surgery performed on an older child does not appear to reduce cancer risk significantly.

Other risk factors include:

- Down syndrome
- abnormal testicle development
- Klinefelter's syndrome (a disorder of the sex chromosomes)
- family history of testicular cancer
- HIV/AIDS
- infertility, may result from genetic factors shared by infertility and testicular cancer
- certain occupations, including miners, oil workers, and utility workers
- carcinoma in situ (CIS), which has no symptoms but which may progress to testicular cancer
- personal history of cancer in one testicle

Demographics

Testicular cancer is uncommon, accounting for less than 2% of all cancers in men; however, it is the most common cancer in young men aged 15–35. The American Cancer Society estimated about 8,820 new testicular cancers and 380 deaths in the United States in 2014. The lifetime risk for testicular cancer is one in 270, and it is one of the most curable cancers. The risk of dying from testicular cancer is very low—about one in 5,000.

The average age of testicular cancer diagnosis is about 33, with only about 6% of cases in infants,

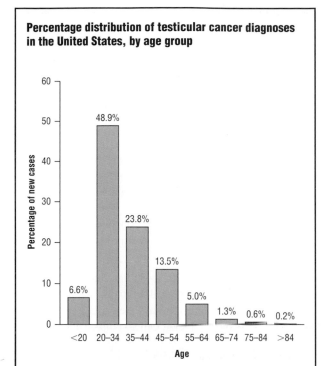

Percentage distribution of testicular cancer diagnoses in the United States, by age group

SOURCE: Data from the National Cancer Institute's Surveillance, Epidemiology, and End Results Program (SEER), 2007–2011 (most recent data available). More information available online at "SEER Stat Fact Sheets: Testis Cancer," http://seer.cancer.gov/statfacts/html/testis.html.

Graph showing the age distribution of testicular cancer diagnoses in the United States. *(Graph by Lumina Datamatics Ltd. © 2015 Cengage Learning®.)*

children, and teens and about 7% in men over 55. Caucasian Americans are four to five times more likely than African Americans and three times more likely than Asian Americans to develop testicular cancer.

The incidence of testicular cancer in the United States has been increasing for several decades, doubling since the 1970s, although the rate of increase has slowed in recent years. Seminomas account for most of the increase. The highest incidences occur in Scandinavian countries; rates of this cancer are also high in Germany and New Zealand, and the rates are lowest in Asia and Africa.

Causes and symptoms

The exact causes of testicular cancer are unknown. Inherited variations in a number of different genes appear to increase the risk, although most men with testicular cancer do not have a family history of the disease. Most testicular cancer cells have extra copies of a part of chromosome 12, a condition known as isochromosome 12p. Sometimes there are also changes in other chromosomes or an abnormal number of chromosomes.

Some researchers believe that environmental chemicals called endocrine disruptors are involved in the development of testicular cancer. Research has suggested associations between endocrine disruptors called phthalates and birth defects, infertility, and testicular cancer. Phthalates are used to soften plastics and are found in food, water, and dust. They appear to interfere with the activity of male hormones. A 2005 study found that mothers with higher levels of phthalates were more likely to give birth to boys with cryptorchidism and a shorter-than-normal distance between the anus and genitals. However, evidence has not been conclusive that environmental exposure to chemicals or injuries to the testicles cause testicular cancer.

Only 25% of men with testicular cancer experience early symptoms. The most typical symptom is a painless mass or lump in either testicle—usually pea-sized, but possibly as large as a marble or an egg. Other symptoms include:

• any enlargement or significant shrinkage of a testicle
• a sensation of heaviness in the scrotum
• dull ache in the groin or lower abdomen
• sudden collection of fluid in the scrotum
• tenderness or enlargement of the breasts
• pain or discomfort in a testicle or the scrotum

Symptoms of advanced cancer that has spread to the lymph nodes in the abdomen, the lungs, and/or the brain include:

• lower back pain
• shortness of breath
• chest pain
• cough
• abdominal pain
• headaches

Diagnosis

Examination

Physicians generally examine the testicles as part of a routine male physical, even in the absence of symptoms. If a lump or other sign is evident, the physician will examine the scrotum, abdomen, lymph nodes, and other parts of the body for any signs of cancer. A complete personal and family medical history will include questions to assess risk factors for testicular cancer.

Tests

Certain blood tests help in the diagnosis of some testicular tumors. Some testicular cancers secrete high

---

KEY TERMS

Alpha-fetoprotein (AFP)—A fetal blood protein found in amniotic fluid and secreted by non-seminomatous testicular cancers.

Carcinoma in situ (CIS)—A noninvasive cancer that may not require treatment; testicular CIS is usually diagnosed from a biopsy performed for another purpose, such as infertility.

Cryptorchidism—The failure of one or both testes to descend normally; a risk factor for testicular cancer.

Endocrine disrupter—A chemical that interferes with the endocrine or hormone system, causing adverse developmental, neurological, reproductive, or immunological effects.

Human chorionic gonadotropin (hCG)—A hormone secreted by the placenta in early pregnancy and produced by some testicular tumors.

Lactate dehydrogenase (LDH)—An enzyme that is a possible tumor marker for testicular cancer.

Non-seminoma—Any germ-cell cancer of the testicle that is not a pure seminoma.

Orchiectomy—Surgical removal of a testis; radical inguinal orchiectomy is the standard treatment for testicular cancer.

Phthalates—Chemicals used in plastic manufacture that are ubiquitous in the environment and may be associated with the development of testicular cancer.

Scrotum—The external sac containing the testes.

Seminoma—A type of testicular germ-cell cancer.

Testes—The paired, hormone- and sperm-producing, male reproductive glands that descend into the scrotum.

Testicle—The testis and its enclosing structures.

TNM—A cancer staging system used for testicular cancer, in which T is the primary tumor size and location, N signifies lymph node involvement, and M is metastases to distant parts of the body.

---

levels of proteins called **tumor markers**. Alpha-fetoprotein (AFP) is produced by non-seminomatous testicular tumors but not by pure seminomas. Human chorionic gonadotropin (hCG) can be secreted by seminomas and non-seminomas. A high level of the enzyme lactate dehydrogenase (LDH) is sometimes associated with testicular cancer. These markers may help identify a tumor that is too small to be felt during a physical examination. Blood tests are also helpful in determining the cancer stage, evaluating response to treatment, and monitoring for cancer recurrence.

Procedures

Procedures for diagnosing testicular cancer, determining whether a cancer has spread (metastasized) or responded to treatment, and monitoring for recurrences include:

- ultrasound, which utilizes sound waves to visualize internal organs and can be useful for distinguishing fluid-filled cysts from a solid mass, which is more likely to be cancerous
- computed tomography (CT) scans of the abdomen, pelvic area, and chest to diagnose malignant germ-cell tumors in undescended testes and to determine whether a cancer has spread to other areas of the body
- chest x-rays to determine whether the cancer has spread to the lungs and/or the lymph nodes in the thoracic area
- occasionally, magnetic resonance imaging (MRI), especially of the brain and spinal cord, and/or positron emission tomography (PET) scans for seminomas
- bone scans

A suspicious growth is surgically removed and examined microscopically for cancer cells by a pathologist. The surgery is usually a radical inguinal **orchiectomy** that removes the entire affected testicle and spermatic cord through an incision in the groin just above the pubic area—not through the scrotum. The spermatic cord contains part of the vas deferens and blood and lymph vessels that could carry cancer to other parts of the body; therefore, these vessels are tied off early in the operation. Biopsies—the typical method for diagnosing most cancers—are rarely performed for a lump in the testicles, since they risk of spreading the cancer; also, the results of blood tumor marker tests and ultrasound are fairly diagnostic for testicular cancer. Rarely, in order to spare the testicle if cancer is not present, it is withdrawn and examined by the pathologist before removal.

Clinical staging

Testicular cancer is classified using the TNM system of the **American Joint Committee on Cancer**. An X following the letter means that the tumor could not be assessed.

- T1–T4 indicate the degree to which the primary tumor has spread to tissues adjacent to the testicle, with T1 confined to the testicle and T4 having spread to the skin of the scrotum. T0 is the absence of a primary tumor, and Tis is CIS (noninvasive).

- N0–N3 indicate the degree to which cancer has spread to nearby lymph nodes, with N0 indicating the absence of lymph node involvement and N3 indicating spread to at least one node that is more than 2 in. (5 cm) across.
- M indicates whether the cancer has or has not to distant lymph nodes or other organs (M1 and M0, respectively).
- S is the serum (blood) levels of tumor markers following testicle removal.

T, N, M, and S are used to stage the cancer:

- Stage 0 is Tis, N0, M0, S0.
- Stage I is cancer confined to the testicle, with no spread to the lymph nodes or distant organs (any T, N0, M0, SX or S0–S3).
- Stage II is cancer that has spread to the lymph nodes in the abdomen, but not to lymph nodes in other parts of the body (any T, N1–N3, M0, SX or S0–S1).
- Stage III is cancer that has spread beyond the lymph nodes in the abdomen and/or is in parts of the body distant from the testicles, such as the lungs or liver (any T, N, M, and S).
- Recurrent disease is cancer that has returned after treatment in the same testicle (if not removed) or some other part of the body.

Treatment

Treatment decisions are based on the stage and cancer cell type, as well as the patient's age and overall health. Before treatment, patients are advised about fertility preservation options, including sperm banking.

Surgery

Radical inguinal orchiectomy is normally the first line of treatment for testicular cancer. Depending on the type and stage, some lymph nodes may be removed at the same time or possibly in a second operation called a retroperitoneal **lymph node dissection**. Some patients experience temporary complications after surgery, including infections and bowel obstruction. If both of the testicles are removed, the man will be unable to produce sperm cells and will be infertile (unable to father a child). Lymph node removal may damage nearby nerves, possibly interfering with the ability to ejaculate. Men undergoing surgery for testicular cancer should discuss nerve-sparing surgery and sperm banking with their doctor.

Radiation

Seminomas are very sensitive to external-beam **radiation therapy**; however, this therapy can destroy nearby healthy tissue as well as cancer cells. Potential side effects include nausea, **diarrhea**, and **fatigue**. A special device that protects an unaffected testicle might preserve fertility.

Chemotherapy

Chemotherapy drugs used for testicular cancer include **carboplatin**, **bleomycin**, **etoposide**, **cisplatin**, **vinblastine**, paclitaxel, and **ifosfamide**. Two or more drugs are administered in various combinations.

Chemotherapy agents can affect normal as well as cancerous cells, resulting in side effects that may include:

- nausea and vomiting
- changes in appetite (anorexia)
- temporary hair loss (alopecia)
- mouth sores
- increased risk of infections
- bleeding or bruising
- fatigue
- diarrhea or constipation

Most side effects disappear after treatment, and several drugs are available to lessen side effects. Some chemotherapy agents for testicular cancer may cause long-term side effects. These include hearing loss, nerve damage, and possible kidney or lung damage. Another potentially serious long-term complication is the increased risk of leukemia. This is a rare side effect, occurring in less than 1% of testicular cancer patients who receive chemotherapy. Chemotherapy may also interfere with sperm production. Although this side effect is sometimes permanent, fertility often returns within a few years.

Stem-cell transplantation

Advanced testicular cancer may be treated with high-dose chemotherapy combined with stem-cell transplantation. Blood-forming cells called stem cells are taken from the patient—either from the bone marrow or filtered from the blood—and frozen. Following chemotherapy, the stem cells are returned via infusion.

Preferred treatment plans by disease stage

Stage 0 (CIS) germ-cell tumors found by testicular **biopsy** may simply be monitored with physical exams, ultrasound, and tumor marker tests. CIS may also be treated with testicle removal or radiation. If diagnosed after testicle removal, CIS tumors require no further treatment.

Stage I seminomas are usually treated by radical inguinal orchiectomy followed by low-dose radiation aimed at the lymph nodes. More than 95% of stage I seminomas are cured with this treatment. One or two cycles of carboplatin are as effective as radiation. However, careful follow-up surveillance is necessary, especially if radiation is not used, since recurrence can occur up to five years or longer after orchiectomy. Radiation or chemotherapy is often delayed in favor of careful surveillance for up to ten years. Stage I nonseminomas are also highly curable with surgery, followed by retroperitoneal lymph node dissection, two to four cycles of chemotherapy, or careful observation for several years.

Stage II testicular cancers are classified as bulky or nonbulky. Nonbulky seminomas (no lymph nodes can be felt in the abdomen) are treated with orchiectomy followed by radiation to the lymph nodes. Bulky seminomas are treated with surgery, followed by three–four cycles of chemotherapy. Nonbulky Stage II non-seminomas are treated with surgery and lymph node removal and sometimes chemotherapy. Bulky non-seminomas are treated with surgery followed by chemotherapy.

Stage III seminomas and non-seminomas are treated with surgery followed by three–four chemotherapy courses. Approximately 80% of patients with advanced seminomas are cured after chemotherapy. Metastasized cancer may require additional surgeries or chemotherapy. Cancer that is resistant to chemotherapy or has spread to many organs may be treated with high-dose chemotherapy followed by a stem-cell transplant or a clinical trial of new chemotherapy agents.

Recurrent or relapsed testicular cancer usually appears in the first two years after treatment. Further surgery or chemotherapy is dependent upon the initial treatment and where the cancer recurs. Many men whose disease recurs after chemotherapy are treated with high-dose chemotherapy followed by autologous stem-cell transplantation.

Sertoli cell and Leydig cell tumors are typically treated with radical inguinal orchiectomy and possibly retroperitoneal lymph node removal. Radiation and chemotherapy are usually ineffective.

Prognosis

Early diagnosis is key. The overall five-year survival rate for testicular cancer is 95%, making it one of the most curable forms of cancer.

- Localized cancer has a five-year survival rate of 99%.
- If the cancer has spread regionally, the five-year survival rate is 96%.
- The survival rate is 74% if the cancer has spread to distant sites.
- Approximately 3%–4% of men whose cancer is cured in one testicle will develop cancer in the other testicle.

QUESTIONS TO ASK YOUR DOCTOR

- How do I perform a testicular self-examination?
- What kind of testicular cancer do I have?
- What treatment choices do I have?
- How long will my treatments last?
- What side effects can I expect from my treatment?
- How long will it take me to recover?
- What are the chances that the cancer will come back?
- Will I be infertile?

Prevention

There are no known preventive measures for testicular cancer. Testicular self-examinations and regular physical exams can help detect the disease at an early stage. Although surgical correction of cryptorchidism in boys is usually recommended for in order to preserve fertility and **body image**, it is unclear whether this significantly reduces the risk of testicular cancer.

Special concerns

Infertility is often an important concern for men with testicular cancer. Assisted reproduction, including in vitro fertilization, can help ensure future fatherhood, even when sperm counts are very low. Sometimes sperm cells from a biopsy specimen can be used.

The testicles are important for body image in many men, and their removal can cause embarrassment, loss of self-esteem, or fear of a partner's reaction. A testicular prosthesis can be implanted in the scrotum. It looks and feels like a real testicle, and the surgical procedure usually leaves only a small scar.

See also Fertility issues; Sexual issues for cancer patients.

Resources

BOOKS

Hasan, Heather. *Testicular Cancer: Current and Emerging Trends in Detection and Treatment.* New York: Rosen, 2012.

Judd, Sandra J. *Men's Health Concerns Sourcebook.* 4th ed. Detroit: Omnigraphics, 2013.

PERIODICALS

Horwich, Alan, David Nicol, and Robert Huddart. "Testicular Germ Cell Tumours." *British Medical Journal* 347, no. 7926 (September 28, 2013): 25.

Hoyt, Michael A., et al. "Health-Related Quality of Life in Young Men with Testicular Cancer: Validation of the Cancer Assessment for Young Adults (CAYA)." *Journal of Cancer Survivorship* 7, no. 4 (December 2013): 630–40.

Ruark, Elise, et al. "Identification of Nine New Susceptibility Loci for Testicular Cancer, Including Variants Near DAZL and PRDM14." *Nature Genetics* 45, no. 6 (June 2013): 686–9.

Stone, Zak. "The End of Male." *Utne* (May/June 2013): 8–12.

WEBSITES

"Testicular Cancer." American Cancer Society. 2014. http://www.cancer.org/cancer/testicularcancer/index (accessed June 27, 2014).

"Testicular Cancer." MedlinePlus. June 23, 2014. http://www.nlm.nih.gov/medlineplus/testicularcancer.html (accessed June 27, 2014).

"Testicular Cancer." National Cancer Institute. http://www.cancer.gov/cancertopics/types/testicular (accessed June 27, 2014).

ORGANIZATIONS

American Cancer Society, 250 Williams Street NW, Atlanta, GA 30303, (800) 227-2345, http://www.cancer.org.

National Cancer Institute, 6116 Executive Boulevard, Suite 300, Bethesda, MD 20892-8322, (800) 4-CANCER (422-6237), http://www.cancer.gov.

Deanna Swartout-Corbeil, R.N.
Rebecca J. Frey, PhD
Melinda Oberleitner, R.N., D.N.S., A.P.R.N., C.N.S.
Margaret Alic, PhD

Testicular self-exam

Definition

A testicular self-examination (TSE) is the procedure by which a man checks the appearance and consistency of his testes. It should be performed by all males past puberty (age 15 or older).

Purpose

Most testicular cancers are first noticed by the man himself, many times after a blow or other injury to the scrotum. Lumps or other suspicious changes may also be noticed by the man's spouse or sexual partner. Men should perform a TSE every month to find out what is normal for them in terms of the size and texture of their testes, and whether the testes contain any suspicious lumps or other irregularities that could be signs of **cancer** or infection.

KEY TERMS

Epididymis—A tube in the back of the testes that transports sperm.

Hydrocele—A benign condition in which fluid collects around a testicle, causing enlargement. Hydroceles are usually painless unless they grow very large.

Scrotum—The pouch containing the testes.

Second cancer—A primary cancer that occurs at least two months after cancer treatment for a previous cancer ends. Second cancers may occur months or years after treatment for a first cancer has concluded.

Testes (singular, testis)—Egg-shaped male gonads located in the scrotum. Testes is the plural form of testis, which is a testicle.

Varicocele—A benign condition in which the veins in the scrotum dilate, causing swelling and lumpiness around the testicle. Varicoceles are usually painless but may cause the scrotum to feel heavy or to feel like "a bag of worms" when the scrotum is examined.

Vas deferens (plural, vasa deferentia)—A tube that is a continuation of the epididymis. This tube transports sperm from the testis to the prostatic urethra.

It is particularly important for adult male survivors of **childhood cancers** to perform TSE on a regular basis, as they are at a greater risk of developing second cancers—including **testicular cancer**. Other groups that have received increased attention in recent years regarding information about and promotion of TSE are older adolescents in high school or college and men in the military.

Description

A TSE should take place during or shortly after a warm shower or bath, when the skin is warm, wet, and soapy. The man should step out of the tub and stand in front of a mirror. The heat from the tub or shower will relax the scrotum (sac containing the testes) and the skin will be softer and thinner, making it easier to feel a lump. It is important to perform the exam very gently.

The man should stand facing the mirror and look for swelling on the scrotum. Using both hands, he should gently lift the scrotum so that the area underneath can be checked.

The next step is the exam by hand. The index and middle fingers should be placed under each testicle with the thumbs on top. The testes should be examined one at a time. The man should roll each testicle between his fingers and thumbs. He should feel for lumps of any size (even as small as a pea or grain of rice) particularly on the front or side of each testicle. He should also look for soreness or irregularities. Next, the epididymis and vas deferens, located on the top and back of each testis, should be felt. The epididymis feels like a cord and should not be tender.

Results

It is normal for one testicle to be larger than the other and for them to hang at different levels, but the size should stay the same from one month to the next. The testes should be free from lumps, pain, irregularities, and swelling.

Abnormal results

A TSE is considered abnormal if any swelling, tenderness, lumps, or irregularities are found. Hard, unmoving lumps are abnormal even if they are painless. A lump could be a sign of an infection or a cancerous tumor. A change in testicle size from one month to the next—particularly a significant loss in size— is also abnormal. A feeling of heaviness in the scrotum is another abnormal sign. A man should check with the doctor if he notices any of the following:

- A sudden buildup of fluid in the scrotum.
- Pain moving from the testicles to the penis, groin, abdomen, or lymph nodes in the groin area.
- Enlargement or soreness of the breasts.
- Blood in the semen during ejaculation or blood in the urine (hematuria).

While these symptoms do not necessarily indicate the presence of cancer—they can be caused by an injury or by such benign conditions as hydroceles or varicoceles— they should be checked by a physician in any case.

Resources

BOOKS

Galsky, Matthew D. *Dx/Rx.: Genitourinary Oncology: Cancer of the Kidneys, Bladders, and Testis*. 2nd ed. Sudbury, MA: Jones and Bartlett Learning, 2012.

Hasan, Heather. *Testicular Cancer: Current and Emerging Trends in Detection and Treatment*. New York: Rosen Publishing, 2012.

Judd, Sandra J., ed. *Men's Health Concerns Sourcebook.* 3rd ed. Detroit, MI: Omnigraphics, 2009.

PERIODICALS

Brown, C. G., P. A. Patrician, and L. R. Brosch. "Increasing Testicular Self-Examination in Active Duty Soldiers: An Intervention Study." *Medsurg Nursing* 21 (March–April 2012): 97–102.

Rovito, M. J., et al. "Perceptions of Testicular Cancer and Testicular Self-Examination among College Men: A Report on Intention, Vulnerability, and Promotional Material Preferences." *American Journal of Men's Health* 5 (November 2011): 500–507.

Wanzer, M.B., et al. "Educating Young Men about Testicular Cancer: Support for a Comprehensive Testicular Cancer Campaign." *Journal of Health Communication* 19 (March 2014): 303–20.

WEBSITES

American Cancer Society (ACS). "Testicular Self-Exam." http://www.cancer.org/cancer/testicularcancer/moreinformation/doihavetesticularcancer/do-i-have-testicular-cancer-self-exam (accessed August 12, 2014).

Nemours Foundation. "How to Perform a Testicular Self-Examination." http://kidshealth.org/teen/sexual_health/guys/tse.html (accessed August 12, 2014).

Testicular Cancer Resource Center (TCRC). "How to Do a Testicular Self Examination." http://tcrc.acor.org/tcexam.html (accessed August 12, 2014).

Testicular Cancer Society. "Testicular Self Exam." http://www.testicularcancersociety.org/testicular-self-exam.html (accessed October 15, 2014).

ORGANIZATIONS

American Cancer Society (ACS), 250 Williams Street NW, Atlanta, GA 30303, (800) 227-2345, http://www.cancer.org/aboutus/howwehelpyou/app/contact-us.aspx, http://www.cancer.org/index.

Testicular Cancer Society (TCS), 1173 Alnetta Drive, Cincinnati, OH 45230, (513) 696-9827, http://www.testicularcancersociety.org.

Rhonda Cloos, RN
Rebecca J. Frey, PhD

Testolactone

Definition

Testolactone is a synthetic drug related to the male hormone **testosterone**. It is used to reduce the size of tumors in some women with advanced **breast cancer**. Testolactone is available in the U.S. under the brand name Teslac.

Purpose

Testolactone is used in treating advanced breast **cancer** in postmenopausal women and in women who have had their ovaries removed. It is never used in treating breast cancer in men.

Description

Testolactone is approved by the United States Food and Drug Administration (FDA), and its cost usually is covered by insurance. It is classified as an antineoplastic agent, which means that it stops or slows the growth of malignant cells. One advantage of testolactone is that, although it is related to testosterone, it does not cause women to develop male characteristics such as a deep voice or facial hair.

As noted above, testolactone is related to the male hormone testosterone. The way in which it inhibits the growth of breast cancer cells is not clear. However, it is known that the hormone estrogen stimulates the growth of some breast cancer cells, and testolactone seems to interfere with estrogen production. The resulting reduction in estrogen levels may slow the growth of breast cancers sensitive to this hormone.

In breast cancer, testolactone is a palliative treatment. This means that it helps relieve symptoms, but does not cure the cancer. It is effective only in about 15% of the women who take it. In these women, however, it helps reduce the size of half or more tumors. Normally testolactone is used along with other **chemotherapy** drugs for fighting advanced breast cancer.

Recommended dosage

Testolactone comes as a 50 mg tablet. The dose will depend on the patient's body weight and her general health, as well as other drugs she may be taking. A standard dose is 250 mg (5 tablets) four times a day for three months. It takes at least several weeks before the drug begins to be effective. Tablets should be stored at room temperature.

Precautions

People with a history of heart or kidney disease should be sure to tell their doctor, as this may affect their use of testolactone.

KEY TERMS

Malignant—Cancerous. Malignant cells tend to reproduce without normal controls on growth and form tumors or invade other tissues.

Ovaries—A pair of female reproductive organs that release eggs. They are the main source of the female hormone estrogen.

Postmenopausal—Older women who no longer menstruate because of their age.

Testosterone—The main male hormone. It is produced in the testes and is responsible for the development of primary and secondary male sexual traits.

Side effects

Testolactone often causes nausea, vomiting, and loss of appetite (**anorexia**). Because testolactone must be taken over many months to be effective, people who experience these symptoms should talk to their doctor about medications to relieve the **nausea and vomiting** so that they can continue to take testolactone.

Other side effects reported with testolactone include numbness or tingling in the toes, fingers, and face; **diarrhea**; swelling and water retention in the feet and legs; swelling of the tongue; hair loss (**alopecia**); and abnormal nail growth. However, since women who take this drug are receiving other chemotherapy drugs and are in an advanced stage of cancer, it is difficult to pinpoint whether testolactone is exclusively responsible for some of these side effects.

Interactions

Many drugs interact with nonprescription (over-the-counter) drugs and herbal remedies. Patients should always tell their health care providers about these remedies, as well as any prescription drugs they are taking. Patients should also mention if they are on a special diet such as low salt or high protein. They should not take calcium supplements, since testosterone already has the potential to increase circulating calcium to dangerous levels.

Testolactone may increase the effect of anticoagulants (blood thinning medication). In women where cancer has spread to the bones, testolactone may increase the circulating level of calcium in the body. Calcium levels need to be tested regularly.

Resources

BOOKS

Chu, Edward, and Vincent T. DeVita Jr. *Physicians' Cancer Chemotherapy Drug Manual 2014*. Burlington, MA: Jones & Bartlett Learning, 2014.

WEBSITES

Micromedex. "Testolactone." Mayo Clinic. http://www.mayo-clinic.org/drugs-supplements/testolactone-oral-route/description/drg-20066287 (accessed November 14, 2014).

U.S. National Library of Medicine. "Testolactone." Pubmed Health. http://pubchem.ncbi.nlm.nih.gov/compound/testolactone#section=Top (accessed November 14, 2014).

Tish Davidson, A.M.

Testosterone

Definition

Synthetic derivatives of the natural hormone testosterone are used to reduce the size of hormone-responsive tumors.

Purpose

Testosterone-related drugs are used to treat advanced disseminated **breast cancer** in women.

Description

Testosterone belongs to a class of hormones called androgens. These are male hormones responsible for the development of the male reproductive system and secondary male sexual characteristics such as voice depth and facial hair. Testosterone is normally produced by the testes in large quantities in men. It also occurs normally in smaller quantities in women.

Several man-made derivatives of testosterone are used to treat advanced disseminated breast **cancer** in women, especially when cancer has spread to the bones. The most common of these testosterone-like drugs are **fluoxymesterone** (Halotestin) and methyltestosterone (Testred). These androgens are used only in women who have late-stage breast cancer and who meet specific criteria. These criteria include:

• The patient is postmenopausal.

• The tumors have been shown to be hormone-dependent.

• The tumors have spread, often to the bone, or recurred after other hormonal cancer treatments.

KEY TERMS

Hormone—A chemical produced by a gland in one part of the body that travels through the circulatory system and affects only specific receptive tissues at another location in the body.

Postmenopausal—Women have stopped menstruating, usually because of their age.

Testes—Egg-shaped male sexual organs contained in the scrotum that produce testosterone and sperm.

Using testosterone derivatives to treat breast cancer is a palliative treatment. This means that the treatment helps relieve symptoms but does not cure the cancer. These drugs are approved by the U.S. Food and Drug Administration (FDA), and their cost is usually covered by insurance.

Recommended dosage

Dosage is individualized and depends on the patient's body weight and general health, as well as the other drugs she is taking and the way her cancer responds to hormones. Halotestin comes in tablets of 2 mg, 5 mg, or 10 mg. A standard dose of Halotestin for inoperable breast cancer is 10 to 40 mg in divided doses daily for several months. Tablets should be stored at room temperature. Testred comes in 10 mg capsules. A standard dose for women with advanced breast cancer is 50 to 200 mg daily.

Precautions

Women who take testosterone derivatives for advanced breast cancer are postmenopausal, so the usual precautions about avoiding pregnancy when receiving androgen therapy do not apply.

Side effects

The most serious side effect of these drugs is **hypercalcemia**, a condition in which too much calcium circulates in the blood. This occurs because these drugs liberate calcium from bones. Calcium levels are monitored regularly, and the drug is discontinued if hypercalcemia occurs. Another serious (but less common) side effect is the development of tumors in the liver. Other side effects include deepening of the voice, development of facial hair and acne, fluid retention, and nausea.

Interactions

As with any course of treatment, patients should alert their physician to any prescription, over-the-counter, or herbal remedies they are taking in order to avoid harmful drug interactions. Patients should also mention if they are on a special diet, such as low salt or high protein. They should not take calcium supplements, since testosterone already has the potential to increase circulating calcium to dangerous levels.

Testosterone derivatives may interact with anticoagulant drugs (blood thinners) such as Coumadin.

Resources

WEBSITES

A.D.A.M. Medical Encyclopedia. "Testosterone." Medline Plus. http://www.nlm.nih.gov/medlineplus/ency/article/003707.htm (accessed November 14, 2014).

American Society of Clinical Oncology. "Prostate Cancer:Risk Factors, and Prevention." Cancer.net. http://www.cancer.net/cancer-types/prostate-cancer/risk-factors-and-prevention (accessed November 14, 2014).

National Cancer Institute. "Prostate Cancer Prevention." http://www.cancer.gov/cancertopics/pdq/prevention/prostate/healthprofessional/page3 (accessed November 14, 2014).

Tish Davidson, A.M.

Tetrahydrocannabinol

Definition

Tetrahydrocannabinol (THC) is the main psychoactive substance found in the hemp plant *Cannabis sativa*, or marijuana.

Purpose

A number of studies indicate medical benefits of THC for **cancer** and AIDS patients by increasing appetite and decreasing nausea, blocking the spread of some cancer-causing **herpes simplex** viruses. It has been shown to assist some glaucoma patients by reducing pressure within the eye, and is used, in the form of cannabis, by a number of multiple sclerosis patients for relieving spasms. Effects include relaxation; euphoria; altered space-time perception; enhancement of visual, auditory, and olfactory senses; disorientation; and appetite stimulation. Synthetic THC, also known under the substance name *dronabinol*, is available as a prescription drug under the trade name Marinol in several countries including the United States, Netherlands, and Germany.

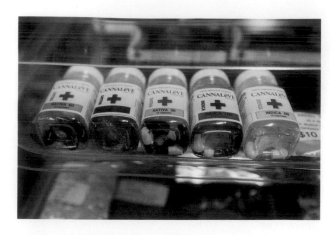

Medical marijuana tablets on display at a dispensary.
(Bloomberg/Getty Images)

Description

The issue of medical uses of THC is politicized in the United States because of its status as a Schedule I drug under the U.S. Controlled Substances Act of 1970. Schedule I drugs are defined as those considered to have high potential for abuse, with no recognized medical use in treatment in the United States. In this drug's case, its recreational use is distinguished from its medical use. Marijuana is Schedule I, but tetrahydrocannabinol (THC, Marinol) is Schedule II.

There have been major advances in THC pharmacology and in the understanding of the cancer disease process. In particular, research has demonstrated the presence of numerous cannabinoid (chemical constituents of marijuana) receptors in the nucleus of the solitary tract, a brain center that is important in the control of vomiting. While other anti-vomiting drugs are equally or more effective than oral THC, Marinol, or smoked cannabis for certain individuals unresponsive to conventional anti-emetic drugs, the use of smoked cannabis can provide relief more effectively than oral preparations, which may be difficult to swallow or be expelled in vomit before having a chance to take effect. The euphoria effect of THC or smoked cannabis improves mood, whereas several conventional tranquilizers, also used in the treatment of psychoses such as schizophrenia, may produce unwanted side effects such as excessive sedation, flattening of mood, and distressing physical symptoms such as uncontrolled or compulsive movements.

There would appear to be growing evidence of direct anti-tumor activity of cannabinoids, specifically CB1 and CB2 agonists, in a range of cancer types, including brain (gliomas), skin, pituitary, prostate, and bowel. The anti-tumor activity has led in laboratory animals and in-vitro human tissues to regression of tumors, reductions in vascularisation (blood supply) and metastases (secondary tumors), as well as direct inducement of death among cancer cells. Indeed, the complex interactions of cannabinoids and receptors contribute to scientific understanding of the mechanisms by which cancers develop. However, smoking of cannabis releases a number of non-cannabinoid **carcinogens** into the lungs and upper respiratory tract, and a number of researchers have identified precancerous changes in lung cells. The failure of these researchers to discover significant evidence of actual cancer cells in the lung may be attributed to these anti-cancer activities of cannabinoids, including THC, counteracting the effects of other carcinogens in smoked cannabis. Some researchers have investigated the link between mental and spiritual state and cancer remission, associating the cannabinoid system with the expression of pleasure on the one hand and stress on the other.

Recommended dosage

The average dose of Marinol is 5–20 mg daily. Most patients respond to 5 mg three or four times daily. Dosage may be escalated during a **chemotherapy** cycle or at subsequent cycles, based upon initial results. Therapy should be initiated at the lowest recommended dosage and increased based on clinical response. Marinol is a small soft gel and is available in three strengths: 2.5, 5, and 10 mg. The pediatric dosage for the treatment of chemotherapy-induced emesis is the same as in adults. Caution is recommended in prescribing Marinol for children because of the psychoactive effects.

Precautions

THC and Marinol should be carefully evaluated in patients with the following medical conditions because of individual variation in response and tolerance to the effects of the drugs: patients with cardiac disorders; patients with a history of **substance abuse**, including alcohol abuse or dependence; mania (a psychiatric disorder characterized by excessive physical activity, rapidly changing ideas, and impulsive behavior); **depression**; or schizophrenia. Marinol and THC should be used with caution in patients receiving sedatives, hypnotics, or other psychoactive drugs because of the potential for additive or synergistic effects on the central nervous system. Marinol should be used with caution in pregnant patients, nursing mothers, or pediatric patients because it has not been studied in these populations.

Side effects

Some negative effects are associated with constant, long-term use, including memory loss, depression, and

KEY TERMS

Cannabinoid—Chemical constituents of marijuana, such as THC.

Carcinogens—Cancer-causing agents.

Chemotherapy—The use of chemical agents to treat diseases, especially cancer.

Glaucoma—An eye disorder marked by abnormally high pressure within the eyeball.

Herpes simplex—Either of two viral diseases marked by clusters of small watery blisters, one affecting the area of the mouth and lips and the other the genitals.

Multiple sclerosis—A serious progressive disease of the central nervous system.

loss of motivation. The long-term effects of THC on humans is highly disputed.

Interactions

No clinically significant drug-to-drug interactions were discovered in Marinol **clinical trials**.

Resources

WEBSITES

American Cancer Society. "Marijuana." http://www.cancer.org/treatment/treatmentsandsideeffects/complementaryandalternativemedicine/herbsvitaminsandminerals/marijuana (accessed November 14, 2014).

Cancer Research UK. "Other Ways of Controlling Sickness." http://www.cancerresearchuk.org/about-cancer/coping-with-cancer/coping-physically/sickness/treatment/other-ways-of-controlling-sickness (accessed November 14, 2014).

National Cancer Institute. "Canabis and Cannabinoids." http://www.cancer.gov/cancertopics/pdq/cam/cannabis/health-professional/page5 (accessed November 14, 2014).

Ken R. Wells,

▌Thalidomide

Definition

Thalidomide, which is also known as Thalomid, is a drug used to fight aggressive cancers, particularly those that have metastasized, or spread. It became infamous as a teratogen in the 1960s for the severe birth defects that it

caused in 46 countries around the world. Thalidomide was never approved for use in the United States but it was widely available elsewhere from 1957 to 1961 as a sedative and treatment for nausea during pregnancy. It was withdrawn from the market in 1961 after what has been called the largest medical tragedy of modern times. The number of children with birth defects caused by thalidomide is estimated to be between 10,000 and 20,000.

Purpose

Thalidomide is given primarily to adult patients to treat either multiple **myeloma** or erythema nodosum, but can be prescribed for children as young as 11 years of age.

Thalidomide is presently classed as an immunomodulatory agent, which means that it is a drug that affects the immune system. It appears to change the levels of certain proteins that the body normally uses to control the activity of cells.

There are many studies, either in progress or recently completed, that suggest thalidomide can slow or stop the spread of **cancer** of the brain, breast, colon, and prostate, as well as **multiple myeloma** (MM: a cancer of the bone marrow). Thalidomide appears to be useful in treating patients with MM who have not benefited from other therapies. Research studies that consider the benefit of thalidomide in treating other cancers are multiplying rapidly. The use of the drug in cancer therapy is likely to increase.

The same action of thalidomide that harms babies makes it useful as a powerful cancer fighter. Thalidomide interferes with the formation of blood vessels, a process known as **angiogenesis**. It is therefore called an antiangiogenic drug as well as an immunomodulator.

Cancers that spread have a lot of blood vessels (are highly vascularized). Thus, when cancer cells are not nourished by a blood supply, they die. One way to stop the spread of cancer is to stop the formation of the blood vessels that carry nourishment to the cancer cells, and that is what thalidomide is thought to do. Researchers also are interested in other activities of thalidomide, particularly the ones that make it capable of eliminating such skin eruptions as sores or ulcers in the mouths of patients with AIDS and leprosy.

Other cancers for which thalidomide is being tested as a therapy include **thyroid cancer** and malignant **melanoma**.

Description

Origins

There is some debate about the origin of the research that led to thalidomide. Although the drug was patented in 1954 by a German company named Grünenthal, some evidence indicates that thalidomide was first developed by a Nazi scientist in 1944 as a possible antidote for nerve gas. Other historians claim that the drug was first synthesized by British scientists working at the University of Nottingham in 1949.

Thalidomide was first introduced under the name of Contergan on the European market in 1957 as a tranquilizer, a medication prescribed particularly for imparting drowsiness and sleep. The drug was sold over the counter; it was not a prescription medication. Ironically, Contergan was considered a safe sedative because unlike barbiturates, it could not be used in high doses to commit suicide. It was then given to pregnant women to provide them with relief from morning sickness. Soon after being given to pregnant women, thalidomide was linked to death or severe disabilities in newborns. Some children who had been exposed to thalidomide while in the womb (in utero) failed to develop limbs or had very short limbs, a condition called phocomelia. Other children were born blind or deaf or with other physical problems.

The connection between thalidomide and birth defects was suspected in 1960 by two doctors, an Australian obstetrician named William McBride (1927–) and a German pediatrician named Widukind Lenz (1919–95). Dr. Lenz was able to prove that the drug was the cause of the birth defects in 1961. Dr. Frances Kelsey (1914–), a Canadian physician who became an American citizen in the 1930s, became a heroine in 1962 for her work in preventing the licensing of Contergan (under the trade name Kevadon) in the United States. Dr. Kelsey began working for the FDA in 1960 and withheld approval of thalidomide because she was not satisfied that it had been tested adequately. Her concern was vindicated by the following year by Dr. Lenz's publications.

Interest in thalidomide as a treatment for leprosy and a skin disease called erythema nodosum (EN) began in Israel in 1964 and was continued by researchers at Rockefeller University in New York in the 1990s. In 1998, the FDA approved the use of thalidomide for leprosy and EN; it approved the use of thalidomide for newly diagnosed multiple myeloma patients in 2006.

Recommended dosage

Thalidomide is given as a capsule taken by mouth. There are four sizes: 50 mg, 100 mg, 150 mg, and 200 mg. Dosages used are highly individualized and depend on the type of cancer or other disease being attacked. For example, in one study of multiple myeloma therapy, a starting dose of 200 mg per day was increased to 800 mg per day over a two-week period.

There is no standard dosage for thalidomide; some patients benefit from low doses of the drug alone, while others need to use it in combination with steroid medications like **dexamethasone**. Selection of an appropriate treatment regimen is made on a case-by-case basis.

In a **colon cancer** study, 400 mg per day of thalidomide were given in combination with the anticancer drug **irinotecan**. The dose of irinotecan was between 300 and 350 mg per day. Used in combination with irinotecan, thalidomide contributed its own cancer-fighting properties and it also seemed to reduce the side effects of irinotecan.

In a trial using thalidomide to treat **prostate cancer**, both low doses (as low as 200 mg per day) and high doses (as high as 1,200 mg per day) were tried. The patients taking high doses fared somewhat better.

Precautions

In 1998, the U.S. Food and Drug Administration (FDA) required the company that sells thalidomide to establish a System for Thalidomide Education and Prescribing Safety (S.T.E.P.S) oversight program. The program includes: limiting prescription and dispensing rights to authorized prescribers and pharmacies; keeping a registry of all patients who are prescribed thalidomide; providing extensive patient education about the risks associated with the drug; and providing periodic pregnancy tests for women who take it.

Thalidomide can also be detected in male sperm; therefore four men who are taking the drug and having sexual relations with women of childbearing age must use latex condoms during and at least four weeks after completing treatment with thalidomide.

Because thalidomide can make people drowsy, patients who take it should avoid driving a car, operating heavy machinery, or performing other tasks that could be made dangerous by sleepiness.

Patients should contact their doctor about any side effects with thalidomide, particularly if they experience peripheral **neuropathy**. The doctor may lower the dosage or take the patient off the drug. Patients should not, however, change their dosage or discontinue the drug on their own but should consult their doctor.

Pediatric

Thalidomide has been used to treat children as young as 11; however, the S.T.E.P.S. program requires that a child or adolescent under 18 years of age must understand the nature of the drug, have received warnings about its risks and possible side effects, show sufficient maturity to comply with contraceptive measures (if applicable), and have a parent or guardian sign a statement guaranteeing the young person's compliance with the program.

Pregnant or breastfeeding

The serious threat thalidomide poses to fetuses cannot be overstated. No pregnant woman and no woman who has any chance of becoming pregnant should take thalidomide. Only women who have had a hysterectomy or who are at the age of menopause and have been in a menopausal state—which is no menses, or periods, for 24 consecutive months—can be considered as having no chance of becoming pregnant.

Side effects

Besides the extreme risk thalidomide poses to fetuses, it also produces side effects in the person taking the drug. The side effects of thalidomide are milder than those of many other **anticancer drugs**, and because the drug poses less discomfort than other cancer-fighting drugs, it is particularly attractive to oncologists, or physicians who treat cancer patients.

Among the side effects are erratic heartbeat, swelling (edema), digestive upsets of all sorts, including both constipation and **diarrhea**, pain in back and neck muscles, low blood pressure, and skin rashes.

More serious side effects include:

- drowsiness
- dizziness
- peripheral neuropathy (tingling sensations or numbness in the arms, legs, hands, or feet)
- leukopenia (low level of white blood cells)
- Stevens-Johnson syndrome and toxic epidermal necrolysis (TEN), life-threatening skin disorders that require immediate medical care; TEN in particular has a death rate of 30%–40%
- increased risk of blood clot formation in the venous circulation, which increases the risk of heart attack or stroke
- seizures

Interactions

Barbiturates, salts, esters used to encourage sleep, and alcohol increase the effect of thalidomide's power of sedation. They should not be taken with the drug. Thalidomide also intensifies the action of chlorpromazine (Thorazine) and reserpine, which are antipsychotic drugs.

Patients taking griseofulvin, rifampin, **carbamazepine**, **phenytoin**, or certain herbal supplements (particularly

St. John's wort) must use at least two other effective methods of contraception or abstain from sexual relations while taking thalidomide, as these other drugs interfere with the effectiveness of oral contraceptives.

Food interferes with the absorption of thalidomide; the drug should therefore be taken only when the stomach is empty.

Results

Thalidomide appears to be most effective in treating newly diagnosed patients with multiple myeloma, with a response rate of 60%–70%. It is also highly effective in treating patients with erythema nodosum, having a higher response rate than prednisolone and other steroid medications.

Treatment team

Patients taking thalidomide will have to be under the care of an oncologist or other specialist authorized to prescribe the drug and experienced in interpreting the results of treatment as well as monitoring the patient for side effects. The patient's pharmacist may be helpful in providing additional information about drug interactions and precautions.

Alternatives

Other prescription drugs that are being used as alternatives to thalidomide include lenalidomide (Revlimid), a derivative of thalidomide made by the same company that manufactures Thalomid; and **bortezomib** (Velcade), a proteasome inhibitor approved by the FDA in 2003. Revlimid was approved by the FDA in 2006 for use with dexamethasone in treating patients with multiple myeloma. Velcade is also used to treat multiple myeloma. Both drugs have the advantage of having fewer side effects than thalidomide itself, particularly a lower risk of blood clot formation.

Another derivative of thalidomide, **pomalidomide** (Actimid), was approved by the FDA in 2013.

Resources

BOOKS

Chabner, Bruce A., and Dan L. Longo, eds. *Cancer Chemotherapy and Biotherapy: Principles and Practice.* 4th ed. Philadelphia: Lippincott Williams and Wilkins, 2006.

Schlich, Thomas, and Ulrich Trohler. *The Risks of Medical Innovation: Risk Perception and Assessment in Historical Context.* New York: Routledge, 2006.

PERIODICALS

Holaday, J.W., and B.A. Berkowitz. "Antiangiogenic Drugs: Insights into Drug Development from Endostatin, Avastin and Thalidomide." *Molecular Interventions* 9 (August 2009): 157–66.

Kaur, I., et al. "Comparative Efficacy of Thalidomide and Prednisolone in the Treatment of Moderate to Severe Erythema nodosum leprosum: A Randomized Study." *Australasian Journal of Dermatology* 50 (August 2009): 181–85.

Laubach, J.P., et al. "Hematology: Thalidomide Maintenance in Multiple Myeloma." *Nature Reviews: Clinical Oncology* 6 (October 2009): 565–66.

Layzer, R., and J. Wolf. "Myeloma-associated Polyneuropathy Responding to Lenalidomide." *Neurology* 73 (September 8, 2009): 812–13.

Lee, S.M., et al. "Anti-angiogenic Therapy Using Thalidomide Combined with Chemotherapy in Small Cell Lung Cancer: A Randomized, Double-blind, Placebo-controlled Trial." *Journal of the National Cancer Institute* 101 (August 5, 2009): 1049–57.

Martin, M.G., and R. Vij. "Arterial Thrombosis with Immunomodulatory Derivatives in the Treatment of Multiple Myeloma: A Single-center Case Series and Review of the Literature." *Clinical Lymphoma and Myeloma* 9 (August 2009): 320–23.

Pretz, J., and B.C. Medeiros. "Thalidomide-induced Pneumonitis in a Patient with Plasma Cell Leukemia: No Recurrence with Subsequent Lenalidomide Therapy." *American Journal of Hematology* 84 (July 16, 2009): 698–99.

Zangari, M., et al. "Thrombotic Events in Patients with Cancer Receiving Antiangiogenesis Agents." *Journal of Clinical Oncology* 27 (October 10, 2009): 4865–73.

ORGANIZATIONS

ASHP (formerly the American Society of Health-System Pharmacists), 7272 Wisconsin Ave., Bethesda, MD 20814, (301) 664-8700, (866) 279-0681, custserv@ashp.org, http://www.ashp.org.

Celgene Corporation (manufacturer of Thalomid), 86 Morris Avenue, Summit, NJ 07901, 908-673-9000, 888-423-5436, http://www.thalomid.com/.

European Medicines Agency (EMEA), 7 Westferry Circus, Canary Wharf, London, United Kingdom E14 4HB, +44 2074188400, Fax: +44 2074188416, http://www.emea.europa.eu/.

International Myeloma Foundation (IMF), 12650 Riverside Drive, Suite 206, North Hollywood, CA 91607-3421, 818-487-7455, 800-452-2873 (U.S. and Canada), Fax: 818-487-7454, TheIMF@myeloma.org, http://myeloma.org/.

Multiple Myeloma Research Foundation (MMRF), 383 Main Avenue, Fifth Floor, Norwalk, CT 06851, 203-229-0464, Fax: 203-229-0572, info@themmrf.org, http://www.multiplemyeloma.org/.

U.S. Food and Drug Administration, 10903 New Hampshire Ave., Silver Spring, MD 20993, (888) INFO-FDA (463-6332), http://www.fda.gov.

Diane M. Calabrese
Rebecca J. Frey, PhD

Thioguanine

Definition

Thioguanine is an anticancer (antineoplastic) agent belonging to the class of drugs called antimetabolites. It also acts as a suppressor of the immune system. It is available only in the generic form in the United States, or under the brand name Lanvis in Canada. Other common designations for thioguanine include 6-thioguanine (6-TG) and TG.

Purpose

Thioguanine is used to treat various forms of acute and nonlymphocytic leukemias. It is usually used in combination with other **chemotherapy** drugs, such as **cyclophosphamide**, **cytarabine**, prednisone, and/or **vincristine**.

Description

Thioguanine chemically interferes with the synthesis of genetic material of **cancer** cells. It acts as a false building block for DNA and RNA, which, when used to copy DNA and RNA, leads to cell death.

Recommended dosage

Thioguanine is administered orally. It is generally given once per day in a dosage of 2 mg per kg (2.2

pounds) of body weight. This dosage may be increased to 3 mg per kg if the patient does not respond to the medication within three weeks.

Precautions

Thioguanine can cause an allergic reaction in some people. Patients with a prior allergic reaction to thioguanine or **mercaptopurine** should not take thioguanine.

Thioguanine can cause serious birth defects if either the man or the woman is taking this drug at the time of conception or if the woman is taking this drug during pregnancy. Because thioguanine is easily passed from mother to child through breast milk, breast feeding is not recommended while thioguanine is being taken.

This drug suppresses the immune system and interferes with the normal functioning of certain organs and tissues. For these reasons, it is important that the prescribing physician is aware of any of the following pre-existing medical conditions:

- a current case of, or recent exposure to, chicken pox
- herpes zoster (shingles)
- a current case, or history of, gout or kidney stones
- all current infections
- kidney disease
- liver disease

Also, because thioguanine is such a potent immunosuppressant, patients receiving this drug must exercise extreme caution to avoid contracting any new infections, and should make an effort to:

- avoid any individual with any type of infection
- avoid bleeding injuries, including those caused by brushing or flossing the teeth
- avoid contact of the hands with the eyes or nasal passages
- avoid contact sports or any other activity that could cause a bruising or bleeding injury

Side effects

A common side effect of thioguanine use is **myelosuppression** with decreases in white blood cell and platelet counts. Other possible side effects include:

- increased susceptibility to infection
- nausea and vomiting
- diarrhea
- mouth sores
- skin rash, itching, or hives
- swelling in the feet or lower legs

A doctor should be consulted immediately if the patient experiences:

- black, tarry or bloody stools
- blood in the urine
- persistent cough
- fever and chills
- pain in the lower back or sides
- painful or difficult urination
- unusual bleeding or bruising

Interactions

Thioguanine should not be taken in combination with any prescription drug, over-the-counter drug, or herbal remedy without prior consultation with a physician. It is particularly important that the prescribing physician be aware of the use of any of the following drugs:

- antithyroid agents
- azathioprine
- chloramphenicol
- colchicine
- flucytosine
- interferon
- plicamycin
- probenecid
- sulfinpyrazone
- zidovudine
- any radiation therapy or chemotherapy medicines

See also Cancer genetics; Chemoprevention; DNA flow cytometry; Drug resistance.

Resources

WEBSITES

American Cancer Society. "Thioguanine." http://www.cancer.org/treatment/treatmentsandsideeffects/guidetocancerdrugs/thioguanine (accessed December 18, 2014).

Paul A. Johnson, EdM

Thioplex *see* **Thiotepa**

Thiotepa

Definition

Thiotepa is a **chemotherapy** drug used to reduce the size of a cancerous tumor and prevent the growth of new **cancer** cells. This drug is sometimes referred by the brand name Thioplex.

Purpose

Thiotepa has been used in the treatment of many types of tumors, but it is most often used as a treatment for the advanced stages of **breast cancer**, **ovarian cancer**, the middle and late stages of **bladder cancer**, and to control body cavity effusions, such as **pleural effusion** and **pericardial effusion**, that occur with some cancers. It is also sometimes used for the treatment of **Hodgkin lymphoma** and other lymph system cancers.

Description

Thiotepa was developed in the 1950s. It has been an approved cancer drug in the United States for over 20 years.

This drug is included in the cancer drug category termed **antineoplastic agents**, which slow or prevent the growth of cancerous tumors. Specifically, thiotepa is among a group of antineoplastic agents that were designed to alter the structure of the DNA in cells, causing a cell to die or to fail to replicate itself. These drugs do not distinguish between normal and cancerous cells and thus affect both equally.

Thiotepa is among several chemotherapy drugs being investigated for use in experimental high-dose chemotherapy, where a cancer patient is given a combination of several chemotherapy drugs at higher than normal dose levels. This treatment approach has been the focus of numerous **clinical trials**, most commonly for advanced breast cancer. One high-dose breast cancer chemotherapy treatment uses a combination of thiotepa, **cyclophosphamide**, and **carboplatin**; however, based on results from studies dating from 1999 to 2000, the effect of high-dose chemotherapy treatments, including those using thiotepa, have not conclusively improved the outcome or quality of life for breast cancer patients.

One approved chemotherapy treatment for advanced stages of breast cancer, where patients have not responded to other chemotherapy treatments or have experienced a relapse after a chemotherapy treatment, is a combination drug therapy of thiotepa, **doxorubicin**, and **vinblastine**. However, the success rates for this and other treatment options for late-stage breast cancer are relatively low—treatment with a combination of chemotherapy drugs results in approximately 10% to 20% of patients

KEY TERMS

DNA (Deoxyribonucleic acid)—The genetic material found in each cell in the body that plays an important role in controlling many of the cell's functions. When a cell divides to create two new cells, an identical copy of its DNA is found in each. If there is an error in a cell's DNA, division may not occur.

Effusion—The collection of fluid in a body cavity or tissue due to the rupture of a blood or other body vessel, resulting from a type of trauma, cancer, or other condition.

Lymph system—This system is involved in preventing bacteria and other infection-causing particles from entering into the bloodstream. It is made up of small organs called lymph nodes, which make and store infection-fighting cells, and thin tubes, or vessels, that branch into all parts of the body.

Myelosuppression—The suppression of bone marrow activity, resulting in reduction in the number of platelets, red cells, and white cells found in the circulation.

showing no signs of cancer, and the duration of this response is usually less than 12 months.

Thiopeta is about as equally effective as the other chemotherapy drugs recommended for treating bladder cancer, including **mitomycin-C**, doxorubicin, ethoglucid, or **epirubicin**. Research results suggest that these drugs may reduce the chance for cancer recurrence but has little effect on reducing the **metastasis** of the disease. After surgical removal of a tumor, thiotepa has been shown to reduce the size of the remaining tumor in 29% of bladder cancer patients.

Body cavity effusions are a known complication for the advanced stages of many cancers, including lung cancer and breast cancer. Fluid in the heart cavity, or pericardial effusion, can be managed with the use of a procedure called a **pericardiocentesis** and the injection of thiotepa into the cavity. This treatment has been shown to result in the absence of pericardial effusion in approximately 70% to 90% of all cancer patients for at least 30 days. In a 1998 study of 23 cancer patients with pericardial effusion, 83% responded to this treatment, and the condition did not worsen for about nine months.

Recommended dosage

Patients are usually given thiotepa intravenously (directly into the vein) either as a rapid injection or through an intravenous (IV) infusion (drip). It can also be administered as an injection into a muscle or into the fluid that surrounds the spinal cord. For the treatment of body cavity effusions, it is injected through a tube into the site where this condition occurs. In bladder cancer patients, it is instilled directly into the bladder.

Each dosage is calculated based on a patient's weight at the start of each treatment. The correct dosage is carefully matched and adjusted to an individual's overall condition and response to the treatment. There is a range of doses for each method used to administer the drug, and the initial dose is usually the higher value in the range. How well the patient tolerates the treatment and the effectiveness of the dosage in treating the cancer will determine the final dosage on which the patient is maintained for the duration of the therapy.

When given intravenously, such as for breast or ovarian cancer, the initial dose is 0.4 milligram per kilogram (mg/kg) of body weight. Once the best dose for an individual patient is determined, it is given every one to four weeks.

For bladder cancer patients, an initial treatment of 60 mg of thiotepa that has been dissolved in 60 milliliters (mL) of sodium chloride is instilled directly into the bladder. If a patient has difficulty retaining this volume for two hours, the dose is reduced to 30 mL. The typical treatment cycle is once a week over a four-week period.

The dosage of thiotepa for the treatment of effusion ranges from 0.6 to 0.8 mg/kg. The dosage and duration of treatment varies with the specific site of the condition, and can be as frequent as one to two times per week.

Because **myelosuppression** is a common reaction to this drug treatment, white blood cell and platelet counts are carefully monitored, usually weekly during the treatment and for three weeks after. This condition may limit the dose level that a patient can tolerate. If blood counts are below a certain level, treatment is either postponed or the dosage is decreased in the next treatment cycle.

Precautions

As with many chemotherapy drugs, vaccines should not be given to patients taking thiotepa, and patients should avoid contact with people who have recently taken the oral polio vaccine. Myelosuppression can increase the chance for infection and bleeding. Contact with people who have an infection should be avoided. To decrease the chance for bleeding, aspirin or aspirin-containing medicines should not be taken. High doses of thiotepa can lead to severe cases of myelosuppression and may increase a patient's chance for a later occurrence of leukemia.

Side effects

Myelosuppression, usually **neutropenia** (decrease of the infection-fighting white cells) or **thrombocytopenia** (decrease of the platelets responsible for blood clotting), is common and usually occurs one to three weeks after each treatment, but may last throughout the therapy. **Nausea and vomiting** are uncommon and are most likely to occur six to twelve hours after the drug is given. Dizziness or a mild headache can occur within the first few hours after a treatment. **Anorexia**, **stomatitis**, **diarrhea**, infertility, **fever**, and **alopecia** are uncommon. Severe myelosuppression, stomatitis, **memory change**, and problems with thinking or speaking may result from high dose treatments. Side effects for bladder cancer treatment can include pain when urinating, blood in the urine, or inflammation of the bladder.

Coping with side effects may require making some life-style changes or in some cases, such as nausea, taking medication. Treatment options for side effects should be discussed with a doctor.

According to reports, Thiotepa conditioning regimen in patients with advanced hematologic neoplasms is associated with renal and hepatic toxicity. Relapse of hematologic malignancies after allogeneic **stem cell transplantation** remains a common problem, in particular for patients who have advanced disease at the time of transplantation. Researchers concluded that this regimen requires modification to reduce toxicity.

Interactions

Thiotepa combined with nitrogen mustard chemotherapy drugs such as cyclophosphamide or combined with **radiation therapy** does not improve the response to this treatment and can intensify some side effects, such as myelosuppression and infertility.

See also Cancer genetics; Chemoprevention; DNA cytometry; Drug resistance.

Resources

WEBSITES

American Cancer Society. "Thiotepa." http://www.cancer.org/treatment/treatmentsandsideeffects/guidetocancerdrugs/thiotepa (accessed December 18, 2014).

Monica McGee, M.S.

Thoracentesis

Definition

Also known as pleural fluid analysis, thoracentesis is a procedure that removes an abnormal accumulation of fluid or air from the chest through a needle or tube.

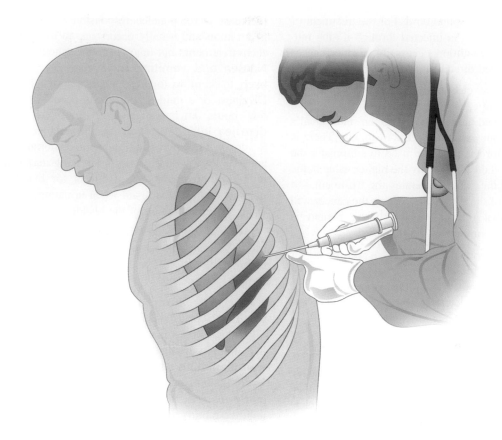

In thoracentesis, a needle is inserted into the back (or below the armpit) to withdraw excess fluid. *(Illustration by Electronic Illustrators Group. © 2015 Cengage Learning®.)*

Purpose

Thoracentesis can be performed as a diagnostic or treatment procedure. For diagnosis, only a small amount of fluid is removed for analysis. For treatment, larger amounts of air or fluid are removed to relieve symptoms.

The lungs are lined on the outside with two thin layers of tissue called pleura. The space between these two layers is called the pleural space. Normally, there is only a small amount of lubricating fluid in this space. Liquid and/or air accumulates in this space between the lungs and the ribs from many conditions. The liquid is called a **pleural effusion**; the air is called a pneumothorax. Most pleural effusions are complications emanating from metastatic malignancy, or the movement of **cancer** cells from one part of the body to another; these are known as malignant pleural effusions. Other causes include trauma, infection, congestive heart failure, liver disease, and renal disease. Most malignant pleural effusions are detected and controlled by thoracentesis.

Symptoms of a pleural effusion include shortness of breath, chest pain, **fever**, **weight loss**, cough, and edema.

Removal of air is often an emergency procedure to prevent suffocation from pressure on the lungs. Negative air pressure within the chest cavity allows normal respiration. The accumulation of air or fluid within the pleural space can eliminate these normal conditions and disrupt breathing and the movement of air within the chest cavity. Fluid removal is performed to reduce the pressure in the pleural space and to analyze the liquid.

Thoracentesis often provides immediate abatement of symptoms; however, fluid often begins to re-accumulate. A majority of patients will ultimately require additional therapy beyond a simple thoracentesis procedure.

Precautions

Thoracentesis should never be performed by inserting the needle through an area with an infection. An alternative site needs to be found in these cases. Before undergoing this procedure, a patient must make their doctor aware of any allergies, bleeding problems or use of anticoagulants, pregnancy, or possibility of pregnancy.

KEY TERMS

Axilla—Armpit.

Catheter—A tube that is moved through the body for removing or injecting fluids into body cavities.

Hypovolemic shock—Shock caused by a lack of circulating blood.

Osmotic pressure—The pressure in a liquid exerted by chemicals dissolved in it. It forces a balancing of water in proportion to the amount of dissolved chemicals in two compartments separated by a semi-permeable membrane.

Pleura—Two thin layers lining the lungs on the outside.

Description

Prior to thoracentesis, the location of the fluid is pinpointed through x-ray, **computed tomography** (CT) scan, or ultrasound. Ultrasound and CT are more accurate methods when the effusion is small or walled off in a pocket (loculated). A sedative may be administered in some cases but is generally not recommended. Oxygen may be given to the patient.

The usual place to tap the chest is below the armpit (axilla) or in the back. Under sterile conditions and local anesthesia, a needle, a through-the-needle-catheter, or an over-the-needle catheter may be used to perform the procedure. Overall, the catheter techniques may be safer. Once fluid is withdrawn, it is sent to the laboratory for analysis. If the air or fluid continue to accumulate, a tube is left in place and attached to a one-way system so that it can drain without sucking air into the chest.

Preparation

Patients should check with their doctor about continuing or discontinuing the use of any medications (including over-the-counter drugs and herbal remedies). Unless otherwise instructed, patients should not eat or drink milk or alcohol for at least four hours before the procedure, but may drink clear fluids like water, pulp-free fruit juice, or tea until one hour before. Patients should not smoke for at least 24 hours prior to thoracentesis. To avoid injury to the lung, patients should not cough, breathe deeply, or move during this procedure.

Aftercare

After the tube is removed, x-rays will determine if the effusion or air is reaccumulating, though some researchers and clinicians believe chest x-rays do not need to be performed after routine thoracentesis.

QUESTIONS TO ASK YOUR DOCTOR

- How will thoracentesis benefit me?
- Will I have to have this procedure more than once?
- How soon after this procedure can I resume my normal activities?
- Will this procedure cure my problem?
- Will I require hospitalization?

Risks

Reaccumulation of fluid or air are possible complications, as are hypovolemic shock (shock caused by a lack of circulating blood) and infection. Patients are at increased risk for poor outcomes if they have a recent history of anticoagulant use, have very small effusions, have significant amounts of fluid, have poor health leading into this condition, have positive airway pressure, or have adhesions in the pleural space. A pneumothorax can sometimes be caused by the thoracentesis procedure. The use of ultrasound to guide the procedure can reduce the risk of pneumothorax.

Thoracentesis can also result in hemothorax, or bleeding within the thorax. In addition, internal structures, such as the lung, diaphragm, spleen, or liver, can be damaged by needle insertion. Repeat thoracenteses can increase the risk of developing hypoproteinemia (a decrease in the amount of protein in the blood).

Resources

PERIODICALS

Dutt, N. "Therapeutic Thoracentesis in Tuberculous Pleural Effusion: Needs More Ammunition to Prove." *Annals of Thoracic Medicine* 8, no. 1 (2013): 65. http://www.ncbi.nlm.nih.gov/pmc/articles/PMC3573564/ (accessed November 14, 2014).

WEBSITES

A.D.A.M. Medical Encylopedia. "Thoracentesis." MedlinePlus. http://www.nlm.nih.gov/medlineplus/ency/article/003420.htm (accessed November 14, 2014).

Johns Hopkins Medicine. "Thoracentesis." http://www.hopkins-medicine.org/healthlibrary/test_procedures/pulmonary/thoracentesis_92,P07761/ (accessed November 14, 2014).

J. Ricker Polsdorfer, M.D.
Mark A. Mitchell, M.D.

Thoracic surgery

Definition

Thoracic surgery is any surgery performed in the chest (thorax).

Purpose

The purpose of thoracic surgery is to treat diseased or injured organs in the thorax, including the esophagus (muscular tube that passes food to the stomach), trachea (windpipe that branches to form the right bronchus and the left bronchus), pleura (membranes that cover and protect the lung), mediastinum (area separating the left and right lungs), chest wall, diaphragm, heart, and lungs.

General thoracic surgery is a field that specializes in diseases of the lungs and esophagus. The field also encompasses accidents and injuries to the chest, esophageal disorders (**esophageal cancer** or esophagitis), lung **cancer**, lung transplantation, and surgery for emphysema.

Description

The most common diseases requiring thoracic surgery include lung cancer, chest trauma, esophageal cancer, emphysema, and lung transplantation.

Lung cancer

Lung cancer is one of the most significant public health problems in the world. According to the American Cancer Society, approximately 224,210 new cases of lung cancer were diagnosed in 2014. It is the second most common type of cancer and the leading cause of cancer deaths among both men and women, contributing to 27% of all cancer-related deaths. The overall five-year survival rate for all types of lung cancer is about 16.3%, as compared to 65.2% for **colon cancer**, 90% for **breast cancer**, and 99.9% for **prostate cancer**.

Lung cancer develops primarily by exposure to toxic chemicals. Cigarette smoking is the most important risk factor responsible for the disease. Other environmental factors that may predispose a person to lung cancer include industrial substances such as arsenic, nickel, chromium, asbestos, radon, organic chemicals, air pollution, and radiation.

Most cases of lung cancer develop in the right lung because it contains the majority (55%) of lung tissue. Additionally, lung cancer occurs more frequently in the upper lobes of the lung than in the lower lobes. The tumor receives blood from the bronchial artery (a major artery in the pulmonary system).

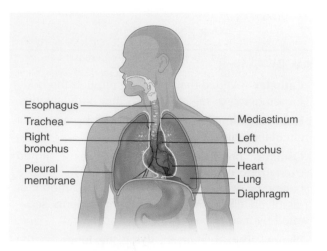

Illustration of the thoracic region. (*Illustration by Electronic Illustrators Group. © 2015 Cengage Learning®.*)

Adenocarcinoma of the lung is the most frequent type of lung cancer, accounting for 45% of all cases. This type of cancer can spread (metastasize) earlier than another type of lung cancer called squamous cell **carcinoma**, which occurs in approximately 30% of lung cancer patients. Approximately 66% of squamous cell carcinoma cases are centrally located. They expand against the bronchus, causing compression. Small-cell carcinoma accounts for 20% of all lung cancers; the majority (80%) are centrally located. Small-cell carcinoma is a highly aggressive lung cancer, with early **metastasis** to distant sites such as the brain and bone marrow—the central portion of certain bones, which produce formed elements that are part of blood.

Most lung tumors are not treated with thoracic surgery since patients seek medical care later in the disease process. **Chemotherapy** increases the rate of survival in patients with limited (not advanced) disease. Surgery may be useful for staging or diagnosis. Pulmonary resection (removal of the tumor and neighboring lymph nodes) can be curative if the tumor is less than or equal to 1.8 in. (3 cm) and presents as a solitary nodule. Lung tumors spread to other areas through neighboring lymphatic channels. Even if thoracic surgery is performed, postoperative chemotherapy may also be indicated to provide comprehensive treatment—i.e., to kill any tumor cells that may have spread via the lymphatic system.

Genetic engineering has provided insights related to the growth of tumors. A genetic mutation called a k-ras mutation frequently occurs, and is implicated in 90% of genetic mutations for adenocarcinoma of the lung. Mutations in the cancer cells make them resistant to chemotherapy, necessitating the use of multiple chemotherapeutic agents.

Esophageal cancer

The number of new cases of esophageal cancer is slowly rising, with about 18,170 people diagnosed in the United States in 2014. While the cause of esophageal cancer is not precisely known, the greatly increased rate of esophageal cancer seems to be tied to the epidemic of obesity in the United States. Obesity results in acid reflux into the esophagus, chronic esophageal irritation, and progression to abnormal cell types that result in esophageal cancer, specifically of adenocarcinoma of the esophagus. Smoking and alcohol seem to also result in chronic esophageal irritation, leading to an association with squamous cell carcinoma of the esophagus.

Difficulty swallowing (dysphagia) is the primary symptom of esophageal cancer. Radiography, endoscopy, **computed tomography** (CT scan), and **ultrasonography** are part of a comprehensive diagnostic evaluation. The standard operation for patients with resectable esophageal carcinoma includes removal of the tumor from the esophagus, a portion of the stomach, and the lymph nodes (within the cancerous region).

Preparation

The surgeon may use two common incisional approaches: sternotomy (incision through and down the breastbone) or via the side of the chest (**thoracotomy**).

An operative procedure known as video-assisted thoracoscopic surgery (VATS) is minimally invasive. During VATS, a lung is collapsed and the thoracoscope and surgical instruments are inserted into the thorax through any of three or four small incisions in the chest wall.

Another approach involves the use of a mediastinoscope or bronchoscope to visualize the internal anatomical structures during thoracic surgery or diagnostic procedures.

Preoperative evaluation for most patients (except emergency cases) must include cardiac tests, blood chemistry analysis, and physical examination. Like most operative procedures, the patient should not eat or drink food 10–12 hours prior to surgery. Patients who undergo thoracic surgery with the video-assisted approach tend to have shorter inpatient hospital stays.

Aftercare

Patients typically experience severe pain after surgery and are given appropriate pain medications. In uncomplicated cases, chest and urine tubes are usually removed within 24–48 hours. A highly trained and comprehensive team of respiratory therapists and nurses is vital for postoperative care that results in improved lung function via deep breathing and coughing exercises.

KEY TERMS

Diaphragm—A membrane in the thorax that moves to assist the breathing cycle.

Dyspnea—Difficulty breathing.

Hemothorax—Blood in the pleural cavity.

Mediastinum—The portion of the thorax that consists of the heart, thoracic parts of the great vessels, and thoracic parts of the trachea, esophagus, thymus, and lymph nodes.

Metastasis—Spread of cancerous cells via lymph or blood to an area of the body remote from the primary tumor.

Risks

Precautions for thoracic surgery include coagulation blood disorders (disorders that prevent normal blood clotting) and previous thoracic surgery. Risks include hemorrhage, myocardial infarction (heart attack), stroke, nerve injury, embolism (blood clot or air bubble that obstructs an artery), and infection. Total lung collapse can occur from fluid or air accumulation, as a result of chest tubes that are routinely placed after surgery for drainage.

Health care team roles

Thoracic surgery is performed in a hospital by a specialist in general surgery who has received advanced training in thoracic surgery.

Resources

BOOKS

Mason, Robert J., et al. *Murray & Nadel's Textbook of Respiratory Medicine.* 5th ed. Philadelphia: Saunders/ Elsevier, 2010.

McKenna, Robert J. Jr., Ali Mahtabifard, and Scott J. Swanson. *Atlas of Minimally Invasive Thoracic Surgery (VATS).* Philadelphia: Saunders/Elsevier, 2011.

PERIODICALS

Nelems, Bill. "Palliative Care Principles for Thoracic Surgery." *Thoracic Surgery Clinics* 23, no. 3 (2013): 443–46. http:// dx.doi.org/10.1016/j.thorsurg.2013.04.006 (accessed October 3, 2014).

Rupp, Michael, Helen Miley, and Kathleen Russell-Babin. "Incentive Spirometry in Postoperative Abdominal/ Thoracic Surgery Patients." *AACN Advanced Critical Care* 24, no. 3 (2013): 255–63. http://dx.doi.org/ 10.1097/NCI.0b013e31828c8878 (accessed October 3, 2014).

WEBSITES

American Cancer Society. "What are the Key Statistics about Cancer of the Esophagus?" http://www.cancer.org/cancer/esophaguscancer/detailedguide/esophagus-cancer-key-statistics (accessed August 20, 2014).

American Cancer Society. "What are the Key Statistics about Lung Cancer?" http://www.cancer.org/cancer/lungcancer-non-smallcell/detailedguide/non-small-cell-lung-cancer-key-statistics (accessed August 20, 2014).

Harvard Medical School. "Video-Assisted Thoracic Surgery." http://www.health.harvard.edu/diagnostic-tests/video-assisted-thoracic-surgery.htm (accessed August 20, 2014).

ORGANIZATIONS

American Association for Thoracic Surgery, 500 Cummings Ctr., Ste. 4550, Beverly, MA 01915, (978) 927-8330, http://aats.org.

American Thoracic Society, 25 Broadway, New York, NY 10004, (212) 315-8600, Fax: (212) 315-6498, atsinfo@thoracic.org, http://www.thoracic.org.

The Society of Thoracic Surgeons, 633 N. Saint Clair St., Fl. 23, Chicago, IL 60611, (312) 202-5800, Fax: (312) 202-5801, http://sts.org.

Laith Farid Gulli, MD, MS
Abraham F. Ettaher, MD
Nicole Mallory, MS, PA-C

Thoracoscopy

Definition

Thoracoscopy is the insertion of an endoscope, a narrow diameter tube with a viewing mirror or camera attachment, through a very small incision (cut) in the chest wall.

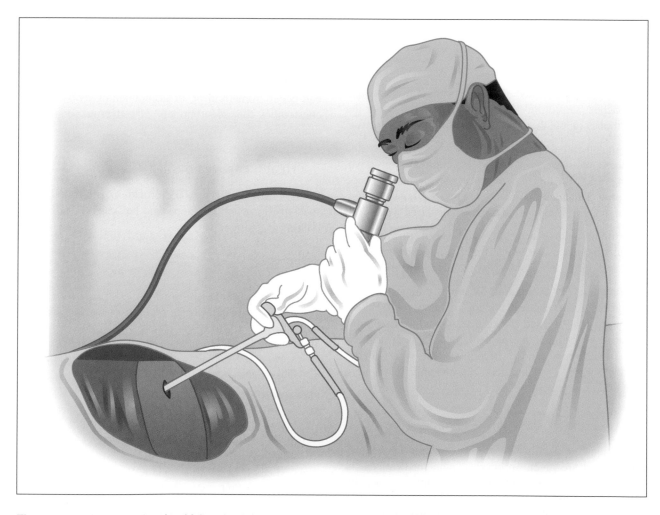

Thoracoscopy is a procedure in which a physician can view the chest cavity and the lungs by inserting an endoscope through the chest wall. Thoracoscopy is less invasive than surgical lung biopsy. *(Illustration by Electronic Illustrators Group. © 2015 Cengage Learning®.)*

Purpose

Thoracoscopy makes it possible for a physician to examine the lungs or other structures in the chest cavity, without making a large incision. It is an alternative to **thoracotomy** (opening the chest cavity with a large incision). Many surgical procedures, especially taking tissue samples (biopsies), can also be accomplished with thoracoscopy. The procedure is done to:

- assess lung cancer
- take a biopsy for study
- determine the cause of fluid in the chest cavity
- introduce medications or other treatments directly into the lungs
- treat accumulated fluid, pus (empyema), or blood in the space around the lungs

For many patients, thoracoscopy replaces thoracotomy. It avoids many of the complications of open chest surgery and reduces pain, hospital stay, and recovery time.

Precautions

Because one lung is partially deflated during thoracoscopy, the procedure cannot be done on patients whose lung function is so poor that they do not receive enough oxygen with only one lung. Patients who have had previous surgery that involved the chest cavity, or who have blood-clotting problems, are not good candidates for this procedure.

Thoracoscopy gives physicians a good but limited view of the organs, such as lungs, in the chest cavity. Endoscope technology is being refined every day, as is what physicians can accomplish by inserting scopes and instruments through several small incisions instead of making one large cut.

Description

Thoracoscopy is most commonly performed in a hospital, and general anesthesia is used. Some of the procedures are moving toward outpatient services and local anesthesia. More specific names are sometimes applied to the procedure, depending on what the target site of the effort is. For example, if a physician intends to examine the lungs, the procedure is often called pleuroscopy. The procedure takes two to four hours.

The surgeon makes two or three small incisions in the chest wall, often between the ribs. By making the incisions between the ribs, the surgeon minimizes damage to muscle and nerves and the ribs themselves. A tube is inserted in the trachea and connected to a ventilator, which is a mechanical device that assists the patient with inhaling and exhaling.

> ## KEY TERMS
>
> **Endoscope**—Instrument designed to allow direct visual inspection of body cavities, a sort of microscope in a long access tube.
>
> **Thoracotomy**—Open chest surgery.
>
> **Trachea**—Tube of cartilage that carries air into and out of the lungs.

The most common reason for a thoracoscopy is to examine a lung that has a tumor or a metastatic growth of **cancer**. The lung to be examined is deflated to create a space between the chest wall and the lung. The patient breathes with the other lung with the assistance of the ventilator.

A specialized endoscope, or narrow diameter tube, with a video camera or mirrored attachment, is inserted through the chest wall. Instruments for taking necessary tissue samples are inserted through other small incisions. After tissue samples are taken, the lung is re-inflated. All incisions, except one, are closed. The remaining open incision is used to insert a drainage tube. The tissue samples are sent to a laboratory for evaluation.

Preparation

Prior to thoracoscopy, the patient will have several routine tests, such as blood, urine, and chest x-ray. Older patients must have an electrocardiogram (a trace of the heart activity) because the anesthesia and the lung deflation put a big load on the heart muscle. The patient should not eat or drink from midnight the night before the thoracoscopy. The anesthesia used can cause vomiting, and, because anesthesia also causes the loss of the gag reflex, a person who vomits is in danger of moving food into the lungs, which can cause serious complications and death.

Aftercare

After the procedure, a chest tube will remain in one of the incisions for several days to drain fluid and release residual air from the chest cavity. Hospital stays range from two to five days. Medications for pain are given as needed. After returning home, patients should do only light lifting for several weeks.

Risks

The main risks of thoracoscopy are those associated with the administration of general anesthesia. Sometimes excessive bleeding, or hemorrhage, occurs, necessitating a thoracotomy to stop it. Another risk comes when the drainage tube is removed, and the patient is vulnerable to lung collapse (pneumothorax).

Resources

BOOKS

Raymond A. Dieter, Jr. *Thoracoscopy for Surgeons: Diagnostic and Therapeutic.* New York: IGAKU-SHOIN, 1995.

WEBSITES

American Cancer Society. "How is Non-Small Cell Lung Cancer Diagnosed?" http://www.cancer.org/cancer/lung-cancer-non-smallcell/detailedguide/non-small-cell-lung-cancer-diagnosis (accessed November 14, 2014).

Canadian Cancer Society. "Thoracoscopy (Pleuroscopy)." http://www.cancer.ca/en/cancer-information/diagnosis-and-treatment/tests-and-procedures/thoracoscopy/?region=on (accessed November 14, 2014).

Tish Davidson, A.M.

Thoracotomy

Definition

Thoracotomy is the process of making of an incision (cut) into the chest wall.

Purpose

A physician gains access to the chest cavity (called the thorax) by cutting through the chest wall. Reasons for the entry are varied. Thoracotomy allows for study of the condition of the lungs; removal of a lung or part of a lung; removal of a rib; and examination, treatment, or removal of any organs in the chest cavity. Thoracotomy also provides access to the heart, esophagus, diaphragm, and the portion of the aorta that passes through the chest cavity.

Lung **cancer** is the most common cancer requiring a thoracotomy. Tumors and metastatic growths can be removed through the incision (a procedure called resection). A **biopsy**, or tissue sample, can also be taken through the incision, and examined under a microscope for evidence of abnormal cells.

A resuscitative or emergency thoracotomy may be performed to resuscitate a patient who is near death as a result of a chest injury. An emergency thoracotomy provides access to the chest cavity to control injury-related bleeding from the heart, cardiac compressions to restore a normal heart rhythm, or to relieve pressure on the heart caused by cardiac tamponade (accumulation of fluid in the space between the heart's muscle and outer lining).

Description

The thoracotomy incision may be made on the side, under the arm (axillary thoracotomy); on the front, through the breastbone (median sternotomy); slanting from the back to the side (posterolateral thoracotomy); or under the breast (anterolateral thoracotomy). The exact location of the cut depends on the reason for the surgery. In some cases, the physician is able to make the incision between ribs (called an intercostal approach) to minimize cuts through bone, nerves, and muscle. The incision may range from just under 5–10 in. (12.7–25 cm).

During the surgery, a tube is passed through the trachea. It usually has a branch to each lung. One lung is deflated for examination and surgery, while the other one is inflated with the assistance of a mechanical device (a ventilator).

A number of different procedures may be commenced at this point. A **lobectomy** removes an entire lobe or section of a lung (the right lung has three lobes and the left lung has two). It may be done to remove cancer that is contained by a lobe. A **segmentectomy**, or wedge resection, removes a wedge-shaped piece of lung smaller than a lobe. Alternatively, the entire lung may be removed during a **pneumonectomy**.

In the case of an emergency thoracotomy, the procedure performed depends on the type and extent of injury. The heart may be exposed so that direct cardiac compressions can be performed; the physician may use one hand or both hands to manually pump blood through the heart. Internal paddles of a defibrillating machine may be applied directly to the heart to restore normal cardiac rhythms. Injuries to the heart causing excessive bleeding (hemorrhaging) may be closed with staples or stitches.

Once the procedure that required the incision is completed, the chest wall is closed. The layers of skin, muscle, and other tissues are closed with stitches or staples.

If the breastbone was cut—as in the case of a median sternotomy—it is stitched back together with wire.

Demographics

Thoracotomy may be performed to diagnose or treat a variety of conditions; therefore, no data exist as to the overall incidence of the procedure. Lung cancer, a common reason for thoracotomy, is diagnosed in approximately 196,000 people each year and affects more men than women—108,355 diagnoses in men compared to 87,897 in women.

Preparation

Patients are told not to eat after midnight the night before surgery. They must tell their physicians about all known allergies so that the safest anesthetics can be selected. Older patients must be evaluated for heart ailments before surgery because of the additional strain on the heart.

Aftercare

Opening the chest cavity means cutting through skin, muscle, nerves, and sometimes bone. It is a major procedure that often involves a hospital stay of five to seven days. The skin around the drainage tube to the thoracic cavity must be kept clean, and the tube must be kept unblocked.

The pressure differences that are set up in the thoracic cavity by the movement of the diaphragm (the large muscle at the base of the thorax) make it possible for the lungs to expand and contract. If the pressure in the chest cavity changes abruptly, the lungs can collapse. Any fluid that collects in the cavity puts a patient at risk for infection and reduced lung function, or even collapse (called a pneumothorax). Thus, any entry to the chest usually requires that a chest tube remain in place for several days after the incision is closed.

The first two days after surgery may be spent in the intensive care unit (ICU) of the hospital. A variety of tubes, catheters, and monitors may be required after surgery.

Risks

The rich supply of blood vessels to the lungs makes hemorrhage a risk; a blood transfusion may become necessary during surgery. General anesthesia carries risks such as nausea, vomiting, headache, blood pressure issues, or allergic reaction. After a thoracotomy, there may be drainage from the incision. There is also the risk of infection; the patient must learn how to keep the incision clean and dry as it heals.

After the chest tube is removed, the patient is vulnerable to pneumothorax. Physicians strive to reduce the risk of collapse by timing the removal of the tube.

Doing so at the end of inspiration (breathing in) or the end of expiration (breathing out) poses less risk. Deep breathing exercises and coughing should be emphasized as an important way that patients can improve healing and prevent **pneumonia**.

Results

The results following thoracotomy depend on the reasons why it was performed. If a biopsy was taken during the surgery, a normal result would indicate that no cancerous cells are present in the tissue sample. The procedure may indicate that further treatment is necessary; for example, if cancer was detected, **chemotherapy**, **radiation therapy**, or more surgery may be recommended.

Morbidity and mortality rates

One study following lung cancer patients undergoing thoracotomy found that 10%–15% of patients experienced heartbeat irregularities, readmittance to the ICU, or partial or full lung collapse; 5%–10% experienced pneumonia or extended use of the ventilator (greater than 48 hours); and up to 5% experienced wound infection, accumulation of pus in the chest cavity, or blood clots in the lung. The mortality rate in the study was 5.8%, with patients dying as a result of the cancer itself or of postoperative complications.

Alternatives

Video-assisted **thoracic surgery** (VATS) is a less invasive alternative to thoracotomy. Also called **thoracoscopy**, VATS involves the insertion of a thoracoscope (a thin, lighted tube) into a small incision through the chest wall. The surgeon can visualize the structures inside the chest cavity on a video screen. Instruments such as a stapler or grasper may be inserted through other small incisions. Although initially used as a diagnostic tool (to visualize the lungs or to remove a sample of lung tissue for further examination), VATS is being increasingly used to remove some lung tumors, and is usually appropriate for those under 2.4 in. (6 cm). In some practices, as many as 8% of all lobectomies are now performed using VATS technique.

An alternative to emergency thoracotomy is a tube thoracostomy, a tube placed through chest wall to drain excess fluid. Over 80% of patients with a penetrating chest wound can be successfully managed with a thoracostomy.

Health care team roles

Thoracotomy may be performed by a thoracic surgeon, a medical doctor who has completed surgical training in the areas of general surgery and surgery of the chest area, or an emergency room physician (in the case of emergency thoracotomy). The procedure is generally performed in a hospital operating room, although emergency thoracotomies may be performed in an emergency department or trauma center.

Resources

BOOKS

Khatri, V. P., and J. A. Asensio. *Operative Surgery Manual.* Philadelphia: Saunders, 2003.

Mason, Robert J., et al. *Murray & Nadel's Textbook of Respiratory Medicine.* 5th ed. Philadelphia: Saunders/Elsevier, 2010.

Townsend, Courtney M., et al. *Sabiston Textbook of Surgery.* 19th ed. Philadelphia: Saunders/Elsevier, 2012.

PERIODICALS

Matsutani, Noriyuki, and Masafumi Kawamura. "Successful Management of Postoperative Pain with Pregabalin after Thoracotomy." *Surgery Today* (September 27, 2013): e-pub ahead of print. http://dx.doi.org/10.1007/s00595-013-0743-x (accessed October 3, 2014).

Yao, S., et al. "Incidence and Risk Factors for Acute Lung Injury after Open Thoracotomy for Thoracic Diseases." *Journal of Thoracic Disease* 5, no. 4 (2013): 455–60. http://dx.doi.org/10.3978/j.issn.2072-1439.2013.08.20 (accessed October 3, 2014).

OTHER

American College of Surgeons. *Thoracotomy in the Emergency Department.* http://www.facs.org/trauma/publications/thoracotomy.pdf (accessed October 3, 2014).

University of Michigan Health System, Department of Thoracic Surgery. *Preparing for Your Thoracotomy.* http://www.med.umich.edu/1libr/surgery/thoracicsurgery/Thoracotomy.pdf (accessed October 3, 2014).

WEBSITES

American Cancer Society. "Lung Cancer." http://www.cancer.org/cancer/lungcancer/index (accessed October 3, 2014).

Brohi, Karim. "Emergency Department Thoracotomy." Trauma.org. http://www.trauma.org/archive/thoracic/EDTintro.html (accessed October 3, 2014).

ORGANIZATIONS

American Cancer Society, 250 Williams St. NW, Atlanta, GA 30303, (800) 227-2345, http://www.cancer.org.

National Cancer Institute, 6116 Executive Blvd., Ste. 300, Bethesda, MD 20892-8322, (800) 4-CANCER (422-6237), http://cancer.gov.

The Society of Thoracic Surgeons, 633 N. Saint Clair St., Fl. 23, Chicago, IL 60611, (312) 202-5800, Fax: (312) 202-5801, http://sts.org.

Diane M. Calabrese
Stephanie Dionne Sherk

Thrombocytopenia

Definition

Thrombocytopenia is a blood disorder characterized by an abnormally low number of circulating platelets (thrombocytes) in the bloodstream. Platelets are blood cell derivatives that help the blood to clot (coagulate) and plug damaged blood vessels. Thrombocytopenia is a common side effect of blood cancers such as leukemia

KEY TERMS

Interleukin-11 (IL-11)—A growth factor that stimulates platelet production in the bone marrow; oprelvekin is a recombinant form of IL-11 that is used to prevent or treat thrombocytopenia.

Megakaryocytes—Platelet precursor cells in the bone marrow.

Metastases—Tumors that arise from cancer cells that have migrated from a primary cancer to other parts of the body.

Platelets—Small cell-like bodies in the blood that are involved in clot formation.

Spleen—An abdominal organ that filters the blood, stores platelets, and has a role in the production of immune-system lymphocytes.

and **lymphoma**. It can also be caused by tumors that spread (metastasize) to the bone and as a side effect of radiation or **chemotherapy** to treat cancers.

Description

Thrombocytopenia causes patients to bruise easily, and it may cause episodes of excessive bleeding (hemorrhage). In addition to leukemia, lymphoma, bone metastases, radiation, and chemotherapy, other causes of thrombocytopenia include aplastic **anemia** and viral infections such as rubella.

Platelets and red and white blood cells are made in the bone marrow, the spongy center of the large bones of the body. Platelets are irregular, disc-shaped fragments of large cells called megakaryocytes. They are the smallest cell-like structures in the blood. When a blood vessel is damaged or punctured, mature platelets aggregate or collect at the site, forming a plug that stops the bleeding. The lifespan of platelets in the blood is relatively short (five to ten days), so the bone marrow of healthy individuals is continually producing new platelets to replace the old ones.

Causes and symptoms

Thrombocytopenia can be caused by:

- decreased production of platelets by the bone marrow
- increased destruction of circulating platelets
- increased trapping of platelets by the spleen
- platelet loss from hemorrhage

The most common cause of thrombocytopenia is a decrease in platelet production by the bone marrow. Abnormalities in the bone marrow can cause the megakaryocytes to lose their ability to produce platelets in sufficient amounts. With leukemia or lymphoma, the abnormal growth of white blood cells in the bone marrow crowds out the normal bone marrow cells, including megakaryocytes and platelets. Rarely, thrombocytopenia is caused by cancers such as breast or prostate cancers that spread to the bone. Radiation and **cancer** chemotherapy drugs can damage the bone marrow, especially when they are used in combination, thereby lowering the production of platelets. Radiation alone does not usually cause thrombocytopenia unless significant levels are directed at the pelvis. Some drugs, such as aspirin or **heparin**, do not cause a decrease in the number of platelets, but rather interfere with the ability of platelets to aggregate.

Platelets can break down in unusually high numbers from abnormalities in blood vessel walls, blood clots, or replacement heart valves. Devices (stents) placed inside blood vessels to keep them from closing—because of weakened walls or fat build-up—can also cause destruction of platelets. Severe microbial infections, infection with the human immunodeficiency virus (HIV)—the virus that causes AIDS—and other changes in the immune system can speed up the removal of platelets from the circulation. In some cases, immune system antibodies are produced that attack and destroy the body's own platelets.

About one-third of the body's platelets are normally stored in the spleen, while the remaining two-thirds of platelets circulate through the blood stream. Liver disease or cancer of the spleen can cause spleen enlargement (splenomegaly) and trap many more platelets than normal, so there are fewer circulating platelets in the blood.

Symptoms of thrombocytopenia often do not appear until the level of platelets is very low. Symptoms include:

- unusual bruising
- small purple or red spots under the skin
- bleeding from the gums or nose
- unusually heavy menstrual bleeding
- black or bloody stool or red or pink urine
- bloody vomit
- severe headaches
- dizziness or weakness
- joint or muscle pain

Diagnosis

Patients are often unaware that they have thrombocytopenia until it is diagnosed with a blood test that shows a low platelet level. Patients with cancers known to cause thrombocytopenia or undergoing cancer treatment known to reduce platelet levels often have regular measurements of their platelet counts. The blood normally contains 150,000–400,000 platelets per microliter (ul). In adults, a platelet count of less than 100,000/ul is considered low, but might not cause symptoms. Abnormal bleeding often occurs at platelet counts below 30,000/ul. If the count falls below 10,000/ul, abnormal external bleeding is usually evident and serious internal bleeding can be life-threatening.

Treatment

Thrombocytopenia does not necessarily require treatment. Thrombocytopenia caused by chemotherapy usually resolves when the therapy ends. Sometimes the chemotherapy dose is lowered, the period between chemotherapy sessions is prolonged, or a different chemotherapy drug is administered. Chemotherapy patients may be treated with **oprelvekin** (Neumega) to stimulate the production of megakaryocytes by the bone marrow. Oprelvekin is a recombinant version of the naturally occurring protein interleukin-11 (IL-11). Cancer surgery may be delayed until platelet counts are restored because of the risk of bleeding.

If a patient's immune system is destroying platelets, a corticosteroid (such as prednisone) or gamma globulin is often used to suppress the **immune response** and help maintain adequate platelet levels.

If an enlarged spleen is the underlying cause of thrombocytopenia, **corticosteroids** or epinephrine may be given to release platelets from the spleen. Surgical removal of the spleen (**splenectomy**) can also raise the platelet level. Lymphoma or cancer that has spread to the spleen from another part of the body must also be treated.

Severe thrombocytopenia that is causing external or internal bleeding may be treated with a platelet transfusion. Platelet transfusions can prevent hemorrhage, but only last for about three days, so multiple transfusions may be necessary.

Alternative and complementary therapies

Many over-the-counter medicines, herbal supplements (such as garlic, ginger, feverfew, and ginkgo biloba), and **vitamins** can affect the ability of platelets to function properly. It is very important to inform one's

---

QUESTIONS TO ASK YOUR DOCTOR

- What could be causing my thrombocytopenia?
- Am I at risk for thrombocytopenia during chemotherapy?
- How will you check for thrombocytopenia?
- Can you give me medication to prevent thrombocytopenia?
- What are the symptoms of thrombocytopenia?

---

physicians as to every drug, over-the-counter remedy, and herb or supplement being used.

Prevention

To prevent bleeding caused by thrombocytopenia, patients should:

- avoid alcohol and any medications that increase bleeding
- use an extra-soft toothbrush and avoid flossing if the gums bleed
- blow the nose gently using a soft tissue
- be particularly careful with sharp objects such as knives, tools, needles, or scissors to prevent injury
- avoid burns while cooking
- shave with an electric razor
- avoid contact sports or other activities that could result in injury

Resources

OTHER

"ASCO Answers Thrombocytopenia." ASCO/Cancer.Net. http://www.cancer.net/sites/cancer.net/files/asco_answers_thrombocytopenia.pdf (accessed August 29, 2014).

WEBSITES

"Thrombocytopenia." Cancer.Net. April 2012. http://www.cancer.net/navigating-cancer-care/side-effects/thrombocytopenia (accessed August 29, 2014).

ORGANIZATIONS

American Cancer Society, 250 Williams Street NW, Atlanta, GA 30303, (800) 227-2345, http://www.cancer.org.

American Society of Clinical Oncology, 2318 Mill Road, Suite 800, Alexandria, VA 22314, (571) 483-1300, Fax: (571) 366-9537, (888) 651-3038, contactus@cancer.net, http://www.asco.org.

Beverly Miller, MT(ASCP)
Dominic De Bellis
Margaret Alic, PhD

Thrombopoietin

Definition

Thrombopoietin is an investigational or experimental drug that may increase the number of platelets in the bloodstream.

Purpose

Thrombopoietin is an experimental drug that may be used to treat **thrombocytopenia** (a reduced number of platelets in the blood).

Description

Thrombocytopenia, or a low number of platelets in the blood, can be a life-threatening condition. Platelets are necessary for the normal process of blood clotting. When someone experiences thrombocytopenia, a cut or bruise might not heal quickly, or at all, without medical intervention. Therefore, patients with a low platelet cell count must take special precautions, and suffer significant risk.

Thrombocytopenia is a common side effect from many common **chemotherapy** agents. These agents temporarily decrease the production of platelets, as well as white blood cells that fight infection and red blood cells that carry oxygen. **Carboplatin** is an example of an agent that has a tendency to lower platelet counts. Like other cells of the blood (white blood cells and red blood cells), the number of platelets will generally increase and return to normal over days and weeks following the administration of chemotherapy.

By reducing the severity of platelet-related side effects, thrombopoietin could allow the antitumor medication to be used at higher doses and/or for longer periods of time. Thrombopoietin may also be used in other situations in which patients have low platelet cell counts.

Thrombopoietin is derived from the gene of the same name. A laboratory-synthesized version of the human gene product encourages the development of platelet cells from precursor cells in the blood.

Thrombopoietin is an investigational, or an experimental, drug in the U.S. Generally, **investigational drugs** are made available through participation in **clinical trials**.

Recommended dosage, precautions, side effects, and interactions

As noted above, investigational drugs generally are prescribed as part of a clinical trial. Clinical trials seek to determine how effective a drug is at treating the targeted condition, the effective dose of the drug, any precautions patients should take before the drug is administered, any side effects the drug may have, and any interactions the investigational drug may have with other drugs. Since thrombopoietin is investigational, it is premature to discuss dosage, precautions, side effects, and interactions.

Resources

PERIODICALS

Hitchcock, I.S., Kaushansky, K. "Thrombopoietin From Beginning to End." *British Journal of Haematolgy* 165, no. 2 (2014). 259–68. http://www.ncbi.nlm.nih.gov/pubmed/24499199 (accessed November 14, 2014).

WEBSITES

Genetics Home Reference. "THPO." http://ghr.nlm.nih.gov/gene/THPO (accessed November 14, 2014).

National Cancer Institute. "Thrombopoietin." http://www.cancer.gov/dictionary?cdrid=46158 (accessed November 14, 2014).

Michael Zuck, PhD

Thrush

Description

Thrush (Candidiasis) is a superficial yeast infection of the mouth and throat. Other names for this common condition include oral candidiasis, oropharyngeal candidiasis, pseudomembranous candidiasis, and mycotic **stomatitis**. Thrush is often a temporary side effect of cancer treatment; it can take up to a year for the immune system to recover from intensive radiation therapy. Thrush that is related to the cancer may be persistent or recurrent.

Thrush itself is a harmless infection; however, *Candida* may spread throughout the body (systemic

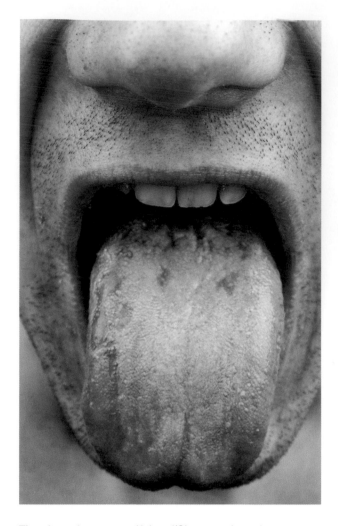

Thrush on the tongue. *(Adam J/Shutterstock.com)*

infection) to the kidneys, lungs, joints, bones, and brain and spinal cord (central nervous system). A systemic infection can be very serious, especially in a **cancer** patient with a weakened immune system.

Causes and symptoms

Causes

Thrush may be caused by several different species of *Candida*. Thrush rarely occurs in healthy persons. Three factors contribute to infection *Candida*: impairment of the immune system (immunosuppression), injury to the tissues (mucosa, mucous membranes) of the mouth, and decrease in saliva flow. In addition, thrush can occur following treatment with **antibiotics**, when normal mouth (oral) bacteria have been eliminated allowing for overgrowth of *Candida*. In addition to standard intravenous chemotherapeutic agents, **corticosteroids**, **cyclosporine** A, and interleukin-2 (**aldesleukin**) suppress the immune system, placing the patient at a higher risk of

infection. Patients who have been treated with myeloablative therapy, as in preparation for **bone marrow transplantation**, are at a very high risk of infection. In addition, certain cancers predispose the patient to developing candidiasis, including **multiple myeloma**, **chronic lymphocytic leukemia**, **hairy cell leukemia**, **Hodgkin lymphoma**, and **adrenal tumors**. Malnutrition, which is not uncommon among cancer patients, also suppresses the immune system.

Patients undergoing **chemotherapy** and/or head and neck radiation are at an increased risk of developing thrush. These therapies target the rapidly dividing cancer cells. The mucosal cells that line the mouth are also rapidly dividing. The skin and mucous membranes make up the first line of defense against invading organisms, and when damaged by cancer treatments, these tissues become susceptible to infection. Chemotherapy can decrease the number of neutrophils, a type of white blood cell, causing a condition called **neutropenia**. Neutropenia significantly increases the patient's risk of infection. **Radiation therapy** reduces the number of white blood cells, which impairs the immune system.

Symptoms

Thrush is characterized by the presence of thick, curd-like white patches on the tongue and inside of the cheeks. The underlying tissue is red and inflamed. The roof and floor of the mouth and the gums may also be affected.

Diagnosis

Thrush may be easily diagnosed by the appearance of the lesion. To confirm the diagnosis, a sample for microscopic analysis may be taken by scraping the lesion with a tongue depressor.

Treatment

Thrush is usually treated with the antifungal drugs clotrimazole, nystatin, or amphotericin. Clotrimazole is taken as a lozenge which is allowed to dissolve slowly in the mouth. The commonly used nystatin is taken as a solution that is swished through the mouth, although recent studies have shown that nystatin may not be as effective as the newer antifungals. Amphotericin is taken as a tablet or solution. The duration of treatment may range from five to 14 days. Often, thrush resolves with local treatment alone, however, systemic medication (such as fluconazole) may be used in some cases.

The patient with thrush should faithfully conduct a daily oral hygiene routine consisting of tooth brushing two to three times, flossing once, utilizing medicated rinses as prescribed by the physician. Brushing and flossing should be performed carefully to prevent damage to the weakened oral mucosa. Dentures and other mouth appliances, which can harbor the yeast and be a source for possible reinfection, need to be disinfected.

Alternative and complementary therapies

Because there is the risk that *Candida* may spread and cause a serious systemic infection, thrush should be treated with antifungal drugs. The patient with thrush can help fight the infection by eating a well-balanced diet to counteract immunosuppression caused by malnutrition. Nutritional supplements may also be useful. Some practitioners claim that herbs (such as goldenseal or garlic) can be used to kill yeasts and boost the immune system. However, these complementary therapies should be discussed with the patient's physician because of thrush's potentially serious threat to the cancer patient.

See also Chemoprevention.

Resources

PERIODICALS

Sivabalan, S., Mahadevan, S., Srinath, M.V. "Recurrent Oral Thrush." *Indian Journal of Pediatrics* 81, no. 4 (2014): 394–6. http://link.springer.com/article/10.1007%2Fs12098-013-1201-x (accessed November 14, 2014).

WEBSITES

A.D.A.M. Medical Encyclopedia. "Thrush - Children and Adults." MedlinePlus. http://www.nlm.nih.gov/medlineplus/ency/article/000626.htm (accessed November 14, 2014).
Micromedex. "Oral Thrush Causes." Mayo Clinic. http://www.mayoclinic.org/diseases-conditions/oral-thrush/basics/causes/con-20022381 (accessed November 14, 2014).

ORGANIZATIONS

National Cancer Institute, 9609 Medical Center Dr., BG 9609 MSC 9760, Bethesda, MD 20892-9760, (800) 4-CANCER (422-6237), http://www.cancer.gov.

Belinda Rowland, PhD

Thymic cancer

Definition

Thymic **cancer** (also called thymus cancer) refers to any of a group of tumors that originate within the thymus, an organ of the immune system.

Description

The thymus is located in the upper chest just below the neck in an area called the mediastinum, which also holds the heart and large heart vessels, esophagus, trachea, phrenic and cardiac nerves, and the lymph nodes of the chest. The thymus is in front of the heart and behind the breastbone (sternum). It is a small organ with two lobes and an outer capsule and its main function is to produce specialized immune system cells called T-cells from stem cells. T-cells are a specific type of white blood cells called T-lymphocytes (in the thymus they are called thymocytes) that are an important part of the body's immune system. Once released from the thymus, lymphocytes travel to lymph nodes throughout the body where they help to fight infection. The thymus gland is largest and most active in the fetus before birth and then during childhood, but becomes smaller in adulthood and is gradually taken over by fatty tissue.

Cancer that develops in the thymus gland is categorized based on the type of cell or tissue in which it originates. The many types of thymic tumors are classified according to detailed criteria developed by the World Health Organization (WHO). Thymic epithelial tumors (e.g., thymomas and thymic carcinomas) develop in the epithelial cells that make up the outer tissue layer of the thymus. Thymomas and thymic carcinomas each include many different types of tumors identified by their cellular characteristics. Neuroendocrine epithelial tumors, for example, are a type of thymic **carcinoma** (thymic carcinoid tumor) that arises in hormone-producing cells known as Kulchitsky cells. **Germ cell tumors** (e.g., seminoma, embryonal carcinoma, choriocarcinoma, and teratoma) develop in the mediastinum. Lymphomas (**Hodgkin lymphoma** and **non-Hodgkin lymphoma**) also arise in the mediastinum in lymphocytes called T-cells and B-cells; these tumors may also be called T-cell lymphomas and B-cell lymphomas. Another category of tumor arising in the mediastinum is called a mesenchymal tumor, including thymolipoma, synovial **sarcoma**, vascular neoplasms, **rhabdomyosarcoma**, and tumors of the peripheral nerves. Extremely rare tumors of the mediastinum may include tumors outside the thymus called ectopic tumors; these may involve the thyroid and parathyroid. Combinations of different types of thymic tumors may also occur.

Epidemiology

Thymic tumors are the most common tumors in the mediastinum of the chest cavity, yet are rare overall. Collectively, thymus cancers represent only from 0.2 to 1.5% of all malignancies. They represent less than 1% of all adult cancers, with an incidence rate of 1 to 5 cases per one million population worldwide. In the United States, 1.5 cases are diagnosed in one million people annually, which equals about 400 cases each year. Thymomas are the most common type of thymic cancer in adults, followed by mediastinal lymphomas. Only 1% of all tumors in children are mediastinal thymic tumors, of which non-Hodgkin **lymphoma** is the most common. Thymomas are rare in children. Thymic carcinoma and thymic carcinoid tumors are exceptionally rare, with fewer than 200 cases of each reported annually.

Demographics

Thymic cancer occurs in adults and children and is most common in middle-aged and older adults. The **National Cancer Institute** (NCI) reports that most patients diagnosed with these cancers are between ages 40 and 60. **Thymoma** and thymic carcinoma affect men and women equally. Thymic carcinoid tumors are found more frequently in men.

Causes and symptoms

The cause of thymic cancer is unknown. Cancer develops when the normal mechanisms that control cell growth become disturbed, causing the cells to grow continually without stopping and thus forming growths or tumors. This is sometimes triggered by damage to the DNA in the cell from toxic exposure or genetic mutations. Thymoma is often associated with autoimmune diseases (e.g., **myasthenia gravis**, rheumatoid arthritis), which involve abnormal T-cells in the blood and in some cases a decrease in circulating B cells, but the exact mechanism behind the relationship is still unknown. **Epstein-Barr virus** has also been thought to play a role in some thymic carcinomas and Hodgkin lymphomas. Although some researchers think that previous exposure to radiation of the upper chest may be a risk factor for thymic cancer, that association has not been established.

Thymic tumors are not usually evident until the enlarged thymus presses on the windpipe (trachea) or blood vessels, which may produce symptoms. The symptoms of thymic cancer vary depending on what type of cancer is present. Symptoms of any thymic tumor may include shortness of breath, swelling of the face, coughing, and chest pain.

Thymic carcinoid tumors and germ cell tumors can release hormones that may cause symptoms. Symptoms of thymic carcinoid tumors may also include warm, reddened (flushed) skin, **diarrhea**, and asthma-like respiratory symptoms.

Approximately 40% of the patients diagnosed with thymoma have no symptoms. The signs and symptoms of thymoma range considerably because they are related to the many disorders associated with thymoma (**paraneoplastic syndromes**), which include autoimmune diseases such as red cell aplasia, myasthenia gravis, rheumatoid

arthritis, and hypogammaglobulinemia. In autoimmune diseases, the immune system attacks normal body cells as though they were foreign cells. About 47% of thymomas are associated with myasthenia gravis. Symptoms of thymoma may also include:

- muscle weakness (especially in the eyes, neck, and chest, resulting in problems with vision, swallowing, and breathing)
- generalized weakness
- dizziness
- shortness of breath
- fatigue

Diagnosis

A complete physical examination will be performed. The physician may be able to feel a fullness or mass in the lower neck region. Routine blood tests will be performed. **Imaging studies** are necessary because the symptoms of thymic cancer can be caused by many other diseases. About half of thymic tumors can be identified by plain-film chest x-ray, while certain other tumors may only be identified by **magnetic resonance imaging** (MRI), and radio-enhanced **computed tomography** (CT), which provide more detailed visualization of soft tissue than **x-rays**. **Positron emission tomography** (PET scan) may be done if a patient with thymic carcinoma shows signs of invasion of other organs in the mediastinum such as regional lymph nodes, liver, or lungs.

A **biopsy** of tumor tissue may be performed, in which a small sample of the tumor is removed, stained in the laboratory and examined under the microscope by a pathologist to identify the type of cells in the tumor. Because of the risk of "seeding" cancerous cells into other parts of the body, biopsies are not routinely performed. However, because other tumors can lie in the mediastinum with the thymus, thymic cancer can be diagnosed only by identification of the cells that make up the tumor, and that requires a tissue biopsy. Biopsy of a thymic tumor can be done by **mediastinoscopy**, in which a tubular, lighted fiberoptic instrument with a camera attached (endoscope) is passed through a small incision in the lower neck. The surgeon can see the tumor on a monitor and can remove small samples for microscopic analysis of cells. Mediastinoscopy is performed under general anesthesia. Alternatively, a needle biopsy can be taken using a long needle that is passed through the skin and into the tumor. Fine needle biopsy uses a thin needle and larger-core needle biopsy uses a wider needle. Needle biopsies are usually performed with CT-guided imaging to help pinpoint the tumor.

Patients who are having difficulty breathing may have a **bronchoscopy** performed to examine the windpipe.

A flexible fiberoptic endoscope, in this case a broncho-scope, is inserted through the mouth and into the windpipe. The physician will look for tumors and may perform biopsies of thymic tissue.

Treatment team

The treatment team for thymic cancer may include a hematologist, pulmonologist, immunologist, oncologist, thoracic surgeon, cardiologist, radiation oncologist, nurse oncologist, psychiatrist, psychological counselor, and social worker.

Clinical staging

More than one type of staging system has been designed for thymic cancer, but the Masaoka system is used most often. This staging system was developed for thymoma; however, it is sometimes used to stage the other thymic cancers as well. Thymic carcinoma is graded (low or high) based on the cell type present in the tumor. Thymoma is categorized into four stages (I, II, III, and IV), which may be further subdivided (A and B) based on the spread of cancerous tissue. The Masaoka staging system is as follows:

- Stage I. The thymoma lies completely within the thymus.
- Stage II. The thymoma has spread out of the thymus and invaded the outer layer of the lung (pleura) or nearby fatty tissue.
- Stage III. The thymoma has spread to other neighboring tissues of the mediastinum, including the outer layer of the heart (pericardium), the lungs, or the main cardiac blood vessels.
- Stage IVA. The thymoma has spread throughout the pericardium and/or the pleura.
- Stage IVB. The thymoma has spread (metastasized) to organs in other parts of the body.

Treatment

The treatment for thymic cancer depends on the type and stage of cancer and the patient's overall health. Because thymic cancers are so rare, treatment is individualized and no defined plan exists. Treatment options include surgery, **radiation therapy**, and/or **chemotherapy**. Surgical removal of the tumor is the preferred treatment, usually performed using video-assisted thoracoscopic tumor resection or thymectomy, and sometimes robotic surgery. Surgery is often the only treatment required for stage I thymic cancers, especially thymoma. Treatment performed to aid the primary treatment is called adjuvant therapy. Thymic carcinoma is a more aggressive tumor and will therefore usually require more aggressive surgical treatment and adjuvant therapies, including chemotherapy using platinum-based compounds and a series of radiation treatments. Stages II, III, and IV thymic cancers are often treated with surgery and some form of adjuvant therapy.

Surgery

Thymic cancer may be treated by resection (surgical removal) of the tumor along with some of the nearby tissue and possibly lymph nodes. Removal of the entire thymus is called a thymectomy. Surgery on the thymus is usually performed through the chest wall by splitting open the breastbone (sternum), a procedure called a median sternotomy. When complete removal of the tumor is impossible, the surgeon will remove as much of the tumor as possible (**debulking surgery**, subtotal resection). In these cases, if the tumor has spread, surgery may include removal of other tissues such as the pleura, pericardium, blood vessels of the heart, lung, and nerves.

Radiation therapy

Radiation therapy uses high-energy radiation from x-rays and gamma rays to kill the cancer cells. Radiation directed from outside the body is called external beam radiation therapy. Radiation therapy is often used as adjuvant therapy following surgery to reduce the chance of cancer recurrence. Radiation may be used to kill cancer cells in cases in which the tumor was only partially removed. It may be used before surgery to shrink a large tumor. Radiation therapy is not considered effective when used alone, although it may be used alone when the patient is too sick to withstand surgery.

The skin in the treated area may become red and dry and may take as long as a year to return to normal. Radiation to the chest may damage the lung, causing shortness of breath and other breathing problems. The tube that goes between the mouth and stomach (esopha-gus) may be irritated by radiation, causing swallowing difficulties. **Fatigue** is a major side effect of radiation therapy and other common complaints are upset stomach, diarrhea, and nausea. Most side effects go away weeks or a few months after radiation therapy has ended.

Chemotherapy

Chemotherapy uses **anticancer drugs** or targeted therapies such as **monoclonal antibodies** to kill the cancer cells. Anticancer drugs are given by mouth (orally) or intravenously, by which they enter the bloodstream and travel to all parts of the body. They attack normal cells as well as cancer cells. Chemotherapy may be given before surgery to shrink a tumor, which is called neoadjuvant therapy. Thymic tumor cells are very sensitive to anticancer drugs, especially **cisplatin**, **doxorubicin**, and **ifosfamide**. Generally, a combination of drugs is given because it has been shown to be more effective than using a single drug in treating thymic cancer.

The side effects of chemotherapy are significant and include stomach upset, **nausea and vomiting**, appetite loss (**anorexia**), hair loss (**alopecia**), mouth sores, and fatigue. Women may experience vaginal sores, menstrual cycle changes, and premature menopause. White blood cell counts can become markedly reduced (leukopenia), which can increase the chance of infection. Red blood cell counts may also be reduced, resulting in **anemia**. Blood cell counts will be monitored regularly.

Alternative and complementary therapies

Although alternative and complementary therapies are used by many cancer patients who report experiencing benefits, the effectiveness of such therapies has not been demonstrated in controlled studies. Mind-body techniques such as prayer, biofeedback, visualization, meditation, and yoga can help reduce stress and lessen some of the side effects of cancer treatments while improving general health status and enhancing treatment.

Clinical studies of hydrazine sulfate and amygdalin (Laetrile) have not shown any direct effects on cancer. Clinical studies suggest that melatonin may increase the survival time and quality of life for cancer patients. Selenium in safe doses may delay the progression of thymic cancer. Laboratory and animal studies suggest that curcumin, the active ingredient of turmeric, has anticancer activity. Maitake mushrooms may boost the immune system, according to laboratory and animal studies.

Prognosis

Thymomas are slower growing than thymic carcinomas or carcinoid tumors and tend to recur locally rather than spread to distant organs. Because they are often completely removed with surgical resection, the prognosis is better than with thymic carcinoma, however, risk of a second malignancy is high. Thymic carcinomas are typically invasive and carry a higher risk of relapse and death. The approximate five-year survival rates are 35% for thymic carcinomas and 60% for thymic carcinoids. The five-year survival rates for thymomas are 96% for stage I, 86% for stage II, 69% for stage III, and 50% for stage IV.

Thymomas rarely spread (metastasize), but thymic carcinomas frequently spread to local and distant organs. Thymic carcinomas spread most often to the pleura, lung, local lymph nodes in the mediastinum, bone, and liver. Thymic carcinoid tumors commonly spread to local lymph nodes.

Thymomas are prone to recurrence, even 10–15 years following surgery. However, recurrence rates for thymomas are drastically reduced and five-year survival rates are significantly increased in patients who receive adjuvant radiation therapy. Recurrence of thymic carcinoid tumors is common. Thymomas also have a significant association with the development of **second cancers**, such as non-Hodgkin lymphoma and soft tissue sarcomas.

Coping with cancer treatment

Patients are advised to consult members of the treatment team regarding any side effects or complications of treatment. Many of the side effects of chemotherapy can be relieved by medications. Patients are also advised to consult a psychotherapist and/or join a support group to deal with the emotional consequences of cancer and its treatment.

Clinical trials

Clinical trials continue to investigate the safety and efficacy of specific therapies for thymic cancers. The National Cancer Institute website has information on continuing studies at: http://www.cancer.gov/clinical-trials/search. Patients can consult with their treatment team to determine if they are candidates for any ongoing studies.

Prevention

Because no known risk factors are associated with the development of thymic cancer, there are no preventive measures. However, studies have suggested a possible association between thymic cancer and exposure of the chest to radiation.

Special concerns

Damage to the lungs and/or esophagus caused by radiation therapy to the upper chest is a concern. Biopsy runs the risk of seeding tumor cells to other parts of the body. Because of the increased risk of tumor recurrence or second malignancies, patients diagnosed with thymomas are advised to have lifelong surveillance. Recurrences can be tracked by measuring interferon-alpha and interleukin-2 antibody levels.

See also Hodgkin lymphoma; Non-Hodgkin lymphoma; Thoracotomy; Thymectomy.

QUESTIONS TO ASK YOUR DOCTOR

- What type of thymic cancer do I have?
- What stage of cancer do I have?
- Has the cancer spread?
- What is the five-year survival rate for patients with this type of cancer?
- Will you perform a biopsy? What type of biopsy?
- What is the risk of spreading cancerous cells during a biopsy?
- What are my treatment options?
- What are the risks and side effects of these treatments?
- What medications can I take to relieve treatment side effects?
- Are there any clinical studies underway that would be appropriate for me?
- What effective alternative or complementary treatments are available for thymic cancer?
- How debilitating is the treatment? Will I be able to continue working?
- What is the chance that the cancer will recur?
- What are the signs and symptoms of recurrence?
- What can be done to prevent recurrence?
- How often will I have follow-up examinations?

Resources

BOOKS

Bruss, Katherine, Christina Salter, and Esmeralda Galan, eds. *American Cancer Society's Complete Guide to Complementary and Alternative Cancer Therapies*, 2nd ed. Atlanta: American Cancer Society, 2009.

Cameron, Robert, Patrick Loehrer, and Charles Thomas Jr. "Neoplasms of the Mediastinum." In *Cancer: Principles and Practice of Oncology*, 9th ed. Vincent T. DeVita, Samuel Hellman, and Steven Rosenberg, eds., 871–881. Philadelphia: Lippincott Williams & Wilkins, 2011.

Raghavan D., M. Brecher, and D. Johnson, et al., eds. "Thymoma and Thymic Tumors." In *Textbook of Uncommon Cancer*. 4th ed. Hoboken, NJ: John Wiley & Sons, 2012.

PERIODICALS

Ruffini E., and F. Venuta. "Management of Thymic Tumors: A European Perspective." *Journal of Thoracic Diseases* Supplement 2 (May 2014): S228–S237.

Syrios, J., N. Diamantis, and E. Fergadis, et al. "Advances in Thymic Carcinoma Diagnosis and Treatment: A Review of the Literature." *Medical Oncology* 31 (Jul 2014): 44–48.

Ye, B., J. C. Tantal, and W. Li, et al. "Video-assisted Thoracoscopic Surgery versus Robotic-assisted Thoracoscopic Surgery in the Surgical Treatment of Masaoka Stage I Thymoma." *World Journal of Surgical Oncology* 11 (Jul 2013): 157–163.

ORGANIZATIONS

American Cancer Society, 1599 Clifton Rd. NE, Atlanta, GA 30329, (800) ACS-2345, http://www.cancer.org.

Cancer Research Institute, National Headquarters, 681 Fifth Ave., New York, NY 10022, (800) 992-2623, http://www.cancerresearch.org.

National Institutes of Health. National Cancer Institute, 9000 Rockville Pike, Bethesda, MD 20982, (800) 4-CANCER (422-6237), http://cancernet.nci.nih.gov.

L. Lee Culvert
Belinda Rowland, PhD
Rebecca J. Frey, PhD

Thymoma

Definition

Thymomas are the most common tumor of the thymus.

Description

The thymus is located in the upper chest just below the neck. It is a small organ that produces certain white blood cells before birth and during childhood. These white blood cells are called lymphocytes and are an important part of the body's immune system. Once released from the thymus, lymphocytes travel to lymph nodes where they help to fight infections. The thymus gland becomes smaller in adulthood and is gradually taken over by fat tissue.

Although rare, thymomas are the most common type of thymic tumor. The term thymoma traditionally refers to a non-invasive, localized (only in the thymus) type of thymic tumor. Thymomas arise from thymic epithelial cells, which make up the covering of the thymus. Thymomas frequently contain lymphocytes, which are noncancerous. Thymomas are classified as either noninvasive (previously called benign) or invasive (previously called malignant). Noninvasive thymomas are those in which the tumor is encapsulated and easy to remove. Invasive thymomas have spread to nearby structures (such as the lungs) and are difficult to remove. Approximately 30% to 40% of thymomas are of the invasive type.

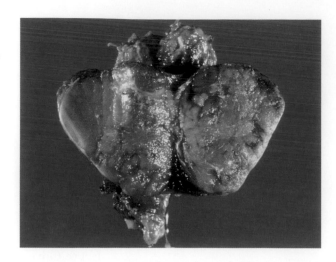

Gross specimen of the human thymus gland cut to show a tumor (thymoma). *(SPL/Science Source)*

Demographics

Thymoma affects men and women equally. It is usually diagnosed between the ages of 40 and 60 years. Thymomas are uncommon in children.

Causes and symptoms

The cause of thymoma is unknown. **Cancer** is caused when the normal mechanisms that control cell growth become disturbed, causing the cells to grow continually without stopping. This is caused by damage to the DNA in the cell.

Approximately 40% of the patients diagnosed with thymoma have no symptoms. The symptoms in the remaining 60% of patients are caused by pressure from the enlarged thymus on the windpipe (trachea) or blood vessels or by **paraneoplastic syndromes**. Paraneoplastic syndromes are collections of symptoms in cancer patients that cannot be explained by the tumor. Seventy-one percent of thymomas are associated with paraneoplastic syndromes. The most common syndromes related to thymoma are pure red cell aplasia (having abnormally low levels of red blood cells), **myasthenia gravis** (a muscular disorder), and hypogammaglobulinemia (having abnormally low levels of antibodies). These conditions are autoimmune diseases, those in which the body mounts an attack against certain normal cells of the body. Regarding myasthenia gravis, 15% of patients with this syndrome have thymomas. Alternately, 50% of patients with thymomas have myasthenia gravis. The relationship between the two entities is not clearly understood, though it is believed that the thymus may give incorrect instructions about the production of acetylcholine receptor antibodies, thus setting the state for faulty neuromuscular transmission. The confirmed presence of either thymomas or myasthenia gravis should prompt investigation for the other condition.

Symptoms of thymoma may include:

- shortness of breath
- swelling of the face
- coughing
- chest pain
- muscle weakness (especially in the eyes, neck, and chest, causing problems with vision, swallowing, and breathing)
- weakness
- dizziness
- shortness of breath
- fatigue

Diagnosis

The physician will conduct a complete physical exam. He or she may be able to feel a fullness in the lower neck region. Routine blood tests may be performed. **Imaging studies** are necessary because the symptoms of thymoma can be caused by many other diseases. Thymomas can be identified by chest x-ray, **magnetic resonance imaging** (MRI), and **computed tomography** (CT).

A **biopsy** may be performed, in which a small sample of the tumor is removed and examined under the microscope; however, because of the risk of "seeding" cancerous cells, biopsies are not routinely performed. There are a few different methods to biopsy a thymoma. For a **mediastinoscopy**, a wand-like lighted camera (endoscope) and special instruments are passed through a small cut in the lower neck. The surgeon can see the tumor on a monitor and can cut off small samples for microscopic analysis. Mediastinoscopy is performed under general anesthesia. Alternatively, a needle biopsy will be taken in which a long needle is passed through the skin and into the tumor. Fine needle biopsy uses a thin needle and larger-core needle biopsy uses a wider needle. Needle biopsies may be performed in conjunction with computed tomography imaging.

Patients who are having difficulty breathing may have a **bronchoscopy** performed to examine the wind pipe. An endoscope, in this case a bronchoscope, is inserted through the mouth and into the windpipe. The physician will look for tumors and may perform biopsies.

Treatment team

The treatment team for thymoma may include a hematologist, pulmonologist, immunologist, oncologist, thoracic surgeon, cardiologist, radiation oncologist, nurse oncologist, psychiatrist, psychological counselor, and social worker.

Clinical staging

There is more than one type of staging system for thymoma but the Masaoka system, a surgical staging system developed in 1981, is used most often. Thymoma is categorized into four stages (I, II, III, and IV) which may be further subdivided (A and B) based on the spread of cancerous tissue. The Masaoka staging system is as follows:

- Stage I. The thymoma lies completely within the thymus.
- Stage II. The thymoma has spread out of the thymus and invaded the outer layer of the lung (pleura) or nearby fatty tissue.
- Stage III. The thymoma has spread to other neighboring tissues of the upper chest including the outer layer of the heart (pericardium), the lungs, or the heart's main blood vessels.
- Stage IVA. The thymoma has spread throughout the pericardium and/or the pleura.
- Stage IVB. The thymoma has spread to organs in other parts of the body.

In 1999, the World Health Organization (WHO) adopted a new classification system for thymic tumors. This system is a histologic classification, which means that it is based on the microscopic features of the cells that make up the tumor. The WHO classification system ranks thymomas into types A, AB, B1, B2, B3, and C, by increasing severity.

Treatment

The treatment for thymoma cancer depends on the stage of cancer and the patient's overall health. Because thymomas are so rare, there are no defined treatment plans. Treatment options include surgery, **radiation therapy**, and/or **chemotherapy**. Surgical removal of the tumor is the preferred treatment. Surgery is often the only treatment required for stage I tumors. Treatment of thymoma often relieves the symptoms caused by paraneoplastic syndromes.

A treatment that is intended to aid the primary treatment is called adjuvant therapy. For instance, chemotherapy may be used along with surgery to treat thymoma. Stages II, III, and IV thymomas are often treated with surgery and some form of adjuvant therapy.

Surgery

Thymoma may be treated by surgically removing (resecting) the tumor and some of the nearby healthy tissue. Removal of the entire thymus gland is called a thymectomy. Surgery on the thymus is usually performed through the chest wall by splitting open the breast bone (sternum), a procedure called a median sternotomy. When complete removal of the tumor is impossible, the surgeon will remove as much of the tumor as possible (**debulking surgery**, sub-total resection). In these cases, if the tumor has spread, surgery may include removal of other tissues such as the pleura, pericardium, blood vessels of the heart, lung, and nerves.

Radiation therapy

Radiation therapy uses high-energy radiation from x-rays and gamma rays to kill the cancer cells. Radiation given from a machine that is outside the body is called external radiation therapy. Radiation therapy is often used as adjuvant therapy following surgery to reduce the chance of cancer recurrence. Radiation may be used to kill cancer cells in cases in which the tumor was only partially removed. It may be used before surgery to shrink a large tumor. Radiation therapy is not very effective when used alone, although it may be used alone when the patient is too sick to withstand surgery.

The skin in the treated area may become red and dry and may take as long as a year to return to normal. Radiation to the chest may damage the lung causing shortness of breath and other breathing problems. Also, the tube that goes between the mouth and stomach (esophagus) may be irritated by radiation causing swallowing difficulties. **Fatigue**, upset stomach, **diarrhea**, and nausea are also common complaints of patients having radiation therapy. Most side effects go away about two to three weeks after radiation therapy has ended.

Chemotherapy

Chemotherapy uses **anticancer drugs** to kill the cancer cells. The drugs are given by mouth (orally) or intravenously. They enter the bloodstream and can travel to all parts of the body. Chemotherapy may be given before surgery to shrink a tumor, which is called neoadjuvant therapy. Thymoma cells are very sensitive to anticancer drugs, especially **cisplatin**, **doxorubicin**, and **ifosfamide**. Generally, a combination of drugs is given because it is more effective than a single drug in treating cancer. **Corticosteroids** are also used to treat thymoma.

The side effects of chemotherapy are significant and include stomach upset, **nausea and vomiting**, appetite loss (**anorexia**), hair loss (**alopecia**), mouth sores, and fatigue. Women may experience vaginal sores, menstrual

Thymoma

cycle changes, and premature menopause. There is also an increased chance of infections.

Alternative and complementary therapies

Although alternative and complementary therapies are used by many cancer patients, very few controlled studies on the effectiveness of such therapies exist. Mind-body techniques such as prayer, biofeedback, visualization, meditation, and yoga have not shown any effect in reducing cancer but they can reduce stress and lessen some of the side effects of cancer treatments. Gerson, macrobiotic, orthomolecular, and Cancell therapies are ineffective treatments for cancer.

Clinical studies of hydrazine sulfate found that it had no effect on cancer and even worsened the health and well-being of the study subjects. One clinical study of the drug amygdalin (Laetrile) found that it had no effect on cancer. Laetrile can be toxic and has caused deaths. Shark cartilage, although highly touted as an effective cancer treatment, is an improbable therapy that has not been the subject of clinical study. Although the results are mixed, clinical studies suggest that melatonin may increase the survival time and quality of life for cancer patients.

Selenium, in safe doses, may delay the progression of cancer. Laboratory and animal studies suggest that curcumin, the active ingredient of turmeric, has anticancer activity. Maitake mushrooms may boost the immune system, according to laboratory and animal studies. The results of laboratory studies suggest that **mistletoe** has anticancer properties; however, clinical studies have not been conducted.

For more comprehensive information, the reader should consult the book on complementary and alternative medicine published by the American Cancer Society listed in the Resources section.

Prognosis

The five-year survival rates for thymomas are 96% for stage I, 86% for stage II, 69% for stage III, and 50% for stage IV. Thorough (radical) surgery is associated with a longer survival rate. Almost 15% of thymoma patients develop a second cancer.

Thymomas rarely spread (metastasize) outside of the chest cavity. **Metastasis** is usually limited to the pleura. Invasive thymomas are prone to recurrence, even 10 to 15 years following surgery. The recurrence rates are drastically reduced and the five-year survival rates are drastically increased in patients who receive adjuvant radiation therapy.

QUESTIONS TO ASK YOUR DOCTOR

- What histologic class of thymoma do I have?
- What stage of cancer do I have?
- Has the cancer spread?
- What is the five-year survival rate for patients with this stage of thymoma?
- Will you perform a biopsy?
- What type of biopsy will you perform?
- What is the risk of seeding during a biopsy?
- What are my treatment options?
- What are the risks and side effects of these treatments?
- What medications can I take to relieve treatment side effects?
- Are there any clinical studies underway that would be appropriate for me?
- What effective alternative or complementary treatments are available for thymoma?
- How debilitating is the treatment? Will I be able to continue working?
- What is the chance that the cancer will recur?
- What are the signs and symptoms of recurrence?
- What can be done to prevent recurrence?
- How often will I have follow-up examinations?

Coping with cancer treatment

The patient should consult his or her treatment team regarding any side effects or complications of treatment. Many of the side effects of chemotherapy can be relieved by medications. Patients should consult a psychotherapist and/or join a support group to deal with the emotional consequences of cancer and its treatment.

Clinical trials

As of 2014, there were 25 active **clinical trials** studying thymoma. The **National Cancer Institute** sponsors these studies. Several were studying different chemotherapy drugs on advanced or recurrent tumors. The National Cancer Institute website provides information on these and other studies at: http://www.cancer.gov/clinicaltrials/search. Patients should consult with their treatment team to determine if they are candidates for these or any other ongoing studies.

Prevention

Because there are no known risk factors for the development of thymoma, there are no preventive measures. However, there may be an association between **thymic cancer** and exposure of the chest to radiation.

Special concerns

Damage to the lungs and/or esophagus caused by radiation therapy to the upper chest is a concern. Biopsy runs the risk of seeding tumor cells to other parts of the body.

See also Thoracotomy.

Resources

PERIODICALS

Sandri, A., et al. "Long-Term Results After Treatment for Recurrent Thymoma: A Multicenter Analysis." *Journal of Thoracic Oncology* 9, no. 12 (2014): 1796–1804. http://www.ncbi.nlm.nih.gov/pubmed/25393792 (accessed November 14, 2014).

WEBSITES

American Society of Clinical Oncology. "Thymoma." Cancer.net http://www.cancer.net/cancer-types/thymoma (accessed November 14, 2014).
National Cancer Institute. "Thymoma and Thymic Carcinoma Treatment." http://www.cancer.gov/cancertopics/pdq/treatment/thymoma/patient/page1 (accessed November 14, 2014).

ORGANIZATIONS

American Cancer Society, 250 Williams St. NW, Atlanta, GA 30303, (800) 227-2345, http://www.cancer.org.
National Cancer Institute, 9609 Medical Center Dr., BG 9609 MSC 9760, Bethesda, MD 20892-9760, (800) 4-CANCER (422-6237), http://www.cancer.gov.

Belinda Rowland, PhD

Thyroid cancer

Definition

Thyroid **cancer** is the abnormal, uncontrolled growth of cells of the thyroid gland into a mass (tumor).

Description

The thyroid is a hormone-producing, two-lobed, butterfly-shaped gland located in the neck at the base of the throat. It uses iodine—a mineral found in some foods—to produce several of its hormones. Thyroid hormones regulate essential body processes, such as heart rate, blood pressure, body temperature, and metabolism, and affect the nervous system, muscles, and other organs.

There are two main types of cells in the thyroid gland: follicular cells produce thyroid hormones, and C cells or parafollicular cells produce **calcitonin**, a hormone that controls calcium levels in the blood. The thyroid gland also contains immune-system lymphocytes and supportive stromal cells.

Types of thyroid cancer

Thyroid cancers are classified by the type of cell in which they develop and their appearance under a microscope. There are four main types that are usually defined clinically as well-differentiated (similar in appearance to normal thyroid tissue) or poorly differentiated.

- Papillary carcinoma, which accounts for about 80% of all thyroid cancers, is a very slow-growing cancer of differentiated follicular cells, usually occurring in one lobe of the gland. It can spread to lymph nodes in the neck. There are several subtypes, of which papillary/follicular carcinoma, containing a mixture of cell types, is most common. Other subtypes tend to grow and spread more rapidly.

- Follicular carcinoma, which accounts for about 10% of thyroid cancers, is a differentiated cancer that develops in follicular cells. It is more common in parts of the world where the population consumes iodine-poor diets. It does not usually spread to the lymph nodes but can spread to other parts of the body, such as the lungs or bones. Hurthle cell carcinoma is a variant of follicular carcinoma with a poorer prognosis. It accounts for about 3% of thyroid cancers.

- Medullary thyroid carcinoma (MTC), which accounts for about 4% of thyroid cancers, develops in C cells. These cancers often release too much calcitonin and a protein called carcinoembryonic antigen (CEA) into the blood. Most MTCs (80%) are sporadic (not inherited); they develop in older adults and affect only one lobe. Familial MTC is inherited, often develops in children or young adults, affects several areas of both lobes, and may spread (metastasize) early.

- Anaplastic carcinoma, which accounts for just 2% of thyroid cancers, is the fastest growing, most aggressive type. It is subdivided into small-cell and giant-cell types.

- Rare thyroid cancers include lymphoma that develops from lymphocytes, sarcoma that develops in supporting cells, and carcinosarcoma.

Risk factors

Risk factors associated with the development of thyroid cancer include:

Thyroid cancers

Cancer type	Characteristics	Prognosis
Papillary	60–80% of thyroid cancers Slow-growing cancer in hormone-producing cells	90% of patients will live for 15 years or longer after diagnosis
Follicular	30–50% of thyroid cancers Found in hormone-producing cells	90% of patients will live for 15 years or longer after diagnosis
Medullary	5–7% of thyroid cancers Found in calcitonin-producing cells Difficult to control as it often spreads to other parts of the body	80% of patients will live for at least 10 years after surgery
Anaplastic	2% of thyroid cancers Fastest growing Rapidly spreads to other parts of the body	3–17% of patients will survive for five years

Characteristics and prognoses of thyroid cancers. *(Table by GGS Creative Resources. © Cengage Learning®.)*

- Gender: Thyroid cancers—like most thyroid diseases—are three times more common in women than in men.

- Age: Diagnoses of thyroid cancer peak in women in their 40s and 50s and in men in their 60s or 70s.

- Diet: Diets low in iodine are associated with the development of follicular carcinoma and also with papillary carcinoma in people exposed to radiation. Most people in the United States get adequate iodine from iodized table salt and other foods.

Radiation exposure, especially in childhood, is a known risk factor for thyroid cancer, with the risk rising with increasing radiation dosage and younger age at exposure. Prior to the 1960s, children were often treated with radiation for minor conditions such as acne, ringworm (a fungal infection of the scalp), and enlarged tonsils or adenoids, as well as for cancers. Today, radiation exposure in children, including x-rays and **computed tomography** (CT) scans, is kept to a minimum. Thyroid cancers were many times more common in children and adults exposed to radiation from the 1986 Chernobyl nuclear power plant accident; increased thyroid cancers have been found among children exposed to fallout from Japan's Fukushima nuclear plant meltdowns, as well as among adult cleanup crews. New York City police working at the site of the World Trade Center 2001 terrorist attack have been shown to be at a tenfold-higher risk for one type of thyroid cancer.

Several inherited conditions or a family history of thyroid cancer are linked to specific types of thyroid cancer. About one-third of MTCs are inherited. Other uncommon inherited conditions that increase the risk of thyroid cancers include familial adenomatous polyposis (FAP), a FAP subtype called Gardner syndrome, Cowden disease, Carney complex type I, and familial nonmedullary thyroid **carcinoma**.

Demographics

Diseases of the thyroid gland affect millions of Americans. The most common are hyperthyroidism (Grave's disease), or an overactive thyroid, and hypothyroidism, or an underactive thyroid. Sometimes lumps or masses develop in the thyroid. Although most (95%) thyroid lumps or nodules are noncancerous (benign), all thyroid growths should be taken seriously.

Thyroid cancer is one of the most treatable forms of cancer, with a five-year overall survival rate of 97%. The American Cancer Society (ACS) estimates that in 2014, approximately 62,980 new cases of thyroid cancer will be diagnosed in the United States—47,790 in women and 15,190 in men—and 1,890 people will die from the disease. Unlike most adult cancers, thyroid cancer is more common in younger adults, with almost two-thirds of cases in people under age 55. Only about 2% of cases occur in children and adolescents. Caucasians are affected more often than are African Americans, but African Americans tend to have more advanced cancer at the time of diagnosis.

Thyroid cancer diagnoses are increasing at a faster rate in the United States than any other cancer, although the death rate has remained fairly stable for many years. Thyroid cancer incidence has almost tripled since 1983. Although much of this increase is attributed to better ultrasound detection of small nodules, a 2013 study indicated that better detection alone could not explain the dramatic increase.

Causes and symptoms

Although the exact causes of thyroid cancer are unknown, a number of genes contribute to susceptibility:

- About 10%–30% of papillary carcinomas have alterations (mutations) in specific portions of the RET gene that convert it into the so-called PTC oncogene, especially

KEY TERMS

Anaplastic thyroid carcinoma—Undifferentiated cancer cells that are aggressive and difficult to treat.

C cells—Parafollicular cells; thyroid gland cells that produce the hormone calcitonin.

Calcitonin—A thyroid hormone that regulates calcium levels in the blood.

Carcinoembryonic antigen (CEA)—A fetal protein that is released into the blood by some medullary thyroid carcinomas.

Familial adenomatous polyposis (FAP)—An inherited disease of the large intestine that is a risk factor for thyroid cancer.

Follicular carcinoma—A well-differentiated cancer that develops in the hormone-producing follicular cells of the thyroid gland.

Medullary thyroid carcinoma (MTC)—A poorly differentiated cancer of C cells.

Papillary carcinoma—The most common type of thyroid cancer, which develops in follicular cells and is well-differentiated.

Thyroid-stimulating hormone (TSH)—A hormone secreted by the pituitary gland that regulates the production and secretion of thyroid hormones.

Thyroidectomy—Surgical removal of the thyroid gland.

in children and/or those exposed to radiation. These changes are usually acquired rather than inherited, so they are not passed on to offspring.

- Many papillary carcinomas, especially those that grow and metastasize faster, have a mutated BRAF gene.

- Mutations in other genes, including NTRK1, are associated with papillary carcinoma.

- Acquired changes in the RAS oncogene are involved in some follicular carcinomas.

- Inherited MTCs have mutations in different regions of the RET gene than those that cause papillary carcinomas.

- Anaplastic thyroid cancers often have the above mutations, as well as changes in the P53 tumor suppressor gene and the CTNNB1 oncogene.

- FAP and Gardner syndrome are caused by defects in the APC gene.

- Carney complex type I, which increases the risk of papillary and follicular carcinomas, is caused by defects in the PRKAR1A gene.

A painless lump or nodule in the neck is the most frequent sign of thyroid cancer. The lymph nodes in the neck may be swollen. Hoarseness may develop as a tumor presses on nerves leading to the voice box. Some patients experience a tight or full feeling in the neck and have difficulty breathing or swallowing.

Diagnosis

Examination

Thyroid tumors are sometimes discovered during routine checkups, and the ACS recommends routine examination of the neck and lymph nodes in the neck area. Some physicians recommend self-exams of the neck twice per year.

Tests

Various tests are used to diagnose thyroid cancer, as well as to screen patients with family history of thyroid cancer or MTC:

- Blood tests for thyroid stimulating hormone (TSH) and the thyroid hormones T3 and T4 are used to assess thyroid function, although these are usually normal in thyroid cancer.

- Excess calcitonin and CEA levels in the blood help diagnose or confirm MTC or its recurrence. Blood calcium levels may also be measured.

- The blood level of the protein thyroglobulin is sometimes used to confirm the removal and/or destruction of all thyroid cells after treatment. A rise in the level may indicate recurrence of the cancer.

- Various blood tests are performed before thyroid surgery and in MTC patients.

- Anyone with a family history of MTC should undergo genetic testing at a young age for MTC-associated gene mutations.

Procedures

Ultrasound of the thyroid is sometimes used to screen people at high risk for thyroid cancer. Ultrasound performed for other medical problems sometimes reveals early cancers. Ultrasound bounces high-frequency sound waves off the thyroid. The pattern of echoes produced by these waves is converted into a computerized image on a screen, which helps determine whether the lumps are benign fluid-filled cysts or solid malignant tumors. CT scans, **magnetic resonance imaging** (MRI), or **positron** emission tomography (PET) scans are also be used to diagnose thyroid cancers.

A radioiodine scan is used to identify abnormal areas of the thyroid. The patient swallows or is injected with a very small amount of radioactive iodine, which accumulates in the thyroid. An x-ray or scan identifies areas—called cold spots—that do not absorb the iodine normally. If a significant amount of iodine concentrates in a nodule, it is termed "hot" and is usually benign. Radioiodine scanning is also performed after surgical removal of the thyroid (thyroidectomy) to check for remaining thyroid cells.

A **biopsy** is the most accurate diagnostic tool. A sample of thyroid tissue is obtained—either by withdrawing it through a needle (such as a fine-needle aspiration biopsy) or by surgical removal of the nodule—and examined under a microscope by a pathologist. A needle biopsy takes a few minutes and is performed by a trained physician, usually a radiologist. A surgical biopsy is performed by a surgeon under general anesthesia and takes a few hours.

If thyroid cancer is diagnosed, further tests help determine the stage of the disease and plan appropriate treatment. A vocal cord exam called a **laryngoscopy** is often performed before surgery to determine involvement of the vocal cords. An octreotide scan may be ordered to detect the spread of MTC.

Clinical staging

Cancer staging determines the type of thyroid cancer (different types vary in their aggressiveness), the tumor size, and whether the cancer has spread to surrounding lymph nodes or metastasized to distant regions. Unlike most cancers, thyroid cancer staging also considers the cancer subtype and the patient's age.

Papillary and follicular (differentiated) carcinomas in patients younger than 45 are categorized as stage I—without evidence of cancer beyond the thyroid, although it may be present in nearby lymph nodes—and stage II—cancer spread beyond the thyroid to one or more distant sites. In patients over 45 with papillary and follicular carcinomas and patients of any age with MTC:

- Stage I tumors are 2 cm (0.3 in.) or less across and have not spread to nearby lymph nodes or distant sites.

- Stage II tumors are 2–4 cm (0.3–0.6 in.) across but have not spread to adjacent lymph nodes or distant sites.

- Stage III tumors are larger than 4 cm (0.6 in.) or have grown slightly beyond of the thyroid but not to lymph nodes or distant sites; stage III tumors also include tumors of any size that have spread to nearby lymph nodes.

- Stage IV tumors have spread beyond the thyroid or outside the thyroid area (distant metastases), most often to the lungs and/or bones. All cases of anaplastic (undifferentiated) thyroid cancer are considered as stage IV, because this type of cancer is extremely aggressive and has a poor prognosis.

Treatment

Treatment depends on the type of cancer and its stage. Optimal results are usually achieved with a combination of two or more therapies.

Surgery

Thyroidectomy is the primary treatment for early-stage papillary, follicular, and medullary thyroid cancers. Small tumors that have not spread may be treated with removal of the affected lobe (**lobectomy**). Adjoining lymph nodes may be removed during surgery for staging and to potentially lower the risk of recurrence. More extensive removal of lymph nodes in the neck is required if the cancer has spread. Subsequent treatment depends on the cancer stage, although surgery alone has an excellent cure rate.

Some experts believe that thyroid cancer is overdiagnosed and surgery is overused. A 2010 Japanese study found that only a small minority of 340 patients who underwent surveillance rather than surgery experienced tumor growth in the following six years.

Radioactive iodine therapy/radiation

Radioactive iodine may be used in addition to surgery for papillary and follicular carcinomas. The patient swallows a drink containing radioactive iodine, which is absorbed and destroyed by any remaining thyroid tissue.

External-beam radiation may be used if radioactive iodine treatment is unsuccessful or if the cancer has spread. It is used for MTC, because these cancers do not take up iodine. It may also be used for anaplastic cancers and as a palliative therapy to increase patient comfort.

Thyroid hormone therapy

Once the thyroid gland is removed, the body no longer produces thyroid hormones. Patients must then take synthetic hormones for the rest of their lives to maintain normal body metabolism. When low levels of thyroid hormones remain, they may stimulate the pituitary gland to produce TSH, which can stimulate the growth of any remaining thyroid cells and promote cancer cell growth. Higher-than-normal doses of thyroid hormones help keep TSH levels very low to slow the growth of any remaining cancer cells and help prevent recurrences.

Targeted therapy

Papillary and follicular carcinomas that do not respond to surgery and radioactive iodine, cancers that have spread, or recurrent cancers may be treated with targeted drugs such as **sorafenib**, **sunitinib**, pazopanib, or vandetanib. Vandetanib stops the growth of advanced MTC for an average of six months but has potentially serious side effects. Cabozantinib stops the growth of MTC for about seven months but has not been shown to extend survival.

Chemotherapy

Chemotherapy may be used for advanced thyroid cancers when surgery is not an option, for recurrent cancer, or for patients who have not responded well to other treatments. There is no standard chemotherapeutic regimen for advanced papillary, follicular, and anaplastic thyroid cancers. Anaplastic cancers may respond locally to **doxorubicin**, which is used as a radiation sensitizer in combination with hyperfractionated **radiation therapy**. Paclitaxel may provide some palliative benefit. Participation in **clinical trials** of chemotherapy drugs is sometimes an option.

Prognosis

Papillary carcinomas are usually treated successfully. Follicular carcinomas generally have high cure rates but are sometimes difficult to control if the cancer has invaded blood vessels or spread to nearby structures in the neck. MTC is more difficult to control, because it often spreads to other parts of the body. Anaplastic thyroid cancer is the fastest growing and tends to respond poorly to all treatments. Five-year relative survival rates are:

- 99.9% for localized cancers confined to the primary site—68% of all thyroid cancers
- 97.6% for all cancers spread to regional lymph nodes—26% of cases
- 54.7% for metastasized cancers—4% of cases
- 88.1% for unknown/unstaged cancers—2% of cases

Prevention

Most people with thyroid cancer have no known risk factors for the disease. Children are no longer treated with radiation if avoidable, and the lowest possible doses are used for necessary x-rays and CT scans. Other sources of radiation should be avoided by

---

QUESTIONS TO ASK YOUR DOCTOR

- What type of thyroid cancer do I have?
- Has it spread beyond my thyroid gland?
- Is my thyroid cancer hereditary? Should other members of my family be tested?
- What treatments do you recommend? Do you recommend a clinical trial?
- What are the advantages, disadvantages, and side effects of this treatment?
- How much experience do you have treating thyroid cancer/performing thyroid surgery?

---

children and adults. Patients treated with radiation to the head and neck should be examined by a physician for thyroid lumps and enlarged lymph nodes every one to two years.

Family members of patients with inherited MTC should receive **genetic testing** and, if positive, be screened for early thyroid cancer. Since nearly all children and adults with RET mutations will eventually develop MTC, most doctors recommend prophylactic thyroidectomy at an early age.

Resources

BOOKS

Freedman, Jeri. *Thyroid Cancer: Current and Emerging Trends in Detection and Treatment.* New York: Rosen, 2012.

Friedman, Theodore C., and Winnie Yu Scherer. *The Everything Guide to Thyroid Disease.* Avon, MA: Adams Media, 2012.

Green, John. *The Fault in Our Stars.* New York: Dutton, 2012.

PERIODICALS

Earl, Evangeline. "In 'The Fault in Our Stars,' My Sister Gets a Sequel." *Washington Post* (June 15, 2014): B1.

Li, Mingsi, et al. "Anaplastic Thyroid Cancer in Young Patients: A Contemporary Review." *American Journal of Otolaryngology* 34, no. 6 (2013): 636–40.

Sawka, Anna M., et al. "Managing Newly Diagnosed Thyroid Cancer." *Canadian Medical Association Journal* 186, no. 4 (March 4, 2014): 269–75.

Whitaker, Phil. "Health Matters." *New Statesman* 143, no. 5193 (January 17–23, 2014): 68.

Zhuang, Yixin, et al. "Common Genetic Variants on FOXE1 Contributes to Thyroid Cancer Susceptibility: Evidence Based on 16 Studies." *Tumor Biology* 35, no. 6 (June 2014): 6159–66.

WEBSITES

"Thyroid Cancer." MedlinePlus. June 16, 2014. http://www.nlm.nih.gov/medlineplus/thyroidcancer.html (accessed June 30, 2014).

"Thyroid Cancer Treatment (PDQ)." National Cancer Institute. June 10, 2014. http://www.cancer.gov/cancertopics/pdq/treatment/thyroid/Patient (accessed June 30, 2014).

"What is Thyroid Cancer?" American Cancer Society. March 20, 2014. http://www.cancer.org/cancer/thyroidcancer/detailedguide/thyroid-cancer-what-is-thyroid-cancer (accessed June 30, 2014).

ORGANIZATIONS

American Cancer Society, 250 Williams Street NW, Atlanta, GA 30303, (800) 227-2345, http://www.cancer.org.

American Thyroid Association, 6066 Leesburg Pike, Suite 550, Falls Church, VA 22041, (703) 998-8890, Fax: (703) 998-8893, thyroid@thyroid.org, http://www.thyroid.org.

National Cancer Institute, 6116 Executive Boulevard, Suite 300, Bethesda, MD 20892-8322, (800) 4-CANCER (422-6237), http://www.cancer.gov.

Lata Cherath, PhD
Kulbir Rangi, D.O.
Melinda Oberleitner, R.N., D.N.S.
Margaret Alic, PhD

Thyroid nuclear medicine scan

Definition

A thyroid nuclear medicine scan is a diagnostic procedure to evaluate the thyroid gland, which is located in the front of the neck and controls the metabolism of the body. A radioactive substance that concentrates in the thyroid is taken orally or injected into a vein (intravenously), or both. There are three types of radioactive iodine used in these scans. A special camera is used to take an image of the distribution of the radioactive substance in and around the thyroid gland. This is interpreted to evaluate thyroid function and to diagnose abnormalities. Although other imaging methods exist for evaluating thyroid disease, thyroid scanning is the most commonly used and is the most cost-effective.

Purpose

A thyroid scan can help assess the overall structure and function of the thyroid. It can be used to identify benign cancers, to assess nodules, to evaluate masses, to locate the source of a painful gland, to assess gland size, to find differentiated carcinomas, and to identify thyroid tissue. A thyroid scan may be ordered by a physician when the gland becomes abnormally large, especially if the enlargement is greater on one side, or when hard lumps (nodules) are felt. The scan can be helpful in determining whether the enlargement is caused by a diffuse increase in the total amount of thyroid tissue or by a nodule or nodules. The thyroid scan plays a critical role in the diagnosis of **thyroid cancer**.

When other laboratory studies show an overactive thyroid (hyperthyroidism) or an underactive thyroid (hypothyroidism), a radioactive iodine uptake scan is often used to confirm the diagnosis. A thyroid scan is often performed in conjunction with this scan. Thyroid radionuclide scanning is being considered as a means to screen individuals at risk for thyroid disease following **radiation therapy**.

Precautions

Women who are pregnant should not have this test. Any person with a history of allergy to iodine, such as those with shellfish allergies, should notify the physician before the procedure is performed.

Description

This test is performed in a radiology facility, either in an outpatient x-ray center or a hospital department. Most often, the patient is given the radioactive substance in the form of a tasteless liquid or capsule. It may be injected into a vein (intravenously) in some instances. Generally, the patient lies on an examination table as the scanning is performed. Images will be taken at a specified amount of time after this, depending on the radioisotope used. Most often, scanning is done 24 hours later, if the radioisotope is given orally. If it is given intravenously, the scan is performed approximately 20 minutes later.

For a thyroid scan, the patient is positioned lying down on his or her back, with the head tilted back. The radionuclide scanner, also called a gamma camera, is positioned above the thyroid area as it scans. This takes 30–60 minutes.

The uptake study may be done with the patient sitting upright in a chair or lying down. The procedure is otherwise the same as described for the thyroid scan. It takes approximately 15 minutes. There is no discomfort involved with either study.

A thyroid scan may also be referred to as a thyroid scintiscan. The name of the radioactive substance used may be incorporated and the study called a technetium thyroid scan or an iodine thyroid scan. The radioactive iodine uptake scan may be called by its initials, an RAIU test, or an iodine uptake test.

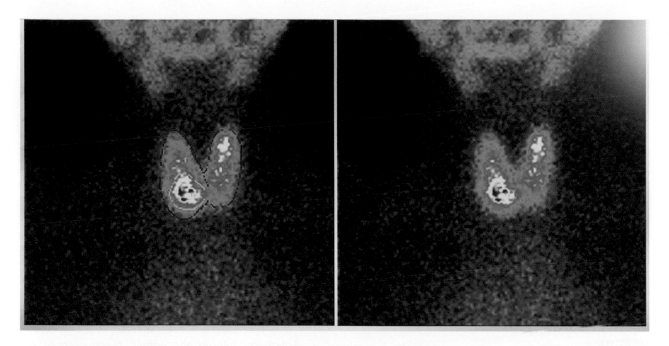

Thyroid nuclear medicine scan (thyroid gland is shown in green). *(Miriam Maslo/Science Source)*

Preparation

Certain medications can interfere with iodine uptake. These include certain cough medicines, some oral contraceptives, non-steroidal anti-inflammatory drugs, epilepsy drugs, and thyroid medications. The patient is usually instructed to stop taking these medications for a period of time before the test. This period may range from several days up to three to four weeks, depending on the amount of time the medicine takes to clear from the body.

Other **nuclear medicine scans** and x-ray studies using contrast material performed within the past 60 days may affect this test. Therefore, patients should tell their doctors if they have had either of these types of studies before the thyroid scan is begun, to avoid inaccurate results.

Thyroid scan test results can be affected by other conditions, such as kidney failure, **cancer**, cancer **chemotherapy**, hepatitis, cirrhosis of the liver, infections, trauma, poor nutrition, and mental illness.

Some institutions prefer that the patient have nothing to eat or drink after midnight on the day before the radioactive liquid or capsule is to be taken. A normal diet can usually be resumed two hours after the radioisotope is taken. Dentures, jewelry, and other metallic objects must be removed before the scanning is performed. No other physical preparation is needed.

The patient should understand that there is no danger of radiation exposure to themselves or others. Only very small amounts of radioisotope are used. The total amount of radiation absorbed is often less than the dose received from ordinary x-rays. The scanner or camera does not emit any radiation, but detects and records it from the patient.

Aftercare

No isolation or special precautions are needed after a thyroid scan. The patient should check with his or her physician about restarting any medications that were stopped before the scan.

Risks

There are no risks with this procedure.

Results

A normal scan will show a thyroid of normal size, shape, and position. The amount of radionuclide uptake by the thyroid will be normal, according to established laboratory figures. There will be no areas where radionuclide uptake is increased or decreased.

Abnormal results

An area of increased radionuclide uptake may be called a hot nodule or "hot spot." This means that a benign growth is overactive. Despite the name, hot nodules are unlikely to be caused by cancer. Increased radionuclide uptake is indicative of hyperthyroidism and may suggest Graves' disease or an active pituitary **adenoma**.

An area of decreased radionuclide uptake may be called a cold nodule, or "cold spot." This indicates that this area of the thyroid gland is underactive. A variety of conditions, including cysts, hypothyroidism, nonfunctioning benign growths, localized inflammation, or cancer, may produce a cold spot. Single nodules that are not functioning are malignant in about 10%–20% of cases. Completely nonfunctioning nodules have a higher probability of being malignant than those that have some degree of function.

A thyroid nuclear medicine scan is rarely sufficient to establish a clear diagnosis. A majority of nonfunctioning nodules are not malignant, but their presence increases the probability of a malignancy. Nodules that are functioning are rarely malignant. Frequently, the information revealed will need to be combined with data from other studies to determine the problem.

Resources

WEBSITES

A.D.A.M. Medical Encyclopedia. "Thyroid Scan." MedlinePlus. http://www.nlm.nih.gov/medlineplus/ency/article/003829.htm (accessed November 14, 2014).

American Cancer Society. "How is Thyroid Cancer Diagnosed." http://www.cancer.org/cancer/thyroidcancer/detailedguide/thyroid-cancer-diagnosis (accessed November 14, 2014).

American Society of Clinical Oncology. "Thyroid Cancer: Diagnosis." Cancer.net http://www.cancer.net/cancer-types/thyroid-cancer/diagnosis (accessed November 14, 2014).

Mark A. Mitchell, M.D.

TNM staging *see* **Tumor staging**

Toposar *see* **Etoposide**

Topotecan

Definition

Topotecan is a drug used to treat certain types of **cancer**. Topotecan is available under the trade name Hycamtin, and may also be referred to as topotecan hydrochloride or topotecan HCl.

Purpose

Topotecan is an antineoplastic agent used to treat **small cell lung cancer**, and certain cancers of the ovary.

As of late 2003, **clinical trials** are underway in Italy and France to test the effectiveness of topotecan in treating tumors of the brain (glioblastomas) and autonomic nervous system (neuroblastomas). In the French study, topotecan is given together with radiotherapy while the Italian trial uses topotecan as part of combination **chemotherapy**. Early results indicate that the drug may be useful in treating cancers of the nervous system as well as ovarian and small-cell lung cancers.

Description

Topotecan is a synthetic derivative of the naturally occurring compound camptothecin. Camptothecin belongs to a group of chemicals called alkaloids, and is extracted from plants such as *Camptotheca acuminata*. Camptothecin was initially investigated as a chemotherapeutic agent due to its anti-cancer activity in laboratory studies. The chemical structure and biological action of topotecan is similar to that of camptothecin and **irinotecan**.

Topotecan inhibits the normal functioning of the enzyme topoisomerase I. The normal role of topoisomerase I is to aid in the replication, recombination, and repair of deoxyribonucleic acid (DNA). Higher levels of topoisomerase I have been found in certain cancer tumors compared to healthy tissue. Inhibiting topoisomerase I causes DNA damage. This damage leads to apoptosis, or programmed cell death.

Topotecan is used in patients whose cancer of the ovary has recurred or progressed after platinum-based treatment such as **cisplatin**. Topotecan is also used to treat relapse of small cell lung cancer that initially responded to other drugs. Increases in survival times have been observed in patients treated with topotecan compared to control populations treated with paclitaxel.

Tumors that are targeted by topotecan sometimes develop resistance to the drug. Although the reasons for this resistance are not fully understood as of late 2003, researchers think that they may be related either to inadequate amounts of drug in the tumor or to alterations in topoisomerase I that make the enzyme resistant to topotecan.

Recommended dosage

Patients should be carefully monitored before and during topotecan treatment for bone marrow function.

Topotecan is administered intravenously over 30 minutes once per day for five consecutive days followed by 16 days of rest. This schedule may be repeated every 21 days. The initial dose of topotecan may be adjusted downward depending on patient tolerance to the toxic side effects of topotecan.

The dose of topotecan may be reduced in patients with kidney dysfunction.

No dose modification is necessary for patients with liver impairment.

No dose modification is necessary for elderly patients.

Precautions

Topotecan should be used only under the supervision of a physician experienced in the use of cancer chemotherapeutic agents. Certain complications will only be possible to manage if the necessary diagnostic and treatment resources are readily available. Topotecan should not be used in patients with bone marrow depression before starting treatment. Skin that comes in contact with topotecan must be washed thoroughly with soap and warm water.

The dose of topotecan may be reduced in patients with moderate kidney dysfunction. Topotecan is not recommended for use in patients with severe kidney dysfunction.

Topotecan should not be administered to pregnant women. Women of child bearing age are advised not to become pregnant during treatment. Women should discontinue nursing prior to taking topotecan.

Side effects

Suppression of bone marrow function is the most serious side effect commonly observed in this treatment and can lead to death. Bone marrow reserves should be monitored by blood cell counts for all patients before and during topotecan treatment. The suppression of bone marrow is not cumulative over time. Additional side effects including **nausea and vomiting**, **anorexia**, **diarrhea**, constipation, headache, and hair loss (**alopecia**) may occur.

Interactions

Suppression of bone marrow is more severe when topotecan is given with platinum drugs. G-CSF (**filgrastim**) may extend the duration of bone marrow suppression. If G-CSF is used, it should not be administered until day six of the 21-day course.

See also Lung cancer, small cell.

Resources

WEBSITES

American Cancer Society. "Topotecan." http://www.cancer.org/treatment/treatmentsandsideeffects/guidetocancerdrugs/topotecan (accessed November 14, 2014).

Cancer Research UK. "Topotecan (Hycamtin, Potactasol)." http://www.cancerresearchuk.org/about-cancer/cancers-in-general/treatment/cancer-drugs/topotecan (accessed November 14, 2014).

The Scott Hamilton CARES Initiative. "Topotecan." Chemocare.com http://chemocare.com/chemotherapy/drug-info/Topotecan.aspx (accessed Novmeber 14, 2014).

ORGANIZATIONS

U.S. Food and Drug Administration, 10903 New Hampshire Ave., Silver Spring, MD 20993, (888) INFO-FDA (463-6332), http://www.fda.gov.

Marc Scanio
Rebecca J. Frey, PhD

Toremifene

Definition

Toremifene, also known as Fareston, is a synthetic compound similar to estrogen. It mimics the action of estrogen on the bones and uterus, but blocks the effects of estrogen on breast tissue.

Purpose

Toremifene is used as adjuvant hormone therapy immediately after surgery in early stages of **breast cancer** and also to treat advanced metastatic breast **cancer** (stages III and above) in postmenopausal women. Postmenopausal women at high risk of developing breast cancer may take toremifene to reduce risk.

Description

Toremifene is similar to **tamoxifen** in structure and action. Toremifene can be given as sole treatment, but it is often given in combination with other chemotherapeutic drugs.

Toremifene belongs to a family of compounds called **antiestrogens**. Antiestrogens are used in cancer therapy by inhibiting the effects of estrogen on target tissues. Estrogen is a steroid hormone secreted by granulosa cells of a maturing follicle within the female ovary. Depending on the target tissue, estrogen can stimulate the growth of female reproductive organs and breast tissue, play a role in the female menstrual cycle, and protect against bone loss by binding to estrogen receptors on the outside of cells within the target tissue. Antiestrogens act selectively against the effects of estrogen on target cells in a variety of ways, thus they are called selective estrogen receptor modulators (SERMs).

Toremifene selectively inhibits the effects of estrogen on breast tissue, while mimicking the effects of estrogen on bone (by increasing bone mineral density) and uterine tissues. The former makes toremifene an excellent therapeutic agent against breast cancer. Although researchers are unclear of the precise mechanism by which toremifene kills breast cancer cells, it is known to compete with estrogen by binding to estrogen receptors, therefore limiting the effects of estrogen on breast tissue. Toremifene also may be involved in other anti-tumor activities affecting oncogene expression, promotion of apoptosis and growth factor secretion.

Recommended dosage

Toremifene is taken orally, and the recommended dose is usually 40 to 60 milligrams once a day, although larger doses are sometimes prescribed. If a dose is missed, patients should not double the next dosage. Instead, they should return to their regular schedule and contact their doctor.

Precautions

Toremifene is not recommended for use in children. Women who are pregnant or nursing should not use this drug since it has several side effects that, although rare, can be severe. It is known to cause miscarriages and birth defects. Women are encouraged to use birth control while taking toremifene. However, oral contraceptives can negatively alter the effects of toremifene, so patients should explore other birth control options.

Great care should be exercised when toremifene is used with **warfarin**, an anticoagulant, because toremifene can amplify the effects of warfarin, prolonging bleeding times. The result could possibly be fatal. Patients who are predisposed to the formation of thromboembolisms should use toremifene with caution, because toremifene can increase the risk.

Side effects

Although toremifene is usually well tolerated by patients, there are some side effects. One of the most serious side effects is development of uterine cancer. Less common effects include eye problems such as retinal lesions, macular edema, and corneal changes (most resolve themselves after use is discontinued); neurological problems such as **depression**, dizziness, confusion, and **fatigue**; and genital problems such as vaginal bleeding, vaginal discharge, and endometriosis. Patients also may experience liver problems.

Interactions

Toremifene can interfere with the anticoagulant drug warfarin, resulting in severe consequences and death. If these two drugs are used together, patients will be monitored closely. Oral contraceptives and estrogen supplements can also interfere with the action of toremifene.

See also Raloxifene.

Resources

WEBSITES

AHFS Consumer Medication Information. "Toremifene." American Society of Health-System Pharmacists. Available from: http://www.nlm.nih.gov/medlineplus/druginfo/meds/a608003.html (accessed November 14, 2014).

National Cancer Institute. "Toremifene." http://www.cancer.gov/cancertopics/druginfo/toremifene (accessed November 14, 2014).

The Scott Hamilton CARES Initiative. "Toremifene." Chemocare.com http://chemocare.com/chemotherapy/drug-info/Toremifene.aspx (accessed Novmeber 14, 2014).

Sally C. McFarlane-Parrott
Teresa G. Odle

Torisel *see* **Temsirolimus**

Tositumomab

Definition

Tositumomab is a mouse monoclonal antibody that directly targets and binds with the CD20 receptor of normal and malignant B-cell lymphocytes. When linked with iodine I-131, Tositumomab creates a radioimmunotherapy agent, Iodine I-131 Tositumomab; also known as the BEXXAR therapeutic regimen. In 2014, BEXXAR was voluntarily withdrawn from the market due to low sales.

Purpose

BEXXAR was used in the treatment of patients with CD20 positive, follicular, **non-Hodgkin lymphoma** (NHL), with or without transformation, whose disease was untreatable with **rituximab** (Rituxan) and relapsed following **chemotherapy**.

Description

Tositumomab, a monoclonal antibody, can recognize and target the protein produced by the CD20 receptor commonly found on the surface of normal and malignant B-cell lymphocytes. Once injected into the body, the monoclonal antibody seeks out and binds with the CD20 receptor. Once attached to the CD20 receptor, the antibody produces a cytotoxic effect and triggers the body's immune system against the **cancer** cell. This, in turn, exposes the cancer cell, making it more susceptible to radiation. When combined with a radioactive substance, the monoclonal antibody allows the ionizing radiation to directly target the cancerous lymphocytes.

Recommended dosage

Intended for a single course of treatment, BEXXAR was administered in two discrete stages over a period of one to two weeks. These stages, the dosimetric stage and the therapeutic stage, were conducted over a period of four hospital visits.

Before treatment began and for two weeks subsequent to the therapeutic stage, the patient was provided with daily iodine supplements, typically in the form of liquid drops or tablets. The supplements protected the patient's thyroid gland from the radioactive I-131 during the treatment.

Precautions

The BEXXAR regimen was contraindicated for patients with known hypersensitivity to murine (mouse) proteins and/or intolerance to thyroid-blocking agents. Patients were screened for human hypersensitivity antibodies (HAMA) to avoid risk of serious reactions, including anaphylaxis.

Due to the radioactive components of this treatment, the BEXXAR regimen was contraindicated for pregnant women. An effective contraceptive had to be used during and for at least a year following therapy to prevent possible birth defects. Iodine I-131 tositumomab possesses the risk of toxic effects on male and female fertility.

Side effects

Clinical studies of the BEXXAR regimen found prolonged and severe cytopenias (low blood cell counts) to be the most common adverse reactions, occurring in 71% of the patients studied. **Thrombocytopenia** and **neutropenia** were the primary forms of cytopenia, documented in 63% and 53% of patients undergoing therapy, respectively. **Anemia** also appeared in 27% of the studied patients.

Allergic reactions (angioedema and bronchospasm), **pneumonia**, secondary leukemia, solid tumors, and myelodysplasia were also observed. The most frequent nonhematological adverse effects observed in patients included asthenia (weakness), **fever**, nausea, gastrointestinal symptoms, chills, and pruritus (intense **itching**). Other known side effects included back pain, constipation, **diarrhea**, dizziness, and headache. The regimen was also associated with further risks of infusion-related reactions, delayed-onset hypothyroidism, and HAMA.

Interactions

Drugs such as aspirin, ibuprofen, ketoprofen, and naproxen could increase the risk of hemorrhaging in patients receiving BEXXAR. Additionally, anticoagulants and agents interfering with platelet function increased the risk of bleeding.

Resources

WEBSITES

National Cancer Institute. "FDA Approval for Tositumomab and Iodine I 131 Tositumomabb." http://www.cancer.gov/cancertopics/druginfo/fda-tositumomab-I131iodine-tositumomab (accessed October 9, 2014).

National Cancer Institute. "Tositumomab and Iodine I 131 Tositumomab." http://www.cancer.gov/cancertopics/druginfo/tositumomab-I131tositumomab (accessed October 9, 2014).

U.S. Food and Drug Administration. "GlaxoSmithKline LLC; Withdrawal of Approval of the Indication for Treatment of Patients With Relapsed or Refractory, Low Grade, Follicular, or Transformed CD20 Positive Non-Hodgkin's Lymphoma Who Have Not Received Prior Rituximab; BEXXAR." U.S. Federal Register. https://www.federalregister.gov/articles/2013/10/23/2013-24840/glaxosmithkline-llc-withdrawal-of-approval-of-the-indication-for-treatment-of-patients-with-relapsed (accessed October 9, 2014).

Jason Fryer

Tracheostomy

A tracheostomy is an artificial airway, which is surgically inserted through the windpipe to allow normal respiration.

The key purpose of a tracheostomy is to provide a patient with an open, functional airway. Normal respiration can become hindered or blocked by an obstruction to the upper respiratory tract; the area between the nose and mouth down through the larynx. When a serious obstruction occurs, normal respiratory techniques, such as oral or nasal intubation, may be inadequate or

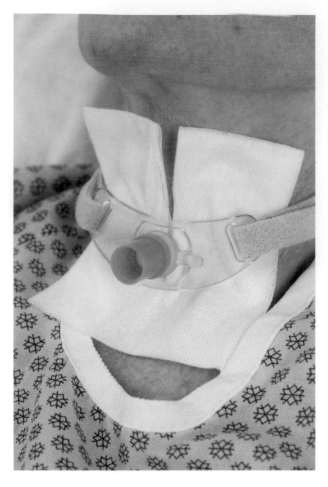

Tracheostomy tube. *(3660 Group/Custom Medical Stock Photo)*

completely ineffective. Obstructions can come from several sources, including foreign bodies, swollen soft tissue, and injury to the larynx and/or trachea. Furthermore, proper respiration can also be obstructed by the growth of malignant tumors in the mouth, larynx, trachea, nasopharynx (the space above and behind the soft palate), and the nasal cavity and paranasal sinuses.

Proper oxygenation of the lungs may also require the use of a tracheostomy. Malignant pulmonary cancers, such as bronchioloalveolar **carcinoma** and **mesothelioma**, can cause serious respiratory problems, including hypoxia (an insufficient oxygen level in the blood and tissues) or hypercapnia (excess levels of carbon dioxide in the blood due to hypoventilation). A tracheostomy can provide the required oxygen levels via the tracheobronchial tree, also known as the bronchia.

A tracheostomy may also be used to clean and remove secretions that build up in the bronchia and throat due to injury, disease, and tumors. This excess fluid can cause obstructions and/or restrict proper oxygenation.

Blood and secretions can be suctioned out through the trachea to relieve breathing problems.

There are no known contraindications for the use of a tracheostomy; however, some surgical modalities, such as removal of malignancies, may be required prior to the tracheotomy procedure.

At the simplest level, a *tracheostomy* is an artificial airway that is inserted into the trachea (windpipe) to bypass the upper airway. The surgical procedure to create this secondary airway is known as a *tracheotomy*. Tracheostomies provide physicians with one of the most effective methods to relieving breathing problems due to obstruction. Indeed, historical evidence reveals that tracheostomies may have been used as far back as 2000 BC Since Antonio Brasavola performed the first documented tracheotomy in the sixteenth century, surgeons and doctors have been developing and refining this effective medical procedure.

The most common form of tracheostomy is a hollow tube of plastic, silicon, or metal, also known as a tracheostomy tube or trach. During a tracheotomy, this tube is surgically inserted into the patient's neck just beneath the larynx to provide access to the trachea, thus acting as a secondary airway. The surgical opening through which the tracheostomy is inserted is also known as the stoma. Depending on the underlying cause of obstruction and/or respiratory distress, a tracheostomy may be temporary or permanent in nature. Tracheostomies are far more effective for suctioning purposes and maintaining respiratory function than other artificial airways. There are three key types of tracheotomies: *Elective*, *Awake*, and *Emergent*.

- Elective—The majority of tracheotomy procedures are elective in nature. Most patients will have already been intubated by this point in time and may require more prolonged and/or more effective form of intubation. These procedures are conducted under controlled conditions, usually performed in a hospital's operating room under the supervision of a surgeon and anesthesiologist.

- Awake—Acute respiratory distress may require an "awake" tracheotomy. These procedures are typically conducted under controlled conditions and using local anesthesia. However, the patient remains conscious throughout the procedure, which can be extremely disconcerting for the patient. The operating surgeon must be prepared for difficulties caused the heightened levels of anxiety the patient will undoubtedly exhibit.

- Emergent—Emergent tracheotomies, sometimes crudely referred to as "slash" tracheostomies, generally should not be considered unless the patient is in extremis and intubation is inadvisable. Even in these extreme cases, a cricothyrotomy is more advisable to relieve respiratory distress than a tracheotomy.

There are several variations of the tracheotomy, but follow a basic guideline. Once the patient is anesthetized, either generally or locally, the neck is cleaned and positioned. Surgical incisions expose the tough cartilage rings that form the trachea's outer wall. An incision is made through two of these rings and a tracheostomy tube is inserted into the windpipe.

Tracheostomy tubes come in a variety of shapes, sizes, and compositions. Tubes are generally designed to meet specific medical requirements, and can be either disposable or reusable in nature. The Universal is the most commonly used tracheostomy tube. Also known as the "double-luman" or "double-cannula" tube, the Universal consists of three parts: the outer cannula (with cuff and pilot tube), the inner cannula, and the obturator. Other commonly used tracheostomy tubes include:

- Single cannula (used for patients with long and/or thin necks)
- Fenestrated (allow speech and improve swallow function)
- Tracheostomy Button (used to wean patients before final removal of tracheostomy tubes or in the treatment of sleep apnea)
- Cuffed tube (used commonly when mechanical ventilation is required and prevents aspiration of secretions)
- Cuffless tube (used in long-term management)

If possible, the patient should fully discuss the procedure and other viable opinions with their physician at length before undergoing a tracheostomy. Additionally, cancers of the upper airway and throat may require the use of other surgical procedures beforehand. In these cases, an effective treatment plan incorporating the tracheostomy should be established. Stabilization of precipitating factors may also be required beforehand.

Successful tracheostomies require effective and thorough postoperative care. Patients may require one to three days to breathe normally following the insertion of a tracheostomy tube. The tube may prevent verbal communication for a prolonged period, and other methods of communication should be utilized. All patients with tracheostomy tubes require humidification to prevent further complications associated with inspired gases. Aftercare modalities should strive to accomplish four key goals:

- Maintain the patient's airway
- Maintain tracheal integrity
- Avoid infections
- Avoid tube displacement

Patients and family members should be educated in aftercare modalities and information as soon as possible. Home nursing service may be required for patients; otherwise, a return to regular home life is encouraged. While outdoors, however, a scarf or similar covering around the throat is indicated.

Directly following the procedure, the trachea will produce excessive secretions due to trauma. In addition to monitoring of these secretions, continual saline irrigation and suctioning will be required. Mucolytic (anti-mucus) agents can be utilized to prevent dangerous obstructions. Assessment of the patient's vital signs should also be maintained, in addition to monitoring for other complications associated with surgery.

Further complications can be encountered at all stages of recovery following a tracheotomy: *immediate*, *early*, and *late*.

Immediate complications can occur directly following the tracheotomy and include:

- Apnea
- Bleeding
- Pneumothorax (accumulation of air or gas in the pleural cavity)
- Pneumomediastinum (escape of air into the pleural tissues)
- Injury to adjacent structures
- Postobstructive pulmonary edema (accumulation of fluid in the lungs)

Early complications typically occur within seven days of the tracheotomy and include:

- Bleeding
- Mucus obstructions
- Inflammation of the trachea
- Inflammation of subcutaneous or connective tissue around the incision
- Tube displacement
- Subcutaneous emphysema (air or gas in subcutaneous tissues)
- Total or partial collapse of the lung

Late complications can occur at any time seven days following the tracheotomy and can include:

- Bleeding
- Tracheomalacia (degeneration of the elastic and connective tissue of the trachea)
- Tracheoesophageal fistula (an abnormal connection between the trachea and the esophagus)
- Tracheocutaneous fistula (an abnormal connection between the trachea and the surface of the neck)

- Granulation and scarring
- Failure to remove the tracheostomy tube

The normal tracheostomy can be used for days, weeks, and even or years with proper treatment; however, tracheostomy tubes should be downsized and removed as quickly as medically viable. Once the tracheostomy is removed, the stoma is sealed and allowed to heal over a period of five to seven days. Typically, a full recovery can be expected within two weeks with little to no scarring.

Several abnormal results of varying seriousness are associated with tracheostomies. Patients should contact local emergency services if their tracheostomy tube is dislodged and cannot be replaced. Additional concerns include:

- Infection
- Fever
- Chills
- Incision site problems, such as swelling, increased pain, and excessive bleeding
- Nausea and/or vomiting
- Shortness of breath and/or cough despite suctioning
- Persistent speech difficulties after tracheostomy removal

Resources

PERIODICALS

Hsu, C.L., K.Y. Chen, C.H. Chang, J.S. Jerng, C.J. Yu, and P.C. Yang. "Timing of Tracheostomy as a Determinant of Weaning Success in Critically Ill Patients: A Retrospective Study." 9, no. 1 (2005): R46–R52.

WEBSITES

Morgan, C., and S. Dixon. "Tracheostomy." http://www.emedicine.com/ent/topic356.htm. (accessed October 16, 2014).
"Tracheostomy Home." http://www.tracheostomy.com/. (accessed October 17, 2014).

Jason Fryer

▌Trametinib

Definition

Trametinib (Mekinist) is a drug for treating advanced melanomas (a type of **skin cancer**) that have specific changes (mutations) in a gene called BRAF. Trametinib is a type of targeted-therapy drug called a kinase inhibitor.

Purpose

Trametinib was approved by the U.S. Food and Drug Administration (FDA) in 2013 to treat melanomas that cannot be surgically removed (are unresectable) or that have spread to other parts of the body (metastasized)—stage IIIC or IV melanomas—and that also have specific mutations in the BRAF gene. These gene mutations change the amino acid at position 600 in the B-raf protein from a valine (V) to either a glutamate (E), known as V600E, or a lysine (K), known as V600K. The mutations are detected by an FDA-approved test. About 40%–60% of advanced melanomas have BRAF V600 mutations. **Clinical trials** showed that trametinib shrunk tumors more and extended life longer than standard **chemotherapy** drugs. Median progression-free survival (PFS) was 4.8 months for the trametinib-treated group, compared with 1.5 months for the patients receiving chemotherapy. Trametinib cannot be used alone to treat patients who have previously been treated with a B-raf inhibitor, since the clinical trial showed no antitumor activity with the drug in such patients.

Trametinib may be used alone or in combination with **dabrafenib**. In January 2014, the FDA gave accelerated approval to the combination therapy. A clinical study of patients with stage IIIC or IV melanomas with BRAF V600E or V600K mutations suggested an improved response rate with the combination treatment: 76% of patients receiving the combined drugs responded for a median duration of 10.5 months, compared with a 54% response rate for 5.6 months in patients administered dabrafenib alone. The combination did not improve disease-related symptoms or overall survival; however, the combination treatment significantly reduced the risk of squamous cell **carcinoma** and keratocanthoma. These are small—usually treatable—skin lesions that commonly develop in patients receiving BRAF inhibitors such as trametinib and dabrafenib. Only 7% of patients receiving the combination developed squamous cell carcinomas or keratoacanthomas, compared with 19% of patients receiving dabrafenib alone. Furthermore, the combination treatment dramatically reduced the development of acneiform dermatitis, a serious skin rash that is a common side effect of trametinib and other MEK inhibitors. A larger clinical trial of the drug combination was ongoing as of 2014. Trametinib and dabrafenib are also being studied for treatment of other types of cancers.

Description

The B-raf protein is a serine/threonine kinase that transmits signals through a chain of other kinases to the cell's control center. The abnormal B-raf kinase

KEY TERMS

BRAF—A gene encoding a serine/threonine kinase protein called B-raf that activates a cell-signaling pathway and is often mutated in melanomas, causing continuous activation of the pathway.

Dabrafenib (Tafinlar)—A drug that targets a different tyrosine kinase in the same pathway as the kinases targeted by trametinib and that may be prescribed in combination with trametinib.

Kinase inhibitor—A drug such as trametinib that inhibits an enzyme called a kinase that adds phosphate to a protein in a signaling pathway.

MEK—Mitogen-activated protein kinase; mitogen/extracellular signal-regulated kinase; an enzyme that adds a phosphate to the enzyme mitogen-activated protein kinase in a cell-signaling pathway controlled by B-raf; the target of trametinib.

Melanoma—A malignant skin tumor that originates in melanocytes (pigmented cells) of normal skin or moles.

Metastasized—Cancer that has spread from its site of origin to other parts of the body.

Progression-free survival (PFS)—The length of time patients survive without their cancer progressing; used in clinical trials to measure the effectiveness of a drug.

Targeted therapy—A drug that interferes with specific molecules involved in cancer cell growth and/or survival.

Tyrosine kinase—An enzyme that adds phosphate to the amino acid tyrosine on a protein as part of a signaling pathway.

Trametinib was the first cancer drug to selectively target MEK kinases. MEK1 and MEK2 can be overactive in various types of cancers, and clinical testing of trametinib is farther along than the testing of any other MEK inhibitors.

Brand names

Trametinib is manufactured by GlaxoSmithKline, LLC, as trametinib dimethyl sulfoxide tablets, with the international trade name Mekinist. The FDA has approved the THxID BRAF assay, manufactured by bioMerieux, Inc., for detection of the BRAF mutations. In 2014, Mekinist was recommended for marketing by the Committee for Medicinal Products for Human Use of the European Union's European Medicines Agency.

Recommended dosage

The recommended dosage of trametinib is 2 milligrams (mg) taken orally once daily, at least one hour before or two hours after a meal, at the same time each day. The trametinib dosage is the same, whether alone or in the combination treatment. In the combination treatment, 150 mg of dabrafenib is taken orally twice per day. The trametinib dose is taken at the same time as either dabrafenib dose. Trametinib is supplied as 0.5 mg, 1 mg, or 2 mg tablets. The different strength tablets are of different colors and have different markings. The trametinib dose, when administered either alone or in combination, may first be reduced to 1.5 mg daily and then to 1 mg daily. It must be permanently discontinued if 1 mg is not tolerated. A missed dose should be taken as soon as possible, but should be skipped if it is less than 12 hours until the next scheduled dose; the regular dosing schedule is then resumed. Double doses should not be taken to make up for a missed dose. Some severe adverse reactions may require withholding one or the other drug for a period of time, or a lower dose; otherwise, the treatment is continued until the cancer progresses or toxicity becomes unacceptable.

Precautions

Most patients taking trametinib develop skin problems, such as rash, redness, infections, or **hand-foot syndrome**. The latter causes pain, numbness, tingling, redness, or swelling in the hands or feet and, in severe cases, peeling, blistering, or open sores. For a few patients, these symptoms are severe enough to require hospitalization.

Trametinib can also:

• impair fertility

produced by the BRAF V600E and V600K mutant genes in **melanoma** cells is continually (constitutively) active so that it continually sends signals for the cell to grow and divide out of control (proliferate). Trametinib inhibits the activity of tyrosine kinases downstream from B-raf in the signaling pathway, so that the signal does not reach the control center. This helps stop the **cancer** cells from proliferating. Trametinib specifically binds to and blocks kinases called MEK1 and MEK2, helping to shut down this pathway. Dabrafenib targets a different downstream tyrosine kinase in the signaling pathway from B-raf, which may enhance the anticancer activity.

- cause heart damage in some people, possibly leading to congestive heart failure, so heart function is checked before and during treatment
- cause severe lung disease in a small number of patients, which may require hospitalization
- cause or worsen high blood pressure, so blood pressure is checked regularly during treatment
- cause eye problems ranging from minor vision changes to blindness
- cause possibly severe diarrhea

Pediatric

The safety and effectiveness of trametinib alone or in combination with dabrafenib in pediatric patients has not been determined.

Geriatric

Clinical trials of trametinib did not include enough subjects aged 65 or older to determine whether older patients respond differently than younger patients.

Pregnant or breastfeeding

Trametinib can harm a fetus at the time of conception or during pregnancy. Women should not become pregnant while taking trametinib or for at least four months afterwards. Women should not breastfeed while taking trametinib.

Other conditions and allergies

Patients should tell their doctors if they are allergic to anything, including drugs, dyes, additives, or foods. They should also inform their doctor if they have:

- heart problems
- high blood pressure
- lung or breathing problems
- any type of liver or kidney disease (which might interfere with clearing the drug from the body)
- eye or vision problems
- other conditions, including bleeding problems, gout, or infections

Side effects

Side effects of trametinib affecting at least 20% of patients are rash, **diarrhea**, and lymphedema (swelling of the face, arms, or legs). Other common side effects are abnormal blood tests for liver function, low blood albumin levels, and **anemia** (low red blood cell counts). The most common side effects of the trametinib/dabrafenib combination are:

- fever
- chills
- night sweats
- fatigue
- rash
- decreased appetite
- nausea
- vomiting
- diarrhea
- constipation
- abdominal pain
- peripheral edema (swelling in the extremities)
- cough
- headache
- joint pain
- muscle pain

Less common side effects of trametinib are:

- mouth sores
- dry skin
- itching
- skin infection around the nails
- serious skin problems, such as infections
- high blood pressure
- abdominal pain
- bleeding
- heart damage

Serious side effects in at least 5% of patients taking the drug combination are severe **fever**, back pain, acute renal failure, and hemorrhage. Other serious adverse reactions to the drug combination are venous thrombo-embolism (a blood clot that breaks free and clogs a blood vessel), a new primary cancer, heart damage, severe skin toxicity, and eye disorders.

Rare side effects of trametinib are:

- dry mouth
- taste changes
- dizziness
- lung damage
- eye problems
- slow heart rate
- muscle breakdown, which can lead to kidney damage

Interactions

As of 2014, trametinib was not known to interact with other drugs, supplements, or foods, but it is possible that other drugs or supplements may affect the levels of

QUESTIONS TO ASK YOUR DOCTOR

- Is trametinib being prescribed alone or in combination with another drug?
- Can you explain the instructions and warnings supplied with my prescription?
- How should I take this medication?
- What side effects can I expect?
- What side effects should I notify my doctor about?

trametinib or that trametinib may affect the levels of other drugs. Patients should tell their doctors about all of their prescription and over-the-counter medicines and supplements, including **vitamins** and herbs.

Resources

PERIODICALS

Kwong, L. N., and M. A. Davies. "Targeted Therapy for Melanoma: Rational Combinatorial Approaches." *Oncogene* 33, no. 1 (January 2, 2014): 1–9.

Shah, Darshil J., and Roxana S. Dronca. "Latest Advances in Chemotherapeutic, Targeted, and Immune Approaches in the Treatment of Metastatic Melanoma." *Mayo Clinic Proceedings* 89, no. 4 (April 2014): 504–19.

OTHER

GlaxoSmithKline. "Full Prescribing Information." U.S. Food and Drug Administration. http://www.accessdata.fda.gov/drugsatfda_docs/label/2014/204114s001lbl.pdf (accessed October 19, 2014).

WEBSITES

"MEK: A Single Drug Target Shows Promise in Multiple Cancers." Cancer Research Updates. National Cancer Institute. June 24, 2013. http://www.cancer.gov/cancertopics/research-updates/2013/MEK (accessed October 19, 2014).

Pazdur, Richard. "FDA Approval for Trametinib." National Cancer Institute. http://www.cancer.gov/cancertopics/druginfo/fda-trametinib (accessed October 19, 2014).

"Trametinib." American Cancer Society. June 12, 2013. http://www.cancer.org/treatment/treatmentsandsideeffects/guidetocancerdrugs/trametinib (accessed October 19, 2014).

"Trametinib." MedlinePlus. October 15, 2013. http://www.nlm.nih.gov/medlineplus/druginfo/meds/a613040.html (accessed October 19, 2014).

ORGANIZATIONS

American Cancer Society, 250 Williams Street NW, Atlanta, GA 30303, (800) 227-2345, http://www.cancer.org.

National Cancer Institute, 6116 Executive Boulevard, Suite 300, Bethesda, MD 20892-8322, (800) 4-CANCER (422-6237), http://www.cancer.gov.

U.S. Food and Drug Administration, 10903 New Hampshire Avenue, Silver Spring, MD 20993-0002, (888) INFO-FDA (463-6332), http://www.fda.gov.

Margaret Alic, PhD

Transderm-Scop *see* **Scopolamine**

Transderm-V *see* **Scopolamine**

Transfusion therapy

Definition

Transfusion therapy is the administration of donated whole blood or blood components.

Purpose

Transfusion therapy is used to restore lost blood or depleted blood components, improve clotting time, and improve the ability of blood to deliver oxygen to the body's tissues. Transfusions may be needed during surgery or to treat injuries or various medical conditions, including **cancer**.

- Some cancers, especially cancers of the digestive system, can cause internal bleeding that leads to anemia or low red blood cell (RBC) counts that may require transfusions.
- Anemia of chronic disease, which can occur in long-term cancer patients, affects the production and lifespan of RBCs and may require transfusions.
- Since blood cells are produced in the bone marrow (the spongy centers of large bones), cancers such as leukemias that originate in the bone marrow, or cancers that spread (metastasize) to bone can crowd out blood-producing cells, leading to low blood counts that require transfusions of clotting factors, platelets, or other blood components.
- Cancers that affect the kidneys or spleen that regulate blood cell levels can require transfusions.
- Most chemotherapy drugs affect the bone marrow, leading to low blood cell counts and increased risk of infection or bleeding.
- Radiation therapy to a large area of bone can damage the bone marrow.
- Cancer surgeries can lead to blood loss and the need for RBC or platelet transfusions.

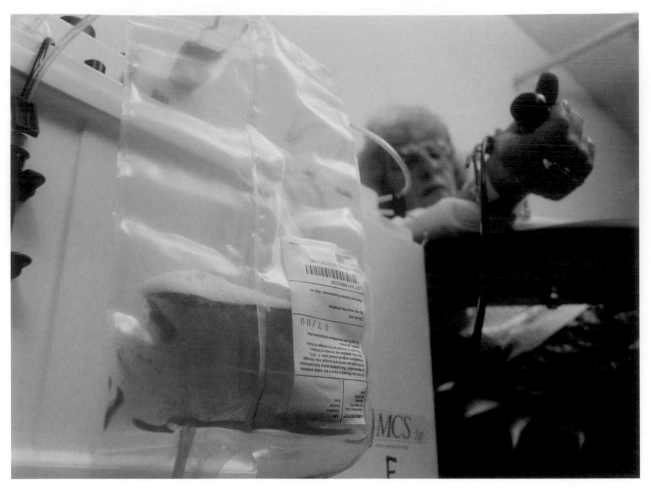

Woman donating blood platelets (yellow) for transfusion. *(James King-Holmes/Science Source)*

• Patients receiving bone marrow or peripheral blood stem-cell transplants are given large doses of chemotherapy and/or radiation that destroys the bone marrow and often require post-procedure transfusions.

Description

Changes in surgery and cancer therapies have significantly reduced the use of transfusions, and most transfusions are of blood components such as plasma, RBCs, platelets, clotting factors, or immunoglobulins, rather than whole blood. A single donation of whole blood is a pint or unit (16 oz. or 473 mL). The blood is usually fractionated into components that can be used to treat multiple patients with only the blood component needed by each. One unit of a blood component is the amount obtained from one unit of whole blood.

Whole blood

Whole-blood transfusions may be administered during or after surgery to replace lost blood. Whole-blood transfusions are rare, because they can overload the circulatory system with fluid, causing high blood pressure and congestive heart failure. Some studies have suggested that certain cancers, including colorectal, prostate, lung, and breast cancers, have worse outcomes if transfusions are administered before or during surgery. Although the reason for this is unknown, it has been suggested that the transfused blood may affect the patient's immune system.

Plasma

Plasma is the clear, pale-yellow liquid portion of blood that contains clotting factors and immunoglobulins (antibodies). After removing the RBCs, plasma or plasma fractions containing clotting factors are usually frozen and can be kept for up to one year. Plasma can also be donated by apheresis or plasmapheresis, in which the donor is hooked to a machine that removes the blood, separates the plasma, and returns the RBCs and other components to the donor's bloodstream.

KEY TERMS

Anemia—A deficiency in red blood cells, in the hemoglobin component of red blood cells, or in total blood volume.

Antibodies—Immune-system proteins that recognize specific antigens, such as disease-causing organisms or proteins on blood cells.

Antigen—A protein or other molecule that evokes a specific immune response.

Apheresis—A process that involves the withdrawal of blood, removal of one or more blood components such as plasma (plasmapheresis) or platelets (plateletpheresis), and return of the blood to the donor's body.

Autologous—Transfusion with the recipient's own previously collected blood or blood components.

Graft-versus-host disease (GVHD)—A life-threatening illness caused by donor T cells (white blood cells) attacking the recipient's cells and tissues.

Hematocrit—The separation of red blood cells from plasma to determine their percent volume in whole blood, normally 35%–47% in females and 42%–52% in males.

Hematopoietic progenitor cells (HPCs)—Hematopoietic stem cells (HSCs); cells in the bone marrow and blood (peripheral blood progenitor cells or PBPCs) that can mature into red and white blood cells and platelets.

Hemoglobin—A protein that binds oxygen as it passes through the lungs and delivers it to the cells of the body.

Human leukocyte antigen (HLA)—Any of the proteins of the histocompatibility complex that are expressed on the surface of white blood cells.

Immunoglobulins—Antibodies.

Neutrophils—The major infection-fighting white blood cells of the immune system.

Plasma—The fluid component of blood.

Platelets—Small cell-like bodies in the blood that are involved in clot formation.

Red blood cells (RBCs)—The cells in the blood that carry oxygen to the tissues of the body.

Transfusion-related acute lung injury (TRALI)—A life-threatening transfusion reaction, especially to antigens in transfused plasma.

Umbilical cord blood (UBC)—Blood collected from the umbilical cord after birth and used as a source of hematopoietic progenitor or stem cells.

Volume expander—Any of several solutions that can be transfused when fluid (but not blood components) is required, as for preventing or treating shock.

White blood cells (WBCs)—Leukocytes; any colorless blood cells that have nuclei and lack hemoglobin; including lymphocytes and neutrophils.

RBCs

RBCs are the most commonly transfused component. RBCs that have been separated from liquid plasma (packed RBCs) have a shelf life of 42 days and are transfused into patients with **anemia** or who have lost a lot of blood. A hematocrit—the percentage of RBCs in a given volume of blood—and a complete blood count that includes the hemoglobin level (the oxygen-carrying capacity of the RBCs) are used to determine the need for a transfusion. Normal hemoglobin levels are 12–18 grams per deciliter (g/dL); a level below 8 g/dL may require an RBC transfusion. Some studies have noted a poorer prognosis when transfusions are given before surgery for breast, colon, and non-small cell lung cancers and sarcomas. It is recommended that transfusions before surgery not be used simply to raise hemoglobin levels above 10 g/dL.

RBC transfusions usually begin at a slow rate to monitor for signs of a transfusion reaction. The patient's vital signs, including temperature, heart rate, blood pressure, and respiration, are checked frequently. An RBC unit is usually transfused over about two hours, and the procedure is completed within four hours. Plasma, platelets, and other components are in smaller volumes and are transfused much faster.

Platelets

Platelets are cell fragments in the blood that are produced from bone marrow cells called megakaryocytes. They function with clotting factors to prevent bleeding. Bone marrow that has been damaged by **chemotherapy** and/or radiation or crowded out by the growth of cancer cells might not produce enough platelets. Depending on the laboratory, normal platelet counts are 150,000–400,000 per mm^3 of blood. Platelet counts below a critical level, often 20,000 per mm^3, can cause dangerous bleeding. Platelet transfusions are often deferred if the patient has no clinical signs of bleeding, but transfusions of platelets might be given at higher platelet counts if the patient requires surgery or is at risk of bleeding.

Platelets and clotting factors are separated from plasma and concentrated. Since a unit of whole blood contains only a small volume of platelets, an adult transfusion requires six to ten units of platelets pooled from different donors. Unlike RBCs, platelets do not have blood types and so can usually be transfused into any patient. Like plasma, platelets can also be obtained from donors by apheresis or plateletpheresis in a procedure that removes the platelets and returns the blood cells and plasma to the donor. This collects enough single-donor platelets so that pooling is unnecessary.

White blood cells (WBCs)

WBC or granulocyte transfusions were once common in cancer patients to help fight infections. Although chemotherapy patients may develop low WBC counts, granulocyte (a type of WBC) transfusions are no longer performed because they cause **fever** and can potentially transmit infections, such as cytomegalovirus, which are particularly dangerous for cancer patients with weakened immune systems. The levels of WBCs called neutrophils are carefully monitored in cancer patients, because neutrophils are very important for fighting multiple types of infection. If neutrophil counts become very low, colony-stimulating factors or growth factors—including granulocyte colony-stimulating factor (G-CSF; **filgrastim** or pegfilgrastim), granulocyte macrophage colony-stimulating factor (GM-CSF; **sargramostim**), and interleukin-3—can stimulate the production of neutrophils in the bone marrow. Immunoglobulins (gamma globulin or immune serum) can also be collected from plasma and transfused to temporarily boost immune systems that have been depressed by cancer, cancer treatments, or other conditions such as HIV/AIDS.

Autologous transfusions

Autologous transfusions are transfusions with a patient's own blood that was either donated prior to surgery or collected ("salvaged") during surgery. This ensures that the blood is an exact match and eliminates the risk of a transfusion reaction or infection, which is particularly important for cancer patients. However, some studies have found tumor cells in salvaged blood. As with other forms of specialized blood donations, there is a processing fee for collection and delivery of each unit of blood, which may not be reimbursed by **health insurance**.

Cell transfusion therapy

Hematopoietic progenitor or stem cells (HPCs or HSCs) in the blood (peripheral blood progenitor cells or PBPCs) and bone marrow can mature into RBCs, platelets, and WBCs. PBPCs are collected by apheresis and used to treat leukemia and **lymphoma**, as well as other diseases. Several days before collection, the patient or other donor is treated with hematopoietic growth factor to increase the number of PBPCs. The PBPCs can be stored or even frozen if there is a delay between apheresis and transfusion. Cell therapies require tissue (HLA) matches between the donor and recipient.

Umbilical cord blood (UCB)—usually 50–200 mL—can be collected as a source of HPCs after the delivery of a baby. The RBCs are removed, and the plasma is frozen and stored in a private/family bank for use by a family member or in a public bank for an unrelated recipient. Because the HPCs in UCB may be less mature, the HLA match between donor and recipient may not need to be as close as with PBPCs. There may also be less risk of life-threatening **graft-versus-host disease** (GVHD). If it often easier to find a suitable UCB match than a PBPC match for patients with rare HLA types.

Alternatives to blood transfusions

Patients who require large volumes of fluids to prevent or treat shock can be given intravenous (IV) volume expanders—such as solutions of normal saline, lactated Ringer's solution, dextrans, albumin, hydroxyethyl starch, or purified protein fractions—that can restore fluid volumes.

Erythropoietin and thrombopoietin stimulate the production of RBCs and platelets, respectively. Interleukin-11 (**oprelvekin**) can also raise platelet levels. However, these drugs carry risks, are expensive, and only slowly raise blood levels of RBCs or platelets, so they are impractical in emergencies. Furthermore, patients with severe bone marrow disease may not have enough blood-producing bone marrow cells to respond to growth factors, and some growth factors can stimulate the rapid growth of some types of cancer cells. Therefore, growth factors are administered for only a short time and are not used in patients who are expected to be cured of their cancer.

Blood donations

About 14,000,000 units of blood are donated each year in the United States. The collection, processing, storage, and transport of blood and blood products are strictly regulated by the Food and Drug Administration (FDA), as well as the American Red Cross, the American Association of Blood Banks, and most states, to ensure quality and prevent the transmission of infectious diseases. Donors are screened for risk factors for infectious diseases, as well as for medication use and certain medical conditions, including cancer. All donated blood and blood products are extensively tested for infectious agents, such as hepatitis virus and HIV.

Plasmapheresis donors may be paid for their plasma, because plasma can be treated for safety in ways that blood cells cannot. This plasma is generally used by pharmaceutical companies to make drugs rather than for transfusions.

Directed donations are donations made by a patient's family or friends for that patient's use. Directed donations follow the same procedures as general blood donations and are added to the general blood supply if not used by the patient. Studies do not indicate that directed donations are safer than the general blood supply.

Precautions

The U.S. blood supply is considered very safe, and blood banks take many precautions. The transfused blood type is matched with that of the recipient. Blood is transfused slowly by gravity flow directly into a vein so that the patient can be observed for signs of adverse reactions. People who have received many transfusions (such as leukemia patients) sometimes develop an **immune response** to factors in foreign blood cells and must be checked for immune reactions before transfusion.

Preparation

Transfusions are usually performed in a hospital or outpatient clinic. Patients who are very ill, unable to travel to a facility, and require frequent transfusions over a long period may receive transfusions at home from a visiting nurse. The patient is made comfortable, and vital signs are checked. The needle-insertion site is washed carefully with a soap-based solution, followed by an iodine-containing antiseptic. The skin is dried and a transfusion needle or catheter connected to tubing is inserted into the vein. During the early stages of a transfusion, the recipient is closely monitored for adverse reactions, and routine monitoring continues for the duration of the transfusion.

Aftercare

A pressure bandage is placed over the needle-insertion site to prevent bleeding, and vital signs continue to be monitored. Acetaminophen (Tylenol) and **diphenhydramine** (Benadryl) are often administered to reduce symptoms of minor transfusion reactions. A hematocrit and hemoglobin and platelet counts are performed to determine if the transfusion was sufficient.

QUESTIONS TO ASK YOUR DOCTOR

- How often will I have a complete blood count?
- Will I need a transfusion before, during, or after my surgery?
- Am I a candidate for autologous transfusion?
- Am I a candidate for a directed donation?
- Am I a candidate for a stem-cell transfusion?

Risks

Transfusion reactions occur when antibodies in the recipient's blood react to proteins or other substances introduced by the transfusion.

- Allergic reactions such as itching or hives are the most common transfusion reaction and are treated with antihistamines. However, hypersensitivity reactions that can cause tissue damage are also possible.

- Reactions to minor factors in a transfusion might include dizziness, fever, headache, rash, swelling, and sometimes breathing difficulties and muscle spasms.

- Febrile reaction—a sudden fever during or within 24 hours of the transfusion, sometimes accompanied by headache, nausea, and chills—is often a response to WBCs. It is more common in patients who have had previous transfusions and in women who have had several pregnancies. People at risk for febrile reactions are usually given leukoreduced blood that has had the WBCs removed.

- Transfusion-related acute lung injury (TRALI) is a rare reaction that is more likely to occur with transfusions containing more plasma. It can occur during or up to six hours after a transfusion. A delayed syndrome can occur up to 72 hours later. Even with breathing and blood pressure support, TRALI is fatal in 5%–10% of cases and in up to 40% of delayed syndromes.

- Acute immune hemolytic reaction is caused by mismatched donor and recipient blood types. It is the most serious transfusion reaction but is very rare because blood-type matches are checked several times before a transfusion begins. Hemolytic reactions occur when the recipient's antibodies attack the donor RBCs, causing them to break open or hemolyze and release harmful substances. Symptoms include chills, fever, chest and back pain, and nausea. The kidneys can be damaged and, if the transfusion is not halted immediately, the recipient can die.

- Delayed hemolytic reactions are caused by the recipient's antibodies slowly attacking donor RBC antigens other than the ABO blood type antigens. The donor RBCs are destroyed over a period of days or weeks. There are usually no symptoms, but the patient's RBC count falls. Delayed reactions usually occur only in recipients who have had previous transfusions.

- GVHD is caused by transfused WBCs attacking the tissues of a patient with a very weak immune system. It is more likely to occur if the donor is a relative or someone with the same HLA type, so that the patient's immune system does not recognize the transfused WBCs as foreign. Fever, rash, diarrhea, and liver problems can develop within a month of the transfusion. Treating donated blood with radiation before transfusion prevents GVHD. Irradiated blood products are often used for cancer patients with weakened immune systems.

Infections from transfusions are extremely rare in the United States due to careful donor and blood screenings. The risk of hepatitis B virus in a unit of donated blood is about one in 800,000 or less; it is one in 1.6 million for hepatitis C virus and about one in two million for HIV. All transfused blood is also tested for syphilis, the HTLV-I and HTLV-II viruses associated with human T-cell leukemia/lymphoma, West Nile virus, and Chagas disease, which is common in Central and South America. Although diseases such as babesiosis, Lyme disease, and malaria can be transmitted through transfusions, donors are screened for health status and travel, and such transmissions are very rare. On rare occasions, blood, especially platelets (which are stored at room temperature), are contaminated with miniscule amounts of skin bacteria that can cause severe illness minutes or hours after the start of transfusion. Routine testing of platelets by blood banks has reduced this problem. Single-donor platelets are less likely to have bacterial contamination than pooled platelets.

Resources

OTHER

"Blood Transfusion and Donation." American Cancer Society. September 7, 2013. http://www.cancer.org/acs/groups/cid/documents/webcontent/002989-pdf.pdf (accessed August 30, 2014).

WEBSITES

"Facts About Cellular Therapies." American Association of Blood Banks. http://www.aabb.org/aabbcct/therapyfacts/Pages/default.aspx (accessed August 30, 2014).

"Hematopoietic Stem Cells." American Association of Blood Banks. http://www.aabb.org/aabbcct/therapyfacts/Pages/hsc.aspx (accessed August 30, 2014).

"Umbilical Cord Blood Donation FAQs." American Association of Blood Banks. http://www.aabb.org/sa/facilities/celltherapy/Pages/cordbloodfaqs.aspx (accessed August 30, 2014).

ORGANIZATIONS

American Association of Blood Banks, 8101 Glenbrook Road, Bethesda, MD 20814-2749, (301) 907-6977, Fax: (301) 907-6895, http://www.aabb.org.

American Cancer Society, 250 Williams Street NW, Atlanta, GA 30303, (800) 227-2345, http://www.cancer.org.

American Red Cross, 2025 E Street NW, Washington, DC 20006, (202) 303-4498, (800) RED CROSS (733-2767), http://www.redcross.org.

America's Blood Centers, 725 15th Street NW, Suite 700, Washington, DC 20005, (202) 393-5725, Fax: (202) 393-1282, (888) USBLOOD, http://www.americasblood.org.

John T. Lohr
Molly Metzler, R.N.
Margaret Alic, PhD

Transitional care

Definition

According to the **National Cancer Institute** (NCI), transitional care may refer either to a patient's movement from one level of **cancer** care to another, or from one place of care to another. Levels of cancer care are defined as active (intended to cure the cancer), supportive (intended to relieve discomfort associated with the symptoms of the cancer or the side effects of treatment), or palliative (intended to manage pain when cure is no longer possible). Places of care are categorized as acute care facilities, subacute care facilities (e.g., rehabilitation centers, nursing homes, and hospices), and home care (usually the patient's or family's house).

Description

Transitional care for cancer patients has become a pressing health care issue in the twenty-first century. One reason is that health care in the United States and Canada has become increasingly specialized in terms of facilities as well as care givers; in addition, the NCI states that almost 90% of care for cancer patients is now given on an outpatient basis. In an acute care hospital or cancer center, a cancer patient may have a health care team that consists of three or more doctors in various medical and surgical specialties as well as nurses, physical therapists, social workers, nutritionists, and others. As the patient undergoes various forms of cancer therapy, his or her response to treatments as well as financial concerns, family issues, and other considerations may lead to transfer to a subacute care facility or to home care.

Another factor that has led to a new understanding of the importance of transitional care is the growing number of long-term survivors of cancer. Although these people may be able to live at home by themselves or return to work, they still require various types of follow-up to monitor the long-term physical and psychological side effects of the cancer treatment they received.

Because of the growing complexity of cancer treatment and the risk that the patient's care may be fragmented or interrupted by changes in caregivers or facilities, medical professionals and policy makers presently emphasize the importance of integrated or "seamless" care. This concern for continuity is reflected both in the NCI's recommendations about changes in patient care and in its use of the biopsychosocial model of health care. The biopsychosocial model is the medical term for understanding the patient as a human being with thoughts, emotions, spiritual needs, and important relationships with family members and friends, as well as physical symptoms related to the cancer. The NCI recommends the use of community liaison nurses and social workers as coordinators of patient care in order to relieve the patient or family members of the stress of relaying information from one health care professional to another, and to prevent the patient's care from being interrupted or weakened during transfers from one care facility to another.

The biopsychosocial model is the basis for the comprehensive assessment that precedes planning for transitional care. The patient's health care team will evaluate his or her needs in each of the following areas:

- Physical. This area includes nutritional status, ability to function, smoking history, and future treatment options as well as the current stage of the patient's disease and symptom profile.

- Demographics of the patient and his or her family. This area includes marital status, other family members at home, primary language, cultural background, and educational level.

- Psychological. This part of the assessment covers the patient's (and family members') attitudes toward the cancer, fears and anxieties, habitual coping patterns, history of psychiatric illness, and overall level of family stability.

- Social. This area includes the patient's social support networks, employment history, insurance coverage, availability of transportation, and the patient's knowledge and use of resources in the community.

- Spiritual. This part of the assessment includes the patient's religious beliefs and the level of importance of religion in their life, the extent of their support network in their faith community, and the ways in which their religious beliefs or practices may affect their cancer treatment.

- Legal. This area concerns such matters as the patient's will, estate planning, living will, end-of-life care directives, etc.

This comprehensive assessment should be made at regular intervals during the patient's treatment in order to make any necessary adjustments due to changes in the patient's physical symptoms and level of functioning, family situation, employment, etc.

Treatment

The treatments given during transitional care are highly individualized; they depend on the specific patient's health status, type of cancer, and the types of treatments (surgery, **chemotherapy**, radiotherapy, etc.) that he or she received in the acute care hospital or cancer center. Advances in medical technology, however, have increased the range and variety of treatments that can be delivered by visiting health care professionals in the patient's home. These advances make transitional care at home a possibility for many cancer patients.

Alternative and complementary therapies

It is usually possible to integrate CAM therapies into transitional care, provided that the patient discusses the specific alternative treatments desired with his or her doctor. Some types of movement or massage therapy may not be suitable immediately following surgery, however, while some herbal preparations or traditional Chinese medicines may interact with the drugs given to treat the cancer itself or to relieve the side effects of treatment.

Special concerns

The NCI notes that some groups of cancer patients are at risk of not receiving adequate treatment planning or transitional care. These patients include low-income and homeless people; members of minority groups living in the inner city; and people living in rural areas.

In addition to consulting with a social worker or other professional coordinator, patients and their families should be actively involved in planning for transitional care. They can gather information about various therapies, care facilities, local support groups, and other resources, and discuss these among themselves as well as with members of the patient's treatment team. The patient and his or her family should not hesitate to ask questions or bring up issues that are not mentioned by the health care team during the patient's evaluation for transitional care.

See also Psycho-oncology.

Resources

PERIODICALS

Manville, M., Klein, M.C., Bainbridge, L. "Improved Outcomes for Elderly Patients Who Received Care on a Transitional Care Unit." *Canadian Family Physician* 60, no. 5 (2014): 263–71. http://www.ncbi.nlm.nih.gov/pmc/articles/PMC4020664/ (accessed November 14, 2014).

Mary Naylor, Stacen A. Keating. "Transitional Care: Moving Patients From One Care Setting to Another." *The American Journal of Nursing* 108, no. 9 (2008): 58–63. http://www.ncbi.nlm.nih.gov/pmc/articles/PMC2768550/#__ffn_sectitle (accessed November 14, 2014).

Sunga, Annette, MD, Margaret M. Eberl, MD, Kevin C. Oeffinger, MD, et al. "Care of Cancer Survivors." *American Family Physician* 71 (February 15, 2005): 699–714.

ORGANIZATIONS

American Cancer Society, 250 Williams St. NW, Atlanta, GA 30303, (800) 227-2345, http://www.cancer.org.

National Cancer Institute, 9609 Medical Center Dr., BG 9609 MSC 9760, Bethesda, MD 20892-9760, (800) 4-CANCER (422-6237), http://www.cancer.gov.

Rebecca Frey, PhD

Transitional cell carcinoma

Definition

Transitional cell **carcinoma** (TCC) is a type of **cancer** that usually originates in the kidney, bladder, or ureter (the tube that carries urine from the kidney to the bladder). It has also been recently recognized as a subtype of **ovarian cancer.**

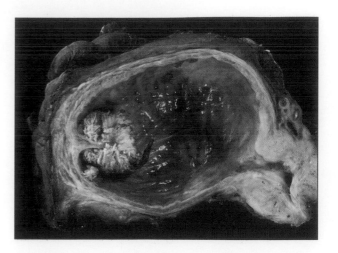

Transitional cell carcinoma of the bladder (shown on the left of the image). *(BIOPHOTO ASSOC/Science Source)*

Description

A transitional cell is intermediate between the flat squamous cell and the tall columnar cell. It is restricted to the epithelium (cellular lining) of the urinary bladder, ureters (tubes that carry urine from the kidneys to the bladder), and the pelvis of the kidney (that portion of the kidney collecting the urine as it leaves the kidneys and enters the ureters). Transitional cell carcinomas have a wide range in their gross appearance depending on their locations. Some of these carcinomas are flat in appearance, some are papillary (small elevation), and others are in the shape of a node. Under the microscope, however, most of these carcinomas have a papillary-like look. There are three generally recognized grades of transitional cell carcinoma. The grade of the carcinoma is determined by particular characteristics found in the cells of the tumor. Transitional cell carcinoma typically affects the mucosa (the moist tissue layer that lines hollow organs or the cavity of the body) in the areas where it originates.

The most common site of transitional cell carcinoma is in the urinary bladder. Transitional cell carcinoma is the form of cancer in about 90% of cancers found in the bladder. The highest grade of transitional cell carcinoma is very likely to spread to other parts of the body. There are two primary ways that transitional cell carcinoma spreads into the surrounding structures. The first is by way of epithelial cells that line the body cavity and many of the passageways that exit the body. The other means of spread is through the lymphatic (network that resembles the circulatory system but transports proteins, salts, water, and other substances) system.

Demographics

Most patients who develop transitional cell carcinoma are older than 40 years of age; the peak age of incidence is 60–70 years of age. The male:female ratio for this type of cancer is about 5:2. About 93% of all bladder cancers in North American are of the transitional cell carcinoma type. Only 8% of all renal cancers are of the transitional cell carcinoma type. According to the American Cancer Society (ACS), 74,690 people in the United States were diagnosed with **bladder cancer** in 2014, with 15,580 deaths from the disease.

Causes and symptoms

The causes and mechanisms of transitional cell carcinoma, like all forms of cancer, are not entirely known or understood. However, researchers have isolated several factors that have been associated with an increased risk for developing this carcinoma.

Cigarette smoking is the strongest risk factor for transitional cell carcinoma. Researchers have found smoking increases the risk for developing this condition by three to seven times. In men with bladder cancer, 50% to 80% have a history of smoking **cigarettes**. Other methods of using tobacco, such as cigar and pipe smoking and chewing tobacco, have been shown to increase the risk of developing this carcinoma but at a reduced rate compared with smoking.

Individuals who have undergone long-term exposure to industrial chemicals, such as the class of compounds known as arylamines, are known to have an increased risk of developing transitional cell carcinoma. One of the most dangerous of these chemicals is one known as 2-naphthylamine. Individuals who develop these carcinomas usually do so anywhere from 15 to 40 years following the first exposure to these chemicals. Arsenic is another chemical that has been recently implicated in the development of TCC.

Individuals who have used analgesics for many years, or have used them excessively in the short-term, are at an increased risk for developing transitional cell carcinoma. Many of these patients have suffered at least some damage to the kidneys before developing the carcinoma. Drugs given to patients to treat an earlier cancer, such as the commonly used **cyclophosphamide**, increase the risk of developing transitional cell carcinoma at a later time.

Researchers believe these factors somehow alter genes that are important in the development of transitional cell carcinoma. These changes most often involve the deletions of certain chromosomes but also may result from mutations.

The most common symptom of transitional cell carcinoma is blood in the urine without accompanying pain. There may also be changes in the urge for the patient to urinate and in the frequency of urination.

In some cases, urine may be partially obstructed by a tumor in the ureter. Rarely, pain occurs in the pelvic region. Physicians rarely detect a tumorous mass by touch during the first examination.

Diagnosis

There are a variety of ways that can be used to help diagnose transitional cell carcinoma. Many of these involve the use of **imaging studies**. In some cases, traditional x-rays may be used to image upper urinary tract tumors. One of the things that physicians look for in patients suspected of having transitional cell carcinoma is the abnormal filling of structures in the urinary system. A type of imaging called excretory urography can help detect such flaws in the system. A different imaging method called retrograde urography can help physicians image the process of urinary collection and detect irregularities. **Computed tomography** (CT), more commonly called the CAT scan, is a very useful tool in the imaging of tumors in the upper tract of the urinary system. CT is more sensitive than traditional x-rays. In some cases, however, small tumors can be missed using this method.

Ultrasound may also be used to help tell the difference between tumors and normal structures in this region. **Magnetic resonance imaging**, more commonly referred to as MRI, has not been found to have any significant advantage over computed tomography in the diagnosis of transitional cell carcinoma.

Cystoscopy is the examination of the bladder using a cystoscope, an instrument that allows the interior imaging of the ureter and bladder. Cystoscopy is usually mandatory in patients suspected of having transitional cell carcinoma and can be helpful in determining the origin of the bleeding in these patients. Patients who are suspected of having transitional cell carcinoma, or other type of cancer in the upper urinary tract, need to have laboratory analysis of the cells in the suspected mass. This cell analysis tells the physician what type and stage of cell is present.

The easiest but least accurate way to study these cells is to have the patient provide urine samples. Patients who have a low-grade tumor in the upper urinary tract will have normal results in up to 80% of cases when urinalysis is used; however, such urinalysis can be more effective in diagnosis of bladder tumors. Obtaining urine samples from the upper urinary tract using a catheter can provide more accurate analysis of upper urinary tract tumors.

A technique called the brush **biopsy** involves the placing of a tiny brush into a catheter. The catheter is then placed in the ureter and moved into the upper urinary tract where the brush scrapes off cells for later analysis. More modern techniques of imaging and sampling use tiny tubes with attached videocameras called endoscopes. These tubes can be moved into the upper urinary tract to locate bleeding and tumors and can be used to obtain biopsy samples.

Treatment team

The treatment team that treats the patient with suspected and confirmed transitional cell carcinoma usually involves a primary care physician who refers to a specialist, such as a urologist or nephrologist (kidney specialist); a radiologist who performs the imaging; a pathologist who studies the sampled cells; an oncologist who monitors the overall course of the cancer; and a surgeon who performs the surgical removal of the carcinoma.

Clinical staging

The International Society of Urological Pathology has developed a classification scheme for grading transitional cell carcinoma. These four grades are urothelial papilloma, urothelial neoplasms of low malignant potential, low-grade urothelial carcinoma, and high-grade carcinoma. Papilloma is usually seen in younger patients and is rare. Neoplasms of low malignant potential are sometimes difficult to differentiate from low-grade urothelial carcinomas. These tumors rarely become invasive to nearby tissue. Low-grade urothelial carcinoma tends to appear in the form of papillomas as well. These tumors can invade nearby tissue but usually do not progress. High-grade carcinomas are flat, papillary, or both. These tumors are larger and are more likely to invade nearby muscle tissue.

Treatment

The most common means to treat papillary transitional cell carcinoma in the bladder is with surgery. When these tumors are classified as low grade, they can typically be removed completely. Unfortunately, these carcinomas recur 50% to 70% of the time. Because of this high rate of cancer recurrence, patients with transitional cell carcinoma have to be carefully monitored following surgery with cystoscopy and regular urinalysis.

Other types of therapy called immunologic therapy (**immunotherapy**) and **chemotherapy** are often used in treating bladder carcinoma. These methods use agents that are directly applied to the bladder. The most commonly used agent in these therapies is called **bacillus Calmette-Guérin** (BCG). When BCG is placed in the bladder, the body begins an **immune response** that sometimes destroys the tumor. Patients usually receive

one treatment per week for six weeks. After this period, a maintenance program involving three-week BCG courses of treatment for up to two years is used. The most common chemotherapy used for transitional cell carcinoma in the past is a combination of the drugs **cisplatin**, **doxorubicin**, **vinblastine**, and **methotrexate**. Newer and less toxic drugs, such as celecoxib, **bortezomib**, ixabepilone, and gallium maltolate are being tested to replace these older agents. A combination regimen of chemotherapy and radiation is being considered as a therapy when the carcinoma invades the muscle surrounding the bladder. The effectiveness of this method has not been studied yet in research studies. **Radiation therapy** alone is not an effective treatment.

Transitional cell carcinoma in the upper urinary tract is also treated with surgical procedures. Affected areas in this region, including the kidney, are sometimes removed. Part or all of the ureter and parts of the bladder are also removed in some cases.

Those with superficial, noninvasive, or nonmalignant disease should receive a cystoscopy and a thorough examination every three months for two years followed by a regimen every six months for an additional two years. In those with advanced disease but who did not receive complete bladder removal, a cystoscopy with a thorough examination should be performed every three months for two years, followed by every six months for an additional two years, and then one per year. These patients should also receive a computed tomography (CT) scan of the pelvis and abdomen every six months for two years. Chest x-rays, liver function tests, and serum creatinine tests should also be performed on this schedule. Those who had bladder removal should have chest x-rays, liver function tests, computed tomography scan of abdomen and pelvis, and serum creatinine tests performed every six months for two years. In addition, an endoscopy of the newly formed bladder structure should be performed.

Prognosis

The noninvasive papilloma rarely recurs once removed. If urothelial neoplasms of low malignant potential recur, they are usually benign tumors; however, in about 3% to 5% of cases, these recurrences are of a higher grade. These carcinomas rarely become invasive, and patients with them have a one-year survival rate of 95% to 98%. Low-grade urothelial carcinomas often show signs of invasion during diagnosis, but are not associated with a high risk for malignancy. High-grade carcinomas have considerable invasiveness into nearby tissue, particularly muscle, and are associated with a very high risk for **metastasis** (movement of cancer cells from one part of the body to another).

Coping with cancer treatment

A variety of issues need to be considered when the patient is receiving cancer treatment. One of the most important of these issues is the ability to cope with the emotion of having cancer in the first place. Several techniques, such as relaxation training, meditation, and biofeedback, may be beneficial to the patient in reducing anxiety. Other issues such as missed work and other daily activities need to be planned before the treatment period to reduce emotional stress. The patient needs to consider worst-case scenarios, such as side effects from chemotherapy, when planning these future events. Participation in cancer support groups helps many patients with the stress of the treatment period.

There are physical issues as well during this period. Pain following surgery can be a significant problem. Fortunately, there are many effective pain medications available to handle most pain events. Nausea and hair loss (**alopecia**) are two of the more notable effects of chemotherapy. Nausea can be effectively treated with drugs in most cases. Hair loss is only a temporary event, but it often has significant psychological effects that can be somewhat alleviated through social support.

Clinical trials

As of 2014, the **National Cancer Institute** (NCI) listed 24 **clinical trials** in progress for treating transitional cell carcinoma. Several drugs were being tested. The best way to obtain the most current information is to call the Cancer Information Service at (800) 4-CANCER or visit the NCI's clinical trials website at: http://www.cancer.gov/clinicaltrials/search.

Prevention

Cigarette smoking is a major risk factor for the development of transitional cell carcinoma. Cigarette smoking has been associated with 25% to 65% of all cases of bladder cancer. Smokers are two to four times more likely to develop transitional cell carcinoma than nonsmokers. Smoking increases the risk of developing tumors that are at a higher grade, in greater number, and of larger size. Those individuals who have abused analgesics are at an increased risk for developing transitional cell carcinoma. Exposure to the **human papillomavirus** type 16 also increases the risk of developing transitional cell carcinoma. Petroleum, dye, textile, tire, and rubber workers are at increased risk for developing this carcinoma. Exposure to chemicals, such as 2-naphthylamine, benzidine, 4-amino-biphenyl, nitrosamines, or O-toluidine can also increase the risk of developing transitional cell carcinoma.

QUESTIONS TO ASK YOUR DOCTOR

- What type of type of tests are necessary to make an accurate diagnosis?
- Are these tests painful?
- How long will it take to get results?
- If the tests are positive for cancer, what happens then?
- If it is transitional cell carcinoma, is the tumor invasive?
- Has the carcinoma spread to other tissues?
- What stage is the carcinoma?
- What treatment alternatives are there?
- If surgery is necessary, what will the surgery entail?
- What is the recuperation period like after the surgery?
- How long will I be in the hospital?
- If radiation is necessary, what sort of side effects are common?
- If chemotherapy or immunotherapy is necessary, what side effects are common?
- Will chemotherapy cause my hair to fall out?
- Are there any clinical trials that I can participate in?
- What type of surveillance schedule will I be on following the initial surgery and therapy?

Eliminating exposure to these substances substantially reduces the risk of developing transitional cell carcinoma.

Resources

WEBSITES

Cancer Research UK. "Transitional Cell Cancer of the Kidney (Renal Pelvis) or Ureter and its Treatment." http://www.cancerresearchuk.org/about-cancer/cancers-in-general/cancer-questions/transitional-cell-cancer-kidney-ureter-treatment (accessed November 14, 2014).

National Cancer Institute. "General Information About Transitional Cell Cancer of the Renal Pelvis and Ureter." http://www.cancer.gov/cancertopics/pdq/treatment/transitional-cell/Patient/page1 (accessed November 14, 2014).

National Cancer Institute. "Transitional Cell Cancer (Kidney/Ureter)." http://www.cancer.gov/cancertopics/types/transitionalcell (accessed November 14, 2014).

ORGANIZATIONS

American Cancer Society, 250 Williams St. NW, Atlanta, GA
    30303, (800) 227-2345, http://www.cancer.org.
National Cancer Institute, 9609 Medical Center Dr., BG 9609
    MSC 9760, Bethesda, MD 20892-9760, (800) 4-CANCER
    (422-6237), http://www.cancer.gov.

Mark Mitchell, M.D.
Rebecca Frey, PhD

Transrectal ultrasound *see* **Endorectal ultrasound**

Transurethral bladder resection

Definition

Transurethral bladder resection is a surgical procedure used to view the inside of the bladder, remove tissue samples, and/or remove tumors. Instruments are passed through a cystoscope (a slender tube with a lens and a light) that has been inserted through the urethra into the bladder.

Purpose

Transurethral resection is the initial form of treatment for bladder cancers. The procedure is performed to remove and examine bladder tissue and/or a tumor. It may also serve to remove lesions, and it may be the only treatment necessary for noninvasive tumors. This procedure plays both a diagnostic and therapeutic role in the treatment of bladder cancers.

Description

Cancer begins in the lining layer of the bladder and grows into the bladder wall. Transitional cells line the inside of the bladder. Cancer can begin in these lining cells.

During transurethral bladder resection, a cystoscope is inserted through the urethra into the bladder. A clear solution is infused to maintain visibility and the tumor or tissue to be examined is cut away using an electric current. A **biopsy** is taken of the tumor and muscle fibers in order to evaluate the depth of tissue involvement, while avoiding perforation of the bladder wall. Every attempt is made to remove all visible tumor tissue, along with a small border of healthy tissue. The resected tissue is examined under the microscope for diagnostic purposes. An indwelling catheter may be inserted to ensure adequate drainage of the bladder postoperatively.

At this time, interstitial **radiation therapy** may be initiated, if necessary.

Demographics

According to the American Cancer Society (ACS), there were 72,570 new cases of **bladder cancer** in the United States in 2013, with approximately 15,210 deaths from the disease.

Industrialized countries such as the United States, Canada, France, Denmark, Italy, and Spain have the highest incidence rates for bladder cancer. Rates are lower in England, Scotland, and Eastern Europe. The lowest rates occur in Asia and South America.

Smoking is a major risk factor for bladder cancer; it increases a person's cancer risk by two to five times and accounts for approximately 50% of bladder cancers found in men and 30% found in women. If cigarette smokers quit, their risk declines in two to four years. Exposure to a variety of industrial chemicals also increases the risk of developing this disease. Occupational exposures may account for approximately 25% of all urinary bladder cancers.

Men have a 1-in-30 chance of developing bladder cancer; women have a 1-in-90 chance of developing bladder cancer. The incidence of bladder cancer in the Caucasian population is almost twice that of the African American population. For other ethnic and racial groups in the United States, the incidence of bladder cancer falls between that of Caucasians and African Americans.

There is a greater incidence of bladder cancer with advancing age. Of newly diagnosed cases in both men and women, approximately 80% occur in people aged 60 years and older.

Diagnosis

If there is reason to suspect a patient may have bladder cancer, the physician will use one or more methods to determine if the disease is actually present. The doctor first takes a complete medical history to check for risk factors and symptoms, and does a physical examination. An examination of the rectum and vagina (in women) may also be performed to determine the size of a bladder tumor and to see if and how far it has spread. If bladder cancer is suspected, the following tests may be performed, including:

- biopsy
- cystoscopy
- urine cytology
- bladder washing
- urine culture

KEY TERMS

Biopsy—The removal and microscopic examination of a small sample of body tissue to see whether cancer cells are present.

Bladder irrigation—To flush or rinse the bladder with a stream of liquid (as in removing a foreign body or medicating).

Bladder tumor marker studies—A test to detect specific substances released by bladder cancer cells into the urine using chemicals or immunology (using antibodies).

Bladder washing—A procedure in which bladder washing samples are taken by placing a salt solution into the bladder through a catheter (tube) and then removing the solution for microscopic testing.

Chemotherapy—The treatment of cancer with anti-cancer drugs.

Cystoscopy—A procedure in which a slender tube with a lens and a light is placed into the bladder to view the inside of the bladder and remove tissue samples.

Immunotherapy—A method of treating allergies in which small doses of substances that a person is allergic to are injected under the skin.

Interstitial radiation therapy—The process of placing radioactive sources directly into the tumor. These radioactive sources can be temporary (removed after the proper dose is reached) or permanent.

Intravenous pyelogram—An x-ray of the urinary system taken after injecting a contrast solution that enables the doctor to see images of the kidneys, ureters, and bladder.

Metastatic—A change of position, state, or form; as a transfer of a disease-producing agency from the site of disease to another part of the body; a secondary growth of a cancerous tumor.

Noninvasive tumors—Tumors that have not penetrated the muscle wall and/or spread to other parts of the body.

Radiation therapy—The use of high-dose x-rays to destroy cancer cells.

Retrograde pyelography—A test in which dye is injected through a catheter placed with a cystoscope into the ureter to make the lining of the bladder, ureters, and kidneys easier to see on x-rays.

Ureters—Two thin tubes that carry urine downward from the kidneys to the bladder.

Urethra—The small tube-like structure that allows urine to empty from the bladder.

Urine culture—A test which tests urine samples in the lab to see if bacteria are present.

Urine cytology—The examination of the urine under a microscope to look for cancerous or precancerous cells.

- intravenous pyelogram

- retrograde pyelography

- bladder tumor marker studies

Most of the time, the cancer begins as a superficial tumor in the bladder. Blood in the urine is the usual warning sign. Based on how they look under the microscope, bladder cancers are graded using Roman numerals 0 through IV. In general, the lower the number, the less the cancer has spread. A higher number indicates greater severity of cancer.

Because it is not unusual for people with one bladder tumor to develop additional cancers in other areas of the bladder or elsewhere in the urinary system, the doctor may biopsy several different areas of the bladder lining. If the cancer is suspected to have spread to other organs in the body, further tests will be performed.

Because different types of bladder cancer respond differently to treatment, the treatment for one patient could be different from that of another person with bladder cancer. Doctors determine how deeply the cancer has spread into the layers of the bladder in order to decide on the best treatment.

Aftercare

As with any surgical procedure, blood pressure and pulse will be monitored. Urine is expected to be blood-tinged in the early postoperative period. Continuous bladder irrigation (rinsing) may be used for approximately 24 hours after surgery. Most operative sites should be completely healed in three months. The patient is followed closely for possible recurrence with visual examination, using a special viewing device (cystoscope) at regular intervals. Because bladder cancer has a high rate of recurrence, frequent screenings are recommended. Normally, screenings would be needed every three to six months for the first three years, and every year after that, or as the physician considers necessary. **Cystoscopy** can catch a recurrence before it progresses to invasive cancer, which is difficult to treat.

Risks

All surgery carries some risk due to heart and lung problems or the anesthesia itself, but these risks are generally extremely small. The risk of death from general anesthesia for all types of surgery, for example, is only about one in 1,600. Bleeding and infection are other risks of any surgical procedure. If bleeding becomes a complication, bladder irrigation may be required postoperatively, during which time the patient's activity is limited to bed rest. Perforation of the bladder is another risk, in which case the urinary catheter is left in place for four to five days postoperatively. The patient is started on antibiotic therapy preventively. If the bladder is lacerated, accompanied by spillage of urine into the abdomen, an abdominal incision may be required.

Results

The results of transurethral bladder resection will depend on many factors, including the type of treatment used, the stage of the patient's cancer before surgery, complications during and after surgery, the age and overall health of the patient, as well as the recurrence of the disease at a later date. The chances for survival are improved if the cancer is found and treated early.

Morbidity and mortality rates

After a diagnosis of bladder cancer, up to 95% of patients with superficial tumors survive for at least five years. Patients whose cancer has grown into the lining of the bladder but not into the muscle itself, and is not in any lymph nodes or distant sites, have a five-year survival rate as high as 85%. The five-year survival rate may be as high as 55% for patients whose tumors have invaded the bladder muscle, but not spread through the muscle into the surrounding fatty tissue. When the cancer has grown totally through the bladder muscle into the surrounding fatty tissue, and perhaps into nearby tissues such as the prostate, uterus, or vagina, the five-year survival rate is about 38%. For patients whose cancer has spread through the bladder wall to the pelvis or abdominal wall or has spread distantly to lymph nodes or other organs (such as the bones, liver, or lungs), the five-year survival rate is 16%.

The five-year survival rate refers to the percentage of patients who live at least five years after their cancer is found, although many people live much longer. Five-year relative survival rates do not take into account patients who die of other diseases. Every person's situation is unique and the statistics cannot predict exactly what will happen in every case; these numbers provide an overall picture.

Mortality rates are two to three times higher for men than women. Although the incidence of bladder cancer in the Caucasian population exceeds that of the African American population, African American women die from the disease at a greater rate. This is due to a larger proportion of these cancers being diagnosed and treated at an earlier stage in the Caucasian population. The mortality rates for Hispanic and Asian men and women are only about one-half those for Caucasians and African Americans. Over the past 30 years, the age-adjusted mortality rate has decreased in both races and genders. This may be due to earlier diagnosis, better therapy, or both.

Alternatives

Surgery, radiation therapy, **immunotherapy**, and **chemotherapy** are the main types of treatment for cancer of the bladder. One type of treatment or a combination of these treatments may be recommended, based on the stage of the cancer.

After the cancer is found and staged, the cancer care team discusses the treatment options with the patient. In choosing a treatment plan, the most significant factors to consider are the type and stage of the cancer. Other factors to consider include the patient's overall physical health, age, likely side effects of the treatment, and the personal preferences of the patient.

In considering treatment options, a second opinion may provide more information and help the patient feel more confident about the treatment plan chosen.

Alternative methods are defined as unproved or disproved methods, rather than evidence-based or proven methods to prevent, diagnose, and treat cancer. For some cancer patients, conventional treatment is difficult to tolerate and they may decide to seek a less unpleasant alternative. Others are seeking ways to alleviate the side effects of conventional treatment without having to take more drugs. Some do not trust traditional medicine, and feel that with alternative medicine approaches, they are more in control of making decisions about what is happening to their bodies.

A cancer patient should talk to the doctor or nurse before changing the treatment or adding any alternative methods. Some methods can be safely used along with standard medical treatment. Others may interfere with standard treatment or cause serious side effects.

QUESTIONS TO ASK YOUR DOCTOR

- What benefits can I expect from this operation?
- What are the risks of this operation?
- What are the normal results of this operation?
- What happens if this operation does not go as planned?
- Are there any alternatives to this surgery?
- What is the expected recovery time?

The American Cancer Society (ACS) encourages people with cancer to consider using methods that have been proven effective or those that are currently under study. They encourage people to discuss all treatments they may be considering with their physician and other health care providers. The ACS acknowledges that more research is needed regarding the safety and effectiveness of many alternative methods. Unnecessary delays and interruptions in standard therapies could be detrimental to the success of cancer treatment.

At the same time, the ACS acknowledges that certain complementary methods such as aromatherapy, biofeedback, massage therapy, meditation, tai chi, or yoga may be very helpful when used in conjunction with conventional treatment.

Health care team roles

Transurethral bladder resections are usually performed in a hospital by a urologist, a medical doctor who specializes in the diagnosis and treatment of diseases of the urinary systems in men and women and also treats structural problems, tumors, and stones in the urinary system. Urologists can prescribe medications and perform surgery. If a transurethral bladder resection is required by a female patient, and there are complicating factors, an urogynecologist may perform the surgery. Urogynecologists treat urinary problems involving the female reproductive system.

Resources

BOOKS

Miller, Ronald D., et al. *Miller's Anesthesia*. 7th ed. Philadelphia: Churchill Livingstone/Elsevier, 2010.

Raghavan, Derek, and Michael Bailey. *Bladder Cancer*. Abingdon, UK: Health Press, 2006.

Wein, Alan J., et al. *Campbell-Walsh Urology*. 10th ed. Philadelphia: Saunders/Elsevier, 2012.

WEBSITES

American Cancer Society. "Surgery for Bladder Cancer." http://www.cancer.org/cancer/bladdercancer/detailedguide/bladder-cancer-treating-surgery (accessed October 3, 2014).

American Cancer Society. "What Are the Key Statistics about Bladder Cancer?" http://www.cancer.org/cancer/bladder-cancer/detailedguide/bladder-cancer-key-statistics (accessed October 3, 2014).

National Cancer Institute. "Bladder Cancer." http://www.cancer.gov/cancertopics/types/bladder (accessed October 3, 2014).

University of Cincinnati Cancer Institute. "Treating Bladder Cancer: TUR (Transurethral Resection)." http://cancer.uc.edu/CancerInfo/TypesOfCancer/BladderCancer/TransurethralResection.aspx (accessed October 3, 2014).

ORGANIZATIONS

American Cancer Society, 250 Williams St. NW, Atlanta, GA 30303, (800) 227-2345, http://www.cancer.org.

National Cancer Institute, 6116 Executive Blvd., Ste. 300, Bethesda, MD 20892-8322, (800) 4-CANCER (422-6237), http://cancer.gov.

National Comprehensive Cancer Network (NCCN), 275 Commerce Dr., Ste. 300, Fort Washington, PA 19034, (215) 690-0300, Fax: (215) 690-0280, http://www.nccn.org.

Kathleen D. Wright, RN
Crystal H. Kaczkowski, MSc
REVISED BY ROSALYN CARSON-DEWITT, MD

Transvaginal ultrasound

Definition

A transvaginal ultrasound, also called transvaginal sonogram (TVS), is an ultrasound that uses an internal probe, or transducer, that enters the vaginal cavity. Either a radiology technician or physician performs the test, and a radiologist interprets the results.

Purpose

An internal probe allows for closer access to the structures that need evaluation. With closer access, higher frequency sound waves can be used, which provides a clearer image due to better resolution. It is often used to evaluate suspected **cancer** or abnormal growths in the female reproductive system.

Precautions

While the transvaginal ultrasound produces a clearer image, it may also create false positive results. This can

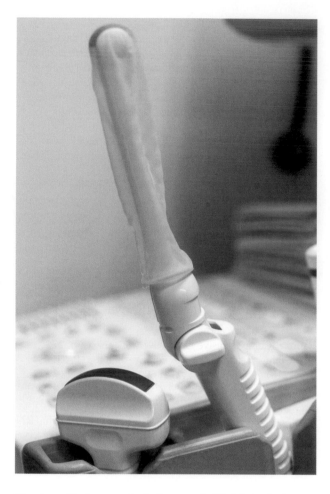

Wand used in transvaginal ultrasound. *(Matt Valentine/ Shutterstock.com)*

lead to unnecessary testing to further evaluate the condition, with its accompanying physical and emotional impact.

Description

The transvaginal ultrasound uses a small, wand-like transducer, or probe, which is inserted into the vagina. The probe emits high-frequency sound waves, which are not audible by humans. These sound waves painlessly bounce off the structures in its path. The returning echo wave is picked up by the probe. This information is fed into an attached computer that then creates an image, or sonogram, on a screen. It can differentiate between structures that are solid, such as a tumor, or filled with fluid, such as a cyst. It can be used to measure the thickness of the lining of the uterus, as well as of other organs.

A technique called color flow Doppler imaging may be used to evaluate the blood flow to certain structures. This can be helpful in establishing whether blood flow has been obstructed or enhanced to an organ. It cannot

tell if a solid mass is malignant or benign. Other tests, such as a **biopsy**, would be needed to gather that information. It is done on an outpatient basis, is less expensive than imaging tests such as **magnetic resonance imaging** (MRI), and is considered safe, using sound waves rather than radiation to generate an image.

Preparation

Little preparation is needed for the transvaginal ultrasound. A woman will need to undress from the waist down, and lie face-up on the examination surface. Legs may be put in stirrups, or a bolster may be placed under the hips to tilt the pelvic area upwards to facilitate use of the probe, both for insertion as well as for the ultrasound process itself. The test is done with an empty bladder, which is more comfortable than the full bladder required for the abdominal ultrasound. This method may be a preferred choice for women who have difficulty with bladder control. A woman may wish to request that she insert the probe herself, which is similar to the insertion of a tampon. Gel that has been warmed will make insertion more comfortable.

Aftercare

Because of the small amount of gel used on the probe for easier insertion, a woman may wish to use a sanitary pad to protect her underpants from any minor leakage after she stands up. After the test a woman will be able to resume her regular scheduled activities.

Risks

The risk involved in using the transvaginal ultrasound is that of obtaining a false positive result, any resulting tests that would be ordered unnecessarily, and their accompanying emotional burden.

Results

The normal results of a transvaginal ultrasound are the finding of the normal shape and size of any structure evaluated, with no abnormal thickness, masses or growths of any kind found.

Abnormal results

Abnormal results include the finding of growths, such as masses or cysts, and any unexpected thickness of the structures evaluated. Because of the risk of false positive results, any abnormal findings should be further evaluated and confirmed before undergoing surgery or treatment for the suspected condition. Magnetic resonance imaging (MRI) is often ordered to further evaluate masses. An endometrial biopsy is performed to further evaluate a thickened uterine lining.

Resources

PERIODICALS

E. Steiner, I. Juhasz-Bösz, G. Emons, H. Kölbl, R. Kimmig, P. Mallmann. "Transvaginal Ultrasound for Endometrial Carcinoma Screening - Current Evidence-Based Data." *Geburtshilfe und Frauenheilkunde* 72, no. 12 (2012): 1088–1091.

WEBSITES

A.D.A.M. Medical Encyclopedia. "Transvaginal Ultrasound." MedlinePlus. http://www.nlm.nih.gov/medlineplus/ency/article/003779.htm (accessed November 14, 2014).

Micromedex. "Transvaginal Ultrasound." http://www.mayoclinic.org/diseases-conditions/pcos/multimedia/transvaginal-ultrasound/img-20007770 (accessed November 14, 2014).

Esther Csapo Rastegari, R.N., B.S.N., Ed.M.

Transverse myelitis

Definition

Transverse myelitis (TM) is an inflammation or infection of the spinal cord in which the effect of the lesion spans the width of the entire spinal cord at a given level.

Description

The spinal cord consists of four regions: the cervical (neck), followed by the thoracic (chest), the lumbar (lower back) and the sacral (lowest back). TM can occur in any of these regions. The disease is uncommon, but not rare, as it occurs in one to five persons per million population in any given year in the United States. It is equally diagnosed in both adults and children. TM may occur by itself or in conjunction with other illnesses such as viral or bacterial infectious diseases, autoimmune diseases such as multiple sclerosis, vascular illnesses such as thrombosis, and **cancer**.

Causes and symptoms

Causes

The exact cause of TM is unknown but research results point to autoimmune deficiencies, meaning that the patient's own immune system abnormally attacks the spinal cord, resulting in inflammation and tissue damage.

There is also evidence suggesting that TM occurs as a result of **spinal cord compression** by tumors or as a result of direct spinal cord invasion by infectious agents, especially the human immunodeficiency virus (HIV) and the human T-lymphotropic virus type I (HTLV-1).

Symptoms

The symptoms of TM depend on the level of spinal cord lesion with sensation usually diminished below the spinal cord level affected. Some patients experience tingling sensations or numbness in the legs with bladder control also being disturbed.

Diagnosis

The condition is usually diagnosed following **magnetic resonance imaging** (MRI) or **computed tomography** (CT) with "spinal taps" (lumbar punctures) taken for additional analysis.

Treatment

There is no specific treatment for transverse myelitis. Treatment of the illness is largely symptomatic, meaning that it depends on the specific symptoms of the patient. The region in which the spinal cord has been infected is critical but a course of intravenous steroids is generally prescribed at the onset of treatment.

Treatment of the bladder function impairment resulting from TM include drugs, external catheters for men, and padding for women, with surgery recommended in certain cases. A common TM side effect is difficulty with stool evacuation and this condition can be treated by diets that include stool softeners and fiber.

As a result of TM, muscle groups below the affected level may become spastic. Treatment of spasticity usually involves prescriptions of drugs such as Baclofen (Lioresal), which stops reflex activity, and Dantrolene sodium (Dantrium), which acts directly on muscle.

A new very well-tolerated drug, Tizanidine, has also recently been introduced in the United States. Muscle pain is generally treated with analgesics such as acetaminophen (Tylenol) or ibuprofen (Naprosyn, Aleve, Motrin). Nerve disorders might be treated with anticonvulsant drugs such as **carbamazepine**, **phenytoin**, or **gabapentin** (Tegretol, Dilantin, Neurontin).

Alternative and complementary therapies

Individuals with TM may experience serious difficulty with common tasks such as dressing, bathing, and eating. Complementary TM therapies may accordingly include a course of **physical therapy** so as to help patients recover mobility. This can be achieved with special exercises, canes, walkers and custom-designed braces.

After the acute phase, people with TM start the rehabilitation process. During this period, the focus of care is shifted from designing an effective TM treatment to learning to cope with a serious disease. TM patients must learn to cope with the loss of abilities which healthy people take for granted and this process is necessarily harder if TM is associated with AIDS or another serious autoimmune disease. Resources that may help this required adjustment are psychological assistance from counselors, relatives and friends, and making contact with TM support groups.

Prognosis

Recovery depends on the general health status of the patient and is usually considered unlikely if no improvement is observed within three months.

See also Imaging studies; Lumbar puncture.

Resources

WEBSITES

Johns Hopkins Medicine. "What is Transverse Myelitis?" http://www.hopkinsmedicine.org/neurology_neurosurgery/centers_clinics/transverse_myelitis/about-tm/what-is-transverse-myelitis.html (accessed November 14, 2014).

Micromedex. "Transverse Myelitis." Mayo Clinic. http://www.mayoclinic.org/diseases-conditions/transverse-myelitis/basics/definition/con-20028884 (accessed November 14, 2014).

National Institute of Neurological Disorders and Stroke. "Transverse Myelitis Fact Sheet." http://www.ninds.nih.gov/disorders/transversemyelitis/detail_transversemyelitis.htm (accessed November 14, 2014).

ORGANIZATIONS

National Institute of Neurological Disorders and Stroke (NINDS), NIH Neurological Institute, PO Box 5801, Bethesda, MD 20824, (301) 496-5751, (800) 352-9424, http://www.ninds.nih.gov.

Transverse Myelitis Association, 1787 Sutter Parkway, Powell, OH 43065-8806, (614) 317-4884, (855) 380-3330, info@myelitis.org, https://myelitis.org.

Monique Laberge, PhD

Trastuzumab

Definition

Trastuzumab is an **immunotherapy** drug used in the treatment of **cancer**. It is formulated as a monoclonal antibody, a type of anti-tumor drug that works to slow or stop the growth of certain cancerous tumors by targeting a specific protein on the surface of the cancer cells.

Purpose

Trastuzumab is used to treat gastric cancers and breast cancers that have spread to other parts of the body

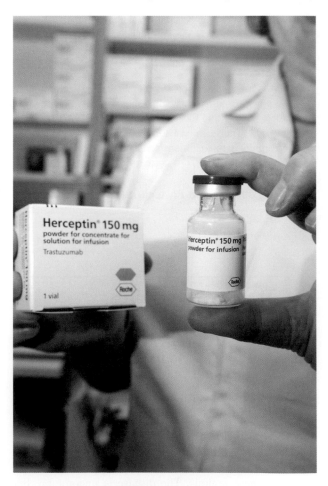

Trastuzumab (Herceptin). *(Gusto/Science Source)*

(metastasized). It is a form of targeted therapy used only in patients whose tumor cells produce an overabundance of a protein known as human epidermal growth factor receptor 2 (HER2). The primary function of trastuzumab is to attach to the epidermal growth factor receptor 2 on tumor cells to block their action in controlling cell growth and division in the tumor. Based on its main function, trastuzumab is known as an epidermal growth factor receptor antagonist.

Description

Trastuzumab (Herceptin, rhuMAb HER2) is an anti-tumor (antineoplastic) drug that works differently than **chemotherapy** or hormonal **anticancer drugs**. As a monoclonal antibody, it is genetically engineered in the laboratory from a single HER2-positive cell to target the HER2 receptors on cancer cell surfaces. Many different types of normal cells and cancer (malignant) cells have epidermal growth factor receptors on their cell surfaces. Epidermal growth factor attaches to epidermal growth factor receptors, producing new proteins that stimulate the cells to grow and divide. This is a natural process in the production and maintenance of normal cells; however, some malignant cells develop too many or overactive epidermal growth factor receptors. This overproduction of growth-regulating proteins in the cell results in the uncontrolled growth and division of malignant cells, which leads to tumor formation. Tumors made up of cells that have the HER2 antigens on their surfaces are known as HER2-positive tumors. The monoclonal antibody trastuzumab targets HER2-positive cancer cells that fuel cancer growth. It works by binding to the HER2 receptors to stop their activity and slow down or stop the cancer cell growth by signaling the cell not to grow and divide.

In addition, when trastuzumab attaches to cancer cell surfaces, it marks these cells, which helps natural killer cells of the immune system to recognize the cells as abnormal and kill them. This boost to the immune system also enhances the activity of first-line chemotherapy drugs. Although trastuzumab and chemotherapy work differently, they work synergistically when used together. Treatment with trastuzumab prevents intracellular DNA repair after the impact of DNA-damaging chemotherapy that stops the tumor cells from growing.

The American Cancer Society reports that approximately 25%–30% of patients who have gastric and breast cancers have higher than normal numbers of HER2 receptors on tumor cell surfaces, which leads the cells to produce too much of the protein and results in uncontrolled tumor growth. Therefore, HER2-positive tumors tend to grow faster and are more likely to recur. The amount of HER2 that is present in a tumor can be

---

measured in the clinical laboratory and only patients with high levels are expected to benefit from treatment with trastuzumab.

Recommended dosage

Trastuzumab is administered intravenously. The first dose is usually infused over 90 minutes to observe for any possible reactions and then it will be administered over a 30-minute period on a weekly basis in a hospital or clinic setting. Based on the patient's body weight, the typical dosage is 2–6 mg per kg of body weight (approximately 0.9–3.6 mg per lb.).

Precautions

Patients with allergies to any substances such as foods or medicines are advised to inform their doctors before beginning to take trastuzumab, because the drug itself is associated with allergic reactions. Patients with a history of (or who are being treated for) kidney or liver disease, heart disease, diabetes, gout or infection may require dosage adjustment for any related medications being taken. Patients who have had congestive heart failure or **radiation therapy** to the chest may be at increased risk of congestive heart failure while taking trastuzumab.

It is unknown whether trastuzumab is safe for women to take during pregnancy. Nonetheless, patients are advised to avoid becoming pregnant while they are taking trastuzumab. Mothers are advised not to breast-feed their babies while they are being treated with trastuzumab, or for at least six months after treatment, because the drug does pass into the breast milk. It is not known whether trastuzumab affects fertility.

Side effects

The two most serious side effects associated with the use of trastuzumab are related to heart and lung function. Damage to the heart muscle, which can lead to heart failure, and lung complications that may cause serious breathing problems, can occur. In both cases, immediate medical attention is required. Whether during or after treatment, patients experiencing difficulty breathing or any of the signs associated with heart failure, including shortness of breath, rapid heartbeat, or swelling in the feet or legs, are advised to contact their physicians as soon as symptoms are noticed. Cardiac side effects are more frequently experienced by older adult patients. Patients receiving trastuzumab are usually monitored carefully and screened prior to their treatment for any lung or heart problems. Treatment may sometimes be discontinued if signs and symptoms of heart or lung problems develop.

Trastuzumab is known to cause allergic reactions, especially with the first treatment. Most are mild, usually consisting of chills and **fever** and will occur less frequently as treatment progresses. However, some patients may have more severe allergic reactions such as low blood pressure, shortness of breath, rashes, and wheezing. These reactions are usually more common in patients who have already been diagnosed with lung disease.

Other common reactions include nausea, vomiting, **diarrhea**, dizziness, sleeplessness, appetite loss, cough, abdominal and back pain, headache, and sore throat. **Depression**, tingling in the hands or feet, fluid retention, sinus irritation, and flu-like symptoms are less commonly reported. Uncommon side effects are acne, cold sores, and urinary infection, as well as pain in the joints, bones, or nerves. Side effects may vary when trastuzumab is used with different chemotherapy agents, and may include reduced red blood cell count (**anemia**), reduced white blood cell count (leukopenia), diarrhea, and infection. Therefore, blood tests may be required more frequently for patients being treated with both trastuzumab and chemotherapy.

Clinical trials

Trastuzumab is being studied in **clinical trials** for its effectiveness in treating other types of cancer, including non-metastatic **breast cancer**, **ovarian cancer**, and cancers of the lung, colon, prostate, and bladder. Only patients with HER2-positive tumors are enrolled in the clinical trials. Researchers also continue to investigate the effectiveness of trastuzumab with and without different chemotherapy agents.

Interactions

Patients who take trastuzumab in combination with anthracycline chemotherapy (i.e., **doxorubicin**, **daunorubicin**, **epirubicin**, or **mitoxantrone**) have a greater risk of heart problems. Patients are advised to discuss any medications they are taking (over-the-counter, herbal, and prescription) with their physician so that an assessment can be made regarding the risk of interactions.

See also Epidermal growth factor receptor antagonists; Immunotherapy.

Resources

PERIODICALS

Satoh, T., Y. J. Bang, and E. A. Gotovkin, et al. "Quality of Life in the Trastuzumab for Gastric Cancer Trial." *The Oncologist* 19 (Jul 2014): 712–719.

Untch, M., P. A. Fasching, and G. E. Konecny, et al. "Pathologic Complete Response After Neoadjuvant Chemotherapy Plus Trastuzumab Predicts Favorable Survival in Human Epidermal Growth Factor Receptor 2-Overexpressing Breast Cancer: Results From the TECHNO Trial of the AGO and GBG Study Groups." *Journal of Clinical Oncology* 29 (Sept 2011): 3351-3357.

Won, E., Y. J. Janjigian, and D. H. Ilson. "HER2 Directed Therapy for Gastric/Esophageal Cancers." *Current treatment Options in Oncology* 15 (Sept 2014): 395–404.

WEBSITES

American Cancer Society. "Trastuzumab." http://www.cancer.org/treatment/treatmentsandsideeffects/guidetocancerdrugs/trastuzumab (accessed October 12, 2014).

ORGANIZATIONS

American Cancer Society, 1599 Clifton Rd., NE, Atlanta GA 30329, (404) 320-3333, (800) ACS-2345, http://www.cancer.org.

National Cancer Institute Public Inquiries Office, 6116 Executive Boulevard, Room 3036A, Bethesda, MD 20892-8322, (800) 4-CANCER (422-6237), http://www.cancer.gov.

L. Lee Culvert
Lee Ann Paradise

Treanda *see* **Bendamustine hydrochloride**

Tretinoin

Definition

Tretinoin, a natural vitamin A metabolite, is an anticancer drug used in the treatment of acute promyelocytic leukemia (APL). Tretinoin is more commonly used to treat such skin disorders as acne, warts, hyperpigmentation, and reactions to sunlight.

Purpose

Tretinoin is given to APL patients with the goal of bringing on a remission. The drug is being investigated as a treatment for **skin cancer**, and it is also available in an acne cream commonly called Retin-A.

Tretinoin has also being investigated as a possible chemopreventive for **breast cancer**.

Description

Tretinoin causes abnormal leukemia cells in the blood to mature into normal cells (granulocytes). The exact mechanism of action is not known. In **clinical trials** 72%–94% of APL patients experienced a complete remission when taking this drug. Tretinoin can be used to induce remission and to maintain remission.

Recommended dosage

The recommended dosage for adults with APL is 45 milligrams per square meter taken by mouth as two evenly divided doses. The physician will calculate the specific dose for each patient. The drug should be discontinued 30 days after remission or 90 days after treatment begins, whichever comes first.

Precautions

Patients who are hypersensitive to vitamin A or other retinoids should not take this drug. People should avoid tretinoin if they are sensitive to parabens, a preservative used in the drug's capsule. Pregnant or breast-feeding women should not take tretinoin. Women of childbearing age should take a pregnancy test to assure that they are not pregnant prior to starting this drug.

Side effects

Tretinoin has a number of side effects. Patients should discuss the risk of complications with their physician. Some side effects resemble symptoms that are common in APL patients. All side effects should be reported to a patient's doctor.

Side effects that are more commonly reported include headache, **fever**, dry skin and mucous membranes, **bone pain**, rash, **itching**, inflamed lips, sweating, **nausea and vomiting**, abdominal pain, **diarrhea**, constipation, indigestion, bloating, irregular heart beat, visual disturbances, earache, hair loss (**alopecia**), skin changes (including formation of inflammatory growths known as granulomas), vision changes, and bone inflammation.

Hemorrhage is a life-threatening complication. Blood coagulation studies are done while the patient is taking the drug to monitor the risk of hemorrhage. Hepatitis is another life-threatening side effect. Liver function tests can be abnormal in 50%–60% of patients taking the drug. Liver function is monitored periodically while a person is taking the drug.

In addition, approximately one-quarter of patients taking tretinoin develop retinoic-acid-APL (RA-APL) syndrome. Symptoms include fever, weight gain, difficulty breathing, and other respiratory disorders. Some patients have cardiac changes and low blood pressure as part of this syndrome. The syndrome can occur two days after treatment begins or three to four weeks later. Symptoms must be reported to the patient's physician immediately so that treatment can begin. In rare cases this syndrome is fatal. Most patients do not need to stop taking tretinoin if the syndrome develops.

Approximately 40% of patients taking tretinoin develop high white blood cell counts (leukocytosis). If the number of white blood cells increases rapidly there is a higher chance of developing life-threatening complications. White blood cell counts are monitored during treatment. As many as 60% of patients taking tretinoin develop increased cholesterol and triglyceride levels. The levels drop when the medication is stopped. Cholesterol and triglyceride levels are monitored while the drug is being taken.

Tretinoin has other side effects that may impact the heart, skin, digestive tract, lungs, central nervous system, and other parts of the body. Patients should report all unusual symptoms to the doctor immediately.

Interactions

Tretinoin interacts with:

- Cimetidine (antipeptic ulcer drug)
- Cyclosporine (immunosuppressant)
- Diltiazem (heart medication)
- Erythromycin (antibiotic)
- Glucocorticoids (steroids)
- Ketoconazole (antifungal drug)
- Phenobarbital (sedative/hypnotic)
- Pentobarbital (sedative/hypnotic)
- Rifampicin (an antituberculosis drug, also known as rifampin)
- Verapamil (heart medication)

See also Acute myelocytic leukemia; Antineoplastic agents.

Resources

BOOKS

Beers, Mark H., MD, and Robert Berkow, MD, editors. "Acne." In *The Merck Manual of Diagnosis and Therapy*. Whitehouse Station, NJ: Merck Research Laboratories, 2007.

Beers, Mark H., MD, and Robert Berkow, MD, editors. "Warts (Verrucae)." In *The Merck Manual of Diagnosis and Therapy*. Whitehouse Station, NJ: Merck Research Laboratories, 2007.

Wilson, Billie Ann, Margaret T. Shannon, and Carolyn L. Stang. *Nurse's Drug Guide 2003*. Upper Saddle River, NJ: Prentice Hall, 2003.

PERIODICALS

Halder, R. M., and G. M. Richards. "Topical Agents Used in the Management of Hyperpigmentation." *Skin Therapy Letter*9 (June-July 2004): 1–3.

Kligman, D. E., and Z. D. Draelos. "High-Strength Tretinoin for Rapid Retinization of Photoaged Facial Skin." *Dermatologic Surgery*30 (June 2004): 864–866.

Simeone, A. M., and A. M. Tari. "How Retinoids Regulate Breast Cancer Cell Proliferation and Apoptosis." *Cellular and Molecular Life Sciences*61 (June 2004): 1475–1484.

Teknetsis, A., D. Ioannides, G. Vakali, et al. "Pyogenic Granulomas Following Topical Application of Tretinoin." *Journal of the European Academy of Dermatology and Venereology*18 (May 2004): 337–339.

ORGANIZATIONS

ASHP (formerly the American Society of Health-System Pharmacists), 7272 Wisconsin Ave., Bethesda, MD 20814, (301) 664-8700, (866) 279-0681, custserv@ashp.org, http://www.ashp.org.

U.S. Food and Drug Administration, 10903 New Hampshire Ave., Silver Spring, MD 20993, (888) INFO-FDA (463-6332), http://www.fda.gov.

Rhonda Cloos, R.N.
Rebecca J. Frey, PhD

Trichilemmal carcinoma

Definition

Trichilemmal **carcinoma** is an uncommon malignant tumor of the hair follicle, and is assumed to be the malignant counterpart of the benign trichilemmoma.

Description

Trichilemmal carcinomas most often occur on part of the skin that has been often exposed to the sun, like the face. The tumors look like tan or flesh-colored spots. They can resemble warts and sometimes have a hair in them. Usually, a trichilemmal carcinoma will occur as an isolated lesion.

Trichilemmal carcinomas are thought to be the malignant form of the non-cancerous tumors called trichilemmomas, which are seen in Cowden syndrome. Cowden syndrome is an inherited disorder that predisposes individuals to breast and **thyroid cancer**. The disease is inherited in an autosomal dominant inheritance pattern. With autosomal dominant inheritance, men and women are equally likely to inherit the syndrome. In addition, children of individuals with the disease are at 50% risk of inheriting it. **Genetic testing** is available for Cowden syndrome, but due to the complexity, genetic counseling should be considered before testing. Although they are thought to be related to trichilemmomas, none of the reports of trichilemmal carcinomas have been seen in patients with Cowden syndrome.

It is important to note that trichilemmal carcinoma is not the same as "malignant proliferating trichilemmal tumor," which is usually seen on the scalp and the back of the neck.

Demographics

Trichilemmal carcinomas are most often seen in older people. They occur with equal frequency in both males and females.

Causes and symptoms

The causes of trichilemmal carcinoma are unknown. The only recognizable symptom is the presence of an unusual, tan or flesh-colored spot on the skin.

Diagnosis

Diagnosis of a trichilemmal carcinoma is very important. Because the tumors are so rare, a physician may not immediately recognize its exact diagnosis. A dermatologist will suspect an abnormality on the skin and have it removed. It is only on the pathologic examination (when a physician examines the abnormality under a microscope) that the tumor can be correctly classified.

Treatment team

The treatment of trichilemmal carcinoma will involve a dermatologist (a physician who specializes in diseases of the skin) and a surgeon (a physician who will surgically remove the tumor).

Treatment

Once a trichilemmal carcinoma has been diagnosed, a surgeon must remove it. It is necessary that documented clear margins are obtained, indicating that the entire tumor has been removed. There is a chance that the tumor will recur (return) locally (in the same spot or near the same spot). If this occurs, the recurrent tumor needs to be surgically removed as well. It is very unlikely that a trichilemmal carcinoma will metastasize (spread to other parts of the body), and further treatment with **chemotherapy** is not needed.

Alternative and complementary therapies

Because trichilemmal carcinoma is easily treated with removal, there are no suggested alterative and/or complementary therapies.

Coping with cancer treatment

The surgical procedure to remove a trichilemmal carcinoma is relatively straightforward and low-risk. Most surgeries will be done on an outpatient basis, requiring no stay in the hospital. A small scar on the skin may be left after the tumor is removed.

Clinical trials

No **clinical trials** for trichilemmal carcinoma could be identified.

Prevention

Because the underlying cause of trichilemmal carcinoma is largely unknown, preventive strategies have not been suggested.

Resources

PERIODICALS

Hamman, M.S., Brian Jiang SI. "Management of Trichilemmal Carcinoma: An Update and Comprehensive Review of the Literature." *Dermatologic Surgery* 40, no. 7 (2014): 711–7. http://www.ncbi.nlm.nih.gov/pubmed/25111341 (accessed November 14, 2014).

Kulahci, Y., Oksuz, S., Kucukodaci, Z., Uygur, F., Ulkur, E. "Multiple Recurrence of Trichilemmal Carcinoma of the Scalp in a Young Adult." *Dermatologic Surgery* 36, no. 4 (2010): 551–4. http://onlinelibrary.wiley.com/doi/10.1111/j.1524-4725.2010.01498.x/abstract (accessed November 14, 2014).

Peryassú, B.C., Peryassú, R.C., Peryassú, M.A., Maceira, J.P., Ramos-E-Silva, M. "Trichilemmal Carcinoma–a Rare Tumor: Case Report." *Acta Dermatovenerologica Croatica* 16, no. 1 (2008): 28–30. http://www.ncbi.nlm.nih.gov/pubmed/18358106 (accessed November 14, 2014).

Kristen Mahoney Shannon, M.S., C.G.C.

Trimethoprim *see* **Antibiotics**

Trimetrexate

Definition

Trimetrexate (Neutrexin) is a drug that was first used to treat bacterial infections, and is now being investigated as a treatment for several different cancers.

Purpose

Trimetrexate is most commonly used to treat **pneumonia** in patients with acquired immunodeficiency syndrome (AIDS); however, it was recently discovered that the drug was able to kill a variety of different **cancer** cells. As a result, trimetrexate is now considered to be an investigational drug for cancer treatment.

Ongoing **clinical trials** are using trimetrexate to treat a number of cancers including advanced colon and rectal cancers, advanced **pancreatic cancer**, and advanced squamous cell cancers of the head and neck. Results from many trials are still preliminary, but trimetrexate appears to be most promising as a treatment for advanced colon and rectal cancers.

Description

Trimetrexate glucoronate works by stopping cells from using **folic acid** (vitamin B9). As a result, cells cannot make essential components they need to survive, and they die. Because trimetrexate is toxic to both cancer cells and healthy cells, it is always used in combination with **leucovorin** (Wellcovorin, citrovorum factor). Leucovorin is a drug that protects healthy cells from the harmful effects of certain types of **chemotherapy**.

Trimetrexate can also enhance the anti-cancer effect of another chemotherapy drug called **fluorouracil** (Adrusil, 5-FU). Fluorouracil is frequently used to treat patients with colon and rectal cancers.

Recommended dosage

In clinical trials, patients with colon and rectal cancers were given trimetrexate, fluorouracil, and leucovorin for eight-week cycles. A cycle consisted of six weeks of treatment followed by two weeks rest with no treatment. Patients received trimetrexate intravenously, with the dose depending on their weight. Twenty-four hours after trimetrexate treatment, patients received intravenous fluorouracil and leucovorin treatment. Some patients also took oral leucovorin every six hours for several days after their intravenous chemotherapy.

Patients with squamous cell cancer of the head and neck received trimetrexate in combination with **cisplatin** (Platinol), leucovorin, and fluorouracil in a 21-day cycle. These patients also received surgery or **radiation therapy**. Pancreatic cancer patients received eight-week cycles of trimetrexate, fluorouracil, and leucovorin, similar to that given to patients with **colon cancer**.

Precautions

Patients who are given oral leucovorin as part of their chemotherapy must take their medication.

Trimetrexate is a toxic drug, and patients who do not take leucovorin may experience severe side effects. Pregnant women should not take trimetrexate because it may harm the fetus. Women who are taking trimetrexate should avoid becoming pregnant. In addition, women should not breast feed while taking this drug. The liver and kidney are used to break down and eliminate trimetrexate from the body. As a result, patients with a history of liver or kidney disease should tell their doctor.

Side effects

Patients taking trimetrexate will have their blood monitored regularly to check for the development of **myelosuppression**. Myelosuppression is a condition where a patient's bone marrow makes fewer blood cells and platelets than normal. As a result of this condition, patients have an increased risk of infection, may bleed more, and may experience symptoms of **anemia**. Trimetrexate may also cause damage to the kidneys and the liver. Some patients also experience **nausea and vomiting**, and may develop a rash or inflammation and sores in their mouths. Taking leucovorin with trimetrexate helps to reduce or eliminate the risk of experiencing many of these side effects.

Interactions

Trimetrexate is known to interact with several other drugs. Some antifungal drugs such as ketoconazole (Nizoral) and fluconazole (Diflucan) interfere with the way the body breaks down trimetrexate. The antibiotic erythromycin also has this effect. Patients taking these drugs will be monitored carefully. The toxic effects of trimetrexate can be increased by other drugs. Patients should therefore tell their doctor about any medication they are taking whether it is prescription or over the counter.

Resources

BOOKS

Chu, Edward, and Vincent T. DeVita Jr. *Physicians' Cancer Chemotherapy Drug Manual 2014.* Burlington, MA: Jones & Bartlett Learning, 2014.

WEBSITES

AHFS Consumer Medication Information. "Trimetrexate Glucuronate." American Society of Health-System Pharmacists. Available from: http://www.nlm.nih.gov/medlineplus/druginfo/meds/a694019.html (accessed November 14, 2014).

Alison McTavish, M.S.

Triple negative breast cancer

Definition

Triple negative **breast cancer** (TNBC) is breast **cancer** in which the abnormal cells have neither estrogen receptors, progesterone receptors, or excess HER2 protein on their surfaces. TNBC is an aggressive form of breast cancer that is more difficult to treat than other types. Also called triple-negative phenotype, the formal name for TNBC is estrogen receptor (ER)-negative, progesterone receptor (PR)-negative, and HER2-negative invasive breast cancer.

Description

TNBC is an invasive ductal **carcinoma** that originates in the lining of the milk ducts. It is estimated that 65%–90% of TNBC cases are of a subtype called basal-like, meaning that the cells resemble the basal cells that line the ducts and normally give rise to mature glandular breast cells. TNBC tends to grow and spread (metastasize) more quickly than other types of breast cancer. When staged, basal-like cancers tend to be more aggressive and of a higher grade—i.e., larger tumor, more lymph nodes involved, and more advanced **metastasis**.

Estrogen and progesterone bind to hormone receptors, signaling the cells to grow. About 75% of breast cancers have cells with estrogen receptors and about 65% have cells with both estrogen and progesterone receptors. Hormone therapies such as **tamoxifen** or **aromatase inhibitors** block these receptors, halting the growth of breast cancer cells. About 20%–30% of breast cancer cells have excess HER2 on their surface and certain drugs such as **trastuzumab** (Herceptin) and **lapatinib** (Tukerb) target HER2, preventing the cancer cells from growing. However, the HER2-negative cells of TNBC may not respond to medications that target HER2. In addition, since TNBC lacks hormone receptors, targeted hormone therapies such as tamoxifen and anastrozole are ineffective against TNBC, making this cancer especially difficult to treat.

Risk factors

The lifetime risk of developing breast cancer is 12% in the United States and the greatest risk is in women aged 60 and older. About 5% of women have a mutation in one of the breast cancer genes (*BRCA1* and *BRCA2*) and women who inherit the *BRCA1* gene mutation are at an increased risk for TNBC. The *BRCA* genes were originally discovered by studying gene mutations in families with a history of early-onset breast cancer, especially among Ashkenazi Jews. Having a first degree rclative with breast cancer may double a woman's risk, and two or more first degree relatives with breast cancer may increase that risk by five times. However, many women with TNBC have no family history of breast cancer. Studies have suggested that women who breast-feed for six months or longer reduce their risk of TNBC.

Lifestyle factors that may increase the risk of breast cancer include:

- having taken birth control pills
- obesity
- gaining weight after menopause, especially after natural menopause or age 60
- excess alcohol consumption
- synthetic hormone-replacement therapy after menopause.

Demographics

Breast cancer is the second most commonly diagnosed cancer among women and the second leading cause of cancer death in women after lung cancer. Among 232,000 new cases of breast cancer diagnosed in the United States in 2013, about 40,000 deaths were recorded. About 10%–20% of all diagnosed breast cancers are TNBC. Only about one-third of breast cancers have cells that lack receptors for both of the female hormones, estrogen and progesterone. One in five breast cancers produces excess human epidermal growth factor receptor 2 (HER2) and the rest are different phenotypes, including HER-2 negative.

TNBC is more likely to occur in women younger than age 40–50, while other breast cancers commonly develop in women aged 60 and older. TNBC is also more commonly diagnosed in women of African descent and in young Hispanic women than it is in Asian and non-Hispanic white women. The incidence of TNBC among African American women has helped to explain, in part, the longstanding observation that African American women are significantly more likely to die of breast cancer than white American women.

Causes and symptoms

The exact cause of TNBC is unknown but the disease is believed to stem from a combination of genetic and environmental factors. Most breast cancers in older women appear to be related to long-term exposure of cells to estrogen. Both genetic and environmental factors influence the amount of estrogen a woman produces, how the estrogen is metabolized, and how many years the breast tissue is exposed to high levels of estrogen. Early-onset menstruation and late-onset menopause increase lifetime exposure and pregnancy and breastfeeding decrease exposure. In addition, two major pathways are associated with the metabolism of estrogen—one leads to a metabolite that increases the risk of breast cancer and the other leads to a metabolite that may actually reduce the risk. Heredity and dietary factors may influence which metabolic pathway is utilized.

Early-stage breast cancer has few symptoms and the early symptoms of TNBC are the same as for other breast cancers:

- a thickening or lump in the breast or underarm
- a change in the size, shape, contour, or feel of the breast, nipple, or areola—the dark area surrounding the nipple
- a change in the appearance of the breast skin or nipple, such as a puckering or dimpling, ridges or pitting, crustiness or scaliness
- nipple tenderness or discharge
- a nipple that is pulled back or inverted

Diagnosis

Breast examination

Most breast cancers, including TNBC, are first detected by screening during:

- a self-examination
- an annual clinical breast exam by a healthcare professional
- an annual or biennial screening mammogram or x-rays of the breasts, which can detect cancers that are too small to feel.

Diagnostic tests

A variety of clinical laboratory tests may be performed, including blood tests and breast tissue cell differentiation, to diagnose and stage breast cancer. For TNBC, the most important tests are those for the presence of estrogen and progesterone receptors and excess HER2. Diagnosis is confirmed by **biopsy** of breast tissue. Cancer cells removed during a biopsy or surgery are evaluated by **immunohistochemistry** (IHC) staining and microscopic evaluation by a pathologist. The IHC staining test uses specific antibodies that bind to estrogen or progesterone receptors to stain the cells and allow microscopic detection. Positive test results for TNBC will indicate the complete absence of both estrogen and progesterone receptors, which will rule out hormone therapy as treatment. IHC staining using specific antibodies that bind to HER2 is used to measure the amount of HER2. The IHC test is scored from 0 to 3+ to indicate amount. If the IHC result is 0 or 1+, the cancer is HER2-negative. Test results of 2+ are considered inconclusive and HER2 is re-measured by fluorescent in situ hybridization (FISH), a more sensitive test. Excess HER2 is caused by extra HER2 genes in cancer cells. FISH uses fluorescence-labeled pieces of DNA that bind to these genes so that they can be counted under the microscope. Various other genetic tests also may be performed on biopsied cancer cells.

Imaging studies

Imaging studies are performed to determine the size of the tumor and whether it has spread to the lymph nodes or other parts of the body. These scanning procedures may include:

• diagnostic mammograms

• magnetic resonance imaging (MRI)

• ultrasound

• a ductogram if nipple discharge is present

Positron emission tomography (PET) scanning may be undertaken if biopsy or other scans indicate spreading of the cancer to lymph nodes or distant sites. Prior to a PET scan, the patient is injected with a type of sugar and a radioactive material; cancer cells will absorb more of this radioactive sugar than normal cells. Suspicious areas of cell growth in lymph nodes or organs anywhere in the body will be highlighted in the PET images, helping radiologists to identify possible cancer sites. PET scans are not used for breast cancer screening, only for evaluating cancer spread in patients once they have been diagnosed.

Clinical staging

Staging of TNBC is based on the results of imaging examinations and biopsies. It applies the TNM (T = tumor, N = lymph nodes, M = metastasis or degree of spread) classification system, which adds TNM numerical scores from 0 to 3 to the four stages (I to IV) of the cancer to designate the grade of the disease. The four stages include:

• Stage O: cancer cells are within a duct and have not invaded surrounding fatty breast tissue (T0, N0, M0).

• Stages I, II, and III may include a tumor of any size (T1, 2 or 3) and will be graded based on whether the cancer has spread to the lymph nodes near the breast and how many nodes are involved (N0 to N3) or to the chest wall and skin (M0 to M2).

• Stage IV: the tumor is advanced (T3) and has spread to more distant lymph nodes (N2 to N3) and other organs (M2 to M3) distant from the breast. The different stages and grades help the oncologist determine the appropriate type and timing of treatment.

Treatment

Although TNBC tends to be more aggressive than other types of breast cancer, it is not necessarily treated more aggressively. For example, a diagnosis of triple-negative breast cancer does not necessarily result in a **mastectomy** rather than a **lumpectomy**. For stage I or stage II TNBC, in which the cancer has not spread to the lymph nodes, the tumor tissue is surgically removed, followed by **chemotherapy** and often localized **radiation therapy** directed at the cancer site. Metastatic TNBC is almost always treated with a combination of surgery, chemotherapy, and radiation therapy.

Surgery

Surgery is the first-line approach to treating TNBC; the type of surgery depends upon the stage and grade of the cancer. Lumpectomy or breast-conserving surgery may be performed to remove only the tumor and a small amount of surrounding tissue. Lumpectomy with radiation is considered to be as effective as mastectomy if the cancer is smaller and limited to only one site in the breast. Mastectomy removes all breast tissue except the muscles under the breast. A lumpectomy or mastectomy may include lymph node removal if a biopsy indicates that the cancer has spread beyond the milk duct. **Breast reconstruction** is performed to rebuild the breast after mastectomy and occasionally even after a lumpectomy. The reconstruction is often performed at the same time as the cancer is removed or later.

Chemotherapy

TNBC often responds better to chemotherapy than hormone receptor-positive breast cancer. Some women with TNBC benefit from receiving primary systemic (neo-adjuvant) chemotherapy prior to surgery. This treatment sometimes eradicates all signs of cancer even though surgery will still be performed to ensure the removal of all cancerous tissue. Some of the chemotherapy drugs used to treat breast cancer include **bevacizumab**, **capecitabine**, **cisplatin**, cyclophosphamide, doxorubicin, exemestane, **gemcitabine**, ixabepilone, letrozole, paclitaxel and tras-tuzumab. Combining anticancer agents is sometimes more effective in treating TNBC. Specific combinations include:

• gemcitabine and carboplatin

• ACT—doxorubicin (Adriamycin), cyclophosphamide, and paclitaxel (Taxol)

• carboplatin and cisplatin for metastatic TNBC

Targeted therapy to block the growth and spread of cancer involves the use of drugs that are synthetic immune system proteins. These drugs target the cancer cells directly and therefore do not harm normal cells. Trastuzumab (Herceptin), for example, is targeted at the HER2 gene in the cancer cells of TNBC. Bevacizumab (Avastin) inhibits a growth-inducing protein called vascular endothelial growth factor (VEGF) and it blocks blood vessel growth to tumors to deplete the cancer cells of nutrients. The anti-leukemia drug **dasatinib** targets enzymes called src kinases that transmit growth and survival signals to tumor cells. These enzymes are overproduced in many types of cancer, including some types of TNBC. TNBC tumor cells often display high levels of epidermal growth factor receptor (EGFR), which may help the cells grow. Drugs such as **cetuximab**, which is used to treat metastatic colorectal cancer, block EGFR and may also be useful against metastatic TNBC. It is important to note that researchers are finding that targeted therapies are not as effective alone as they are in combination with certain chemotherapy agents. HER-2 negative tumors have shown sensitivity to anthracycline-based chemotherapy and related drugs are being studied in TNBC patients.

Immunotherapy is a form of targeted therapy that is designed to activate immune system cells to fight the cancer. **Monoclonal antibodies** are immune system proteins that can be directed to attack a specific part of a cancer cell. **Cancer vaccines** are also in process of development to trigger an **immune response** against the cancer. Other immunotherapies such as interleukins and **interferons** that normally occur as cytokines in immune system cells, boost the immune system in a more general way to increase activity against cancer cells.

Prognosis

Breast cancers without estrogen and progesterone receptors have a poorer prognosis than cancers that are ER+ and PR+ and basal-like tumors have a poorer prognosis than non-basal cell tumors. TNBC also is more likely than other breast cancers to invade other parts of the body. However the majority of women with stage I or stage II TNBC that has not yet spread to distant areas are cancer-free for many years following treatment and many patients with stage III or stage IV lymph-node-positive TNBC also respond well to chemotherapy. Studies conducted in patients with TNBC and other subtypes of breast cancer indicate that patients who have a pathologic complete response to neoadjuvant chemotherapy have a good prognosis, regardless of the molecular subtype of the cancer. Basal-like tumors have a significantly higher rate of distant lymph node involvement, which is associated with a poorer prognosis.

Five-year-survival rates tend to be lower for TNBC than for non-TNBC disease, but the rate of death after five years is no greater than that of other breast cancer

patients. Studies of women with all stages of breast cancer found that 77% with TNBC survived for five years, compared with 93% of women with other types of breast cancer. TNBC is more likely than other breast cancers to recur after treatment. Disease recurrence within five years is about 32% for TNBC compared with only about 15% for other types of breast cancer. The average length of survival after recurrence is 7 to 13 months compared to more than 20 months for patients with non-TNBC; the risk of recurrence is greatest in the first few years after treatment. Studies indicate that TNBC is more likely to recur outside of the breasts only in the first three years following treatment; after three years, the risk of recurrence is similar to that of other breast cancers.

Coping with cancer treatment

Sufficient rest and good nutrition are important for relieving the side effects of treatment for breast cancer. A healthy, low-fat diet, regular exercise, and limited alcohol consumption are important to maximize the effectiveness of breast cancer treatment. Support groups may be helpful to deal with the emotional effects of treatment.

Clinical trials

Researchers are investigating chemotherapeutic agents and combinations of chemotherapy agents that may be more effective in the treatment of TNBC. In early clinical studies, a potent oral poly (ADP-ribose) polymerase (PARP) inhibitor called olaparib given in combination with paclitaxel has shown an encouraging response rate in treating TNBC; however, further study of dosing was indicated and **clinical trials** for olaparib are still underway. Ongoing efforts are underway to define appropriate targets for directed TNBC-specific therapy, including microRNA-200b, which has been shown to suppress TNBC metastasis. The **National Cancer Institute** and other cancer organizations will often help patients and their families find suitable clinical trials.

Prevention

Genetic testing is available for identifying BRCA mutations that increase the risk of TNBC. Since early detection is very important for the prognosis of TNBC and other breast cancers, women with a *BRCA* mutation should use augmented breast cancer surveillance techniques:

• monthly breast self-examinations beginning at age 18
• clinical breast examinations performed by a physician or nurse breast specialist every 6–12 months beginning at age 18

- mammograms every 6–12 months, beginning at age 25–35, or at least five years before the youngest age that breast cancer was diagnosed in a family member

Mammograms do not detect some breast cancers, especially in younger women such as those who are at risk due to *BRCA* mutations.

Risk-reducing, prophylactic or preventive mastectomy—the removal of the breasts and as much at-risk tissue as possible—in healthy women with a *BRCA* mutation reduces the risk of breast cancer by 90%. However, it is not clear whether women undergoing this procedure are at any less risk of dying from breast cancer than are women who use careful surveillance methods.

Resources

BOOKS

Hirshaut, Yashar, and Peter I. Pressman. *Breast Cancer: The Complete Guide*. 5th ed. New York: Bantam, 2008.

Miller, Kenneth D. *Choices in Breast Cancer Treatment: Medical Specialists and Cancer Survivors Tell You What You Need to Know*. Baltimore: Johns Hopkins University Press, 2008.

PERIODICALS

Bauer, K. R., et al. "Descriptive Analysis of Estrogen Receptor (ER)-Negative, Progesterone Receptor (PR)-Negative, and HER2-Negative Invasive Breast Cancer, the So-Called Triple-Negative Phenotype: A Population-Based Study from the California Cancer Registry." *Cancer* 109, no. 9 (May 1, 2007): 1721–28.

Dent, Rebecca A., et al. "Phase I Trial of the Oral PARP Inhibitor Olaparib in Combination with Paclitaxel for First- or Second-Line Treatment of Patients with Metastatic Triple-Negative Breast Cancer." *Breast Cancer Research* 15 (May 2013): R88.

Humphries, B., et al. "MicroRNA-200b Targets Protein Kinase C-Alpha and Suppresses Triple Negative Breast Cancer Metastasis." *Carcinogenesis* 35, no. 10 (2014): 2254–63.

Kennecke, H., et al. "Metastatic Behavior of Breast Cancer Subtypes." *Journal of Clinical Oncology* 28 (2010): 3271–77.

Köster, Frank, et al. "Triple-Negative Breast Cancers Express Receptors for Growth Hormone-Releasing Hormone (GHRH) and Respond to GHRH Antagonists with Growth Inhibition." *Breast Cancer Research and Treatment* 116, no. 2 (July 2009): 273–79.

Miyoshi, Y., et al. "Predictive Factors for Anthracycline-Based Chemotherapy for Human Breast Cancer." *Breast Cancer* 17 (April 2010): 103–9.

Viale, Giuseppe, et al. "Invasive Ductal Carcinoma of the Breast with the 'Triple-Negative' Phenotype: Prognostic Implications of EGFR Immunoreactivity." *Breast Cancer Research and Treatment* 116, no. 2 (July 2009): 317–28.

WEBSITES

American Cancer Society. "What Is Breast Cancer?" http://www.cancer.org/docroot/CRI/content/CRI_2_4_1X_What_is_breast_cancer_5.asp (accessed December 17, 2014).

Lebrasseur, Nicole, and Heather L. Van Epps. "Targeting the Triple Threat." CureToday. http://www.curetoday.com/index.cfm/fuseaction/article.show/id/2/article_id/1235 (accessed December 17, 2014).

"Triple-Negative Breast Cancer." Breastcancer.org. http://www.breastcancer.org/symptoms/diagnosis/trip_neg/ (accessed December 17, 2014).

ORGANIZATIONS

American Cancer Society, 1599 Clifton Road NE, Atlanta, GA 30329-4251, (800) ACS-2345, http://www.cancer.org.

Breakthrough Breast Cancer, Weston House, 246 High Holborn, London, England WC1V 7EX, 020 7025 2400, 08080 100 200, Fax: 020 7025 2401, info@breakthrough.org.uk, http://breakthrough.org.uk/.

Breastcancer.org, 7 East Lancaster Avenue, Third Floor, Ardmore, PA 19003, http://www.breastcancer.org.

National Cancer Institute, NCI Public Inquiries Office, 6116 Executive Boulevard, Room 3036A, Bethesda, MD 20006, (800) 4-CANCER, http://www.cancer.gov.

Triple Negative Breast Cancer Foundation, PO Box 204, Norwood, NJ 07648, (646) 942-0242, (877) 870-TNBC (8622), info@tnbcfoundation.org, http://www.tnbcfoundation.org.

L. Lee Culvert

REVISED BY MARGARET ALIC, PhD
REVIEWED BY MELINDA GRANGER OBERLEITNER, RN, DNS, APRN, CNS

Triptorelin pamoate

Definition

Triptorelin pamoate is a synthetic luteinizing hormone-releasing hormone (LHRH) agonist, which is a substance that reduces the level of sexual hormones in the system.

Purpose

Since its approval by the FDA (Food and Drug Administration) in June of 2000, triptorelin pamoate has been recognized as a successful option in the treatment of long-term **cancer** of the prostate gland. The prostate gland is a solid, chestnut-shaped organ surrounding the male urethra. It produces secretions that become part of seminal fluid. In the case of cancer of the prostate gland, it is advantageous to reduce prostate gland cell activity. One way to do this is to reduce the amount of hormones circulating in the system that will stimulate prostate activity. LHRH-agonists, such as triptorelin, are indicated when either **orchiectomy** (surgical removal of one of both testes) or the administration of the female hormone estrogen is either inadvisable or considered unacceptable by the person suffering from the cancer.

Triptorelin pamoate has been successfully used to alleviate symptoms in cases of such advanced **prostate cancer**, and is now being used and researched as a treatment for:

- all prostate cancers
- ovarian cancer
- *in vitro* fertilization
- endometriosis, or chronic disease of the mucous membrane lining the uterus
- uterine leiomyoma, also called uterine fibroids, a non-cancerous growth on the smooth muscle of the uterine wall
- precocious puberty, a condition in which children of either sex may undergo pubescent changes at an abnormally early age
- fibrocystic breast disease, or the presence of one or more benign tumors in the breast

Description

The human body provides balance in the provision of all chemicals necessary to its function. The pituitary gland and hypothalamus in the brain interact to release substances called gonadotropins, which trigger and regulate the production of estrogen (female) and androgen (male) hormones. Synthetic LHRH medications (similar in chemical makeup to natural LHRH enzymes) reduce the quantity of natural gonadotropins released. This reduces cell activity occurring in organs affected by these hormones, such as the prostate gland, ovaries, testes, uterus, and breasts, therefore slowing the growth of cancerous cells.

Triptorelin is a potent synthetic LHRH medication, effectively reducing gonadotropins if administered to maintain a continuous, therapeutic level in the body. Initially, there is often a temporary surge in circulating amounts of both male and female hormones, but usually within two to four weeks of beginning therapy, there is a marked reduction of these sex hormones. In men, there is a reduction in **testosterone** in the blood stream comparable to the level usually seen in surgically castrated men. Consequently, cells that rely upon these hormones for stimulation become less active. In most cases, the effect of triptorelin pamoate on sexual hormones is reversible once treatment is completed.

Recommended dosage

For advanced prostate cancer, the most common application for triptorelin, the usual dose is 3.75 milligrams (mg) given once per month as a single intramuscular injection. This will normally maintain a therapeutic level. If necessary, this medication may also be given intravenously.

Precautions

In the treatment of prostate cancer, there have been reported flare-ups of the disease at the onset of therapy. Patients with a prostate tumor affecting the spinal cord or urinary flow should use caution, as an increase in tumor activity may initially worsen symptoms. Triptorelin pamoate is capable of causing harm to fetuses if administered to pregnant women. During long-term treatment of endometriosis or uterine fibroids, bone loss has been reported.

Side effects

The following side effects have either been reported or were observed:

- nausea and vomiting
- hot flashes
- vaginal dryness
- impotence
- loss of sex drive
- breakthrough bleeding
- sleep disturbance
- diarrhea
- fatigue
- hair loss (alopecia)
- mouth sores
- breast tenderness
- weight gain
- pain at injection site
- increases in cholesterol
- headache

Interactions

Because triptorelin pamoate has only had FDA approval since the early 2000s, not all information is known regarding its interactions with other medicines. Currently, no drug interactions have been reported.

Resources

BOOKS

Chu, Edward, and Vincent T. DeVita Jr. *Physicians' Cancer Chemotherapy Drug Manual 2014*. Burlington, MA: Jones & Bartlett Learning, 2014.

WEBSITES

The Scott Hamilton CARES Initiative. "Triptorelin Pamoate." Chemocare.com http://chemocare.com/chemotherapy/drug-info/triptorelin-pamoate.aspx (accessed November 13, 2014).

U.S. Food and Drug Administration. "Safety Information: Trelstar (Triptorelin Pamoate for Injectable Suspension)." http://www.fda.gov/Safety/MedWatch/SafetyInformation/ucm347049.htm (accessed November 14, 2014).

Joan Schonbeck, R.N.

Trisenox *see* **Arsenic trioxide**

Trousseau syndrome *see* **Hypercoagulation disorders**

Tube enterostomy

Definition

Tube enterostomy, or tube feeding, is a form of enteral or intestinal site feeding that employs a stoma or semi-permanent surgically placed tube to the small intestines.

Purpose

Many patients are unable to take in food by mouth, esophagus, or stomach. A number of conditions can render a person unable to take in nutrition through the normal pathways. Neurological conditions or injuries, injuries to the mouth or throat, obstructions of the stomach, **cancer** or ulcerative conditions of the gastrointestinal tract, and certain surgical procedures can make it impossible for a person to receive oral nutrition. Tube feeding is indicated for patients unable to ingest adequate nutrition by mouth, but who may have a cleared passage in the esophagus and stomach, and even partial functioning of the gastrointestinal tract. Enteral nutrition procedures that utilize the gastrointestinal tract are

---

KEY TERMS

Enteral nutritional support—Nutrition utilizing an intact gastrointestinal tract, but bypassing another organ such as the stomach or esophagus.

Parenteral nutritional support—Intravenous nutrition that bypasses the intestines and its contribution to digestion.

Stoma—A portal fashioned from the side of the abdomen that allows for ingestion into or drainage out of the intestines or urinary tract.

Tube feeding—Feeding or nutrition through a tube placed into the body through the esophagus, nose, stomach, intestines, or via a surgically constructed artificial orifice called a stoma.

---

preferred over intravenous feeding or parenteral nutrition because they maintain the function of the intestines, provide for immunity to infection, and avoid complications related to intravenous feeding.

Tube enterostomy, a feeding tube placed directly into the intestines or jejunum, is one such enteral procedure. It is used if the need for enteral feeding lasts longer than six weeks, or if it improves the outcomes of drastic surgeries such as removal or resection of the intestines. Recently, it has become an important technique for use in surgery in which a gastrectomy—resection of the intestinal link to the esophagus—occurs. The procedure makes healing easier, and seeks to retain the patient's nutritional status and quality of life after **reconstructive surgery**. Some individuals have a tube enterostomy surgically constructed, and successfully utilize it for a long period of time.

There are a variety of enteral nutritional products, liquid feedings with the nutritional quality of solid food. Patients with normal gastrointestinal function can benefit from these products. Other patients must have nutritional counseling, monitoring, and precise nutritional diets developed by a health care professional.

Description

Tube enterostomy refers to placement via a number of surgical approaches:

- laparoscopy
- esophagostomy (open surgery via the esophagus)
- stomach (gastrostomy or PEG)
- upper intestines or jejunum (jejunostomy)

The appropriate method depends on the clinical prognosis, anticipated duration of feeding, risk of aspirating or inhaling gastric contents, and patient preference. Whether through a standard operation or with laparoscopic surgical techniques, the surgeon fashions a stoma or opening into the esophagus, stomach, or intestines, and inserts a tube from the outside through which nutrition will be introduced. These tubes are made of silicone or polyurethane, and contain weighted tips and insertion features that facilitate placement. The surgery is fairly simple to perform, and most patients have good outcomes with stoma placement.

Demographics

Tube enterostomy provides temporary enteral nutrition to patients with injuries as well as inflammatory, obstructive, and other intestinal, esophageal, and abdominal conditions. Other uses include patients with pediatric abnormalities and those who have had surgery for cancerous tumors of the gastroesophageal junction (many of these cases are associated with Barrett's epithelium). Intestinal cancers in the United States have declined since the 1950s. However, this endemic form of gastric cancer is one of the most common causes of death from malignant disease, with an estimated 798,000 annual cases worldwide and 21,900 in the United States. As gastric cancer has declined, esophageal cancers have increased, requiring surgeries that resect and reconstruct the passage between the esophagus and intestine.

Preparation

A number of conditions necessitate tube enterostomy for **nutritional support**. Many are chronic and require a complete medical evaluation including history, physical examination, and extensive imaging tests. Some conditions are critical or acute, and may emerge from injuries or serious inflammatory conditions in which the patient is not systematically prepared for the surgery. In many cases, the patient undergoing this type of surgery has been ill for a period of time. Sometimes the patient is a small child or adult who accidentally swallowed a caustic substance. Some are elderly patients who have obstructive **carcinoma** of the esophagus or stomach.

Optimal preparation includes an evaluation of the patient's nutritional status, and his or her potential requirements for blood transfusions and **antibiotics**. Patients who do not have gastrointestinal inflammatory or obstructive conditions are usually required to undergo bowel preparation that flushes the intestines of all material. The bowel preparation reduces the chances of infection.

The patient's acceptance of tube feeding as a substitute for eating is of paramount importance. Health care providers must be sensitive to these problems, and offer early assistance and feedback in the self-care that the tube enterostomy requires.

In preparation for surgery, patients learn that the tube enterostomy will be an artificial orifice placed outside the abdomen through which they will deliver their nutritional support. Patients are taught how to care for the stoma, cleaning and making sure it functions optimally. In addition, patients are prepared for the loss of the function of eating and its place in their lives. They must be made aware that their physical body will be altered, and that this may have social implications and affect their intimate activities.

Aftercare

Tube enterostomy requires monitoring the patient for infection or bleeding, and educating him or her on the proper use of the enterostomy. According to the type of surgery—minimally invasive or open surgery—it may take several days for the patient to resume normal functioning. Fluid intake and urinary output must be monitored to prevent dehydration.

Risks

Tube enterostomies are not considered high risk surgeries. Insertions have been completed in over 90% of attempts. Possible complications include **diarrhea**, skin irritation due to leakage around the stoma, and difficulties with tube placement.

Tube enterostomy is becoming more frequent due to great advances in minimally invasive techniques and new materials used for stoma construction. However, one recent radiograph study of 289 patients who had jejunostomy found that 14% of patients suffered one or more complications, 19% had problems related to the location or function of the tube, and 9% developed thickened small-bowel folds.

Results

Recovery without complications is the norm for this surgery. The greatest challenge is educating the patient on proper stoma usage and types of nutritional support that must be used.

Morbidity and mortality rates

Some feeding or tube stomas have the likelihood of complications. A review of 1,000 patients indicated that PEG tube placement has mortality in 0.5%, with major complications (stomal leakage, peritonitis [infection in

Nutrition and Intravenous Glucose in Cancer Patients Enrolled in Specialized Palliative Care." *Nutrients* 5, no. 1 (2013): 267–82. http://dx.doi.org/10.3390/nu5010267 (accessed October 3, 2014).

Rajab, T. K., and J. Watkins. "Anatomic Site of Tube Feeding Influences Glycemic Control—An Evidence-Based Hypothesis." *Surgery* 153, no. 5 (2013): 608–10. http://dx.doi.org/10.1016/j.surg.2012.08.069 (accessed October 3, 2014).

OTHER

California Dietetic Association. *The Selection and Care of Enteral Feeding Tubes.* http://www.dietitian.org/d_cvd/docs/kc_enteral_feeding.pdf (accessed October 3, 2014).

WEBSITES

ALS Association. "Information About Feeding Tubes." http://www.alsa.org/als-care/resources/publications-videos/fact-sheets/feeding-tubes.html (accessed October 3, 2014).

ORGANIZATIONS

American Society for Parenteral and Enteral Nutrition, 8630 Fenton St., Ste. 412, Silver Spring, MD 20910, (301) 587-6315, (800) 727-4567, aspen@nutr.org, https://www.nutritioncare.org.

United Ostomy Associations of America, Inc. (UOAA), PO Box 512, Northfield, MN 55057-0512, (800) 826-0826, info@ostomy.org, http://www.ostomy.org.

Nancy McKenzie, PhD

Tumor debulking *see* **Debulking surgery**

QUESTIONS TO ASK YOUR DOCTOR

- How long will the tube enterostomy remain in place?
- How much assistance will be given in adjusting to the stoma and the special diet?
- If the condition does not improve, what other surgical alternatives are available?
- How long can a person live safely and comfortably with a tube enterostomy?

the abdomen], traumatized tissue of the abdominal wall, and gastric [stomach] hemorrhage) in 1% of cases. Wound infection, leaks, tube movement or migration, and **fever** occurred in 8% of patients. In a review of seven published studies, researchers found that a single intravenous dose of a broad-spectrum antibiotic was very effective in reducing infections with the stoma. Open surgery always carries with it a small percentage of cardiac complications, blood clots, and infections. Many gastric stoma patients have complicated diseases that increase the likelihood of surgical complications.

Alternatives

Oral routes are always the preferred method of providing nutritional intake. Intravenous fluid intake can be used as an eating substitute, but only for a short period of time. It is the preferred alternative when adequate protein and calories cannot be provided by oral or other enteral routes, or when the gastrointestinal system is not functioning.

Health care team roles

Gastrointestinal surgeons and surgical oncologists perform this surgery in general hospital settings.

Resources

BOOKS

Feldman, M., et al. *Sleisenger & Fordtran's Gastrointestinal and Liver Disease.* 9th ed. Philadelphia: Saunders/Elsevier, 2010.

Townsend, Courtney M., et al. *Sabiston Textbook of Surgery.* 19th ed. Philadelphia: Saunders/Elsevier, 2012.

PERIODICALS

Best, C. "Maintaining Hydration in Enteral Tube Feeding." *Nursing Times* 109, no. 26 (2013): 16–17.

Orrevall, Ylva, et al. "A National Observational Study of the Prevalence and Use of Enteral Tube Feeding, Parenteral

Tumor grading

Definition

Tumor grading is an estimate of a tumor's malignancy and aggressiveness based on how the tumor cells appear under a microscope and the number of malignant characteristics they possess. It is a way to predict how quickly a tumor is likely to grow and spread in the body, and is used when planning a specific treatment plan for a **cancer** patient. Different tumor grading systems are used depending on the type of cancer being described.

Purpose

Tumor grading, together with the stage of the tumor, assists doctors in planning treatment strategies. Grading is a part of describing most cancers, and it is extremely important in helping to determine the course of treatment for specific cancers such as soft tissue sarcomas, **brain tumors**, lymphomas, and breast and **prostate cancer**.

Gleason tumor scoring system

Gleason X	Cannot be determined
Gleason 2–6	Well differentiated
Gleason 7	Moderately differentiated
Gleason 8–10	Poorly differentiated or undifferentiated

SOURCE: National Cancer Institute, "Tumor Grade," National Institutes of Health. Available online at: http://www.cancer.gov/cancertopics/factsheet/Detection/tumor-grade.

One example of a tumor grading system is the Gleason system, used to grade prostate cancer. *(Illustration by PreMediaGlobal. © Cengage Learning®.)*

Generally, higher grade and higher stage tumors require more intensive therapy than lower grade and lower stage tumors. Tumor grade and stage also help doctors estimate the prognosis for the patient. Patients with lower grade and stage tumors usually have a more positive prognosis than patients with higher grade and stage tumors. Patients should thoroughly discuss the grade and stage of their tumor with their physician and ask about necessary treatments and prognosis.

Description

Before a tumor can be assigned a grade, a sample of tissue must be removed for microscopic evaluation. Tissue samples can be obtained through one of various types of **biopsy** or through exfoliative **cytology** (e.g., Pap smear). A pathologist analyzes various characteristics of the tissue, such as the size and shape of the nucleus, the ratio of the volume of the nucleus to the volume of the cytoplasm, the relative number of dividing cells (the mitotic index), the organization of the tissue, the boundary of the tumor, and how well-differentiated the cells appear—how close to normal the cells seem in maturity and function.

Benign tumors have normal-looking cells. That is, they have small and regular-shaped nuclei, small nuclear volume relative to the rest of the cellular volume, a relatively low number of dividing cells, and normal and well-differentiated tissue that has a well-defined tumor boundary. Malignant tumors generally have all or several of the following characteristics: large and pleomorphic (irregular-shaped) nuclei, large nuclear volume compared to the rest of the cellular volume, a high number of dividing cells, and disorganized and anaplastic (poorly differentiated) tissue that has a poorly defined tumor boundary.

Depending on the number of malignant characteristics present, the American Joint Commission on Cancer

KEY TERMS

Anaplasia—The loss of distinctive cell features, which is a distinct characteristic of malignant neoplasms, or tumors.

Mitotic—Relating to mitosis, or the process by which a cell divides into two cells, each with identical sets of chromosomes.

Pathologist—A medical professional who studies and diagnoses diseases.

Tubule—Small tubular part of an animal.

Tumor—An uncontrolled mass of body cells that may be benign or malignant.

recommends that tumors be given a grade using G0 through G4:

- G0: A benign lesion or tumor.
- G1: Well-differentiated (Low-grade and less aggressive).
- G2: Moderately well-differentiated (Intermediate-grade and moderately aggressive).
- G3: Poorly differentiated (High-grade and moderately aggressive).
- G4: Undifferentiated (High-grade and aggressive).

Alternatively, Roman numerals I through IV, respectively, may be used. Low-grade tumors are assigned lower Roman numerals (e.g., grade I), indicating that the tumor is less aggressive. High-grade tumors are assigned higher Roman numerals (e.g., grade IV), indicating that the tumor is very aggressive, growing and spreading quickly. This description is stated as:

- I: Well-differentiated (Low-grade and less aggressive).
- II: Moderately well-differentiated (Intermediate-grade and moderately aggressive).
- III: Poorly differentiated (High-grade and moderately aggressive).
- IV: Undifferentiated (High-grade and aggressive).

Some cancers have their own specific grading convention. For example, the Gleason system is a unique grading system that was developed to describe **adenocarcinoma** of the prostate. Pathologists analyze prostate tissue and give a Gleason score ranging from 2 to 10, subject to the number of malignant characteristics observed. Well-differentiated, less aggressive prostate tumors with only a few malignant characteristics are given lower Gleason numbers, while poorly differentiated, more aggressive prostate tumors that possess many malignant characteristics are assigned higher Gleason numbers.

Breast cancer tumors

Breast cancers are graded using a system called the Nottingham system. It is also called the Bloom-Richardson grading system, a modification of the Bloom-Richardson-Elston grading system (sometimes known as the modified Bloom-Richardson-Elston system) that originated in 1957. The Nottingham system also goes by such names as the Modified Bloom-Richardson, Scarff-Bloom-Richardson, SBR Grading, and BR Grading. Breast tumors, specifically the cells and tissue structure of the breast, are assessed to determine the state of the cancer. A pathologist examines a sample of breast tissue under a microscope, and the tumors are analyzed (and scored) based on the following three features:

- degree of tubule (gland) formation—the amount of tubule structure that is present
- nuclear grade (pleomorphism)—cell size and appearance, and uniformity of individual cells
- mitotic rate—amount of activity of cell division

Each feature is assigned a score from 1 to 3 based on the following:

- 1: slow cell growth rate
- 2: intermediate cell growth rate
- 3: fast cell growth rate

Cells and tissue structure that look normal are assigned lower scores, while abnormal-looking cells and structure are given higher scores. The scoring, based on the above three features, ranges from 3 (least serious) to 9 (most serious) on the Nottingham system. The total feature score is graded as follows:

- total points 3 to 5: grade 1 tumor—well-differentiated, appears normal, growing slowly, not aggressive
- total points 6 to 7: grade 2 tumor—moderately differentiated, appears semi-normal, growing moderately fast

- total points 8 to 9: grade 3 tumor—poorly differentiated, appears abnormal, growing quickly, aggressive

As an example, the pathologist might give 1 point to degree of tubule formation, 2 points for nuclear grade, and 1 point for mitotic rate, for a total of 4 points. In this case, the tumor is classified as a grade 1 tumor. The higher-grade tumors are treated more aggressively, because they spread faster and are associated with a lower survival rate. Lower-grade tumors have a much higher survival rate for women, so they are treated in a less aggressive manner.

Results

Once a grading system has been used to determine the severity of the tumor, doctors will use that tumor grade, along with other relevant information, to develop a treatment plan for the patient. The grading system also helps to determine a prognosis for the patient, including how aggressive the treatment needs to be, the likely chance for recovery, the likelihood that the cancer will reoccur, and other important concerns. Once a tumor's grade has been determined, it is important that patients discuss these results with their doctor so an effective course of action can be taken.

Resources

BOOKS
Damjanov, Ivan, and Fang Fan, eds. *Cancer Grading Manual.* Berlin: Springer, 2013.

Epstein, Jonathan I. *The Gleason Grading System: A Complete Guide for Pathologists and Clinicians.* Philadelphia: Wolters Kluwer Health/Lippincott Williams & Wilkins, 2013.

Weinberg, Robert A. *The Biology of Cancer.* New York: Garland Science, 2014.

WEBSITES
American Brain Tumor Association. "Grading and Staging." http://www.abta.org/understanding-brain-tumors/diagnosis/grading-and-staging.html (accessed September 27, 2013).

California Cancer Registry. "Bloom-Richardson Grade for Breast Cancer." http://www.ccrcal.org/DSQC_Pubs/V1_2013_Online_Manual/Part_V_Tumor_Data/V_3_5_8_Bloom_Richardson_Grade_for_Breast_Cancer.htm (accessed September 25, 2013).

Johns Hopkins Medicine, Johns Hopkins University. "Overview of Histologic Grade: Nottingham Histologic Score (Elston Grade)." http://pathology.jhu.edu/breast/grade.php (accessed September 25, 2013).

National Cancer Institute. "Tumor Grade." http://www.cancer.gov/cancertopics/factsheet/detection/tumor-grade (accessed September 25, 2013).

Susan G. Komen Foundation. "Tumor Grade." http://ww5.komen.org/BreastCancer/TumorGrade.html (accessed September 27, 2013).

ORGANIZATIONS

American Cancer Society, 250 Williams St. NW, Atlanta, GA 30303, (800) 227-2345, http://www.cancer.org.

Cancer Research Institute, One Exchange Plz., 55 Broadway, Ste. 1802, New York, NY 10006, (212) 688-7515, (800) 99-CANCER (992-2623), http://cancerresearch.org.

National Cancer Institute, 6116 Executive Blvd., Ste. 300, Bethesda, MD 20892-8322, (800) 4-CANCER (422-6237), http://cancer.gov.

Sally C. McFarlane-Parrott
REVISED BY WILLIAM A. ATKINS, BB, BS, MBA

⎸ Tumor lysis syndrome

Definition

Tumor lysis syndrome is a life-threatening metabolic emergency that complicates the treatment of certain types of tumors (neoplasms).

Description

Concentrations of intracellular electrolytes, those that are within the cell, differ from extracellular electrolytes, or those that are outside the cell and in the bloodstream. In tumor lysis syndrome, tumor cells lyse, or break apart, releasing their contents into the blood stream. The result is a dangerous alteration in the normal balance of serum electrolytes—potassium, phosphate, and uric acid levels are elevated, while calcium levels are decreased. The changes occur so quickly and can be so dramatic that immediate death can result.

Demographics

Many factors contribute to the development of tumor lysis syndrome. Most of the research performed to date revolves around high-grade **non-Hodgkin lymphoma** cases, 40% of which demonstrate laboratory evidence of tumor lysis syndrome. An estimated 6% demonstrate clinical evidence of the syndrome. Tumors that carry the highest risk of the development of tumor lysis syndrome are those that are large and bulky, usually greater than eight to ten cm (3-4 in.), and comprised of rapidly dividing cells. In addition, tumors that respond well to treatment are associated with tumor lysis syndrome because treatment results in rupture of a large number of cells.

Most often, the syndrome is associated with blood-based (hematologic) tumors—such as non-Hodgkin **lymphoma** and particularly Burkitt lymphoma—and

acute leukemia. Though less likely because of lower rates of cell division, tumor lysis syndrome can also occur in solid tumors such as **breast cancer**. The Washington Manual of Medical Therapeutics associates the following **cancer** types with tumor lysis syndrome:

- non-Hodgkin lymphoma (NHL)
- acute lymphocytic leukemia (ALL)
- acute myelocytic leukemia (AML)
- chronic lymphocytic leukemia (CLL)
- chronic myelocytic leukemia (CML)
- breast cancer
- testicular cancer
- medulloblastoma
- merkel cell carcinoma
- neuroblastoma
- small cell carcinoma of the lung

Causes and symptoms

Usually, tumor lysis syndrome develops after the administration of combination **chemotherapy** regimens, but it may also occur spontaneously or as a result of radiation or corticosteroid therapy. Lactic acid dehydrogenase (LDH) is an enzyme found in cells of body tissues. An increase in the LDH level is considered a marker of bulky disease that correlates with the risk of tumor lysis syndrome.

Patients with underlying kidney (renal) dysfunction and/or decreased urine output are at a higher risk of developing tumor lysis syndrome. Without optimal kidney functioning, waste products that build up cannot be excreted in the urine at a high enough rate. Patients with cancer may be predisposed to conditions that increase the risk of renal failure due to increased uric acid buildup. For example, a patient undergoing chemotherapy may experience **nausea and vomiting**, and may, as a result, be dehydrated, increasing the risk. The same patient may have decreased white blood cell counts, making him or her more susceptible to infections. Many **antibiotics** adversely affect the kidneys, also increasing the risk.

In some cases, the patient does not manifest any symptoms of tumor lysis syndrome. Instead, the electrolyte derangements are noted on blood testing. In other cases, the derangements may be extreme enough to cause overt signs and symptoms, such as:

- Bloody urine
- Flank pain
- High blood pressure
- Decreased urine output

- Lethargy
- Sleepiness
- Muscle cramps and twitching
- Heart arrhythmias
- Fainting
- Nausea
- Vomiting
- Severe diarrhea
- Sudden death
- Confusion
- Seizures
- Coma

Treatment

Treatment is aimed at prevention and supportive care, with the main goals being to prevent renal failure and severe electrolyte imbalances. Patients at risk receive treatment on an inpatient basis to allow for close monitoring by medical personnel. At all times, patients should have reliable intravenous access. Prior to initiating treatment, a patient's hydration status and electrolyte levels are carefully evaluated. If there are abnormalities, a treatment delay may be considered, though this is not always an option.

Laboratory tests are done frequently to monitor levels of calcium, potassium, phosphate, magnesium, and uric acid. A typical hospital protocol may require blood be drawn for these tests every two to six hours over the course of two to three days. Following are prevention and management strategies for each of the major electrolyte imbalances, hyperuricemia, hyperkalemia, hyperphosphatemia, and **hypocalcemia**.

Hyperuricemia is a medical term used to describe an abnormal increase of uric acid levels in the blood that can lead to acute renal failure. There are several methods employed to prevent kidney damage—aggressive hydration being a major focus. Intravenous (IV) hydration is started before treatment and continues throughout to maintain a urine output of 100 to 200 milliliters per hour (mL/hr). Medications called diuretics, such as furosemide or acetazolamide, are given to help increase urine output when necessary.

Urine may be alkalized to prevent uric acid buildup. Alkalization can be accomplished by adding sodium bicarbonate to the patient's IV fluid. For example, the basic maintenance IV fluid may consist of 5% dextrose in 0.25 normal saline, to which sodium bicarbonate, in amounts ranging from 50 to 200 milliequivalents (mEq— the total number of charges of electrolytes in solution), may be added. Urine pH is routinely tested, and the sodium bicarbonate is periodically increased or decreased to maintain a pH level between 7 and 8.

Urine alkalinization is somewhat controversial. If urine is too alkaline, calcium phosphate crystal formation may occur, increasing the likelihood of renal failure. It is generally believed that if urine output levels are appropriately maintained, calcium phosphate will be diluted, and the possibility of crystal formation will diminish.

Patients at risk for tumor lysis syndrome may also be given **allopurinol** prophylactically. One dose of 600 milligrams (mg) may be given the day before treatment, followed by 300 mg once a day for the remainder of treatment days. Allopurinol is effective because it inhibits the formation of uric acid. In 2004, a new drug called rasburicase became available in the United States. It prevents the damaging effects of tumor lysis syndrome with fewer side effects.

Hyperkalemia is a medical term used to describe an abnormal increase of potassium levels in the blood that can cause dangerous abnormalities in heart rhythms, heart attack, and muscle weakness. Frequent monitoring with electrocardiography (EKG) is recommended in patients at risk for tumor lysis syndrome so that alterations in the electrical activity of the heart can be caught early. Potassium-rich foods may also be restricted to prevent already elevated levels from increasing. Sometimes, medications such as Kayexalate are administered to help reduce potassium levels.

Hyperphosphatemia is a medical term used to describe an abnormal increase on phosphate levels in the blood that can cause neuromuscular irritability and worsen kidney function. Malignant cells may contain up to four times as much phosphate as non-malignant cells. Patients experiencing acute tumor lysis syndrome may be instructed to reduce their dietary intake of phosphate. In addition, they may be given medications that bind to phosphate, thereby inhibiting its absorption in the intestines.

Hypocalcemia is a medical term used to describe an abnormal decrease in calcium levels in the blood that can cause muscle spasms (tetany), muscle cramps, and seizures. A calcium supplement may be required.

Dialysis is a procedure used to normalize electrolyte imbalances through the diffusion and ultrafiltration of fluid. Potassium, for example, can be separated and filtered from fluid, bringing levels back to a safer range. Hemodialysis is a procedure that removes waste products through the blood. Dialysis can alternatively be performed through the peritoneum, the tissue that lines the abdominal area and surrounds the organs in what is called peritoneal dialysis. Because peritoneal dialysis does not clear phosphate and urate as efficiently, and because it is not feasible in patients with abdominal tumors, hemodialysis is the preferred method. A doctor who specializes in nephrology will generally examine a high-risk patient before cancer treatment begins, to prepare for the possibility of dialysis treatment. In some cases, dialysis is started as a preventive measure, either before or during chemotherapy treatment.

Prognosis

The prognosis of tumor lysis syndrome is good, as long as the problem is identified and treated early in its course. If the process is allowed to continue unchecked, the syndrome can prove life-threatening.

Prevention

Patients who are going to be treated for tumors known to have high rates of tumor lysis syndrome (such as lymphomas and leukemias) should be given medications to prevent the production and/or buildup of uric acid, such as allopurinol or Rasburicase. Patients should be monitored carefully for the advent of electrolyte changes that could suggest that they are at risk for developing full-blown tumor lysis syndrome.

Resources

BOOKS

Goldman, Lee, and Andrew I. Schafer. *Goldman's Cecil Medicine.* 24th ed. Philadelphia: Saunders/Elsevier, 2012.
Hoffman R., et al. *Hematology: Basic Principles and Practice.* 5th ed. Philadelphia: Elsevier, 2008.
Marx, John A., et al. *Rosen's Emergency Medicine.* 6th ed. St. Louis, MO: Mosby, Inc., 2006.

Tamara Brown, R.N.
Teresa G. Odle

Tumor markers

Definition

Tumor markers, also called biomarkers, are substances (usually proteins) in tissue, blood, urine, or other body fluids that can be associated with certain cancers. As of 2014, there were more than 20 tumor markers in clinical use, and tumor markers were a major focus of **cancer research**.

Purpose

Tumor markers are most often used to monitor the effects of **cancer** treatment. Tumor markers measured in blood or urine can be easily followed before, during, and for many years after treatment to detect recurrences. Tumor-marker testing is far less invasive and expensive than imaging techniques. Decreases in tumor marker levels indicate that the cancer is responding to treatment; stable or increasing levels indicate that the cancer is not responding and that a different treatment may be necessary. The exception to this is a temporary increase in a tumor marker during treatment, as dying cancer cells release them into the circulation. Periodic tumor-marker testing can sometimes detect a cancer recurrence months earlier than other diagnostic methods. Tumor markers on cancer cells that are not detectable in body fluids are usually measured only once, to confirm a diagnosis and inform treatment choices.

Tumor markers are rarely specific enough to diagnose cancer. They may be used clinically to:

- screen people who are at high risk for certain cancers
- confirm a cancer diagnosis in conjunction with other clinical findings
- stage cancers or help to determine the extent of a cancer—higher tumor-marker levels may indicate more advanced cancer and a poorer prognosis
- help determine where a metastasized cancer originated, which is important for identifying the type of cancer and guiding its treatment
- plan primary and adjuvant treatments, including choosing chemotherapy and targeted drugs
- predict responses to treatment and prognosis
- monitor the progression of advanced cancer

Description

Tumor markers are either produced by cancer cells (tumor-derived) or by the body in response to cancer cells (tumor-associated). Although most tumor markers are also produced by normal cells, cancer cells may produce markers in greater amounts and leak them into the blood, urine, or stool as the cells grow and multiply. The utility of tumor markers depends on their specificity and sensitivity. Some tumor markers are associated with many types of cancer as well as with noncancerous (benign) conditions; others are associated with just one or a few cancers. Some tumor markers are always elevated in specific cancers; however, most are less predictable. There is no "universal" tumor marker for all types of cancer.

Most tumor markers are proteins, including antigens on the surfaces of or secreted by cancer cells, hormones, growth-factor and hormone receptors, enzymes, and immunoglobulins (antibodies). Some tumor markers—such as alpha-fetoprotein (AFP), carcinoembryonic antigen (CEA), and cancer antigen (CA) 72-4—are proteins

KEY TERMS

Alpha-fetoprotein (AFP)—A fetal blood protein found in amniotic fluid and secreted by some cancers.

Antibodies—Immune-system proteins that recognize specific antigens, such as proteins on tumor cells.

Antigen—A protein or other molecule that evokes a specific immune response.

Beta-2 microglobulin (B2M)—A small membrane protein that may be elevated in some cancers.

Biopsy—The removal of a small piece of tissue for examination and testing.

Cancer antigen (CA)—Marker proteins for some types of cancer.

Carcinoembryonic antigen (CEA)—A fetal protein that is present at high levels in the blood with some types of cancer, such as breast or digestive system cancers.

Epidermal growth factor receptor (EGFR)—EGFR1 (HER1); a cell-surface protein that initiates growth and proliferation and is a tumor marker for certain cancers.

Estrogen receptor (ER)—A cell-surface protein that binds the female hormone estrogen; present on ER-positive breast cancer cells.

HER2—Human epidermal growth factor receptor 2 (EGFR2), which is overproduced in HER2-positive breast cancers.

Human chorionic gonadotropin (hCG)—A hormone secreted by the placenta in early pregnancy and produced by some tumors; beta-hCG is a tumor marker for some germ-cell cancers.

Immunoglobulins (Igs)—Antibodies; some types of immunoglobulins or portions of immunoglobulins called light chains, including the Bence-Jones protein, can be used as markers for some types of cancer.

Lactate dehydrogenase (LDH)—An enzyme that can be a tumor marker in the blood for some cancers.

Neuron-specific enolase (NSE)—An enzyme that may be elevated in tumors originating in neuroendocrine cells.

Polymerase chain reaction (PCR)—A method used to directly detect and quantify specific DNA or RNA in blood or tissue.

Progesterone receptor (PR)—A protein on the surface of cells that binds the female hormone progesterone; a marker on PR-positive breast cancer cells.

Prostate specific antigen (PSA)—A biomarker used as a preliminary screen for prostate cancer.

Receptor—A molecule, usually a protein, inside or on the surface of a cell that binds a specific chemical group or molecule, such as a hormone or growth factor, to initiate a sequence of events.

---

normally produced during embryonic development that decrease soon after birth. They are produced by many types of cancer cells that have dedifferentiated—reverted to immature cell types—and, thus, are very nonspecific. However, they are useful for monitoring cancer progression and response to treatment.

Tumor markers are most often measured in laboratories by immunological tests. A blood or tissue sample is reacted with antibodies specific for the tumor marker. The amount of antibody bound to markers in the sample is measured. Results are usually available within a few days. Tumor markers in blood or urine are measured repeatedly to assess the effects of treatment or detect cancer recurrence. Tumor-marker tests are approved by the U.S. Food and Drug Administration (FDA), and guidelines for their use are established by organizations such as the American Society of Clinical Oncology (ASCO). Not all tumor marker tests are widely available nor are they all widely accepted.

Newer tumor markers being studied as of 2014 include:

- protein profiles or "signatures"—multiple proteins that are increased in specific cancers
- autoantibodies—antibodies that the immune system produces against proteins produced in high amounts by tumor cells
- gene changes (mutations) in cancer cells
- epigenetic changes—alterations to cancer cell genes that do not involve changes or mutations in the DNA sequence of the gene
- specific RNAs that can be detected in the blood

Prostate-specific antigen (PSA)

PSA, a blood screen for **prostate cancer**, is the most widely used tumor marker and the only tumor marker used to screen a general population—men over age 50 and high-risk men over 40. PSA is tissue-specific—it is produced only by the prostate gland and may be overproduced by prostate cancers. Once prostate cancer is diagnosed, PSA levels can help determine the cancer stage and are very useful for monitoring response to treatment and recurrence. Any PSA detected following **prostatectomy** indicates residual prostate tissue and possibly **metastasis**; however, PSA is also increased in benign prostatic hyperplasia (BPH), an enlarged prostate condition common in older men, and in prostatitis (inflammation of the prostate). Further, although prostate cancer usually causes high PSA levels, men with healthy prostates can have high levels, and normal levels do not mean the absence of cancer. Therefore, many doctors do not believe that all men should be screened for PSA. Two large randomized controlled trials have indicated that PSA screening leads to only a small reduction in deaths from prostate cancer. It is unclear whether the benefits of PSA screening outweigh the harm of follow-up tests and treatment for cancers that would never become life-threatening.

PSA can be detected in blood serum in two states—bound and free. Measuring both can increase specificity and reduce unnecessary biopsies. Since the percentage of free PSA is greater with BPH than with prostate cancer, a **biopsy** may be indicated only when total PSA is above 4.0 nanograms/milliliter (ng/mL) and free PSA is less than 25% of the total.

Prostatic acid phosphatase (PAP) was once thought to be a blood marker for prostate cancer, but it has been replaced by PSA. However, PAP may help diagnose **multiple myeloma** and lung cancer.

Alpha-fetoprotein (AFP) and human chorionic gonadotropin (hCG)

AFP is produced in high amounts by fetal tissue and is elevated during pregnancy. AFP in blood is the most widely used marker for primary **liver cancer** and germ-cell tumors, including some testicular cancers and rare types of **ovarian cancer**. AFP levels are high in 70% of liver cancers and are used for screening in China, which has a high rate of liver cancer. A biopsy is still necessary for diagnosis, since benign liver conditions moderately increase AFP levels. AFP is used to stage liver and germ-cell cancers, monitor treatment responses, and screen for cancer recurrences.

hCG is normally produced by the placenta during pregnancy. It consists of two protein subunits, alpha and beta, and it is the beta subunit that is increased in serum and urine during early pregnancy and with some germ-cell tumors. Tumors that secrete beta-hCG are typically ovarian and testicular tumors with embryonal tissue, as well as **gestational trophoblastic tumors**, such as choriocarcinoma. Such tumors may also secrete AFP, and hCG and AFP tests are often used in combination.

Very high AFP or beta-hCG levels in **testicular cancer** indicate aggressive disease and poor prognosis.

Carcinoembryonic antigen (CEA)

High blood plasma levels of CEA are most often associated with colorectal cancer. CEA levels are used to monitor patients with colorectal cancer, evaluate the success of surgery, diagnose metastases, and help with prognosis and early detection of recurrence. CEA levels are also used in **breast cancer** to assess response to treatment and diagnose recurrence. CEA is very nonspecific and can be increased in many types of cancer as well as in some benign conditions. CEA levels also may be elevated in elderly people and smokers.

Cancer antigens

CA 15-3/CA 27.29 are different blood tests for the same antigen and are used to assess response to breast cancer treatment and monitor for recurrence. CA 27.29 is elevated in 80% of women with breast cancer; however, neither test can detect early breast cancer. Furthermore, both tests can be positive with various other cancers and noncancerous conditions, including pregnancy and lactation.

CA 125 is the standard blood marker that is followed during and after treatment for the most common type of ovarian cancer, as well as fallopian tube and primary peritoneal cancers. Although CA 125 is produced by a number of cell types, 80% of women with ovarian cancer and more than 90% of those with advanced cancer have elevated levels. However, CA 125 levels may also increase during menstruation and pregnancy and with various other cancers and benign conditions. Since ovarian cancer is somewhat rare, high CA 125 is more likely to be caused by some other condition.

CA 19-9 was developed as a colorectal cancer blood marker but is more often used for **pancreatic cancer**, where higher levels are associated with more advanced disease. It is used to monitor the course of pancreatic cancer and response to treatment, as well as to determine the aggressiveness of **bladder cancer**. CA 19-9 is related to the Lewis blood group, and so only patients positive for the Lewis blood group antigen will test positive for CA 19-9. Higher CA 19-9 is also associated with other digestive tract and abdominal cancers and with some benign conditions.

CA 72-4 is slightly elevated with most carcinomas, but is primarily associated with **stomach cancer**.

Receptors and hormones

Human epidermal growth factor receptor 2 (HER2; also called HER2/neu, erbB-2, or EGFR2) is a tumor marker that is measured in biopsy tissue, either by immunological assays or polymerase chain reaction (PCR) to quantify its DNA. HER2-positive breast cancers, as well as stomach and esophageal cancers, can be treated with the targeted drug **trastuzumab** (Herceptin). Cancer cells with normal amounts of HER2 will not respond to trastuzumab. HER2-positive cancers usually grow and spread faster than other types of cancer. About 20% of breast cancers are HER2-positive.

All breast tumor biopsy samples are tested for estrogen receptors (ER) and progesterone receptors (PR) as well as for HER2. Most breast cancers in postmenopausal women are ER-positive and grow in response to estrogen. ER- and PR-positive breast cancers can be treated with hormonal therapies, such as **tamoxifen** that blocks the receptor or **aromatase inhibitors** that reduce estrogen in the body. About two-thirds of breast cancers are positive for at least one of these receptors. They tend to grow more slowly and have a better prognosis than other breast cancers. Some **gynecologic cancers** are also tested for hormone receptors.

Epidermal growth factor receptor (EGFR or HER1) may be increased on some cancer tissues and is a sign of a fast growing and spreading, hard-to-treat cancer that may be aggressively treated with drugs that block EGFR. Some lung cancers—especially those in women, Asians, and nonsmokers—have EGFR gene mutations that make it more likely that certain drugs will be effective.

Endocrine-gland tumors over-secrete their corresponding hormones, and serial measurements can be used to monitor treatment.

• Medullary thyroid carcinoma (MTC) can secrete calcitonin, which normally regulates calcium levels. Calcitonin is one of the few tumor markers that can help detect early cancer and can be used to screen for MTC, which, although rare, is often inherited. Calcitonin blood levels can be used to aid diagnosis and assess treatment response and recurrence.

• Pituitary gland tumors may secrete growth hormone or cortisol.

• Carcinoid tumors secrete serotonin.

• Some pancreatic tumors secrete insulin.

• Breast cancer cells may secrete prolactin and estrogen.

• Pheochromocytomas secrete catecholamines.

• Blood levels of inhibin can be high with a rare type of ovarian cancer.

Enzymes

Neuron-specific enolase (NSE) is found mainly in neurons and neuroendocrine cells and is elevated in tumors derived from these tissues, including **neuroblastoma** and **small cell lung cancer**. NSE blood levels can provide information about the extent of disease, prognosis, and response to treatment.

Several serum enzymes can help detect cancer metastases. Tumors that metastasize to the liver increase serum levels of alkaline phosphatase, gamma-glutamyltransferase, and transaminases. Tumors that metastasize to bone sometimes secrete elevated alkaline phosphatase.

Lactate dehydrogenase (LDH) is an enzyme found throughout the body, and high levels occur with many conditions. LDH blood levels can be used to assess the stage, prognosis, and response to treatment of testicular and other germ-cell cancers, as well as **Ewing sarcoma**, **non-Hodgkin lymphoma**, and some types of leukemia.

Other proteins

The Bence-Jones protein was the first identified tumor marker, found in the urine of patients with multiple **myeloma** and **Waldenström macroglobulinemia**. It is the light-chain portion of an immunoglobulin (Ig) known as monoclonal Ig or M protein. M or Bence-Jones proteins (also called free light chains), as well as the amounts of each Ig class, can be measured in the blood to assist in diagnose and guide treatment.

Beta-2 microglobulin (B2M) is a small membrane protein measured in blood, urine, or cerebrospinal fluid for prognosis and monitoring treatment responses in multiple myeloma, chronic lymphocytic leukemia, and some lymphomas. B2M levels are higher in patients with poorer prognosis.

• Chromogranin A (CgA) can be secreted into the blood by some neuroendocrine tumors such as small cell lung cancer, neuroblastoma, and carcinoid tumors. High levels are detected in about one-third of patients with localized cancer and about two-thirds of those with advanced cancer.

• Fibrin or fibrinogen can be measured in urine to monitor progression of bladder cancer and response to treatment.

• Nuclear matrix protein 22 in the urine is used to monitor treatment response in bladder cancer.

• Thyroglobulin in the blood is used to monitor treatment response and recurrence of thyroid cancers. Antibodies against thyroglobulin are often measured as well.

• Urokinase plasminogen activator (uPA) and plasminogen activator inhibitor (PAI-1) are used to determine breast cancer tumor aggressiveness and guide treatment.

• Some ovarian cancers have multiple HE4 genes and make more HE4 protein that can be measured in the blood and used to guide treatment, most often in patients with normal CA 125 levels.

- Squamous cell carcinoma (SCC) antigen was first identified in cervical cancers and is a marker for squamous cell cancers of the cervix, head and neck, lung, and skin.
- The amount of CD20 on blood cells is used to determine whether targeted therapy is appropriate for non-Hodgkin lymphoma.
- Cytokeratin fragment 21-1 in the blood can help detect lung cancer recurrence.
- S-100 is present in most melanoma cells. Biopsy samples may be tested to help with diagnosis, and blood levels are sometimes used to diagnose metastasized melanoma.
- Soluble mesothelin-related peptide (SMRP) is sometimes used as a blood screen in people at high risk for mesothelioma or to detect recurrence.
- A five-protein signature known as Ova1 in the blood is used to assess suspected ovarian cancer before surgery.

Genes

The BCR-ABL fusion gene is formed when the ABL gene from chromosome 9 breaks off and joins the BCR gene on chromosome 22 to form the Philadelphia chromosome. This occurs in most chronic myelogenous leukemias and some acute lymphoblastic and acute myelogenous leukemias. The fusion can be detected in the blood or bone marrow by PCR and is used to confirm diagnosis, monitor disease status, and guide treatment.

The KRAS gene is mutated in 30%–40% of colorectal tumors. ASCO recommends that people with metastasized **colon cancer** be tested for KRAS mutations, since cancer with these mutations cannot be treated with **cetuximab** (Erbitux) and **panitumumab** (Vectibix) that target the EGFR protein in advanced colorectal cancer. KRAS mutation analysis is also used for **non-small cell lung cancer**, since cancers with KRAS mutations do not respond to the drugs **erlotinib** (Tarceva) and **gefitinib** (Iressa).

Rearrangements in the ALK gene that codes for anaplastic **lymphoma** kinase can be detected in tumor tissue and are used to help determine treatment and prognosis of non-small cell lung cancer and anaplastic large cell lymphoma. ALK gene mutations that cause lung cancer cells to grow out of control can be targeted with a drug such as crizotinib (Xalkori).

A specific mutation (V600E) in the BRAF gene in tumor tissue makes a protein that may increase the growth and spread of cancer cells, especially cutaneous **melanoma** and colorectal cancer. An altered BRAF

protein can be targeted with a drug such as vemurafenib (Zelboraf). Colorectal cancers with BRAF mutations cannot be treated with drugs that target EGFR.

Mutation analysis of EGFR on tumor cell surfaces can help determine treatment and prognosis for non-small cell lung cancer.

A 21-gene signature known as Oncotype DX and a 70-gene signature called the Mammaprint are used to analyze breast cancer tumors for risk of recurrence.

Chromosomes 3, 7, 17, and 9p21 in the urine can be used to help monitor recurrence of bladder cancer.

Precautions

Tumor markers are most useful for choosing targeted drugs, monitoring the effects of treatment, and detecting recurrences. They are rarely useful for detecting early cancers. Furthermore, false positives can lead to emotional distress and unnecessary tests, and false negatives can result in patients foregoing additional testing or treatment that might be beneficial. Tumor marker usefulness has been limited because:

- Most people have small amounts of tumor markers in their blood.
- Markers in blood tend to be high only with advanced cancer.
- Some people with cancer never have high tumor-marker levels.
- Many other conditions can cause high tumor-marker levels.

Only tumor markers that were elevated before treatment should be used for monitoring during or after treatment. Timing of the tests is also important. Each tumor marker has a unique lifespan in the blood, and to monitor treatment effectiveness, enough time must have passed for the marker to be cleared from the blood. Normal and high ranges for many tumor markers vary significantly between testing labs. If possible, serial testing should always be performed by the same lab so that results are comparable. It is also important to ensure that the results are in the same measurement units.

Commercial labs have tests for many more tumor markers. However, some advertised tests have not been proven effective, and others have been taken off the market at the request of the FDA.

Preparation

Tumor-marker tests usually require 5–10 mL of blood obtained in a routine blood draw. Urine tests typically require collecting all urine for 24 hours—usually about 1.5 quarts (L) or more. Other tumor markers require tissue samples from a needle biopsy or surgery.

QUESTIONS TO ASK YOUR DOCTOR

- Will you test for any tumor markers?
- How will the tumor-marker tests be performed?
- Will I have tumor-marker tests throughout and after treatment?
- What information will the tests provide?
- How accurate are the tumor-marker tests?

Aftercare

Blood draws usually require no aftercare. Aftercare of a biopsy depends on the procedure.

Results

Normal values for some tumor markers include:

- PSA—increases with age, but typically less than 4 nanograms per milliliter (ng/mL) means prostate cancer is unlikely
- AFP—less than 15 ng/mL in 99% of nonpregnant individuals and less than 6 ng/mL in 95%
- beta-HCG—less than 2.5 international units per liter (IU/L) in males; less than 5.0 IU/L in nonpregnant females
- CEA—less than or equal to 5 ng/mL
- CA 15-3—less than 30–40 U/mL but may be as high as 100 U/mL in women without cancer
- CA 27.29—less than or equal to 38–40 U/mL
- CA 125—less than 35 U/L
- CA 19-9—less than 37–40 U/mL
- calcitonin—below 5–12 picograms (pg)/mL
- B2M—below 2.5 mg/L

Abnormal results

Abnormal values for some tumor markers include:

- PSA—about one in four men with 4–10 ng/mL has prostate cancer; cancer is likely above 10 ng/mL
- AFP—above 400 ng/mL is associated with cancer or another pathology
- CEA—above 5.5 ng/mL; the higher the level, the more advanced the colorectal cancer
- calcitonin—above 100 pg/mL with medullary thyroid carcinoma
- NSE—above 9 micrograms (ug)/mL

Resources

BOOKS

Barh, Debmalya, et al. *Cancer Biomarkers: Minimal and Noninvasive Early Diagnosis and Prognosis.* Boca Raton, FL: CRC/Taylor & Francis Group, 2014.

Georgakilas, Alexandros. *Cancer Biomarkers.* Boca Raton, FL: Taylor & Francis/CRC, 2013.

Lenz, Heinz-Josef, ed. *Biomarkers in Oncology: Prediction and Prognosis.* New York: Springer, 2013.

PERIODICALS

Ballehaninna, Umashankar K., and Ronald S. Chamberlain. "Biomarkers for Pancreatic Cancer: Promising New Markers and Options Beyond CA 19-9." *Tumor Biology* 34, no. 6 (December 2013): 3279–92.

Jerónimo, Carmen, and Rui Henrique. "Epigenetic Biomarkers in Urological Tumors: A Systematic Review." *Cancer Letters* 342, no. 2 (January 28, 2014): 264–74.

Ng, Lui, et al. "Biomarkers for Predicting Future Metastasis of Human Gastrointestinal Tumors." *Cellular and Molecular Life Sciences* 70, no. 19 (October 2013): 3631–56.

Ogino, S., et al. "Discovery of Colorectal Cancer PIK3CA Mutation as Potential Predictive Biomarker: Power and Promise of Molecular Pathological Epidemiology." *Oncogene* 33, no. 23 (June 5, 2014): 2949–55.

Russo, N., et al. "A Novel Approach to Biomarker Discovery in Head and Neck Cancer Using an Autoantibody Signature." *Oncogene* 32, no. 42 (October 17, 2013): 5026–37.

Wang, Gangping, et al. "Nipple Discharge of CA15-3, CA125, CEA and TSGF as a New Biomarker Panel for Breast Cancer." *International Journal of Molecular Sciences* 15, no. 6 (2014): 9546–65.

OTHER

American Cancer Society. "Tumor Markers." http://www.cancer.org/acs/groups/cid/documents/webcontent/003189-pdf.pdf (accessed August 30, 2014).

WEBSITES

American Society of Clinical Oncology. "Tumor Marker Tests." Cancer.Net. http://www.cancer.net/navigating-cancer-care/diagnosing-cancer/tests-and-procedures/tumor-marker-tests (accessed August 30, 2014).

National Cancer Institute. "Proteomics Video Tutorial." http://proteomics.cancer.gov/whatisproteomics/videotutorial (accessed August 30, 2014).

National Cancer Institute. "Tumor Markers." http://www.cancer.gov/cancertopics/factsheet/detection/tumor-markers (accessed August 30, 2014).

ORGANIZATIONS

American Cancer Society, 250 Williams Street NW, Atlanta, GA 30303, (800) 227-2345, http://www.cancer.org.

American Society of Clinical Oncology, 2318 Mill Road, Suite 800, Alexandria, VA 22314, (571) 483-1300, Fax: (571) 366-9537, (888) 651-3038, contactus@cancer.net, http://www.asco.org.

National Cancer Institute, 6116 Executive Boulevard, Suite 300, Bethesda, MD 20892-8322, (800) 4-CANCER (422-6237), http://www.cancer.gov.

Nancy J. Nordenson
REVISED BY MARGARET ALIC, PhD
REVIEWED BY MELINDA GRANGER OBERLEITNER, RN, DNS, APRN, CNS

Tumor necrosis factor

Definition

Tumor necrosis factor is a protein produced by several of the body's cell types, such as white blood cells, red blood cells, and other cells that line the blood vessels. It promotes the destruction of some types of **cancer** cells.

Description

In the 1970s, researchers took **sarcoma** cells in culture and exposed them to a protein produced by white blood cells. The protein caused necrosis (death) of the sarcoma cells but had little effect on normal cells in the culture. Hence, the protein was called "tumor necrosis factor" (TNF).

TNF is a type of cytokine released by white blood cells. Cytokines are a group of molecules that are released by many different cells to communicate with other cells and regulate the duration of an **immune response**. There are many different kinds of cytokines, each with a different effect on specific target cells. Once a cell releases the cytokines, they bind to corresponding receptors located on target cells, thus causing a change to take place within the target cell. Tumor necrosis factor is released by special white blood cells called macrophages. Although researchers are still investigating the exact mechanism by which TNF kills cancer cells, it is clear that TNF binds to receptors located on the surface of cancer cells, causing a change and then death of the cell. This was found to be true in animal models. As a result, researchers thought TNF might enhance the reaction of the human immune system to cancer cells.

In the mid-1980s, TNF became available in recombinant form and was analyzed in clinical human trials. At that time, researchers discovered that TNF administered systemically was toxic to humans' normal tissues at the maximum doses required to kill all of the cancer cells, thus limiting its usefulness. At maximum doses required to kill cancer cells, patients experienced **fever**, loss of appetite (**anorexia**), and cachexia (severe weight loss, malnutrition, and wasting away of the body).

TNF can be effectively combined with other systemic chemotherapeutic drugs such as **doxorubicin** and **etoposide**. TNF in conjunction with the above drugs enhances DNA breakage in tumor cells, contributing to their death. In addition to administering TNF systemically, TNF (with or without other chemotherapeutic drugs) can be forced through the blood at the capillary beds at or near the site of the tumor. The regional perfusion of TNF allows larger dosages to be administered only in the area requiring the treatment. Therefore, less normal and healthy tissue is disrupted before reaching the maximum tolerable limits. Research performed in 1998 (by Lejeune, et al.) found regional perfusion to be especially successful in the case of melanomametastasis, resulting in complete remission of 70% to 80% of patients.

Although TNF is valuable in killing cells in **melanoma** and sarcoma tumors, it can promote growth of other kinds of cancers. Therefore, the action of TNF is continually under research with the hope of increasing its effectiveness on killing cancer cells, while decreasing the toxic side effects on healthy tissue.

Resources

PERIODICALS

Wajant, H. "The Role of TNF in Cancer." *Results and Problems in Cell Differentiation* 49 (2009): 1–15. http://link.springer.com/chapter/10.1007%2F400_2008_26 (accessed November 13, 2014).

Waters, J.P., Pober, J.S., Bradley, J.R. "Tumour Necrosis Factor and Cancer." *The Journal of Pathology* 230, no. 3 (2013): 241–8. http://onlinelibrary.wiley.com/doi/10.1002/path.4188/abstract;jsessionid=EAD462406A26DC2643-CE2E41E68F9147.f03t02 (accessed November 13, 2014).

WEBSITES

National Cancer Institute. "Tumor Necrosis Factor." http://www.cancer.gov/dictionary?cdrid=45290 (accessed November 13, 2014).

Sally C. McFarlane-Parrott

Tumor removal

Definition

A tumor is an abnormal growth in the body that is caused by the uncontrolled division of cells. Benign tumors do not have the potential to spread to other parts

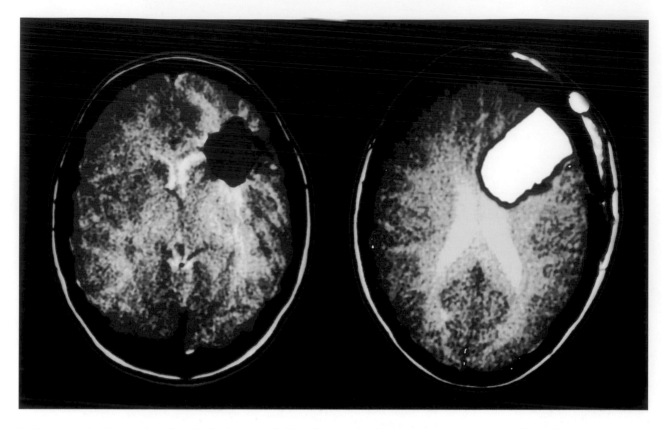

Brain scans showing the location of a brain tumor (left) and the brain after the tumor was removed. *(Scott Camazine/Science Source)*

of the body (a process called **metastasis**) and are curable by surgical removal. Malignant or cancerous tumors, however, may metastasize to other parts of the body and will ultimately result in death if not successfully treated by surgery and/or other methods.

Purpose

Surgical removal is one of four main ways that tumors are treated; the other treatment options include **chemotherapy**, **radiation therapy**, and biological therapy. There are a number of factors used to determine which methods will best treat a tumor. Because benign tumors do not have the potential to metastasize, they are often treated successfully with surgical removal alone. Malignant tumors, however, are most often treated with a combination of surgery and chemotherapy and/or radiation therapy (in about 55% of cases). In some instances, non-curative surgery may make other treatments more effective. Debulking a cancer—making it smaller by surgical removal of a large part of it—is thought to make radiation and chemotherapy more effective.

Surgery is often used to accurately assess the nature and extent of a **cancer**. Most cancers cannot be adequately identified without examining a sample of the abnormal tissue under a microscope. Such tissue samples are procured during a surgical procedure. Surgery may also be used to determine exactly how far a tumor has spread and to establish its margins.

There are a few standard methods of comparing one cancer to another for the purposes of determining appropriate treatments and estimating outcomes. These methods are referred to as staging. The most commonly used method is the TNM system:

- **T** stands for tumor, and reflects the size of the tumor.

- **N** represents the spread of the cancer to lymph nodes, largely determined by those nodes removed at surgery that contain cancer cells. Since cancers spread mostly through the lymphatic system, this is a useful measure of a cancer's ability to disperse.

- **M** refers to metastasis, and indicates if metastases are present and how far they are from the original cancer.

Staging is particularly important with such lymphomas as **Hodgkin lymphoma**, which may appear in many places in the lymphatic system. Surgery is a useful tool for staging such cancers and can increase the chance of a successful cure, since radiation treatment is often curative if all the cancerous sites are located and irradiated.

KEY TERMS

Aspiration—A technique for obtaining a piece of tissue for biopsy by using suction applied through a needle attached to a syringe.

Biopsy—The removal of living tissue from the body, done in order to establish a diagnosis.

Debulking—Surgical removal of a major portion of a tumor so that there is less of the cancer left for later treatment by chemotherapy or radiation.

Mammogram—A set of x-rays taken of the front and side of the breast; used to diagnose various abnormalities of the breast.

Metastasis (plural, metastases)—A growth of cancer cells at a site in the body distant from the primary tumor.

Oncologist—A physician who specializes in the diagnosis and treatment of tumors.

Palliative—Offering relief of symptoms, but not a cure.

Pap test—The common term for the Papanicolaou test, a simple smear method of examining stained cells to detect cancer of the cervix.

Staging—The classification of cancerous tumors according to the extent of the tumor.

Description

Surgery may be used to remove tumors for diagnostic or therapeutic purposes.

Diagnostic tumor removal

A **biopsy** is a medical procedure that obtains a small piece of tissue for diagnostic testing. The sample is examined under a microscope by a doctor who specializes in the effects of disease on body tissues (a pathologist) to detect any abnormalities. A definitive diagnosis of cancer cannot be made unless a sample of the abnormal tissue is examined histologically (under a microscope).

There are four main biopsy techniques used to diagnose cancer:

- In an aspiration biopsy, a needle is inserted into the tumor and a sample is withdrawn. This procedure may be performed under local anesthesia or with no anesthesia at all.
- For a needle biopsy, a special cutting needle is inserted into the core of the tumor and a core sample is cut out. Local anesthesia is most often administered.

- With an incisional biopsy, a portion of a large tumor is removed, usually under local anesthesia in an outpatient setting.
- In an excisional biopsy, an entire cancerous lesion is removed along with surrounding normal tissue (called a clear margin). Local or general anesthesia may be used.

Therapeutic tumor removal

Once surgical removal has been decided, a surgical oncologist will remove the entire tumor, taking with it a large section of the surrounding normal tissue. The healthy tissue is removed to minimize the risk that abnormal tissue is left behind. Tumors may be removed by cutting with steel instruments, by the use of a laser beam, by **radiofrequency ablation** (the use of radiofrequency energy to destroy tissue), by cryoablation (the use of extreme cold to freeze and thus destroy the tumor), or by injecting alcohol into the tumor.

When surgical removal of a tumor is unacceptable as a sole treatment, a portion of the tumor is removed to debulk the mass; this process is called cytoreduction. Cytoreductive surgery aids radiation and chemotherapy treatments by increasing the sensitivity of the tumor and decreasing the number of necessary treatment cycles.

Certain types of skin tumors can be removed by a technique called Mohs micrographic surgery, developed in the late 1930s by Dr. Frederic E. Mohs. The Mohs method involves four steps: surgical removal of the tumor, making a slide of the removed tissue and examining it for cancer cells (called mapping the tissue), interpreting the microscope slides and removing more tissue if necessary until no more cancer cells are found, and performing **reconstructive surgery** to cover the wound.

A newer technique for removing some tumors of the spinal cord involves the use of a suction tip rather than a scalpel. The newer technique appears to have a wider margin of safety when working around the delicate structures of the central nervous system.

In some instances, the purpose of tumor removal is not to cure the cancer, but to relieve the symptoms of a patient who cannot be cured. This approach is called palliative surgery. For example, a patient with advanced cancer may have a tumor causing significant pain or bleeding; in such a case, the tumor may be removed to ease the patient's pain or other symptoms even though a cure is not possible.

Seeding

The surgical removal of malignant tumors demands special considerations. There is a danger of spreading cancerous cells during the process of removing abnormal tissue (called seeding). Presuming that cancer cells can implant elsewhere in the body, the surgeon must minimize the dissemination of cells throughout the operating field or into the bloodstream.

Special techniques called block resection and no-touch are used. Block resection involves taking the entire specimen out as a single piece. The no-touch technique involves removing a specimen by handling only the normal tissue surrounding it; the cancer itself is never touched. These approaches prevent the spread of cancer cells into the general circulation. The surgeon takes great care to clamp off the blood supply first, preventing cells from leaving by that route later in the surgery.

Demographics

The American Cancer Society estimates that approximately 1,665,540 cases of cancer will be diagnosed in the United States in 2014. Seventy-eight percent of cancers are diagnosed in men and women over the age of 55, although cancer may affect individuals of any age. Men develop cancer more often than women; one in two men will be diagnosed with cancer during his lifetime, compared to one in three women. Additionally, men are more likely to die of cancer. Cancer affects individuals of all races and ethnicities, although incidence may differ among these groups by cancer type.

Diagnosis

A tumor may first be palpated (felt) by the patient or by a healthcare professional during a physical examination. A tumor may be visible on the skin or protrude outward from the body. Still other tumors are not evident until their presence begins to cause such symptoms as **weight loss**, **fatigue**, or pain. In some instances, tumors are located during routine tests (e.g., a yearly mammogram or Pap smear).

Aftercare

Retesting and periodical examinations are necessary to ensure that a tumor has not returned or metastasized after total removal.

Risks

Each tumor removal surgery carries certain risks that are inherent to the procedure. There is always a risk of misdiagnosing a cancer if an inadequate sample was procured during biopsy, or if the tumor was not properly located. There is a chance of infection of the surgical site, excessive bleeding, or injury to adjacent tissues. The possibility of metastasis and seeding are risks that have to be considered in consultation with an oncologist.

QUESTIONS TO ASK YOUR DOCTOR

- What type of tumor do I have and where is it located?
- What procedure will be used to remove the tumor?
- Is there evidence that the tumor has metastasized?
- What diagnostic tests will be performed prior to tumor removal?
- What method of anesthesia/pain relief will be used during the procedure?
- Will the tumor recur?
- When will I be able to return to normal activities?

Results

The results of a tumor removal procedure depend on the type of tumor and the purpose of the treatment. Most benign tumors can be removed successfully with no risk of the abnormal cells spreading to other parts of the body and little risk of the tumor returning. Malignant tumors are considered successfully removed if the entire tumor can be removed, if a clear margin of healthy tissue is removed with the tumor, and if there is no evidence of metastasis. The normal results of palliative tumor removal are a reduction in the patient's symptoms with no impact on length of survival.

Morbidity and mortality rates

The recurrence rates of benign and malignant tumors after removal depend on the type of tumor and its location. The rate of complications associated with tumor removal surgery differs by procedure, but is generally very low.

Despite low rates of complication for the actual tumor removal procedures, cancer itself remains the second most frequent cause of death among Americans, responsible for about 25% of all deaths. In 2014, about 585,720 people in the United States were expected to die of cancer.

Alternatives

If a benign tumor shows no indication of harming nearby tissues and is not causing the patient any symptoms, surgery may not be required to remove it. Chemotherapy, radiation therapy, and biological therapy are treatments that may be used alone or in conjunction with surgery.

Health care team roles

Tumors are usually removed by a general surgeon or surgical oncologist. The procedure is frequently done in a hospital setting, but specialized outpatient facilities may sometimes be used.

Resources

BOOKS

Niederhuber, John E., et al. *Abeloff's Clinical Oncology*. 5th ed. Philadelphia: Saunders/Elsevier, 2013.

PERIODICALS

Arata, Jumpei, et al. "Neurosurgical Robotic System for Brain Tumor Removal." *International Journal of Computer-Assisted Radiology and Surgery* 6, no. 3 (2011): 375–85. http://dx.doi.org/10.1007/s11548-010-0514-8 (accessed September 19, 2013).

WEBSITES

MedlinePlus. "Benign Tumors." U.S. National Library of Medicine, National Institutes of Health. http://www.nlm.nih.gov/medlineplus/benigntumors.html (accessed September 19, 2013).

MedlinePlus. "Cancer." U.S. National Library of Medicine, National Institutes of Health. http://www.nlm.nih.gov/medlineplus/cancer.html (accessed September 19, 2013).

ORGANIZATIONS

American Cancer Society, 250 Williams St. NW, Atlanta, GA 30303, (800) 227-2345, http://www.cancer.org.

National Cancer Institute, 6116 Executive Blvd., Ste. 300, Bethesda, MD 20892-8322, (800) 4-CANCER (422-6237), http://cancer.gov.

Society of Surgical Oncology, 9525 W. Bryn Mawr Ave., Ste. 870, Rosemont, IL 60018, (847) 427-1400, info@surgonc.org, http://surgonc.org.

J. Ricker Polsdorfer, MD

REVISED BY STEPHANIE DIONNE SHERK
REVISED BY REBECCA FREY, PhD

Tumor staging

Definition

Tumor staging is the process of defining at what point in the natural history of the malignant disease the patient is when the diagnosis is made. The organ and cell type in which the malignancy has developed defines the type of malignancy. For example, **adenocarcinoma** of

Example of TNM staging (pancreatic cancer)

Stage 0	Cancer has been identified in the top layer of cells but has not reached deeper tissues.
Stage IA	The cancer is no larger than 2 cm and has not spread beyond the pancreas.
Stage IB	The cancer has grown larger than 2 cm but has not spread.
Stage IIA	The cancer has spread beyond the pancreas but has not reached large blood vessels or lymph nodes.
Stage IIB	The cancer has spread to nearby lymph nodes but not to large blood vessels, nerves, or other parts of the body.
Stage III	The cancer has spread to large blood vessels or nerves but has not reached other parts of the body.
Stage IV	The cancer has spread to other parts of the body.

SOURCE: American Cancer Society, "How is Pancreatic Cancer Staged?" Available online at: http://www.cancer.org/cancer/pancreaticcancer/detailedguide/pancreatic-cancer-staging.

Example of TNM staging for pancreatic cancer. (*Illustration by PreMediaGlobal. © Cengage Learning®.*)

the lung defines that the **cancer** originated in the mucus-secreting cells lining the airways of the lung. Staging is different than defining the type of cancer; it is the process of defining the degree of advancement of the specific type of malignancy in the patient at the time of presentation (the time when the diagnosis is made). Because there are many different types of malignancy arising from many different organs in the body, the specifics of staging systems vary.

Purpose

Staging fulfills an organizational role that is central to the treatment of cancer. After the tumor is staged, the treatment team knows to what degree the cancer has evolved in its natural history. This knowledge will provide the information necessary to formulate a plan of treatment and will allow an estimate of the success of that treatment (prognosis). Finally, by establishing uniform criteria for staging, people with the same type of malignancy presenting at the same stage can be treated equivalently. If a new treatment is tested that improves the long-term prognosis then that treatment will become the new standard of care. Thus, staging is vital to the processes of research and scientific reporting.

Prognosis

The first question that most patients want answered when they find they have cancer is "What am I going to do?" They want to know the ultimate outcome—their prognosis. Because of the existing research on the natural history, or progression of the disease, this information is available on a statistical basis. Staging, then, helps define the patient's prognosis. Intuitively, one would think that those presenting with an earlier stage have a better prognosis. For the most part, that is correct.

Scientific reporting and research

When a patient develops a life-threatening disease such as cancer, the physicians and other members of the treatment team intervene in an effort to improve the prognosis. Treatment regimens are defined as good or bad based on how they influence the prognosis of the disease. Staging allows medical professionals to interpret whether or not their efforts are favorably influencing the natural history of the disease. Once a patient's cancer stage has been established, a baseline exists against which to measure the efficacy of the cancer treatment that follows for that patient.

Staging plays a similar "baseline" role when considering a large group of cancer patients. In order to gauge accurately the effectiveness of any cancer treatment, researchers must know if the patients' conditions really are comparable. If they are, comparisons between treatments are fair. If the patients' conditions vary at the outset of a study, then comparing the outcomes of different treatments is not useful.

Staging provides that useful, objective standard so that researchers can accurately compare specific treatments in certain stages of particular cancers. Staging allows uniformity in treatment protocol and reporting of the data related to outcome. As new treatment protocols are developed, they can be tested on patients with the same type and stage of cancer and the two groups compared. If there is improvement with a new treatment protocol, that treatment regimen will be adopted as standard. Physicians can use these established best practices to determine treatments for their patients.

Criteria for staging

As it became apparent to medical professionals that staging of malignancies was necessary for accurate assessment of treatment regimens and defining the treatment recommendations themselves, criteria for staging needed to be developed. Initially this was done for individual tumors separately. Because of the need for uniformity, a universal set of criteria was desired. The TNM system of staging has been adopted for the most part for this reason. It has been developed and updated by The **American Joint Committee on Cancer** (AJCC). Some of the types of malignancy do not fit well into the TNM criteria and others have older systems that are still in use because they are effective and are deeply established in scientific literature.

TNM system

This system of staging is the general format used for staging cancer of all types and is updated and maintained

---

---

by the AJCC. The "T" stands for tumor size. The "N" stands for spread to lymph nodes (nodal **metastasis**). The "M" stands for metastasis (spread of the cancer to sites in the body other than the organ of origin). When the diagnosis of cancer is made, a physical examination, along with laboratory testing and **imaging studies**, will be performed to define the TNM status of the patient. The TNM status will define the stage.

The tumor size, "T," will be assessed by physical examination or various imaging modalities depending on the accessibility of the tumor. The "T" value is generally defined as 1 through 4 on the basis of size and whether or not the tumor is invading structures that surround it. In cancer so early that it is felt to be incapable of spreading, it is assigned a "T" value of 0. The "T" value is, in essence, a description of the tumor in its local place of origin. As time passes and the staging system is continually updated, the "T" value is being subdivided in certain types of cancer. The subdivisions are indicated by letters "a" through "d" and also have a graduated value system. For example: T1 **breast cancer** is a tumor sized 2 cm or less in greatest dimension. T1a is less than 0.5 cm, T1b is 0.5 to 1.0 cm, and T1c is 1.0 to 2.0 cm.

In many cancers, there seems to be a progression from the place of primary origin, then to the regional lymph nodes, and then throughout the body. Lymph nodes can be thought of as filters that drain tissue fluid coming from a particular organ. If that organ has developed a cancer and some of the cells flow away with the tissue fluid to the lymph node filter that is draining that organ, the cancer may begin to grow there also. Assessment of lymph node involvement thus becomes the next step in staging and defines the "N" value. Since the word metastasis means that the cancer has spread from its point of origin to somewhere else in the body and the lymph nodes are in the region, the "N" value defines presence of regional metastasis. The assessment is performed by physical examination and imaging studies of the region involved. "N" is assigned a value of 0 for no nodes involved, or depending on the anatomic nature of the region, values 1 through 3.

"M" stands for distant metastasis. As mentioned previously, metastasis is the spread of the primary tumor to elsewhere in the body. When that spread or metastasis is outside the region of the primary tumor, the patient has distant metastasis. The "M" value is assessed by physical exam, laboratory studies, and imaging studies. Different cancers have different typical patterns of metastasis. Common areas of metastatic involvement are lung, liver, bone, and brain. The "M" value is assigned either 0 or 1. Another term used to describe the patient who has distant metastasis is having systemic disease. In the TNM system, virtually all patients with an "M" value of 1 have stage IV disease. The "M" value may also have a subscript defining the organ of metastatic involvement.

After the values for TNM have been determined as accurately as possible, the values are grouped together and a stage value is assigned. The stage value is usually I through IV (written in Roman numerals). Each stage may be subdivided if it is useful for treatment recommendations and reporting. In general, stage I implies the tumor is confined to its source of origin and stage IV implies distant metastasis or systemic disease. Because of different anatomical, prognostic, and treatment considerations, the intermediate stages are defined by different tumor sizes, the presence or absence of local invasion of the tumor into surrounding structures, or the number and/ or presence of involved lymph nodes. Treatment recommendations and expected outcome are both defined to a large extent by stage. The specific criteria for each stage are contained in the *AJCC Cancer Staging Manual*.

Special staging systems

In the development of staging systems it has been recognized that some malignancies do not fit well into the scheme of the TNM system or that the system in place reflects the same information as the TNM system. Thus, there are a few special staging systems in use for specific organs of involvement. The goal is the same for these schema as for TNM—to define the point in the natural history of the cancer at presentation, to allow establishment of prognosis and treatment recommendations, and to facilitate scientific research and reporting.

OVARIAN CANCER. Ovarian cancer is staged using FIGO, which stands for the International Federation of Gynecology and Obstetrics. This organization developed staging criteria for the various gynecologic malignancies and ovarian cancer. In the FIGO system, ovarian cancer is staged I through IV similar to the TNM scheme, and then each stage is subdivided into A, B, or C, depending on defined criteria. TNM may also be used, but FIGO is more common.

LYMPHOMA. Anatomically, the lymph system and its nodes are found throughout the body. Malignancies involving the lymph system (lymphomas), do not fit the typical TNM scheme well. The Ann Arbor staging criteria are instead utilized to classify this group of malignancies. The goals of the Ann Arbor **lymphoma** staging system are to define the degree of advancement of the disease so that treatment recommendations can be made, prognosis can be estimated, and consistent reporting and research can be facilitated.

The Ann Arbor system classifies lymphoma into four stages based on anatomic lymph nodal group involvement. Disease confined to one nodal group or location defines stage I. Disease limited to one side of the diaphragm (the muscle separating the chest from the abdomen) defines stage II. Stage III patients have disease on both sides of the diaphragm and stage IV patients once again have disseminated disease. Consideration of involvement of the liver, spleen, and bone marrow are also considered in this system. Finally, the stage is subdivided into categories of A and B depending on the presence of symptoms of **itching**, **weight loss**, **fever**, and **night sweats**. Those having symptoms receive the designation "B" and have a worse prognosis.

LEUKEMIA. Leukemia is a type of malignancy that begins in the cells of the marrow that produce the cellular components of blood, the progenitor cells. These malignancies are truly systemic from their outset and do not fit any form of the TNM system. Still, there is a need to categorize the presenting features of the patients with these diseases to help make treatment recommendations, estimate prognosis, and to facilitate scientific research and reporting. The type of method used depends on the type of leukemia:

• Acute lymphocytic leukemia (ALL) is classified based upon the lymphocyte of origin (B-cell or T-cell).

- Acute myeloid leukemia is classified using the French-American-British (FAB) classification system. The World Health Organization (WHO) has developed a new system that takes more factors into consideration, but FAB is still common.
- Chronic lymphocytic leukemia is staged using the Rai system in the United States and the Binet system in Europe.
- Chronic myeloid leukemia is described as being in various phases rather than stages. Classification is based on a variety of factors, including disease progression, patient age, and white blood cell count.

LUNG CANCER, SMALL CELL. Unlike other types of lung cancer, the staging of **small cell lung cancer** is relatively simple. This is because approximately 70% of patients already have metastatic disease when they are diagnosed, and small differences in the amount of tumor found in the lungs do not change the prognosis. Small cell lung cancer is usually divided into three stages:

- Limited stage: The cancer is found only in one lung and in lymph nodes close to the lung.
- Extensive stage: The cancer has spread beyond the lungs to other parts of the body.
- Recurrent stage: The cancer has returned following treatment.

Defining the stage

The process of defining a stage is quite simple. First, the diagnosis is established by study of the patient and by tissue **biopsy**. Once the cell type and organ of origin are established, the staging criteria are reviewed. The patient will undergo a series of diagnostic tests to define the various parameters of the staging criteria. The results of these tests define the extent of the disease and establish the stage. The known typical natural history of the disease dictates the types of testing done. The tests differ for each type of malignancy.

Special concerns

Clinical vs. pathological stage

The stage of the patient's disease may be categorized into clinical or pathological. As mentioned, the known natural history of the disease and the staging criteria are utilized to define the stage of the patient at the time of presentation. The investigations performed often involve an initial degree of uncertainty when they are based on clinical grounds alone. For example, the physical exam or the imaging of a particular group of lymph nodes may show that they are enlarged, but the enlargement may not accurately define whether they are truly involved with cancer. This issue may only be resolved by removing some or all of the suspect enlarged nodes, sometimes by biopsy before treatment or sometimes by the removal of the questionable nodes at the time of definitive treatment. The evaluation under the microscope of the clinically enlarged nodes will define whether they are really involved with cancer or merely enlarged. When staging criteria are based on clinical assessment alone, it is referred to as the clinical stage. Once the results of the microscopic evaluation are known, the true stage or pathologic stage may be assigned.

Stage is uniform and accurate

One of the main goals of staging is to facilitate communication so that like patients are compared to like patients. It is imperative that the adopted staging criteria are rigidly adhered to or inaccurate comparisons may be made and the results of research to develop better treatment regimens will be difficult to interpret.

Tumor grade

When the tissue obtained for diagnosis is evaluated under the microscope for cell type, another index called grade is often defined. As the pathologist analyzes the malignant cells, attention will be given to how close to a normal cell the malignant cells appear to be. If they are very similar, the malignant cells are not felt to be too aggressive and a low grade value is assigned. The more atypical the malignant cells appear to be, the more aggressive the tumor is and a higher grade value is assigned. Grade is usually assigned a value of I through IV, though more levels can be assigned depending on the particular cancer.

The estimate of grade is just that—an estimation. It is subjective in nature and cannot be determined quantitatively. Though useful in predicting prognosis, the correlation is not exact. Rather, grade is included as only one of the factors influencing prognosis. Grade may be included as part of the actual staging criteria; however, it usually is not part of the scheme.

Tumor boards

A tumor board is a body of specialists in the treatment of cancer that convenes to discuss the aspects of patients presenting with cancer. The AJCC encourages the development of tumor boards throughout the nation to facilitate the use of staging and reporting of cancer statistics from region to region throughout the country. In addition to allowing the collection of vital cancer statistics, local tumor boards create a forum where the clinical aspects of a patient's cancer may be discussed to provide recommendations or to play a role in education.

QUESTIONS TO ASK YOUR DOCTOR

- What do my results mean?
- What are my treatment options?
- What are the side effects of treatment?

Resources

BOOKS

Casciato, Dennis A., ed. *Manual of Clinical Oncology.* 7th ed. Philadelphia: Lippincott Williams & Wilkins, 2012.

Compton, Caryolyn C., et al, eds. *AJCC Cancer Staging Atlas: A Companion to the Seventh Editions of the AJCC Cancer Staging Manual and Handbook.* 2nd ed. New York: Springer, 2012.

DeVita, Vincent T. Jr., et al, eds. *DeVita, Hellman, and Rosenberg's Cancer: Principles and Practice of Oncology.* 9th ed. Philadelphia: Lippincott Williams & Wilkins, 2011.

Edge, Stephen R., et al, eds. *AJCC Cancer Staging Handbook.* 7th ed. New York: Springer, 2010.

PERIODICALS

Al-Hawary, Mahmoud M., et al. "Staging of Pancreatic Cancer: Role of Imaging." *Seminars in Roentgenology* 48, no. 3 (2013): 245–52. http://dx.doi.org/10.1053/j.ro.2013.03.005 (accessed September 25, 2013).

"Current FIGO Staging for Cancer of the Vagina, Fallopian Tube, Ovary, and Gestational Trophoblastic Neoplasia." *International Journal of Gynaecology and Obstetrics* 105, no. 1 (2009): 3–4.

Ghafoori, M., et al. "Value of MRI in Local Staging of Bladder Cancer." *Urology Journal* 10, no. 2 (2013): 866–72.

Heitz, F., P. Harter, and A. du Bois. "Staging Laparoscopy for the Management of Early-Stage Ovarian Cancer: A Metaanalysis." *American Journal of Obstetrics & Gynecology* (June 2013): e-pub ahead of print. http://dx.doi.org/10.1016/j.ajog.2013.06.035 (accessed September 25, 2013).

Nordholm-Carstensen, Andreas, et al. "Indeterminate Pulmonary Nodules at Colorectal Cancer Staging: A Systematic Review of Predictive Parameters for Malignancy." *Annals of Surgical Oncology* (June 2013): e-pub ahead of print. http://dx.doi.org/10.1245/s10434-013-3062-y (accessed September 25, 2013).

Peng, Chun-Wei, et al. "Evaluation of the Staging Systems for Gastric Cancer." *Journal of Surgical Oncology* (June 28, 2013): e-pub ahead of print. http://dx.doi.org/10.1002/jso.23360 (accessed September 25, 2013).

WEBSITES

American Cancer Society. "How is Acute Lymphocytic Leukemia Classified?" http://www.cancer.org/cancer/leukemia-acutelymphocyticallinadults/detailedguide/leukemia-acute-lymphocytic-classified (accessed September 25, 2013).

American Cancer Society. "How is Acute Myeloid Leukemia Classified?" http://www.cancer.org/cancer/leukemia-acutemyeloidaml/detailedguide/leukemia-acute-myeloid-myelogenous-classified (accessed September 25, 2013).

American Cancer Society. "How is Chronic Lymphocytic Leukemia Staged?" http://www.cancer.org/cancer/leukemia-chroniclymphocyticcll/detailedguide/leukemia-chronic-lymphocytic-staging (accessed September 25, 2013).

American Cancer Society. "How is Chronic Myeloid Leukemia Staged?" http://www.cancer.org/cancer/leukemia-chronic-myeloidcml/detailedguide/leukemia-chronic-myeloid-myelogenous-staging (accessed September 25, 2013).

American Cancer Society. "How is Colorectal Cancer Staged?" http://www.cancer.org/cancer/colonandrectumcancer/detailedguide/colorectal-cancer-staged (accessed September 25, 2013).

American Cancer Society. "Staging." http://www.cancer.org/treatment/understandingyourdiagnosis/staging (accessed September 25, 2013).

American Joint Committee on Cancer. "What Is Cancer Staging?" https://cancerstaging.org/references-tools/Pages/What-is-Cancer-Staging.aspx (accessed February 5, 2015).

American Lung Association. "Staging." http://www.lung.org/lung-disease/lung-cancer/learning-more-about-lung-cancer/diagnosing-lung-cancer/staging.html (accessed September 25, 2013).

BreastCancer.org "Stages of Breast Cancer." http://www.breastcancer.org/symptoms/diagnosis/staging (accessed September 25, 2013).

National Cancer Institute. "Cancer Staging." http://www.cancer.gov/cancertopics/factsheet/detection/staging (accessed September 25, 2013).

Target Ovarian Cancer. "Stages and Grades." http://www.targetovariancancer.org.uk/about-ovarian-cancer/what-ovarian-cancer/stages-and-grades (accessed February 5, 2015).

ORGANIZATIONS

American Cancer Society, 250 Williams St. NW, Atlanta, GA 30303, (800) 227-2345, http://www.cancer.org.

American Joint Committee on Cancer (AJCC), 633 N. St. Clair St., Chicago, IL 60611-3211, (312) 202-5205, ajcc@facs.org, http://www.cancerstaging.org.

Cancer Research Institute, One Exchange Plz., 55 Broadway, Ste. 1802, New York, NY 10006, (212) 688-7515, (800) 99-CANCER (992-2623), http://cancerresearch.org.

International Federation of Gynecology and Obstetrics (FIGO), FIGO House, Ste. 3, Waterloo Ct., 10 Theed St., London, SE1 8ST, United Kingdom, +44 20 7928 1166, http://www.figo.org.

National Cancer Institute, 6116 Executive Blvd., Ste. 300, Bethesda, MD 20892-8322, (800) 4-CANCER (422-6237), http://cancer.gov.

Richard A. McCartney, MD

Tumor suppressor genes *see* **Cancer genetics**
2-CdA *see* **Cladribine**

Ultrasonography

Definition

Ultrasonography is the study of internal organs or blood vessels using high-frequency sound waves. The actual test is called an ultrasound scan or sonogram. Duplex ultrasonography uses Doppler technology to study blood cells moving through major veins and arteries. There are several types of ultrasound. Each is used in diagnosing specific parts of the body.

Purpose

An ultrasound is a noninvasive, safe method of examining a patient's eyes, pelvic or abdominal organs, breast, heart, or arteries and veins. It is often used to diagnosis disease, locate the source of pain, or look for stones in the kidney or gallbladder. Ultrasound produces images in real time. Images appear on the screen instantly. It may also be used to guide doctors who are performing a needle **biopsy** to locate a mass—needle biopsies are often used to obtain a sample of breast tissue to test for **cancer** cells. Duplex/Doppler ultrasound aids in diagnosing a blockage in or a malformation of the vessel. Different color flows aid in identifying problem areas in smaller vessels. Endoscopic ultrasound combines a visual endoscopic exam, during which a flexible tube called an endoscope is threaded down the throat, with an ultrasound test. The ultrasound probe is attached to the end of the endoscope. An endoscopic ultrasound is helpful in determining how deeply a tumor has grown into normal tissues or the gastrointestinal tract. During a **transvaginal ultrasound**, the ultrasound probe is inserted into the vagina to obtain better images of the ovaries and uterus. Color flow Doppler imaging using a transvaginal probe is being performed to detect abnormal blood flow patterns associated with **ovarian cancer**.

Description

The patient will be asked to lie still on an exam table in a darkened room. The darkness helps the technician see images on a screen, which is similar to a computer monitor. Sometimes the patients are positioned so they can watch the screen. The technician will apply a lubricating gel to the skin over the area to be studied. Ultrasound uses high-frequency sound waves to produce an image. A small wand-like device called a transducer produces sound waves that are sent into the body when the device is pressed against the skin. The gel helps transmit the sound waves, which do not travel through the air. Neither the patient nor the technician can hear the sound waves. The technician moves the device across the skin in the area to be studied. The sound waves bounce off the fluids and tissues inside the body. The transducer picks up the return echo and records any changes in the pitch or direction of the sound. The image is immediately visible on the screen. The technician may print a still picture of any significant images for later review by the radiologist.

Precautions

Ultrasound is considered safe with no known risks or precautions. The exam uses no radiation. Under normal circumstances the exam is normally painless. If the patient has a full bladder, pressure exerted during the exam may feel uncomfortable. An ultrasound conducted in conjunction with an invasive exam carries the same risks as the invasive exam.

Preparation

Depending on the type of ultrasound ordered, patients may not need to do anything prior to the test. Other ultrasound studies may require that the patient not eat or drink anything for up to 12 hours prior to the exam, in order to decrease the amount of gas in the bowel. Intestinal gas may interfere in obtaining accurate results.

The patient must have a full bladder for some exams and an empty bladder for others.

Aftercare

Remove any gel still left on the skin. No other aftercare is required following an ultrasound.

Risks

Standard, diagnostic ultrasound is considered risk-free. Risks may be associated with invasive tests conducted at the same time, such as an endoscopic ultrasound or an ultrasound-guided needle biopsy.

Results

An ultrasound scan is considered normal when the image depicts normally shaped organs or normal blood flow.

Abnormal results

Abnormal echo patterns may represent a condition requiring treatment. Any masses, tumors, enlarged organs or blockages in the blood vessel are considered abnormal. Additional testing may be ordered.

See also Upper gastrointestinal endoscopy.

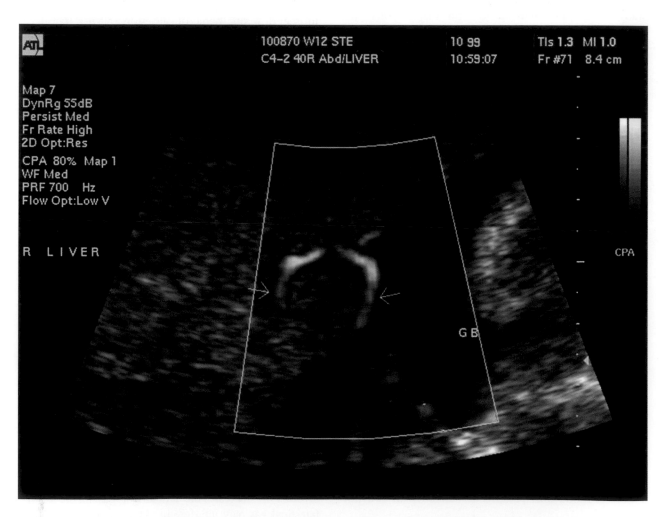

Ultrasound revealing cancer in the liver. The orange spots indicate increased blood flow to the tumor. *(Simon Fraser/Science Source)*

Resources

WEBSITES

American Cancer Society. "Ultrasound." http://www.cancer.org/treatment/understandingyourdiagnosis/examsandtest-descriptions/imagingradiologytests/imaging-radiology-tests-ultrasound (accessed November 13, 2014).

American Society of Clinical Oncology. "Ultrasound." Cancer.net http://www.cancer.net/navigating-cancer-care/diagnosing-cancer/tests-and-procedures/ultrasound (accessed November 13, 2014).

Cancer Research UK. "Ultrasound Scan." http://www.cancer-researchuk.org/about-cancer/cancers-in-general/tests/ultrasound-scan (accessed November 13, 2014).

Debra Wood, R.N.

Upper gastrointestinal endoscopy

Definition

Upper gastrointestinal endoscopy is a procedure that allows the doctor to visually examine the upper portions of the gastrointestinal tract, using a flexible tool called an endoscope. The endoscope has a light source and projects an image on a video screen. An endoscope may also be used to assist with other diagnostic exams and procedures. For instance, an ultrasound probe can be placed on the end of the endoscope to evaluate how deeply a tumor has penetrated the esophagus or wall of the stomach. An endoscope may be used to assist with placement of a permanent feeding tube or to treat a bleeding ulcer.

Purpose

An upper gastrointestinal endoscopy aids in the investigation of the source of pain, difficulty swallowing, bleeding or other symptoms of an upper abdominal problem. During an endoscopy the doctor can obtain samples of tissue for **biopsy**, to check for the presence of **cancer** cells or the bacteria responsible for most stomach ulcers. Various instruments can be passed through the endoscope to treat problems, such as controlling bleeding due to an ulcer. The procedure may be performed on patients who have had stomach surgery to assess for cancer or the return of an ulcer. It may also be used to monitor patients at high risk for upper **gastrointestinal cancers**.

Description

An endoscopy may take place in the physician's office or in a hospital. An intravenous (IV) line will be started in a vein in the arm. Through the IV line, the patient generally receives a sedative and a pain-killer if needed. The medication will help the patient feel relaxed and drowsy. A local anesthetic is usually sprayed into the throat to prevent a gag reflex. Dentures are removed. A mouthpiece will help to keep the mouth open. Patients are positioned onto their sides. The doctor slowly advances the lubricated endoscope down the throat, into the stomach. Air will be passed through the endoscope to make it easier for the doctor to see the lining of the gastrointestinal tract. The endoscope will be repositioned to see different parts of the stomach and the small intestine. The exam usually takes less than an hour. The patient is able to breathe independently during the exam. In some cases a biopsy may be taken. Biopsy forceps or a brush used to secure cells are passed through the endoscope. The tissue sample is taken and then removed through the endoscope.

Precautions

Patients with a history of heart and lung disease and those with blood-clotting problems require special precautions. For instance, a patient with artificial heart valves or a history of infection of the lining of the heart will need **antibiotics** to prevent infection. Patients with an intestinal perforation, or puncture in the gastrointestinal tract, should not have an upper gastrointestinal endoscopy. Patients must be able to cooperate during the procedure. Those who are not able to cooperate are not good candidates for an endoscopy.

Preparation

The doctor should be informed of any allergies as well as all the medications that the patient is currently taking. The doctor may instruct the patient not to take certain medications, like aspirin and anti-inflammatory drugs that interfere with clotting, for a period of time prior to the procedure. The patient should not eat or drink anything for at least eight hours prior to the endoscopy. The doctor should be informed if the patient has had heart valves replaced or a history of an inflammation of the inside lining of the heart, so that appropriate

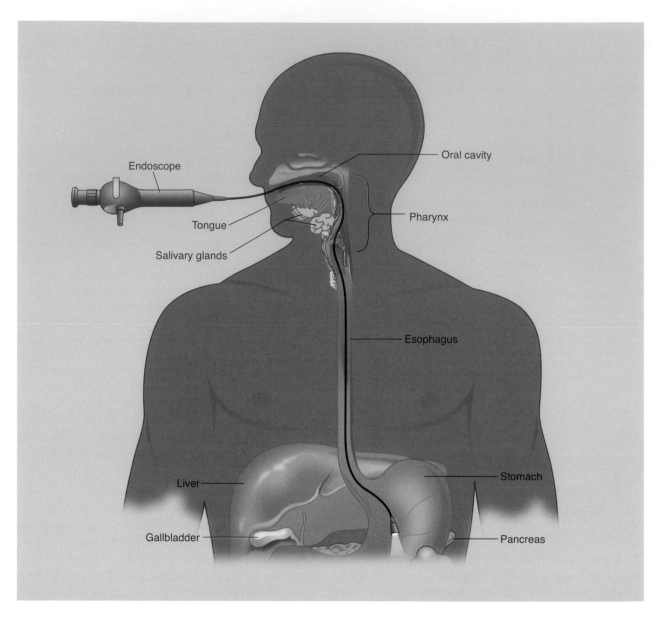

Upper gastrointestinal endoscopy. *(Illustration by Electronic Illustrators Group. © 2015 Cengage Learning®.)*

antibiotics can be administered to prevent any chance of infection. Risks and benefits of the procedure will be explained to the patient. The patient will be asked to sign a consent form.

Aftercare

The patient will be monitored for an hour or two after the procedure, while the effects of the medication wear off. Due to the sedative, the patients will need to arrange for someone to drive them home after the procedure.

Patients may feel bloated due to the air that is introduced into the stomach during the procedure, and may have a sore throat for a couple of days. Patient should contact the doctor if they develop difficulty swallowing, chest pain, severe abdominal pain, throat soreness that becomes more severe or rectal bleeding.

Risks

Endoscopy is usually considered safe when performed by a specially trained physician. As with any invasive procedure it is not risk-free. Complications include bleeding and perforation (puncturing a hole in the lining of the gastrointestinal tract). Scopes are cleaned and disinfected between patients so any risk of transmitting infectious disease from one patient to another by the endoscope would be negligible.

KEY TERMS

Biopsy—Removal of a tissue sample for examination under a microscope to check for cancer cells.

Duodenum—The first portion of the small intestine.

Endoscope—A thin, flexible, lighted tube that is passed down the throat and enables the doctor to view the esophagus, stomach lining and duodenum.

Perforation—Puncture or tear.

Staging—Determination of how advanced the cancer is.

Ultrasound—The study of internal organs using high-frequency sound waves.

QUESTIONS TO ASK YOUR DOCTOR

- Did you see any abnormalities?
- How soon will you know the results of the biopsy (if one was done)?
- When can I resume any medications that were stopped?
- What future care will I need?
- Which problems should prompt me to call you?

Results

A pale reddish pink lining with no abnormal-looking masses or ulcerations is considered a normal result.

Abnormal results

Evidence of an ulcer or other lesion would be considered an abnormal result. If the biopsy determines the presence of cancer cells, a diagnosis of cancer is made. The appearance of the lesion, including its size or if there are multiple lesions, often helps with staging and treatment plans. An ultrasound probe attached to the endoscope also may help with staging.

Resources

PERIODICALS

Vradelis, S., et al. "Quality Control in Upper Gastrointestinal Endoscopy: Detection Rates of Gastric Cancer in Oxford 2005–2008." *Postgraduate Medical Journal* 87, no. 1027 (2011): 335–9.

WEBSITES

American Cancer Society. "How is Stomach Cancer Diagnosed." http://www.cancer.org/cancer/stomachcancer/detailedguide/stomach-cancer-diagnosis (accessed November 13, 2014).

American Society of Clinical Oncology. "Upper Endoscopy." Cancer.net. http://www.cancer.net/navigating-cancer-care/diagnosing-cancer/tests-and-procedures/upper-endoscopy (accessed November 13, 2014).

ORGANIZATIONS

American College of Gastroenterology, 6400 Goldsboro Rd., Ste. 200, Bethesda, MD 20817, (301) 263-9000, http://gi.org.

American Gastroenterological Association, 4930 Del Ray Avenue, Bethesda, MD 20814, (301) 654-2055, Fax: (301) 654-5920, member@gastro.org, http://www.gastro.org.

Debra Wood, R.N.

Upper gastrointestinal series

Definition

An upper gastrointestinal (GI) examination is a fluoroscopic examination (a type of x-ray imaging) of the upper gastrointestinal tract, including the esophagus, stomach, and upper small intestine (duodenum).

Purpose

An upper GI series is frequently requested when a patient experiences unexplained symptoms of abdominal pain, difficulty in swallowing (dysphagia), regurgitation, **diarrhea**, or **weight loss**. It is used to help diagnose disorders and diseases of, or related to, the upper gastrointestinal tract, including cases of hiatal hernia, diverticuli, ulcers, tumors, obstruction, **enteritis**, gastroesophageal reflux disease, Crohn's disease, and pulmonary aspiration.

Precautions

Because of the risks of radiation exposure to the fetus, pregnant women are advised to avoid this procedure. Patients with an obstruction or perforation in their bowel should not ingest barium—a radioactive substance used to show contrast in the images—for an upper GI, but may still be able to undergo the procedure if a water-soluble contrast medium is substituted for the barium.

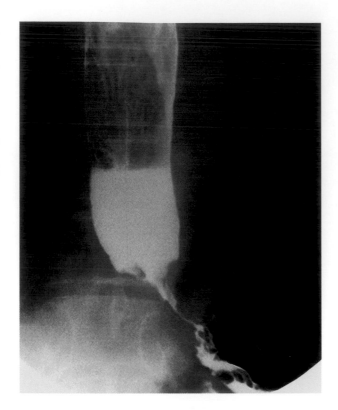

X-ray of the upper gastrointestinal (GI) tract. There is a cancerous tumor at the junction between the esophagus and small intestine. *(Living Art Enterprises/Science Source)*

Glucagon, a medication sometimes given prior to an upper GI procedure, may cause nausea and dizziness.

Description

An upper GI series takes place in a hospital or clinic setting and is performed by an x-ray technician and a radiologist. A radiologist typically is in attendance to oversee the procedure and view and interpret the fluoroscopic pictures. Before the test begins, the patient is sometimes administered an injection of glucagon, a medication that slows stomach and bowel activity, to allow the radiologist to get a clearer picture of the gastrointestinal tract. In order to further improve the clarity of the upper GI pictures, the patient may be given a cup of baking soda crystals to swallow, which distend the stomach by producing gas.

Once these preparatory steps are complete, the patient stands against an upright x-ray table, and a fluoroscopic screen is placed in front of him. The patient will be asked to drink from a cup of flavored barium sulfate, a thick and chalky-tasting liquid that allows the radiologist to see the digestive tract, while the radiologist views the esophagus, stomach, and duodenum on the fluoroscopic screen. The patient will be asked to change positions frequently in order to coat the entire surface of the gastrointestinal tract with barium. The technician or radiologist may press on the patient's abdomen in order to spread the barium. The x-ray table will also be moved several times throughout the procedure. The radiologist will ask the patient to hold his breath periodically while exposures are being taken. The entire procedure may take up to 45 minutes.

In some cases, in addition to the standard upper GI series, a doctor may request a detailed intestine, or small bowel, radiography and fluoroscopy series; it is also called a small bowel follow-through (SBFT). Once the preliminary upper GI series is complete, the patient will be escorted to a waiting area while the barium travels down the rest of the small intestinal path. Every 15 to 30 minutes, the patient will return to the x-ray suite for additional x-rays. Once the barium has traveled down the small bowel tract, the test is complete. This procedure can take anywhere from one to four hours.

Esophageal radiography, also called a barium esophagram or a barium swallow, is a study of the esophagus only, and is usually performed as part of the upper GI series. It is commonly used to diagnose the cause of difficulty in swallowing (dysphagia) and for detecting hiatal hernia. A barium sulfate liquid, and sometimes pieces of food covered in barium or a barium tablet, are given to the patient to drink and eat while a radiologist examines the swallowing mechanism on a fluoroscopic screen. The test takes approximately 30 minutes.

Preparation

Patients must not eat, drink, or smoke for eight hours prior to undergoing an upper GI examination. Longer dietary restrictions may be required, depending on the type and diagnostic purpose of the test. Patients undergoing a small bowel follow-through exam may be asked to take **laxatives** the day prior to the test. Upper GI

QUESTIONS TO ASK YOUR DOCTOR

- What is the purpose of this examination?
- When will I know the results?
- How will I be notified of the results?
- How will the examination results help to determine the next step in the management of my condition?
- What are the alternatives to this diagnostic exam?

patients are typically required to wear a hospital gown, or similar attire, and to remove all jewelry, so the camera has an unobstructed view of the abdomen. Patients who are severely ill may not be able to tolerate the procedure.

Aftercare

No special aftercare treatment or regimen is required for an upper GI series. The patient may eat and drink as soon as the test is completed. The barium sulfate may make the patient's stool white for several days, and patients are encouraged to drink plenty of fluids in order to eliminate it from their system.

Risks

Because the upper GI series is an x-ray procedure, it does involve minor exposure to ionizing radiation. Unless the patient is pregnant or multiple radiological or fluoroscopic studies are required, the small dose of radiation incurred during a single procedure poses little risk. However, multiple studies requiring fluoroscopic exposure that are conducted in a short time period have been known, on rare occasions, to cause skin death (necrosis) in some individuals. This risk can be minimized by careful monitoring and documentation of cumulative radiation doses administered to these patients.

Another risk is barium impaction, which occurs when the patient is unable to completely expel the barium contrast agent before it eventually dries and hardens. The risk of barium impaction is greatest in elderly patients and those with colon obstruction or colon motility disorder.

Results

A normal upper GI series will show a healthy, functioning, and unobstructed digestive tract.

Abnormal results

Obstructions or inflammation, including ulcers of the esophagus, stomach, or small intestine, or irregularities in the swallowing mechanism are some of the possible abnormalities that may show up on an upper GI series. Other abnormalities may include polyps, foreign bodies, or congenital anomalies. Upper GI series are helpful in the diagnosis of gastric (stomach) **cancer**.

Resources

WEBSITES

Canadian Cancer Society. "Upper Gastrointestinal (GI) Series." http://www.cancer.ca/en/cancer-information/diagnosis-and-treatment/tests-and-procedures/upper-gi-series/?region=on (accessed November 13, 2014).

Johns Hopkins Medicine. "Upper Gastrointestinal Series." http://www.ncbi.nlm.nih.gov/pubmed/18856015 (accessed November 13, 2014).

National Cancer Institute. "Upper GI Series." http://www.cancer.gov/dictionary?cdrid=46637 (accessed November 13, 2014).

Paula Anne Ford-Martin

Ureterosigmoidostomy

Definition

Ureterosigmoidostomy is a surgical procedure that treats urinary incontinence by joining the ureters to the lower colon, thereby allowing urine to evacuate through the rectum.

Purpose

The surgery is indicated when there is resection (surgical removal), malformation, or injury to the bladder. The bladder disposes of wastes passed to it from the kidneys, which is the organ that does most of the blood filtering and retention of needed glucose, salts, and minerals.

Wastes from the kidneys drip through the ureters to the bladder and on to the urethra, where they are expelled via urination. Waste from the kidneys is slowed or impaired when the bladder is diseased because of ulcerative, inflammatory, or malignant conditions; is malformed; or if it has been removed. In these cases, the kidney is unable to get rid of the wastes, resulting in hydronephrosis (distention of the kidneys). Over time, this leads to kidney deterioration. Saving the kidneys by bladder diversion is as important as restoring urinary continence.

The surgical techniques for urinary and fecal diversion fall into two categories: continent diversion and conduit diversion. In continent diversion, an internal reservoir for urine or feces is created, allowing natural evacuation from the body. In urinary and fecal conduit diversion, a section of existing tissue is altered to serve as a passageway to an external reservoir or ostomy. Both continent and conduit diversions reproduce bladder or colon function that was impaired due to surgery, obstruction, or a neurogenically (nerve dysfunction) created condition. Both the continent and conduit diversion methods have been used for years, with advancements in minimally invasive surgical techniques and biochemical improvements in conduit materials and ostomy appliances.

Catheterization was the original solution for urinary incontinence, especially when major organ failure or removal was involved. But catheterization was found to have major residual back flow of urine into the kidneys over the long term. With the advent of surgical anastomosis—the grafting of vascularizing tissue for the repair and expansion of organ function—and with the ability to include flap-type valves to prevent back-up into the kidneys, major continent restoring procedures have become routine in urologic surgery. Catheterization has been replaced as a permanent remedy for persistent incontinence. Continent surgical procedures developed since the 1980s offer the possibility of safely retaining natural evacuation functions in both colonic (intestinal) and urinary systems.

Quality of life issues associated with urinary diversion are increasingly important to patients and, along with medical requirements, put an optimal threshold on the requirements for the surgical procedure. The bladder substitute or created reservoir must offer the following advantages:

• maintain continence

• maintain sterile urine

• empty completely

• protect the kidneys

• prevent absorption of waste products

• maintain quality of life

Ureterosigmoidostomy is one of the earliest continent diversions for a resected bladder, bladder abnormalities, and dysfunction. It is one of the more difficult surgeries, and has significant complications. Ureterosigmoidostomy does have a major benefit; it allows the natural expelling of wastes without the construction of a stoma—an artificial conduit—by using the rectum as a

urinary reservoir. When evacuation occurs, the urine is passed along with the fecal matter.

Ureterosigmoidostomy is a single procedure, but there are additional refinements that allow rectal voiding of urine. A procedure known as the Mainz II pouch has undergone many refinements in attempts to lessen the complications that have traditionally accompanied ureterosigmoidostomy. This surgery is indicated for significant and serious conditions of the urinary tract, including:

• Cancer or ulceration of the bladder that necessitates a radical cystectomy or removal of the bladder, primarily occurring in adults, particularly those of advanced age.

• Various congenital abnormalities of the bladder in infants, especially eversion of part or all of the bladder. Eversion (or exstrophy) is a malformation of the bladder in which the wall adjacent to the abdomen fails to close. In some children, the bladder plate may be too small to fashion a closure.

Description

The most basic ureterosigmoidostomy modification is the Mainz II pouch. There is a 2.4 in. (6 cm) cut along antimesenteric border of the colon, both on the proximal and distal sides of the rectum/sigmoid colon junction. The ureters are drawn down into the colon. A special flap technique is applied by folding the colon to stop urine from refluxing back to the kidneys. After the colon is closed, the result is a small rectosigmoid reservoir that holds urine without refluxing it back to the upper urinary tract. Some variations of the Mainz II pouch include the construction of a valve, as in the Kock pouch, that confines urine to the distal segment of the colon.

Ureterosigmoidostomy is typically performed in patients with complex medical problems, often those who have had numerous surgeries. Ureterosigmoidostomy as a continent diversion technique relies heavily upon an intact and functional rectal sphincter. The treatment of pediatric urinary incontinence due to bladder eversion or other anatomical anomalies is a technical challenge, and is not always the first choice of surgeons. In Europe, early urinary diversion with ureterosigmoidostomy is used widely for most exstrophy patients. Its main advantage is the possibility for spontaneous emptying by evacuation of urine and stool.

Demographics

Bladder cancer affects over 50,000 people annually in the United States. The average age at diagnosis is 68 years. It accounts for approximately 10,000 deaths per year. Bladder **cancer** is the fifth leading cause of cancer deaths among men older than 75 years. Male bladder cancer is three times more prevalent than female bladder cancer.

In the United States, radical **cystectomy** (total removal of the bladder) is the standard treatment for muscle-invading bladder cancer. The operation usually involves removal of the bladder (with oncology staging) and pelvic lymph node, and prostate and seminal conduits with a form of urinary diversion. Ureterosigmoidostomy is one option that restores continence.

Pediatric ureterosigmoidostomy is performed primarily for bladder abnormalities occurring at birth. Classic bladder exstrophy occurs in 3.3 per 100,000 births, with a male to female ratio of 3 to 1 (6 to 1 in some studies).

Diagnosis

A number of tests are performed as part of the presurgery diagnostic workup for bladder conditions such as cancer, ulcerative or inflammatory disease, or pediatric abnormalities. Tests may include:

• cystoscopy (bladder inspection with a laparoscope)
• CT scan
• liver function
• renal function
• rectal sphincter function evaluation

The rectal sphincter will be a critical factor in urination after the surgery, and it is important to determine its ability to function. Adult patients are often asked to have an oatmeal enema and sit upright for a period of time to test sphincter function.

Preparation

In adult patients, a discussion of continent diversion is conducted early in the diagnostic process. Patients are asked to consider the possibility of a conduit urinary diversion if the ureterosigmoidostomy proves impossible to complete. Educational sessions on specific conduit alternatives take place prior to surgery. Topics include options for placement of a stoma, and appliances that may be a part of the daily voiding routine after surgery. Many doctors provide a stomal therapist to consult with the patient.

Aftercare

After surgery, patients may remain in the hospital for a few days to undergo blood, renal, and liver tests, and monitoring for **fever** or other surgical complications. In pediatric patients, a cast keeps the legs abducted (apart) and slightly elevated for three weeks. Bladder and kidneys are fully drained via multiple catheters during the first few weeks after surgery. **Antibiotics** are continued after surgery. Permanent follow-up with the urologist is essential for proper monitoring of kidney function.

Results

Good results have been reported, especially in children; however, ureterosigmoidostomy offers some severe morbid complications. Postsurgical bladder function and continence rates are very high. However, many newly created reservoirs do not function normally; some deteriorate over time, creating a need for more than one diversion surgery. Many patients have difficulty voiding after surgery. Five-year survival rates for bladder surgery patients are 50%–80%, depending on the grade, depth of bladder penetration, and nodal status.

Morbidity and mortality rates

The continence success rate with ureterosigmoidostomy and its variants is higher than 95% for exstrophy; however, long-term malignancy rates are quite high. **Adenocarcinoma** is the most common of these malignancies, and may be caused by chronic irritation and inflammation of exposed mucosa of the exstrophic bladder. In one series of studies, adenocarcinoma was reported in more than 10% of patients; however, the malignancy is actually higher in untreated patients whose bladders are left exposed for years before surgery.

Upper urinary tract deterioration is a potential complication, caused by reflux of urine back to the kidneys, resulting in febrile infections.

Alternatives

Other options include construction of a full neo-bladder in certain carefully defined circumstances, and bladder enhancement for congenitally shortened or abnormal bladders. Surgical bladder resection is often followed by continent operations using other parts of the colon, and by various conduit surgeries that utilize an external ostomy appliance.

Health care team roles

Ureterosigmoidostomy is usually performed by a urological surgeon with advanced training in urinary continent surgeries, often in consultation with a neonatologist (in newborn patients) or an oncological surgeon. The surgery takes place in a general hospital.

Resources

BOOKS

Wein, Alan J., et al. *Campbell-Walsh Urology*. 10th ed. Philadelphia: Saunders/Elsevier, 2012.

PERIODICALS

Pettersson, Louise, et al. "Half Century of Followup After Ureterosigmoidostomy Performed in Early Childhood." *The Journal of Urology* 189, no. 5 (2013): 1870–75. http://dx.doi.org/10.1016/j.juro.2012.11.179 (accessed October 4, 2013).

Tollefson, Matthew K., et al. "Long-Term Outcome of Ureterosigmoidostomy: An Analysis of Patients with >10 Years of Follow-Up." *BJU International* 105, no. 6 (2010): 860–63. http://dx.doi.org/10.1111/j.1464-410X.2009.08811.x (accessed October 4, 2013).

OTHER

University of North Carolina Health Care. *Living with Your Ureterosigmoidostomy: A Guide to Home Care*. http://www.unchealthcare.org/site/Nursing/servicelines/wocn/patient%20educational%20materials_new/LLWOCNWebEdUSig.pdf (accessed October 14, 2014).

WEBSITES

Ochsner. "Ureterosigmoidostomy." http://healthlibrary.ochsner.org/Library/HealthSheets/3,S,41095 (accessed October 4, 2013).

ORGANIZATIONS

National Institute of Diabetes and Digestive and Kidney Diseases (NIDDK), Bethesda, MD 20892-2560, (301) 496-3583, http://www.niddk.nih.gov.

Society for Pediatric Urology, 500 Cummings Ctr., Ste. 4550, Beverly, MA 01915, (978) 927-8330, Fax: (978) 524-8890, http://spuonline.org.

Urology Care Foundation, 1000 Corporate Blvd., Linthicum, MD 21090, (410) 689-3700, (800) 828-7866, Fax: (410) 689-3998, info@urologycarefoundation.org, http://www.urologyhealth.org.

Nancy McKenzie, PhD

Ureterostomy, cutaneous

Definition

A cutaneous ureterostomy, also called ureterocutaneostomy, is a surgical procedure that detaches one or both ureters from the bladder, and brings them to the surface of the abdomen with the formation of an opening (stoma) to allow passage of urine.

Purpose

The bladder is the membranous pouch that serves as a reservoir for urine. Contraction of the bladder results in urination. A ureterostomy is performed to divert the flow of urine away from the bladder when the bladder is not functioning or has been removed. The following conditions may result in a need for ureterostomy.

- bladder cancer
- spinal cord injury
- malfunction of the bladder
- birth defects, such as spina bifida

Description

Urostomy is the generic name for any surgical procedure that diverts the passage of urine by re-directing the ureters (fibromuscular tubes that carry the urine from the kidney to the bladder). There are two basic types of urostomies. The first features the creation of a passage called an "ileal conduit." In this procedure, the ureters are detached from the bladder and joined to a short length of the small intestine (ileum). The other type of urostomy is cutaneous ureterostomy. With this technique, the surgeon detaches the ureters from the bladder and brings one or both to the surface of the abdomen. The hole created in the abdomen is called a stoma, a reddish, moist abdominal protrusion. The stoma is not painful; it has no sensation. Since it has no muscles to regulate urination, urine collects in a bag.

There are four common types of ureterostomies:

- single ureterostomy—brings only one ureter to the surface of the abdomen
- bilateral ureterostomy—brings both ureters to the surface of the abdomen, one on each side
- double-barrel ureterostomy—brings both ureters to the same side of the abdominal surface
- transuretero urctcrostomy (TUU)—brings both ureters to the same side of the abdomen, through the same stoma

Demographics

Bladder disorders afflict millions of people in the United States. According to the American Cancer Society (ACS), there were 72,570 new cases of **bladder cancer** in the United States in 2013, with approximately 15,210 deaths from the disease.

Preparation

Ureterostomy patients may have the following tests and procedures as part of their diagnostic work-up:

- renal function tests, including blood, urea, nitrogen (BUN) and creatinine
- blood tests, including complete blood count (CBC) and electrolytes
- imaging studies of the ureters and renal pelvis

The quality, character, and usable length of the ureters is usually assessed using any of the following tests:

- Intravenous pyelogram (IVP) is a special diagnostic test that follows the time course of excretion of a contrast dye through the kidneys, ureters, and bladder after it is injected into a vein.
- Retrograde and antegrade pyelograms are x-ray studies of the kidneys and urinary tract.
- Computed tomography (CT) is a special imaging technique that uses a computer to collect multiple x-ray images into a two-dimensional cross-sectional image.
- Magnetic resonance imaging (MRI) with intravenous gadolinium is a special technique used to image internal structures of the body, particularly the soft tissues. An MRI image is often superior to a routine x-ray image.

KEY TERMS

Anastomosis—An opening created by surgical, traumatic, or pathological means between two separate spaces or organs.

Cecum—The pouch-like start of the large intestine (colon) at the end of the small intestine.

Gastrointestinal (GI) tract—The entire length of the digestive tract, from the stomach to the rectum.

Ileum—The last portion of the small intestine that communicates with the large intestine.

Large intestine—Also called the colon, this structure has six major divisions: cecum, ascending colon, transverse colon, descending colon, sigmoid colon, and rectum.

Ostomy—General term meaning a surgical procedure in which an artificial opening is formed to either allow waste (stool or urine) to pass from the body, or to allow food into the GI tract. An ostomy can be permanent or temporary, as well as single-barreled, double-barreled, or a loop.

Small intestine—The small intestine consists of three sections: duodenum, jejunum, and ileum.

Spina bifida—A congenital defect in the spinal column, characterized by the absence of the vertebral arches through which the spinal membranes and spinal cord may protrude.

Stent—A tube made of metal or plastic that is inserted into a vessel or passage to keep it open and prevent closure.

Stoma—A surgically created opening in the abdominal wall.

Ureter—The fibromuscular tube that transports the urine from the kidney to the bladder.

The presurgery evaluation also includes an assessment of overall patient stability. The surgery may take from two to six hours, depending on the health of the ureters, and the experience of the surgeon.

Aftercare

After surgery, the condition of the ureters is monitored by IVP testing, repeated postoperatively at six months, one year, and then yearly.

Following ureterostomy, urine needs to be collected in bags. Several designs are available. One popular type features an open bag fitted with an anti-reflux valve, which prevents the urine from flowing back toward the stoma. A urostomy bag connects to a night bag that may be attached to the bed at night. Urostomy bags are available as one- and two-piece bags:

- With one-piece bags, the adhesive and the bag are sealed together. The advantage of using a one-piece appliance is that it is easy to apply, and the bag is flexible and soft.

- For two-piece bags, the bag and the adhesive are two separate components. The adhesive does not need to be removed frequently from the skin, and can remain in place for several days while the bag is changed as required.

Risks

The complication rate associated with ureterostomy procedures is less than 5%–10%. Risks during surgery include heart problems, pulmonary (lung) complications, development of blood clots (thrombosis), blocking of arteries (embolism), and injury to adjacent structures, such as bowel or vascular entities. Inadequate ureteral length may also be encountered, leading to ureteral kinking and subsequent obstruction. If plastic tubes need inserting, their malposition can lead to obstruction and eventual breakdown of the opening (anastomosis). Anastomotic leak is the most frequently encountered complication.

Results

Normal results for a ureterostomy include the successful diversion of the urine pathway away from the bladder, and a tension-free, watertight opening to the abdomen that prevents urinary leakage.

Morbidity and mortality rates

The outcome and prognosis for ureterostomy patients depends on a number of factors. The highest rates of complications exist for those who have pelvic cancer or a history of **radiation therapy**.

In one study, a French medical team followed 69 patients for a minimum of one year (an average of six years) after TUU was performed. They reported one complication per four patients (6.3%), including a case requiring open drainage, prolonged urinary leakage, and common ureteral death (necrosis). Two complications occurred three and four years after surgery. The **National Cancer Institute** performed TUU for pelvic malignancy in 10 patients. Mean follow-up was 6.5 years. Complications include common ureteral narrowing (one patient); subsequent kidney removal, or **nephrectomy** (one patient); recurrence of disease with ureteral obstruction (one patient); and disease progression in a case of

---

QUESTIONS TO ASK YOUR DOCTOR

- Why is ureterostomy required?
- What type will be performed?
- How long will it take to recover from the surgery?
- When can normal activities be resumed?
- How many ureterostomies does the surgeon perform each year?
- What are the possible complications?

---

inflammation of blood vessels, or vasculitis (one patient). One patient died of sepsis (infection in the bloodstream) due to urine leakage at the anastomosis, one died after a heart attack, and three died from **metastasis** of their primary cancer.

Alternatives

There are several alternative surgical procedures available:

- In an ileal conduit urostomy, also known as "Bricker's loop," the two ureters that transport urine from the kidneys are detached from the bladder, and then attached so that they will empty through a piece of the ileum. One end of the ileum piece is sealed off and the other end is brought to the surface of the abdomen to form the stoma. It is the most common technique used for urinary diversion.

- With cystostomy, the flow of urine is diverted from the bladder to the abdominal wall. It features placement of a tube through the abdominal wall into the bladder, and is indicated in cases of blockage or stricture of the ureters. It can be temporary or permanent.

- An Indiana pouch refers to the construction of a pouch from the end part of the ileum and the first part of the large intestine (cecum). The remaining ileum is first attached to the large intestine to maintain normal digestive flow. A pouch is then created from the removed cecum, and the attached ileum is brought to the surface of the abdominal wall to create a stoma.

- Percutaneous nephrostomy diverts the flow of urine from the kidneys to the abdominal wall. Tubes are placed within the kidney to collect the urine as it is generated, and transport it to the abdominal wall. This procedure is usually temporary; however, it may be permanent for cancer patients.

Health care team roles

Ureterostomy is performed in a hospital setting by experienced surgeons trained in urology, the branch of medicine concerned with the diagnosis and treatment of diseases of the urinary tract and urogenital system. Specially trained nurses called wound ostomy continence nurses (WOCN) are commonly available for consultation in most major medical centers.

Resources

BOOKS

Door Mullen, Barbara, and Kerry Anne McGinn. *The Ostomy Book: Living Comfortably With Colostomies, Ileostomies, and Urostomies*. 3rd ed. Boulder, CO: Bull Publishing, 2008.

Graham, Sam D., and Thomas E. Keane, eds. *Glenn's Urologic Surgery*. Philadelphia: Wolters Kluwer/Lippincott Williams & Wilkins, 2010.

PERIODICALS

Rodríguez, Alejandro R., et al. "Cutaneous Ureterostomy Technique for Adults and Effects of Ureteral Stenting: An Alternative to the Ileal Conduit." *The Journal of Urology* 186, no. 5 (2011): 1939–43. http://dx.doi.org/10.1016/j.juro.2011.07.032 (accessed October 3, 2014).

Zilberman, D. E., et al. "Long-Term Urinary Bladder Function following Unilateral Refluxing Low Loop Cutaneous Ureterostomy." *Korean Journal of Urology* 53, no. 5 (2012): 355–59.

WEBSITES

American Cancer Society. "What Are the Key Statistics about Bladder Cancer?" http://www.cancer.org/cancer/bladder-cancer/detailedguide/bladder-cancer-key-statistics (accessed October 3, 2014).

National Kidney and Urologic Diseases Information Clearinghouse. "Urostomy and Continent Urinary Diversion." National Institute of Diabetes and Digestive and Kidney Diseases. http://www.kidney.niddk.nih.gov/kudiseases/pubs/urostomy (accessed October 3, 2014).

ORGANIZATIONS

National Institute of Diabetes and Digestive and Kidney Diseases (NIDDK), 31 Center Dr., MSC 2560, Bldg. 31, Rm. 9A06, Bethesda, MD 20892-2560, (301) 496-3583, http://www2.niddk.nih.gov.

United Ostomy Associations of America, Inc. (UOAA), PO Box 512, Northfield, MN 55057-0512, (800) 826-0826, info@ostomy.org, http://www.ostomy.org.

Urology Care Foundation, 1000 Corporate Blvd., Linthicum, MD 21090, (410) 689-3700, (800) 828-7866, Fax: (410) 689-3998, info@urologycarefoundation.org, http://aua-foundation.org.

Monique Laberge, PhD

Urethral cancer

Definition

Urethral **cancer** is a rare form of cancer that develops in the urethra that carries urine, and in men, semen out of the body.

Description

The urethra connects the bladder to its opening outside the body (urinary meatus) for the purpose of removing fluids from the body. Urethral cancer can affect both women and men. In women, the urethra is a short tube that passes directly from the bladder to an opening outside the body just above the vaginal opening. In men, the urethra is a much longer tube that originates at the bladder and passes through the prostate gland and penis before it opens outside the body. It carries semen as well as urine. Several different types of urethral cancer can develop in different cells and different parts of the urethra. The main types are squamous cell **carcinoma**, **transitional cell carcinoma**, **adenocarcinoma** that develops in glands near the urethra, and two extremely rare types: **melanoma** that develops in pigment-producing skin cells, and **sarcoma**, which develops in blood vessels, smooth muscle and connective tissue.

Urethral cancer has a tendency to invade local and nearby soft tissues. Late diagnosis is common, and as a result, the majority of urethral tumors are advanced and have already spread to local organs, which may result in a poor prognosis despite aggressive treatment. Urethral cancer rarely spreads (metastasizes) to distant locations. In women, the most common sites of tumor invasion are the vagina and bladder, and in men, tumor invasion most commonly occurs in the deep tissues of the perineum, the prostate, and the penile and scrotal skin. Most urethral tumors are of the squamous-cell type, which accounts for 80% of cases in men and 60% of cases in women. The second most common type is transitional-cell carcinoma.

Demographics

Urethral cancer is very rare and makes up fewer than 1% of all malignancies; only about 2,000 cases have been reported. Urethral cancer occurs more often in women than in men. Although people of any age can be diagnosed with urethral cancer, the incidence is highest in people in their 60s. Urethral cancer is more common in Caucasians than in African Americans; however, African Americans tend to have a poorer prognosis after urethral cancer has been diagnosed.

KEY TERMS

Adjuvant therapy—A treatment that is intended to aid primary treatment.

Biopsy—Removal of a small piece of tissue for microscopic examination. This is done under local anesthesia and removed by either using a scalpel or a punch, to acquire a small cylindrical portion of tissue.

Metastasis—The migration of cancer cells from a primary cancer site to another organ either nearby or distant through the lymph system or blood circulation.

Pelvic exenteration—Surgical removal of the organs of the true pelvis, which includes the uterus, vagina, and cervix.

Causes and symptoms

The precise cause of urethral cancer is unknown. Patients with a history of **bladder cancer** have an increased risk of developing urethral cancer. Two types of **human papillomavirus** (HPV) and other sexually transmitted diseases are also shown to be associated with increased risk of urethral cancer. Chronic urinary tract infection or chronic irritation from childbirth or sexual intercourse may increase risk as well. In addition, cigarette smoking and exposure to certain chemicals, including solvents used in the rubber industry and dry cleaning, are known to contribute to the development of bladder cancer, and bladder cancer, in turn, increases the risk for urethral cancer.

Symptoms typically appear late, resulting in late diagnosis. Often the first symptom of urethral cancer is blood in the urine, although it may be present in such small amounts that it can only be detected in a microscope. Sometimes, however, the urine may be visibly red. Pelvic pain and a reduced flow of urine due to obstruction (urethral stricture) may make urination difficult. At the same time, frequent urination and increased nighttime urination (nocturia) are common symptoms as the disease progresses. There may be **itching** and incontinence, as well as pain during or after sexual intercourse (dyspareunia). A lump may be found on the urethra and swollen glands may develop in the groin in advanced cases. In women, tiny growths that bleed may be present at the external opening of the urethra.

Diagnosis

To diagnose urethral cancer, a physician will conduct a physical examination, including examining the patient for any lumps in the groin area. A urinalysis will be done to check for red blood cells and white blood cells under the microscope, which can indicate possible bleeding or infection, respectively. **Cystoscopy** will usually be required to thoroughly examine the urethra and bladder. In adults, the procedure is usually done under local anesthesia injected into the area around the urethral opening. The cystoscope, a long, lighted, flexible fiberoptic tube with a lens and tiny camera attached, is inserted through the urethra so the physician can examine the area through a scope, and sometimes on a video monitor. A **biopsy** will be done, removing a small sample of the urethral tissue with surgical instruments passed through the cystoscope. The sample will then be stained in the laboratory and viewed under a microscope by a pathologist to check for cells suggestive of cancer. If the biopsy is positive, imaging tests such as x-ray, **computed tomography** (CT scan), and **magnetic resonance imaging** (MRI scan) are done to determine the staging of the cancer and extent of **metastasis**; MRI is the most sensitive method for evaluating urethral cancer.

Treatment team

The treatment team comprises physicians from a variety of medical specialties, including the patient's primary care physician, a urologist, an oncologist, an oncology radiologist, surgeon, and **pain management** specialist. Women may also seek the advice of their gynecologist. Caretakers in the home may also be part of the treatment team, providing important physical and emotional support to the patient. Physicians and patients who value a holistic approach to fighting cancer may add a variety of other advisors to the treatment team, such as psychologists, religious advisors, and alternative medicine specialists.

Clinical staging

After a diagnosis of cancer has been made and imaging results are evaluated, the urethral cancer will be staged to determine whether the cancer has spread to other areas of the body. The stage of urethral cancer is determined by the cancer's location and whether it has metastasized. The **National Cancer Institute** staging criteria describes the different stages of urethral cancer as:

• Anterior urethral cancer: the cancer is located on the urethra near the outside of the body.

• Posterior urethral cancer: the cancer is located on the urethra near the bladder.

• Urethral cancer associated with invasive bladder cancer: the cancer has spread to the urethra because of the presence of bladder cancer.

Another staging system uses: stage 0 to represent abnormal cells in the lining of the urethra, but no actual tumor (carcinoma in situ); stage A in which a tumor has formed and spread into the layer of tissue just under the urethral lining; stage B in which cancer is found in the muscle tissue around the urethra or, in men, penile tissue; stage C represents the spread of cancer beyond the urethral tissue itself, which may be found in the vagina, vaginal lips, or muscle in women, and in men may be found in the penis or nearby muscle tissue; stage D is subdivided into D1, in which the cancer has spread to nearby lymph nodes in the pelvic area, or D2 in which it has spread to distant lymph nodes or organ systems such as lungs, liver, and bone.

Treatment

Treatment for urethral cancer depends on the disease stage and location of the tumor, as well as the patient's age, gender, and overall health status. The treatment options include surgery, **radiation therapy**, and **chemotherapy**. If tumors are not larger than two centimeters, they can sometimes be treated with radiation alone, surgery alone, or a combination of the two treatment options. Surgery is the primary treatment because urethral cancer is usually invasive. Several different procedures may be used for early-stage cancer, including electrofulguration that applies electric current to kill the cancer cells, and laser therapy that focuses a narrow beam of powerful light on the tumor to kill the cancer cells.

More advanced cancer will receive more aggressive surgical treatment, with one of several procedures based on tumor location. The main procedures for advanced urethral cancer include:

• Cystourethrectomy, removal of the bladder and urethra.

• Partial penectomy, removal of part of the penis.

• Radical penectomy, removal of the penis, urethra, and penile root.

• Cystoprostatectomy, removal of the bladder and prostate.

• Lymph node dissection, removal of nearby cancerous lymph nodes.

• Anterior extenteration, removal of the bladder, urethra, and vagina.

The individual surgical options may also have certain additional requirements. Removing the urethra requires the surgeon to create a urinary diversion, which simply means that another way to urinate will need to be constructed. If a penectomy, partial or radical, is done, the patient will need plastic surgery to create a new penis from the patient's own skin. In women, surgery to remove the vagina will require plastic surgery to create a new vagina using local tissue.

When a patient's bladder and urethra are removed, the surgeon may use part of the small intestine to create a tube to replace the urethra so that the patient can urinate. A mouth-like opening called a stoma will also be made surgically on the outside of the body. This procedure is called an ostomy. The patient then uses a special glue to connect a bag designed especially to connect to the stoma. As a patient urinates, the urine collects in the bag. The patient can then discard the bag and replace it with a new one. The bag is hidden under the patient's clothing. Ostomy patients can be prone to infection and some patients with sensitive skin may experience occasional skin irritation due to the glue that holds the bag in place.

Some patients have difficulty accepting their ostomy psychologically. Fears of having "accidents" or "smelling bad" sometimes overwhelm ostomy patients. Support groups and special counseling can be very helpful to patients who are having a difficult time adjusting to their new situation.

Based on the severity and extent of the cancer, adjuvant radiation and/or chemotherapy treatments after surgery may be recommended to help destroy cancer cells in the pelvic area or elsewhere in the body in an effort to prevent new cancer development. Radiation may be given as external beam radiotherapy or as surgically implanted radioactive seeds or pellets, a procedure called brachytherapy. Sometimes the two types of radiation are used together. Chemotherapy provides systemic destruction of cancer cells throughout the body. Chemotherapy drugs may be administered orally or intravenously. The most commonly used drugs are **cisplatin** (Plantinol), **vincristine** (Oncovin), and **methotrexate** (Trexall), which may be used singly or in combination. Both radiation and chemotherapy are associated with side effects, including **fatigue**, **diarrhea**, and inflammation of the bladder (cystitis) after radiation, and **anemia**, **nausea and vomiting**, hair loss, mouth sores, and increased risk of infection with chemotherapy. Certain medications may be given to help reduce or alleviate side effects.

Complications of surgery can include adverse reactions to anesthesia, bowel obstruction, infection, and incontinence. A narrowing of the urethra (stricture) may result in abnormal passage of urine, a condition called fistula. Recurrence of cancer is likely in about half of all cases receiving surgery. About 1%–2% of patients will die as a result of surgical complications.

Prognosis

The prognosis of urethral cancer depends on the tumor's size and location, as well as the extent of the

QUESTIONS TO ASK YOUR DOCTOR

- How advanced is my cancer? Has it spread to other locations?
- What are my treatment options?
- What are the side effects of that treatment?
- How will having a penectomy affect my survival time?
- When is it safe for me to resume sexual relations?
- How successful is the reconstructive surgery?
- How will the treatment affect my ability to have children?
- How will my ability to urinate be affected if I have an ostomy?
- Are there any clinical trials that may be appropriate for me?

cancer and the patient's general health. The 5-year survival rates for noninvasive urethral cancer that has been treated with radiation or surgery are about 60%. For advanced urethral tumors, the 5-year survival rate drops to 45%. Early diagnosis and treatment leads to the best cure rates, but the recurrence rates for invasive cancer that has been treated aggressively with surgery, chemotherapy, and radiation combined are still higher than 50%.

Coping with cancer treatment

Patients having difficulty coping with the pain associated with cancer and chemotherapy might find it helpful to be referred to a physician who specializes in pain management or a pain clinic. Physicians specializing in the treatment of pain come from a variety of medical backgrounds, such as anesthesiology, urology, and surgery. Because of the complicated nature of cancer and cancer-related pain, ideally a pain management team should be formed that works with the patient's primary care physician, oncologist, and radiologist to provide comprehensive care to the patient.

Besides coping with the physical side effects of cancer treatment, patients with urethral cancer also face emotional challenges associated with their treatment. Men and women may be concerned about how the treatment will affect their sexual relations. They may have to deal with a variety of psychological issues, including **body image** versus self-image, and how to manage living with an ostomy. Patients having difficulty

dealing with the emotional aspects of their cancer may find it useful to see a psychologist who may provide a variety of coping mechanisms that can help them adjust and improve their quality of life.

It is important for cancer patients to understand that they are not alone. Support groups exist to help patients cope not only with the physical aspects of having cancer, but with the psychological ones as well. Talking about their concerns may help patients cope. The positive support provided by caregivers can help to improve a patient's comfort and quality of life. In addition, online support groups make it possible for patients, even those in rural or remote areas, to reach out to one another in ways that allow anonymity.

Resources

BOOKS

D. Raghavan, M. Brecher, and D. Johnson, et al., eds. "Urethral Cancer, Ch. 3." In *Textbook of Uncommon Cancer*. 4th ed. Hoboken, NJ: John Wiley & Sons, 2012.

PERIODICALS

Dayyani, F., K. Hoffman, and P. Eifel, et al. "Management of Advanced Primary Urethral Carcinomas." *British Journal of Urology International* 114 (Apr 2014): 25–31.

Tritschler, S., K. Lellig, A. Roosen, A. Horng, and C. Stief. "Organ and Function Preservation in Urethral Cancer." *Urologe A* 53 (Aug 2014): 1310–1315.

WEBSITES

National Cancer Institute. "Urethral Cancer Treatment (PDQ®)" 23 July 2014. http://www.cancer.gov/cancertopics/pdq/treatment/urethral/HealthProfessional/page1 (accessed October 25, 2014).

United Ostomy Association, Inc. "What is an Ostomy?" http://www.ostomy.org/Ostomy_Information.html (accessed October 25, 2014).

L. Lee Culvert
Lee Ann Paradise

Urostomy

Definition

Urostomy is a surgical procedure that creates an opening (stoma) in the abdominal wall through which urine leaves the body.

Purpose

Doctors perform urostomy when a patient has **bladder cancer**, spinal cord injury, specific types of

KEY TERMS

Bladder neck—The narrowest part of the bladder.

Cystoscopy—Diagnostic procedure that allows the doctor to view the entire bladder wall.

Kidney failure—Inability of the kidneys to excrete waste and maintain a proper chemical balance. Also called renal failure.

birth defects, or when the bladder is not functioning properly and must be removed.

Description

Urostomy is a form of urinary diversion. Surgeons perform this reconstructive procedure when disease, infection, injury, or congenital abnormality makes it necessary to remove a patient's bladder and create a new channel (conduit) for urine to leave the body.

Surgeons perform urostomy by separating a short piece of the large or small intestine from the rest of the intestine. They attach the separated intestine to the two thick tubes (ureters) that carry urine from the kidneys to the bladder and connect the ureters to the stoma.

Continent and incontinent diversions

An incontinent ostomy drains continuously into a small pouch fitted over the stoma and worn under the patient's clothes. The patient wears a collection pouch at all times and empties it several times a day.

To perform a continent urinary diversion, the surgeon uses a piece of the patient's intestine to create an internal reservoir to store urine. The patient does not wear an ostomy pouch but empties the reservoir four to six times a day by inserting a drainage tube (catheter) into the stoma.

Types of urostomy

The most common types of urostomy are the ileal conduit, which uses a piece of the small intestine (ileum), and the colonic conduit, which uses a piece of the large intestine (colon). Orthotopic neobladder is a new type of continent diversion that channels urine into the tube that drains urine from the bladder (urethra) and enables the patient to urinate almost normally.

Temporary urostomy does not involve severing the ureters and is most often performed in children.

Doctors consider the likelihood of disease recurring in the pelvis or urethra as well as the patient's gender to determine which type of urostomy is most appropriate. Neobladders are not appropriate for female patients whose **cancer** involves the bladder neck or male patients with problems affecting the right colon or small bowel.

If bladder cancer has metastasized or cannot be surgically removed, the surgeon may perform a urostomy without removing the patient's bladder.

Precautions

In an individual who is obese or who has folds in the skin or scars in the abdominal wall, an internal collection sac (reservoir) the patient can empty (catheterize) works better than a passage that lets urine flow out of the body into a collection bag (pouch) worn next to the skin under the clothes.

Preparation

Before undergoing a urostomy, the patient learns where on the abdomen the stoma will be created, what type of collection device (if any) will be worn, and what changes in appearance the operation may cause.

Nurses encourage the patient preparing to undergo an incontinent urostomy to become familiar with the collection device that will be worn after the operation. They may arrange to have someone who has already had the operation (ostomate) reassure the patient preparing for either an incontinent or continent procedure and answer questions about life after the surgery.

Preoperative restrictions

The patient may be told not to eat certain foods before surgery and must fast for eight hours and have a cleansing enema before the operation.

Fluid and **antibiotics** may be given to a patient who is frail.

Aftercare

A patient who has undergone an incontinent diversion wears a collection device that is odor-free, not visible under clothing, disposable or reusable, and available at drug stores or medical supply houses or through the mail.

To prevent urine leakage, infection, skin irritation, and odor, the patient should re-measure the stoma and make any necessary adjustments in the size of the flat sponge-like patch that covers and protects it. This should be done during the first few months after the operation (when shrinkage occurs) or whenever gaining or losing weight. Measuring devices and instructions are included in every box of collection pouches.

Some doctors recommend taking Vitamin C to prevent infection- and odor-causing bacteria from accumulating in the urine. Other recommendations include drinking eight to ten glasses of water a day to reduce the likelihood of kidney infection.

Risks

Because tumors sometimes develop in neobladders, a patient who undergoes this procedure must have a **cystoscopy** within five years.

Results

A patient who has had a urostomy can:

• Shower or bathe with or without the collection pouch

• Usually wear the clothes worn before the operation

• Return to work shortly after leaving the hospital (although a doctor's permission is required before doing heavy lifting)

• Enjoy intimate relationships

• Participate in athletic activities, but should avoid strenuous contact sports like football or wrestling

Dietary restrictions are rare.

A woman who has undergone a urostomy should talk with her doctor before becoming pregnant.

Abnormal results

Almost half (40%) of patients who undergo continent diversions and 24.1% of those who undergo ileal or colonic conduits require subsequent surgery to repair leaks or obstructions and correct other surgery-related problems.

A patient who has had a urostomy may also experience:

• kidney damage, infection, or failure

• swelling, shrinkage (stenosis), or displacement (prolapse) of the stoma

• infections of the stoma or urinary tract

• fever

QUESTIONS TO ASK YOUR DOCTOR

• What type of urostomy will I have?

• Will I have to wear a pouch after the operation?

• Will I be able to take care of myself after the operation?

• Will other people be able to tell that I have had a urostomy?

• hernia

• diarrhea

• urinary problems

• chills

• pain in the leg or abdomen

• blood or pus in the urine

Resources

PERIODICALS

Nazarko, L. "Caring For a Patient With a Urostomy in a Community Setting." *British Journal of Community Nursing* 13, no. 8 (2008): 354, 356, 358. http://www.ncbi.nlm.nih.gov/pubmed/18856015 (accessed November 13, 2014).

WEBSITES

American Cancer Society. "Urostomy." http://www.cancer.org/treatment/treatmentsandsideeffects/physicalsideeffects/ostomies/urostomyguide/urostomy-guide-toc (accessed November 13, 2014).

ORGANIZATIONS

United Ostomy Associations of America, 2489 Rice St, Suite 275, Roseville, MN 55113-3797, (800) 826-0826, http://www.ostomy.org.

Maureen Haggerty

Uterine cancer *see* **Endometrial cancer**

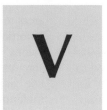

Vaginal cancer

Definition

Vaginal **cancer** refers to a cancerous growth in the tissues of the birth canal (vagina).

Description

Vaginal cancer is rare and accounts for only 1% to 2% of all **gynecologic cancers**. About 1 in every 1,100 women will develop vaginal cancer. As of 2014, approximately 3,170 new cases of vaginal cancer were projected to be diagnosed in the United States, with approximately 880 deaths from the disease. Vaginal cancer that originates in the vagina is called primary vaginal cancer; if cancer spreads to the vagina from another site, it is called metastatic cancer. About 80% of vaginal cancers are metastatic. Metastatic cancers carry the name of the primary cancer site. For instance, cancer that has spread from the cervix to the vagina would be called metastatic **cervical cancer** rather than vaginal cancer.

The vagina is a short tube (3–4 inches) that extends from the outer female genitalia (vulva) to the opening to the uterus (cervix). It serves to receive the penis during sexual intercourse, as an outlet for shed tissue and blood during menstruation, and as a passageway for the baby during childbirth. Most cancers are located in the upper third of the vagina.

Squamous cells line the vagina and squamous cell **carcinoma** is the most common type of vaginal cancer, accounting for 70% of cases. Less common types of vaginal cancer include adenocarcinomas that begin in gland cells, melanomas that develop in pigment-producing cells, and sarcomas that come from deep within the vaginal wall. About 9 of every 100 cases of vaginal cancer are melanomas, and 4 of every 100 vaginal cancers are sarcomas. Adenocarcinomas account for about 15% of cases and are usually found in young women (ages 12 to 30 years). Squamous cell cancer (squamous carcinoma) is usually found in older women (ages 60 to 80 years). Although vaginal melanomas can occur in adult women of any age, the average age at diagnosis is somewhere in the forties.

Demographics

Vaginal cancer is most common in women between the ages of 60 and 80, with 50% of vaginal tumors diagnosed in women age 70 and older. Only 15% of cases are found in women younger than age 40.

Causes and symptoms

Cancer is caused when the normal mechanisms that control cell growth become disturbed, causing cells to grow and divide without stopping. This is usually the result of damage to the genetic material of the cell (deoxyribonucleic acid, or DNA). Although the precise cause of vaginal cancer is not known, risk factors for developing vaginal cancer include: age over 70; previous use of a hormonal drug called diethylstilbestrol (DES), or being the daughter of a woman who took the drug; previous diagnosis of a type of **human papillomavirus** (HPV); positive for human immunodeficiency virus (HIV); having cervical cancer or precancerous cervical dysplasia; and a history of smoking or excessive alcohol consumption. Chronic vaginal irritation either from sexual intercourse or the use of a pessary for vaginal prolapse is thought to increase the risk of developing squamous cell vaginal cancer.

Symptoms of vaginal cancer appear when the cancer has become more advanced. Approximately 20% of women with vaginal cancer have no symptoms (asymptomatic) and are diagnosed after they have abnormal **Pap test** results. Symptoms of vaginal cancer include:

- abnormal vaginal bleeding or discharge
- pain during intercourse
- pain in the pelvic area
- difficult or painful urination
- constipation

KEY TERMS

Adjuvant therapy—A treatment that is intended to aid the primary treatment. Adjuvant treatments for vaginal cancer are radiation therapy and chemotherapy.

Biopsy—Removal of a small piece of tissue for microscopic examination. This is done under local anesthesia and removed by either using a scalpel or a punch to acquire a small cylindrical portion of tissue.

Colposcope—An instrument used for examination of the vagina and cervix. The instrument includes a light and magnifying lens for better visualization.

Intracavitary radiation—Radiation therapy for vaginal cancer in which a cylindrical container holding a radioactive substance is placed into the vagina for one or two days.

Metastasis—The migration of cancer cells from a primary tumor site to nearby (local) tissues or organs or to distant organs either through the lymph system or blood circulation.

Pelvic exenteration—Surgical removal of the organs of the pelvis, including the uterus, vagina, and cervix.

Squamous cells—Scale-like cells that cover certain organ surfaces and body cavities.

Vaginectomy—Surgical removal of the vagina. An artificial vagina can be constructed using grafts of skin or intestinal tissue.

Diagnosis

The diagnosis of vaginal cancer is made by physical examination, including pelvic examination, and laboratory analysis of vaginal tissue samples. During the pelvic examination, the physician will place one or two fingers into the vagina and press down on the lower abdomen with his or her free hand to feel (palpate) the reproductive organs and any masses. During a routine speculum examination, the physician will obtain a sample of cervical and vaginal cells (using a swab, brush, or wooden applicator) for laboratory analysis (Pap test).

A special magnifying instrument called a colposcope may be used to view the vagina and cervix. Additionally, the surface of the vagina may be treated with a diluted solution of acetic acid, which causes some abnormal areas to turn white. Squamous carcinoma and **adenocarcinoma** usually appear as growths on the surface of the vagina. Squamous carcinoma may present as an open sore (ulcer). Adenocarcinoma may lie deeper so that it is not visible and detected only by palpation. Vaginal **melanoma** appears as a brown or black skin tag (polypoid), a growth attached to the vaginal wall by a stem (pedunculated), a nipple-like growth (papillary), or a fungus-like growth (fungating). Sarcomas often appear as a grape-like mass.

If any area appears abnormal, a tissue sample (**biopsy**) will be taken. The biopsy can be performed in the doctor's office with the use of local anesthetic. A small piece of tissue containing the suspect lesion, some surrounding normal skin, and underlying skin layers and connective tissue will be removed. Small lesions may be removed in their entirety (excisional biopsy). The diagnosis of cancer depends on a microscopic analysis of this tissue by a pathologist.

Chest **x-rays** and routine blood work are commonly performed in the diagnosis of any cancer. Endoscopic examination of the bladder (**cystoscopy**) and/or rectum (proctoscopy) may be performed if it is suspected that the cancer has spread to these organs.

Treatment team

The treatment team for vaginal cancer may include a gynecologist, gynecologic oncologist, radiation oncologist, plastic surgeon, gynecologic nurse oncologist, sexual therapist, psychiatrist, psychological counselor, and social worker.

Clinical staging

The clinical staging system of the International Federation of Gynecology and Obstetrics (FIGO) is applied by most gynecologic oncologists to stage vaginal cancer. The system categorizes the cancer in one of five stages (0, I, II, III, and IV) that may be further subdivided (A and B) based on the depth or spread of cancerous tissue. The FIGO stages for vaginal cancer are:

• Stage 0. Cancer is confined to the outermost layer (epithelium) of vaginal cells and is called carcinoma *in situ* or vaginal intraepithelial neoplasia (VAIN).

• Stage I. Cancer is confined to the vagina.

• Stage II. Cancer has spread to the tissues near the vagina.

• Stage III. Cancer has spread to the bones of the pelvis, local lymph nodes, and/or other reproductive organs.

• Stage IV. Cancer has spread to the bladder, rectum, or other parts of the body.

Treatment

The treatment of vaginal cancer varies considerably and depends on the type of cancer, stage of cancer, and the patient's age and overall health. Surgery is the most common treatment for vaginal cancer. **Radiation therapy** and **chemotherapy** are often used as adjuvant therapy to complement the surgical treatment by killing any remaining cancer cells.

Surgery

The amount of tissue removed depends upon the stage and type of cancer. The local lymph nodes may also be removed (lymphadenectomy). Laser surgery may be used to destroy the cancerous cells in stage 0 vaginal cancer. Wide local excision may be applied for stages 1–2 to completely excise the cancerous tissue and some surrounding healthy tissue. Wide local excisions may require skin grafts to repair the vagina.

For more extensive tumors, the vagina may be removed (vaginectomy). Following vaginectomy, skin grafts and plastic surgery are used to create an artificial vagina. Vaginal cancer that has spread to the other reproductive organs is usually treated by radical hysterectomy in which the uterus, fallopian tubes, and ovaries are removed. Cancer that has spread beyond the reproductive organs may be treated by pelvic **exenteration**, in which the vagina, cervix, uterus, fallopian tubes, and ovaries are removed; if necessary, the lower colon, bladder, or rectum may also be removed.

Potential surgical complications include reactions to anesthesia, urinary tract infections, wound infection, temporary nerve injury, fluid accumulation (edema) in the legs, urinary incontinence, falling or sinking of the genitals (genital prolapse), and blood clots (thrombi).

Radiation therapy

Radiation therapy may be used as the sole treatment for vaginal cancer or as an adjuvant therapy to complement surgery. Radiation therapy uses high-energy radiation from x-rays and gamma rays to kill the cancer cells. Radiation applied externally is called external beam radiation therapy. Radiation applied internally is called internal radiation therapy or brachytherapy. Sometimes applicators containing radioactive compounds are placed inside the vagina (intracavitary radiation) or directly into the cancerous lesion (interstitial radiation). External and internal radiation may be used in combination to treat vaginal cancer.

The skin in the treated area may become red and dry and may take as long as a year to return to normal. **Fatigue**, upset stomach, **diarrhea**, and nausea are also common complaints of women undergoing radiation therapy. Radiation therapy in the pelvic area may cause the vagina to become narrow as scar tissue forms. This phenomenon, known as vaginal stenosis, makes intercourse painful.

Chemotherapy

Chemotherapy is not very a very successful treatment of vaginal cancer and is generally reserved for patients with advanced disease. Chemotherapy uses **anticancer drugs** to kill the cancer cells. The drugs are usually given by mouth (orally) or intravenously. They enter the bloodstream and can travel to all parts of the body to kill cancer cells. Generally, a combination of drugs is given because it is more effective than a single drug in treating cancer. For vaginal cancer, anticancer drugs may be put into the vagina (intravaginal chemotherapy).

The side effects of chemotherapy are significant and include stomach upset, vomiting, appetite loss (**anorexia**), hair loss (**alopecia**), mouth or vaginal sores, fatigue, menstrual cycle changes, and premature menopause. There is also an increased chance of infections.

Alternative and complementary therapies

Although alternative and complementary therapies are used by many cancer patients, very few controlled studies on the effectiveness of such therapies exist. Mind-body techniques such as prayer, biofeedback, visualization, meditation, and yoga have not shown any effect in reducing cancer, but they may help reduce stress and lessen some of the side effects of cancer treatments.

Clinical studies of hydrazine sulfate found that it had no effect on cancer and even worsened the health and well-being of the study subjects. One clinical study of the drug amygdalin (Laetrile) found that it had no effect on cancer. Laetrile can be toxic and has caused death. Shark cartilage, although highly touted as an effective cancer treatment, is an improbable therapy that has not been the subject of clinical study.

The American Cancer Society has found that "metabolic diets" pose serious risk to the patient. The effectiveness of the macrobiotic, Gerson, and Kelley diets, as well as Manner metabolic therapy, has not been scientifically proven. The U.S. Food and Drug Administration (FDA) has been unable to substantiate the anticancer claims made about the popular Cancell treatment.

There is no evidence for the effectiveness of most over-the-counter herbal cancer remedies. However, some herbals have shown anticancer effects. Some studies have shown that polysaccharide krestin (PSK), a substance from the mushroom *Coriolus versicolor*, has some effectiveness against cancer. In a small study, the green alga *Chlorella pyrenoidosa* has been shown to have anticancer activity. In a few small studies, evening primrose oil has shown some benefit in the treatment of cancer. However, herbals can have a negative impact on conventional treatment, and patients must discuss herbal use with a physician.

Prognosis

Survival is related to the stage and type of vaginal cancer. The five-year survival rates for squamous carcinoma and adenocarcinoma of the vagina are: 96%, stage 0; 73%, stage I; 58%, stage II; 36%, stage III; and 36%, stage IV. With a five-year survival rate of less than 20%, melanoma has a poor prognosis. Vaginal cancer most commonly spreads (metastasizes) to the lungs, but may spread to the liver, bone, or other sites.

Coping with cancer treatment

The patient should consult with her treatment team regarding any side effects or complications of treatment. Vaginal stenosis can be prevented and treated by vaginal dilators, gentle douching, and sexual intercourse. A water-soluble lubricant may be used to make sexual intercourse more comfortable. Women with a reconstructed vagina will need to use a water-soluble lubricant during sexual intercourse. Many of the side effects of chemotherapy can be relieved by medications. Women may wish to consult a psychotherapist and/or join a support group to deal with the emotional consequences of cancer and vaginectomy.

Clinical trials

As of 2014, a variety of studies were under way to examine the connection between vaginal cancer and human papillomavirus, to improve radiation and surgical techniques for treatment, to assess the efficacy and safety of new chemotherapeutic agents, and to improve modalities of supportive care for women with vaginal cancer. Women should consult with their treatment team to determine if they are candidates for any ongoing studies.

Prevention

The only preventive measure for vaginal cancer is avoiding known risk factors. Risk factors for vaginal cancer include:

- Diethylstilbestrol (DES). Young women whose mothers took DES during pregnancy (prescribed between 1945 and 1970) are at a higher risk of developing vaginal cancer, particularly clear cell carcinoma.

- Cervical cancer. Women with a history of cervical cancer have a high risk of developing vaginal cancer.

QUESTIONS TO ASK YOUR DOCTOR

- What type of cancer do I have?
- What type and what stage is my cancer?
- What is the five-year survival rate for women with this type and stage of cancer?
- Has the cancer spread?
- What are my treatment options?
- How much tissue will you be removing? Can you remove less tissue and complement my treatment with adjuvant therapy?
- What are the risks and side effects of these treatments?
- What medications can I take to relieve treatment side effects?
- Are there any clinical studies under way that would be appropriate for me?
- How debilitating is the treatment? Will I be able to continue working?
- Are there any restrictions regarding sexual activity?
- How is a vaginal reconstruction performed?
- How will a vaginal reconstruction affect my sexual functioning?
- Are there any local support groups for vaginal cancer patients?
- What is the chance that the cancer will recur?
- Is there anything I can do to prevent recurrence?
- How often will I have follow-up examinations?

- Hysterectomy. Up to half of all patients with vaginal cancer have had a hysterectomy, and vaginal cancer may be metastatic cervical cancer that spread prior to radical hysterectomy.

- Chronic irritant vaginitis. Chronic irritation to the vagina, such as from sexual intercourse or use of a vaginal pessary to support the uterus in uterine prolapse, is associated with vaginal cancer.

- Vaginal adenosis. This condition, in which cells that resemble those of the uterus are found in the vaginal lining, places a woman at a higher risk of developing vaginal cancer.

- Human papillomavirus (HPV) infection. Infection by this sexually transmitted virus, the cause of genital warts, increases a woman's risk of developing squamous cell carcinoma.

- Smoking. There is believed to be an association between tobacco use and vaginal cancer.

All women, even those who have had a hysterectomy or are past menopause, should get an annual pelvic examination and Pap test. Women who had a hysterectomy because of cancer may benefit from more frequent Pap tests. The earlier that precancerous abnormalities or vaginal cancer are detected, the better the prognosis. Women whose mothers took DES during pregnancy and those with vaginal adenosis should be screened regularly. Women can reduce the risk of contracting HPV by avoiding sexual intercourse with individuals who have had many sexual partners, limiting their number of sexual partners, and delaying first sexual activity until an older age. Avoiding tobacco products may reduce a woman's risk of developing vaginal cancer.

Special concerns

Of special concern to women undergoing treatment for vaginal cancer is the effect surgery and/or radiation therapy may have on sexual functioning. Women of childbearing age may worry about their fertility and whether or not they will be able to bear children. **Depression** may occur as a result of the effects of surgery on **body image** and sexuality. In addition, short- and long-term complications after extensive surgical treatment of vaginal cancer are not uncommon.

See also Fertility issues; Vulvar cancer.

Resources

BOOKS

Abeloff, M. D., et al. *Clinical Oncology*, 5th ed. New York: Churchill Livingstone, 2014.

Bruss, Katherine, Christina Salter, and Esmeralda Galan, eds. *American Cancer Society's Complete Guide to Complementary and Alternative Cancer Therapies*, 2nd ed. Atlanta: American Cancer Society, 2009.

Eifel, Patricia, Jonathan Berrek, and M. A. Markman. "Cancer of the Cervix, Vagina, and Vulva." In *Cancer: Principles & Practice of Oncology*, 9th ed., edited by Vincent T. DeVita, Samuel Hellman, and Steven Rosenberg, 1311–1344. Philadelphia: Lippincott Williams & Wilkins, 2011.

Garcia, Agustin, and J. Tate Thigpen. "Tumors of the Vulva and Vagina" In *Textbook of Uncommon Cancer*, edited by D. Raghavan, M. Brecher, and D. Johnson, et al. 4th ed. Hoboken, NJ: John Wiley & Sons, 2012.

Katz V. L., et al. *Comprehensive Gynecology*, 6th ed. St. Louis: Mosby, 2012.

Lentz, S. G., et al. *Comprehensive Gynecology*, 6th ed. Philadelphia: Elsevier, Inc., 2013.

Niederhuber, J. E., et al. *Clinical Oncology*, 5th ed. Philadelphia: Elsevier, 2014.

PERIODICALS

Lee, L. J., A. Jhingran, and E. Kidd, et al. "American College of Radiology (ACR) Appropriateness Criteria Management of Vaginal Cancer." *Oncology (Willston Park)* 27 (Nov 2013): 1166–1173.

McCallum, M., L. Jolicoeur, and M. Lefebvre, et al. "Supportive Care Needs After Gynecologic Cancer: Where Does Sexual Health Fit In?" *Oncology Nursing Forum* 41 (May 2014): 297–306.

ORGANIZATIONS

American Cancer Society, 1599 Clifton Rd. NE, Atlanta, GA 30329, (800) ACS-2345, http://www.cancer.org.

Cancer Research Institute, 681 Fifth Ave., New York, NY 10022, (800) 992-2623, http://www.cancerresearch.org.

Gynecologic Cancer Foundation, 401 North Michigan Ave., Chicago, IL 60611, (312) 644-6610 (800) 444-4441, http://www.wcn.org/gcf.

National Institutes of Health, National Cancer Institute, 9000 Rockville Pike, Bethesda, MD 20982, (800) 4-CANCER (422-6237), http://cancernet.nci.nih.gov..

L. Lee Culvert
Belinda Rowland, PhD

Valacyclovir HCl *see* **Antiviral therapy**

Valium *see* **Diazepam**

Valrubicin

Definition

Valrubicin (also known as Valstar) is a chemotherapeutic drug that interferes with the metabolism of DNA, thus disrupting the proliferation of cells, including **cancer** cells.

Purpose

Valrubicin is an antineoplastic drug that is used as a treatment for a form of **bladder cancer** called papillary bladder cancer when the bladder cannot be surgically removed due to increased risk of morbidity or mortality. It is also being tested as treatment for several other types of **carcinoma** *in situ*.

Description

The U.S. Food and Drug Administration approved valrubicin for bladder cancer treatment in 1998. It has also been tested in **clinical trials** for both bladder and **ovarian cancer** treatments. It is an anthracycline-like compound that acts by penetrating cells and disrupting the dividing cell cycle by interfering with DNA metabolism. Valrubicin acts by inhibiting nucleoside incorporation into nucleic acids, thus causing major damage to DNA. Research performed in 1999 indicated that valrubicin entered cells faster than **doxorubicin**, another anthracycline. Research has also shown that complete response is seen in one in five patients.

Recommended dosage

Valrubicin is available in instillation form and can be administered only under the supervision of a physician. During initial clinical trials, patients received doses ranging from 200 milligrams to 900 milligrams each week. The normal dose is 800 milligrams once a week for six weeks. However, dosing may vary from patient to patient. The drug is administered intravesically (directly into the bladder) through a catheter tube that penetrates into the bladder wall. Once delivered to the bladder, the solution should be maintained in the bladder for approximately two hours.

During clinical trials for ovarian cancer, valrubicin is administered through the abdomen.

Precautions

There are other bladder problems that may affect the use of valrubicin. Patients with bladder irritation can have an increased risk of unwanted effects. Patients with perforated bladders should not take this medication. Patients with small bladders could have trouble holding all of the medication. Finally, if patients have urinary tract infections, they should use caution when taking this medication.

Valrubicin has not been studied in pregnant women, but it has been studied in pregnant animals. In animals it can cause birth defects. Therefore, women who are pregnant or breast-feeding should not take valrubicin. Additionally, women should not become pregnant while on this medication. Men taking this medication should not engage in procreative activities. Both men and women should use appropriate forms of contraception to avoid causing pregnancy.

There have not been appropriate studies done specifically on children or the elderly to determine the risk of using this medication in these populations. However, this drug is not expected to act differently in the elderly than it does in younger adults.

Side effects

During the six-week course of treatment patients could experience one or more side effects. The most common are loss of bladder control, increased frequency of urination, and blood in the urine. Other less common and rare side effects are bladder pain, pelvic pain, urethral pain, and loss of the sense of taste.

Interactions

Valrubicin may raise the risk of infection in patients who are also taking immunosuppressive drugs such as azathioprine (Imuran) or the chemotherapy drugs cladribine (Leustatin) or omacetaxine (Synribo). Vitamin E supplements may reduce the effectiveness of valrubicin. Patients should consult with their physicians before taking any drugs or supplements.

See also Daunorubicin; Taste alteration.

Sally C. McFarlane-Parrott

Valstar *see* **Valrubicin**

Vancomycin *see* **Antibiotics**

Vascular access

Definition

Vascular access is the use of a flexible tube (catheter) inserted into a blood vessel for the infusion of **antibiotics**, **chemotherapy**, pain medications, transfusions of blood or blood products, fluids, or **nutritional support**, as well as the withdrawal of blood samples. An external catheter in a vein in the arm or hand is called a peripheral line. A vascular access device (VAD) is a catheter that remains inserted for weeks or months. Peripherally inserted central catheters (PICCs) are external VADs inserted into an arm and threaded into a larger chest vein. A central line or central venous catheter (CVC) is an internal catheter in a larger vein in the neck or chest.

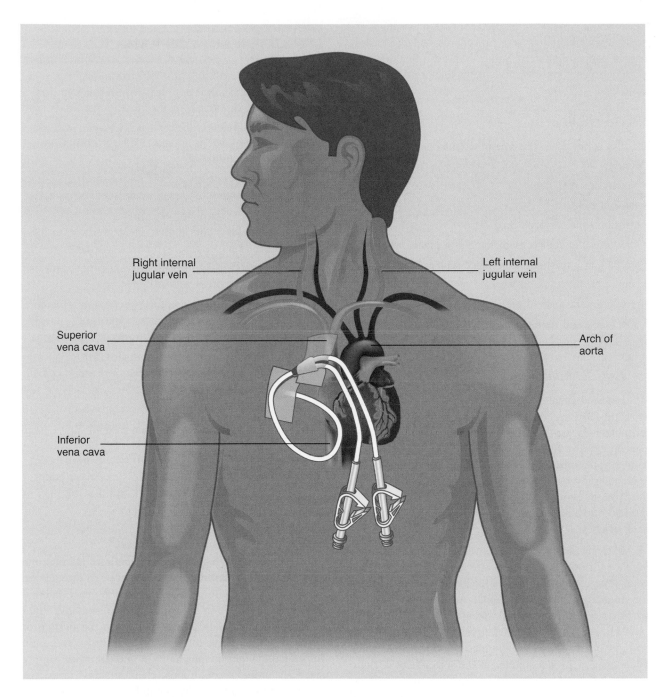

Right internal
jugular vein

Left internal
jugular vein

Superior
vena cava

Arch of
aorta

Inferior
vena cava

Vascular access uses slim tubes (catheters) to administer chemotherapy drugs or other fluids directly into a patient's blood vessels. *(Illustration by Electronic Illustrators Group. © 2015 Cengage Learning®.)*

Purpose

Vascular access is required for **cancer** patients who need intravenous (IV) chemotherapy drugs infused into the bloodstream and/or testing that requires frequent blood samples. Some chemotherapy drugs cannot be taken by mouth because they are irritants or are not absorbed by the digestive system. Some patients may be unable to swallow liquids or pills, have severe vomiting or **diarrhea** that prevents taking oral medications, or are unable to remember when and how to take oral medications. Vascular access is also needed to administer multiple drugs simultaneously. VADs that remain in place save the patient from the discomfort of and protect veins from the trauma of repeated punctures, as well as prevent the accidental release of harsh chemical agents into skin and subcutaneous tissues. PICCs are especially useful for administering fluids or medications that irritate vessel walls. VADs can be used for both intermittent and continuous treatments and procedures and can reduce patient pain and anxiety. Some VADs can function for a year or longer and are less likely than IV lines to be dislodged.

Description

Decisions about the type of vascular access are based on:

- patient age and size
- catheter purpose
- infusion time for each drug dose
- how long the catheter will remain in place
- the patient's previous experience with vascular access
- condition of the blood vessels
- physician and patient preferences
- VAD cost and required care
- any special patient circumstances or needs

External catheters

External catheters are usually made of polyurethane for short-term use and silicone for long-term use. Long-term devices are surrounded with an internal cuff to prevent catheter movement and infection. They have one to three openings called lumens. One might be used for chemotherapy, the second for nutritional support, and the third for drawing blood samples. The catheter can be inserted into a peripheral arm vein or a central vein in the neck or chest.

External central catheters that are designed to remain in place for only a week or so are inserted directly into a vein. Longer-term devices, which may remain in place for months, are tunneled under the skin to the point where they enter a central blood vessel, such as the cephalic, jugular, or subclavian vein. A PICC may limit arm movement and is usually placed in the patient's less dominant arm; for example, in the left arm of a right-handed patient. However, if a procedure such as breast surgery has been performed on one side, the PICC will most likely be inserted into the arm on the other side. Midline catheters are also placed in an arm vein but are not threaded as far as a PICC. External catheters require care and regular flushing.

Internal catheters

Internal catheters are also called implantable venous access ports. The catheter in a large or central vein connects to a drum-shaped port made of plastic, stainless steel, or titanium with a silicone septum over the top. It is surgically implanted under the skin, either in the chest or

upper arm. Although the system is entirely internal, the port is located near the surface and accessed through the skin and septum with a needle. Over the years, internal VADs have become smaller and more comfortable. Fluid flow is regulated by a pump located on the outside or implanted internally during the surgical procedure. Implanted titanium pumps have an internal power supply and can provide continuous chemotherapy infusions. External pumps are usually portable.

There are many different types of CVCs with different types of catheters and ports. Each type has advantages and potential problems and complications. Some may restrict certain activities. The port does not require routine care, although it may require flushing if it is not used for a month.

Preparation

The choice of appropriate vascular access can have a profound effect on quality of life, and patient involvement in the decision can improve outcomes. Blood tests

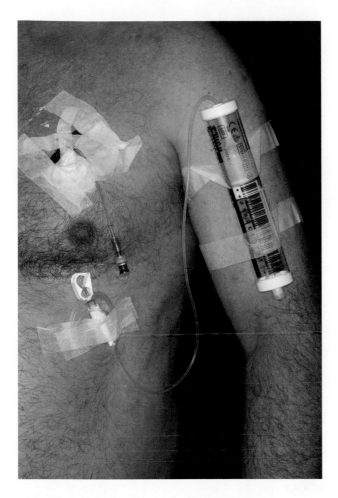

This patient is fitted with a catheter to administer chemotherapy drugs. (P. Marazzi/Science Source)

are performed to assess kidney function and blood clotting. Patients may need to discontinue blood thinners or other medications that interfere with clotting, and they are often instructed not to eat or drink for several hours before the procedure.

External long-term indwelling catheters, such as Hickmans, and internal catheters, such as Port-a-Caths, are inserted in a surgical or radiologic setting in a treatment center, clinic, or hospital. Patients are positioned with their legs elevated during the procedure. Some VAD insertion procedures are more involved than others. Heart rate and blood pressure are monitored during the procedure. The insertion site—usually the arm for PICCs and the upper chest for tunneled catheters—is shaved, sterilized, covered with a surgical drape, and numbed with a local anesthetic. A peripheral IV line may be inserted, and the patient may be sedated. PICC insertion does not usually require sedation. Ultrasound or x-rays and fluoroscopy are typically used to identify a suitable vein for catheter placement and for the insertion

of the guide wire and catheter. A midline catheter and some PICC lines are inserted through a vein near the elbow and threaded through a large vein in the upper arm at the patient's bedside without imaging.

A small needle is used to advance a guide wire. The catheter is advanced over the guide wire and positioned in a large central vein, and the guide wire is then removed. A chest x-ray confirms correct catheter position. The catheter is secured to the skin with a suture, and the insertion site is covered with a dressing. Tunneled catheters and subcutaneous ports require surgical insertion with two small incisions. The catheter is placed through the tunnel. The end of the tunnel is stitched to help hold the catheter in place.

Aftercare

X-ray imaging confirms that the VAD is correctly positioned, and fluid is injected through the catheter to confirm that the device is functioning properly. Patients must be driven home and should rest for the remainder of the day. They can resume normal activities the following day, while avoiding heavy lifting. Pain medication may be taken for any bruising, swelling, or tenderness. The catheter site must be kept clean and dry for the first week and may require cleaning with peroxide, application of an antibiotic ointment, and bandages. Patients can shower after one week, with plastic wrap covering the catheter site. The catheter is often flushed with **heparin** to prevent clotting.

A nurse or technician can remove a PICC or non-tunneled CVC. Tunneled and port catheters are removed by a physician, with the skin numbed. Removal takes about 15 minutes. The site must be kept dry until the incision has completely healed.

Special concerns

VADs must be cleaned daily and handled carefully. They are flushed with heparin or saline, usually every day or every other day, depending on the device, to prevent clotting. Specific care of indwelling catheters depends on the device. Most VADs eventually need replacement. The reservoir septa of implanted ports must be replaced after about 1,000 punctures.

Risks

There are various risks and potential complications associated with vascular access:

• Although pneumothorax (air in the pleural cavity) or hemothorax (blood in the pleural cavity) is rare, ultrasound or fluoroscopy-guided insertion can reduce the risk even further.

- Damage to the blood vessel can cause bruising or bleeding at the puncture site or infection.

- Even with normal blood clotting, blood sometimes leaks from a vein and causes problems.

- Disturbances of heart rhythm are usually temporary and rarely serious.

- Rarely, the catheter enters an artery instead of a vein. The catheter is removed, and the artery normally heals itself.

As many as 50% of patients have vascular access complications, some of which can be serious or life-threatening. Displacement or clogging are the most common complications with peripheral catheters.

- Blockage in the tubing is a common problem. The first sign is usually difficulty withdrawing blood. A blockage can be confirmed with a chest x-ray and can sometimes be cleared with flushing.

- The catheter can leak due to a defect or from being pinched between the collarbone and rib.

- The catheter can move over time. To replace a dislodged catheter, patients are sometimes instructed to raise their arms or attempt other maneuvers. If catheter movement continues, the device will malfunction and may need to be removed.

- Blood clots are a risk. Treatment can be as simple as changing an arm position. In more serious cases, the catheter might require removal. Although blood clots sometimes produce no symptoms, they can break loose and form emboli that travel through the bloodstream and are potentially fatal.

- A catheter that is not taped or sutured to the skin may move or pull out.

- When not in use, the catheter should always be clamped and caps screwed on tight to prevent air from entering the bloodstream. A large volume of air in the catheter can be an emergency situation.

Infection is the most common complication associated with long-term vascular access. Infections can occur on the surface or internally along the tubing itself. A surface infection is usually red, tender to the touch, and may have discharge. Gram-positive bacteria, such as staphylococcus, are the most common causes of infection, although other bacteria can also cause infection. Treatment is determined by the seriousness of the infection, the site of the problem, and the type of catheter. A minor infection is often treated with a topical antibiotic. In more severe cases, such as infections along the tubing, in the bloodstream, or in an implantable port, a course of antibiotics will be prescribed. Cleanliness when handling the catheter, careful changing of dressings, checking of the

---

QUESTIONS TO ASK YOUR DOCTOR

- What type of vascular access will be used?
- Why was this particular method or type selected?
- What treatments will I receive through the catheter?
- Will insertion be an outpatient procedure or require a hospital stay?
- Who will insert the catheter?
- How should I prepare for insertion?
- What are the risks of a complication during insertion?
- What special care does the device require?
- What are the symptoms of a catheter problem?
- Will the catheter cause any physical limitations?
- How long will my catheter remain in place?
- How will the catheter be removed?

---

skin at each dressing change, and use of sterile technique minimize the risk of infection.

Resources

BOOKS

Nakae, Hajime. "Vascular Access Catheters: Types, Applications, and Potential Complications." In *Catheters: Types, Applications, and Potential Complications*, edited by Robert C. Diggery and Daniel T. Grint. New York: Nova Science, 2012.

Phillips, Lynn Dianne, and Lisa A. Gorski. *Manual of I.V. Therapeutics: Evidence-Based Practice for Infusion Therapy.* 6th ed. Philadelphia: F. A. Davis, 2014.

Sansivero, Gail Egan, Gary Siskin, and David Singh. "Role of Ultrasound in Central Vascular Access Device Placement." In *Diagnostic Medical Sonography: The Vascular System*, edited by Ann Marie Kupinski. Philadelphia: Wolters Kluwer/Lippincott Williams & Wilkins, 2013.

PERIODICALS

Chen, Wenfeng, et al. "A Comprehensive Intervention Program on the Long-Term Placement of Peripherally Inserted Central Venous Catheters." *Journal of Cancer Research and Therapeutics* 10, no. 2 (April–June 2014): 359–62.

Hemmati, Hossein, et al. "Ultrasound Guided Port-A-Cath Implantation." *Surgical Science* 5, no. 4 (April 2014): 159–63.

Odabas, Hatice, et al. "Effect of Port-Care Frequency on Venous Port Catheter-Related Complications in Cancer Patients." *International Journal of Clinical Oncology* 19, no. 4 (August 2014): 761–6.

Rosen, Jennifer, et al. "Massage for Perioperative Pain and Anxiety in Placement of Vascular Access Devices." *Advances in Mind-Body Medicine* 27, no. 1 (Winter 2013): 12–23.

WEBSITES

"How is Chemotherapy Given?" American Cancer Society. February 7, 2013. http://www.cancer.org/treatment/treatmentsandsideeffects/treatmenttypes/chemotherapy/chemotherapyprinciplesanin-depthdiscussionofthetechniquesanditsroleintreatment/chemotherapy-principles-how-is-chemo-given (accessed August 31, 2014).

Larson, Shawn D. "Vascular Access Overview." Medscape. July 31, 2012. http://emedicine.medscape.com/article/1018395-overview#showall (accessed August 31, 2014).

"Vascular Access Procedures." RadiologyInfo.org. August 5, 2013. http://www.radiologyinfo.org/en/info.cfm?pg=vasc_acccss&bhcp=1&mobilebypass=1 (accessed August 31, 2014).

ORGANIZATIONS

American Cancer Society, 250 Williams Street NW, Atlanta, GA 30303, (800) 227-2345, http://www.cancer.org.

American College of Radiology, 1891 Preston White Drive, Reston, VA 20191, (703) 648-8900, info@acr.org, http://www.acr.org.

Radiology Society of North America, 820 Jorie Boulevard, Oak Brook, IL 60523-2251, (630) 571-2670, Fax: (630) 571-7837, (800) 381-6660, http://www.rsna.org.

U.S. Food and Drug Administration, 10903 New Hampshire Avenue, Silver Spring, MD 20993-0002, (888) INFO-FDA (463-6332), http://www.fda.gov.

Rhonda Cloos, R.N.
Margaret Alic, PhD

Vectibix *see* **Panitumumab**

Velban *see* **Vinblastine**

Velcade *see* **Bortezomib**

Velsar *see* **Vinblastine**

Venoocclusive disease *see* **Bone marrow transplantation**

VePesid *see* **Etoposide**

Vidaza *see* **Azacitidine**

Vinblastine

Definition

Vinblastine is a drug used to treat certain types of **cancer**. Vinblastine is available under the trade names Velban and Velsar, and may also be referred to as

---

KEY TERMS

Alkaloid—A nitrogen-containing compound occurring in plants.

Microtubules—A tubular structure located in cells that help them to replicate.

Therapeutic index—A ratio of the maximum tolerated dose of a drug divided by the dose used in treatment.

---

vinblastine sulfate. The drug was previously known as vincaleukoblastine or VLB.

Purpose

Vinblastine is an antineoplastic agent used to treat **Hodgkin lymphoma**, non-Hodgkin lymphomas, **mycosis fungoides**, cancer of the testis, **Kaposi sarcoma**, Letterer-Siwe disease, as well as other cancers.

Description

Vinblastine was approved by the U.S. Food and Drug Administration (FDA) in 1961.

Vinblastine is a naturally occurring compound that is extracted from periwinkle plants. It belongs to a group of chemicals called alkaloids. The chemical structure and biological action of vinblastine is similar to **vincristine** and **vinorelbine**.

Vinblastine prevents the formation of microtubules in cells. One of the roles of microtubules is to aid in the replication of cells. By disrupting this function, vinblastine inhibits cell replication, including the replication the cancer cells.

Vinblastine is one the most effective treatments for Hodgkin **lymphoma** and is typically used in combination with **doxorubicin**, **bleomycin**, and **dacarbazine**. It is also used to treat non-Hodgkin lymphomas, mycosis fungoides, and Letterer-Siwe disease. Vinblastine is also used to treat cancer of the testis in combination with other cancer drugs, and Kaposi **sarcoma** alone or in combination with other drugs. Vinblastine is used less frequently to treat other types of cancer.

Recommended dosage

Vinblastine is administered by intravenous injection at intervals of at least seven days. Blood tests may be necessary every seven days to ensure that enough white blood cells are present to continue treatment. The initial dose of vinblastine may be adjusted upward or downward depending on patient tolerance to the toxic side effects of treatment. The minimum recommended treatment duration is four to six weeks.

Precautions

Vinblastine must only be administered by individuals experienced in the use of this cancer chemotherapeutic agent. Vinblastine must only be administered intravenously (directly into a vein). Accidental administration of vinblastine into spinal cord fluid is a medical emergency that may result in death. Vinblastine has a low therapeutic index; it is unlikely there will be therapeutic benefit without toxic side effects. Certain complications can only be managed by a physician experienced in the use of cancer chemotherapeutic agents.

Because vinblastine is administered intravenously, the site of infusion and surrounding tissue should be monitored for signs of inflammation and irritation.

Adverse side effects are more likely in patients with malnutrition or skin ulceration.

Blood tests may be necessary to ensure that the number of white blood cells is adequate for treatment to continue. Vinblastine is not recommended for use in patients with low white blood cell levels. Infections should also be controlled before vinblastine treatment.

Patients should inform their physician if they experience sore throat, **fever**, chills, or sore mouth and any serious medical event.

Vinblastine may cause harm to a fetus when administered to pregnant women. Only in life-threatening situations should this treatment be used during pregnancy. Women of childbearing age are advised not to become pregnant during treatment. Breast-feeding mothers should stop nursing before beginning treatment due to the potential for serious adverse side effects in the nursing infants.

Side effects

The side effects of vinblastine treatment are usually related to the dose of drug and are generally reversible. Toxic side effects are more common in patients with poor liver function. Studies have also shown that patients with advanced **prostate cancer** experienced toxic side effects of **estramustine** phosphage (EMP) plus vinblastine (VBL) and from EMP alone.

A decrease in the number of white blood cells is the principal adverse side effect associated with vinblastine treatment. Blood tests will allow a doctor to determine if there are an adequate number of white blood cells to begin or continue treatment. **Nausea and vomiting** may occur, for which antiemetic agents are usually effective. Shortness of breath is a potentially severe side effect that patients should report to their doctor.

Additional side effects, including loss of appetite (**anorexia**), **diarrhea**, constipation, pain, rectal bleeding, dizziness, hearing impairment, and hair loss (**alopecia**) may occur.

Interactions

Drugs that may alter the metabolism of vinblastine, particularly itraconazole, should be used with caution due to the potential for interactions. Hearing impairment may be enhanced when vinblastine is used with other drugs that affect the ear. These drugs include platinum-containing **antineoplastic agents**, such as **cisplatin**. Seizures have been reported in patients taking vinblastine and **phenytoin**. The doses of vinblastine and phenytoin may need to be adjusted to decrease the chance of this problem.

Resources

BOOKS

Chu, Edward, and Vincent T. DeVita Jr. *Physicians' Cancer Chemotherapy Drug Manual 2014*. Burlington, MA: Jones & Bartlett Learning, 2014.

WEBSITES

AHFS Consumer Medication Information. "Vinblastine." American Society of Health-System Pharmacists. Available from: http://www.nlm.nih.gov/medlineplus/druginfo/meds/a682848.html (accessed November 13, 2014).
American Cancer Society. "Vinblastine." http://www.cancer.org/treatment/treatmentsandsideeffects/guidetocancer-drugs/vinblastinc (accessed November 13, 2014).

Marc Scanio

Vincasar *see* **Vincristine**

Vincrex *see* **Vincristine**

Vincristine

Definition

Vincristine is a drug used to treat certain types of **cancer**. Vincristine is available under the trade names Oncovin, Vincasar, and Vincrex, and may also be referred to as vincristine sulfate, or VCR. The drug was previously known as leurocristine, or LCR.

Purpose

Vincristine is an antineoplastic agent used to treat leukemia, **Hodgkin lymphoma**, malignant lymphomas, **neuroblastoma**, **rhabdomyosarcoma**, and **Wilms tumor**, as well as other cancers.

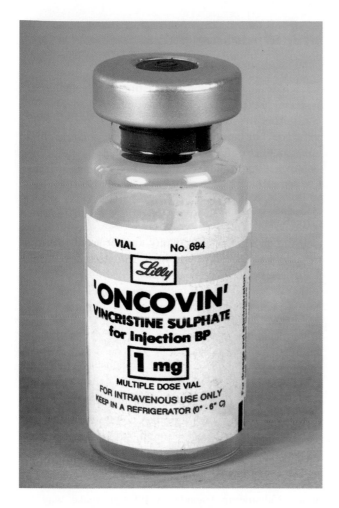

Vial of vincristine (Oncovin). *(MedicImage/Alamy)*

Description

Vincristine was approved by the U.S. Food and Drug Administration (FDA) in 1984.

Vincristine is a naturally occurring compound that is extracted from periwinkle plants. It belongs to a group of chemicals called alkaloids. The chemical structure and biological action of vincristine is similar to **vinblastine** and **vinorelbine**.

Vincristine prevents the formation of microtubules in cells. One of the roles of microtubules is to aid in the replication of cells. By disrupting this function, vincristine inhibits cell replication, including the replication of the cancer cells.

Vincristine is used in combination with other drugs to treat leukemia. It is also used in combination with other drugs, such as **mechlorethamine**, **procarbazine**, and prednisone, to treat Hodgkin **lymphoma**, and is used in combination to treat non-Hodgkin lymphomas, neuroblastoma, rhabdomyosarcoma, and Wilms tumor.

Vincristine is used less frequently to treat other types of cancer.

Recommended dosage

Vincristine is administered by intravenous injection once per week and is usually capped at a maximum of 2 milligrams (mg) per dose. The initial dose of vincristine may be adjusted upward or downward depending on patient tolerance to the toxic side effects of treatment.

Precautions

Vincristine must only be administered by individuals experienced in the use of this cancer chemotherapeutic agent. Vincristine must be administered intravenously—that is, directly into a vein. Accidental administration of vincristine into the spinal cord fluid is a medical emergency that may result in death. Vincristine has a low therapeutic index. It is unlikely there will be therapeutic benefit without toxic side effects. Certain complications can only be managed by a physician experienced in the use of cancer chemotherapeutic agents.

Because vincristine is administered intravenously and is extremely irritating, the site of infusion and surrounding tissue should be monitored for signs of inflammation.

Some experts recommend blood tests to ensure that the number of white blood cells is adequate for treatment to continue. Infections should also be controlled before vincristine treatment starts.

Vincristine is not recommended for use in patients with the demyelinating form of Charcot-Marie-Tooth syndrome.

Vincristine is not recommended for patients receiving **radiation therapy** though a port in the liver.

Vincristine may cause harm to a fetus when administered to pregnant women. Only in life-threatening situations, should this treatment be used during pregnancy. Women of childbearing age are advised not to become pregnant during treatment. Breast-feeding women should stop nursing before beginning treatment due to the potential for serious adverse side effects in the nursing infants.

Side effects

The side effects of vincristine treatment are usually related to the dose of drug and are generally reversible. Toxic side effects may be more common in patients with poor liver function.

Toxicity of the nervous system is the principal adverse side effect associated with vincristine treatment. This toxicity may cause numbness; pain, especially of the jaw; tingling; and headaches. Lengthy treatment at high doses may cause even more severe toxicity. Constipation is a common side effect. **Laxatives** and enemas are typically used to prevent severe constipation. Shortness of breath is a potentially severe side effect that patients should report to their doctor. Additional side effects, including rash, an increase or decrease in blood pressure, dizziness, **nausea and vomiting**, hearing impairment, and hair loss (**alopecia**) may occur.

Interactions

Drugs that may alter the metabolism of vincristine, particularly itraconazole, should be used with caution due to the potential for interactions. Hearing impairment may be enhanced when vincristine is used with other drugs that affect the ear. These drugs include platinum-containing **antineoplastic agents**, such as **cisplatin**. Seizures have been reported in patients taking vincristine and **phenytoin**. The doses of vincristine and phenytoin may need to be adjusted to decrease the chance of this problem.

Resources

BOOKS

Chu, Edward, and Vincent T. DeVita Jr. *Physicians' Cancer Chemotherapy Drug Manual 2014.* Burlington, MA: Jones & Bartlett Learning, 2014.

WEBSITES

American Cancer Society. "Vincristine." http://www.cancer.org/treatment/treatmentsandsideeffects/guidetocancerdrugs/vincristine (accessed November 13, 2014).

Cancer Research UK. "Vincristine." http://www.cancerresearchuk.org/about-cancer/cancers-in-general/treatment/cancer-drugs/vincristine (accessed November 13, 2014).

Marc Scanio

Vindesine

Definition

Vindesine (desacetyl **vinblastine** amide sulfate) is a synthetic derivative of vinblastine. Vindesine is a **chemotherapy** drug that is given as a treatment for some types of **cancer**. This drug belongs to the group of **anticancer drugs** known as vinca alkaloids. Vindesine is also called vindesine sulfate, desacetylvinblastine amide, DAVA, DVA, or VDS, and by its brand name, Eldisine.

Purpose

Vindesine is used primarily to treat **acute lymphocytic leukemia**. Less frequently, it is prescribed for use in **breast cancer**, blast crisis of **chronic myelocytic leukemia**, colorectal cancer, **non-small cell lung cancer**, and renal cell cancer (**kidney cancer**).

Description

Vindesine binds to particular proteins and causes cell arrest or cell death. Metabolized by the liver, vindesine is primarily excreted through the biliary system.

Vindesine is used in other countries around the world such as Britain, South Africa, and several European countries, but it is not approved by the U.S. Food and Drug Administration and is thus not commercially available in the United States. Eli Lilly discontinued Eldisine in Canada in 1998 to make way for newer, more effective vinca alkaloid drugs.

For acute lymphocytic leukemia (ALL), vindesine is effective in both adult and pediatric populations. As an agent used alone, vindesine has produced response rates ranging from 5% to 63% in several clinical studies. Vindesine has been used in combination therapy using the following drugs: **daunorubicin**, **asparaginase**, prednisone, **cytarabine**, and **etoposide**.

The clinical response rate in children (41%) is better than in adults (26%) for treatment of ALL. Vindesine with combination therapy has shown very high response rates in childhood ALL.

For treatment during the blast crisis of chronic myelocytic (or myelogenous) leukemia, overall response rates of 51% have been reported in adults when vindesine was used alone or in combination therapy with prednisone. Efficacy has not been demonstrated in pediatric groups.

Vindesine may be effective in treating breast cancer. When used alone, one clinical trial reported that vindesine showed an overall response rate of approximately 19% in treating advanced breast cancer.

KEY TERMS

Acute lymphocytic leukemia—A rapidly progressing disease where too many immature infection-fighting white blood cells called lymphoblasts are found in the blood and bone marrow. It is also known as ALL or acute lymphoblastic leukemia.

Intravenous (or intravenously)—Into a vein.

Vinblastine—A vinca alkaloid.

Vinca alkaloid—A group of cytotoxic alkaloids extracted from a flower called Madagascar periwinkle. Cytotoxic chemotherapy kills cells, especially cancer cells. Vinca alkaloids are cell cycle phase specific; they exert their effect during the M phase of cell mitosis and cause metaphase cell arrest and death. These drugs are for antineoplastic therapy (chemotherapy) for cancer treatment. Other vinca alkaloids include vinblastine, vincristine, vindesine, and vinorelbine.

Vindesine in combination with **cisplatin** is one of the most active treatments for non-small lung cancer, but **vinorelbine** substituted for vindesine has shown higher response rates in treating non-small lung cancer.

Vindesine is not effective for treating acute non-lymphocytic leukemia.

Recommended dosage

There are many dosing schedules that depend on the type of cancer, response to treatment, and other drugs that may be coprescribed. Dosing guidelines also consider the white blood cell count.

Vindesine is injected intravenously through a fine needle (cannula). Alternatively, it may be given through a central line that is inserted under the skin into a vein near the collarbone.

- Intravenous administration for adults: Each one to two weeks a dose of 2–4 mg/m^2 is given, or each three to four weeks 1.5 mg/m^2/day is administered as a continuous infusion for five to seven days.
- Intravenous administration for children: Once a week with 4 mg/m^2 or twice weekly with 2 mg/m^2.

Precautions

Vindesine may cause fertility problems in men and women. In addition, it may harm the fetus or may damage sperm; therefore, it is not recommended for women to use vindesine during pregnancy or for men to father a child while taking this drug. The physician should be alerted immediately if pregnancy occurs. Due to possible secretion into breast milk, breast-feeding is not recommended.

Other considerations include:

- Vindesine is potentially mutagenic or carcinogenic (cancer-causing).
- Vindesine may cause death if injected intrathecally (into the spinal cord). It is for intravenous use only.
- Prior injection sites should be carefully inspected because tissue damage may occur days or weeks after administration.
- Hepatic dysfunction increases the neurotoxic potential of this drug.
- Alert doctors or dentists about vindesine therapy before receiving any treatment.

Side effects

Possible side effects of vindesine therapy include:

- Pain or tenderness may occur at the injection site.
- Hair loss (alopecia) is common.
- Vindesine can damage the surrounding tissue if it leaks into the tissue around the vein. If vindesine leaks under the skin, a burning or stinging sensation may be felt. Alert the doctor immediately if burning or stinging occurs while the drug is administered or if fluid is leaking from the site where the needle was inserted. Also tell the doctor if the area around the injection site becomes red or swollen at any time.
- Constipation or abdominal cramps; these can be alleviated by drinking plenty of water, eating a high-fiber diet, and light exercise.
- A temporary decrease in white blood cell count and platelets may occur.
- Numbing of the fingers or toes may occur over the course of treatment. It may take several months to return to normal.
- Diarrhea occurs infrequently.
- Mouth sores and ulcers may form.
- Nausea and vomiting rarely occurs.
- Anaphylaxis is rare.
- Jaw pain may be severe, but it is rare.
- Thrombocytopenia (a decrease in the number of platelets in the blood) or thrombocytosis; these conditions are also rare.

Interactions

Vindesine may interact with **mitomycin-C** (brand name Mutamycin), causing acute bronchospasm within minutes or hours following administration. **Phenytoin** (brand name Dilantin) may also interact with vindesine, leading to decreased serum levels of phenytoin.

Other drug interactions may occur with:

• Itraconazole

• Live virus and bacterial vaccines; when taking immune suppressing chemotherapy drugs, live vaccinations should not be given.

• Quinupristin/dalfopristin

• Rotavirus vaccine

• Warfarin

Resources

PERIODICALS

Liu L., Sun Y., Si Y., Lin G., Zhang X., Zhao G., Zhang Y., Wu D. "Vindesine Induces Rhabdomyolysis in Patients With Acute Lymphoblastic Leukemia." *Chinese Medical Journal* 127, no. 21 (2014): 3835–36. http://www.cmj.org/ch/reader/view_abstract.aspx?volume=127&issue=21&start_-page=3835 (accessed November 13, 2014).

WEBSITES

Cancer Research UK. "Vindesine (Eldisine)." http://www.cancerresearchuk.org/about-cancer/cancers-in-general/treatment/cancer-drugs/vindesine#general (accessed November 13, 2014).

National Cancer Institute. "Vindesine." http://www.cancer.gov/drugdictionary?CdrID=39732 (accessed November 13, 2014).

Crystal Heather Kaczkowski, MSc.

Vinorelbine

Definition

Vinorelbine is a drug used to treat certain types of lung **cancer**. Vinorelbine is available under the trade name Navelbine. The drug may also be referred to as vinorelbine tartrate or didehydrodeoxynorvincaleukoblastine.

Purpose

Vinorelbine is an antineoplastic agent used to treat non-small cell lung **carcinoma**.

More recently, vinorelbine has been used in the palliative treatment of patients with advanced **esophageal cancer** and advanced **breast cancer**. Early reports of its effectiveness are encouraging.

Description

Vinorelbine was approved by the U.S. Food and Drug Administration (FDA) in 1994.

Vinorelbine is a semisynthetic derivative of **vinblastine**, a naturally occurring compound that is extracted from periwinkle plants. It belongs to a group of chemicals called vinca alkaloids. The chemical structure and biological action of vinorelbine is similar to vinblastine and **vincristine**.

Vinorelbine prevents the formation of microtubules in cells. One of the roles of microtubules is to aid in the replication of cells. By disrupting this function vinorelbine inhibits cell replication, including the replication the cancer cells.

Vinorelbine is used alone and in combination with **cisplatin** (another anticancer drug) to treat non-small cell lung carcinoma. It has been used in combination with other drugs to treat breast cancer. Vinorelbine has also been studied as a treatment for **cervical cancer**.

Recommended dosage

Vinorelbine is administered by intravenous injection (directly into a vein) once per week. The initial dose may be adjusted downward depending on patient tolerance to the toxic side effects of treatment. If toxic effects are severe, vinorelbine treatment may be delayed or discontinued.

Precautions

Vinorelbine must be administered only by individuals experienced in the use of this cancer chemotherapeutic agent.

Vinorelbine must only be administered intravenously. Accidental administration of vinorelbine into the spinal cord fluid is a medical emergency that may result in death. Vinorelbine has a low therapeutic index, which means it is unlikely there will be therapeutic benefit without toxic side effects. Certain complications can only be managed by a physician experienced in the use of cancer chemotherapeutic agents.

Because vinorelbine is administered intravenously and is extremely irritating, the site of infusion and surrounding tissue should be monitored for signs of inflammation.

Blood tests are recommended to ensure that bone marrow function and the number of white blood cells are adequate for treatment to continue. Infections should also be controlled before vinorelbine treatment starts. Special caution should be used with patients whose bone marrow reserves have been reduced by previous radiation or **chemotherapy** treatment.

Vinorelbine may cause harm to a fetus when administered to pregnant women. Only in life-threatening situations should this treatment be used during pregnancy. Women of childbearing age are advised not to become pregnant during treatment. Breast-feeding women should stop nursing before beginning treatment due to the potential for serious adverse side effects in the nursing infants.

The safety of vinorelbine in children under 18 years of age has not been established.

Side effects

The side effects of vinorelbine treatment are usually related to the dose of drug and are generally reversible. It is possible that toxic side effects may be more common in patients with poor liver function and should be used with caution in those patients.

Decreased bone marrow function is the principal adverse side effect. This can reduce the number of white blood cells and increase the chance of infections. Patients should report **fever** or chills to their doctors immediately. Patients should also inform their doctor if they experience abdominal pain, constipation, or an increase in shortness of breath.

Toxicity of the nervous system is another side effect. Shortness of breath is a potentially severe side effect that patients should report to their doctor. Additional side effects, including fever, **anemia**, an increase or decrease in blood pressure, dizziness, **nausea and vomiting**, hearing impairment, and hair loss (**alopecia**) may occur.

Several cases of heart attacks related to vinorelbine have been reported. A group of French researchers estimates that about 1% of patients treated with vinorelbine will develop heart problems; however, vinorelbine does not appear to have a higher rate of these side effects than other drugs in its class.

Interactions

The use of vinorelbine in combination with another anticancer drug, **mitomycin-C**, has caused severe shortness of breath. Patients taking vinorelbine and cisplatin are more likely to experience a decrease in the number of white blood cells. This side effect should be carefully monitored to ensure that the number of white blood cells is adequate for treatment to continue. Patients taking vinorelbine and another anticancer drug, paclitaxel, may be more likely to experience toxicity of the nervous system, and should be carefully monitored for this. Drugs that may alter the metabolism of vinorelbine should be used with caution due to the potential for interactions.

Patients who are treated with vinorelbine during or following radiotherapy may become hypersensitive to radiation treatment.

Resources

BOOKS

Beers, Mark H., MD, and Robert Berkow, MD, editors. "Bronchogenic Carcinoma." In *The Merck Manual of Diagnosis and Therapy*. Whitehouse Station, NJ: Merck Research Laboratories, 2007.

WEBSITES

American Cancer Society. "Vinorelbine." http://www.cancer.org/treatment/treatmentsandsideeffects/guidetocancer-drugs/vinorelbine (accessed November 13, 2014).

Cancer Research UK. "Vinorelbine (Navelbine)." http://www.cancerresearchuk.org/about-cancer/cancers-in-general/treatment/cancer-drugs/vinorelbine (accessed November 13, 2014).

ORGANIZATIONS

ASHP (formerly the American Society of Health-System Pharmacists), 7272 Wisconsin Ave., Bethesda, MD 20814, (301) 664-8700, (866) 279-0681, custserv@ashp.org, http://www.ashp.org.

U.S. Food and Drug Administration, 10903 New Hampshire Ave., Silver Spring, MD 20993, (888) INFO-FDA (463-6332), http://www.fda.gov.

Marc Scanio
Rebecca J. Frey, PhD

Viruses *see* **AIDS-related cancers; Epstein-Barr virus; Human papillomavirus**

Vitamins

Definition

Vitamins are compounds that are essential in small amounts for proper body function and growth. Vitamins are either fat soluble (A, D, E, and K) or water soluble (B and C). The B vitamins include vitamins B_1 (thiamine), B_2 (riboflavin), B_6 (pyridoxine), and B_{12} (cobalamin); pantothenic acid; niacin; biotin; and **folic acid** (folate). Vitamins also may be referred to as micronutrients.

Purpose

Specific nutrients have been linked to prevention of several cancers of the colon, breast, prostate, stomach, and other types of tumors. A high intake of fruits and vegetables as well as fiber appears particularly protective, while a diet high in fat has been implicated as a cancer risk.

Description

A guide to the amount an average person needs each day to remain healthy has been determined for each vitamin. In the United States, this is called the recommended dietary allowance (RDA). Consuming too little of certain vitamins may lead to a nutrient deficiency. Consuming too much of certain vitamins may lead to nutrient toxicity.

Consumption of a wide variety of foods that have adequate vitamins and minerals is the basis of a healthy diet. Good nutrition may assist in the prevention of **cancer** or may help cancer patients to feel better and fight infection during treatments. Obtaining nutrients through food remains the best method for obtaining vitamins; however, requirements may be higher because of the tumor or cancer therapy. Therefore, supplements may be necessary.

Benefits

The following vitamins are important in a healthy diet and also may assist in **cancer prevention**. Their roles in maintaining health and the best food sources vary.

VITAMIN A (RETINAL, CAROTENE). Vitamin A plays a role in the growth and repair of body tissues. It supports vision and immune function. The best sources of vitamin A include eggs; dark green, red, orange, and yellow fruits and vegetables; low-fat dairy products; and liver.

VITAMIN B_6 (PYRIDOXINE). Vitamin B_6 plays a role in the formation of antibodies. It is important in carbohydrate and protein metabolism, the formation of

red blood cells, and nerve function. Vitamin B_6 is found in lean meat, fish, poultry, whole grains, and potatoes.

FOLIC ACID (FOLATE). Folic acid assists in red blood cell formation and is important in protein metabolism and growth and cell division. It is found in green leafy vegetables, poultry, dried beans, fortified cereals, nuts, and oranges.

VITAMIN C (ASCORBIC ACID). Vitamin C helps fight infection and contributes to wound healing. It is important in collagen maintenance, strengthening blood vessels, and maintaining healthy gums. The best sources of vitamin C include citrus fruits, tomatoes, melons, broccoli, green and red peppers, and berries.

VITAMIN E (TOCOPHEROL). Vitamin E may assist in immune function and is important in preventing oxidation of red blood cells and cell membranes. It is found in vegetable oils, wheat germ, nuts, dark green vegetables, beans, and whole grains.

Vitamins important for cancer prevention

Antioxidant vitamins are believed to protect the body from harmful free radicals that can contribute to diseases such as cancer. Antioxidant vitamins include vitamins A, C, and E. However, doses too high may increase oxidative stress and therefore increase cancer risk.

A diet rich in fruits and vegetables (containing B_6, folate, and niacin) appears to protect against **stomach cancer**, particularly intestinal cancer.

One study reported that cruciferous vegetables, especially broccoli, brussels sprouts, cauliflower, and cabbage were associated with a decreased risk of **prostate cancer**. Other foods, such as carrots, beans, and cooked tomatoes, also were associated with a lower risk.

A component of vitamin E, tocotrienol, has been linked to a decreased risk of **breast cancer** in lab animals. Tocotrienol has been shown to readily kill tumor cells grown in cultures. Tocotrienol is not the same type of substance found in generic vitamin E supplements but is plentiful in palm oil; lower concentrations of tocotrienol are found in rice bran oil and wheat bran oil. In 2004, research showed that the nutrients calcium and vitamin D worked together, not separately, to lower risk of colorectal cancer. As of 2014, the **National Cancer Institute** reported that all of the data on vitamin D does not establish whether taking supplements of the vitamin can help prevent cancer. Researchers continue to study whether doses of vitamin D can help prevent prostate, colorectal, and lung cancer.

Researchers state that no single nutrient is the answer, but that the effects of nutrient consumption are cumulative and depend on eating a variety of fruits and vegetables. Because there are many more nutrients available in foods such as fruits and vegetables than in vitamin supplements, food is the best source for acquiring needed vitamins and minerals. Fresh fruits and vegetables also provide fiber and help individuals maintain a balanced diet.

Special concerns

For many years, debate has continued regarding taking vitamin supplements to prevent cancer. In 2004, the U.S. Preventive Services Task Force concluded that the evidence was inadequate to recommend supplementation of vitamins A, C, or E; multivitamins with folic acid; or antioxidant combinations to decrease the risk of cancer. Beta-carotene supplements should not be used in patients with no symptoms because there is no evidence of risk reduction and some evidence that excessive dosages may cause harm. In general, people who have cancer or want to prevent cancer can benefit some from ensuring they consume plenty of foods with **antioxidants**, but vitamin requirements for cancer patients and survivors are the same as those of the general population.

There are concerns regarding antioxidant levels during **chemotherapy** and **radiation therapy**. Researchers report that large amounts of Vitamin C are consumed by cancerous tumors during chemotherapy in studies with mice. Vitamin C is an antioxidant that consumes free radicals and is thought to perhaps interfere with the process of killing cancer cells during chemotherapy or radiation therapy. Cancer patients undergoing chemotherapy are advised to discuss any use of dietary supplements with their doctors when undergoing chemotherapy and other cancer treatments.

Smokers are advised not to consume a diet high in beta-carotene (vitamin A) because research has shown a link to increased lung cancer incidence.

Alternative and complementary therapies

There are a great many claims about particular vitamins and/or antioxidants having beneficial health effects. Proper nutrition with an adequate diet is the best way to obtain vitamins, but a supplement may be required when intake is inadequate, such as if a cancer patient is experiencing **nausea and vomiting** and is not eating normally. It is important to check with a dietitian or doctor before taking nutritional supplements or alternative therapies because they may interfere with cancer medications or treatments.

Resources

BOOKS

Dasgupta, Amitava, and Kimberly Klein. *Antioxidants in Food, Vitamins and Supplements: Prevention and Treatment of Disease.* San Diego, CA; London; Waltham, MA: Elsevier, 2014.

PERIODICALS

Dueregger, A., et al. "The Use of Dietary Supplements to Alleviate Androgen Deprivation Therapy Side Effects during Prostate Cancer Treatment." *Nutrients* 6, no. 10 (2014): 4491–519.

Ho, W. J., et al. "Antioxidant Micronutrients and the Risk of Renal Cell Carcinoma in the Women's Health Initiative Cohort." *Nutrients* (October 9, 2014): e-pub ahead of print. http://dx.doi.org/10.1002/cncr.29091 (accessed November 6, 2014).

Hu, Fulan, et al. "The Plasma Level of Retinol, Vitamins A, C and α-tocopherol Could Reduce Breast Cancer Risk? A Meta-Analysis and Meta-Regression." *Journal of Cancer Research and Clinical Oncology* (October 15, 2014): e-pub ahead of print. http://dx.doi.org/10.1007/s00432-014-1852-7 (accessed November 6, 2014).

WEBSITES

American Society of Clinical Oncology. "Vitamins and Minerals." Cancer.Net. http://www.cancer.net/navigating-cancer-care/prevention-and-healthy-living/diet-and-nutrition/vitamins-and-minerals (accessed September 26, 2014).

National Cancer Institute. "Antioxidants and Cancer Prevention." http://www.cancer.gov/cancertopics/factsheet/prevention/antioxidants (accessed September 26, 2014).

National Cancer Institute. "Vitamin D and Cancer Prevention." http://www.cancer.gov/cancertopics/factsheet/prevention/vitamin-D (accessed September 26, 2014).

The Scott Hamilton CARES Initiative. "Vitamins and Cancer: What About Taking Diet Supplements and Vitamins." Chemocare.com. http://chemocare.com/chemotherapy/health-wellness/vitamins-and-cancer.aspx (accessed November 6, 2014).

ORGANIZATIONS

National Cancer Institute, 9609 Medical Center Drive, Bethesda, MD 20892, (800) 422-6237, http://www.cancer.gov.

National Center for Complementary and Alternative Medicine, 9000 Rockville Pike, Bethesda, MD 20892, (888) 644-6226, http://nccam.nih.gov.

Office of Cancer Complementary and Alternative Medicine (OCCAM), 9609 Medical Center Dr., Rockville, MD 20850, (240) 276-6595, ncioccam1-r@mail.nih.gov, http://cam.cancer.gov.

Crystal Heather Kaczkowski, MSc.
Teresa G. Odle

Von Hippel-Lindau disease

Definition

Von Hippel-Lindau disease (VHL) is a rare familial **cancer** syndrome. A person with VHL can develop both benign and malignant tumors and cysts in many different organs in the body. Tumors and cysts most commonly develop in the brain and spine, eyes, kidneys, adrenal glands, pancreas, and inner ear.

Description

Tumors in the brain and spine, or central nervous system, are called hemangioblastomas. Hemangioblastomas are benign growths (not cancerous), but they may cause such symptoms as headaches and balance problems if they are growing in tight spaces and pressing on surrounding tissues or nerves. The eye tumors in VHL are called retinal angiomas or retinal hemangioblastomas, and they may cause vision problems and blindness if they are not treated. Kidney cysts rarely cause problems, but the kidney tumors can be malignant (renal cell carcinoma). Tumors in the adrenal glands are called pheochromocytomas. Pheochromocytomas are usually not malignant, but they can cause serious medical problems if untreated. This is because pheochromocytomas secrete hormones that can raise blood pressure to dangerous levels, causing heart attacks or strokes. Benign cysts can

KEY TERMS

Benign—Not cancerous; not able to spread to new places in the body.

Cyst—A fluid-filled sac that can be normal or abnormal.

Hemangioblastoma—A benign tumor caused by the abnormal growth of blood vessels.

Malignant—Cancerous; able to spread to new places in the body.

Mutation—A change in the DNA code.

Tumor—An abnormal growth caused by the uncontrolled reproduction of cells.

be found in the pancreas, and pancreatic islet cell tumors can also occur. These tumors grow very slowly and are rarely malignant. Tumors that grow in the ear are called endolymphatic sac tumors, which can result in hearing loss if untreated. Occasionally men and women with VHL will have infertility problems if cysts are present in certain places in the reproductive organs, such as the epididymis (a duct in the testes)in men or the fallopian tubes in women. A few male patients with VHL develop large testicular masses that can be treated successfully with steroid therapy.

Risk factors

The U.S. National Institutes of Health (NIH) has determined risk ranges for a person with VHL to develop certain tumors. Persons with VHL have a 21–72% chance of developing hemangioblastomas of the brain or spinal cord, a 43–60% chance of developing retinal angiomas, a 24–45% chance of developing cysts and tumors of the kidney, an 8–37% chance of developing pancreatic cysts, and an 8–17% chance of developing pancreatic islet cell tumors. It has been proposed that VHL be divided into subtypes depending on the types of tumors present in a family. It is likely that in the future, specific risk figures will be available for the different types of tumors depending on the specific genetic mutation in a family.

Causes and symptoms

Causes

VHL is a genetic disease caused by a mutation of the VHL tumor suppressor gene on chromosome three. It is inherited as an autosomal dominant condition, which means that a person with VHL has a 50% chance of passing it on to each of his or her children. Usually a person with VHL will have a family history of VHL (a parent or sibling who also has VHL), but occasionally he or she is the first person in the family to have VHL. Screening and/or genetic testing of family members can help establish who is at risk for developing VHL. Identification of a person with VHL in a family may result in other family members with more mild symptoms being diagnosed, and subsequently receiving appropriate screening and medical care.

Symptoms

VHL does not have a predictable set of symptoms. VHL affects approximately 1 in 35,000 people, and affects men and women equally. Some families may have different symptoms than other families. Even within a family, there may be people with very mild signs of VHL, and others with more severe medical problems. In one study of a Chinese family with 47 members, 4 were diagnosed as carriers of the VHL gene while 18 others were diagnosed as having VHL itself. Of these 18 patients, 10 had renal cell **carcinoma**, 9 had central nervous system hemangioblastomas, and 7 had multiple pancreatic cysts. The age when symptoms develop can range from infancy to late adulthood, although most people with VHL will have some clinical symptoms by age 65. It is important for a person with VHL to have regular physical examinations to check for signs of VHL in all areas of the body that may be affected

Diagnosis

A clinical diagnosis of VHL can be made in a person with a family history of VHL if he or she has a single retinal angioma, central nervous system hemangioblastoma, or **pheochromocytoma**, or if he or she has renal cell carcinoma. If there is no known family history of VHL, two or more retinal or central nervous system hemangioblastomas must be present, or one retinal or central nervous system hemangioblastoma and one other feature of VHL. Melmon and Rosen published these criteria in 1964, when they first described VHL as a disease with a specific set of features. Because not all people with VHL will meet these diagnostic criteria, VHL may be an underdiagnosed disease. **Genetic testing** can confirm a diagnosis of VHL in a person with clinical symptoms, who may or may not meet the above diagnostic criteria.

Genetic testing

Almost 100% of people with VHL will have an identifiable mutation in the VHL gene. There have been many different mutations found in the VHL gene, but all

persons with VHL in the same family will have the same mutation. If a mutation is known in a family, genetic testing can be done on family members who have not had any symptoms of VHL. A person who tests positive for the family mutation is at risk for developing symptoms of VHL and can pass the mutation on to his or her children. A person who tests negative for the family mutation is not at risk for developing symptoms of VHL, and his or her children are not at risk for developing VHL. Screening is needed for people who test positive for a VHL mutation, and people who are found not to have the family mutation can be spared from lifelong screening procedures. Genetic testing can also be used to determine if a pregnant woman is carrying a fetus affected with VHL. Other techniques may become available that allow selection of an unaffected fetus prior to conception. Families work with a physician, geneticist, or genetic counselor familiar with the most up-to-date information on VHL when having genetic testing, in order to understand the risks, benefits, and current technological limitations prior to testing.

Treatment

Regular screening and monitoring of tumors in people with VHL allows early detection and treatment before serious complications can occur. A physician familiar with all aspects of VHL can coordinate screening with a variety of specialists, such as an ophthalmologist for eye examinations. Ultrasounds, **computed tomography** scans (CT), and **magnetic resonance imaging** (MRI) may be used to screen and detect tumors and cysts. Whether or not treatment is necessary depends on the size of the tumor, where it is growing, what the symptoms are, and if the tumor is benign or malignant. Treatment for benign tumors may include surgery or laser treatments. Cancer in people with VHL is treated just as it would be in someone in the general population with that type of cancer. People with VHL who develop cancer have a better prognosis if the cancer is detected at an earlier stage before it has spread. Urine tests, ultrasound, CT and/or MRI may be used to screen for pheochromocytomas. It is especially important to screen for pheochromocytomas prior to surgery, because an undiagnosed pheochromocytoma can cause complications during surgery. Prior to becoming pregnant, a woman should have a full physical examination looking for all signs of VHL, but most importantly pheochromocytomas. It is best for a woman to avoid VHL-related surgery while she is pregnant unless medically necessary. Pregnancy itself does not seem to make VHL worse or make the tumors grow faster, but any tumors that are present should be evaluated, and a plan for surgical removal or monitoring should be in place.

See also Cancer genetics; Familial cancer syndrome; Kidney cancer.

Resources

BOOKS

Beers, Mark H., MD, and Robert Berkow, MD, editors. "Adrenal Disorders." In *The Merck Manual of Diagnosis and Therapy*. Whitehouse Station, NJ: Merck Research Laboratories, 2007.

Beers, Mark H., MD, and Robert Berkow, MD, editors. "Cancer Genetics." In *The Merck Manual of Diagnosis and Therapy*. Whitehouse Station, NJ: Merck Research Laboratories, 2007.

WEBSITES

American Society of Clinical Oncology. "Von Hippel-Lindau Syndrome." Cancer.Net. http://www.cancer.net/cancer-types/von-hippel-lindau-syndrome (accessed November 14, 2014).

ORGANIZATIONS

VHL Alliance, 2001 Beacon St., Suite 208, Boston, MA 02135-7787, (617) 277-5667, (800) 767-4845, Fax: (866) 209-0288, info@vhl.org, http://www.vhl.org.

Laura L. Stein, M.S., C.G.C.
Rebecca J. Frey, PhD

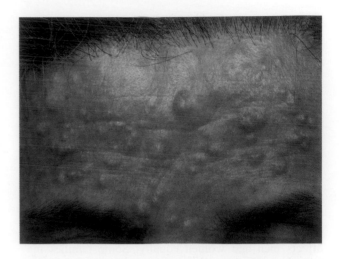

Lesions caused by von Recklinghausen neurofibromatosis. *(Girand/Science Source)*

Von Recklinghausen neurofibromatosis

Definition

Von Recklinghausen neurofibromatosis is also called von Recklinghausen disease, or simply neurofibromatosis (NF). It is an autosomal dominant hereditary disorder. NF is the most common neurological disorder caused by a single gene. Patients develop multiple soft tumors (neurofibromas) and very often skin spots (freckling and café au lait spots). The tumors occur under the skin and throughout the nervous system. The disease is named for Friedrich Daniel von Recklinghausen (1833–1910), a German pathologist, although cases of it have been described in European medical publications since the sixteenth century.

Description

There are three types of neurofibromatosis, although some researchers have proposed as many as eight categories. The two main types of neurofibromatosis are neurofibromatosis 1 (NF1), which affects about 85% of patients diagnosed with neurofibromatosis, and neurofibromatosis 2 (NF2), which accounts for another 10% of patients. NF1 affects approximately 1 in 2,000 to 1 in 5,000 births worldwide. NF2 affects 1 in 35,000 to 1 in 40,000 births worldwide. Recently, schwannomatosis has been recognized as a rare form of NF. Since NF is the most common neurological disorder, NF is more prevalent than the number of people affected by cystic fibrosis, hereditary muscular dystrophy, Huntington disease, and Tay-Sachs disease combined. In addition to skin and nervous system tumors and skin freckling, NF can lead to disfigurement, blindness, deafness, skeletal abnormalities, loss of limbs, malignancies, and learning disabilities. How much a person is affected by a particular form of neurofibromatosis may vary greatly among patients.

Causes and symptoms

A defective gene causes NF1 and NF2. NF1 is due to a defect on chromosome 17q. NF2 results from a defect on chromosome 22. Both neurofibromatosis disorders are inherited in an autosomal dominant fashion. In an autosomal dominant disease, one copy of a defective gene will cause the disease. However, family pattern of NF is only evident for about 50% to 70% of all NF cases. The remaining cases of NF are due to a spontaneous mutation (a change in a person's gene rather than a mutation inherited from a parent). As with an inherited mutated gene, a person with a spontaneously mutated gene has a 50% chance of passing the spontaneously mutated gene to any offspring.

NF1 has a number of possible symptoms:

- Five or more light brown skin spots (café au lait spots, a French term meaning "coffee with milk"). The skin spots measure more than 0.2 inches (5 millimeters) in diameter in patients under the age of puberty or more than 0.6 inches (15 millimeters) in diameter across in adults and children over the age of puberty. Nearly all NF1 patients display café au lait spots.

- Multiple freckles in the armpit or groin area.
- Ninety percent of patients with NF1 have tiny tumors in the iris (colored area of the eye) called Lisch nodules (iris nevi).
- Two or more neurofibromas distributed over the body. Neurofibromas are soft tumors and are the hallmark of NF1. Neurofibromas occur under the skin, often located along nerves or within the gastrointestinal tract. Neurofibromas are small and rubbery, and the skin overlying them may be somewhat purple in color.
- Skeletal deformities, such as a twisted spine (scoliosis), curved spine (humpback), or bowed legs.
- Tumors along the optic nerve, which cause visual disturbances in about 20% of patients.
- The presence of NF1 in a patient's parent, child, or sibling.

There are very high rates of speech impairment, learning disabilities, and attention deficit disorder in children with NF1. Other complications include the development of a seizure disorder, or the abnormal accumulation of fluid within the brain (hydrocephalus). A number of cancers are more common in patients with NF1. These include a variety of types of malignant **brain tumors**, as well as leukemia, and cancerous tumors of certain muscles (**rhabdomyosarcoma**), the adrenal glands (**pheochromocytoma**), or the kidneys (**Wilms tumor**). Symptoms are often visible at birth or during infancy, and almost always by the time a child is about 10 years old.

In contrast to patients with NF1, patients with NF2 have few, if any, café au lait spots or tumors under the skin. Patients with NF2 most commonly have tumors (schwannomas) on the eighth cranial nerve (one of 12 pairs of nerves that enter or emerge from the brain), and occasionally on other nerves. The location of the schwann cell–derived tumors determines the effect on the body. The characteristic symptoms of NF2 include dysfunction in hearing, ringing in the ears (tinnitus), and body balance. The common characteristic symptoms of NF2 are due to tumors along the acoustic and vestibular branches of the eighth cranial nerve. Tumors that occur on neighboring nervous system structures may cause weakness of the muscles of the face, headache, dizziness, numbness, and weakness in an arm or leg. Cloudy areas on the lens of the eye (called cataracts) frequently develop at an early age. As in NF1, the chance of brain tumors developing is unusually high. Symptoms of NF2 may not begin until after puberty.

Multiple schwannomas on cranial, spinal, and peripheral nerves characterize schwannomatosis. People with schwannomatosis usually have greater problems with pain than with neurological disability. The first symptom of schwannomatosis is usually pain in any part of the body without any source. It can be several years before a tumor is found. About one-third of patients with schwannomatosis have tumors in a single part of the body, such as an arm, leg, or segment of spine. People with schwannomatosis do not develop vestibular tumors or any other kinds of tumors (such as meningiomas, ependymomas, or astrocytomas), do not go deaf, and do not have learning disabilities.

Diagnosis

Diagnosis of a form of neurofibromatosis is based on the symptoms outlined above. Although a visual inspection may be sufficient for inspection of tumors for a clinical diagnosis of neurofibromatosis, **magnetic resonance imaging** (MRI) is the most useful type of imaging study for early diagnosis of tumors while CT scans are better for detecting skeletal abnormalities. Diagnosis of NF1 requires that at least two of the above listed symptoms are present. A slit lamp is used to visualize the presence of any Lisch nodules in a person's eye. A person with a parent, sibling, or child with NF1 is another tool used to diagnose a person with NF1.

NF2 can be diagnosed three different ways and with symptoms different from NF1 symptoms:

- The presence of bilateral cranial eighth nerve tumors.
- A person who has a parent, sibling, or child with NF2 and a unilateral eighth nerve tumor (vestibular schwannoma or acoustic neuroma).
- A person who has a parent, sibling, or child with NF2 and any two of the following: glioma, meningioma, neurofibroma, schwannoma, or an early-age cataract.

The presence of multiple schwannomas may be a symptom of NF2 or schwannomatosis. An older person with multiple schwannomas and no hearing loss probably does not have NF2. A high-quality MRI scan should be used to detect any possible vestibular tumors to differentiate between NF2 and schwannomatosis in a younger person with multiple schwannomas or any person with hearing loss and multiple schwannomas.

In prepubertal children, a yearly assessment including blood pressure measurement, eye examination, development screening, and neurologic examination is recommended.

Monitoring the progression of neurofibromatosis involves careful testing of vision and hearing (audiometry). X-ray studies of the bones are frequently done to

KEY TERMS

Audiometry—Testing a person's hearing by exposing the ear to sounds in a soundproof room.

Autosomal dominant—Genetic information on a single non-sex chromosome that is expressed with only one copy of a gene. A child of an affected parent has a 50% chance of inheriting an autosomal dominant gene.

Cancer—Abnormal and uncontrolled growth of cells that can invade surrounding tissues and other parts of the body. Although some cancers are treatable, recurrence and death from cancer can occur.

Cataract—Condition in which the lens of eye loses transparency and becomes cloudy. The cloudiness blocks light rays entering the eye and can lead to blindness.

Chromosome—A structure within the nucleus of every cell that contains genetic information governing the organism's development. There are 22 non-sex chromosomes and one sex chromosome.

Ependymoma—Tumor that grows from cells that line the cavities of the brain ventricles and spinal cord.

Gamma knife—A type of highly focused radiation therapy.

Gene—Piece of information contained on a chromosome. A chromosome is made of many genes.

Magnetic resonance imaging (MRI)—Magnetic resonance imaging measures the response of tissues to magnetic fields to produce detailed pictures of the body, including the brain.

Meningioma—Tumor that grows from the protective brain and spinal cord membrane cells (meninges).

Mutation—A permanent change to the genetic code of an organism. Once established, a mutation can be passed on to offspring.

Neurofibroma—A soft tumor usually located on a nerve.

Radiation therapy—Exposing tumor cells to controlled doses of x-ray irradiation for treatment. Although tumor cells are susceptible to irradiation, surrounding tissues will also be damaged. Radiation therapy alone rarely cures a tumor but can be useful when used in conjunction with other forms of therapy or when a patient cannot tolerate other forms of therapy.

Schwannoma—Tumor that grows from the cells that line the nerves of the body (Schwann cells).

Tinnitus—Noises in the ear that can include ringing, whistling, or booming.

Tumor—An abnormally multiplying mass of cells. Tumors that invade surrounding tissues and other parts of the body are malignant and considered a cancer. Non-malignant tumors do not invade surrounding tissues and other parts of the body. Malignant and non-malignant tumors can cause severe symptoms and death.

watch for the development of deformities. CT scans and MRI scans are performed to track the progression of tumors in the brain and along the nerves. Auditory-evoked potentials (the electric response evoked in the cerebral cortex by stimulation of the acoustic nerve) may be helpful to determine involvement of the acoustic nerve, and EEG (electroencephalogram, a record of electrical currents in the brain) may be needed for patients with suspected seizures.

Treatment

There are no cures for any form of neurofibromatosis. To some extent, the symptoms of NF1 and NF2 can be treated individually. Skin tumors can be surgically removed. Some brain tumors and tumors along the nerves can be surgically removed or treated with drugs (**chemotherapy**) or x-ray treatments (**radiation therapy**, including gamma knife therapy). Twisting or curving of the spine and bowed legs may require surgical treatment or the wearing of a special brace.

Prognosis

Prognosis varies depending on the types of tumors that an individual develops. In general, however, patients with neurofibromatosis have a shortened life expectancy; the average age at death is 55–59 years, compared with 70–74 years for the general U.S. population. As tumors grow, they begin to destroy surrounding nerves and structures. Ultimately, this destruction can result in blindness, deafness, increasingly poor balance, and increasing difficulty with the coordination necessary for walking. Deformities of the bones and spine can also interfere with walking and movement. When cancers develop, prognosis worsens according to the specific type of **cancer**.

Clinical trials

As of 2014, the **National Cancer Institute** (NCI) was sponsoring 11 clinical trials regarding neurofibromatosis. More information is available online at: http://www.cancer.gov/clinicaltrials/search.

Prevention

There is no known way to prevent the cases of NF that are due to a spontaneous change in the genes (mutation). Since genetic tests for NF1 and NF2 are available, new cases of inherited NF can be prevented with careful genetic counseling. A person with NF can be made to understand that each of his or her offspring has a 50% chance of also having NF. When a parent has NF, and the specific genetic defect causing the parent's disease has been identified, prenatal tests can be performed on the fetus during pregnancy. Amniocentesis and chorionic villus sampling are two techniques that allow small amounts of the baby's cells to be removed for examination. The tissue can then be examined for the presence of the parent's genetic defect. Some families choose to use this information in order to prepare for the arrival of a child with a serious medical problem. Other families may choose not to continue the pregnancy. **Genetic testing** may also be useful for evaluating individuals with a family history of neurofibromatosis who do not yet show symptoms.

Resources

BOOKS

Beers, Mark H., MD, and Robert Berkow, MD, editors. "Disorders of the Peripheral Nervous System." In *The Merck Manual of Diagnosis and Therapy.* Whitehouse Station, NJ: Merck Research Laboratories, 2007.

PERIODICALS

K. B. Gupta, Vipul Kumar, Sanjeev Tandon, and Meenu Gill. "Primary Carcinoma of the Lung in Von Recklinghausen Neurofibromatosis." *Lung India* 26, no. 4 (2009): 130–132.

WEBSITES

John Hopkins Medicine. "Neurofibromatosis Type 1 (NF1)." http://www.hopkinsmedicine.org/neurology_neurosurgery/centers_clinics/neurofibromatosis/nf1/ (accessed November 13, 2014).

ORGANIZATIONS

Children's Tumor Foundation, 120 Wall Street, 16th Floor, New York, NY 10005-3904, (212) 344-6633, info@ctf.org, http://www.ctf.org.

March of Dimes National Office, 1275 Mamaroneck Avenue, White Plains, NY 10605, (914) 997-4488, http://www.marchofdimes.org.

National Cancer Institute, 9609 Medical Center Dr., BG 9609 MSC 9760, Bethesda, MD 20892-9760, (800) 4-CANCER (422-6237), http://www.cancer.gov.

National Institute of Neurological Disorders and Stroke (NINDS), NIH Neurological Institute, PO Box 5801, Bethesda, MD 20824, (301) 496-5751, (800) 352-9424, http://www.ninds.nih.gov.

Neuro Foundation, HMA House, 78 Durham Rd., London, England United KingdomSW20 0TL, 020 8439 1234, Fax: 020 8439 1200, info@nfauk.org, http://www.nfauk.org.

Neurofibromatosis Network, 213 S. Wheaton Ave., Wheaton, IL 60187, (630) 510-1115, (800) 942-6825, Fax: (630) 510-8508, admin@nfnetwork.org, http://www.nfnetwork.org.

Rosalyn S. Carson-DeWitt, M.D.
Laura Ruth, PhD
Rebecca J. Frey, PhD

Vorinostat

Definition

Vorinostat (Zolinza) is a histone deacetylase inhibitor manufactured by Merck & Co., Inc. It is used to treat **cutaneous T-cell lymphoma** that has failed to respond to other drug treatments.

Purpose

Vorinostat is used to treat cutaneous T-cell **lymphoma** (CTCL). CTCL is a rare (about 4 cases per 1,000,000 population) type of **non-Hodgkin lymphoma** that affects the skin, most often in individuals ages 40–60 years. Vorinostat is a second-line treatment used in progressive, persistent, or recurrent CTCL after two systemic therapies, one of which must have contained the drug **bexarotene** (Targetrin), have failed.

Description

Vorinostat is sold both in the United States and internationally under the brand name Zolinza. It is a white or light orange water-soluble powder contained in a white hard gelatin capsule. Vorinostat has orphan drug status in both the United States and the European Union, which means that it is approved to treat a rare condition. It was approved for the treatment of CTCL in October 2006 and has also been studied for use against other cancers.

Vorinostat belongs to a class of drugs called histone deacetylase (HDAC) inhibitors. Histones are proteins around which deoxyribonucleic acid (DNA) is coiled. Too much HDAC activity causes DNA to coil up too tightly. When it is tightly coiled, some of the genes that control cell division and programmed cell death (apoptosis) do not function. This allows abnormal (malignant) T cells to reproduce wildly and uncontrollably. Vorinostat inhibits (slows) HDAC activity so that the DNA becomes less tightly coiled and these genes can function again. Allowing the genes that control cell reproduction and cell death to function slows the spread of the **cancer**.

Recommended dosage

Vorinostat comes only in 100 mg capsules that should be stored at room temperature. The standard dose for all patients is 400 mg by mouth once a day. This can be reduced to 300 mg once a day or 300 mg five days a week if the standard dose causes toxicity. Vorinostat is always taken with food. Capsules should not be opened or crushed.

There are no special dosage recommendations for use of vorinostat in the elderly, those with liver (hepatic) impairment, or those with kidney (renal) impairment, although caution is urged when prescribing for these groups. The safety and effectiveness of this drug have not been established in children.

Precautions

Precautions should be taken concerning the following adverse reactions.

- Monitoring should be done for pulmonary embolism and deep vein thrombosis.
- Decrease in the number of blood platelets (thrombocytopenia) may reduce the ability of the blood to clot, and a decrease in the number of red blood cells (anemia) also may occur. Blood count should be monitored regularly. In severe cases, medication may need to be reduced or discontinued.

- Blood glucose (sugar) levels may rise (hyperglycemia). Individuals with diabetes are especially at risk; diet and insulin intake may need to be modified.
- Vomiting and diarrhea may be severe enough to require replacement fluids and electrolytes. Blood chemistries should be monitored regularly

Pregnant or breastfeeding

Vorinostat is a pregnancy category D drug. Women who are pregnant or who might become pregnant should not use vorinostat. It is not known whether the drug is excreted in breast milk. Women taking this drug who are or who want to breast-feed should discuss the risks and benefits with their doctor and err on the side of caution, as there is the potential for this drug to cause serious adverse effects in nursing infants.

Side effects

The most serious side effect in clinical trials was pulmonary embolism in 3.5– 4.7% of patients.

More common but somewhat less serious side effects included:

- loss of appetite
- fatigue
- nausea and vomiting
- weight loss
- diarrhea
- fever
- anemia
- distortion or loss of sense of taste (dysgeusia)

Interactions

When taken with warfarin-based anticoagulants (blood thinners such as Coumadin), blood clotting time is increased.

When taken with other HDAC inhibitor drugs (e.g., valproic acid), severe gastrointestinal bleeding and severe decrease in platelets may occur.

Resources

OTHER

"Vorinostat (Zolinza) for Cutaneous T-cell Lymphoma—Second Line." National Institute for Health Research, National Horizon Scanning Centre, University of Birmingham (UK). http://www.haps.bham.ac.uk/publichealth/horizon/outputs/documents/2008/january/Vorinostat.pdf (accessed October 15, 2014).

WEBSITES

Cancer Research UK. "What Is Cutaneous T Cell Lymphoma (CTCL)?" http://www.cancerhelp.org.uk/help/default.asp?page=3962 (accessed October 14, 2014).

Pazdur, Richard. "FDA Approval for Vorinostat." National Cancer Institute. http://www.cancer.gov/cancertopics/druginfo/fda-vorinostat (acessed October 15, 2014).

ORGANIZATIONS

American Cancer Society, 250 Williams St. NW, Atlanta, GA 30303, (800) 227-2345, http://www.cancer.org.

Leukemia & Lymphoma Society, 1311 Mamaroneck Avenue, Suite 310, White Plains, NY 10605, (800) 955-4572, http://www.leukemia-lymphoma.org.

National Cancer Institute, 9609 Medical Center Dr., BG 9609 MSC 9760, Bethesda, MD 20892-9760, (800) 4-CANCER (422-6237), http://www.cancer.gov.

National Organization for Rare Diseases (NORD), 55 Kenosia Avenue, Danbury, CT 06813-1968, (203) 744-0100, (800) 999-NORD (6673), http://www.rarediseases.org.

Tish Davidson, A.M.

Vulvar cancer

Definition

Vulvar **cancer** refers to an abnormal cancerous growth in the tissues of the external female genitalia.

Description

Vulvar cancer is a rare disease in which malignant cells are found in the tissues of the external female genitalia, which includes the rounded hair-covered area in front of the pubic bones (mons pubis), labia (inner and outer vaginal lips), the opening of the vagina, the clitoris between the lips, and the space between the vaginal opening and the anus (perineum). The outer lips (labia) meet to protect the vaginal opening and the tubular urethra that connects to the bladder. The outer, more prominent folds of skin are called labia majora, and the smaller, inner skin folds are called labia minora. Vulvar cancer can affect any part of the female genitalia, but usually affects the outer vaginal lips. Vulvar cancer is slow growing, with abnormal cells growing in the vulvar skin for a long time. As a result, vulvar cancer is

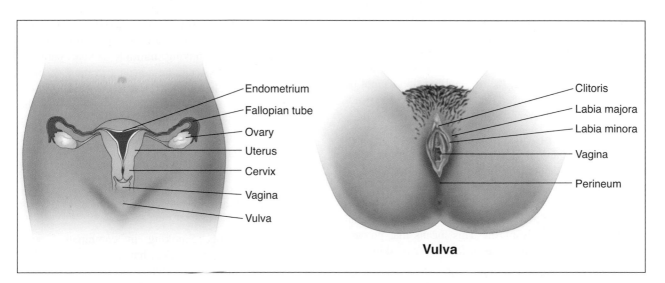

Illustration showing the female reproductive anatomy (left) and the anatomy of the vulva (right). *(Illustration by Electronic Illustrators Group. © Cengage Learning®.)*

KEY TERMS

Adjuvant therapy—A treatment that is intended to aid primary treatment. Adjuvant treatments for vulvar cancer are radiation therapy and chemotherapy.

Biopsy—Removal of a small piece of tissue for microscopic examination. This is done under local anesthesia and removed by either using a scalpel or a punch to acquire a small cylindrical portion of tissue.

Colposcope—An instrument used for examination of the vagina and cervix. Part of the instrument includes a magnifying lens for better visualization.

Metastasis—The migration of cancer cells from a primary cancer site to another organ, either nearby or distant, through the lymph system or blood circulation.

Pelvic exenteration—Surgical removal of the organs of the true pelvis, which includes the uterus, vagina, and cervix.

Sentinel lymph node—The first lymph node to receive lymph fluid from a tumor. If the sentinel node is cancer-free, then it is likely that the cancerous cells have not metastasized.

diagnosed most often in older adult women, with a median age at diagnosis of 65 to 70 years.

Vulvar cancer represents about 5% of all cancers affecting the female genital system. Approximately 50% of vulvar cancers involve the labia majora, 15% to 20% affect the labia minora, 15% to 20% involve the clitoris, and 15% to 20% involve the perineum. In approximately 5% of the cases, the cancer develops at more than one location. In approximately 10% of women, cancer affects so much of the vulva that the original location cannot be determined. Vulvar cancer can spread to nearby structures, including the anus, vagina, and urethra.

About 90% of vulvar cancers are squamous cell carcinomas. Squamous cells are the main cell type of the skin. Squamous cell **carcinoma** often begins at the edges of the labia majora or labia minora or the area around the vagina. This type of cancer may begin with a precancerous condition referred to as vulvar intraepithelial neoplasia (VIN), or dysplasia. This means that precancerous cells are present in the surface layer of skin.

Other even more rare types of vulvar cancer are melanomas, basal cell carcinomas, adenocarcinomas, Paget's disease of the vulva, and tumors of the connective tissue under the skin. **Melanoma**, a cancer that develops from the cells that produce the pigment that determines the skin's color, can occur anywhere on the skin, including the vulva. Melanoma is the second most common type of vulvar cancer and accounts for 5% to 10% of cases. Half of all vulvar melanomas involve the labia majora. **Basal cell carcinoma**, which is the most common type of cancer that occurs on parts of the skin exposed to the sun, very rarely occurs on the vulva. Adenocarcinomas develop in glands, including the glands at the opening of the vagina (Bartholin's glands) that produce a mucus-like lubricating fluid.

Demographics

Vulvar cancer is rare, accounting for only 1% of all cancers in women. It occurs most commonly in women between the ages of 65 and 75 years old. In the United States, there are approximately 4,850 new cases of vulvar cancer diagnosed each year, 1,030 women die from the disease. Approximately 5% of all **gynecologic cancers** develop in the vulva. For unknown reasons, the incidence of vulvar cancer appears to be rising.

Causes and symptoms

Cancer is caused when the normal mechanisms that control cell growth become disturbed, causing the cells to grow continually without stopping. This is usually the result of damage to the DNA in the cell. Although the exact cause of vulvar cancer is unknown, studies have identified several factors that increase the risk for developing vulvar cancer. These include:

- Vulvar intraepithelial neoplasia (VIN). This abnormal growth of the surface cells of the vulva can sometimes progress to cancer.
- Infection with human papillomavirus (HPV). This virus is sexually transmitted and can cause genital warts, and is associated with having multiple sexual partners. Although HPV DNA can be detected in most cases of vulvar intraepithelial neoplasia, it is detected in fewer than half of all cases of vulvar cancer. Therefore, the link between HPV infection and vulvar cancer is unclear, but some researchers believe that two classes of vulvar cancer exist: one that is associated with HPV infection and one that is not.
- Herpes simplex virus 2 (HSV2). This sexually transmitted virus is also associated with increased risk for vulvar cancer.
- Cigarette smoking. Smoking in combination with infection by HPV or HSV2 has been shown to be strongly associated with vulvar cancer.
- Infection with human immunodeficiency virus (HIV). This virus that causes AIDS can decrease the body's

immune system functioning, leaving it vulnerable to a variety of diseases, including vulvar cancer.

- Chronic vulvar inflammation. Long-term chronic irritation and inflammation of the vulva and vagina, which may be caused by poor hygiene, can increase the risk of developing vulvar cancer.

- A history of cervical cancer. Many cases of vulvar cancer are actually metastatic cervical cancer. This may not be determined in older women who have had radical hysterectomies.

- Abnormal Pap smears. Women who have had abnormal Pap smears are at an increased risk of developing vulvar cancer.

- Chronic immunosuppression. Women who have had long-term suppression of their immune system caused by disease (such as certain cancers) or immunosuppressive medications (such as those taken after organ transplantation or for treatment of certain autoimmune diseases) have an increased risk of developing vulvar cancer.

The hallmark symptom of vulvar cancer is **itching** (pruritus), which is experienced by 90% of the women who develop this cancer. The cancerous lesion is usually readily visible. Women sometimes delay medical assessment of vulvar abnormalities because of embarrassment or denial. Women are advised to report any abnormalities to their gynecologist as soon as possible.

Squamous cell vulvar cancer may appear as a raised red, pink, or white bump (nodule). It is often accompanied by pain, bleeding, vaginal discharge, and painful urination. Malignant melanoma of the vulva usually appears as a pigmented, ulcerated growth. Other types of vulvar cancer may appear as a distinct mass of tissue, sore and scaly areas, or cauliflower-like growths that look like warts.

Diagnosis

A gynecological examination will be performed to visually observe the suspected area. During this examination, the physician may use a special magnifying instrument called a colposcope to view the vulva, vagina, and cervix more closely. Additionally, the area may be treated with a diluted solution of acetic acid, which causes some abnormal areas to turn white, making them easier to see. During this examination, if any area is suspected of being abnormal, a tissue sample (**biopsy**) will be taken. The biopsy can be performed in the doctor's office with the use of local anesthesia. A small, wedge-shaped piece of tissue containing the suspect lesion, some surrounding normal skin, underlying skin layers, and connective tissue will be removed. Small lesions will be removed in their entirety (excisional

biopsy). The diagnosis of cancer depends on microscopic analysis of this tissue by a pathologist.

The diagnosis of vulvar cancer includes determining how advanced the cancer is and how much it has spread. This depends on the size of the tumor and how deeply it has invaded the surrounding tissues and organs, including spreading to the lymph nodes. It will also be determined if the cancer has metastasized, or spread to other organs. Imaging examinations using **x-rays**, **computed tomography** (CT scan), or **magnetic resonance imaging** (MRI) may be done to visualize the pelvic organs and distant organs such as the lungs and liver for possible metastases. Endoscopic examination of the bladder (**cystoscopy**) and/or rectum (proctoscopy) may be performed if it is suspected that the cancer has spread to these organs.

Treatment team

The treatment team for vulvar cancer may include a gynecologist, gynecologic oncologist, radiation oncologist, gynecologic nurse oncologist, sexual therapist, psychiatrist, psychological counselor, and social worker.

Clinical staging

The staging system of the International Federation of Gynecology and Obstetrics (FIGO) is used by most gynecologists to stage vulvar cancer. The stage of cancer is determined after surgery when the extent of the cancer is known. Vulvar cancer is categorized into five stages (0, I, II, III, and IV) and may be further subdivided (A and B) based on the depth or spread of cancerous tissue. The FIGO stages for vulvar cancer are:

- Stage 0. Vulvar intraepithelial neoplasia (precancerous cells).

- Stage I. Cancer is confined to the vulva and perineum. The lesion is less than 2 cm (about 0.8 in.) in size.

- Stage II. Cancer is confined to the vulva and perineum. The lesion is larger than 2 cm (larger than 0.8 in.) in size.

- Stage III. Cancer has spread to the vagina, urethra, anus, and/or the lymph nodes in the groin (inguinofemoral).

- Stage IV. Cancer has spread to the bladder, bowel, pelvic bone, pelvic lymph nodes, and/or other parts of the body.

Treatment

Treatment for vulvar cancer will depend on its stage and the patient's general state of health. Surgery is the firstline treatment for most cases of vulvar cancer.

Surgery

Treatment for vulvar intraepithelial neoplasia, Stage 0 of vulvar cancer, involves surgical removal of single lesions or wide local excision. Laser surgery or ultrasound surgical aspiration may be used to treat the most superficial layer of tissue. A procedure called a skinning vulvectomy may be done, with or without a follow-up skin graft. Surgical resection is the primary treatment for stage I and stage II vulvar cancer. A wide local excision is done for lesions less than one millimeter deep, and a radical local excision with removal of nearby lymph nodes is performed for deeper lesions. The choice will depend on the extent of cancer spread. If a large area of the vulva is removed, it is called a vulvectomy. Radical vulvectomy removes the entire vulva. A vulvectomy may require skin grafts from other areas of the body to cover the wound and make an artificial vulva. Because of the significant morbidity and the psychosexual consequences of radical vulvectomy, the amount of tissue excised will usually be minimized. The specific inguinofemoral lymph node that is closest to the vulvar lesion (sentinel node) and would be the first to receive lymph fluid from the cancerous lesion may be exposed for surgical examination (sentinel **lymph node dissection** and biopsy) or removed (lymphadenectomy) if cancer cells are found. Surgery may be followed by **chemotherapy** and/or **radiation therapy** to kill remaining cancer cells in nearby organs and throughout the body. Radiation can be applied to pelvic nodes to avoid further surgery, and radical radiation therapy may be used in patients unable to tolerate surgery because of the extent of disease and poor overall health status.

Surgical treatment of stage III and stage IV vulvar cancer is much more complex. Extensive surgery is necessary to completely remove the cancerous tissue, including excision of pelvic organs (pelvic **exenteration**), radical vulvectomy, and lymphadenectomy. Because this extensive surgery comes with a substantial risk of complications, some cases of advanced vulvar cancer may be treated with less extensive surgery combined with radiation therapy and/or chemotherapy as supportive treatment (adjuvant therapy). Chemoradiation is the preferred approach for older adult women with very advanced vulvar cancer.

Identifying the sentinel node may help to minimize the extent of surgery since nodes that are negative for cancer will not be removed. If the sentinel node is negative, then more distant nodes will most likely not be affected. Lymphoscintigraphy, an intraoperative technique that is used to identify the sentinel node in **breast cancer** and melanoma, is sometimes performed during surgery for vulvar cancer, allowing the surgeon to immediately identify the sentinel node. A radioactive compound (e.g.,

technetium 99m sulfur colloid) is injected into the cancerous lesion approximately two hours prior to surgery. This injection may cause only some minor discomfort, so local anesthesia is not required. During surgery, the scintillation counter that detects radioactivity is used to locate the sentinel node and possibly other nodes to which cancer has spread. Positive nodes will then be removed or, in some cases, irradiated.

The most common complication of vulvectomy is the development of a tumor-like collection of clear liquid (wound seroma). Other surgical complications include urinary tract infection, wound infection, temporary nerve injury, fluid accumulation (edema) in the legs, urinary incontinence, falling or sinking of the genitals (genital prolapse), and blood clots (thrombi).

Radiation therapy

Radiation therapy uses high-energy radiation from x-rays and gamma rays to kill the cancer cells. The skin in the treated area may become red and dry and may take as long as a year to return to normal. **Fatigue**, upset stomach, **diarrhea**, and nausea are also common complaints of women having radiation therapy. Radiation therapy in the pelvic area may cause the vagina to become narrow as scar tissue forms. This side effect, known as vaginal stenosis, makes intercourse painful.

Chemotherapy

Chemotherapy uses **anticancer drugs** to kill the cancer cells. The drugs are given by mouth (orally) or intravenously for a specified period of days and weeks. They enter the bloodstream and travel to all parts of the body to kill cancer cells. Although no standard chemotherapy regimen has been used for treating vulvar cancer, regimens for other squamous cell cancers have been used, including 5-fluorouracil, **cisplatin**, **mitomycin-C**, or **bleomycin**. Generally, a combination of drugs is given because it has been shown to be more effective than using a single drug in treating cancer. However, chemotherapy has not improved the overall prognosis of vulvar cancer. The side effects of chemotherapy are significant and include **nausea and vomiting**, appetite loss (**anorexia**), hair loss (**alopecia**), mouth or vaginal sores, fatigue, menstrual cycle changes, and premature menopause. The immunosuppressive action of the drugs may also increase the risk of developing infection. Because so many patients with vulvar cancer are elderly, patient tolerance is a primary factor in deciding whether to employ chemotherapy.

Alternative and complementary therapies

Although alternative and complementary therapies are used by many cancer patients who report experiencing benefits, very few controlled studies have been conducted on the effectiveness of such therapies. Mind-body techniques such as meditation, prayer, biofeedback, visualization, acupuncture, and yoga are sometimes used to reduce stress and lessen some of the side effects of cancer treatments. A clinical study of the drug amygdalin (Laetrile) found that it had no effect on cancer.

Certain herbs have demonstrated anticancer effects in clinical studies. Polysaccharide krestin, from the mushroom *Coriolus versicolor*, has significant effectiveness against cancer. In a small study, the green alga *Chlorella pyrenoidosa* has been shown to have anticancer activity. In a few small studies, evening primrose oil has shown some benefit in the treatment of cancer. However, patients are advised to discuss the use of any alternative or complementary therapies with their doctor.

Prognosis

Factors associated with disease outcome include the diameter and depth of the cancerous lesion, involvement of local lymph nodes, cell types, HPV status, and age and general health status of the patient. Vulvar cancers that are HPV positive have a better prognosis than those that are HPV negative. The overall survival rate for treated vulvar cancer is 90%, but the five-year survival rate for vulvar cancer with nodal involvement is 50% to 60%. The survival rate drops steadily as the number of affected lymph nodes increases. The five-year survival rate is 75% for patients with one or two nodes, 36% for those with three or four, and 24% for those with five or six involved lymph nodes.

Vulvar cancer can spread locally to encompass the anus, vagina, and urethra. Because of the anatomy of the vulva, it is not uncommon for the cancer to spread to the local lymph nodes. Advanced stages of vulvar cancer can affect the pelvic bone. The lungs are the most common site for vulvar cancer **metastasis**. Metastasis occurs primarily through the lymph system and spreading through the blood (hematogenous spread) is uncommon.

Coping with cancer treatment

Patients are advised to consult their treatment teams regarding any side effects or complications of treatment or concerns about sexuality. Vaginal stenosis can be prevented and treated by vaginal dilators, gentle douching, and sexual intercourse. A water-soluble lubricant may be used to make sexual intercourse more comfortable. Many of the side effects of chemotherapy can be relieved by medications. Women are advised to consult a psychotherapist and/or join a support group to deal with the emotional consequences of cancer and vulvectomy.

QUESTIONS TO ASK YOUR DOCTOR

- What type of cancer do I have?
- What type and stage of cancer do I have?
- Has the cancer spread?
- What are my treatment options?
- How much tissue will you be removing? Can you remove less tissue and complement my treatment with adjuvant therapy?
- What are the risks and side effects of these treatments?
- What medications can I take to relieve treatment side effects?
- Are there any clinical studies under way that would be appropriate for me?
- How debilitating is the treatment? Will I be able to continue working?
- What is the five-year survival rate for women with my type and stage of cancer?
- How will the treatment affect my sexuality?
- Are there any restrictions regarding sexual activity?
- How realistic will a vulvar reconstruction look?
- Are there any local support groups for vulvar cancer patients?
- What is the chance that the cancer will recur?
- Is there anything I can do to prevent recurrence?
- How often will I have follow-up examinations?

Clinical trials

Long-term **clinical trials** for the diagnosis and treatment of vulvar cancer are ongoing, including some sponsored by the **National Cancer Institute**. One trial was testing the effectiveness of the chemotherapeutic agent cisplatin in combination with radiation therapy. This treatment study was open to patients with stage I, II, or III squamous cell carcinoma of the vulva. Women are advised to consult with their treatment team to determine if they are candidates for specific clinical studies. The National Cancer Institute has a list of ongoing trials.

Prevention

The risk of vulvar cancer can be decreased by avoiding established risk factors, most of which involve lifestyle choices. Specifically, to reduce the risk of vulvar cancer, women are advised to not smoke or engage in unsafe sexual behavior. Good hygiene of the genital area is necessary to prevent infection and inflammation, which may also reduce the risk of developing vulvar cancer.

Because vulvar cancer is highly curable in its early stages, women are advised to consult a physician as soon as any vulvar abnormality is detected. Regular gynecological examinations are necessary to detect precancerous conditions that can be treated before the cancer becomes invasive. Because some vulvar cancer is a type of **skin cancer**, the American Cancer Society also recommends self-examination of the vulva using a mirror. If moles are present in the genital area, women should employ the ABCD rule:

- Asymmetry. A cancerous mole may have two halves of unequal size.

- Border irregularity. A cancerous mole may have ragged or notched edges.

- Color. A cancerous mole may have variations in color.

- Diameter. A cancerous mole may have a diameter wider than 6 mm (1/4 in).

Special concerns

Surgical removal of the cancerous lesion may remove some or all of the vulva. Vulvectomy alters the appearance of the vulva and affects sexual function. **Depression**, due to the effects of surgery on appearance and sexuality, may occur. Short-term and long-term complications following extensive surgical treatment of vulvar cancer are not uncommon. Women of childbearing age are advised to discuss future fertility with their physician.

Resources

BOOKS

Bruss, Katherine, Christina Salter, and Esmeralda Galan, eds. *American Cancer Society's Complete Guide to Complementary and Alternative Cancer Therapies*. 2nd ed. Atlanta: American Cancer Society, 2009.

Eifel, Patricia, Jonathan Berrek, and M. A. Markman. "Cancer of the Cervix, Vagina, and Vulva." In *Cancer: Principles & Practice of Oncology*. 9th ed., edited by Vincent DeVita, Samuel Hellman, and Steven Rosenberg, 1311–1344. Philadelphia: Lippincott Williams & Wilkins, 2011.

Garcia, Agustin, and J. Tate Thigpen. "Tumors of the Vulva and Vagina, Ch. 41." In *Textbook of Uncommon Cancer*, edited by D. Raghavan, M. Brecher, and D. Johnson, et al. 4th ed. Hoboken, NJ: John Wiley & Sons, 2012.

PERIODICALS

Fuh, K. C., and J. S. Berek. "Current Management of Vulvar Cancer." *Hematology and Oncology Clinics of North America* 26 (February 2012): 45–62.

Hampl, M., P. Hantschmann, W. Michels, and P. Hillemanns: German Multicenter Study Group. "Validation of the Accuracy of the Sentinel Lymph Node Procedure in Patients with Vulvar Cancer: Results of a Multicenter Study in Germany." *Gynecologic Oncology* 111 (Nov. 2008): 282–288.

WEBSITES

National Cancer Institute. "Vulvar Cancer Treatment (PDQ®)." http://www.cancer.gov/cancertopics/pdq/treatment/vulvar/patient (accessed February 5, 2015).

ORGANIZATIONS

American Cancer Society, 1599 Clifton Rd. NE, Atlanta, GA 30329, (800) ACS-2345, http://www.cancer.org.

Cancer Research Institute, 681 Fifth Ave., New York, NY 10022, (800) 992-2623, http://www.cancerresearch.org.

Gynecologic Cancer Foundation, 401 North Michigan Ave., Chicago, IL 60611, (312) 644-6610, (800) 444-4441, http://www.wcn.org/gcf.

National Institutes of Health, National Cancer Institute, 9000 Rockville Pike, Bethesda, MD 20982, (800) 4-CANCER (422-6237), http://cancernet.nci.nih.gov.

L. Lee Culvert
Cindy L. Jones, PhD
Belinda Rowland, PhD

Vumon *see* **Teniposide**

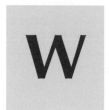

Waldenström macroglobulinemia

Definition

Waldenström macroglobulinemia is a rare, chronic **cancer** of the immune system that is characterized by hyperviscosity, or thickening, of the blood.

Description

Waldenström (Waldenström, Waldenstroem's) macroglobulinemia (WM) is a **lymphoma**, or cancer of the lymphatic system. It was first identified in 1944, by the Swedish physician Jan Gosta Waldenström, in patients who had a thickening of the serum, or liquid part, of the blood. Their blood serum contained a great deal of a very large molecule called a globulin. Thus, the disorder is called macroglobulinemia.

Lymphomas are cancers that originate in tissues of the lymphatic system. All lymphomas other than **Hodgkin lymphoma**, including WM, are known collectively as non-Hodgkin lymphomas. There are 13 major types of non-Hodgkin lymphomas, and others that are very rare. Other names that are sometimes used for WM include: lymphoplasmacytic lymphoma, lymphoplasmacytic leukemia, macroglobulincmia of Waldenström, primary macroglobulinemia, Waldenström syndrome, Waldenström purpura, or hyperglobulinemic purpura. Purpura refers to purple spots on the skin, resulting from the frequent bleeding and bruising that can be a symptom of WM.

WM is classified as a low-grade or indolent form of lymphoma because it is a slow-growing cancer that produces fewer symptoms than other types of lymphomas. WM most often affects males over the age of 65. Frequently, this disease produces no symptoms and does not require treatment. It has not been studied as extensively as other types of lymphoma.

The lymphatic system

The lymphatic system is part of the body's immune system, for fighting disease, and part of the blood-producing system. It includes the lymph vessels and nodes, the spleen, bone marrow, and thymus. The narrow lymphatic vessels carry lymphatic fluid from throughout the body. The lymph nodes are small, pea-shaped organs that filter the lymphatic fluid and trap foreign substances, including viruses, bacteria, and cancer cells. The spleen, located in the upper left abdomen, removes old cells and debris from the blood. The bone marrow, the spongy tissue inside the bones, produces new blood cells.

B lymphocytes or B cells are white blood cells that recognize disease-causing organisms. They circulate throughout the body in the blood and lymphatic fluid. Each B lymphocyte recognizes a specific foreign substance, or antigen. When it encounters its specific antigen, the B cell begins to divide and multiply, producing large numbers of identical (monoclonal), mature plasma cells. These plasma cells produce large amounts of antibody that are specific for the antigen. Antibodies are large proteins called immunoglobulins (Igs) that bind to and remove the specific antigen.

A type of Ig, called IgM, is part of the early **immune response**. The IgM molecules form clusters in the bloodstream. When these IgM clusters encounter their specific antigen, usually a bacterium, they cover it so that it can be destroyed by other immune system cells.

Plasma cell neoplasm

WM is a type of plasma cell neoplasm or B-cell lymphoma. These are lymphomas in which certain plasma cells become abnormal, or cancerous, and begin to grow uncontrollably. In WM, the cancerous plasma cells overproduce large amounts of identical (monoclonal) IgM antibody. This IgM also is called M protein, for monoclonal or **myeloma** protein.

KEY TERMS

Anemia—Any condition in which the red blood cell count is below normal.

Antibody—Immunoglobulin produced by immune system cells that recognizes and binds to a specific foreign substance (antigen).

Antigen—Foreign substance that is recognized by a specific antibody.

Autosomal dominant—Genetic trait that is expressed when present on only one of a pair of non-sex-linked chromosomes.

B cell (B lymphocyte)—Type of white blood cell that produces antibodies.

Bence-Jones protein—Light chain of an immunoglobulin that may be overproduced in Waldenström macroglobulinemia; it is excreted in the urine.

Biopsy—Removal of a small sample of tissue for examination under a microscope; used in the diagnosis of cancer.

Cryoglobulinemia—Condition in which protein in the blood forms particles in the cold, blocking blood vessels and leading to pain and numbness of the extremities.

Hyperviscosity—Thick, viscous blood, caused by the accumulation of large proteins, such as immunoglobulins, in the serum.

Immunoelectrophoresis—Use of an electrical field to separate proteins in a mixture (such as blood or urine), on the basis of the size and electrical charge of the proteins; followed by the detection of an antigen (such as IgM), using a specific antibody.

Immunoglobulin (Ig)—Antibody such as IgM; large protein produced by B cells that recognizes and binds to a specific antigen.

Interferon alpha—Potent immune-defense protein; used as an anti-cancer drug.

Lymphatic system—The vessels, lymph nodes, and organs, including the bone marrow, spleen, and thymus, that produce and carry white blood cells to fight disease.

Lymphoma—Cancer that originates in lymphatic tissue.

M protein—Monoclonal or myeloma protein; IgM that is overproduced in Waldenström macroglobulinemia and accumulates in the blood and urine.

Monoclonal—Identical cells or proteins; cells (clones) derived from a single, genetically distinct cell, or proteins produced by these cells.

Plasma cell—Type of white blood cell that produces antibodies; derived from an antigen-specific B cell.

Plasmapheresis—Plasma exchange transfusion; the separation of serum from blood cells to treat hyperviscosity of the blood.

Platelet—Cell that is involved in blood clotting.

Stem cell—Undifferentiated cell that retains the ability to develop into any one of numerous cell types.

Macroglobulinemia refers to the accumulation of this M protein in the serum of the blood. This large amount of M protein can cause the blood to thicken, causing hyperviscosity. The malignant plasma cells of some WM patients also produce and secrete partial immunoglobulins called light chains, or Bence-Jones proteins. The malignant plasma cells can invade various tissues, including the bone marrow, lymph nodes, and spleen, causing these tissues to swell.

Demographics

WM accounts for about 1%–2% of non-Hodgkin lymphomas. It is estimated that it may affect about five out of every 100,000 people. It usually affects people over the age of 50, and most often develops after age 65. It is more common in men than in women. In the United States, WM is more common among Caucasians than among African Americans. The disease can run in families.

Causes and symptoms

The cause of WM is not known.

Many individuals with WM have no symptoms of the disease. This is known as asymptomatic macroglobulinemia. When symptoms of WM are present, they may vary greatly from one individual to the next.

Hyperviscosity syndrome

At least 50% of individuals with WM have hyperviscosity syndrome, an increased viscosity or thickening of the blood caused by the accumulation of

IgM in the serum. Hyperviscosity can cause a slowing in the circulation through small blood vessels. This condition can lead to a variety of symptoms:

- fatigue
- weakness
- rash
- bruising
- nose bleeds
- gastrointestinal bleeding
- weight loss
- night sweats
- increased and recurrent infections
- poor blood circulation in the extremities

Poor blood circulation, or Raynaud's phenomenon, can affect any part of the body, but particularly the fingers, toes, nose, and ears.

Cold weather can cause additional circulatory problems, by further thickening the blood and slowing down circulation. In some cases, the excess blood protein may precipitate out of the blood in the cold, creating particles that can block small blood vessels. This is called cryoglobulinemia. The extremities may turn white, or a patchy red and white. The hands, feet, fingers, toes, ears, and nose may feel cold, numb, or painful.

Hyperviscosity may affect the brain and nervous system, leading to additional symptoms. These symptoms include:

- peripheral neuropathy, caused by changes in the nerves, leading to pain or numbness in the extremities
- dizziness
- headaches
- vision problems or loss of vision
- mental confusion
- poor coordination
- temporary paralysis
- mental changes

Hyperviscosity can clog the tubules that form the filtering system of the kidneys, leading to kidney damage or kidney failure. Existing heart conditions can be aggravated by WM. In extreme cases, WM may result in heart failure. Late-stage WM also may lead to mental changes that can progress to coma.

Anemia

The accumulation of IgM in the blood causes an increase in the volume of the blood plasma. This effectively dilutes out the red blood cells and other blood components. The lowered concentration of red blood cells can lead to **anemia** and cause serious **fatigue**. Likewise, a deficiency in platelets (**thrombocytopenia**), which cause the blood to clot, can result in easy bleeding and bruising. As the cancer progresses, there may be abnormal bleeding from the gums, nose, mouth, and intestinal tract. There may be bluish discoloration of the skin. In the later stages of the disease, leukopenia, a deficiency in white blood cells, also can develop.

Organ involvement

In 5%–10% of WM cases, the IgM may be deposited in tissues; thus, some individuals with WM have enlargement of the lymph nodes, the spleen, and/or the liver.

If Bence-Jones proteins are produced by the malignant plasma cells, they may be deposited in the kidneys. There they can plug up the tiny tubules that form the filtering system of the kidneys. This can lead to kidney damage and kidney failure.

Diagnosis

Since many individuals with WM have no symptoms, the initial diagnosis may result from blood tests that are performed for some other purpose. Blood cell counts may reveal low red blood cell and platelet levels. A physical examination may indicate enlargement of the lymph nodes, spleen, and/or liver. A retinal eye examination with an ophthalmoscope may show retinal veins that are enlarged or bleeding.

Blood and urine tests

Serum **protein electrophoresis** is used to measure proteins in the blood. In this laboratory procedure, serum proteins are separated in an electrical field, based on the size and electrical charge of the proteins. Serum **immunoelectrophoresis** uses a second antibody that reacts with IgM. A spike in the Ig fraction indicates a large amount of identical or monoclonal IgM in individuals with WM.

Normal serum contains 0.7–1.6 gm per deciliter (g/dL) of Ig, with no monoclonal Ig present. At serum IgM concentrations of 3–5 g/dl, symptoms of hyperviscosity often are present; however, some individuals remain asymptomatic with IgM levels as high as 9 g/dL.

Urinalysis may indicate protein in the urine. A urine Bence-Jones protein test may indicate the presence of these small, partial Igs.

Bone marrow

Abnormal blood tests usually are followed by a **bone marrow biopsy**. In this procedure, a needle is inserted into a bone and a small amount of marrow is removed. Microscopic examination of the marrow may reveal elevated levels of lymphocytes and plasma cells. However, less than 5% of patients with WM have lytic bone lesions, caused by cancerous plasma cells in the bone marrow that are destroying healthy cells. Bone lesions can be detected with x-rays.

Treatment team

WM usually is diagnosed and treated by a hematologist/oncologist, a specialist in diseases of the blood. Asymptomatic macroglobulinemia is followed closely by the patient's physician for the development of symptoms.

Clinical staging

Clinical staging, to define how far a cancer has spread through the body, is the common method for choosing a cancer treatment. However, there is no generally accepted staging system for WM.

Treatment

There also is no generally accepted course of treatment for WM. Treatment may not be necessary for asymptomatic macroglobulinemia. If IgM serum levels are very high, treatment may be initiated even in the absence of symptoms. If symptoms are present, treatment is directed at relieving symptoms and retarding the disease's development. Of major concern is the prevention or alleviation of blood hyperviscosity. Therefore, the initial treatment depends on the viscosity of the blood at diagnosis.

Hyperviscosity

Plasmapheresis, or plasma exchange transfusion, is a procedure for thinning the blood. In this treatment, blood is removed and passed through a cell separator that removes the plasma, containing the IgM, from the red and white blood cells and platelets. The blood cells are transfused back into the patient, along with a plasma substitute or donated plasma. Plasmapheresis relieves many of the acute symptoms of WM. Individuals with WM may be given fluid to counter the effects of hyperviscous blood.

Low blood cell counts

Treatments for low blood cell levels include:

• the drug Procrit to treat anemia
• transfusions with packed red blood cells to treat anemia in later stages of the disease
• antibiotics to treat infections caused by a deficiency in white blood cells
• transfusions with blood platelets

Chemotherapy

Chemotherapy, the use of anti-cancer drugs, helps to slow the abnormal development of plasma cells, but does not cure WM. It can reduce the amount of IgM in the bone marrow. In particular, chemotherapy is used to treat severe hyperviscosity and anemia that are caused by WM.

Chlorambucil (Leukeran), possibly in combination with prednisone, is the typical chemotherapy choice for WM. This treatment is effective in 57% of cases. These drugs are taken by mouth. Prednisone is a corticosteroid that affects many body systems. It has anti-cancer and anti-inflammatory effects and is an immune system suppressant. Other drug combinations that are used to treat WM include **cyclophosphamide** (Cytoxan), **vincristine**, and prednisone, with or without **doxorubicin**. **Fludarabine**, 2-chlorodeoxyadenosine, and **corticosteroids** also may be used.

Side effects of chemotherapy may include:

• mouth sores
• nausea and indigestion
• hair loss (alopecia)
• increased appetite
• nervousness
• insomnia

These side effects disappear after the chemotherapy is discontinued.

The long-term management of WM usually is accomplished through a combination of plasmapheresis and chemotherapy.

Alternative and complementary therapies

Biological therapy or **immunotherapy**, with the potent, immune system protein interferon alpha, is used to relieve the symptoms of WM. Interferon alpha works by boosting the body's immune response. Interferon can cause flu-like symptoms, such as **fever**, chills, and fatigue. It also can cause digestive problems and may affect blood pressure.

The drug **rituximab**, an antibody that is active against antibody-producing cells, is effective in about 30% of individuals with WM. Rituximab is a monoclonal antibody produced in the laboratory. Monoclonal antibody treatment may cause a an allergic reaction in some people.

Prognosis

There is no cure for WM. In general, patients go into partial or complete remission following initial treatments;

however, the disease is not cured and follow-up treatment may be necessary.

The prognosis for this cancer depends on an individual's age, general health, and genetic (hereditary) makeup. Males, individuals over age 60, and those with severe anemia have the lowest survival rates. The Revised European American Lymphoma (REAL) classification system gives WM a good prognosis following treatment, with an average five-year survival rate of 50%–70%; however, many people with WM live much longer, some without developing any symptoms of the disease. About 16%–23% of individuals with WM die of unrelated causes.

Clinical trials

Clinical studies for the treatment of WM are ongoing. These studies are focusing on new anti-cancer drugs, new combinations of drugs for chemotherapy, and new biological therapies to boost the immune system. The drug **thalidomide** is a promising new treatment for WM. Its mode of action is unclear; the drug appears to have various effects on the immune system and may inhibit cancerous plasma cells, both directly and indirectly. If thalidomide is taken during pregnancy, it can cause severe birth defects or death of the fetus.

Biological therapies in clinical trial include **monoclonal antibodies** that contain radioactive substances (radioimmunotherapy), in combination with autologous peripheral blood stem cell rescue or transplantation (PBSCT). With PBSCT, the patient's peripheral blood stem cells (immature bone marrow cells found in the blood) are collected and frozen prior to radioimmunotherapy, which destroys bone marrow cells. A procedure called apheresis is used to collect the stem cells. Following the therapy, the stem cells are reinjected into the individual. The procedure is autologous because it utilizes the individual's own cells. A similar procedure that utilizes chemotherapy with PBSCT also is being tested.

Prevention

There is no known prevention for WM.

Special concerns

WM is a rare disorder and many physicians and even hematologists may not have had experience with it. Furthermore, there is not a clear consensus among professionals as to what constitutes a diagnosis of WM; nor is there a defined course of treatment or accurate prognosis. Thus, it is important that the patient obtain all available information, including seeking second opinions and additional consultations.

QUESTIONS TO ASK YOUR DOCTOR

- Why have you diagnosed Waldenström macroglobulinemia?
- Is my disease likely to progress?
- Do you recommend treatment, and if so, why?
- What are my treatment options?
- What is my prognosis?

See also Bone marrow transplantation; Immunotherapy; Pheresis; Transfusion therapy.

Resources

BOOKS

Morie A. Gertz, S. Vincent Rajkumar, eds. *Multiple Myeloma: Diagnosis and Treatment*. New York: Springer, 2014.

WEBSITES

A.D.A.M Medical Encyclopedia. "Macroglobulinemia of Waldenstrom." MedlinePlus. http://www.nlm.nih.gov/medlineplus/ency/article/000588.htm (accessed November 13, 2014).

American Cancer Society. "What is Waldenstrom Macroglobulinemia?" http://www.cancer.org/cancer/waldenstrommacroglobulinemia/detailedguide/waldenstrom-macroglobulinemia-w-m (accessed November 13, 2014).

ORGANIZATIONS

International Waldenstrom's Macroglobulinemia Foundation, 6144 Clark Center Ave., Sarasota, FL 34238, (941) 927-4963, Fax: (941) 927-4467, info@iwmf.com.

Leukemia & Lymphoma Society, 1311 Mamaroneck Ave., Ste. 310, White Plains, NY 10605, (914) 949-5213, Fax: (914) 949-6691, infocenter@lls.org, http://www.lls.org.

Lymphoma Research Foundation, 115 Broadway, Suite 1301, New York, NY 10006, (212) 349-2910, Fax: (212) 349-2886, LRF@lymphoma.org, http://www.lymphoma.org.

J. Ricker Polsdorfer, M.D.
Margaret Alic, PhD

Warfarin

Definition

Warfarin is a vitamin K antagonist that belongs to the family of drugs called anticoagulants, also known as blood thinners. The brand name of warfarin in the United States is Coumadin.

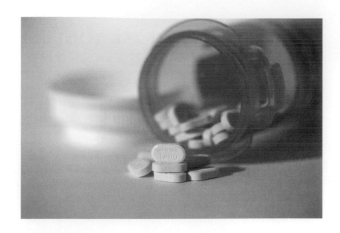

Warfarin tablets. *(Brian Green/Alamy)*

Purpose

Warfarin is used to decrease the clotting ability of the blood and to help prevent harmful clots from forming in the blood vessels. It is also used for the long-term treatment of thromboembolic disease, a common side effect of **cancer**.

One of the most common hematological complications is disordered coagulation. Approximately 15% of all cancer patients are affected by thromboembolic disease, and it is the second leading cause of death for cancer patients. However, thromboembolic disease may represent only one of many complications in end-stage patients. Thromboembolic disease includes superficial and deep vein thrombosis, pulmonary embolism, thrombosis of venous access devices, arterial thrombosis, and embolism. The cancer itself or cancer treatments may induce coagulation. For example, **tamoxifen**, a drug prescribed to treat **breast cancer**, increases the chance of developing pulmonary embolism or deep vein thrombosis.

Cancer and its treatment can affect all three causes of thromboembolic disease including the alteration of blood flow; damage to the cells in blood vessels or endothelial cells; and enhancing procoagulants, which are precursors, such as fibrinogen or prothrombin, that mediate coagulation. Cancer can affect blood flow by mechanically affecting blood vessels close to a tumor. In addition, tumors cause **angiogenesis**, which may create complexes of blood vessels with a disordered appearance and flow, varying in magnitude and direction. **Chemotherapy** or tumors may directly damage endothelial cells. Procoagulants may be secreted into the blood stream by cancer cells or can be increased on the surface of cancer cells.

Description

Warfarin will not dissolve an existing blood clot, but it may prevent it from getting larger. When warfarin is taken orally, it is absorbed quickly from the gastrointestinal tract. It reaches a maximal plasma concentration in 90 minutes and stays in the bloodstream (i.e., its half-life) 36–42 hours. Warfarin circulates in the bloodstream attached to plasma proteins—in particular, a protein called albumin. The response or effects of a warfarin dose vary from person to person.

Whether anticoagulants like warfarin may also improve cancer survival rates independent of their effect on thromboembolism has been investigated. There is suggestive evidence that warfarin may actually enhance cancer survival rates. Animal studies show that warfarin and other agents such as **heparin**, fibrinolytics, and even antiplatelet agents inhibit tumor growth and **metastasis**.

Recommended dosage

A doctor may prescribe a dosage based on laboratory blood tests that determine a patient's clotting time. This blood test, called prothrombin time, is conducted usually weekly or monthly as suggested by a physician and should always be done at the same time of day. Based on the clotting time, the doctor determines the dose and/or whether the dose should be adjusted. Warfarin is normally prescribed to be taken once a day, and it should be taken at the same time every day.

Precautions

Following certain precautions when taking warfarin may reduce the risk of side effects and improve the effectiveness of the medication. The rate of blood clotting is affected by illness, diet, medication changes, and physical activities. If an individual has other medical problems, this may affect the use of warfarin. Of particular importance are bleeding ulcers, heavy menstrual periods, infections, high blood pressure, and liver or kidney problems. The doctor should be informed of any changes in these conditions so dose alterations can be made, if necessary. If a patient using warfarin is scheduled for surgery or dental work, the doctor or dentist should be informed that the patient is taking this medication. Warfarin should not be prescribed if an allergic reaction has occurred in the past, during pregnancy or while breastfeeding, or if pregnancy is planned. Anyone taking warfarin should exercise extra care not to cut him/herself and not to sustain injuries that can result in bruising or bleeding.

In addition, patients taking warfarin should watch their intake of vitamin K, since too much vitamin K may alter the way in which warfarin works. The amount of foods high in vitamin K—such as broccoli, spinach, and turnip greens—eaten each week should be kept stable. Grapefruit juice should be avoided because it may intensify the effects of this medication. Alcohol should also be avoided while taking warfarin because it interferes with warfarin's effectiveness.

In order to determine a safe and effective dose, regular blood tests to check prothrombin time should be done while taking this medicine. Individuals taking warfarin frequently require dose adjustments.

Side effects

The most common complication of long-term warfarin therapy is bleeding. The intensity of anticoagulant therapy, age, kidney function, and unidentified diseases of the gastrointestinal and genitourinary tracts all directly influence the risk of bleeding. Patients taking warfarin should be aware of the signs and symptoms that may indicate a bleeding problem. These signs and symptoms include:

- bleeding from the gums or nose
- red or black bowel movements
- coughing up blood (hemoptysis)
- heavy bleeding from cuts or wounds that will not stop
- unusually heavy menstrual bleeding
- blood in the urine
- easy bruising or purple spots on the skin
- severe headache

The patient should inform his/her doctor immediately if any of these symptoms is present.

Other side effects that may occur with warfarin treatment include:

- mild stomach cramps
- upset stomach
- hair loss (alopecia)
- poor appetite (anorexia)
- cough or hoarseness
- fever or chills
- skin rash, hive, or itching
- painful or difficult urination

The occurrence of any of these side effects should also be reported to the doctor.

Interactions

Some medications should not be combined. The patient should check with the doctor monitoring the warfarin treatment before taking any new medication, including over-the-counter medication or medication prescribed by another doctor.

Among the medications and dietary supplements that may alter the way warfarin works are:

KEY TERMS

Angiogenesis—The formation of new blood vessels that occurs naturally under certain circumstances, for example, in the healing of a cut.

Anticoagulant—A medication that prevents the formation of new blood clots and keeps existing blood clots from growing larger.

Arterial thrombosis—A condition characterized by a blood clot in an artery.

Blood clot—A clump of blood that forms in or around a vessel as a result of coagulation. The formation of blood clots when the body has been cut is essential because without blood clots to stop the bleeding, a person would bleed to death from a relatively small wound.

Coagulation—The blood's natural tendency to clump and stick.

Embolism—An obstruction in a blood vessel due to a blood clot or other foreign matter that gets stuck while traveling through the bloodstream.

Embolus—A blood clot, gas bubble, piece of tumor tissue, or other foreign matter that moves through the bloodstream from its site of origin to obstruct a blood vessel.

Endothelial cells—The cells lining the inside of blood vessels.

Fibrinolytics—Agents that decompose fibrin, a protein produced in the clotting process.

Pulmonary embolism—A blockage of the pulmonary artery by foreign matter such as a blood clot.

Thromboembolic disease—A condition in which a blood vessel is obstructed by an embolus carried in the bloodstream from the site of formation.

Thrombosis—A condition in which a clot develops in a blood vessel.

Vein thrombosis—A condition characterized by a blood clot in a vein.

- other prescription medications
- nonprescription medications such as aspirin or nonsteroidal anti-inflammatory drugs (i.e., ibuprofen)
- cough or cold remedies
- herbal products and nutritional supplements
- products containing vitamin K

Studies have shown that warfarin along with cranberry juice can be big trouble. The volume of the case studies included glasses of cranberry juice daily, not gallons. This drug-food interaction was shown to cause an increased risk of bleeding. This risk prompted the UK's Committee on Safety of Medicines and the Medicines and Healthcare Products Regulatory Agency to warn patients of warfarin to limit consumption of cranberry juice or avoid it altogether. According to Dr. Jacci Bainbrigde of the University of Colorado, Denver, "A cranberry juice/warfarin interaction is biologically plausible. Warfarin is metabolized chiefly by cytochrome P-450 in the liver, and the antioxidant flavonoids contained in the juice are known to inhibit the enzyme pathway." Limited consumption is advised.

See also Low molecular weight heparin.

Resources

WEBSITES

AHFS Consumer Medication Information. "Warfarin." American Society of Health-System Pharmacists. http://www.nlm.nih.gov/medlineplus/druginfo/meds/a682277.html (accessed November 18, 2014).

Crystal Heather Kaczkowski, MSc.

Weight loss

Definition

Weight loss is a reduction in body mass characterized by a loss of body fat and skeletal muscle.

Description

Unintentional weight loss is the most common symptom of **cancer** and often a side effect of cancer treatments. A poor response to cancer treatments, reduced quality of life, and shorter survival time may result from substantial weight loss. The patient's body may become weaker and less able to tolerate cancer therapies. As body weight decreases, body function declines and may lead to malnutrition, illness, infection, and perhaps death.

Most cancer patients in the United States expect to suffer weight loss during treatment for their disease; a study of 938 patients from 17 communities in upstate New York reported in 2004 that weight loss was the fourth most commonly expected side effect of cancer therapy, after **fatigue**, nausea, and sleep disturbances. Approximately 40% of patients experience some weight loss when they are diagnosed with cancer, and 80% of patients with advanced cancer have weight loss that is

---

KEY TERMS

Anorexia—A condition frequently observed in cancer patients characterized by a loss of appetite or desire to eat.

Cachexia—A condition in which the body weight "wastes" away, characterized by a constant loss of weight, muscle, and fat.

Cancer—A group of diseases in which abnormal cells divide without control. Cancer cells can invade nearby tissues and can spread through the bloodstream and lymphatic system to other parts of the body.

Chemotherapy—Chemotherapy kills cancer cells using drugs taken orally or by needle in a vein or muscle. Most chemotherapy is a systemic treatment, meaning it travels through the bloodstream and kills cancer cells throughout the body.

Enteral nutrition—Feedings administered through a nose tube (or surgically placed tubes) for patients with eating difficulties.

Parenteral nutrition—Feeding administered most often by an infusion into a vein. It can be used if the gut is not functioning properly or due to other reasons that prevent normal or enteral feeding.

Protein-calorie malnutrition—A lack of sufficient protein and calories to sustain the body's composition, resulting in weight loss and muscle wasting.

Radiation therapy—Also called radiotherapy; uses high-energy rays to kill cancer cells.

Wasting—When inadequate calories are consumed, it can lead to depletion of body mass. Wasting results in weight loss in tissues such as skeletal muscle and adipose tissue (fat).

---

severe enough to lose muscle mass, which is called cachexia or wasting.

Severe malnutrition is typically defined in two ways: functionally (increased risk of morbidity and/or mortality) and by degree of weight loss (greater than 2% per week, 5% per month, 7.5% per three months, and 10% per six months). Without considering a specific time course, grading is as follows:

• Grade 0 = less than 5.0% weight loss

• Grade 1 = 5.0% to 9.9%

• Grade 2 = 10.0% to 19.9%

• Grade 3 = greater than 20.0%

- Grade 4 (life-threatening) is not specifically defined. Paying attention to weight loss at an early stage is necessary to prevent deterioration of weight, body composition, and performance status.

Malnutrition in cancer patients is a poor prognostic sign, increasing complications, risk of death, and functional debilitation.

Causes and symptoms

There are many reasons for weight loss in cancer patients, including appetite loss because of the effect of cancer treatments (**chemotherapy**, **radiation therapy**, or biological therapy) or psychological factors such as **depression**. Patients may suffer from **anorexia** and lose the desire to eat, thus consuming less energy. They may have less appetite or have side effects such as nausea, mouth sores, or problems swallowing. When inadequate calories are consumed, it can lead to "wasting" of body stores (muscle and adipose tissue). Weight loss may be temporary or may continue at a life-threatening pace.

Weight loss may be also be a consequence of an increased requirement for calories (energy) due to infection, **fever**, or the effects of the tumor or cancer treatments. If infection or fever is present, it is necessary to consider that there is an increased caloric need of approximately 10% to 13% per degree above 98.6°F (37°C). Therefore, energy intake has to be increased to account for this rise in body temperature.

Weight loss may be a result of a common problem in cancer called cachexia. Cachexia is a wasting syndrome that induces metabolic changes leading to a loss of muscle and fat. It has been proposed that cachexia may be from the effects of a tumor, but some patients with very large tumors do not experience cachexia, while others have wasting even though their tumors are less than 0.01% of body mass. Cachexia is most common in patients with pancreatic and gastric cancer. Approximately 83% to 87% of these patients experience weight loss. Cachexia is characterized by such symptoms as decreased appetite, fatigue, and poor performance status. It can occur in individuals who consume enough food, but cannot absorb enough nutrients because of disease complications. Although energy expenditure is sometimes increased, cachexia can occur even with normal energy expenditure. Cachexia is multifactorial in nature and associated with mechanical factors, psychological factors, changes in taste, and cytokines. It should be distinguished from anorexia, in which there is a loss of desire to eat, resulting in weight loss. Cachexia is a serious complication in cancer patients and is thought to be responsible for as many as 20% of all deaths from cancer.

Treatment

Nutritional problems related to side effects should be addressed to ensure adequate nutrition and prevent weight loss. In particular, cancer patients should maintain an adequate intake of calories and protein to prevent protein-calorie malnutrition. The patient's caloric requirements can be calculated by a dietitian or doctor since nutrient requirements vary considerably from patient to patient. Moreover, patient education about nutrition is vitally important. Patients who do not receive help with nutrition and weight loss should ask their cancer treatment team for assistance.

The following dietary tips may help patients to reduce weight loss:

- Eat more when feeling the hungriest.
- Eat foods that are enjoyed the most.
- Eat several small meals and snacks instead of three large meals. A regular meal schedule should be kept so meals are not missed.
- Have ready-to-eat snacks on hand such as cheese and crackers, granola bars, muffins, nuts and seeds, canned puddings, ice cream, yogurt, and hard-boiled eggs.
- Eat high-calorie foods and high-protein foods.
- Take a small meal as to enjoy the satisfaction of finishing a meal. Have seconds if still hungry.
- Eat in a pleasant atmosphere with family and friends if desired.
- Make sure to consume at least eight to ten glasses of water per day to maintain fluid balance.
- Consider commercial liquid meal replacements such as Ensure, Boost, Carnation, and Sustacal.

An appetite stimulant such as **megestrol acetate** or **dexamethasone** may be given in order to prevent further weight loss. In **clinical trials**, both these medications appear to have similar and effective appetite stimulating effects with megestrol acetate having a slightly better toxicity profile. **Fluoxymesterone** has shown inferior efficacy and an unfavorable toxicity profile.

A group of compounds known as cannabinoids for the treatment of cachexia and vomiting has been shown to help patients undergoing cancer treatment. The best-known natural cannabinoids are derived from marijuana. As of fall 2014, 21 states and the District of Columbia had laws legalizing marijuana in some form, mostly for medical purposes only.

Further research is needed in order to devise an effective treatment for the loss of muscle tissue in cachexia. As of 2014, there were no medications, nutritional supplements, or other treatments that were even moderately successful in reversing the wasting of muscle tissue in

QUESTIONS TO ASK YOUR DOCTOR

- How can I improve my appetite when many foods taste awful to me?
- Is there any benefit to weight loss for cancer prevention?
- Is there any benefit to weight loss if I am diagnosed with cancer?
- What are some nutritious foods that also help me gain weight?
- Can I have a consultation with a dietitian?
- Are you willing to prescribe medical marijuana to relieve my nausea from treatment?

cachexia. The only way to manage the problem is to attempt to increase appetite with the use of substances such as **corticosteroids** or cannabiniboids.

Alternative and complementary therapies

Depression may affect approximately 15%–25% of cancer patients, particularly if the prognosis for recovery is poor. If anorexia is due to depression, there are antidepressant choices available through a physician. Counseling may be also be sought through a psychologist or psychiatrist to cope with depression.

It is important to check with a dietitian or doctor before taking nutritional supplements or alternative therapies because they may interfere with cancer medications or treatments. St. John's Wort has been used as a herbal remedy for treatment of depression, but it and prescription antidepressants are a dangerous combination that may cause symptoms such as nausea, weakness, and may cause one to become incoherent.

Special concerns

To allow normal tissue repair following aggressive cancer therapies, patients require adequate calories and macronutrients in the form of protein, carbohydrates, and fat. Inadequate consumption of food and/or poor nutrition may impair the ability of a patient to tolerate a specific therapy. If a low tolerance to therapy necessitates a decrease in dose, the therapy's effectiveness could be compromised. Wound healing may also be impaired with poor nutrition and inadequate energy intake.

Research has demonstrated that men often experience significantly more weight loss than women over the course of the disease and lose weight much faster. On average, survival time for men is shorter than for women. Significant predictors of patient survival are stage of disease, initial weight-loss rate, and gender.

Because depression can also decrease appetite, leading to weight loss, it is important that a careful assessment be conducted to ascertain whether a patient is experiencing depression.

See also Taste alteration.

Resources

BOOKS

Abeloff, M. D., et al. *Clinical Oncology.* 5th ed. New York: Churchill Livingstone, 2013.

Niederhuber, J. E., et al. *Clinical Oncology.* 5th ed. Philadelphia: Elsevier, 2014.

PERIODICALS

Baicus, C., et al. "Cancer and Involuntary Weight Loss: Failure to Validate a Prediction Score." *PLoS One* 9, no. 4 (2014): e95286. http://dx.doi.org/10.1371/journal.pone.0095286 (accessed November 10, 2014).

Kiss, N., et al. "The Prevalence of Weight Loss during (Chemo) radiotherapy Treatment for Lung Cancer and Associated Patient- and Treatment-Related Factors." *Clinical Nutrition* (November 27, 2013): e-pub ahead of print. http://dx.doi.org/10.1016/j.clnu.2013.11.013 (accessed November 10, 2014).

Lena, M., and L. Pernilla. "Risk Factors for Weight Loss among Patients Surviving 5 Years after Esophageal Cancer Surgery." *Annals of Surgical Oncology* (August 14, 2014): e-pub ahead of print. http://dx.doi.org/10.1245/s10434-014-3973-2 (accessed November 10, 2014).

WEBSITES

American Society of Clinical Oncology. "Weight Loss." Cancer.Net. http://www.cancer.net/navigating-cancer-care/side-effects/weight-loss (accessed November 3, 2014).

Szafranski, Michele. "Weight Loss During Chemo." American Cancer Society. http://www.cancer.org/cancer/news/expertvoices/post/2012/01/24/weight-loss-during-chemo.aspx (accessed November 3, 2014).

ORGANIZATIONS

American Society for Nutrition, 9650 Rockville Pike, Bethesda, MD 20814, (301) 634-7050, http://www.nutrition.org/.

National Cancer Institute, 9609 Medical Center Drive, Bethesda, MD 20892, (800) 422-6237, http://www.cancer.gov.

National Center for Complementary and Alternative Medicine, 9000 Rockville Pike, Bethesda, MD 20892, (888) 644-6226, http://nccam.nih.gov/.

Crystal Heather Kaczkowski, MSc.
Rebecca J. Frey, PhD
REVISED BY TERESA G. ODLE

Wellcovorin *see* **Leucovorin**

Whipple procedure

Definition

A Whipple procedure, or pancreaticoduodenectomy, is a surgical procedure that generally removes the head of the pancreas, the majority of the duodenum (the first part of the small intestine), part or all of the common bile duct, and possibly the gallbladder. It sometimes includes removal of part of the stomach or the body of the pancreas. It is most often performed to treat **pancreatic cancer**.

Purpose

A Whipple procedure is the most common surgery for **cancer** of the pancreas. It may also be performed for cancer of the duodenum, cancer of the bile duct (cholangiocarcinoma), cancer of the ampulla (the area where the bile and pancreatic ducts enter the small intestine), and for chronic pancreatitis and benign (noncancerous) tumors involving the pancreatic head.

Description

The pancreas is an organ located near the liver on the right side of the body. The exocrine pancreas produces digestive juices, and the endocrine pancreas produces hormones such as insulin, which is involved in the regulation of blood sugar and overall metabolism. Pancreatic cancer most often affects the exocrine pancreas, and the Whipple procedure is the most common surgery for removing tumors of the exocrine pancreas. It is also sometimes used to treat cancers of the endocrine pancreas.

Procedure

Although it was originally described by an Italian surgeon in 1898, the Whipple procedure is named after Dr. Alan O. Whipple, an American surgeon who developed an improved form of the surgery in 1935 and subsequently devised multiple refinements. It is a lengthy and complex operation, lasting between four and ten hours. It is only performed by experienced and skilled surgeons. General anesthesia is required.

A classic Whipple procedure requires a large abdominal incision; however, a minimally invasive laparoscopic Whipple procedure is also available. Laparoscopic surgery is performed through four small abdominal incisions, using a fiber-optic laparoscope and miniaturized surgical instruments, with or without robotic assistance.

There are several varieties of Whipple procedures. A standard Whipple procedure removes the head of the pancreas, the gallbladder, part of the duodenum, the small bottom portion of the stomach known as the pylorus (where the stomach empties into the duodenum), part of the common bile duct, and the lymph nodes near the head of the pancreas. Sometimes the body of the pancreas is also removed. A classic Whipple procedure removes 40% of the stomach as well. After the head of the pancreas has been removed, three important connections (anastomoses) must be made: the small intestine must be connected to the remains of the pancreas, to the remaining bile duct, and to the stomach. These anastomoses must be very carefully performed, so that pancreatic digestive enzymes, bile, and the contents of the stomach flow into the small intestine. Any leak may cause pancreatic juices to enter the abdomen, with the risk of severe complications. A pylorus-preserving Whipple leaves the pylorus intact. During a Whipple procedure, a jejunostomy tube (j-tube) may be inserted temporarily into the digestive tract to maintain nutrition during recovery.

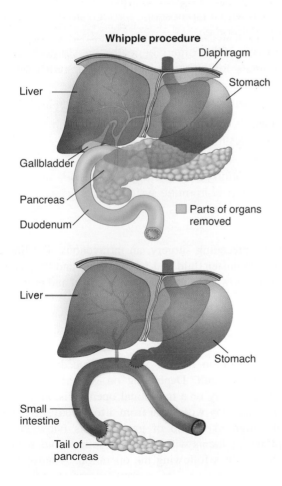

Whipple procedure

Diaphragm
Stomach
Liver
Gallbladder
Pancreas
Duodenum
Parts of organs removed

Liver
Stomach
Small intestine
Tail of pancreas

In a Whipple procedure, the gallbladder, duodenum, and pancreatic head are removed. The tail of the pancreas is attached to the remainder of the small intestine. *(Illustration by Electronic Illustrators Group. © 2015 Cengage Learning®.)*

Demographics

The American Cancer Society estimates that 43,920 cases of pancreatic cancer were diagnosed in the United States in 2012, affecting approximately equal numbers of males and females. An estimated 34,290 people died of pancreatic cancer in 2012. The incidence of pancreatic cancer has been increasing at a rate 1.5% per year since 2004. Most people diagnosed with pancreatic cancer are over age 60.

Risk factors for the development of pancreatic cancer include smoking, a history of diabetes, a family history of pancreatic cancer, and a personal history of chronic pancreatitis. Environmental factors, such as certain workplace exposures or a high-fat diet, may also increase an individual's risk of pancreatic cancer.

Precautions

A Whipple procedure is very complex surgery, and experienced surgeons and hospitals are associated with better outcomes. For the best outcome, patients are advised to choose a surgeon who has performed many such operations at a hospital that performs at least 20 Whipple procedures per year.

Potentially curative Whipple procedures usually treat cancers at the head of the pancreas. Since these cancers are near the bile duct, they may cause jaundice. If they are detected at an early enough stage to be completely removed by surgery, the cancer can be cured. Whipple procedures that involve other parts of the pancreas are generally only performed if all of the cancer can potentially be removed.

Preparation

Pancreatic cancer initially causes only vague symptoms and, thus, is often not diagnosed until later stages of the disease. Furthermore, pancreatic cancer spreads very quickly, so that the cancer has often widely metastasized by the time it is finally diagnosed. Symptoms of pancreatic cancer can include pain in the upper abdomen, often radiating to the back; jaundice (yellow eyes and skin); decreased appetite; **weight loss**; and **depression**.

A candidate for a Whipple procedure meets with the surgeon to discuss the details of the surgery and receive instructions on preoperative and postoperative care. Patients having their spleen removed during the procedure are often given certain vaccines prior to surgery, since their bodies will be less able to fight infection. Blood tests to evaluate bleeding time and an electrocardiogram (EKG) to evaluate heart function may be performed several days prior to the operation.

Directly preceding surgery, an intravenous (IV) line is set to administer fluid and medications, and the patient is given a bowel prep to cleanse the bowel and prepare it for surgery.

Aftercare

Recuperation from a Whipple procedure may be slow and difficult. Depending on whether minimally invasive surgery or a traditional open incision is used, the hospital stay will range from 5 to 14 days. Because of the high likelihood of gastroparesis (slow gastric emptying), patients will remain on intravenous feeding for 5 or 6 days following the operation. A nasogastric tube may be required to remove excess stomach acid and juices that accumulate. The dietary advancement from clear liquids to full liquids, soft foods, and a regular diet is slow, with the time frame depending on the patient's tolerance of each new step. Some patients take as long as four to six weeks for normal stomach emptying to return. A feeding tube that delivers a nutritional formula directly into the jejunum (the section of the small intestine below the duodenum) may be used if recovery is overly slow.

Following a Whipple procedure, the remaining portion of the pancreas often produces little or no digestive enzymes, and patients are prescribed pancreatic enzymes to be taken with all meals and snacks. Patients who have undergone surgery for pancreatic cancer usually must avoid large meals and fatty, greasy, or fried foods. Many patients must adhere to a low-fat diet containing 1.4–2.1 oz. (40–60 g) of fat per day for the long term. Small sips of fluids with meals can help prevent bloating, gas, abdominal cramping, and **diarrhea**. Patients should eat five or six small meals and snacks of nutrient-rich foods daily, with at least eight cups (237 mL) of fluids daily, taken an hour before or after meals. Nutrient beverages such as juices, smoothies, or food supplements may be taken with meals. Alcohol should be avoided. Vitamin supplements may be necessary.

A daily food journal is helpful. The amounts of specific foods, daily body weight, doses of pancreatic enzymes, bowel movements, and possibly blood glucose readings should be recorded. Such a journal can assist a physician or dietitian in making additional dietary recommendations.

Risks

Whipple procedures have a high risk of complications—30%–50%. Some of these complications may be fatal. Loss of 5%–10% of pre-surgical body weight is common. Digestive difficulties and other complications may be long term.

The most common complication of a Whipple procedure is delayed gastric emptying, in which the stomach takes too long to empty after meals, affecting approximately 19% of patients. Generally, the stomach begins to function properly after seven to ten days; however, if gastroparesis persists, a supplemental feeding tube may be necessary. The most serious potential complication of a Whipple procedure is leakage of pancreatic juices into the abdomen at the point where the pancreas connects with the intestine or other connections with the intestine. This occurs in approximately 10% of patients. Such leakage can cause infection or digestion of internal organs by the pancreatic enzymes: this can result in perforations (holes) in the intestine, stomach, or other nearby organs; abnormal connections between organs (fistulas); or necrosis (cell death) within an affected organ. Whipple procedures can also result in complications due to general anesthesia or cause excessive bleeding or diabetes.

Results

Although recuperation times may be long, most patients return to their previous level of functioning and quality of life after a Whipple procedure. However, the risk of further advancement of the pancreatic cancer and death is very high, even though many patients receive **chemotherapy** and radiation treatments in addition to the surgery.

Morbidity and mortality

Whipple procedures have high rates of morbidity and mortality. When performed in cancer centers by experienced surgeons, less than 5% of patients die as a direct result of surgical complications; however, in small hospitals or with less experienced surgeons, fatality rates from the procedure may exceed 15%.

Only about 10% of pancreatic cancers appear to be contained entirely within the pancreas at the time of diagnosis, and once surgery has commenced, only about half of these contained cancers are truly resectable. Even when all of the cancer appears to have been removed, cancer cells have usually escaped from the pancreas and eventually affect other parts of the body. Nevertheless, surgery is the only curative option for **exocrine pancreatic cancer**. About 20% of all Whipple procedure patients survive for five years after their initial diagnosis of pancreatic cancer. Patients with no lymph node involvement at the time of surgery have a higher five-year survival rate of about 40%, compared with a five-year survival rate of only 5% with chemotherapy alone.

Certain conditions have better prognoses. Periampullary **carcinoma** that causes early obstructive jaundice, for example, has a Whipple procedure mortality rate of 3%–5%, a complete cancer removal rate of 70%, and a five-year survival rate of 20%–40%. Pancreatic **neuroendocrine tumors** are much more likely to be cured by a Whipple procedure than other types of pancreatic cancer; however, this treatment may involve removing the spleen, making patients more susceptible to infection.

Health care team roles

A Whipple procedure is performed in a hospital operating room. It is considered one of the most technically difficult operations and should be performed only by experienced, skilled surgeons who have successfully performed many such procedures. General surgeons, surgical gastroenterologists, and surgical oncologists usually perform Whipple procedures.

Resources

PERIODICALS

Fisher, William E., et al. "Assessment of the Learning Curve for Pancreaticoduodenectomy." *American Journal of Surgery* 206, no. 6 (June 2012): 684–90.

WEBSITES

American Cancer Society. "Surgery for Pancreatic Cancer." http://www.cancer.org/cancer/pancreaticcancer/detailed-guide/pancreatic-cancer-treating-surgery (accessed October 3, 2014).

Pancreatic Cancer Action Network. "Nutrition After a Whipple Procedure." http://www.pancan.org/section_facing_pancreatic_cancer/learn_about_pan_cancer/diet_and_nutrition/After_Whipple_procedure.php (accessed October 3, 2014).

Pancreatic Cancer Action Network. "Whipple Procedure." http://www.pancan.org/section_facing_pancreatic_cancer/learn_about_pan_cancer/treatment/surgery/Whipple_procedure.php (accessed October 3, 2014).

Venugopal, Roshni L. "Pylorus-Preserving Pancreaticoduodenectomy (Whipple Procedure)." Medscape Reference. http://emedicine.medscape.com/article/1893199-overview (accessed October 3, 2014).

ORGANIZATIONS

American Cancer Society, 250 Williams St. NW, Atlanta, GA 30303, (800) 227-2345, http://www.cancer.org.

Pancreatic Cancer Action Network, 1500 Rosecrans Ave., Ste. 200, Manhattan Beach, CA 90226, (310) 725-0025, (877) 272-6226, Fax: (310) 725-0029, info@pancan.org, http://www.pancan.org.

Rosalyn Carson-DeWitt, MD
REVISED BY MARGARET ALIC, PhD

Whole brain radiotherapy

Definition

Whole brain radiotherapy or **radiation therapy** (WBRT) is a type of conventional radiotherapy in which an external radiation source is aimed at the entire brain for treating **cancer**.

Purpose

WBRT is most often used to treat multiple **brain tumors** or metastatic cancer that has spread to the brain. Its purpose is to shrink multiple tumors throughout the brain, both large and small, with one procedure, rather than targeting individual tumors. It also can treat tumors deep in the brain that are inaccessible to surgery. In the past WBRT generally was used only for patients who were expected to live no more than one to two years and for whom no other treatment existed.

WBRT may be:

- the sole form of treatment for brain cancer
- performed in advance of other types of radiotherapy or microsurgery
- performed after surgery to reduce the risk of tumor recurrence

WRBT is most often performed:

- following surgery to treat primitive neuroectodermal tumors (PNETs) in adults and in children over age three
- following surgery and/or radiosurgery to treat single or multiple metastatic (secondary) tumors that have spread to the brain from other parts of the body
- to prevent metastasized cancer from spreading to the brain
- to treat HIV/AIDS-related primary central nervous system (CNS) lymphoma

Description

WBET delivers an even dose of high-energy x-rays to the entire brain from two beams of radiation. Unlike radiosurgery or conformal radiotherapy, there is a maximum radiation dose for WBRT. This dose is usually 6,000 gray (Gy). Treatment is divided into daily sessions to allow the healthy tissues surrounding the tumors to repair themselves.

Demographics

- Metastatic brain tumors—cancers that have spread to the brain from other parts of the body, most often the lung or breast—are the most common type of brain tumor, with an annual incidence more than four times

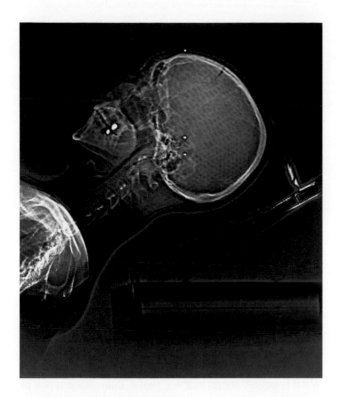

Colored computed tomography (CT) scan of the head of a patient being treated with radiotherapy for brain cancer. *(Zephyr/Science Source)*

greater than that of primary tumors that originate in the brain.

• It is estimated that every year more than 150,000 cancer patients will develop symptoms of a metastatic tumor in the brain or spinal cord.

• Medulloblastomas/embryonal/primitive tumors represent just 1% of all primary brain tumors.

Pediatric

Embryonal/primitive neuroectodermal tumors/medulloblastomas are the most common brain tumors in children from birth to age four, with an incidence of 0.92 per 100,000.

Geriatric

The number of elderly patients receiving WBRT for brain metastases is expected to increase in the future.

Precautions

WBRT is the most damaging of all radiation treatments and causes the most severe long-term side effects. It can lead to long-term disability including neurological deterioration and dementia. Furthermore, new brain tumors can begin to develop within a few months of completing WBRT. Therefore this treatment may only benefit patients in the near-short term. WBRT may not be the best option for patients who are expected to live at least 18 months. These patients may have the option of radiosurgery or multi-session stereotactic radiotherapy. These treatments have few or no side effects from damage to healthy brain tissue and, if necessary, can be repeated to treat either the original tumors or new tumors. An increasing amount of research suggests that radiosurgery and stereotactic radiotherapy can be as effective as WBRT without the side effects. A study published in 2009 found that patients suffered more memory and learning difficulties when WBRT was performed in addition to standard stereotactic radiosurgery (SRS). The study was halted early when it was found that patients receiving both SRS and WBRT were 96% more likely to experience declines in function and memory after four months than patients treated with SRS alone.

Pediatric

Children are extremely susceptible to the side effects of WBRT because their brains are still developing. Treatment with radiation is delayed as long as possible, at least until the age of three. PNETs in children under age three may be treated with **chemotherapy** following surgery to reduce or delay the need for WBRT.

Preparation

WBRT is performed over a period of two to six weeks. Because hair loss is a side effect of WBRT, patients may want to purchase a wig or have a wig made from their own hair before beginning treatment. Corticosteroid treatment is often started at the outset of radiotherapy and continued throughout to help prevent some of the acute side effects.

Aftercare

Acute reactions to WBRT are caused by radiation-induced brain swelling (edema) and intracranial pressure and may include:

• muscle weakness
• headache
• nausea
• vomiting
• speech problems
• double vision

These reactions are temporary and are usually relieved by **corticosteroids** such as **dexamethasone**.

Other neurotoxic side effects of WBRT may include:

• fever
• hair loss (alopecia)

- damage to the skin and scalp (radiation dermatitis)
- hearing loss
- memory loss
- seizures
- lethargy
- fatigue

Some of these effects are transient; however, hair loss, dermatitis, and hearing loss can persist for months. **Fatigue** following WBRT can be severe, but usually lessens within a few weeks after completing treatment.

Early delayed or sub-acute reactions occur a few weeks or months after the completion of WBRT and may include loss of appetite and an increase in pre-existing neurologic symptoms, in addition to lethargy and fatigue. These symptoms usually last about six weeks, but can persist for several months.

Leukoencephalopathy is a type of early delayed reaction that occurs from irritation to the white matter (myelinated tissue) of the brain from the radiation or from dead tumor cells. The severity of the symptoms depends on the amount of tissue damage. Leukoencephalopathy may be reversible and is usually treated with steroids.

Methods for managing acute and early delayed side effects of WBRT include:

- antiemetics, relaxation, imagery, and/or biofeedback to help control nausea and vomiting
- cutting the hair short before treatment and using satin pillowcases, an infant comb and brush, only mild shampoo as the hair begins to grow back, and avoiding strong hair products and appliances
- avoiding the sun to protect damaged skin
- eating a balanced diet despite changes in appetite

Late reactions to WBRT are due to changes in the white matter and brain atrophy and tissue death (necrosis) caused by radiation-damaged blood vessels and the buildup of dead tumor cells. Symptoms can occur months to years after therapy is completed. Although symptoms vary from mild to severe, they are permanent and may become progressively worse. Late reactions can include:

- decreased intellectual abilities
- memory impairment
- confusion
- personality changes
- stroke-like symptoms
- general neurological deterioration
- dementia

Severe reactions such as tumor necrosis may require surgery to remove dead tissue.

QUESTIONS TO ASK YOUR DOCTOR

- How long will the WBRT take?
- What are the potential side effects of WBRT?
- What are the risks associated with WBRT?
- Are there alternatives to WBRT that may be appropriate for me?
- Should I get a second or third opinion before undergoing WBRT?

Risks

WBRT may worsen neurological symptoms such as memory loss and problems with concentration and cognition. Severe radiation-induced dementia following WBRT is estimated to occur in 11% of patients who survive for one year and in up to 50% of those who survive for two years after treatment. Finally, since WBRT targets more healthy tissue than other types of radiotherapy, there is a risk that it will result in the development of new tumors.

Results

New brain tumors can begin to develop within a few months of completing WBRT. A 2009 study of patients with one to three brain metastases, who were treated with SRS alone or with both SRS and WBRT, found that after one year 73% of the SRS plus WBRT patients were recurrence-free; in contrast, only 27% of the patients treated with SRS alone had no tumor recurrence. However, four months after treatment 29% of the SRS plus WBRT patients had died, compared with 13% of the SRS-only patients.

Geriatric

Most elderly patients with brain metastases have an unfavorable prognosis. Although WBRT improves symptoms in about 50% of these patients, long-term survivors are at serious risk for neurotoxic effects and dementia.

Resources

PERIODICALS

Aoyama, H., et al. "Stereotactic Radiosurgery Plus Whole-Brain Radiation Therapy vs. Stereotactic Radiosurgery Alone for Treatment of Brain Metastases: A Randomized Controlled Trial." *Journal of the American Medical Association* 295 (2006): 2483–91.

Fraser, Ginny. "A Life in the Day." *Sunday Times (London)* (January 29, 2006): 86.

"Health Beat." *USA Today* 137, no. 2765 (February 2009): 3.

Nieder, Carsten, et al. "Is Whole-Brain Radiotherapy Effective and Safe in Elderly Patients with Brain Metastases?" *Oncology* 72, no. 5/6 (February 2008): 326–29.

OTHER

National Brain Tumor Foundation and Lung Cancer Alliance. "Understanding Brain Metastasis: A Guide for Patient and Caregiver." http://www.lungcanceralliance.org/assets/docs/lco/brain_metastases.pdf (accessed February 5, 2015).

WEBSITES

American Brain Tumor Association. "Help with Side Effects— Radiation Therapy." http://www.abta.org/index.cfm?contentid=105 (accessed October 14, 2014).

International RadioSurgery Association. "Radiation Injury to the Brain." http://www.irsa.org/radiation_injury.html (accessed October 1, 2014).

Preidt, Robert. "Focused Radiation Protects Tumor Patients' Brain Function." *HealthDay.* http://abcnews.go.com/Health/Healthday/focused-radiation-protects-tumor-patients-brain-function/story?id=8754268 (accessed February 5, 2015).

ORGANIZATIONS

American Brain Tumor Association, 8550 W. Bryn Mawr Ave., Ste. 550, Chicago, IL 60631, (773) 577-8750, (800) 886-2282, Fax: (773) 577-8738, info@abta.org, http://www.abta.org.

American Cancer Society, 250 Williams St. NW, Atlanta, GA 30303, (800) 227-2345, http://www.cancer.org.

American College of Radiology, 1891 Preston White Drive, Reston, VA 20191, (703) 648-8900, (800) 227-5463, info@acr.org, http://www.acr.org.

American Society for Radiation Oncology, 8280 Willow Oaks Corporate Drive, Suite 500, Fairfax, VA 22031, (703) 502-1550, (800) 962-7876, Fax: (703) 502-7852, http://www.astro.org.

International RadioSurgery Association, 3002 N. 2nd Street, Harrisburg, PA 17110, (717) 260-9808, http://www.irsa.org.

National Brain Tumor Society, 55 Chapel St., Ste. 200, Newton, MA 02458, (617) 924-9997, http://www.braintumor.org.

National Cancer Institute, 9609 Medical Center Dr., BG 9609 MSC 9760, Bethesda, MD 20892-9760, (800) 4-CANCER (422-6237), http://www.cancer.gov.

Margaret Alic, PhD

Wilms tumor

Definition

Wilms tumor is a cancerous tumor of the kidney that usually occurs in young children. It is named for Max Wilms, a German surgeon (1867–1918), and is also known as a nephroblastoma.

Description

When an unborn baby is developing, the kidneys are formed from primitive cells. Over time, these cells become more specialized. The cells mature and organize into the normal kidney structure. Sometimes, clumps of these cells remain in their original, primitive form. If these cells begin to multiply after birth, they may ultimately form a large mass of abnormal cells. This is known as a Wilms tumor.

Wilms tumor is a type of malignant tumor. This means that it is made up of cells that are significantly immature and abnormal. These cells are also capable of invading nearby structures within the kidney and traveling out of the kidney into other structures. Malignant cells can even travel through the body to invade other organ systems, most commonly the lungs and brain. These features of Wilms tumor make it a type of **cancer** that, without treatment, eventually causes death. However, advances in medicine during the last 20 years have made Wilms tumor a very treatable form of cancer.

Demographics

Wilms tumor occurs almost exclusively in young children. The average patient is about three to four years old, although cases have been reported in infants younger than six months and adults in their early twenties. Girls are only slightly more likely than boys to develop Wilms tumors. In the United States, only about 500 cases of Wilms tumors are diagnosed each year. The rate is higher among African Americans and lower among Asian Americans. Wilms tumors are found more commonly in patients with other types of birth defects. These defects include:

- absence of the colored part (the iris) of the eye (aniridia)
- enlargement of one arm, one leg, or half of the face (hemihypertrophy)
- certain birth defects of the urinary system or genitals
- certain genetic syndromes (WAGR syndrome, Denys-Drash syndrome, and Beckwith-Wiedemann syndrome)

Causes and symptoms

The cause of Wilms tumor is not completely understood. It is clear that having an inherited genetic alteration increases the risk of developing a Wilms tumor. A genetic syndrome known as WAGR syndrome has been identified in some patients on chromosome 11. The tendency to develop a Wilms tumor can run in families. In fact, about 1.5% of all children with a Wilms tumor have family members who have also had a Wilms tumor. The genetic mechanisms associated with the

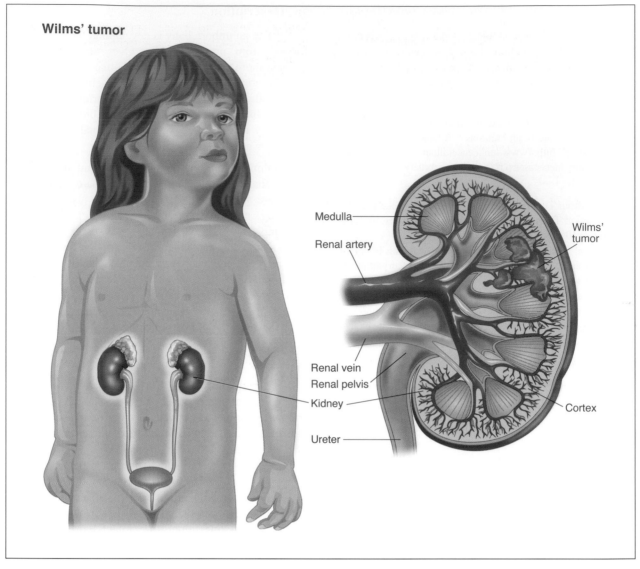

Wilms' tumor

Medulla

Renal artery

Renal vein

Renal pelvis

Kidney

Ureter

Wilms' tumor

Cortex

Wilms tumor is a type of kidney cancer that is most common in young children. *(Illustration by Electronic Illustrators Group. © Cengage Learning®.)*

disease are unusually complex; it is thought that the tumor develops because the defective gene fails to stop its growth. If a child has WAGR syndrome, the child has a 30% to 50% chance of having a Wilms tumor. Other genes that have been linked to Wilms tumor are located on chromosomes 16q, 7p15, and 17q12.

Some patients with Wilms tumor experience abdominal pain, nausea, vomiting, high blood pressure, or blood in the urine; however, the parents of many children with this type of tumor are the first to notice a firm, rounded mass in their child's abdomen. This discovery is often made while bathing or dressing the child and frequently occurs before any other symptoms appear. Rarely, a Wilms tumor is diagnosed after there has been bleeding into the tumor, resulting in sudden swelling of the abdomen and a low red blood cell count (**anemia**).

About 4%–5% of Wilms tumor cases involve both kidneys during the initial evaluation. The tumor appears on either side equally. When pathologists look at these tumor cells under the microscope, they see great diversity in the types of cells. Some types of cells are associated with a more favorable outcome in the patient than others. In about 15% of cases, physicians find some degree of cancer spread (**metastasis**). The most common sites in the body where metastasis occurs are the liver and lungs.

Researchers have found evidence that certain types of lesions occur before the development of the Wilms tumor. These lesions usually appear in the form of stromal, tubule, or blastemal cells.

Diagnosis

Children with Wilms tumor generally first present to physicians with a swollen abdomen or with an obvious abdominal mass. The physician may also find that the child has **fever**, bloody urine, or abdominal pain. The physician will order a variety of tests before imaging is performed. These tests mostly involve blood analysis in the form of a complete blood cell count, and serum calcium evaluation. Liver and kidney function testing will also be performed, as well as a urinalysis.

Initial diagnosis of Wilms tumor is made by looking at the tumor using various imaging techniques. Ultrasound and **computed tomography** scans (CT scans) are helpful in diagnosing Wilms tumor. Intravenous pyelography, where a dye injected into a vein helps show the structures of the kidney, can also be used in diagnosing this type of tumor. Final diagnosis, however, depends on obtaining a tissue sample from the mass (**biopsy**), and examining it under a microscope in order to verify that it has the characteristics of a Wilms tumor. This biopsy is usually done during surgery to remove or decrease the size of the tumor. Other studies (chest x-rays, CT scan of the lungs, **bone marrow biopsy**) may also be done in order to see if the tumor has spread to other locations.

Treatment

In the United States, treatment for Wilms tumor almost always begins with surgery to remove or decrease the size of the kidney tumor. Except in patients who have tumors in both kidneys, this surgery usually will require complete removal of the affected kidney. During surgery, the surrounding lymph nodes, the area around the kidneys, and the entire abdomen will also be examined. While the tumor can spread to these surrounding areas, it is less likely to do so compared to other types of cancer. In cases where the tumor affects both kidneys, surgeons will try to preserve the kidney with the smaller tumor by removing only a portion of the kidney, if possible. Additional biopsies of these areas may be done to see if the cancer has spread. The next treatment steps depend on whether/where the cancer has spread. Samples of the tumor are also examined under a microscope to determine particular characteristics of the cells making up the tumor.

Information about the tumor cell type and the spread of the tumor is used to decide the best kind of treatment for a particular patient. Treatment is usually a combination of surgery, medications used to kill cancer cells (**chemotherapy**), and x-rays or other high-energy rays used to kill cancer cells (**radiation therapy**). These therapies are called adjuvant therapies, and this type of combination therapy has been shown to substantially improve outcomes in patients with Wilms tumor. It has long been known that Wilms tumors respond to radiation therapy. New radiation therapy techniques use advanced imaging to target the tumor more precisely and minimize the amount of radiation that strikes healthy tissue near the cancer. Likewise, some types of chemotherapy have been found to be effective in treating Wilms tumor. A combination of effective drugs often includes **dactinomycin** and **vincristine**. For more advanced tumors or those that recur (return), doctors might use **doxorubicin**, **cyclophosphamide** and other chemotherapy drugs. In rare cases, **bone marrow transplantation** may be used.

Because Wilms tumor is such a rare cancer, children should be treated and operated on by specialists familiar with **childhood cancers** and specifically with Wilms tumors. Specialized cancer centers often participate in **clinical trials** to test new approaches to treatment. These may include new targeted or biologic therapy. Also called **immunotherapy**, biologic therapy is a kind of treatment that helps the patient's immune system fight cancer. Clinical trials were underway in 2014 to identify biomarkers, or substances that can be measured to predict how aggressive the tumors may be.

The Children's Oncology Group is the system used most often in the United States to describe Wilms tumors. All of the stages assume that surgical removal of the tumor has occurred. Stage I involves Wilms tumor cells in only one kidney and not invading blood vessels in or near the kidney. Nearly half of all Wilms tumors fall into this early stage. Stage II tumors involve growth of the tumor past the kidney into nearby blood vessels or fatty tissue, but not into lymph nodes, and complete removal with surgery. Stage III tumors are not completely removed with surgery and have spread to lymph nodes, nearby organs that make it too difficult to remove, or into areas in the abdomen. The tumor might have been removed by the surgeon, but in several sections because of its spread. Stage IV disease is the most advanced, when the cancer has spread to distant organs such as the brain or bone, or is found in lymph nodes far from the kidneys. Stage V is a finding of Wilms tumor in both kidneys when the cancer is diagnosed.

Prognosis

The prognosis for patients with Wilms tumor is quite good, compared to the prognosis for most types of cancer. As many as 90% of patients with these tumors now can be treated successfully. The patients who have the best prognosis are usually those who have a small-sized tumor, a favorable cell type, are young (especially under two years old), and have an early stage of cancer that has not spread. Modern treatments have been especially effective in the treatment of this cancer.

QUESTIONS TO ASK YOUR DOCTOR

- What kinds of diagnostic studies will be required to ascertain the type and spread of this tumor?
- Could there be a genetic component to this tumor? Should other family members be tested?
- What types of treatments are available?
- What types of side effects from treatments can my child expect? What are your recommendations to help deal with those side effects?
- Is my child eligible for any clinical trials? Would these be helpful to consider?
- Are there foods my child should avoid?
- How often should my child be checked after treatment has ended?
- Is there a support group that I can join to hear about other people's experiences with this disorder?

Prevention

There are no known ways to prevent a Wilms tumor, although it is important that children with birth defects associated with Wilms tumor be carefully monitored.

Resources

BOOKS

Abeloff, M. D., et al. *Clinical Oncology*. 5th ed. New York: Churchill Livingstone, 2013.

Behrman R. E., et al. *Nelson Textbook of Pediatrics*. 19th ed. Philadelphia: Saunders, 2011.

Niederhuber, J. E., et al. *Clinical Oncology*. 5th ed. Philadelphia: Elsevier, 2014.

Wein, A. J., et al. *Campbell-Walsh Urology*. 10th ed. Philadelphia: Saunders, 2012.

PERIODICALS

Charlton, J., et al. "Methylome Analysis Identifies a Wilms Tumor Epigenetic Biomarker Detectable in Blood." *Genome Biology* 15, no. 8 (2014): 434.

Dean, J. B., and J. S. Dome. "Breast Cancer in Wilms Tumor Survivors: New Insights into Primary and Secondary Prevention." *Cancer* (October 27, 2014): e-pub ahead of print. http://dx.doi.org/10.1002/cncr.28906 (accessed November 10, 2014).

Gleason, J. M., et al. "Innovations in the Management of Wilms' Tumor." *Therapeutic Advances in Urology* 6, no. 4 (2014): 165–76.

OTHER

American Cancer Society. "Wilms' Tumor." http://www.cancer.org/acs/groups/cid/documents/webcontent/003149-pdf.pdf (accessed November 4, 2014).

WEBSITES

National Cancer Institute. "General Information About Childhood Kidney Tumors." http://www.cancer.gov/cancertopics/pdq/treatment/wilms/HealthProfessional (accessed November 4, 2014).

ORGANIZATIONS

American Cancer Society, 1599 Clifton Rd., NE, Atlanta, GA 30329, (800) 227-2345, http://www.cancer.org.

March of Dimes Birth Defects Foundation, 1275 Mamaroneck Avenue, White Plains, NY 10605, (914) 997-4488, http://www.marchofdimes.org.

National Cancer Institute, 9609 Medical Center Drive, Bethesda, MD 20892, (800) 422-6237, http://www.cancer.gov.

National Wilms Tumor Study, 1100 Fairview Avenue N, MJ-A876, Seattle, WA 98109-1024, (800) 553-4878, Fax: (206) 667-4842, nwtsg@fhcrc.org, http://www.nwtsg.org/.

Mark A. Mitchell, M.D.

REVISED BY REBECCA J. FREY, PhD
REVISED BY TERESA G. ODLE
REVIEWED BY ROSALYN CARSON-DEWITT, MD

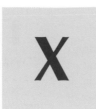

Xeloda *see* **Capecitabine**

Xerostomia

Definition

Xerostomia, also known as dry mouth, is marked by a significant reduction in the secretion of saliva. Xerostomia makes the mouth less able to neutralize acid, clean the teeth and gums, and protect itself from infection. This lack of saliva can lead to the development of gum disease and cavities.

Description

Saliva is necessary for carrying out the normal functions of the oral cavity, such as taste, speech, and swallowing. Saliva provides calcium and phosphate, minerals that protect the teeth against softening. It also contains substances inhibiting the production of bacteria that cause tooth decay. In addition, saliva buffers the acids produced when leftover food particles are broken down by bacteria.

Xerostomia causes the following mouth changes that can contribute to discomfort for the patient, and an increased risk of oral lesions:

- Saliva becomes thick and is less able to lubricate the mouth.
- Acids in the mouth cannot be neutralized, leading to mineral loss from the teeth.
- There is an increased risk of cavities because the mouth is less able to control bacteria.
- Plaque becomes thicker and heavier because of the patient's difficulty in maintaining good oral hygiene.
- The acid produced after eating or drinking sugary foods leads to further mineral loss from the teeth, causing even more tooth decay.

Causes and symptoms

Causes

Xerostomia in **cancer** patients is primarily caused by the effects of **radiation therapy** on the salivary glands, usually the result of radiation to the head and neck area. These changes may occur rapidly and cannot normally be reversed, especially if the salivary glands themselves are irradiated. Within one week of starting radiation treatment, the production of saliva drops and continues to decrease as treatment continues. The severity of xerostomia is dependent upon the radiation dose and how many salivary glands are irradiated. Typically, the salivary glands inside the upper back cheeks (the parotid glands) are more affected than others. Salivary glands that are not irradiated may become more active as a way of compensating for the loss of saliva from the destroyed glands.

A number of medications can cause xerostomia, including many drugs used in the management of cancer or cancer treatment side effects. Some of these are: atropine, **amitriptyline**, **carbamazepine**, **diphenhydramine**, **gabapentin**, haloperidol, loperamide, **lorazepam**, and **scopolamine**, among several others.

Symptoms

Signs and symptoms of xerostomia include:

- dryness of the mouth
- cracked lips, cuts, or cracks at the corners of the mouth
- taste changes
- a burning sensation of the tongue
- changes in the surface of the tongue
- difficulty wearing dental appliances (like dentures)
- difficulty swallowing fluids accompanied by an increase in thirst

Treatment

A number of **clinical trials** are investigating drugs called radioprotectors, which are given at the time of radiation therapy in an attempt to prevent xerostomia. If xerostomia has already developed, there are a number of measures that may help to both alleviate the symptoms of dry mouth and prevent cavities and gum disease. These measures include:

- cleaning the mouth well at least four times per day (after every meal and at bedtime)
- rinsing the mouth immediately after every meal
- using fluoride toothpaste to brush the teeth
- sipping water frequently
- rinsing the mouth with a salt and baking soda solution four to six times per day (1/2 tsp. salt, 1/2 tsp. baking soda, and 8 oz. of water)
- avoiding foods and liquids containing large amounts of sugar
- avoiding mouthwashes containing alcohol
- using moisturizer on the lips
- using saliva substitutes to help relieve discomfort
- using a sialogogue such as pilocarpine (Salagen), which can stimulate saliva secretion from the remaining salivary glands
- applying a prescription-strength fluoride gel daily at bedtime to clean the teeth

Xerostomia usually cannot be reversed when the cause is the destruction of the salivary glands by radiation treatments. It may be reversible if related to a medication. All treatment measures serve to increase the level of comfort, decrease the chance for oral lesions, and reduce the occurrence of gum disease and cavities.

Resources

WEBSITES

American Society of Clinical Oncology. "Dry Mouth or Xerostomia." Cancer.net. http://www.cancer.net/navigating-cancer-care/side-effects/dry-mouth-or-xerostomia (accessed November 13, 2014).

Cancer Research UK. "Types and Causes of Mouth Problems." http://www.cancerresearchuk.org/about-cancer/coping-with-cancer/coping-physically/mouth/types-and-causes-of-mouth-problems (accessed November 13, 2014).

National Cancer Institute. "Managing Oral Complications During and After Chemotherapy or Radiation Therapy." http://www.cancer.gov/cancertopics/pdq/supportivecare/oralcomplications/Patient/page4 (accessed November 18, 2014).

Deanna Swartout-Corbeil, R.N.
Rebecca J. Frey, PhD

Xgeva *see* **Denosumab**

X-rays

Definition

X-rays are a type of radiation used in imaging and therapy made up of short-wavelength energy beams capable of penetrating most substances except heavy metals.

Purpose

Diagnostic x-rays are some of the most powerful medical imaging tools available. Based on the symptoms presented by the patient, the physician can request specific x-ray examinations (such as chest x-rays), also called radiography, to help diagnose many types of cancers, including sarcomas, lymphomas, and lung cancers. Using x-rays, a physician can see and evaluate internal body structures and functions with little or no invasive procedures. In the past, examinations using x-rays captured images on photographic film. Today, the images can be digitized for the radiologist to view on a special high-resolution monitor.

Mammograms are x-ray images specifically designed to screen for or diagnose **breast cancer**. They are performed on units dedicated for breast imaging. For more complex and detailed information, **computed tomography** (CT) scans, fluoroscopy, or **angiography** might be used. CT takes cross-sectional images of the body using x-rays, and fluoroscopy uses pulses of x-rays to capture movie-like images. Angiography is a method used to study and even treat diseases of the blood vessels, usually with the use of fluoroscopy or CT scanning and

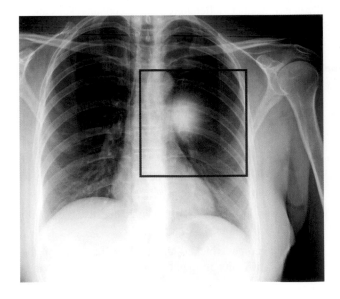

X-ray revealing a cancerous tumor in the lungs.
(Shutterstock.com)

KEY TERMS

Angiography—A radiographic technique in which an opaque contrast material is injected into a blood vessel for the purpose of identifying its anatomy on x-ray.

Computed tomography (CT)—A special radiographic technique that uses a computer to convert multiple x-ray images into a multidimensional cross-sectional image.

Contrast dye—A radiopaque dye that allows enhancement of the anatomy demonstrable with conventional x-ray.

Fluoroscopy—X-ray imaging of moving anatomic structures.

Gene therapy—The delivery of normal genes or genetically altered cells to the site of a tumor.

Interventional radiography—Diagnostic and therapeutic x-ray procedures that are invasive or surgical in nature but do not require the use of general anesthesia.

Pleural effusion—The accumulation of fluid in the pleural space, the region between the outer surface of each lung.

Radiologist—A physician specially trained in the use of x-rays for diagnostic and therapy purposes.

an injected contrast material to highlight key areas. Other imaging techniques that do not use x-rays include **magnetic resonance imaging** (MRI) and **ultrasonography**. Nuclear medicine imaging, including **positron emission tomography** (PET) scanning, uses no x-rays, but special cameras take photos of areas highlighted by injected **radiopharmaceuticals** that have small amounts of radiation in them.

Radiation therapy often uses an x-ray beam aimed at a patient from outside the patient's body to destroy **cancer** cells or shrink tumors. The radiation used in therapy is at a much higher energy level or dose than that used in diagnostic examinations. Some radiation therapy comes from other types of energy or from tiny seeds implanted in the tumor bed.

Description

X-ray examinations are administered in a hospital or outpatient clinical setting. The time required for the examination may vary from a few minutes to more than an hour. There is little or no discomfort associated with

diagnostic x-rays. The general procedure for diagnostic x-rays include:

- proper positioning and shielding of the patient
- administering contrast dyes, if necessary
- administering radiation
- review of the images by a radiologic technologist to ensure proper imaging
- sending the images for evaluation and interpretation by a radiologist (if fluoroscopy or angiography are used, however, the procedure is dynamic [in motion], and the radiologist is present during the x-ray administration)
- dismissal of the patient

Precautions

Before consenting to any x-ray procedure, the patient should consider the impact of existing medical conditions or medications. Sensitivities to contrast dyes may produce allergic reactions. Pregnant women or those who suspect they might be pregnant should consult a physician before having x-ray examinations to avoid injury to the fetus. Nursing mothers may be required to store enough milk to last for 48 hours following certain procedures. Patient age should always be taken into consideration when choosing the type and intensity of x-ray. In particular, children who need repeated x-ray examinations or radiation therapy may be susceptible to effects from the radiation, including increased risk of some cancers. Patients should be aware that some prescribed cancer medications act as radiosensitizers and amplify the effect of x-rays. Any patient with a suppressed immune system or diabetes may require special x-ray procedures.

Preparation

Diagnostic x-rays require little preparation. The patient may be required to abstain from food and liquids for a certain period prior to the examination. For some x-rays, enemas may be necessary or a contrast agent may be administered immediately before or during the exam.

Aftercare

For noninvasive diagnostic x-ray procedures, the patient is dismissed immediately after the images have been reviewed, and little or no aftercare is necessary.

Risks

A general rule for x-rays suggests that the beneficial effects of x-rays far exceed the risks involved. Each state has laws regarding training and certification of radiologic technologists. When hospitals and imaging centers

QUESTIONS TO ASK YOUR DOCTOR

- What type of imaging examination is best to diagnose my condition?
- Will the examination or procedure hurt?
- How long will it take each time and how many treatments are required?
- What are my chances for a complete recovery?
- Are these examinations covered by insurance?
- If my child needs x-rays or radiation therapy, are there alternatives to minimize radiation exposure?

hire registered radiologic technologists, risks from the procedure are extremely rare. However, for any x-ray procedure, radiation exposure is always a concern, and although uncommon, the risk of infection during invasive techniques cannot be discounted.

Results

Screening x-rays can help indicate early signs of cancer. Diagnostic x-rays provide detailed information that the physician can use to determine the best approach to correct or control a medical problem. They often provide initial information for cancer diagnoses and help monitor response to treatment or follow up a cancer survivor's continued freedom from the return of cancer. Normal results indicate no existing abnormalities or tumors.

Abnormal results

Abnormal results would indicate irregularities such as a tumor, an enlarged lymph node, or **pleural effusion**. Although highly unlikely, diagnostic x-ray images can be misread and the wrong diagnosis made. Some cancers cannot be seen on radiographs.

See also Barium enema; Bone survey; CT-guided biopsy; Imaging studies; Intravenous urography; Lymphangiography; Nephrostomy; Pain management; Percutaneous transhepatic cholangiography; Radiation therapy; Stereotactic needle biopsy; Upper GI series.

Resources

BOOKS

Abeloff, M. D., et al. *Clinical Oncology*. 5th ed. New York: Churchill Livingstone, 2013.
Grainger, R. G., et al. *Grainger & Allison's Diagnostic Radiology: A Textbook of Medical Imaging*. 6th ed. Philadelphia: Saunders, 2015.
Mettler, F. A. *Essentials of Radiology*. 3rd ed. Philadelphia: Saunders, 2013.
Niederhuber, J. E., et al. *Clinical Oncology*. 5th ed. Philadelphia: Elsevier, 2014.

WEBSITES

American Cancer Society. "Radiographic Studies (Regular X-rays and Contrast Studies)." http://www.cancer.org/treatment/understandingyourdiagnosis/examsandtestdescriptions/imagingradiologytests/imaging-radiology-tests-xrays (accessed November 3, 2014).
Radiological Society of North America. "X-Ray (Radiography), Chest." RadiologyInfo.org. http://www.radiologyinfo.org/en/info.cfm?pg=chestrad (accessed November 10, 2014).

Jane Taylor-Jones, MS
REVISED BY TERESA G. ODLE
REVIEWED BY ROSALYN CARSON-DEWITT, MD

Z

Zanosar *see* **Streptozocin**

Zevalin *see* **Ibritumomab**

Zinecard *see* **Dexrazoxane**

Zoladex *see* **Goserelin acetate**

Zoledronate

Definition

Zoledronate, which is also known as zoledronic acid, is a treatment for **hypercalcemia** (high levels of calcium in the blood) caused by tumors. It is sold under the brand name Zometa. New laboratory evidence suggests that zoledronate may have direct anticancer effects.

Purpose

Tumor-induced hypercalcemia is also known as hypercalcemia of malignancy. Tumor-induced hypercalcemia may be caused by a tumor spreading to and causing breakdown of bone, or by chemicals released from some tumors. The result is high levels of calcium in the blood. High levels of calcium may cause changes in mental status, constipation, and kidney damage.

Zoledronate was approved by the Food and Drug Administration (FDA) in 2002 as a treatment for **multiple myeloma** and bone metastases. Bone metastases may develop if cells from breast, lung, or other cancers are transferred to bone by the disease process. Bone **metastasis** may cause pain, compression of the nerves of the spine, and bone fractures.

Other drugs in the same class as zoledronate are used to prevent pain or fractures in people with bone metastases. Zoledronate appears to be effective for this use as well, particularly in men being treated for **prostate cancer**. In addition, these drugs (the class of **bisphosphonates**) are being studied to see whether they prevent the development of bone metastases in the first place.

Description

Zoledronate is one of a group of medicines known as bisphosphonates. Bisphosphonates prevent bone destruction by inhibiting the action of osteoclasts, cells that break down bone. Zoledronate is one of the most potent bisphosphonates approved for use in the United States.

Recommended dosage

The recommended dosage of zoledronate is 4 mg, given intravenously over a 15-minute period. This short infusion period gives zoledronate an advantage over other drugs in the bisphosphonate class; one study done in Australia found that patients preferred zoledronate to other intravenous bisphosphonates for this reason. The frequency of administration of zoledronate for hypercalcemia depends on the patient's calcium blood level.

Side effects

The most common side effects due to zoledronate that have been reported to date are **fever**, low blood concentration of phosphate, and low blood calcium (not low enough to cause symptoms). Long-term use of zoledronate and other biphosphonates has been associated with osteonecrosis of the jaw, a condition in which the bones of the jaw do not receive enough blood.

Resources

BOOKS

Karch, Amy Morrison. *2014 Lippincott's Pocket Drug Guide for Nurses*. Philadelphia: Wolters Kluwer/Lippincott Williams & Wilkins Health, 2014.

Otto, Sven, ed. *Drug-Induced Osteonecrosis of the Jaw: Bisphosphonates, Denosumab, and New Agents*. New York: Springer, 2014.

KEY TERMS

Bisphosphonates—A class of drugs that inhibit the action of osteoclasts—the cells that dissolve or break down bone.

Bone metastases—The spread of tumor cells from the primary site of origin to bone. Bone metastases from breast cancer, for example, represent breast cancer cells that have invaded bone. They are not the same as bone cancer cells that originate in bone.

Hypercalcemia of malignancy—Also called tumor-induced hypercalcemia; high levels of calcium in the blood from the dissolving of bone, either directly by cancer cells or indirectly by chemicals released from cancer cells.

PERIODICALS

Chern, B., D. Joseph, D. Joshua, et al. "Bisphosphonate Infusions: Patient Preference, Safety and Clinic Use." *Supportive Care in Cancer*12 (June 2004): 463–466.

Patel, C. G., et al., "Biomarkers of Bone Remodeling in Multiple Myeloma Patients to Tailor Bisphosphonate Therapy." *Clinical Cancer Research 20* (August 1, 2014): 3955–3961.

Rosen, L. S., D. Gordon, N. S. Tchekmedyian, et al. "Long-Term Efficacy and Safety of Zoledronic Acid in the Treatment of Skeletal Metastases in Patients with Nonsmall Cell Lung Carcinoma and Other Solid Tumors: A Randomized, Phase III, Double-Blind, Placebo-Controlled Trial." *Cancer*100 (June 15, 2004): 2613–2621.

Saad, F., D. M. Gleason, R. Murray, et al. "Long-Term Efficacy of Zoledronic Acid for the Prevention of Skeletal Complications in Patients with Metastatic Hormone-Refractory Prostate Cancer." *Journal of the National Cancer Institute*96 (June 2, 2004): 879–882.

ORGANIZATIONS

ASHP (formerly the American Society of Health-System Pharmacists), 7272 Wisconsin Ave., Bethesda, MD 20814, (301) 664-8700, (866) 279-0681, custserv@ashp.org, http://www.ashp.org.

U.S. Food and Drug Administration, 10903 New Hampshire Ave., Silver Spring, MD 20993, (888) INFO-FDA (463-6332), http://www.fda.gov.

Bob Kirsch
Rebecca J. Frey, PhD

Zolinza *see* **Vorinostat**

Zollinger-Ellison syndrome

Definition

In Zollinger-Ellison syndrome (ZES), a tumor (a gastrinoma) secretes the hormone gastrin, which stimulates the secretion of gastric acid. This condition leads to the development of ulcers in the stomach and duodenum (the first part of the small intestine).

Description

In normal individuals, the stomach secretes the hormone gastrin after food enters the stomach. Gastrin is carried by the bloodstream to other parts of the stomach. The main effect of gastrin is to stimulate the parietal cells of the stomach. Parietal cells are stomach cells that secrete gastric acid to aid in digestion. This acid plays a vital role in the digestion of food. This process is highly regulated so that the stomach produces gastrin in significant amounts only when necessary, as when there is food in the stomach.

The underlying entity of ZES is a tumor called a gastrinoma which secretes gastrin inappropriately. Marked overproduction of gastrin leads to hypersecretion of gastric acid by the parietal cells. The end result is severe ulcers of the stomach and duodenum that are more difficult to treat than common ulcers.

Gastrinomas are generally small tumors located in the pancreas or duodenum. They often occur in multiples in the same patient. More than half of all gastrinomas are malignant, with the potential to spread to nearby lymph nodes and also to the liver and other organs by way of **metastasis**. The malignant potential of a gastrinoma is ultimately more life-threatening than the associated ulcers.

The ulcers in ZES are frequently located further down the gastrointestinal tract than common ulcers, and they may be multiple.

About 25% of patients with ZES also demonstrate other tumors of the endocrine system in a syndrome called **multiple endocrine neoplasia** (MEN) syndrome.

Demographics

ZES occurs slightly more frequently in males than females. The average age of onset is between 30 and 50 years of age. It is difficult to determine the prevalence of ZES, but it is not a common syndrome.

Causes and symptoms

The symptoms of ZES are chiefly related to the ulcer disease. The main symptom is abdominal pain, present in the vast majority of patients. Ulcers can also cause

KEY TERMS

Angiography—Radiographic examination of blood vessels after injection with a special dye.

Computed tomography—A radiology test in which images of cross-sectional planes of the body are obtained.

Duodenum—The first portion of the small intestine in continuity with the stomach.

Endoscopy—Examination of the interior of a hollow part of the body by means of a special lighted instrument.

Gastric—Of or relating to the stomach.

Gastrin—Hormone normally secreted by the stomach that stimulates secretion of gastric acid.

Gastrinoma—Tumor that secretes the hormone gastrin.

Magnetic resonance imaging—A radiology test that reconstructs images of the body based on magnetic fields.

Malignant—In reference to cancer, having the ability to invade local tissues and spread to distant tissues by metastasis.

Metastasis—The spread of tumor cells from one part of the body to another.

Parietal cells—Stomach cells that secrete gastric acid to aid in digestion.

Scintigraphy—A radiology test that involves injection and detection of radioactive substances to create images of body parts.

Ultrasound—A radiology test utilizing high frequency sound waves.

nausea, vomiting, and heartburn. Compared with patients with common ulcers, patients with ZES generally have more severe and persistent symptoms that are more difficult to control. In some cases, the ulcers can bleed or actually perforate completely through the walls of the stomach or duodenum.

Many patients also suffer **diarrhea** in addition to ulcer pain. In fact, diarrhea is the only symptom in a small fraction of patients, and the diarrhea may precede the development of ulcers in the stomach and duodenum.

Diagnosis

A number of clinical circumstances suggest that a patient's ulcer disease may be due to ZES:

- ulcer disease resistant to conventional medical treatment
- recurrent ulcers after surgery intended to cure the ulcer disease
- ulcer disease in the absence of the usual risk factors for ulcers
- ulcers located in abnormal locations in the gastrointestinal tract
- multiple ulcers
- ulcers accompanied by diarrhea
- strong family history of ulcer disease

Diagnosis of ZES must be confirmed by observing abnormally high levels of gastrin in the blood. This is the hallmark of the disease. But it must be mentioned that the gastrinoma of ZES is not the only cause of hypersecretion of gastrin. ZES is distinguished from these other conditions by the presence of appropriate symptoms and high levels of gastrin and gastric acid. In cases in which the diagnosis is not clear, several provocative tests can help determine whether the patient has ZES. In the intravenous secretin injection test, a standard dose of the hormone secretin is injected intravenously. If the blood levels of gastrin respond by increasing a certain amount, the diagnosis is ZES. Similarly, in the intravenous calcium infusion test, a dose of calcium is injected and gastrin levels are measured. A substantial increase in the gastrin level points to ZES. A newer test measures the response in gastrin level to the ingestion of a standard meal. For example, the standard meal might be one slice of bread, one boiled egg, 200 mL of milk, and 50 gm of cheese.

Treatment team

The surgeon and a gastroenterologist are the chief members of the treatment team. Radiologists play a vital role in the localization of the gastrinoma before surgery. Oncologists may be involved after surgery or if surgery is not indicated.

Treatment

The goal of treatment for ZES is the elimination of excess gastrin production, acid hypersecretion, ulcer disease, and malignant potential. This result is achieved only by complete surgical removal of all gastrinomas. An attempt at surgical cure is offered to most patients, with the exception of those who already have widespread metastasis to the liver or who are too ill to undergo surgery. It is important to locate the gastrinoma(s) and any possible areas of metastasis before surgery. This can be accomplished with tests such as **computed tomography** (CT), ultrasound, **magnetic resonance imaging**

(MRI), **angiography**, scintigraphy, and endoscopy. But as gastrinomas may be small, multiple, and hidden in atypical positions, finding the exact locations of all cancerous tissue can be challenging and sometimes impossible. In that case, surgeons will still proceed and attempt to find the tumor(s) at the time of operation. All identified gastrinoma should be removed if possible, including involved lymph nodes. Metastatic lesions in the liver can sometimes be safely removed, but only when they are restricted to one part of the liver.

Chemotherapy is sometimes able to reduce tumor size, which may relieve some symptoms due to local invasion or massive growth of the tumor. But it has not been shown to consistently prolong survival.

Medical therapy plays a vital role in the treatment of ZES. A group of drugs known as proton pump inhibitors, which includes omeprazole (a drug used to treat common ulcers), is effective in decreasing acid secretion and promoting ulcer healing in patients with ZES. Omeprazole acts by blocking the last biochemical step in acid production. Omeprazole should be prescribed immediately after diagnosis. If surgery is not attempted or is ultimately unsuccessful, omeprazole is also useful for long-term treatment. For reasons that are not fully known, sometimes patients still require omeprazole after successful surgery. Another drug called octreotide is also effective in reducing acid secretion.

Prognosis

The prognosis for ZES depends primarily on whether the gastrinoma can be completely removed. If the **cancer** has spread diffusely to the liver, surgical cure is nearly impossible. The gastrinoma tissue is completely removed in about 40% of patients, resulting in reduced acid secretion and resolution of ulcer disease or diarrhea. These patients should expect a normal life expectancy, although they should undergo regular testing thereafter and may also require long-term omeprazole treatment. The prognosis is poor for patients in whom all the gastrinoma cannot be removed.

Clinical trials

In 2014 there were 13 **clinical trials** recruiting patients with Zollinger-Ellison syndrome. These trials were studying various aspects of treatment for the syndrome, including several different chemotherapy drugs. For further information about ongoing clinical trials, patients may consult the National Institutes of Health clinical trials website at: http://clinicaltrials.gov/.

See also Multiple endocrine neoplasia syndromes.

Resources

BOOKS

Friesen, Stanley R. *Zollinger-Ellison Syndrome*. Chicago: Year Book Medical Publishers, 1972.

PERIODICALS

Ito T., Igarashi H., Uehara H., Jensen RT. "Pharmacotherapy of Zollinger-Ellison Syndrome." *Expert Opinion on Pharmacotherapy* 14, no. 3 (2013): 307–21. http://www.ncbi.nlm.nih.gov/pmc/articles/PMC3580316/ (accessed November 12, 2014).

WEBSITES

A.D.A.M. Medical Encyclopedia. "Zollinger-Ellison Syndrome." MedlinePlus. http://www.nlm.nih.gov/medlineplus/ency/article/000325.htm (accessed November 12, 2014).

Kevin O. Hwang, M.D.

Zolpidem

Definition

Zolpidem is a medicine that helps a person get to sleep and stay asleep. The brand name of zolpidem in the United States is Ambien.

Purpose

Zolpidem is a sleep medication. It is intended for the short-term treatment of insomnia. Zolpidem may be particularly useful for people who have trouble falling asleep.

Description

Sleep medications are called sedatives or hypnotics. Zolpidem affects brain chemicals, resulting in sleep. It is somewhat similar in its actions on inducing sleep to the group of drugs known as **benzodiazepines**. Zolpidem is only intended for short-term use (7–10 days). Although there is some information published about effectiveness with longer use, some side effects may increase with longer use.

Recommended dosage

The dose recommended to avoid side effects is 5 mg before bedtime for women and 5–10 mg for men. Extended-release forms have slightly higher dosages: 6.25 mg for women and 6.25–12.5 mg for men. The onset of effect occurs within about 30 minutes, and the effects on sleep last for 6–8 hours.

Precautions

It is suggested that zolpidem not be discontinued abruptly after regular use (that is, daily use for even as short a time as one week). Instead, the drug should be gradually tapered. The tapering is recommended to avoid the possibility of a withdrawal syndrome as well as to avoid the possibility of a rebound worsening of insomnia.

Side effects

The most common side effects of zolpidem include drowsiness, dizziness, and headache. Drowsiness, of course, is desirable when it occurs at bedtime. Daytime drowsiness that is left over from the night before would be considered a side effect. Other side effects include **diarrhea**, **nausea and vomiting**, and muscle aches. Rarely, amnesia, confusion, falls, and tremor are seen. Falls probably result from the drowsiness or dizziness. There is also a reported study of a patient sleepwalking when taking zolpidem along with valproic acid. It is possible that the interactions between the two might have resulted in sleepwalking.

Interactions

Increased effects of zolpidem (e.g., more drowsiness, confusion) may be seen with alcohol consumption, SSRI antidepressants, antipsychotic medications, and with other drugs known to cause drowsiness.

Resources

BOOKS

Chu, Edward, and Vincent T. DeVita Jr. *Physicians' Cancer Chemotherapy Drug Manual 2014.* Burlington, MA: Jones & Bartlett Learning, 2014.

WEBSITES

Healthwise. "Zolpidem." Norris Cotton Cancer Center, Dartmouth. http://cancer.dartmouth.edu/pf/health_encyclopedia/d00910a1 (accessed November 12, 2014).

U.S. Food and Drug Administration. "Zolpidem Containing Products: Drug Safety Communication—FDA Requires Lower Recommended Doses." http://www.fda.gov/safety/medwatch/safetyinformation/safetyalertsforhumanmedicalproducts/ucm334738.htm (accessed November 12, 2014).

Bob Kirsch

Zometa *see* **Zoledronate**

Zyloprim *see* **Allopurinol**

ORGANIZATIONS: NATIONAL CANCER INSTITUTE–DESIGNATED COMPREHENSIVE CANCER CENTERS

Comprehensive Cancer Centers have been designated as such by the National Cancer Institute. They are required to have basic laboratory research in several fields; to be able to transfer research findings into clinical practice; to conduct clinical studies and trials; to research cancer prevention and control; to offer information about cancer to patients, the public, and healthcare professionals; and to provide community service related to cancer control. The list of NCI-designated cancer centers is available online at: http://www.cancer.gov/researchandfunding/extramural/cancercenters/find-a-cancer-center.

Alabama

UAB Comprehensive Cancer Center
University of Alabama at Birmingham, 1802 Sixth Avenue South
Birmingham, AL 35294
Phone: (205) 934-5077
Toll free: (800) 822-0933 (UAB-0933)
Web site: http://www3.ccc.uab.edu/

Arizona

Arizona Cancer Center
University of Arizona, 1515 North Campbell Avenue
Tucson, AZ 85724
Phone: (520) 626-7685
Toll free: (800) 524-5928 (patient care and appointments)
Web site: http://azcc.arizona.edu/

California

Chao Family Comprehensive Cancer Center
University of California at Irvine, 101 The City Drive, Building 56, Rt. 81, Room 216L
Orange, CA 92868
Phone: (714) 456-8000 (appointments)
Toll free: (877) 824-3627 (physician referral service)
Web site: http://www.cancer.uci.edu/

City of Hope Comprehensive Cancer Center
1500 East Duarte Road
Duarte, CA 91010
Phone: (626) 256-HOPE (4673)
Toll free: (800) 826-4673 (new patient services)
Web site: http://www.cityofhope.org/

Jonsson Comprehensive Cancer Center
University of California Los Angeles (UCLA), 8-684 Factor Building, 10833 Le Conte Avenue
Los Angeles, CA 90095
Phone: (310) 825-5268
Toll free: (888) 662-8252
Web site: http://www.cancer.ucla.edu/

Salk Institute Cancer Center
10100 North Torrey Pines Road
La Jolla, CA 92037
Phone: (858) 453-4100
Web site: http://www.salk.edu/faculty/cancer_center.html

Sanford-Burnham Medical Research Institute
10901 North Torrey Pines Road
La Jolla, CA 92037
Phone: (858) 646-3100
Web site: http://www.sanfordburnham.org/research/centers/cancer/Pages/Home.aspx

Stanford Cancer Institute
Stanford University, Lorry Lokey Stem Cell Building, 265 Campus Drive, Suite G2103
Stanford, CA 94305
Phone: (650) 498-6000 (referral center)
Toll free: (877) 668-7535
Web site: http://cancer.stanford.edu/

UC Davis Comprehensive Cancer Center
University of California at Davis, 4501 X Street, Suite 3003
Sacramento, CA 95817
Phone: (916) 734-5959
Phone: (916) 703-5210 (new patient referral)
Web site: http://www.ucdmc.ucdavis.edu/cancer/

UC San Diego Moores Cancer Center
University of California at San Diego, 3855 Health Sciences Drive
La Jolla, CA 92093
Phone: (858) 822-6100 (appointments)
Toll free: (866) 773-2703
Web site: http://cancer.ucsd.edu/Pages/default.aspx

UCSF Helen Diller Family Comprehensive Cancer Center
University of California San Francisco, 1450 3rd Street, Box 0128
San Francisco, CA 94115
Phone: (415) 885-3693
Toll free: (415) 353-8489 (international)
Web site: http://cancer.ucsf.edu/

USC/Norris Comprehensive Cancer Center
University of Southern California, 1441 Eastlake Avenue
Los Angeles, CA 90089
Phone: (323) 865-3000
Toll free: (800) 872-2273 (USC-CARE)
Web site: http://ccnt.hsc.usc.edu/

Colorado

University of Colorado Cancer Center
13001 East 17th Place
Aurora, CO 80045
Phone: (720) 848-0300 (adult)
Phone: (720) 777-6688 (pediatric)
Web site: https://www.uchealth.org/pages/services/colorado-cancer-center.aspx

Connecticut

Yale Cancer Center
Yale University School of Medicine, 333 Cedar Street

New Haven, CT 06520
Phone: (203) 785-4191
Toll free: (866) 925-3226
    (YALECANCER)
Web site: http://www.yalecancercenter.
    org/

District of Columbia

**Georgetown Lombardi
    Comprehensive Cancer Center**
Georgetown University, 3970 Reservoir
    Road NW
Washington, DC 20007
Phone: (202) 444-4000
Phone: (202) 444-2223 (appointments)
Web site: http://lombardi.georgetown.
    edu/

Florida

Moffitt Cancer Center
12902 Magnolia Drive, MCC-CEO
Tampa, FL 33612
Phone: (813) 745-4673 (745-HOPE)
Toll free: (888) 860-2778 (patient
    referral)
Web site: http://moffitt.org/

Georgia

Winship Cancer Institute
Emory University, 1365C Clifton Road
Atlanta, GA 30322
Phone: (404) 778-1900
Toll free: (888) 946-7447 (WINSHIP)
Web site: https://winshipcancer.emory.
    edu/

Hawaii

University of Hawaii Cancer Center
701 Ilalo Street, Suite 600
Honolulu, HI 96813
Phone: (808) 586-3010
Web site: http://www.uhcancercenter.org/

Illinois

**Robert H. Lurie Comprehensive
    Cancer Center**
Northwestern University, 303 East
    Superior Street
Chicago, IL 60611
Phone: (312) 695-0990

Toll free: (866) 587-4322 (LURIE-CC)
Web site: http://cancer.northwestern.
    edu/home/index.cfm

**University of Chicago Comprehensive
    Cancer Center**
5841 South Maryland Avenue, MC 2115
Chicago, IL 60637
Phone: (773) 702-6808 (pediatric
    appointments)
Phone: (855) 702-8222 (adult
    appointments)
Web site: http://cancer.uchicago.edu/

Indiana

**Indiana University Melvin and Bren
    Simon Cancer Center**
535 Barnhill Drive
Indianapolis, IN 46202
Phone: (317) 944-5000
Phone: (317) 944-0920 (appointments
    and referrals)
Toll free: (800) 600-4822
Web site: http://www.cancer.iu.edu/

**Purdue University Center for Cancer
    Research**
Hansen Life Sciences Research Building,
    201 South University Street
West Lafayette, IN 47907
Phone: (765) 494-9129
Web site: http://www.cancerresearch.
    purdue.edu/

Iowa

**Holden Comprehensive Cancer
    Center**
University of Iowa, 200 Hawkins Drive,
    5970Z JPP
Iowa City, IA 52242
Phone: (319) 356-4200
Toll free: (800) 237-1225
Web site: http://www.uihealthcare.org
    /HoldenComprehensiveCancerCenter/

Kansas

**The University of Kansas Cancer
    Center**
University of Kansas, 3901 Rainbow
    Boulevard
Kansas City, KS 66160
Phone: (913) 588-1227
Toll free: (800) 332-6048
Web site: http://www.kucancercenter.
    org/

Kentucky

Markey Cancer Center
University of Kentucky, CC140 Roach
    Building, 800 Rose Street
Lexington, KY 40536-0096
Phone: (859) 257-4500
Toll free: (866) 340-4488
Web site: http://ukhealthcare.uky.edu/
    Markey/

Maine

Jackson Laboratory Cancer Center
600 Main Street
Bar Harbor, ME 04609
Phone: (207) 288-6000
Web site: http://www.jax.org/

Maryland

**Sidney Kimmel Comprehensive
    Cancer Center**
Johns Hopkins University, 401 North
    Broadway
Baltimore, MD 21231
Phone: (410) 955-5222
Phone: (410) 955-8964 (appointments
    and referrals)
Web site: http://www.hopkinsmedicine.
    org/kimmel_cancer_center

**University of Maryland Marlene and
    Stewart Greenebaum Cancer
    Center**
22 South Greene Street
Baltimore, MD 21201
Phone: (410) 328-7904
Toll free: (800) 888-8823
Web site: http://www.umgcc.org/

Massachusetts

Dana-Farber/Harvard Cancer Center
450 Brookline Avenue
Boston, MA 02115
Phone: (617) 632-3000
Phone: (617) 632-3673 (Spanish)
Toll free: (866) 408-3324 (408-DFCI)
Web site: http://www.dfhcc.harvard.edu/

**David H. Koch Institute for Integrative
    Cancer Research at MIT**
Massachusetts Institute of Technology,
    77 Massachusetts Avenue, 76-158
Cambridge, MA 02139
Phone: (617) 253-6403
Web site: http://ki.mit.edu/

Michigan

The Barbara Ann Karmanos Cancer Institute
Wayne State University School of
    Medicine, 4100 John R
Detroit, MI 48201
Toll free: (800) KARMANOS (527-6266)
Toll free: (313) 576-8630
Web site: http://www.karmanos.org/home

University of Michigan Comprehensive Cancer Center
1500 East Medical Center Drive
Ann Arbor, MI 48109
Toll free: (800) 865-1125
Web site: http://www.mcancer.org/

Minnesota

Masonic Cancer Center
University of Minnesota, 420 Delaware
    Street SE
Minneapolis, MN 55455
Phone: (612) 624-2620
Phone: (612) 672-7422 (appointments)
Web site: http://www.cancer.umn.edu/

Mayo Clinic Cancer Center
200 First Street SW
Rochester, MN 55905
Phone: (507) 284-2511
Web site: http://www.mayoclinic.org/
    departments-centers/mayo-clinic-
    cancer-center

Missouri

Alvin J. Siteman Cancer Center
Washington University School of
    Medicine and Barnes-Jewish
    Hospital, 660 South Euclid Avenue,
    Campus Box 8109
St. Louis, MO 63110
Phone: (314) 747-7222
Toll free: (800) 600-3606
Web site: http://www.siteman.wustl.edu/

Nebraska

Fred and Pamela Buffett Cancer Center
University of Nebraska Medical Center,
    985950 Nebraska Medical Center
Omaha, NE 68198
Phone: (402) 559-6500
Toll free: (800) 922-0000 (referrals)

Web site: http://www.unmc.edu/
    cancercenter/

New Hampshire

Norris Cotton Cancer Center at Dartmouth
Dartmouth-Hitchcock Medical Center,
    One Medical Center Drive
Lebanon, NH 03756
Phone: (603) 653-9000
Toll free: (800) 639-6918
Web site: http://cancer.dartmouth.edu/

New Jersey

The Cancer Institute of New Jersey
Rutgers University, 195 Little Albany
    Street
New Burnswick, NJ 08903
Phone: (732) 235-2465
Toll free: (732) 235-8515
Web site: http://www.cinj.org/

New Mexico

University of New Mexico Cancer Center
1201 Camino de Salud NE
Albuquerque, NM 87131
Phone: (505) 272-4946
Toll free: (800) 432-6806
Web site: http://cancer.unm.edu/

New York

Albert Einstein Cancer Center
Yeshiva University, 1300 Morris Park
    Avenue
Bronx, NY 10461
Phone: (718) 430-2302
Web site: http://www.einstein.yu.edu/
    centers/cancer/

Cold Spring Harbor Laboratory Cancer Center
1 Bungtown Road
Cold Spring Harbor, NY 11724
Phone: (516) 367-8800
Web site: http://www.cshl.edu/

Herbert Irving Comprehensive Cancer Center
Columbia University, 1130 St. Nicholas
    Avenue, Room 508
New York, NY 10032
Phone: (212) 305-2500
Toll free: (877) 697-9355

Web site: http://hiccc.columbia.edu/

Laura and Isaac Perlmutter Cancer Center at NYU Langone
NYU Langone Medical Center, 550
    First Avenue, 1201 Smilow Building
New York, NY 10016
Phone: (212) 731-6000
Toll free: (88) 769-8633 (referrals)
Web site: http://cancer.med.nyu.edu/

Memorial Sloan-Kettering Cancer Center
1275 York Avenue
New York, NY 10065
Phone: (212) 639-2000
Phone: (212) 639-5954 (Pediatric)
Toll free: (800) 525-2225 (Referrals)
Toll free: (888) 675-7722 (International)
Web site: http://www.mskcc.org/

Roswell Park Cancer Institute
Elm and Carlton Streets
Buffalo, NY 14263
Phone: (716) 845-2300
Toll free: (877) 275-7724 (ASK-RPCI);
    Referrals: (800) 767-9355
    (ROSWELL)
Web site: http://www.roswellpark.org/

North Carolina

The Comprehensive Cancer Center of Wake Forest University
Medical Center Boulevard
Winston-Salem, NC 27157
Phone: (336) 716-7971
Phone: (336) 716-WAKE (9253)
Web site: http://www.wakehealth.edu/
    Comprehensive-Cancer-Center/

Duke Cancer Institute
Duke University Medical Center, Box
    2714, 2424 Erwin Road
Durham, NC 27710
Toll free: (888) 275-3853 (ASK-DUKE)
Web site: http://www.
    dukecancerinstitute.org/

UNC Lineberger Comprehensive Cancer Center
450 West Drive, CB 7295
Chapel Hill, NC 27599
Phone: (919) 966-3036
Toll free: (866) 869-1856
Web site: http://unclineberger.org/

Ohio

Case Comprehensive Cancer Center
Case Western Reserve University,
    11100 Euclid Avenue, Wearn 151

Cleveland, OH 44106
Phone: (216) 844-8797
Web site: http://cancer.case.edu/

The Ohio State University Comprehensive Cancer Center
James Cancer Hospital and Solove Research Institute, 300 West 10th Avenue, Suite 159
Columbus, OH 43210
Phone: (614) 293-5066
Toll free: (800) 293-5066
Web site: http://cancer.osu.edu/Pages/index.aspx

Oregon

Knight Cancer Institute
Oregon Health and Science University, 3181 SW Sam Jackson Park Road
Portland, OR 97239
Phone: (503) 494-1617
Web site: http://www.ohsu.edu/xd/

Pennsylvania

Abramson Cancer Center
University of Pennsylvania, 3400 Spruce Street
Philadelphia, PA 19104
Phone: (215) 615-5858
Toll free: (800) 789-7366 (Referrals)
Web site: http://www.penncancer.org/

Fox Chase Cancer Center
333 Cottman Avenue
Philadelphia, PA 19111
Phone: (215) 728-2570
Toll free: (888) 369-2427 (FOX-CHASE)
Web site: http://www.fccc.edu/

Sidney Kimmel Cancer Center at Thomas Jefferson University
Thomas Jefferson University, 233 South 10th Street
Philadelphia, PA 19107
Phone: (215) 503-5692
Web site: http://www.kcc.tju.edu/

University of Pittsburgh Cancer Institute
5150 Centre Avenue
Pittsburgh, PA 15232
Phone: (412) 647-2811
Web site: http://www.upci.upmc.edu/index.cfm

The Wistar Institute Cancer Center
3601 Spruce Street
Philadelphia, PA 19104

Phone: (215) 898-3700
Web site: http://www.wistar.org/

South Carolina

Hollings Cancer Center
Medical University of South Carolina, 86 Jonathan Lucas Street
Charleston, SC 29425
Phone: (843) 792-0700
Toll free: (800) 424-6872 (424-MUSC)
Web site: http://hcc.musc.edu/

Tennessee

St. Jude Children's Research Hospital
262 Danny Thomas Place
Memphis, TN 38105
Phone: (901) 595-3300
Toll free: (866) 278-5833 (2STJUDE)
Web site: http://www.stjude.org/

Vanderbilt-Ingram Cancer Center
691 Preston Research Building
Nashville, TN 37232
Phone: (615) 936-VICC (8422)
Toll free: (877) 936-VICC (8422)
Web site: http://www.vicc.org/

Texas

Cancer Therapy & Research Center
University of Texas Health Science Center, 7979 Wurzbach Road, Urschel Tower, Room U627
San Antonio, TX 78229
Phone: (210) 450-1000
Toll free: (800) 340-2872
Web site: http://www.ctrc.net/

Dan L. Duncan Cancer Center
Baylor College of Medicine, One Baylor Place, MS BCM305
Houston, TX 77030
Phone: (713) 798-1354
Web site: https://www.bcm.edu/healthcare/care-centers/cancer-center/

Harold C. Simmons Cancer Center
University of Texas Southwestern Medical Center, 2201 Inwood Road
Dallas, TX 75390
Phone: (214) 645-HOPE (4673)
Toll free: (866) 460-HOPE (4673)
Web site: http://www.utswmedicine.org/conditions-specialties/cancer/

The University of Texas MD Anderson Cancer Center
1515 Holcombe Boulevard, Unit 91
Houston, TX 77030
Phone: (713) 792-6161
Toll free: (877) 632-6789 (MDA-6789)
Web site: http://www.mdanderson.org/

Utah

Huntsman Cancer Institute
University of Utah, 2000 Circle of Hope
Salt Lake City, UT 84112
Phone: (801) 585-0303
Toll free: (877) 585-0303
Web site: http://healthcare.utah.edu/huntsmancancerinstitute/

Virginia

Massey Cancer Center
Virginia Commonwealth University, PO Box 980037, 401 College Street
Richmond, VA 23298
Phone: (804) 828-0450
Toll free: (877) 462-7739 (4-MASSEY)
Web site: http://www.massey.vcu.edu/

University of Virginia Cancer Center
6171 West Complex
Charlottesville, VA 22908
Phone: (434) 924-3627
Toll free: (800) 223-9173
Web site: http://www.medicine.virginia.edu/research/research-centers/cancer-center

Washington

Fred Hutchinson/University of Washington Cancer Consortium
PO Box 19024, D1-060
Seattle, WA 98109
Phone: (206) 288-7222
Web site: http://www.fredhutch.org/en.html

Wisconsin

University of Wisconsin Carbone Cancer Center
1111 Highland Avenue, Room 7057
Madison, WI 53705
Phone: (608) 263-8600
Toll free: (800) 622-8922
Web site: http://www.uwhealth.org/uw-carbone-cancer-center/cancer/10252

ORGANIZATIONS: SUPPORT GROUPS, GOVERNMENT AGENCIES, AND RESEARCH GROUPS

The following is an alphabetical compilation of relevant organizations listed in the *Resources* sections of the main body entries. Although the list is comprehensive, it is by no means exhaustive. It is a starting point for gathering further information. Many of the organizations listed provide information for multiple disorders and have links to additional related websites. E-mail addresses and web addresses listed were provided by the associations; Gale, Cengage Learning is not responsible for the accuracy of the addresses or the contents of the websites.

A

AABB (American Association of Blood Banks)
8101 Glenbrook Road
Bethesda, MD 20814-2749
Phone: (301) 907-6977
Fax: (301) 907-6895
E-mail: aabb@aabb.org
Website: http://www.aabb.org/

ABCD (After Breast Cancer Diagnosis)
5775 N. Glen Park Road, Suite 201
Glendale, WI 53209
Phone: (414) 977-1780
Toll-free: (800) 977-4121
E-mail: abcdinc@abcdmentor.org
Website: http://www.
  abcdbreastcancersupport.org/

Academy of Nutrition and Dietetics
120 S. Riverside Plaza, Suite 2000
Chicago, IL 60606-6995
Phone: (312) 899-0040
Toll-free: (800) 877-1600
E-mail: amacmunn@eatright.org
Website: http://www.eatright.org/

Acoustic Neuroma Association
600 Peachtree Parkway, Suite 108
Cumming, GA 30041-6899
Phone: (770) 205-8211
Toll-free: (877) 200-8211
Fax: (770) 205-0239
E-mail: info@anausa.org
Website: https://www.anausa.org/

Acoustic Neuroma Association of Canada
PO Box 193
Buckhorn, Ontario K0L 1J0
Canada
Toll-free: (800) 561-2622
Website: http://www.anac.ca

Action on Bladder Cancer (ABC)
Barley Mow Centre, 10 Barley Mow Passage
London W4 4PH
United Kingdom
E-mail: abc@rightangleuk.com
Website: http://www.
  actiononbladdercancer.org/

Aging With Dignity
PO Box 1661
Tallahassee, FL 32302
Phone: (850) 681-2010
Toll-free: (888) 594-7437
Fax: (850) 681-2481
E-mail: fivewishes@agingwithdignity.
  org
Website: http://www.agingwithdignity.
  org/

Alliance for Cancer Gene Therapy
96 Cummings Point Road
Stamford, CT 06902
Phone: (203) 358-8000
Website: http://www.acgtfoundation.org/

American Academy of Allergy, Asthma & Immunology
555 E. Wells Street, Suite 1100
Milwaukee, WI 53202-3823
Phone: (414) 272-6071
Website: http://www.aaaai.org/

American Academy of Child and Adolescent Psychiatry
3615 Wisconsin Avenue NW
Washington, DC 20016-3007
Phone: (202) 966-7300
Fax: (202) 966-2891
Website: http://www.aacap.org/

American Academy of Dermatology (AAD)
PO Box 4014
Schaumburg, IL 60168
Phone: (847) 240-1280

Toll-free: (866) 503-SKIN
Fax: (847) 240-1859
Website: http://www.aad.org/

American Academy of Facial Plastic and Reconstructive Surgery (AAFPRS)
310 S. Henry Street
Alexandria, VA 22314
Phone: (703) 299-9291
Fax: (703) 299-8898
E-mail: info@aafprs.org
Website: http://www.aafprs.org/

American Academy of Family Physicians (AAFP)
11400 Tomahawk Creek Parkway
Leawood, KS 66211-2680
Phone: (913) 906-6000
Toll-free: (800) 274-2237
Fax: (913) 906-6075
Website: http://www.aafp.org/

American Academy of Hospice and Palliative Medicine (AAHPM)
8735 W. Higgins Road, Suite 300
Chicago, IL 60631
Phone: (847) 375-4712
Fax: (847) 375-6475
E-mail: info@aahpm.org
Website: http://aahpm.org/

American Academy of Neurology
201 Chicago Avenue
Minneapolis, MN 55415
Phone: (612) 928-6000
Toll-free: (800) 879-1960
Fax: (612) 454-2746
E-mail: memberservices@aan.com
Website: http://www.aan.com/

American Academy of Ophthalmology
655 Beach Street
San Francisco, CA 94109
Phone: (415) 561-8500

Fax: (415) 561-8533
Website: http://www.aao.org/

**American Academy of Orthopaedic
Surgeons (AAOS)**
9400 W. Higgens Road
Rosemont, IL 60018-4262
Phone: (847) 823-7186
Fax: (847) 823-8125
E-mail: pemr@aaos.org
Website: http://www.aaos.org/

**American Academy of
Otolaryngology—Head and Neck
Surgery**
1650 Diagonal Road
Alexandria, VA 22314-2857
Phone: (703) 836-4444
Website: http://www.entnet.org/

**American Academy of Pain Medicine
(AAPM)**
8735 W. Higgins Road, Suite 300
Chicago, IL 60631-2738
Phone: (847) 375-4731
Fax: (847) 375-6477
E-mail: info@painmed.org
Website: http://www.painmed.org/

**American Academy of Pediatrics
(AAP)**
141 Northwest Point Boulevard
Elk Grove Village, IL 60007-1098
Phone: (847) 434-4000
Fax: (847) 434-8000
Website: http://www.aap.org/

**American Association for Cancer
Research (AACR)**
615 Chestnut Street, 17th Floor
Philadelphia, PA 19106-4404
Phone: (215) 440-9300
Toll-free: (866) 423-3965
Fax: (215) 440-9313
E-mail: aacr@aacr.org
Website: http://www.aacr.org/Pages/
Home.aspx

**American Association for Clinical
Chemistry**
1850 K Street NW, Suite 625
Washington, DC 20006
Toll-free: (800) 892-1400
Fax: (202) 833-4576
E-mail: custserv@aacc.org
Website: http://www.aacc.org/

**American Association for
Respiratory Care**
9425 N. MacArthur Boulevard, Suite
100
Irving, TX 75063-4706
Phone: (972) 243-2272
E-mail: info@aarc.org
Website: http://www.aarc.org/

**American Association for Thoracic
Surgery**
500 Cummings Center, Suite 4550
Beverly, MA 01915
Phone: (978) 927-8330
Website: http://aats.org/

American Association of Blood Banks
8101 Glenbrook Road
Bethesda, MD 20814-2749
Phone: (301) 907-6977
Fax: (301) 907-6895
Website: http://www.aabb.org/

**American Association of Clinical
Endocrinologists**
245 Riverside Avenue, Suite 200
Jacksonville, FL 32202
Phone: (904) 353-7878
Fax: (904) 353-8185
Website: https://www.aace.com/

**American Association of Neurological
Surgeons**
5550 Meadowbrook Drive
Rolling Meadows, IL 60008-3852
Phone: (847) 378-0500
Toll-free: (888) 566-AANS (2267)
Fax: (847) 378-0600
E-mail: info@aans.org
Website: http://aans.org/

**American Board of Colon and Rectal
Surgery**
20600 Eureka Road, Suite 600
Taylor, MI 48180
Phone: (734) 282-9400
Fax: (734) 282-9402
E-mail: admin@abcrs.org
Website: http://www.abcrs.org/

American Board of Plastic Surgery
7 Penn Center, Suite 400, 1635 Market
Street
Philadelphia, PA 19103-2204
Phone: (215) 587-9322
E-mail: info@abplsurg.org
Website: https://www.abplsurg.org/

American Board of Urology
600 Peter Jefferson Parkway, Suite 150
Charlottesville, VA 22911
Phone: (434) 979-0059
Fax: (434) 979-0266
Website: http://www.abu.org/

**American Brain Tumor Association
(ABTA)**
8550 W. Bryn Mawr Avenue, Suite 550
Chicago, IL 60631
Phone: (773) 577-8750
Toll-free: (800) 886-2282
Fax: (773) 577-8738
E-mail: info@abta.org
Website: http://www.abta.org/

American Cancer Society (ACS)
250 Williams Street NW
Atlanta, GA 30303
Toll-free: (800) 227-2345
Website: http://www.cancer.org/

**American Childhood Cancer
Organization (ACCO; formerly
Candlelighters)**
PO Box 498
Kensington, MD 20895-0498
Phone: (301) 962-3520
Toll-free: (855) 858-2226
Fax: (301) 962-3521
Website: http://www.acco.org/

American Chronic Pain Association
PO Box 850
Rocklin, CA 95677
Toll-free: (800) 533-3231
Fax: (916) 632-3208
E-mail: ACPA@theacpa.org
Website: http://www.theacpa.org/

American College of Chest Physicians
2595 Patriot Boulevard
Glenview, IL 60062-2348
Phone: (224) 521-9800
Toll-free: (800) 343-2227
Fax: (224) 521-9801
Website: http://www.chestnet.org/

**American College of Clinical
Pharmacy (ACCP)**
13000 W. 87th Street Parkway
Lenexa, KS 66215-4530
Phone: (913) 492-3311
Fax: (913) 492-0088
E-mail: accp@accp.com
Website: http://www.accp.com/index.
aspx

**American College of Emergency
Physicians**
1125 Executive Circle
Irving, TX 75038-2522
Phone: (972) 550-0911
Toll-free: (800) 798-1822
Fax: (972) 580-2816
E-mail: membership@acep.org
Website: http://www.acep.org/

**American College of
Gastroenterology (ACG)**
6400 Goldsboro Road, Suite 200
Bethesda, MD 20817
Phone: (301) 263-9000
E-mail: info@acg.gi.org
Website: http://gi.org/

**American College of Medical
Genetics (ACMG)**
7220 Wisconsin Avenue, Suite 300
Bethesda, MD 20814
Phone: (301) 718-9603
Fax: (301) 718-9604

E-mail: acmg@acmg.net
Website: https://www.acmg.net

American College of Mohs Surgery (ACMS)
555 E. Wells Street, Suite 1100
Milwaukee, WI 53202
Phone: (414) 347-1103
Toll-free: (800) 500-7224
E-mail: info@mohscollege.org
Website: http://www.mohscollege.org/

American College of Nuclear Medicine
1850 Samuel Morse Drive
Reston, VA 20190-5316
Phone: (703) 326-1190
Fax: (703) 708-9015
Website: http://www.acnmonline.org/

American College of Physicians
190 N. Independence Mall West
Philadelphia, PA 19106-1572
Phone: (215) 351-2400
Toll-free: (800) 523-1546
Website: http://www.acponline.org/

American College of Radiology (ACR)
1891 Preston White Drive
Reston, VA 20191
Phone: (703) 648-8900
E-mail: info@acr.org
Website: http://www.acr.org/

American College of Surgeons
633 N. Saint Clair Street
Chicago, IL 60611-3211
Phone: (312) 202-5000
Toll-free: (800) 621-4111
Fax: (312) 202-5001
E-mail: postmaster@facs.org
Website: http://www.facs.org/

American Congress of Obstetricians and Gynecologists (ACOG)
409 12th Street SW
Washington, DC 20024-2188
Phone: (202) 638-5577
Toll-free: (800) 673-8444
E-mail: resources@acog.org
Website: http://www.acog.org/

American Dental Association (ADA)
211 E. Chicago Avenue
Chicago, IL 60611-2678
Phone: (312) 440-2500
Website: http://www.ada.org/en

American Diabetes Association
1701 N. Beauregard Street
Alexandria, VA 22311
Toll-free: (800) DIABETES (342-2383)
E-mail: AskADA@diabetes.org
Website: http://www.diabetes.org/

American Gastroenterological Association
4930 Del Ray Avenue
Bethesda, MD 20814
Phone: (301) 654-2055
Fax: (301) 654-5920
E-mail: member@gastro.org
Website: http://www.gastro.org/

American Heart Association
7272 Greenville Avenue
Dallas, TX 75231
Toll-free: (800) AHA-USA-1 (242-8721)
Website: http://www.hcart.org/

American Institute for Cancer Research
1759 R Street NW
Washington, DC 20009
Phone: (202) 328-7744
Toll-free: (800) 843-8114
Fax: (202) 328-7226
E-mail: aicrweb@aicr.org
Website: http://www.aicr.org/

American Institute of Stress
6387B Camp Bowie Boulevard #334
Fort Worth, TX 76116
Phone: (682) 239-6823
Fax: (817) 394-0593
E-mail: info@stress.org
Website: http://www.stress.org/

American Joint Committee on Cancer (AJCC)
633 N. Saint Clair Street
Chicago, IL 60611-3211
Phone: (312) 202-5205
E-mail: ajcc@facs.org
Website: http://www.cancerstaging.org/

American Liver Foundation
39 Broadway, Suite 2700
New York, NY 10005
Phone: (212) 668-1000
Toll-free: (800) GO-LIVER
Fax: (212) 483-8179
Website: http://www.liverfoundation.org/

American Lung Association
55 W. Wacker Drive, Suite 1150
Chicago, IL 60601
Toll-free: (800) LUNG-USA (586-4872)
Fax: (202) 452-1805
Website: http://www.lung.org/

American Medical Association
330 N. Wabash Avenue
Chicago, IL 60654
Toll-free: (800) 621-8335
Website: http://www.ama-assn.org/ama

American Osteopathic Colleges of Otolaryngology—Head and Neck Surgery
4764 Fishburg Road, Suite F
Huber Heights, OH 45424
Toll-free: (800) 455-9404
E-mail: info@aocoohns.org
Website: http://www.aocoohns.org/

American Pain Foundation
201 N. Charles Street, Suite 710
Baltimore, MD 21201-4111
Toll-free: (888) 615-PAIN (7246)
E-mail: info@painfoundation.org
Website: http://www.painfoundation.org/

American Pain Society
8735 W. Higgins Road, Suite 300
Chicago, IL 60631
Toll-free: (847) 375-4715
E-mail: info@americanpainsociety.org
Website: http://www.americanpainsociety.org/

American Physical Therapy Association
1111 N. Fairfax Street
Alexandria, VA 22314-1488
Phone: (703) 684-2782
Toll-free: (800) 999-APTA (2782)
Fax: (703) 684-7343
Website: http://www.apta.org/

American Prostate Society
10 E. Lee Street, Suite 1504
Baltimore, MD 21202
Phone: (410) 837-3735
Fax: (410) 837-8510
E-mail: info@americanprostatesociety.com
Website: http://americanprostatesociety.com/

American Psychiatric Association
1000 Wilson Boulevard, Suite 1825
Arlington, VA 22209
Phone: (703) 907-7300
Toll-free: (888) 35-PSYCH (77924)
E-mail: apa@psych.org
Website: http://www.psychiatry.org/

American Psychosocial Oncology Society
154 Hansen Road, Suite 201
Charlottesville, VA 22811
Phone: (434) 293-5350
Toll-free: (866) APOS-4-HELP (276-7443)
Fax: (434) 977-1856
E-mail: info@apos-society.org
Website: http://www.apos-society.org/

American Red Cross
2025 E Street NW
Washington, DC 20006

Phone: (202) 303-4498
Toll-free: (800) RED CROSS (733-2767)
Website: http://www.redcross.org/

American Sexual Health Association
PO Box 13827
Research Triangle Park, NC 27709
Phone: (919) 361-8400
Fax: (919) 361-8425
E-mail: info@ashasexualhealth.org
Website: http://www.ashasexualhealth.org/

American Social Health Association
PO Box 13827
Research Triangle Park, NC 27709
Phone: (919) 361-8400
Toll-free: (800) 227-8922
Fax: (919) 361-8425
Website: http://www.ashastd.org/

American Society for Aesthetic Plastic Surgery (ASAPS)
11262 Monarch Street
Garden Grove, CA 92841
Phone: (562) 799-2356
Toll-free: (800) 364-2147
Fax: (562) 799-1098
E-mail: asaps@surgery.org
Website: http://www.surgery.org/

American Society for Blood and Marrow Transplantation (ASBMT)
85 W. Algonquin Road, Suite 550
Arlington Heights, IL 60005
Phone: (847) 427-0224
Fax: (847) 427-9656
E-mail: mail@asbmt.org
Website: http://asbmt.org/

American Society for Dermatologic Surgery
5550 Meadowbrook Drive, Suite 120
Rolling Meadows, IL 60008
Phone: (847) 956-0900
Website: http://www.asds.net/

American Society for Gastrointestinal Endoscopy
3300 Woodcreek Drive
Downers Grove, IL 60515
Phone: (630) 573-06515
Toll-free: (866) 353-ASGE (2743)
Fax: (630) 963-8332
E-mail: info@asge.org
Website: http://www.asge.org/

American Society for Mohs Surgery
6475 E. Pacific Coast Highway, Box 700
Long Beach, CA 90803-4201
Phone: (714) 379-6262
Toll-free: (800) 616-ASMS (2767)
Fax: (714) 379-6272

E-mail: info@mohssurgery.org
Website: http://www.mohssurgery.org/

American Society for Nutrition
9650 Rockville Pike
Bethesda, MD 20814
Phone: (301) 634-7050
Fax: (301) 634-7894
Website: http://www.nutrition.org/

American Society for Parenteral and Enteral Nutrition
8630 Fenton Street, Suite 412
Silver Spring, MD 20910
Phone: (301) 587-6315
Toll-free: (800) 727-4567
E-mail: aspen@nutr.org
Website: https://www.nutritioncare.org/

American Society for Pharmacology and Experimental Therapeutics
9650 Rockville Pike
Bethesda, MD 20814-3995
Phone: (301) 634-7060
Fax: (301) 634-7061
Website: http://www.aspet.org/

American Society for Radiation Oncology
8280 Willow Oaks Corporate Drive, Suite 500
Fairfax, VA 22031
Phone: (703) 502-1550
Toll-free: (800) 962-7876
Fax: (703) 502-7852
Website: http://www.astro.org/

American Society of Clinical Oncology (ASCO)
2318 Mill Road, Suite 800
Alexandria, VA 22314
Phone: (571) 483-1300
Toll-free: (888) 651-3038
Fax: (571) 366-9537
E-mail: contactus@cancer.net
Website: http://www.asco.org/

American Society of Colon and Rectal Surgeons
85 W. Algonquin Road, Suite 550
Arlington Heights, IL 60005
Phone: (847) 290-9184
Fax: (847) 290-9203
E-mail: ascrs@fascrs.org
Website: http://www.fascrs.org/

American Society of Gene & Cell Therapy
555 E. Wells Street, Suite 1100
Milwaukee, WI 53202
Phone: (414) 278-1341
Fax: (414) 276-3349
E-mail: info@asgct.org
Website: http://www.asgct.org/

American Society of Hematology (ASH)
2021 L Street NW, Suite 900
Washington, DC 20036
Phone: (202) 776-0544
Fax: (202) 776-0545
Website: http://www.hematology.org/

American Society of Plastic Surgeons
444 E. Algonquin Road
Arlington Heights, IL 60005
Website: http://www.plasticsurgery.org/

American Society of Radiologic Technologists (ASRT)
15000 Central Avenue SE
Albuquerque, NM 87123-3909
Phone: (505) 298-4500
Toll-free: (800) 444-2778
Fax: (505) 298-5063
E-mail: memberservices@asrt.org
Website: http://www.asrt.org/

American Thoracic Society
25 Broadway
New York, NY 10004
Phone: (212) 315-8600
Fax: (212) 315-6498
E-mail: atsinfo@thoracic.org
Website: http://www.thoracic.org/

American Thyroid Association
6066 Leesburg Pike, Suite 550
Falls Church, VA 22041
Phone: (703) 998-8890
Fax: (703) 998-8893
E-mail: thyroid@thyroid.org
Website: http://www.thyroid.org/

American Urological Association (AUA)
1000 Corporate Boulevard
Linthicum, MD 21090
Toll-free: (866) RING-AUA (746-4282)
Phone: (410) 689-3700
Website: http://www.auanet.org/

Americans for Nonsmokers' Rights
2530 San Pablo Avenue, Suite J
Berkeley, CA 94702
Phone: (510) 841-3032
Website: http://www.no-smoke.org/

America's Blood Centers
725 15th Street NW, Suite 700
Washington, DC 20005
Phone: (202) 393-5725
Toll-free: (888) USBLOOD (872-5663)
Fax: (202) 393-1282
Website: http://www.americasblood.org/

Amputee Coalition
9303 Center Street, Suite 100
Manassas, VA 20110

Toll-free: (888) 267-5669
Website: https://www.amputee-
coalition.org/

**Aplastic Anemia and MDS
International Foundation**
100 Park Avenue, Suite 108
Rockville, MD 20850
Phone: (301) 279-7202
Toll-free: (800) 747-2820
E-mail: help@aamds.org
Website: http://www.aamds.org/

**ASHP (formerly the American
Society of Health-System
Pharmacists)**
7272 Wisconsin Avenue
Bethesda, MD 20814
Phone: (301) 664-8700
Toll-free: (866) 279-0681
E-mail: custserv@ashp.org
Website: http://www.ashp.org/

**Association for Clinical Pastoral
Education (ACPE)**
One West Court Square, Suite 325
Decatur, GA 30030
Phone: (404) 320-1472
Fax: (404) 320-0849
E-mail: acpe@acpe.edu
Website: http://www.acpe.edu/

**Association of periOperative
Registered Nurses (AORN)**
2170 S. Parker Road, Suite 400
Denver, CO 80231-5711
Phone: (303) 755-6300
Toll-free: (800) 755-2676
Fax: (800) 847-0045
E-mail: custsvc@aorn.org
Website: http://www.aorn.org/

**Asthma and Allergy Foundation of
America**
8201 Corporate Drive, Suite 1000
Landover, MD 20785
Toll-free: (800) 7-ASTHMA (727-8462)
E-mail: info@aafa.org
Website: http://aafa.org/

AVERT
4 Brighton Road
Horsham, West Sussex RH13 5BA
United Kingdom
Phone: +44 (0)1403 210202
E-mail: info@avert.org
Website: http://www.avert.org/

 B

**BMT InfoNet (Blood and Marrow
Transplant Information Network)**
2310 Skokie Valley Road, Suite 104
Highland Park, IL 60035

Phone: (847) 433-3313
Toll-free: (888) 597-7674
Fax: (847) 433-4599
E-mail: help@bmtinfonet.org
Website: http://www.bmtinfonet.org/

Bone and Cancer Foundation
PO Box 287452
New York, NY 10128-0025
E-mail: bcfdn@aol.com
Website: http://www.boneandcancer
foundation.org/

Bone Marrow Donors Worldwide
Plesmanlaan 1-b
2333 BZ Leiden
The Netherlands
Phone: +31 71 5685300
Fax: +31 71 5210457
E-mail: BMDW@Europdonor.NL
Website: http://www.bmdw.org/

Breakthrough Breast Cancer
Weston House, 246 High Holborn
London WC1V 7EX
England
Phone: 020 7025 2400
Toll-free: 08080 100 200
Fax: 020 7025 2401
E-mail: info@breakthrough.org.uk
Website: http://breakthrough.org.uk/

Breastcancer.org
7 E. Lancaster Avenue, 3rd Floor
Ardmore, PA 19003
Phone: (610) 642-6550
Fax: (610) 642-6559
Website: http://www.breastcancer.org/

Burkitt's Lymphoma Society
E-mail: admin@burkittslymphoma.org
Website: http://
burkittslymphomasociety.com/

C

**Cancer Center at Walter Reed
Bethesda**
Building 19 (America), 8901 Wisconsin
Avenue
Bethesda, MD 20889-5600
Phone: (301) 295-4000
Toll-free: (800) 526-7101
E-mail: WRNMMC.
CancerCenter@health.mil
Website: http://www.wrnmmc.capmed.
mil/CancerCenter/SitePages/Home.aspx

**Cancer Research and Prevention
Foundation**
1600 Duke Street, Suite 500
Alexandria, VA 22314
Phone: (703) 836-4412
Toll-free: (800) 227-2732

E-mail: info@preventcancer.org
Website: http://www.preventcancer.org/

Cancer Research Institute
55 Broadway Suite 1802
New York, NY 10006
Toll-free: (800) 992-2623
Website: http://www.cancerresearch.org/

Cancer Support Community
1050 17th Street NW, Suite 500
Washington, DC 20036
Phone: (202) 659-9709
Toll-free: (888) 659-9709
Website: http://www.
cancersupportcommunity.org/

Cancer Survivors Network
Website: http://csn.cancer.org/

Cancer Treatment Centers of America
6000 Broken Sound Parkway NW
Boca Raton, FL 33487
Toll-free: (800) 615-3055
Website: http://www.cancercenter.com/

Cancer*Care*
275 Seventh Avenue
New York, NY 10001
Toll-free: (800) 813-HOPE (4673)
E-mail: info@cancercare.org
Website: http://www.cancercare.org/

**Candlelighters Childhood Cancer
Family Alliance**
8323 Southwest Freeway, Suite 435
Houston, TX 77074
Phone: (713) 270-4700
Fax: (713) 270-9802
Website: https://www.candle.org/

Carcinoid Cancer Foundation
333 Mamaroneck Avenue No. 492
White Plains, NY 10605
Toll-free: (888) 722-3132
Website: http://www.carcinoid.org/

**Cardiovascular and Interventional
Radiological Society of Europe
(CIRSE)**
Neutorgasse 9/6
1010 Vienna
Austria
Phone: +43 1 904 2003
Fax: +43 1 904 2003 30
E-mail: info@cirse.org
Website: http://www.cirse.org/

**Caregiver Action Network (CAN;
formerly the National Family
Caregivers Association)**
2000 M Street NW, Suite 400
Washington, DC 20036
Phone: (202) 772-5050
E-mail: info@caregiveraction.org
Website: http://www.caregiveraction.org/

Celgene Corporation
86 Morris Avenue
Summit, NJ 07901
Phone: (908) 673-9000
Toll-free: (888) 423-5436
Website: http://www.celgene.com/

Center for Cancer Research (CCR), National Cancer Institute (NCI)
Building 31, Room 3A11, 31 Center Drive
Bethesda, MD 20892
Phone: (301) 496-4345
E-mail: NCICCRInfoRequests@mail. nih.gov
Website: https://ccr.cancer.gov/home

Center to Advance Palliative Care (CAPC)
55 W. 125th Street, 13th Floor, Suite 1302
New York, NY 10027
Phone: (212) 201-2670
Website: http://www.capc.org/

Centers for Disease Control and Prevention (CDC), Division of Cancer Prevention and Control
c/o CDC Warehouse, 3719 N. Peachtree Road, Building 100 MS F-76
Chamblee, GA 30341
Toll-free: (800) 232-4636
Website: http://www.cdc.gov/cancer/ index.htm

Childhood Brain Tumor Foundation
20312 Watkins Meadow Drive
Germantown, MD 20867
Phone: (301) 515-2900
Toll-free: (877) 217-4166
E-mail: cbtf@childhoodbraintumor.org
Website: http://www. childhoodbraintumor.org/

Childhood Cancer Survivor Study
Street Jude Children's Research Hospital, Department of Epidemiology, Mail Stop 735, 262 Danny Thomas Place
Memphis, TN 38105-3678
Toll-free: (800) 775-2167
E-mail: ccss@stjude.org
Website: https://ccss.stjude.org/

Children's Brain Tumor Foundation
274 Madison Avenue, Suite 1004
New York, NY 10016
Toll-free: (866) 228-4673
Website: http://www.cbtf.org/

Children's Cancer and Blood Foundation
333 E. 38th Street, Suite 830
New York, NY 10016
Phone: (212) 297-4336
Fax: (212) 297-4340

E-mail: info@childrenscbf.org
Website: http://www.childrenscbf.org/

Children's Craniofacial Association
13140 Coit Road, Suite 517
Dallas, TX 75240
Phone: (214) 570-9099
Toll-free: (800) 535-3643
Fax: (214) 5708811
E-mail: contactCCA@ccakids.com
Website: http://www.ccakids.com/

Children's Oncology Group (COG)
222 E. Huntington Drive, Suite 100
Monrovia, CA 91016
Phone: (626) 447-0064
Fax: (626) 445-4334
E-mail: HelpDesk@childrenson cologygroup.org
Website: http://www.children soncologygroup.org/

Children's Tumor Foundation
120 Wall Street, 16th Floor
New York, NY 10005-3904
Phone: (212) 344-6633
E-mail: info@ctf.org
Website: http://www.ctf.org/

Chordoma Foundation
PO Box 2127
Durham, NC 27702
Phone: (919) 809-6779
Fax: (866) 367-3910
Website: http://www. chordomafoundation.org/

CIBMTR (Center for International Blood and Marrow Transplant Research)
Froedtert and the Medical College of Wisconsin Clinical Cancer Center, 9200 W. Wisconsin Avenue, Suite C5500
Milwaukee, WI 53226
Phone: (414) 805-0700
Fax: (414) 805-0714
E-mail: contactus@cibmtr.org
Website: http://www.cibmtr.org/

ClinicalTrials.gov., a service of the U.S. National Institutes of Health
8600 Rockville Pike
Bethesda, MD 20894
Website: http://clinicaltrials.gov/

Coalition of Cancer Cooperative Groups
1818 Market Street, Suite 1100
Philadelphia, PA 19103
Phone: (215) 789-3600
Fax: (215) 789-3655
E-mail: info@cancertrialshelp.org
Website: http://www.cancertrialshelp. org/

Colon Cancer Alliance
1025 Vermont Avenue NW, Suite 1066
Washington, DC 20005
Phone: (202) 628-0123
Toll-free: (877) 422-2030
Fax: (866) 304-9075
Website: http://ccalliance.org/

Colostomy Association (UK)
Enterprise House, 95 London Street
Reading, Berkshire RG1 4QA
United Kingdom
Phone: +44 118 939 1537
Toll-free: (800) 328-4257
Website: http://www. colostomyassociation.org.uk/

Crohn's & Colitis Foundation of America
386 Third Avenue, Suite 510
New York, NY 10017
Toll-free: (800) 932-2423
E-mail: info@ccfa.org
Website: http://www.ccfa.org/

CureSearch for Children's Cancer
4600 East-West Highway, Suite 600
Bethesda, MD 20814
Toll-free: (800) 458-6223
Fax: (301) 718-0047
E-mail: info@curesearch.org
Website: http://www.curesearch.org/

Cutaneous Lymphoma Foundation
PO Box 374
Birmingham, MI 48012
Phone: (248) 644-9014
Website: http://www.clfoundation.org/

D

Delete Blood Cancer
100 Broadway, 6th Floor
New York, NY 10005
Phone: (212) 209-6700
E-mail: info@dkmsamericas.org
Website: https://www. deletebloodcancer.org/

E

European Medicines Agency (EMEA)
30 Churchill Place Canary Wharf
London E14 5EU
United Kingdom
Phone: +44 20 3660 6000
Fax: +44 20 3660 5555
Website: http://www.ema.europa.eu/

F

Family Caregiver Alliance (FCA)
785 Market Street, Suite 750
San Francisco, CA 94103
Toll-free: (800) 445-8106
Website: https://www.caregiver.org/

Fanconi Anemia Research Fund, Inc.
1801 Willamette Street, Suite 200
Eugene, OR 97401
Phone: (541) 687-4658
Toll-free: 888-FANCONI (326-2664)
E-mail: info@fanconi.org
Website: http://www.fanconi.org/

FORCE: Facing Our Risk of Cancer Empowered
16057 Tampa Palms Boulevard W., PMB #373
Tampa, FL 33647
Toll-free: (866) 288-RISK (7475)
Fax: (954) 827-2200
E-mail: info@facingourrisk.org
Website: http://www.facingourrisk.org/

Foundation for Women's Cancer
230 W. Monroe, Suite 2528
Chicago, IL 60606-4902
Phone: (312) 578-1439
Toll-free: (800) 444-4441
Fax: (312) 578-9769
E-mail: info@foundationforwomens cancer.org
Website: http://www.foundationfor womenscancer.org/

G

Genetic Alliance, Inc.
4301 Connecticut Avenue NW, Suite 404
Washington, DC 20008-2369
Phone: (202) 966-5557
E-mail: info@geneticalliance.org
Website: http://www.geneticalliance. org/

GIST Support International
12 Bomaca Drive
Doylestown, PA 18901
Phone: (215) 340-9374
E-mail: gsi@gistsupport.org
Website: http://www.gistsupport.org/

Gynecologic Cancer Foundation
230 Monroe, Suite 2528
Chicago, IL 60606
Phone: (312) 578-1439
Toll-free: (800) 444-4441

Website: http://www. foundationforwomenscancer.org/

H

Hairy Cell Leukemia Foundation
790 Estate Drive, Suite 180
Deerfield, IL 60015
Phone: (224) 355-7201
E-mail: info@hairycellleukemia.org
Website: http://www.hairycellleukemia. org/

Harvard School of Public Health
677 Huntington Avenue
Boston, MA 02115
Phone: (617) 495-1000
Website: http://www.hsph.harvard.edu/

HealthCare Chaplaincy Network
65 Broadway, 12th Floor
New York, NY 10006-2503
Phone: (212) 644-1111
E-mail: comm@healthcarechaplaincy. org
Website: http://www. healthcarechaplaincy.org/

HealthyWomen
157 Broad Street, Suite 200
Red Bank, NJ 07701
Toll-free: (877) 986-9472
Fax: (732) 530-3347
E-mail: info@healthywomen.org
Website: http://www.healthywomen. org/

Hope for Two . . . The Pregnant with Cancer Network
PO Box 253
Amherst, NY 14226
Toll-free: (800) 743-4471
E-mail: info@hopefortwo.org
Website: http://www. pregnantwithcancer.org/

Hospice Foundation of America
1710 Rhode Island Avenue NW, Suite 400
Washington, DC 20036
Phone: (202) 457-5811
Toll-free: (800) 854-3402
Website: http://hospicefoundation.org/

I

Infectious Diseases Society of America (IDSA)
1300 Wilson Boulevard, Suite 300
Arlington, VA 22209
Phone: (703) 299-0200
Fax: (703) 299-0204

Website: http://www.idsociety.org/ Index.aspx

International Agency for Research on Cancer (IARC)
150 Cours Albert Thomas
69372, Lyon CEDEX 08
France
Phone: +33 0 4 72 73 84 85
Website: http://www.iarc.fr/

International Association of Laryngectomees (IAL)
925B Peachtree Street NE, Suite 316
Atlanta, GA 30309
Phone: (866) 425-3678
Website: http://www.theial.com/

International Association of Living Organ Donors
Website: http://www. livingdonorsonline.org/

International Castleman's Disease Organization
Santa Fe, NM 87508
Website: http://www.castlemans.org/

International Clinical Hyperthermia Society (ICHS)
12099 W. Washington Boulevard #304
Los Angeles, CA 90066
Phone: (310) 398-0013
E-mail: inforequest@hyperthermia-ichs. org
Website: http://www.hyperthermia-ichs. org/

International Federation of Gynecology and Obstetrics (FIGO)
FIGO House, Suite 3, Waterloo Court, 10 Theed Street
London SE1 8ST
United Kingdom
Phone: +44 20 7928 1166
Website: http://www.figo.org/

International Foundation for Functional Gastrointestinal Disorders
700 W. Virginia Street, #201
Milwaukee, WI 53204
Phone: (414) 964-1799
Toll-free: (888) 964-2001
Fax: (414) 964-7176
E-mail: iffgd@iffgd.org
Website: http://www.iffgd.org/

International Meningioma Society
E-mail: info@meningiomasociety.org
Website: http://meningiomasociety.org/

International Myeloma Foundation (IMF)
12650 Riverside Drive, Suite 206

North Hollywood, CA 91607-3421
Toll-free: (800) 452-CURE
Website: http://www.myeloma.org/

**International RadioSurgery
Association (IRSA)**
PO Box 5186
Harrisburg, PA 17110
Phone: (717) 260-9808
Website: http://www.irsa.org/

**International Society for Magnetic
Resonance in Medicine**
2030 Addison Street, 7th Floor
Berkeley, CA 94704
Phone: (510) 841-1899
Fax: (510) 841-2340
E-mail: info@ismrm.org
Website: http://www.ismrm.org/

**International Society of Limb Salvage
(ISOLS)**
c/o Vienna Medical Academy, Alser
    Strasse 4
Vienna 1090
Austria
Phone: +43 1 405 13 83 21
E-mail: office@isols.info
Website: http://isols.info/web/

**International Society of Travel
Medicine (ISTM)**
315 W. Ponce de Leon Avenue,
    Suite 245
Decatur, GA 30030
Phone: (404) 373-8282
Fax: (404) 373-8283
E-mail: istm@istm.org
Website: http://www.istm.org/

**International Waldenstrom's
Macroglobulinemia Foundation**
6144 Clark Center Avenue
Sarasota, FL 34238
Phone: (941) 927-4963
Fax: (941) 927-4467
Website: http://www.iwmf.com/

Interstitial Cystitis Association (ICA)
7918 Jones Branch Drive, Suite 300
McLean, VA 22102
Phone: (703) 442-2070
Fax: (703) 506-3266
E-mail: ICAmail@ichelp.org
Website: http://www.ichelp.org/

Joint Commission
One Renaissance Boulevard
Oakbrook Terrace, IL 60181
Phone: (630) 792-5800
Fax: (630) 792-5005

Website: http://www.jointcommission.
    org/

Kidney Cancer Association
PO Box 96503
Washington, DC 20090
Phone: (202) 280-2371
Website: http://www.kidneycancer.
    org/

Kushi Institute
198 Leland Road
Becket, MA 01223
Phone: (413) 623-5741
Toll-free: (800) 975-8744
Website: http://www.kushiinstitute.
    org/

Leukemia & Lymphoma Society
1311 Mamaroneck Avenue, Suite 310
White Plains, NY 10605
Phone: (914) 949-5213
Toll-free: (800) 955-4572
Website: https://www.lls.org/

**Linus Pauling Institute, Oregon State
University**
307 Linus Pauling Science Center
Corvallis, OR 97331
Phone: (541) 737-5075
Fax: (541) 737-5077
E-mail: lpi@oregonstate.edu
Website: http://lpi.oregonstate.edu/
    infocenter

Look Good . . . Feel Better (LGFB)
Toll-free: (800) 395-LOOK (5665)
Website: http://lookgoodfeelbetter.
    org/

Lung Cancer Alliance
888 16th Street NW, Suite 150
Washington, DC 20006
Phone: (202) 463-2080
Toll-free: (800) 298-2436
E-mail: info@lungcanceralliance.org
Website: http://www.
    lungcanceralliance.org/

Lymphoma Research Foundation
115 Broadway, Suite 1301
New York, NY 10006
Phone: (212) 349-2910
Toll-free: (800) 500-9976
Fax: (212) 349-2886
E-mail: LRF@lymphoma.org
Website: http://www.lymphoma.org/

**March of Dimes Birth Defects
Foundation**
1275 Mamaroneck Avenue
White Plains, NY 10605
Phone: (914) 997-4488
Website: http://www.marchofdimes.
    org/

MDS Foundation
4573 S. Broad Street, Suite 150
Yardville, NJ 08620
Toll-free: (800) MDS-0839
Website: http://www.mds-foundation.
    org/

Melanoma Research Foundation
1411 K Street NW, Suite 800
Washington, DC 20005
Phone: (202) 347-9675
Toll-free: (800) 673-1290
Fax: (202) 347-9678
E-mail: info@melanoma.org
Website: http://www.melanoma.org/

Men's Health Network
PO Box 75972
Washington, DC 20013
Phone: (202) 543-MHN-1 (6461
E-mail: info@menshealthnetwork.org
Website: http://www.
    menshealthnetwork.org/

**MPN (Myeloproliferative
Neoplasms)-Net**
Website: http://mpdinfo.org/xmpd-net.
    php

**Multinational Association of
Supportive Care in Cancer
(MASCC)**
c/o Åge Schultz, Herredsvejen 2
Hillerød, Denmark, DK-3400
Phone: +45 48 20-7022
Fax: +45 48 21-7022
E-mail: aschultz@mascc.org
Website: http://www.mascc.org/

**Multiple Myeloma Research
Foundation**
383 Main Avenue, 5th Floor
Norwalk, CT 06851
Phone: (203) 229-0464
E-mail: info@themmrf.org
Website: http://www.themmrf.org/

**National Adrenal Diseases
Foundation**
505 Northern Boulevard
Great Neck, NY 11021

Phone: (516) 487-4992
E-mail: nadfsupport@nadf.us
Website: http://www.nadf.us/

National Alliance on Mental Health
3803 N. Fairfax Drive, Suite 100
Arlington, VA 22203
Phone: (703) 524-7600
Toll-free: (800) 950-NAMI
Fax: (703) 524-9094
Website: http://www.nami.org/

National Association for Continence (NAFC)
Toll-free: (800) BLADDER (252-3337)
Website: http://www.nafc.org/

National Association for Home Care & Hospice
228 Seventh Street SE
Washington, DC 20003
Phone: (202) 547-7424
Fax: (202) 547-3540
Website: http://www.nahc.org/

National Association for Proton Therapy
1301 Highland Drive
Silver Spring, MD 20910
Phone: (301) 587-20910
Website: http://www.proton-therapy.org/

National Bone Marrow Donor Program
3001 Broadway Street NE, Suite 100
Minneapolis, MN 55413-1753
Toll-free: (800) 627-7692
Website: http://bethematch.org/

National Bone Marrow Transplant Link
20411 W. 12 Mile Road, Suite 108
Southfield, MI 48076
Phone: (248) 358-1886
Toll-free: (800) LINK-BMT (546-5268)
Fax: (248) 358-1889
E-mail: info@nbmtlink.org
Website: http://nbmtlink.org/

National Brain Tumor Society
55 Chapel Street, Suite 200
Newton, MA 02458
Phone: (617) 924-9997
Website: http://www.braintumor.org/

National Breast Cancer Coalition
1010 Vermont Avenue, NW Suite 900
Washington, DC 20005
Phone: (202) 296-7477
Toll-free: (800) 622-2838
Fax: (202) 265-6854
Website: http://www.
    breastcancerdeadline2020.org/

National Breast Cancer Foundation
2600 Network Boulevard, Suite 300

Frisco, TX 75034
Website: http://www.
    nationalbreastcancer.org/

National Cancer Institute
BG 9609 MSC 9760, 9609 Medical
    Center Drive
Bethesda, MD 20892-9760
Toll-free: (800) 4-CANCER (422-6237)
Website: http://www.cancer.gov/

National Cancer Institute (NCI) Office of Cancer Survivorship
BG 9609 MSC 9760, 9609 Medical
    Center Drive
Bethesda, MD 20892-9760
Phone: (240) 276-6690
Website: http://cancercontrol.cancer.
    gov/ocs/index.html

National Center for Complementary and Alternative Medicine (NCCAM)
9000 Rockville Pike
Bethesda, MD 20892
Toll-free: (888) 644-6226
Website: http://nccam.nih.gov/

National Cervical Cancer Coalition (NCCC)
PO Box 13827
Research Triangle Park, NC 27709
Toll-free: (800) 685-5531
Website: http://www.nccc-online.org/

National Children's Cancer Society (NCCS)
500 N. Broadway, Suite 800
Street Louis, MO 63102
Phone: (314) 241-1600
Website: http://www.thenccs.org/

National Coalition for Cancer Survivorship (NCCS)
1010 Wayne Avenue, Suite 315
Silver Spring, MD 20910
Toll-free: (877) 622-7937
E-mail: info@canceradvocacy.org
Website: http://www.canceradvocacy.
    org/

National Comprehensive Cancer Network (NCCN)
275 Commerce Drive, Suite 300
Fort Washington, PA 19034
Phone: (215) 690-0300
Fax: (215) 690-0280
Website: http://www.nccn.org/

National Digestive Diseases Information Clearinghouse (NDDIC)
2 Information Way
Bethesda, MD 20892-3570
Toll-free: (800) 891-5389
TTY: (866) 569-1162

Fax: (703) 738-4929
E-mail: info@niddk.nih.gov
Website: http://digestive.niddk.nih.
    gov/

National Endocrine and Metabolic Diseases Information Service
6 Information Way
Bethesda, MD 20892-3569
Toll-free: (888) 828-0904
TTY: (866) 569-1162
Fax: (703) 738-4929
E-mail: endoandmeta@info.niddk.nih.
    gov
Website: http://www.endocrine.niddk.
    nih.gov/

National Eye Institute Information Office
31 Center Drive, MSC 2510
Bethesda, MD 20992-3655
Phone: (301) 496-5248
E-mail: 2020@nei.nih.gov
Website: http://www.nei.nih.gov/

National Heart, Lung, and Blood Institute
31 Center Drive MSC 2486, Building
    31, Rm. 5A52
Bethesda, MD 20892
Phone: (301) 592-8573
E-mail: nhlbiinfo@nhlbi.nih.gov
Website: http://www.nhlbi.nih.gov/

National Hemophilia Foundation
116 W. 32nd Street, 11th Floor
New York, NY 10001
Phone: (212) 328-3700
Fax: (212) 328-3777
Website: https://www.hemophilia.org/

National Hospice and Palliative Care Organization (NHPCO)
1731 King Street, Suite 100
Alexandria, VA 22314
Phone: (703) 837-1500
Fax: (703) 837-1233
Website: http://www.nhpco.org/

National Human Genome Research Institute (NHGRI)
National Institutes of Health,
    Building 31, Room 4B09, 31
    Center Drive, MSC 2152, 9000
    Rockville Pike
Bethesda, MD 20892-2152
Phone: (301) 402-0911
Fax: (301) 402-2218
Website: http://www.genome.gov/

National Institute for Occupational Safety and Health, U.S. Centers for Disease Control and Prevention
1600 Clifton Road
Atlanta, GA 30333

Toll-free: (800) CDC-INFO (232-4636)
Website: http://www.cdc.gov/niosh/

National Institute of Allergy and Infectious Diseases, Office of Communications and Government Relations
5601 Fishers Lane, MSC 9806
Bethesda, MD 20892-9806
Phone: (301) 496-5717
Toll-free: (866) 284-4107
TDD: (800) 877-8339
Fax: (301) 402-3573
Website: http://www3.niaid.nih.gov/

National Institute of Biomedical Imaging and Bioengineering
9000 Rockville Pike, Building 31, Room 1C14
Bethesda, MD 20892-8859
Phone: (301) 469-8859
E-mail: info@nibib.nih.gov
Website: http://www.nibib.gov/

National Institute of Diabetes and Digestive and Kidney Diseases (NIDDK)
Bethesda, MD 20892-2560
Phone: (301) 496-3583
Website: http://www.niddk.nih.gov/

National Institute of Environmental Health Sciences
111 T.W. Alexander Drive
Research Triangle Park, NC 27709
Phone: (919) 541-3345
E-mail: webcenter@niehs.nih.gov
Website: http://www.niehs.nih.gov/

National Institute of Mental Health
6001 Executive Boulevard, Room 8184, MSC 9663
Bethesda, MD 20892-9663
Phone: (301) 443-4513
Toll-free: (866) 615-6464
Fax: (301) 443-4279
E-mail: nimhinfo@nih.gov
Website: http://www.nimh.nih.gov/

National Institute of Neurological Disorders and Stroke (NINDS)
NIH Neurological Institute, PO Box 5801
Bethesda, MD 20824
Phone: (301) 496-5751
Toll-free: (800) 352-9424
Website: http://www.ninds.nih.gov/

National Institute on Alcohol Abuse and Alcoholism
5635 Fishers Lane, MSC 9304
Bethesda, MD 20892-9304
Phone: (301) 443-3860
E-mail: niaaaweb-r@exchange.nih.gov
Website: http://www.niaaa.nih.gov/

National Institute on Deafness and Other Communication Disorders (NIDCD)
NIDCD Office of Health Communication and Public Liaison, 31 Center Drive, MSC 2320
Bethesda, MD 20892-2320
Phone: (301) 496-7243
Toll-free: (800) 241-1044
TTY: (800) 241-1055
Fax: (301) 402-0018
E-mail: nidcdinfo@nidcd.nih.gov
Website: http://www.nidcd.nih.gov/

National Institute on Drug Abuse (NIDA)
Office of Science Policy and Communications, Public Information and Liaison Branch, 6001 Executive Boulevard, Rm. 5213, MSC 9561
Bethesda, MD 20892-9561
Phone: (301) 443-1124
Website: http://www.drugabuse.gov/

National Institutes of Health
9000 Rockville Pike
Bethesda, MD 20892
Phone: (301) 496-4000
TTY: (301) 402-9612
E-mail: NIHinfo@od.nih.gov
Website: http://nih.gov/

National Jewish Health's Lung Line
Toll-free: (800) 222-LUNG (222-5864)
E-mail: lungline@njhealth.org
Website: http://www.nationaljewish.org/about/contact/lung-line/

National Kidney and Urologic Diseases Information Clearinghouse
3 Information Way
Bethesda, MD 20892-3580
Toll-free: (800) 891-5390
TTY: (866) 569-1162
Fax: (703) 738-4929
E-mail: nkudic@info.niddk.nih.gov
Website: http://kidney.niddk.nih.gov/

National Kidney Foundation
30 E. 33rd Street
New York, NY 10016
Toll-free: (800) 622-9010
Fax: (212) 689-9261
E-mail: info@kidney.org
Website: http://www.kidney.org/

National Lung Health Education Program
18000 W. 105th Street
Olathe, KS 66061
Phone: (913) 895-4631
E-mail: nlhep@goamp.com
Website: http://www.nlhep.org/

National Lymphedema Network
225 Bush Street, Suite 357
San Francisco, CA 94104
Phone: (415) 908-3681
Toll-free: (800) 541-3259
Fax: (415) 908-3813
E-mail: nln@lymphnet.org
Website: http://lymphnet.org/

National Marrow Donor Program (NMDP)
3001 Broadway Street NE, Suite 100
Minneapolis, MN 55413-1753
Toll-free: (800) MARROW2 (627-7692)
E-mail: patientinfo@nmdp.org
Website: http://bethematch.org/

National Multiple Sclerosis Society
Website: http://www.nationalmssociety.org/

National Organization for Rare Diseases (NORD)
55 Kenosia Avenue
Danbury, CT 06810
Phone: (203) 744-0100
Fax: (203) 798-2291
Website: http://www.rarediseases.org/

National Palliative Care Research Center (NPCRC)
Brookdale Department of Geriatrics & Adult Development, Icahn School of Medicine, One Gustave L. Levy Place
New York, NY 10029
Phone: (212) 241-7447
Fax: (212) 241-5977
E-mail: npcrc@mssm.edu
Website: http://www.npcrc.org/

National Pancreas Foundation
3 Bethesda Metro Center, Suite 700
Bethesda, MD 20814
Phone: (301) 961-1508
Toll-free: (866) 726-2737
Fax: (301) 657-9776
E-mail: info@pancreasfoundation.org
Website: http://www.pancreasfoundation.org/

National Parkinson Foundation, Inc.
200 SE 1st Street, Suite 800
Miami, FL 33131
Toll-free: (800) 4PD-INFO (473-4636)
Fax: (305) 537-9901
E-mail: contact@parkinson.org
Website: http://www.parkinson.org/

National Rehabilitation Information Center
8400 Corporate Drive, Suite 500
Landover, MD 20785
Toll-free: (800) 346-2742
TTY: (301) 459-5984

Fax: (301) 459-4263
E-mail: naricinfo@heitechservices.com
Website: http://www.naric.com/

National Society of Genetic Counselors (NSGC)
330 N. Wabash Avenue, Suite 2000
Chicago, IL 60611
Phone: (312) 321-6834
E-mail: nsgc@nsgc.org
Website: http://www.nsgc.org/

National Toxicology Program (NTP)
PO Box 12233, MD K2-03
Research Triangle Park, NC 27709
Phone: (919) 541-0530
Website: http://ntp.niehs.nih.gov/

National Wilms Tumor Study
Fred Hutchinson Cancer Research Center, 1100 Fairview Avenue N, MJ-A876
Seattle, WA 98109-1024
Phone: (206) 667-4842
Toll-free: (800) 553-4878
Fax: (206) 667-4842
E-mail: nwtsg@fredhutch.org
Website: http://www.nwtsg.org/

National Women's Health Network (NWHN)
1413 K Street NW, 4th Floor
Washington, DC 20005
Phone: (202) 682-2640
Fax: (202) 682-2648
E-mail: nwhn@nwhn.org
Website: http://www.nwhn.org/

Neuro Foundation
HMA House, 78 Durham Road
London SW20 0TL
United Kingdom
Phone: +44 020 8439 1234
Fax: +44 020 8439 1200
E-mail: info@nfauk.org
Website: http://www.nfauk.org/

Neurofibromatosis Network
213 S. Wheaton Avenue
Wheaton, IL 60187
Phone: (630) 510-1115
Toll-free: (800) 942-6825
Fax: (630) 510-8508
E-mail: admin@nfnetwork.org
Website: http://www.nfnetwork.org/

Nicotine Anonymous
6333 E. Mockingbird #147-817
Dallas, TX 75214
Toll-free: (877) TRY-NICA (879-6422)
E-mail: info@nicotine-anonymous.org
Website: http://www.nicotine-anonymous.org/

O

Occupational Safety & Health Administration, U.S. Department of Labor
200 Constitution Avenue NW
Washington, DC 20210
Toll-free: (800) 321-OSHA (6742)
Website: https://www.osha.gov/

Office of Cancer Complementary and Alternative Medicine (OCCAM)
9609 Medical Center Drive, Room 5-W-136
Rockville, MD 20850
Phone: (240) 276-6595
Fax: (240) 276-7888
E-mail: ncioccam1-r@mail.nih.gov
Website: http://cam.cancer.gov/

Office of Rare Diseases Research, National Center for Advancing Translational Sciences
National Institutes of Health, 6701 Democracy Boulevard, Suite 1001, MSC 4874
Bethesda, MD 20892
Phone: (301) 402-4336
Fax: (301) 480-9655
E-mail: ordr@nih.gov
Website: http://rarediseases.info.nih.gov/

Oral Cancer Foundation
3419 Via Lido #205
Newport Beach, CA 92663
Phone: (949) 723-4400
Website: http://oralcancerfoundation.org/

Ovarian Cancer National Alliance
1101 14th Street NW, Suite 850
Washington, DC 20005
Phone: (202) 331-1332
Toll-free: (866) 399-6262
Fax: (202) 331-2292
E-mail: ocna@ovariancancer.org
Website: http://www.ovariancancer.org/

P

Pancreatic Cancer Action Network
1500 Rosecrans Avenue, Suite 200
Manhattan Beach, CA 90226
Phone: (310) 725-0025
Toll-free: (877) 272-6226
Fax: (310) 725-0029
E-mail: info@pancan.org
Website: http://www.pancan.org/

Parkinson's Disease Foundation
1359 Broadway, Suite 1509
New York, NY 10018

Phone: (212) 923-4700
Toll-free: (800) 457-6676
Fax: (212) 923-4778
E-mail: info@pdf.org
Website: http://www.pdf.org/

Prevent Cancer Foundation
1600 Duke Street, Suite 500
Alexandria, VA 22314
Phone: (703) 836-4412
Toll-free: (800) 227-2732
Fax: (703) 836-4413
E-mail: pcf@preventcancer.org
Website: http://preventcancer.org/

Prostate Cancer Foundation (PCF)
1250 Fourth Street
Santa Monica, CA 90401
Phone: (310) 570-4700
Toll-free: (800) 757-CURE (2873)
Fax: (310) 570-4701
E-mail: info@pcf.org
Website: http://www.pcf.org/

Pulmonary Paper
PO Box 877
Ormond Beach, FL 32175-0877
Toll-free: (800) 950-3698
E-mail: info@pulmonarypaper.org
Website: https://www.pulmonarypaper.org/

R

Radiological Society of North America (RSNA)
820 Jorie Boulevard
Oak Brook, IL 60523-2251
Phone: (630) 571-2670
Toll-free: (800) 381-6660
Fax: (630) 571-7837
Website: http://www.rsna.org/

Retinoblastoma International
18030 Brookhurst Street, Box 408
Fountain Valley, CA 92708
E-mail: info@retinoblastoma.net
Website: http://www.retinoblastoma.net/

S

San Francisco AIDS Foundation
1035 Market Street, Suite 400
San Francisco, CA 94103
Phone: (415) 487-3000
E-mail: feedback@sfaf.org
Website: http://sfaf.org/

Sarcoma Alliance
775 E. Blithedale #334
Mill Valley, CA 94941

Phone: (415) 381-7236
Fax: (415) 381-7235
E-mail: info@sarcomaalliance.org
Website: http://sarcomaalliance.org/

Skin Cancer Foundation
149 Madison Avenue, Suite 901
New York, NY 10016
Phone: (212) 725-5176
Website: http://www.skincancer.org/

Society for Immunotherapy of Cancer (SITC)
555 E. Wells Street, Suite 1100
Milwaukee, WI 53202-3823
Phone: (414) 271-2456
Fax: (414) 276-3349
E-mail: info@sitcancer.org
Website: http://www.sitcancer.org/

Society for Neuro-Oncology (SNO)
PO Box 273296
Houston, TX 77277-3296
E-mail: linda@soc-neuro-onc.org
Website: http://www.soc-neuro-onc.org/

Society for Pediatric Urology
500 Cummings Center, Suite 4550
Beverly, MA 01915
Phone: (978) 927-8330
Fax: (978) 524-8890
Website: http://spuonline.org/

Society of American Gastrointestinal Endoscopic Surgeons (SAGES)
11300 W. Olympic Boulevard, Suite 600
Los Angeles, CA 90064
Phone: (310) 437-0544
E-mail: webmaster@sages.org
Website: http://www.sages.org/

Society of Gynecologic Oncology (SGO)
230 W. Monroe Street, Suite 710
Chicago, IL 60606-4703
Phone: (312) 235-4060
Fax: (312) 235-4059
E-mail: sgo@sgo.org
Website: https://www.sgo.org/

Society of Interventional Radiology
3975 Fair Ridge Drive, Suite 400 North
Fairfax, VA 22033
Phone: (703) 691-1805
Toll-free: (800) 488-7284
Fax: (703) 691-1855
Website: http://www.sirweb.org/

Society of Laparoendoscopic Surgeons
7330 SW 62nd Pl., Suite 410
Miami, FL 33143-4825
Phone: (305) 665-9959

Fax: (305) 667-4123
E-mail: info@SLS.org
Website: http://www.sls.org/

Society of Nuclear Medicine and Molecular Imaging
1850 Samuel Morse Drive
Reston, VA 20190
Phone: (703) 708-9000
Fax: (703) 708-9015
E-mail: feedback@snmmi.org
Website: http://snmmi.rd.net/index.aspx

Society of Surgical Oncology (SSO)
9525 W Bryn Mawr Avenue, Suite 870
Rosemont, IL 60018
Phone: (847) 427-1400
Fax: (847) 427-1411
E-mail: info@surgonc.org
Website: http://www.surgonc.org/

The Society of Thoracic Surgeons
633 N. Saint Clair Street, Floor 23
Chicago, IL 60611
Phone: (312) 202-5800
Fax: (312) 202-5801
Website: http://sts.org/

Society of Urologic Nurses and Associates
E. Holly Avenue, Box 56
Pitman, NJ 08071-0056
Toll-free: (888) 827-7862
E-mail: suna@ajj.com
Website: http://suna.org/

Support for People with Oral and Head and Neck Cancer (SPOHNC)
PO Box 53
Locust Valley, NY 11560-0053
Toll-free: (800) 377-0928
Fax: (516) 671-8794
E-mail: info@spohnc.org
Website: http://www.spohnc.org/

Susan G. Komen Foundation
5005 LBJ Freeway, Suite 250
Dallas, TX 75244
Toll-free: (877) GO-KOMEN (465-6636)
Website: http://ww5.komen.org/

T

Testicular Cancer Society (TCS)
1173 Alnetta Drive
Cincinnati, OH 45230
Phone: (513) 696-9827

Website: http://www.testicularcancersociety.org/

Transverse Myelitis Association
1787 Sutter Parkway
Powell, OH 43065-8806
Phone: (614) 317-4884
Toll-free: (855) 380-3330
E-mail: info@myelitis.org
Website: https://myelitis.org/

Triple Negative Breast Cancer Foundation
Toll-free: (877) 870-TNBC (8622)
E-mail: info@tnbcfoundation.org
Website: http://www.tnbcfoundation.org/

U

United Network for Organ Sharing (UNOS)
700 N. 4th Street
Richmond, VA 23219
Phone: (804) 782-4800
Toll-free: (888) 894-6361
Website: http://www.unos.org/

United Ostomy Associations of America (UOAA)
2489 Rice St, Suite 275
Roseville, MN 55113-3797
Toll-free: (800) 826-0826
Website: http://www.ostomy.org/Home.html

University of Chicago Medicine, Comer Children's Hospital
5721 S. Maryland Avenue
Chicago, IL 60637
Phone: (773) 702-1000
Toll-free: (888) 824-0200
Website: https://www.uchicagokidshospital.org/

University of Southern California Center for Pancreatic and Biliary Diseases
Healthcare Consultation Center, Suite 430, 1510 San Pablo Street
Los Angeles, CA 90033
Phone: (855) 724-7874
E-mail: PancreasDiseases@surgery.usc.edu
Website: http://www.surgery.usc.edu/divisions/tumor/pancreasdiseases

Urology Care Foundation
1000 Corporate Boulevard
Linthicum, MD 21090
Phone: (410) 689-3700
Toll-free: (800) 828-7866
Fax: (410) 689-3998

E-mail: info@urologycarefoundation.org

Website: http://www.urologyhealth.org/

U.S. Environmental Protection Agency (EPA)

1200 Pennsylvania Avenue NW

Washington, DC 20460

Phone: (202) 272-0167

TTY: (202) 272-0165

Website: http://www2.epa.gov/

U.S. Food and Drug Administration (FDA)

10903 New Hampshire Avenue

Silver Spring, MD 20993

Toll-free: (888) INFO-FDA (463-6332)

Website: http://www.fda.gov/default.htm

V

VHL Alliance

2001 Beacon Street, Suite 208

Boston, MA 02135-7787

Phone: (617) 277-5667

Toll-free: (800) 767-4845

Fax: (866) 209-0288

E-mail: info@vhl.org

Website: http://www.vhl.org/

Visiting Nurse Associations of America

2121 Crystal Drive, Suite 750

Arlington, VA 22202

Phone: (571) 527-1520

Toll-free: (888) 866-8773

Fax: (571) 527-1521

E-mail: vnaa@vnaa.org

Website: http://vnaa.org/

W

World Health Organization (WHO)

Avenue Appia 20

1211 Geneva 27, Switzerland

Phone: +41 22 791 21 11

Fax: + 41 22 791 31 11

E-mail: info@who.int

Website: http://www.who.int/en

Wound, Ostomy and Continence Nurses Society (WOCN)

1120 Rt. 73, Suite 200

Mount Laurel, NJ 08054

Toll-free: (888) 224-9626

Fax: (856) 439-0525

E-mail: wocn_info@wocn.org

Website: http://www.wocn.org/

GLOSSARY

The glossary is an alphabetical compilation of terms and definitions listed in the *Key Terms* sections of the main body entries. Although the list is comprehensive, it is by no means exhaustive.

A

ABCDE. A simple way to remember suspicious signs on the skin that could suggest melanoma; stands for Asymmetry, Border, Color, Diameter, and Evolving.

ABDOMEN. A part of the body that lies between the thorax and the pelvis. It contains a cavity (abdominal cavity) that holds organs including the pancreas, stomach, intestines, liver, and gallbladder. It is enclosed by the abdominal muscles and the vertebral column (backbone).

ABDOMINOPERINEAL (AP) RESECTION. Surgical removal of the lower colon and rectum (and possibly other organs) to treat colon cancer.

ABLATION. The removal of a tumor or other material from the surface of a body tissue or organ by vaporization, abrasion, or a similar process. In radiofrequency ablation (RFA), tissue is removed with the heat generated by a high-frequency alternating current.

ABO ANTIGEN. Protein molecules located on the surfaces of red blood cells that determine a person's blood type: A, B, or O.

ABSCESS. A localized collection of pus or infection that is walled off from the rest of the body.

ACANTHOSIS NIGRICANS. A poorly defined brownish-black hyperpigmentation of the skin found in body folds (under the armpits, the groin, the folds of the neck, and similar areas).

ACE INHIBITORS. A group of drugs used to treat high blood pressure. These drugs work by decreasing production of a certain chemical in the kidneys that causes constriction of blood vessels.

ACETALDEHYDE. A toxic and carcinogenic substance produced by the breakdown of alcohol in the body.

ACHALASIA. Failure of the lower end of the esophagus (or another tubular valve) to open.

ACINAR CELL CARCINOMA. A malignant tumor arising from the acinar cells of the pancreas.

ACINAR CELLS. Cells that comprise small sacs terminating the ducts of some exocrine glands.

ACQUIRED IMMUNE DEFICIENCY SYNDROME (AIDS). A disease caused by infection with the human immunodeficiency virus (HIV). In people with this disease, the immune system breaks down, increasing vulnerability to other infections and some types of cancer.

ACQUIRED MUTATION. A mutation that occurs in cells outside the reproductive cells and is not passed on to an organism's offspring. It is also called a somatic mutation. Most cancers result from this type of mutation.

ACROLEIN. A breakdown product of the chemotherapy drugs ifosfamide and cyclophosphamide that concentrates in the bladder. It irritates the bladder lining and causes bleeding.

ACROMEGALY. Hormonal disorder causing progressive enlargement of hands and feet, elongation of the face, headache, muscle pain, and visual and emotional disturbances in middle-aged men and women.

ACTINIC KERATOSIS. A precancerous skin condition in which skin exposed to the sun forms thick, scaly, or crusty patches. Untreated actinic keratosis has a 20% chance of progressing to skin cancer.

ACUTE. Having a sudden onset and lasting a short time.

ACUTE LYMPHOCYTIC LEUKEMIA (ALL). A rapidly progressing disease where too many immature infection-fighting white blood cells called lymphoblasts are found in the blood and bone marrow. It is also known as acute lymphoblastic leukemia.

ACUTE MYELOGENOUS LEUKEMIA (AML). A type of cancer of the blood, characterized by the rapid growth of abnormal white blood cells that accumulate in the bone marrow and interfere with the production of normal blood cells.

ACUTE PAIN. Short-term pain in response to injury or other stimulus that resolves when the injury heals or the stimulus is removed.

ACUTE PULMONARY EDEMA. An abrupt collection of fluid in the lungs due to failure of the heart muscle to pump blood properly.

ACUTE-PHASE PROTEINS. Proteins produced during the acute-phase response, a set of physiological changes that occur in response to biologic stress such as trauma or sepsis.

ACYCLOVIR. An antiviral drug used to treat infections such as chickenpox, herpes zoster (shingles), and genital herpes.

ADAPTIVE IMMUNE SYSTEM. A subsystem of the immune system that comprises highly specialized cells and processes that inhibit the growth of disease organisms. It is also known as the acquired immune system.

ADDICTION. The use of a drug or other substance in increasing amounts and in a manner that is out of control, compulsive, and continued despite the risk of harm to the user.

ADDISON'S DISEASE. A potentially life-threatening condition that results when adrenocortical function fails.

ADENOCARCINOMA. A type of cancer that develops in the gland-like cells of epithelial tissue, which is the tissue that lines the inner and exterior surfaces of body organs.

ADENOIDS. Common name for the pharyngeal tonsils, which are lymph masses in the wall of the air passageway (pharynx) just behind the nose.

ADENOMA. A type of noncancerous (benign) tumor that often involves the overgrowth of certain cells of the type normally found within glands.

ADENOPATHY. Large or swollen lymph glands.

ADHESION. A band of internal scar tissue that develops after injury or surgery.

ADIPOKINES. Cytokines and growth factors secreted by adipose (fat) cells.

ADIPONECTIN. A hormone secreted by fat cells that regulates glucose and lipid metabolism.

ADIPOSE TISSUE. Fat tissue.

ADJUNCTIVE. Any form of therapy that is considered to help or assist a patient's primary treatment.

ADJUVANT. A treatment or therapy in addition to the primary treatment.

ADJUVANT CHEMOTHERAPY. Treatment of a cancer with drugs after surgery to kill as many of the remaining cancer cells as possible.

ADJUVANT THERAPY. Therapy given in addition to the primary treatment. In cancer treatment, adjuvant therapy usually refers to chemotherapy or radiation therapy given after surgery to prevent recurrence of the cancer.

ADJUVANT TREATMENT. An additional treatment that is added to increase effectiveness of the primary treatment.

ADRENAL GLAND. Gland located above each kidney, consisting of an outer wall (cortex) that produces steroid hormones and an inner section (medulla) that produces other important hormones, such as adrenaline and noradrenaline. Also called suprarenal glands.

ADRENAL MEDULLA. The central core of the adrenal gland.

ADRENALCORTICOID TUMORS. Cancerous tumors that arise on the outer surface of the adrenal glands.

ADRENOCORTEX. Adrenal cortex; the outer part of the adrenal gland that sits on top of the kidneys.

ADRENOCORTICOTROPIC HORMONE (ACTH). A pituitary hormone that stimulates the cortex of the adrenal glands to produce adrenal cortical hormones.

ADULT RESPIRATORY DISTRESS SYNDROME (ARDS). A lung disease characterized by widespread lung abnormalities, fluid in the lungs, shortness of breath, and low oxygen levels in the blood.

ADVANCE DIRECTIVE. A legal document in which a person states the type of care that he or she wishes or does not wish to receive in the event of losing his or her ability to make decisions or express them. "Do not resuscitate" (DNR) orders and living wills are types of advance directives.

ADVANCED BREAST BIOPSY INSTRUMENT (ABBI). A rotating circular knife and thin heated electrical wire used to remove a large cylinder of abnormal breast tissue.

AFLATOXIN. A substance produced by molds that grow on rice and peanuts. Exposure to aflatoxin is thought to explain the high rates of primary liver cancer in Africa and parts of Asia.

AGE-STANDARDIZED RATE (ASR). The cancer rate that a population would have if it was composed of a standard range of ages; used to compare populations with different age distributions.

AGEUSIA. Impairment or absence of the sense of taste.

AGONIST. A drug that binds to cell receptors and stimulates activities normally stimulated by naturally occurring substances.

AIDS. Acquired immune deficiency syndrome.

ALBUMIN. A blood protein produced in the liver that helps to regulate water distribution in the body.

ALCOHOL DEHYDROGENASE (ADH). The enzyme that converts alcohol to acetaldehyde; some forms of the ADH gene, especially in people of Asian descent, are highly active and cause acetaldehyde to build up in the body.

ALDRIN. An organochlorine insecticide that breaks down to dieldrin, a possible carcinogen. Although aldrin was banned by 1987, dieldrin persists in the environment and is associated with cancer.

ALKALINE PHOSPHATASE. A body protein, measurable in the blood, that often appears in high amounts in patients with osteosarcoma. However, many other conditions also elevate the level of alkaline phosphatase.

ALKALOID. Any of a large group of bitter-tasting alkaline substances containing nitrogen that are found in plants. Capsaicin is an example of an alkaloid.

ALKYLATING AGENT. A chemical that alters the composition of the genetic material of rapidly dividing cells, such as cancer cells, causing selective cell death.

ALLELE. One of a number of alternative forms of the same gene or the same genetic locus.

ALLOGENEIC. Referring to transplants or transfusions between two different, genetically dissimilar people.

ALLYL SULFIDES. Phytochemicals in garlic and onions that may have a role in cancer prevention.

ALPHA-FETOPROTEIN (AFP). A protein in blood serum that is found in abnormally high concentrations in most patients with primary liver cancer.

ALTERNATIVE. A form of treatment outside mainstream medicine that is used instead of standard treatments.

ALTERNATIVE THERAPY. A form of therapy used instead of conventional treatments.

ALVEOLAR RHABDOMYOSARCOMA (ARMS). A soft tissue sarcoma in the large muscles of the arms, legs, or trunk that primarily affects older children.

AMBULATION. Moving from place to place.

AMNIOCENTESIS. Prenatal testing performed at 16–20 weeks of gestation by inserting a needle through the mother's abdomen and obtaining a small sample of amniotic fluid containing fetal cells for biochemical and/or DNA testing.

AMYLOIDOSIS. A complication in which amyloid protein accumulates in the kidneys and other organs, tissues, and blood vessels.

ANAL. Pertaining to the anus, which is the terminal orifice of the digestive—or alimentary—canal.

ANALGESIC. Any drug that is given to relieve pain.

ANALOG. A chemical compound with a structure similar to another chemical, but differing in a certain way.

ANAPHYLACTIC SHOCK. Acute systemic allergic reaction that can be life-threatening.

ANAPHYLACTOID PURPURA. A short-term allergic condition of blood vessels, found chiefly in children, that is characterized by wet sores on the skin of the buttocks, legs, and lower abdomen. Joint pain, stomach bleeding, and blood in the urine are also common findings. The disease, also called Henoch-Schonlein (Schonlein-Henoch) purpura, usually lasts for about six weeks and has no long-term effects unless kidney involvement is severe.

ANAPHYLAXIS. A severe allergic reaction to a foreign substance (antigen) that a patient has had previous contact with, characterized by redness and swelling, itching, water buildup, and, in severe cases, extremely low blood pressure, lung spasms, and shock.

ANAPLASIA. Characteristics of a cell, such as shape and orientation, that make it identifiable as a cancer cell.

ANAPLASTIC ASTROCYTOMA. The advanced stage of a rapidly growing brain tumor. This type of tumor originates in the brain, unlike other brain tumors that may occur due to the spreading of cancer from another part of the body.

ANAPLASTIC OLIGODENDROGLIOMA. A form of oligodendroglioma that does not have a well-defined shape and grows very rapidly and aggressively.

ANAPLASTIC THYROID CARCINOMA. Undifferentiated cancer cells located in the thyroid that are aggressive and difficult to treat.

ANASTOMOSIS. The surgical connection of sections of vessels, tubes, or ducts, such as two sections of intestine.

ANATOMY. Structure of the body and of the relationship between its parts.

ANDROGEN. Any substance that promotes the development of masculine characteristics in a person. Testosterone is one type of androgen; others are produced in the adrenal glands located above the kidneys.

ANDROGEN-DEPRIVATION THERAPY (ADT). Also called androgen-suppression therapy; a type of hormone therapy that lowers levels of the male hormone androgen to treat prostate cancer.

ANEMIA. A condition in which there are too few red blood cells, too many abnormal red blood cells, or too little iron-containing hemoglobin for normal oxygen transport in the body. Its symptoms are general weakness and lack of energy, dizziness, shortness of breath, headaches, and irritability.

ANESTHESIA. A combination of drugs administered to provide sedation, amnesia, analgesia (pain relief), and immobility adequate for the accomplishment of a surgical procedure with minimal discomfort, and without injury, to the patient.

ANESTHETIC. A drug that causes loss of sensation. It is used to lessen the pain of surgery and medical procedures.

ANEUPLOID. An abnormal number of chromosomes or amount of DNA in a cell.

ANEURYSM. The bulging of the blood vessel wall. Aneurysms can burst and cause bleeding.

ANGINA. Ischemic heart disease that produces chest pain.

ANGIOEDEMA. A sudden painless swelling of short duration that can affect the face, neck, lips, throat, hands, feet, genitals, or abdominal organs; also called angio-neurotic edema.

ANGIOGENESIS. Physiological process involving the growth of new blood vessels from pre-existing blood vessels; used by some cancers to create their own blood supply.

ANGIOGENESIS INHIBITOR. A substance that prevents the growth of new blood vessels.

ANGIOGRAM. A diagnostic test that makes it possible for blood vessels to be seen on film; the vessels are filled with a contrast substance or dye that appears on x-rays.

ANGIOGRAPHY. A radiographic technique in which an opaque contrast material is injected into a blood vessel for the purpose of identifying its anatomy on x-ray.

ANGIOSARCOMA. A malignant tumor that develops either from blood vessels or from lymphatic vessels.

ANGIOSTATIN. A naturally occurring inhibitor of angiogenesis.

ANGIOTENSIN-CONVERTING ENZYME (ACE) INHIBITORS. Medications that lower blood pressure and reduce the workload of the heart muscle.

ANN ARBOR SYSTEM. A system of tumor staging used to classify non-Hodgkin lymphomas in adults. It specifies four stages, which can be further defined by the use of letters to identify general physical symptoms and the parts of the body affected by the lymphoma. The corresponding staging system in children is the St. Jude Children's Research Hospital system.

ANORECTAL. Pertaining to the anus and rectum.

ANOREXIA. A condition characterized by a loss of appetite or desire to eat.

ANTAGONIST. A drug that binds to a cellular receptor for a hormone, neurotransmitter, or another drug. Antagonists block the action of the substance without producing any physiologic effect itself.

ANTHELMINTIC. An agent destructive to worms. Many anthelmintic drugs are toxic and should be given with care; the patient should be observed carefully for toxic effects after the drug is given.

ANTHOCYANINS. Plant pigments with antioxidant activities.

ANTHRACYCLINES. A group of chemotherapy medicines that are used to treat cancer. They have similar characteristics and are known for their ability to cause heart damage. The drugs included as anthracyclines are doxorubicin, daunorubicin, idarubicin, and epirubicin.

ANTIANDROGEN. A substance that blocks the action of androgens, the hormones responsible for male characteristics. Used to treat prostate cancers that require male hormones for growth.

ANTIANGIOGENIC AGENT. A drug that inhibits angiogenesis.

ANTIBIOTIC. An antimicrobial agent used to kill bacteria.

ANTIBODIES. Proteins normally produced by the immune system to fight infection or rid the body of foreign material. The material that stimulates the production of antibodies is called an antigen. Specific antibodies are produced in response to each different antigen and can only inactivate that particular antigen.

ANTIBODY-DRUG CONJUGATE (ADC). A medication consisting of both an antibody for targeting cancer cells and a drug that kills the cells.

ANTICHOLINERGIC AGENT. Drug that slows the action of the bowel by relaxing the muscles; reduces stomach acid.

ANTICOAGULANT. An agent preventing the coagulation (clotting) of blood.

ANTICONVULSANT. A type of medication given to prevent seizures.

ANTIDIURETIC HORMONE (ADH). A peptide hormone, also called vasopressin, synthesized in the hypothalamus and released by the posterior pituitary gland in response to decreased blood volume. ADH stimulates capillary muscles and concentrates and reduces the elimination of urine.

ANTIDOTE. A drug given to reverse the negative effects of another drug.

ANTIEMETIC. A drug that prevents or alleviates nausea and vomiting.

ANTIESTROGEN. A drug, such as tamoxifen, that prevents the hormone estrogen from influencing the behavior of specific types of cells.

ANTIGEN. A substance that can cause an immune response, resulting in production of an antibody, as part of the body's defense against infection and disease. Many antigens are foreign proteins not found naturally in the body and include germs, toxins, and tissues from another person used in organ transplantation.

ANTIGEN-PRESENTING CELL (APC). An immune-system cell that ingests antigens and exposes them to other cells to evoke a specific immune response to that antigen.

ANTIHISTAMINE. Agent that blocks or counteracts the action of histamine, which is released during an allergic reaction.

ANTIHYPERCALCEMIC. Type of drug that lowers the levels of calcium in the blood.

ANTIMETABOLITE. Anti-cancer drug that prevents cells from growing and dividing by blocking the chemical reactions required in the cell to produce DNA.

ANTIMICROBIAL. Any of a large class of drugs used to kill disease organisms or inhibit their growth. Antimicrobials include antibiotics, antivirals, antiparasitic drugs, and antifungal drugs.

ANTIMYCOTICS. Another name for antifungal drugs.

ANTINEOPLASTIC. An agent that inhibits or prevents the maturation and proliferation of malignant cells.

ANTINEOPLASTON. A substance isolated from normal human blood and urine and tested as a type of treatment for some tumors and AIDS.

ANTIOXIDANT. A molecule that prevents oxidation. In the body, antioxidants attach to other molecules called free radicals and prevent the free radicals from causing damage to cell walls, DNA, and other parts of the cell.

ANTIPERISTALTIC AGENT. Drug that slows the contraction and relaxation (peristalsis) of the intestines.

ANTIPROTOZOAL. An agent destructive to protozoa.

ANTITUMOR ANTIBIOTICS. Chemotherapy drugs derived from natural substances that interfere with cellular functions.

ANTRECTOMY. A surgical procedure for ulcer disease in which the antrum, a portion of the stomach, is removed.

ANTRUM. The lower part of the stomach that lies between the pylorus and the body of the stomach. It is also called the gastric antrum or antrum pyloricum.

ANUS. The terminal orifice of the gastrointestinal (GI) or digestive tract that includes all organs responsible for getting food in and out of the body.

AORTA. The major artery carrying blood away from the heart.

APHERESIS. A process that involves the withdrawal of blood, removal of one or more blood components such as plasma (plasmapheresis) or platelets (plateletpheresis), and return of the blood to the donor's body.

APHONIA. Loss of voice.

APLASTIC ANEMIA. A disorder in which the body produces inadequate amounts of red blood cells and hemoglobin due to underdeveloped or missing bone marrow.

APOPTOSIS. Cell self-destruction, usually brought about by irreparable damage to the cell's DNA.

APPENDICITIS. Inflammation of the appendix.

APUDOMA. A tumor capable of Amine Precursor Uptake and Decarboxylation (APUD).

AREOLA. The pigmented area on the male or female breast that surrounds the nipple.

ARGININE. An essential amino acid derived from dietary protein; sometimes used in combination with glutamine to boost the immune system.

AROMATASE. An enzyme that converts an androgen to an estrogen.

AROMATASE INHIBITOR (AI). A medication for preventing or treating breast cancer in postmenopausal women by inhibiting the body's production of estrogen.

ARRHYTHMIA. Any of a group of conditions in which the heart beats irregularly or faster or slower than normal.

ARSENIC. A poisonous element and known carcinogen that was a common pesticide ingredient prior to 1993.

ARTERIAL THROMBOSIS. A condition characterized by a blood clot in an artery.

ARTERIOGRAM. An x-ray study of an artery that has been injected with a contrast dye.

ARTERIOVENOUS MALFORMATION. Abnormal, direct connection between the arteries and veins. Arteriovenous malformations can range from very small to large.

ASBESTOS. A silicate (containing silica) mineral that occurs in a variety of forms; it is characterized by a fibrous structure and resistance to fire. When inhaled, it can cause lung diseases including cancer and mesothelioma.

ASCITES. Abnormal accumulation of fluid in the abdomen.

ASPERGILLOSIS. A fungal infection that can be life-threatening to patients with weakened immune systems.

ASPIRATION. A procedure to withdraw fluid and cells from the body.

ASTHENIA. A feeling of extreme weakness and fatigue.

ASTHMA. Disorder involving chronic inflammation in which the airways are narrowed in a reversible manner making it difficult to breathe normally, especially during acute exacerbations known as asthma attacks.

ASTROCYTOMA. A type of brain tumor that arises from the astrocytes, specialized brain cells that regulate the chemical environment of the brain and form the blood-brain barrier. These types of tumors are often mixed with oligodendrogliomas to form oligoastrocytomas.

ATAXIA. The inability to perform voluntary, coordinated muscular movements.

ATHEROSCLEROSIS. A chronic condition characterized by thickening and hardening of the arteries and the buildup of plaque on the arterial walls. Atherosclerosis can slow or impair blood circulation.

ATLAS. In anatomy, a collection of medical illustrations of one specific subject, such as the brain or heart. Detailed atlases of the brain are important guides for surgeons performing stereotactic neurosurgery.

ATROPHIC GASTRITIS. A chronic inflammation of the gastric mucosa caused either by an autoimmune process or by infection with *Helicobacter pylori*. It is a risk factor for the development of gastric cancer.

AUDIOMETRY. Testing a person's hearing by exposing the ear to sounds in a soundproof room.

AURA. A field of subtle energy that surrounds the human body, according to external energy therapists.

AUTOANTIBODIES. Antibodies that the immune system produces against the body's own proteins.

AUTOIMMUNE DISEASE. A disease in which the body produces an immunologic reaction against itself.

AUTOIMMUNE DISORDER. A condition in which antibodies are formed against the body's own tissues.

AUTOIMMUNE HEMOLYTIC ANEMIA. Type of anemia in which the immune system of the body attacks its own red blood cells and destroys them in a process known as hemolysis.

AUTOIMMUNE THROMBOCYTOPENIA. Condition in which the immune system of the body attacks its own blood system, resulting in a decreased number of platelets than is necessary for normal blood clotting.

AUTOLOGOUS. From the same person; an autologous breast reconstruction uses the woman's own tissues, while an autologous blood transfusion is blood removed then transfused back to the same person at a later time.

AUTOLOGOUS BLOOD DONATION. Donation of the patient's own blood, made several weeks before elective surgery.

AUTOLOGOUS TRANSPLANTATION. Transplantation in which the individual's own stem cells or bone marrow are removed and then transplanted back into the individual later. Autologous transplantation removes the risk of rejection of the transplanted material.

AUTOPSY. Postmortem surgical procedure performed to examine body tissues and determine the cause of death.

AUTOSOMAL DOMINANT. A gene located on a chromosome other than the X or Y sex chromosomes and whose expression is dominant over that of a second copy of the same gene.

AUTOSOMAL RECESSIVE. A gene located on a chromosome other than the X or Y sex chromosomes and carrying a trait that is not expressed unless the second copy of the same gene inherited from the other parent is also recessive or mutated.

AXILLA. Armpit.

AXILLARY. Pertaining to the armpit.

AXILLARY LYMPH NODES. The glands of the lymphatic system located under the arms; also referred to as axillary nodes.

AXILLARY VEIN. A blood vessel located near the armpit that takes blood from tissues back to the heart to receive oxygenated blood.

AZOTEMIA. A condition in which the blood contains abnormally high levels of nitrogen-rich compounds. It usually results from insufficient filtering of the blood by the kidneys.

B

B CELL. Type of lymphocyte (white blood cell) that creates antibodies to fight infection; also referred to as a B-cell lymphocyte.

BABESIOSIS. Infection transmitted by the bite of a tick and characterized by fever, headache, nausea, and muscle pain.

BALANITIS. Inflammation of the skin of the glans penis. It may be caused by viral, bacterial, or fungal infections; irritation resulting from poor personal hygiene; or poorly controlled diabetes.

BARIATRIC SURGERY. Weight-loss surgery.

BARIUM ENEMA. An x-ray test of the bowel performed after giving the patient an enema of a white chalky substance (barium) that outlines the colon and the rectum.

BARIUM SULFATE. A barium compound used during a barium enema to block the passage of x-rays during the exam.

BARIUM SWALLOW. An x-ray series of the upper gastrointestinal tract used to define the anatomy of the upper digestive tract; the test involves filling the esophagus, stomach, and small intestines with a white liquid material (barium).

BARRETT'S ESOPHAGUS. A precancerous condition of the esophagus that may develop as a complication of gastroesophageal reflux disease (GERD).

BASAL CELL. A keratinocyte in the basal layer, the deepest of the five layers of cells in the epidermis.

BASAL CELL CANCER. The most common form of skin cancer, usually appearing as one or several nodules with a central depression; it rarely spreads (metastasizes) but is locally invasive.

BASAL CELL CARCINOMA (BCC). Cancer originating in basal cells of the skin.

BASEMENT MEMBRANE. A specialized layer of extracellular matrix that separates epithelial tissue from underlying connective tissue; cancer cells must break through the basement membrane to migrate to other parts of the body and form metastases.

BASIC FIBROBLAST GROWTH FACTOR (BFGF). A factor that promotes angiogenesis.

BASOPHIL. A type of white blood cell.

BCD. The combined chemotherapy treatment of bleomycin, cyclophosphamide, and dactinomycin.

B-CELL LYMPHOCYTE. A type of lymphocyte (white blood cell). B cells react to the presence of antigens by dividing and maturing into plasma cells.

B-CELL LYMPHOMAS. Non-Hodgkin lymphomas (cancers of the blood) that arise from B cells.

BENCE-JONES PROTEIN. Light chain of an immunoglobulin that is overproduced in multiple myeloma and is excreted in the urine.

BENIGN. Not malignant; noncancerous.

BENIGN INTRACRANIAL HYPERTENSION. Also called pseudotumor cerebri or meningeal hydrops; a condition of swelling of the optic nerve and mild paralysis of the cranial nerves accompanied by headache, nausea, and vomiting.

BENIGN PROSTATIC HYPERPLASIA (BPH). Noncancerous swelling of the prostate.

BENIGN TUMOR. A growth that is noncancerous.

BENZENE. A toxic and carcinogenic hydrocarbon used in pesticide manufacturing and other industries.

BETA BLOCKERS. Medications that relax blood vessels and slow the heart rate.

BETA-HCH. Beta-hexachlorocyclohexane; a lindane byproduct that persists in the soil and water and accumulates in biological systems.

BETA-HYDROXY-BETA-METHYLBUTYRATE (HMB). A nutritional supplement used to build up muscles and treat muscle-wasting caused by disease.

BETA-2 MICROGLOBULIN (B2M). A small membrane protein that may be elevated in some cancers.

BEVACIZUMAB (AVASTIN). A monoclonal antibody that binds VEGF and prevents it from activating its receptor; the first anti-angiogenic agent approved for treating cancer.

BILATERAL. Affecting both sides.

BILATERAL RETINOBLASTOMA. Tumors affecting both eyes.

BILE. A bitter yellowish-brown fluid secreted by the liver that contains bile salts, bile pigments, cholesterol, and other substances. It helps the body to digest and absorb fats.

BILE DUCTS. Passages external to the liver for the transport of bile.

BILIARY. Relating to bile.

BILIRUBIN. A pigment produced when the liver processes waste products. A high bilirubin level causes yellowing of the skin.

BIOAVAILABILITY. A term used in describing the amount of a medication taken that is actively available to the targeted body area. Bioavailability can be affected by factors such as the rate at which a tablet or capsule dissolves, binding products used in formulating the medication, and the person's ability to break down and use the medication.

BIOETHICIST. A professional concerned with the moral and societal implications of medical research and treatments.

BIOINFORMATICS. An interdisciplinary field that makes use of engineering, computer science, mathematics, and statistics to understand and process biological data.

BIOLOGIC THERAPY. Targeted therapy.

BIOLOGICAL RESPONSE MODIFIERS (BRMS). Substances that stimulate the body to respond to an infection. Some are produced naturally in the body while others are synthesized in laboratories. BRMs include monoclonal antibodies, interferons, interleukins, and colony-stimulating factors. Some of them have the side effect of increasing fatigue in cancer patients.

BIOLOGICS. Drugs or other medical products made from biological sources.

BIOMARKER. A protein or other molecule that is indicative of a process, condition, or disease, such as a protein secreted by a tumor.

BIOPSY. Removal of a small sample of tissue for examination under a microscope; used for the diagnosis and treatment of cancer and precancerous conditions.

BIPOLAR DISORDER. A mood disorder in which the patient experiences both periods of mania and periods of depression.

BISPHENOL A (BPA). A chemical widely used in food packaging that can leach into foods.

BISPHOSPHONATES. A class of drugs that inhibit the action of osteoclasts—the cells that dissolve or break down bone.

BLADDER. A structure located in the lower part of the abdomen that collects urine for temporary storage and is emptied from time to time by urinating.

BLADDER EXSTROPHY. A bladder and urinary congenital abnormality. It occurs when the wall of the bladder fails to close in embryonic development and remains exposed to the abdominal wall.

BLADDER IRRIGATION. To flush or rinse the bladder with a stream of liquid (as in removing a foreign body or medicating).

BLADDER NECK. The narrowest part of the bladder.

BLADDER TUMOR MARKER STUDIES. A test to detect specific substances released by bladder cancer cells into the urine using chemicals or immunology (using antibodies).

BLADDER WASHING. A procedure in which bladder washing samples are taken by placing a salt solution into the bladder through a catheter (tube) and then removing the solution for microscopic testing.

BLAST CELLS. Immature cells of the bone marrow that normally develop into various types of blood cells.

BLAST PHASE. Stage of chronic myelogenous leukemia where large quantities of immature cells are produced by the marrow; not responsive to treatment.

BLASTOMA. An abnormal growth of embryonic cells.

BLOOD CELLS. Cells found in the blood, including red blood cells that carry oxygen, white blood cells that fight infections, and platelets that help the blood to clot.

BLOOD CLOT. A clump of blood that forms in or around a vessel as a result of coagulation. The formation of blood clots when the body has been cut is essential because without blood clots to cease the bleeding, a person would bleed to death from a relatively small wound.

BLOOD ELECTROLYTES. Ions present in the blood such as sodium and potassium that are necessary for health.

BLOOD PLATELETS. Blood component responsible for normal blood clotting to seal wounds.

BLOOD TRANSFUSION. The transfer of stored blood or blood components into a patient through a vein.

BLOOD TYPING. Technique for determining compatibility between donated blood products and transfusion recipients.

BLOOD UREA NITROGEN (BUN). A measurement of the waste product urea in the bloodstream; patients with kidney failure have high BUN levels.

BLOOD-BRAIN BARRIER. The blood vessel network surrounding the brain that blocks the passage of foreign substances into the brain.

BODY IMAGE. A person's sense of his or her physical appearance, often shaped by social standards of attractiveness as well as personal experiences.

BODY MASS INDEX (BMI). A measure of body fat: the ratio of weight in kilograms to the square of height in meters.

BODY SURFACE AREA (BSA). A measurement, based on a patient's height and weight, that helps determine appropriate chemotherapy dosages.

BONE MARROW. A spongy tissue located within flat bones, including the hip and breast bones and the skull. This tissue contains stem cells, the precursors of platelets, red blood cells, and white blood cells.

BONE MARROW ASPIRATION. A common technique used to obtain a bone marrow sample from a patient. A needle is inserted into a marrow-containing bone, such as the hip (iliac crest) or sternum (breast bone) and a small amount of liquid bone marrow is removed for examination.

BONE MARROW BIOPSY. A common technique used to obtain a bone marrow sample from a patient. Like bone marrow aspiration, it is performed with a needle, but a larger one is used and a small piece of bone is removed as well as bone marrow.

BONE MARROW SUPPRESSION. Disorder often caused by anticancer drugs in which the bone marrow no longer produces enough of the blood cells necessary for oxygen transport and the immune system, often causing anemia and life-threatening infections.

BONE MARROW TRANSPLANT (BMT). The destruction of bone marrow by high-dose chemotherapy or radiation and its replacement with healthy bone marrow taken from the patient prior to chemotherapy or from a donor.

BONE METASTASES. The spread of tumor cells from the primary site of origin to bone. Bone metastases from breast cancer, for example, represent breast cancer cells that have invaded bone. They are not the same as bone cancer cells that originate in bone.

BONE SCAN. An x-ray study in which patients are given an intravenous injection of a small amount of a radioactive material that travels in the blood. When it reaches the bones, it can be detected by x-ray to provide an image of their internal structure.

BONE-MINERAL DENSITY (BMD). A measure of bone strength.

BOWEL LUMEN. The space within the intestine.

BOWEL PREPARATION. A procedure done to clean out the colon prior to surgery or certain medical tests; may involve the use of cathartics, laxatives, and/or enemas, as well as a period of fasting.

BPH. Benign prostatic hyperplasia (or hypertrophy), a very common noncancerous cause of prostatic enlargement in older men.

BRACHYTHERAPY. A form of radiation therapy in which small pellets of radioactive material are placed inside or near the area to be treated. It is also known as internal radiation therapy or sealed-source radiotherapy.

BRAF. A gene encoding a serine/threonine kinase protein called B-raf that activates a cell-signaling pathway and is often mutated in melanomas, causing continuous activation of the pathway.

BRAIN SCAN. A general term that can include computed tomography (CT) scans, magnetic resonance imaging (MRI), seldom-used radionuclide scanning (use of radioactive isotopes), or ultrasounds.

BRCA1 AND *BRCA2.* Breast cancer susceptibility genes; specific mutations in these genes greatly increase the risk of breast and ovarian cancers.

BREAKTHROUGH PAIN. Intense, short-lived pain that is experienced despite being medicated for chronic or persistent pain.

BREAST BIOPSY. A procedure in which suspicious tissue is removed and examined by a pathologist for cancer or other disease. The breast tissue may be obtained by open surgery or through a needle.

BREAST-CONSERVING SURGERY. Breast cancer treatment, such as a lumpectomy or partial mastectomy, that removes only the cancerous tissue rather than the entire breast.

BRONCHI (SINGULAR BRONCHUS). The network of tubular passages that carry air to the lungs and allow air to be expelled from the lungs.

BRONCHIOLES. Small airways extending from the bronchi into the lobes of the lungs.

BRONCHOALVEOLAR LAVAGE. A method of obtaining a sample of fluid from the airways by inserting a flexible tube through the windpipe.

BRONCHODILATOR. A drug that relaxes bronchial muscles, resulting in expansion of the bronchial air passages.

BRONCHOPLEURAL FISTULA. An abnormal connection between an air passage and the membrane that covers the lungs.

BRONCHOSCOPE. A thin, flexible, lighted tube that is used to view the air passages in the lungs.

BRONCHOSCOPY. A procedure in which a thin, flexible, lighted tube is threaded through the airways to view the air passages in the lungs.

BRONCHOSPASM. Spasm of the smooth muscles surrounding the bronchi causing constriction and obstructed airways.

BUCCAL. Pertaining to the mouth or cheeks. It is derived from the Latin word for cheek.

BUPROPION (ZYBAN). An antidepressant medication given to smokers for nicotine withdrawal symptoms.

BUSPIRONE (BUSPAR). An anti-anxiety medication that is also given for nicotine withdrawal symptoms.

C

C CELLS. Parafollicular cells; thyroid gland cells that produce the hormone calcitonin.

CACHEXIA. A condition in which the body weight "wastes" away, characterized by a constant loss of weight, muscle, and fat.

CALCIFICATION. A deposit of calcium within cells or tissues. Calcifications in the brain are often visible on imaging studies of SPNETs.

CALCITONIN. A thyroid hormone that regulates calcium levels in the blood.

CALICHEAMICIN. An antitumor drug that binds to DNA within the tumor cells, causing breaks in the strands and killing the cell.

CANCER. A term for diseases in which abnormal cells divide without control. Cancer cells can invade nearby tissues and spread through the bloodstream and lymphatic system to other parts of the body.

CANCER ANTIGEN (CA). Marker proteins for some types of cancer.

CANCER REGISTRY. A recording of all cancer deaths in a given population, including personal characteristics of patients and clinical and pathological characteristics of the cancers; the primary source for cancer epidemiologic research and planning and evaluation of health services.

CANCER SCREENING. An examination designed to detect cancer even though a person has no symptoms, often performed using an imaging technique.

CANCER SURGERY. Surgery in which the goal is to excise a tumor and the surrounding malignant tissue.

CANCER SUSCEPTIBILITY GENE. The type of gene involved in cancer. If a mutation is identified in this type of gene it does not diagnose the cancer, but reveals that an individual is at increased risk of developing a new or recurring cancer in the future.

CANCER VACCINES. A treatment that uses the patient's immune system to attack cancer cells.

CANDIDIASIS. A yeast-like fungal infection occurring on the skin or mucous membranes; for example, in the mouth.

CANNABINOID. Chemical constituents of marijuana, such as THC.

CANNULA. A small tube or hollow needle designed for insertion into a duct.

CAPSAICIN. An active ingredient from hot chili peppers that may have cancer-preventive activity.

CAPSULAR CONTRACTURE. Thick scar tissue around a breast implant, which may tighten and cause discomfort and/or firmness.

CAPSULE. A general medical term for a structure that encloses another structure or body part.

CARBAMATES. Neurotoxic insecticides such as carbaryl (1-naphthyl methylcarbamate); used on a wide variety of crops.

CARCINOEMBRYONIC ANTIGEN (CEA). A fetal protein that is present in high levels in the blood of patients with some forms of cancer, such as breast or digestive system cancers.

CARCINOGEN. A substance or agent that promotes cancer, either directly or following activation in the body.

CARCINOGENIC. A substance that can cause the development of cancer.

CARCINOID. A tumor that develops from neuroendocrine cells.

CARCINOID SYNDROME. Rare malignant disease characterized by facial flushing, abdominal cramps, diarrhea, breathlessness, and other symptoms. Affects fewer than 10% of patients with carcinoid tumors.

CARCINOMA. A cancer that originates in cells that developed from epithelial tissue, a tissue that forms layers and often specializes to cover and protect organs.

CARCINOMA IN SITU (CIS). Cancer that is confined to the cells in which it originated and has not spread to other tissues.

CARCINOMA OF UNKNOWN PRIMARY ORIGIN (CUP). Metastatic cancer in which the type of cancer or site of origin is unknown.

CARDIAC TAMPONADE. Compression of the heart by large amounts of fluid or blood.

CAREGIVER BURDEN. The high level of emotional and physical stress experienced by a person who is caring for someone (most often a family member) with a long-term serious illness.

CARNEY COMPLEX. A genetic disorder characterized by myxomas, spotty pigmentation of the skin and mucous membranes, and endocrine overactivity.

CAROTENES. Pro-vitamin A carotene; orange or red carotenoids such as beta-carotene that can be converted to vitamin A.

CAROTENOIDS. Red or yellow plant pigments and phytonutrients with various biological activities in the human body.

CAROTID ARTERY. An artery located in the neck.

CASTRATION. Removal or destruction by radiation of both testicles (in a male) or both ovaries (in a female), making the individual incapable of reproducing.

CAT. Computerized axial tomography, also called computed tomography.

CATARACT. Formation on the lens of the eye that causes cloudy vision.

CATHARTIC. A general term for any agent that causes the bowel to empty. Cathartics are also known as purgatives.

CATHETER. Tube inserted into a body cavity or blood vessel to allow drainage of fluids (as in a urinary catheter), injection of drugs, or insertion of a surgical instrument.

CAUTERIZE. To use heat or chemicals to stop bleeding, prevent the spread of infection, or destroy tissue.

CBC. Complete blood count; a blood test that measures red cells, white cells and platelets.

CD20. A surface protein on B cells that is the target of obinutuzumab.

CECUM. The pouch-like start of the large intestine (colon) at the end of the small intestine.

CELL CYCLE. The events that take place during cell multiplication and division, also called replication.

CENTRAL NERVOUS SYSTEM (CNS). The brain and spinal cord.

CENTRAL VENOUS CATHETER (CVC). Vascular access device (VAD); a catheter in a larger vein in the neck or chest for delivering chemotherapy.

CEREBELLUM. The part of the brain that lies within the lower back portion of the skull behind the brain stem. The cerebellum helps to coordinate voluntary movements.

CEREBRAL ANEURYSM. An abnormal, localized bulge in a blood vessel that is usually caused by a congenital weakness in the wall of the vessel.

CEREBROSPINAL FLUID (CSF). The fluid surrounding the brain and spinal cord.

CEREBROVASCULAR ACCIDENT. Terminology that may be used to describe a stroke.

CEREBRUM. The largest part of the brain in humans, occupying the upper part of the skull cavity.

CERVICAL CRYOTHERAPY. A type of surgery that freezes and destroys abnormal cervical cells (dysplasia).

CERVICAL INTRAEPITHELIAL NEOPLASIA (CIN). A precancerous condition in which abnormal cells grow on the cervix, but do not extend into the deeper layers of tissue.

CERVIX. Opening of the uterus (womb) that leads into the vagina.

CESAREAN DELIVERY. Infant delivery through an incision in the abdominal wall and uterus.

CHAGAS DISEASE. Acute or chronic infection caused by the bite of a tick and characterized by fever, swollen glands, rapid heartbeat, and other symptoms.

"CHEMO BRAIN." A term used to describe problems with memory, concentration, or thinking clearly following chemotherapy.

CHEMOPROTECTIVE. The ability of a drug or other substance to protect healthy tissues from the toxic effects of chemotherapy drugs.

CHEMOTHERAPY. Administration of special cell-killing drugs into the body by injection or orally where they will circulate and kill cancer cells. Targeted chemotherapy kills only cancer cells; other types of chemotherapy also kill normal cells.

CHEST X-RAY. Brief exposure of the chest to radiation to produce an image of the chest and its internal structures.

CHILDHOOD CANCER SURVIVOR STUDY (CCSS). The National Cancer Institute's long-term study of the health of many thousands of survivors of childhood cancer.

CHIMERIC ANTIGEN RECEPTOR (CAR) CELLS. Immune cells that are genetically modified with receptors that bind a specific cancer-cell antigen; the binding activates the immune cell to destroy the cancer cell.

CHLORAMBUCIL (CLB). A chemotherapy drug used to treat chronic lymphocytic leukemia.

CHLORDANE. A banned organochlorine insecticide that persists in the environment.

CHLOROPHYLLIN. A semi-synthetic chlorophyll derivative that may help protect against the fungal carcinogen aflatoxin.

CHOLANGIOCARCINOMA. The medical name for bile duct cancer.

CHOLANGIOGRAPHY. Radiographic examination of the bile ducts after injection with a special dye. Used to determine whether the bile ducts are enlarged, narrowed, or blocked.

CHOLANGITIS. Inflammation of the bile duct.

CHOLECYSTECTOMY. The medical term for surgical removal of the gallbladder.

CHOLECYSTITIS. Inflammation of the gallbladder, usually due to infection.

CHOLESTEATOMA. A destructive and expanding sac that develops in the middle ear or mastoid process.

CHOLESTEROL. A steroid alcohol found in human cells and body fluids, implicated in the onset of heart disease.

CHORDOMA. A type of bone cancer.

CHORIOCARCINOMA. A malignant tumor that typically develops in the uterus following pregnancy, miscarriage, or abortion, especially in association with a hydatidiform mole.

CHORIONIC VILLUS SAMPLING (CVS). Prenatal testing performed at 10–12 weeks of gestation for biochemical and/or DNA testing of fetal cells.

CHOROID PLEXUS. Tissues of the brain that produce the fluid that coats the brain and spinal cord.

CHOROID PLEXUS CARCINOMA (CPC). A malignant tumor of the choroid plexus that often invades the underlying brain tissues and can spread to other parts of the body.

CHOROID PLEXUS PAPILLOMA (CPP). A benign tumor of the choroid plexus that does not invade the underlying brain tissues and does not spread to other parts of the body.

CHROMOSOME. A structure within the nucleus of every cell that contains genetic information governing the organism's development. There are 22 pairs of non-sex chromosomes and one pair of sex chromosomes.

CHRONIC. Pain that endures beyond the term of an injury or painful stimulus, including cancer pain.

CHRONIC FATIGUE SYNDROME. A term used for a group of debilitating disorders that last for a minimum of six months in adults and are characterized by persistent fatigue that is not caused by another medical disorder and is not relieved by normal sleep or rest. Chronic fatigue syndrome should not be confused with cancer-related fatigue.

CHRONIC LYMPHOCYTIC LEUKEMIA (CLL). A cancer characterized by an abnormal increase in mature lymphocytes, especially B cells, that primarily affects older adults.

CHRONIC MYELOGENOUS LEUKEMIA (CML). Also called chronic myelocytic leukemia; a malignant disorder that involves abnormal accumulation of white cells in the marrow and bloodstream.

CHRONIC PHASE. The initial phase of Chronic myelogenous leukemia (CML).

CHYLOUS ASCITES. A form of ascites in which chyle, a milky fluid formed in the small intestine from lymph and partially digested fats, leaks into the peritoneal cavity from damaged lymphatic vessels.

CIRCULATORY SYSTEM. Made up of the heart and blood vessels. It serves as the body's transportation system.

CIRCUMCISION. The practice of surgically removing the foreskin of the penis shortly after birth, usually for cultural or religious reasons.

CIRRHOSIS. A chronic degenerative disease of the liver, in which normal cells are replaced by fibrous tissue. Cirrhosis is a major risk factor for the later development of liver cancer.

CISPLATIN. A platinum-containing chemotherapy drug that acts as an alkylating agent and increases the risk of developing difficult-to-treat leukemia.

CLEARANCE. A measure of the rate at which a drug or other substance is removed from the blood.

CLINICAL TRIAL. A study to determine the efficacy and safety of a drug or medical procedure. This type of study is often called an experimental or investigational procedure.

C-MYC. An oncogene that is a master regulator of cell-cycle progression, apoptosis, and cellular transformation.

COAGULATION. The blood's natural tendency to clump and stick.

COLLIMATOR. A metal tube designed to control the size and direction of a beam of radiation.

COLON. The large intestine.

COLONOSCOPE. A thin, flexible, hollow, lighted tube that is inserted through the anus and rectum to the colon to enable a physician to view the entire lining of the colon.

COLONOSCOPY. An examination of the rectum and colon performed by inserting a colonoscope (a thin, flexible, lighted tube) through the anus.

COLORECTAL CANCER. Cancer of the colon and rectum.

COLOSTOMY. Surgical connection of the colon to an opening in the abdominal wall to create an artificial anus.

COLPOSCOPE. An instrument used for examination of the vagina and cervix. The instrument includes a light and magnifying lens for better visualization.

COLPOSCOPY. Diagnostic procedure using a hollow lighted tube (colposcope) to look inside the cervix and uterus.

COMPASSIONATE USE. A type of legal exemption that allows patients with life-threatening illnesses access to investigational drugs or alternative therapies when all other treatments have failed.

COMPETENT. Duly qualified; having sufficient ability or authority; possessing all the requirements of law.

COMPLEMENT. A group of complex proteins of the beta-globulin type in the blood that bind to antibodies during anaphylaxis. In the complement cascade, each complement interacts with another in a pattern that causes fluid build-up in cells, leading to lysis (cell destruction).

COMPLEMENTARY. Any form of treatment outside the mainstream that is not considered a cure, but is given to ease symptoms or contribute to general well-being.

COMPLEMENTARY THERAPY. A therapy used in addition to conventional treatments.

COMPLETE BLOOD COUNT (CBC). A blood test that measures red cells, white cells and platelets.

COMPLETE BLOOD COUNT (CBC) WITH DIFFERENTIAL. Counts of red blood cells and platelets, the types and numbers of white blood cells, the amount of hemoglobin in red blood cells, and a hematocrit (the proportion of red cells in the blood); used to screen for second cancers.

COMPLETE REMISSION (CR). The total elimination of all diseased cells detectable following therapy.

COMPLETE RESPONSE. Another term for complete remission; the absence of cancer cells in response to treatment.

COMPUTED TOMOGRAPHY (CT). An imaging technique that produces three-dimensional pictures of organs and structures inside the body using a 360° x-ray beam.

CONDITIONING. Process of preparing a patient to receive marrow donation, often through the use of chemotherapy and radiation therapy.

CONDUIT DIVERSION. A surgical procedure that restores urinary and fecal continence by diverting these functions through a constructed conduit leading to an external waste reservoir (ostomy).

CONGENITAL. Existing at birth.

CONGESTIVE HEART FAILURE. A condition that results from inadequate pumping action of the heart muscle, causing fluid buildup in lungs and tissues.

CONIZATION. Cone biopsy; removal of a cone-shaped section of tissue from the cervix for diagnosis or treatment.

CONJUNCTIVA. A clear membrane that covers the inside of the eyelids and the outer surface of the eye.

CONNECTIVE TISSUE. Cells such as fibroblasts, and material such as collagen and reticulin, that unite one part of the body with another.

CONSCIOUS SEDATION. A level of sedation during which the patient remains awake but very relaxed.

CONSERVATION SURGERY. Surgery that preserves the aesthetics of the area to be worked on.

CONSOLIDATION THERAPY. A stage in treatment of acute lymphocytic leukemia (ALL) that follows induction of remission. The purpose of this stage is to eliminate remaining cancer cells that cannot be detected by usual methods.

CONSTIPATION. Difficult or infrequent bowel movements.

CONTRAST AGENT. A substance introduced into the body that allows radiographic visualization of certain tissues. Often used in MRI and CT imaging scans to emphasize the contrast between healthy and cancerous cells.

CONTRAST DYE. A radiopaque dye that allows enhancement of the anatomy demonstrable with conventional x-ray.

CONTRAST MEDIUM. A substance that highlights the tissue or organ being filmed.

CONVENTIONAL THERAPY. Treatments that are widely accepted and practiced by the mainstream medical community.

CORTICOSTEROIDS. A class of drugs, related to hormones produced by glands in the body, that suppress the immune system. Prednisone (Deltasone) and cortisone are examples of corticosteroids.

CORTISOL. A steroid hormone produced in the cortex of the adrenal gland and released in response to stress.

COSMETIC SURGERY. A form of plastic surgery performed to alter normal tissue to change its appearance.

COWDEN SYNDROME. A rare inherited disorder in which people are at increased risk of both benign and malignant breast tumors, as well as tumors in the digestive tract, ovaries, and thyroid gland.

COX-2 INHIBITOR. An anti-inflammatory drug that blocks the enzyme cyclooxygenase (COX)-2 and that may help prevent colon cancer.

CRANIAL NERVES. The set of 12 nerves found on each side of the head and neck that control the sensory and muscle functions of a number of organs, including the eyes, nose, tongue, face, and throat.

CRANIOCAUDAL. Refers to an x-ray beam placed directly over the part being examined.

CRANIOTOMY. A surgical procedure in which a piece of the skull is removed temporarily to provide access to the brain.

CRANIUM. Skull; the bony framework that holds the brain.

CROHN'S DISEASE. A chronic inflammatory disease that generally starts in the gastrointestinal tract and causes the immune system to attack its own body.

CRYOABLATION. The selective freezing of cancerous tissue in order to kill it.

CRYOGEN. A substance with a very low boiling point, such as liquid nitrogen, used in cryotherapy treatment.

CRYOGLOBULINEMIA. Condition triggered by exposure to low temperatures in which protein in the blood forms particles, blocking blood vessels and leading to pain and numbness of the extremities.

CRYOSURGERY. The use of a very low-temperature probe to freeze and thereby destroy tissue.

CRYOTHERAPY. A procedure that destroys a tumor or other abnormal tissue by freezing.

CRYPTOCOCCOSIS. A fungal infection that can cause meningitis.

CRYPTORCHIDISM. A developmental defect marked by the failure of the testes to descend into the scrotum.

CT SCAN. An imaging technique that uses a computer to combine multiple x-ray images into a two-dimensional cross-sectional image.

CURCUMIN. Phytonutrients in turmeric that have antioxidant and possibly anticancer activities.

CURETTAGE. Surgical method in which a tumor is scraped away from the healthy tissue.

CUSHING SYNDROME. Hormonal disorder characterized by a round face, mental or emotional instability, high blood pressure, weight gain, or abnormal growth of facial and body hair in women.

CUTANEOUS T-CELL LYMPHOMA. A type of skin cancer originating from T lymphocytes.

CYANOSIS. Bluish discoloration of the skin.

CYCLOOXYGENASE. A chemical important for the normal functioning of the human body. The body produces cyclooxygenase 1 (COX 1) and cyclooxygenase 2 (COX 2).

CYCLOOXYGENASE 1 (COX 1). The cyclooxygenase that helps the stomach, kidneys, and blood function.

CYCLOOXYGENASE 2 (COX 2). The cyclooxygenase that helps mediate inflammation and helps the brain feel pain and regulate fever.

CYCLOOXYGENASE-2 INHIBITOR. A type of drug, such as Celebrex, that reduces pain and inflammation. Also called a COX-2 inhibitor.

CYCLOTRON. A machine that accelerates charged atomic particles within a constant magnetic field.

CYP3A4. An enzyme that is predominately responsible for the metabolism of imatinib mesylate.

CYST. An abnormal sac containing fluid or semi-solid material.

CYSTECTOMY. The surgical resection of part or all of the bladder.

CYSTIC TUMOR. A tumor that consists of a sac filled with fluid.

CYSTITIS. An irritation of the bladder lining.

CYSTOSCOPE. Endoscope especially designed for urological use to examine the bladder, lower urinary tract, and prostate gland.

CYSTOSCOPY. A diagnostic procedure in which a hollow lighted tube (cystoscope) is used to look inside the bladder and the urethra.

CYTOCHROME P450. Enzymes present in the liver that metabolize drugs.

CYTOCHROME P450 2E1 (CYP2E1). A secondary pathway for metabolizing alcohol that generates reactive oxygen species that may promote cancer development.

CYTOKINE. A protein secreted by cells of the lymph system that affects the activity of other cells and is important in controlling inflammatory responses. Interleukin-2 is a cytokine.

CYTOLOGY. The study of cells.

CYTOMEGALOVIRUS. A viral disease caused by a herpes virus, generally rare but often seen in cancer patients. It can cause life-threatening pneumonia as well as blindness.

CYTOMETER. An instrument that measures cells.

CYTOPATHOLOGY. Another name for cytology; the study of cells or cell types.

CYTOPENIA. Deficiencies of certain elements in blood, such as red blood cells, white blood cells and/or platelets.

CYTOPLASM. The organized complex of organic and inorganic substances external to the nuclear membrane of a cell.

CYTOREDUCTION. Another term for debulking.

CYTOSTATIC. Inhibiting or suppressing cellular growth and multiplication.

CYTOTOXIC. A term that refers to chemicals that are directly toxic to a cell, preventing the growth or reproduction of the cell.

CYTOTOXIC DRUG. An anticancer drug that acts by killing or preventing the division of cells.

D

DABRAFENIB (TAFINLAR). A drug that targets a different tyrosine kinase in the same pathway as the kinases targeted by trametinib and that may be prescribed in combination with trametinib.

DDE. Dichlorodiphenyldichloroethylene; a common breakdown product of the insecticide DDT that can build up in agricultural soils and the body fat of animals (including humans).

DDT. Dichlorodiphenyltrichloroethane; a toxic organochlorine insecticide widely used for mosquito control but banned in the United States since 1972.

DEBULKING. The surgical removal of part of a cancerous tumor that cannot be completely excised, in order to improve the effectiveness of radiation therapy or chemotherapy.

DEEP VEIN THROMBOSIS. Also known as DVT, a condition in which a blood clot (thrombus) formed in one part of the circulation, becomes detached and lodges at another point (usually in one of the veins of the legs or arms). People may feel pain, redness, and swelling at the site where the blood clot lodges. This condition is treated with blood thinning drugs such as low molecular weight heparins (LMWHs), heparin, or warfarin.

DEFECATION. The act of having a bowel movement.

DEGENERATIVE DISEASES. Diseases characterized by progressive degenerative changes in tissue, including arteriosclerosis, diabetes mellitus, and osteoarthritis.

DELETION. A piece missing from a chromosome.

DELIRIUM. A mental state in which a person is confused, disoriented, and unable to think clearly. The person may also become agitated or have hallucinations.

DENDRITIC CELLS. Antigen-presenting cells that are effective in stimulating T cells.

DEOXYCYTIDINE. Component of DNA, the genetic material of a cell, that is similar in structure to gemcitabine.

DEOXYRIBONUCLEIC ACID (DNA). The genetic material in cells that holds the inherited instructions for growth, development, and cellular functioning.

DEPENDENCE. A strong desire or sense of compulsion to take a drug, combined with difficulty in controlling or stopping the use of the drug. Dependence may be physical, psychological, or both.

DEPERSONALIZATION. An alteration in the perception of self.

DERMATITIS. A skin disorder that causes inflammation; that is, redness, swelling, heat, and pain.

DERMATOFIBROSARCOMA PROTUBERANS (DFSP). A low-grade cancer of fibrous tissue under the skin, usually in the limbs or trunk.

DERMATOLOGIST. A doctor who specializes in skin care and treatment.

DERMATOSIS. A noninflammatory skin disorder.

DERMIS. A layer of skin sandwiched between the epidermis and the fat under the skin. It contains the blood vessels, nerves, sweat glands, and hair follicles.

DESMOID TUMORS. Fibrous tumors that can develop anywhere in the body and may or may not be cancerous.

DETOXIFICATION. Ridding the body of digestive wastes considered toxic through fasting, drinking large quantities of juice, or colonic irrigation.

DEXAMETHASONE. A corticosteroid that may be prescribed in combination with pomalidomide.

DIABETES. A degenerative disease characterized by inadequate production or absorption of insulin, excessive urine production, and excessive amounts of sugar in the blood and urine.

DIALYSIS. A technique used to remove waste products from the blood and excess fluid from the body as a treatment for kidney failure.

DIAPHRAGM. The large flat muscle that runs horizontally across the bottom of the chest cavity.

DIARRHEA. Frequent, watery stools.

DIETHYLSTILBESTROL (DES). A medication used between 1945 and 1970 to prevent miscarriage.

DIFFERENTIATED. Refers to cancer cells that multiply slowly and are closer in structure to normal cells. These cells carry a lower risk of recurrence than poorly differentiated or undifferentiated cells, which spread quickly and do not reach the matured state of normal cells.

DIFFERENTIATION. A change to a more mature phenotype or appearance.

DIFFUSE NEUROENDOCRINE SYSTEM. Concept developed by Feyrter, a German pathologist, more than 60 years ago, to unify tumors that occur in various parts of the body and possess secretory activity as well as similar properties when examined under a microscope.

DIFFUSION TENSOR IMAGING (DTI). A refinement of magnetic resonance imaging that allows the doctor to measure the flow of water and track the pathways of white matter in the brain. DTI is able to detect abnormalities in the brain that do not show up on standard MRI scans.

DIGESTION. The conversion of food in the stomach and intestines into substances capable of being absorbed by the blood.

DIGESTIVE SYSTEM. Organs and paths responsible for processing food in the body. These are the mouth, esophagus, stomach, liver, gallbladder, pancreas, small intestine, colon, and rectum.

DIGITAL RECTAL EXAMINATION (DRE). Procedure in which the physician inserts a gloved finger (digit) into the rectum to examine the rectum and the prostate gland for signs of cancer.

DIHYDROXYACETONE (DHA). A chemical used for staining the skin to simulate a tan.

DIOXINS. Toxic and carcinogenic environmentally persistent contaminants of pesticides and other chemicals.

DIPLOID. A cell with two sets of 23 chromosomes (the normal number in humans).

DISSEMINATED. Spread throughout the body.

DISTRESS. In general, an acute feeling of pain, anxiety, or sadness; in psycho-oncology, any unpleasant emotion that interferes with a cancer patient's ability to cope with symptoms and treatment.

DIURETIC. A drug that promotes the excretion of urine.

DIVERTICULITIS. A condition of the diverticulum of the intestinal tract, especially in the colon, where inflammation may cause distended sacs extending from the colon and pain.

DIVERTICULOSIS. A condition that involves the development of sacs that bulge through the large intestine's muscular walls, but are not inflamed. It may cause bleeding, stomach distress, and excess gas.

DIVERTICULUM (PLURAL, DIVERTICULA). A sac or pouch in the colon wall that is usually asymptomatic (without symptoms), but may cause difficulty if it becomes inflamed.

DM1. The chemotherapy drug mertansine.

DNA. Deoxyribonucleic acid; the genetic material found in each cell in the body that plays an important role in controlling many cell functions. When a cell divides to create two new cells, an identical copy of its DNA is found in each. If there is an error in a cell's DNA, division may not occur.

DNA REPAIR GENES. A type of gene that usually corrects the common mistakes that are made by the body as DNA copies itself. If these genes are themselves mutated and cannot correct these mistakes, the mistakes may accumulate and lead to cancer.

DNA SEQUENCE. The relative order of nucleotides, the chemical subunits of a DNA molecule.

DNA TESTING. Genetic testing for gene mutations.

DOCETAXEL. An anticancer drug, belonging to the drug family called mitotic inhibitors, that was the standard treatment for recurrent non-small cell lung cancer prior to pemetrexed.

DONOR. A healthy person who contributes an organ or bone marrow for transplantation.

DOPAMINE. A neurotransmitter that is a chemical messenger in the brain.

DOUBLE-BLIND STUDY. A study where neither the participant nor the physician know who has received the drug in question.

DOXORUBICIN. An extremely effective anticancer drug isolated from the *Streptomyces peucetius* bacteria.

DRUG CLEARANCE. The amount of a drug that is removed from the body through urination.

DRUG MISUSE. The use of a drug for purposes other than those for which the drug is intended. The recreational use of prescription painkillers is an example of drug misuse.

DUAL DIAGNOSIS. A term used to describe patients who suffer from a diagnosed mental disorder and comorbid substance abuse.

DUCTAL ADENOCARCINOMA. A malignant tumor arising from the duct cells within a gland.

DUCTAL CARCINOMA. Breast cancer that originates in the lining of the milk duct; ductal carcinoma in situ (DCIS) is ductal cancer that has not become invasive.

DUCTOGRAM. A special type of mammogram used to diagnose the cause of abnormal nipple discharges.

DUODENUM. The first part of the small intestine that connects the stomach above and the jejunum below.

DURA MATER. The tough membrane that encases the nerves of the spinal cord.

DYSGEUSIA. Taste dysfunction.

DYSKINESIA. A condition that causes a person to make abnormal, involuntary movements.

DYSPHAGIA. Difficulty in eating as a result of disruption in the swallowing process. Dysphagia can be a serious health threat because of the risk of aspiration pneumonia, malnutrition, dehydration, weight loss, and airway obstruction.

DYSPLASIA. The abnormal change in size, shape, or organization of adult cells.

DYSPLASTIC NEVUS SYNDROME. A familial syndrome characterized by the presence of multiple atypical appearing moles, often at a young age.

DYSPNEA. Difficulty breathing.

E

ECTOCERVIX. The part of the cervix closest to the vagina, covered primarily with squamous cells.

ECTOPIC. In an abnormal position.

ECTOPIC PREGNANCY. A pregnancy that occurs outside the uterus, most commonly in a fallopian tube.

ECZEMA. A superficial inflammation of the skin, generally with itching and a red rash.

EDEMA. An accumulation of watery fluid that causes swelling of the affected tissue.

EFFUSION. The collection of fluid in a body cavity or tissue due to the rupture of a blood or other body vessel, resulting from a type of trauma, cancer, or other condition.

EJECTION FRACTION. The percentage of the blood sitting in the heart between heartbeats that gets pumped to the body with each heartbeat.

ELECTROCARDIOGRAPHY (ECG). Recording of electrical potential during heartbeats.

ELECTROFULGURATION. A procedure in which a high-energy laser beam is used to burn cancerous tissue.

ELECTROLYTE LEVELS. In the bloodstream, electrolyte levels are the amounts of certain acids, bases, and salts. Abnormal levels of certain electrolytes can be life-threatening.

ELECTROLYTES. Elements normally found in the body (sodium, potassium, calcium, magnesium, phosphorus, chloride, and acetate) that are important to maintain the many cellular functions and growth.

ELECTROMAGNETIC SPECTRUM. The entire range of wavelengths or frequencies of radiation, extending from high-energy gamma rays to extremely low-frequency radio waves, including visible light and radiofrequency energy.

ELECTRON BEAM. A type of radiation composed of electrons. Electrons are tiny, negatively charged particles found in atoms.

ELECTROPHORESIS. Use of an electrical field to separate proteins in a mixture (such as blood or urine), on the basis of the size and electrical charge of the proteins.

ELECTROSURGICAL DEVICE. A medical device that uses electrical current to cauterize or coagulate tissue during surgical procedures, often used in conjunction with laparoscopy, colonoscopy, or sigmoidoscopy.

ELLAGIC ACID. A phenolic antioxidant in many fruits and vegetables.

ELUTE. In chemistry, to remove by dissolving or washing. A drug-eluting stent is one that contains a medication to reduce inflammation.

EMASCULATION. Another term for castration of a male.

EMBOLISM. A blood clot, air bubble, or clot of foreign material that travels and blocks the flow of blood in an artery. When blood supply to a tissue or organ is blocked by an embolism, infarction (death of the tissue the artery feeds) occurs. Without immediate and appropriate treatment, an embolism can be fatal.

EMBOLIZATION. A treatment in which foam, silicone, or other substance is injected into a blood vessel in order to close it off.

EMBOLUS (PLURAL, EMBOLI). A clump of tumor cells that breaks off from a primary tumor to travel through the circulatory system and lodge in a capillary in another part of the body.

EMBRYO. A developing human from the time of conception to the end of the eighth week after conception.

EMBRYONAL RHABDOMYOSARCOMA (ERMS). The most common type of RMS in children; it usually occurs in the head, neck, or genitourinary tract and resembles fetal skeletal-muscle tissue.

EMESIS. The expelling of stomach contents, also called vomiting.

EMESIS BASIN. A basin used to collect sputum or vomit.

EMETOGENIC. The relative tendency or likelihood of a drug to produce vomiting in patients receiving it.

EMPHYSEMA. Abnormal lung condition characterized by breathing problems, cough, and rapid heartbeat. Later stages are characterized by restlessness, weakness, confusion, and increased breathlessness. The condition may cause fluid to collect around the lungs (pulmonary edema) and lead to congestive heart failure.

EMPYEMA. An accumulation of pus in the lung cavity, usually as a result of infection.

EMTANSINE. The DM1 and MCC linker portion of ado-trastuzumab emtansine.

ENCEPHALITIS. An inflammation or infection of the brain and spinal cord caused by a virus or as a complication of another infection.

ENCEPHALOPATHY. Syndrome of global brain disease or injury.

ENDEMIC. Present in a specific population or geographical area at all times.

ENDOCERVICAL CURETTAGE. Biopsy performed with a curette to scrape the mucous membrane of the cervical canal.

ENDOCERVIX. The part of the cervix closest to the uterus, covered primarily with glandular cells.

ENDOCRINE. A term used to describe the glands that produce hormones in the body.

ENDOCRINE DISRUPTER. A chemical that interferes with the endocrine or hormone system, causing adverse developmental, neurological, reproductive, or immunological effects.

ENDOCRINE GLAND. A gland that makes hormones and secretes them into the bloodstream.

ENDOCRINOLOGIST. A doctor who specializes in diagnosing and treating disorders that affect the balance of hormones in the body or the organs that produce these hormones.

ENDOMETRIAL CANCER. Cancer of the uterus.

ENDOMETRIAL HYPERPLASIA. A condition in which the endometrium produces an overgrowth of cells during the menstrual cycle. It is not cancerous in itself but is a risk factor for endometrial cancer.

ENDOMETRIAL POLYPS. Growths in the lining of the uterus (endometrium) that may cause bleeding and can develop into cancer.

ENDOMETRIAL TISSUE. The tissue lining the uterus that is sloughed off during a woman's menstrual period.

ENDOMETRIOSIS. A disease involving occurrence of endometrial tissue (lining of the uterus) outside the uterus in the abdominal cavity; often diagnosed and treated using laparoscopy.

ENDOMETRIUM. The inner mucous membrane that lines the uterus in humans and other mammals.

ENDORECTAL PROBE. Instrument which sends sound waves through the prostrate. Sound echoes are then recorded as an image.

ENDORPHINS. A class of peptides in the brain that bind to opiate receptors, resulting in pleasant feelings and pain relief.

ENDOSCOPE. An instrument with a light source attached that allows the doctor to examine the inside of the digestive tract or other hollow organ.

ENDOSCOPIC RETROGRADE CHOLANGIOPANCREATOGRAPHY (ERCP). A procedure to x-ray the ducts (tubes) that carry bile from the liver to the gallbladder and from the gallbladder to the small intestine.

ENDOSCOPIC TUBE. A tube that is inserted into a hollow organ permitting a physician to see inside it.

ENDOSCOPIC ULTRASONOGRAPHY (EUS). Diagnostic imaging technique where an ultrasound probe is inserted down a patient's throat to determine if a tumor is present.

ENDOSCOPIC ULTRASOUND. A radiologic test utilizing a thin, flexible endoscope with a built-in miniature ultrasound probe that emits high frequency sound waves to create images of the gastrointestinal tract.

ENDOSCOPY. A medical examination in which an instrument called an endoscope is passed into an area of the body (the bladder or intestine, for example). The endoscope usually has a fiberoptic camera, which allows a greatly magnified image to be projected onto a video screen, to be viewed by the operator. Many endoscopes also allow the operator to retrieve a small sample (biopsy) of the area being examined, in order to more closely view the tissue under a microscope.

ENDOSTATIN. A naturally occurring polypeptide that inhibits endothelial cell proliferation, angiogenesis, and tumor growth.

ENDOTHELIAL CELLS. The cells lining the inside of blood vessels.

ENDOTRACHEAL. Placed within the trachea, also known as the windpipe.

ENDOTRACHEAL TUBE. A hollow tube that is inserted into the windpipe to administer anesthesia.

ENEMA. Insertion of a tube into the rectum to infuse fluid into the bowel and encourage a bowel movement or to infuse contrast dye for x-rays of the gastrointestinal tract.

ENGRAFTMENT. The process of transplanted stem cells reproducing new cells.

ENTERAL NUTRITION. Feedings administered through a nose tube (or surgically placed tubes) for patients with eating difficulties.

ENTERAL NUTRITIONAL SUPPORT. Nutrition utilizing an intact gastrointestinal tract, but bypassing another organ such as the stomach or esophagus.

ENUCLEATION. Surgical removal of an eye.

ENZYME. A protein in the body that breaks down substances, such as food or medicines, into simpler substances that the body can use.

EPENDYMOMA. A tumor that begins in the tissue that lines the central canal of the spinal cord and the ventricles of the brain.

EPIDEMIOLOGY. The branch of medicine concerned with studying the incidence and prevalence of outbreaks of disease in large groups of people, the factors that affect the frequency or spread of disease, and detection of the sources or causes of epidemics.

EPIDERMAL GROWTH FACTOR. Natural body chemical involved in cellular processes of growth and development.

EPIDERMAL GROWTH FACTOR RECEPTOR (EGFR). A protein on the cell surface that can initiate growth and proliferation.

EPIDERMIS. The outer covering of skin in mammals. In humans, it consists of five layers of cells.

EPIDIDYMIS. A tube in the back of the testes that transports sperm.

EPIDURAL. A type of regional anesthetic delivered by injection into the area around the patient's lower spine. An epidural numbs the body below the waist but allows the patient to remain conscious throughout the procedure.

EPIGENETIC. Changes in gene expression caused by chemical or other outside factors.

EPIGENETICS. The study of changes in genes that do not affect the order in which those genes occur within a segment of DNA. Certain chemical reactions can cause a gene to "turn on" or "turn off" without any changes in the underlying DNA sequence. Epigenetics is the study of these changes.

EPILEPSY. Neurological disorder characterized by recurrent seizures.

EPINEPHRINE. A medication used to treat heart failure and severe allergic reactions.

EPIPHYSIS. The end of long tubular bones such as the femur in the leg and the humerus in the arm. Initially separated from the main bone by a layer of cartilage that eventually allows the parts to fuse.

EPITHELIAL CELLS. Cells that cover the surface of the body and line its cavities.

EPITHELIAL TISSUE. The collection of cells that cover the exterior and line the interior surfaces of the body.

EPITHELIOID HEMANGIOENDOTHELIOMA (EHE). A rare bone tumor that occurs most commonly in adults.

EPITHELIUM. A thin layer of tissue that covers organs, glands, and other structures within the body.

EPITOPE. A portion of a protein or other molecule that is recognized by specific antibodies.

EPSTEIN-BARR VIRUS (EBV). A type of herpesvirus (human herpesvirus 4), first identified in 1964, that causes infectious mononucleosis. It is found in most patients with the endemic form of Burkitt lymphoma, though its role in the disease is still unclear.

ERECTILE DYSFUNCTION (ED). Sexual disorder involving the inability to develop or maintain a penile erection.

ERYTHROCYTE. Red blood cell.

ERYTHRODERMA. An abnormal reddening of the entire skin surface.

ERYTHROMELALGIA. A condition characterized by warmth, redness, and pain in the hands and especially the feet.

ERYTHROPLAKIA. A flat red patch or lesion in the mouth.

ERYTHROPOIESIS. The ongoing production of red blood cells by the bone marrow.

ERYTHROPOIETIN. A drug that stimulates the bone marrow to make more red blood cells. It is also known as epoetin alfa.

ESOPHAGECTOMY. Surgical removal of the esophagus.

ESOPHAGUS. The upper portion of the digestive system, a tube that carries food and liquids from the mouth to the stomach.

ESTROGEN. The primary female sex hormone, responsible for the buildup of endometrial tissue, the development of secondary sexual characteristics in women, and regulation of other aspects of the menstrual cycle.

ESTROGEN RECEPTOR (ER). A cell-surface protein that binds the female hormone estrogen; present on ER-positive breast cancer cells.

ETHICS. The branch of philosophy that discusses and analyzes what is the best way for humans to live, and which actions may be right or wrong in specific circumstances. The English word is derived from the Greek word for habit or custom.

EUPHORIA. A state of intense pleasure, elation, or feelings of well-being that can be produced by normal human experiences but can also result from taking opioids or other psychoactive drugs. Euphoria induced by drugs is often referred to as a "high."

EUTHANASIA. The practice of intentionally ending life to relieve prolonged pain or suffering.

EWING SARCOMA. A highly malignant primary bone tumor most often found in young adults under the age of 30.

EX VIVO. Combined gene and cell-transfer therapy, in which cells are removed from the patient's blood, genetically modified, and returned to the patient.

EXCISION. Surgical removal.

EXENTERATION. Extensive surgery to remove the uterus, ovaries, pelvic lymph nodes, part or all of the vagina, and the bladder, rectum, and/or part of the colon.

EXOCRINE. A term used to describe organs that secrete substances outward through a duct.

EXOCRINE GLAND. A gland that secretes substances outwardly through a duct into a body cavity or onto a body surface (e.g., sweat glands and salivary glands).

EXTRACELLULAR MATRIX. A collection of connective-tissue proteins and fibers that supports and nourishes body tissues. The extracellular matrix forms a physical barrier to the movement of tumor cells.

EXTRACORPOREAL PHOTOCHEMOTHERAPY. A treatment procedure in which the white blood cells are exposed to a chemical called psoralen, which is removed from the blood and treated with UVA light, then reinfused into the body.

EXTRAMAMMARY PAGET DISEASE. Paget disease that is located anywhere on the body, excluding the breasts.

EXTRAOCULAR RETINOBLASTOMA. Cancer that has spread beyond the eye.

EXTRAOSSEOUS EWING TUMOR (EOE). A soft tissue tumor outside of bone tissue with some characteristics of embryonic nerve tissue.

EXTRAPYRAMIDAL. Referring to movement disorders that are associated with the use of certain drugs that act on the central nervous system and are also experienced by patients with central nervous system diseases such as Parkinson disease.

EXTRAVASATION. Passage or leakage from a blood vessel into the surrounding tissue.

F

FALLOPIAN TUBES. Slender tubes that carry ova from the ovaries to the uterus.

FALSE NEGATIVE. Test results showing no problem when one exists.

FALSE POSITIVE. Test results showing a problem when one does not exist.

FAMILIAL ADENOMATOUS POLYPOSIS (FAP). An inherited disease of the large intestine that is a risk factor for thyroid cancer.

FEBRILE NEUTROPENIA. A reduced neutrophil count (less than 0.5×10^9/l) accompanied by fever (an elevated oral temperature greater than $101.3°F$ [$38.5°C$]).

FEMORAL ARTERY. An artery located in the groin area.

FIBER. Roughage; bulk; indigestible material in food that may reduce the risk of colorectal cancer; insoluble fiber moves through the digestive system, giving bulk to stool; soluble fiber dissolves in water and helps keep stool soft.

FIBEROPTICS. Bundles of specially treated glass or plastic fibers that intensify light from a light source by internal reflection.

FIBRINOLYTICS. Agents that decompose fibrin, a protein produced in the clotting process.

FIBROADENOMA. A benign breast growth made up of fibrous tissue. It is the most common mass in women under 35 years of age, and is found in both breasts in 3% of cases.

FIBROID. A benign smooth muscle tumor of the uterus.

FIBROSIS. A condition characterized by the presence of scar tissue, or reticulin and collagen proliferation in tissues to the extent that it replaces normal tissues.

FINE-NEEDLE ASPIRATION (FNA). Use of a very thin type of needle to withdraw cells and body fluid for examination.

FISSURE. Any cleft or groove, normal or otherwise, especially a deep fold in the anus.

FISTULA (PLURAL, FISTULAE). An abnormal passage that develops either between two organs inside the body or between an organ and the surface of the body.

FIXATIVE. A chemical that preserves tissue without destroying or altering the structure of the cells.

FIXED. Chemically preserved dead tissue.

FLAP. A section of tissue moved from one area of the body to another.

FLAP SURGERY. A procedure in which a portion of living tissue is moved from one part of a patient's body to another to restore shape and/or function to the targeted location.

FLAVONOIDS. A large group of aromatic compounds, including many plant pigments and antioxidants.

FLUDARABINE. A drug that inhibits a blood cell's ability to produce DNA, eliminating native cells from FA patients so they can undergo BMT.

FLUORESCEIN DYE. An orange dye used to illuminate the blood vessels of the retina in fluorescein angiography.

FLUORESCENCE. Light absorbed at one wavelength and emitted at another so that it glows.

FLUORESCENT-ACTIVATED CELL SORTING (FACS). Flow cytometry or immunophenotyping.

FLUOROSCOPE. An imaging device that displays "moving x-rays" of the body.

FLUOROSCOPY. Also called radioscopy, this procedure involves the examination of internal body structures using x-rays and projecting images on a fluorescent screen.

FLUOROURACIL. A prescription drug used to treat actinic keratoses, solar keratoses, and various forms of cancer.

FOLATE. Folic acid; a B-complex vitamin that is required for normal fetal development and may help prevent cancer.

FOLIC ACID. Vitamin B9.

FOLIC ACID ANTAGONIST. A drug that interferes with the action of folic acid.

FOLLICULAR CARCINOMA. A well-differentiated cancer that develops in the hormone-producing follicular cells of the thyroid gland.

FOOD AND DRUG ADMINISTRATION. A government agency that oversees public safety in relation to drugs and medical devices. The FDA gives approval to pharmaceutical companies for commercial marketing of their products in the United States.

FORESKIN. The ring of smooth tissue that covers the glans penis in uncircumcised men.

FORMALIN. A clear solution of diluted formaldehyde that is used to preserve liver biopsy specimens until they can be examined in the laboratory.

FRACTIONATED. In radiotherapy, treatment that is divided into several sessions of smaller doses of radiation rather than one large dose delivered in a single session.

FRACTIONATION. A procedure for dividing a dose of radiation into smaller treatment doses.

FREE FLAP. A section of tissue that is detached from its blood supply, moved to another part of the body, and reattached by microsurgery to a new blood supply.

FREE RADICAL. An unstable, highly reactive molecule that occurs naturally as a result of cellular metabolism, but can be increased by environmental toxins, ultraviolet rays, and nuclear radiation. Free radicals damage cellular DNA and are thought to play a role in aging, cancer, and other diseases. Free radicals can be neutralized by antioxidants.

FREE RADICAL SCAVENGERS. Another name for antioxidants.

FRONTAL LOBES. The two lobes of the cerebrum of the brain that are responsible for cognitive thought processes (knowing, thinking, learning, and judging).

FUNCTIONAL SILO SYNDROME. A term used to refer to a closed-off information system incapable of interacting with other related systems. In cancer research, "silo" is often used to describe a pattern of storing research data or qualitative findings without sharing the information with other researchers.

G

GADOLINIUM. A very rare metallic element useful for its sensitivity to electromagnetic resonance, among other things. Traces of it can be injected into the body to enhance MRI images.

GALLBLADDER. The sac that stores bile from the liver.

GALLIUM. A form of radionuclide that is used to help locate tumors and inflammation; specifically referred to as GA67 citrate.

GAMMA KNIFE. A specific type of radiosurgery that uses highly focused cobalt-60 radiation to destroy cancerous tissue in the brain. It is not a knife in the conventional sense.

GAMMA RAYS. Short wavelength, high energy electromagnetic radiation emitted by radioactive substances.

GANTRY. A name for the portion of a CT scanner that houses the x-ray tube and detector array used to capture image information and send it to a computer.

GASTRECTOMY. A surgical procedure in which all or a portion of the stomach is removed.

GASTRIC. Of or relating to the stomach.

GASTRIC JUICE. An acidic secretion of the stomach that breaks down the proteins contained in ingested food, prior to digestion.

GASTRIN. Hormone normally secreted by the stomach that stimulates secretion of gastric acid.

GASTRINOMA. Tumor that arises from the gastrin-producing cells in the pancreas.

GASTRODUODENOSTOMY. A surgical procedure in which a new connection between the stomach and the duodenum is created.

GASTROESOPHAGEAL JUNCTION. The connection between the esophagus (the muscular tube extending from the pharynx) and the stomach.

GASTROESOPHAGEAL REFLUX DISEASE (GERD). A condition of excess stomach acidity in which stomach acid and partially digested food flow back into the esophagus during or after eating.

GASTROINTESTINAL (GI). Pertaining to the stomach and intestine.

GASTROINTESTINAL STROMAL TUMOR (GIST). Tumor of the gastrointestinal tract derived from connective tissue.

GASTROINTESTINAL TRACT. A group of organs and related structures that includes the esophagus, stomach, liver, gallbladder, pancreas, small intestine, large intestine, rectum, and anus.

GASTROJEJUNOSTOMY. A surgical procedure where the stomach is surgically connected to the jejunum.

GASTROPARESIS. Partial paralysis of the stomach, as can occur after a Whipple procedure.

GAZYVA/CHLORAMBUCIL (GCLB). Combined treatment with obinutuzumab and chlorambucil.

GENDER IDENTITY DISORDER (GID). A condition in which a person strongly identifies with the other sex and feels uncomfortable with his or her biological sex. It occurs more often in males than in females.

GENDER REASSIGNMENT SURGERY. The surgical alteration and reconstruction of a person's sex organs to resemble those of the other sex as closely as possible; it is sometimes called sex reassignment surgery.

GENE. A building block of inheritance, made up of a compound called DNA (deoxyribonucleic acid) and containing the instructions for the production of a particular protein. Each gene is found on a specific location on a chromosome.

GENE AMPLIFICATION. The presence of multiple copies of a small segment of chromosome containing one or more genes as a separate chromosome or as part of an otherwise normal chromosome.

GENE REARRANGEMENT. A change in the structure of a chromosome that changes the order of genes.

GENE THERAPY. The use of genes to treat cancer and other diseases.

GENERAL ANESTHESIA. Method used to completely sedate a patient and stop pain from being felt during an operation. General anesthesia is generally used only for major operations such as brain, neck, chest, abdomen, and pelvis surgery.

GENES. Packages of DNA that control the growth, development and normal function of the body.

GENETIC COUNSELOR. A specially trained health care provider who helps individuals understand whether a disease (such as cancer) runs in their family and their risk of inheriting this disease. Genetic counselors also discuss the benefits, risks and limitations of genetic testing with patients.

GENETIC TEST. A test to determine the presence of specific genes or the presence of mutations on specific genes.

GENETICALLY ENGINEERED. An organism that has been modified by the intervention of humans, usually by the addition of DNA, or hereditary material, from one species to the DNA of another species.

GENETICALLY MODIFIED (GM OR GMO) CROPS. Crops that contain genes from other organisms that confer resistance to herbicides.

GENETICALLY MODIFIED (GM OR GMO) FOODS. Foods from crops that contain genes from other organisms.

GENOME. The DNA sequences of all of the genes in a cell.

GENOMICS. The branch of science that deals with genomes and their functions.

GERM CELLS. Cells that are involved in reproduction. These cells are usually located in the gonads. Sometimes they fail to move to the gonads during embryonic development and cause tumors in other parts of the body.

GERMLINE. A genetic trait such as a mutation that is carried in the egg or sperm and transmitted to offspring.

GERMLINE MUTATION. A mutation that affects the germ cells (sperm or eggs) of an organism that reproduces by sexual reproduction. This type of mutation is inherited but is responsible for only a small minority of cancers.

GESTATIONAL TROPHOBLASTIC CANCER. A pregnancy-associated cancer in which a grape-like mole develops in the uterus instead of a fetus.

GESTATIONAL TROPHOBLASTIC DISEASE (GTD). A group of related, rare tumors that arise during pregnancy or after childbirth from embryonic tissue and include hydatidiform mole, choriocarcinoma, and placental-site trophoblastic tumors.

GLAND. A collection of cells whose function is to release certain chemicals (hormones) that are important to the functioning of other, sometimes distantly located, organs or body systems.

GLANS PENIS. The bulb of sensitive skin at the lower end of the penis. It is sometimes simply called the glans.

GLAUCOMA. An eye disorder marked by abnormally high pressure within the eyeball and vision disturbances.

GLEASON GRADING SYSTEM. A method of predicting the tendency of a tumor in the prostate to metastasize based on how similar the tumor is to normal prostate tissue; the higher the number the greater the predicted tendency of the tumor to metastasize.

GLIOBLASTOMA. Most aggressive and common type of primary brain tumor.

GLIOMA. Any tumor that arises from the supporting cells in the brain called glial cells.

GLOBULINS. A group of proteins in blood plasma whose levels can be measured by electrophoresis in order to diagnose or monitor a variety of serious illnesses.

GLUCOCORTICOID. An adrenocortical steroid hormone that is stimulated by the anterior pituitary. The three naturally occurring types are hydrocortisone, corticosterone, and cortisone.

GLUCOCORTICOID THERAPY. Treatment using corticoids that are anti-inflammatory and immunosuppressive.

GLUCONEOGENESIS. The formation of glucose from non-carbohydrates such as protein or fat.

GLUCOSINOLATES. Sulfur-containing phytonutrients in cruciferous plants that are metabolized to bioactive compounds such as isothiocyanates and indoles that may be anticarcinogenic.

GLUTAMINASE. The enzyme that breaks down glutamine; high glutaminase activity may be correlated with the proliferation of cancer cells.

GLUTATHIONE (GSH). A three-amino-acid tripeptide that reduces harmful oxygen radicals and activates some proteins, including natural killer cells.

GLYCOENGINEERING. The production of drugs, such as monoclonal antibodies, with specific sugar molecules attached to enhance their activity.

GONADOTROPIN-RELEASING HORMONE (GNRH). A hormone produced in the brain that controls the release of other hormones that are responsible for reproductive function.

GONADS. The male and female reproductive organs, which produce sperm (testes) and ovum (ovaries).

GONIOMETER. An instrument for measuring angles of a joint.

GONZALEZ REGIMEN. An alternative therapy for pancreatic cancer that includes a special diet, nutritional supplements, pancreatic enzymes, and coffee enemas.

GORLIN SYNDROME. A rare genetic condition in which a child is born with a predisposition to develop basal cell carcinoma. It is named for Robert Gorlin (1923–2006), the researcher who first described it in 1960.

GOUT. Disease caused by elevated levels of uric acid in the bloodstream that deposit as crystals in joints, tendons, and the big toe, causing painful arthritic attacks.

GRADE. As a noun: a classification of the cancerous qualities of an individual tumor. A higher grade indicates a more serious disease than does a lower grade. As a verb: to classify the cancerous qualities of an individual tumor.

GRAFT-VERSUS-HOST DISEASE (GVHD). A life-threatening complication of bone marrow transplants in which the donated marrow causes an immune reaction against the recipient's body.

GRAM-NEGATIVE. Types of bacteria that do not retain Gram stain.

GRAM-POSITIVE. Types of bacteria that retain Gram stain.

GRANULOCYTE. Any of three types of white blood cells (neutrophils, eosinophils, and basophils) that contain visible granules.

GRANULOCYTE COLONY-STIMULATING FACTOR (G-CSF). A protein and a type of hormone called a growth factor that stimulates the bone marrow to make neutrophils and some other types of white blood cells. Pharmaceutical granulocyte colony-stimulating factors are filgrastim (Neupogen) and lenograstim (Granisetron).

GRANULOCYTE-MACROPHAGE COLONY-STIMULATING FACTOR (GM-CSF). A growth factor that stimulates the bone marrow to make neutrophils and some other types of white blood cells. Pharmaceutical GM-CSFs are sargramostim and molgramostim.

GRANULOMATOUS DISEASE. A disease characterized by growth of tiny blood vessels and connective tissue.

GRANULOSA CELLS. Cells that form the wall of the ovarian follicle and produce various steroid hormones.

GROWTH FACTOR. A hormone that can stimulate body cells to grow or stimulate the bone marrow to make more cells. Growth factors are found naturally in the body, but synthetic versions can also be manufactured as drugs.

GUIDE WIRE. A wire that is inserted into an artery to guide a catheter to a certain location in the body.

GUILLAIN-BARRÉ SYNDROME. An inflammation involving nerves that affects the extremities and may spread to the face, arms, and chest.

GYNECOMASTIA. Benign enlargement of breast tissue in men. It may result from hormonal changes during puberty, the decline of testosterone production in older men, metabolic disorders, obesity, or Klinefelter's syndrome.

H

HAIRY CELL LEUKEMIA. A rare form of cancer in which hairy cells grow out of control in the blood, liver, and spleen.

HALF-LIFE. Length of time for the decay of one half of the radiation in a sample of a given radioactive isotope.

HEALTH CARE PROVIDER. A doctor, hospital, lab, or other professional person or facility offering health care services.

HEALTH CARE PROXY. A document in which a person appoints someone else (known as an agent) to make health care decisions in the event of the loss of the ability to do so.

HEALTH INSURANCE CLAIM. A bill for health care services that is submitted to the health insurance company for payment.

HEART MURMUR. Abnormal heart sound heard through a stethoscope.

HELICOBACTER PYLORI. A rod-shaped bacterium found in the stomach and associated with an increased risk of stomach cancer.

HEMANGIOBLASTOMA. A tumor composed of capillaries and disorganized clumps of capillary cells or angioblasts.

HEMANGIOENDOTHELIOMA. A low-grade sarcoma of the blood vessels of soft tissues or internal organs such as the lungs or liver.

HEMANGIOMA. A benign tumor consisting of a mass of blood vessels.

HEMATOCRIT. The separation of red blood cells from plasma to determine their percent volume in whole blood, normally 35%–47% in females and 42%–52% in males.

HEMATOLOGIC. Relating to blood.

HEMATOLOGIST. A specialist who treats diseases and disorders of the blood and blood-forming organs.

HEMATOMA. An accumulation of blood, often clotted, in a body tissue or organ, usually caused by a break or tear in a blood vessel.

HEMATOPOIETIC. Referring to proteins that cause growth and maturity in blood cells.

HEMATOPOIETIC STEM CELLS (HSCS). Cells that have the potential to mature into red blood cells, white blood cells, or platelets; also called hematopoietic progenitor cells (HPCs).

HEMATOPORPHYRIN. A dark reddish-purple pigment found in blood. A purified form of hematoporphyrin is used in the compounding of porfimer sodium.

HEMATURIA. The presence of blood in the urine.

HEMICOLECTOMY. Surgical removal of half of the large intestine.

HEMODIALYSIS. The removal of blood from an artery for purification and its return to a vein.

HEMOGLOBIN. A respiratory pigment in the red blood cells that combines with and transports oxygen around the body.

HEMOLYSIS. Also called hematolysis, the breakage of red blood cells and concomitant liberation of hemoglobin.

HEMOLYTIC ANEMIA. Type of anemia involving destruction of red blood cells.

HEMOPTYSIS. The expectoration of blood or of sputum containing blood.

HEMORRHAGE. Very severe, massive bleeding that is difficult to control.

HEMORRHAGIC CYSTITIS. Irritation of the bladder lining that causes bleeding.

HEMOSTASIS. Slowing down or stoppage of bleeding.

HEMOTHORAX. Blood in the pleural cavity.

HEPARIN. A medication that prevents blood clotting.

HEPATIC. Of the liver.

HEPATIC CAPSULE. The membranous bag enclosing the liver.

HEPATIC INTRA-ARTERIAL INFUSION. Injection of medicine into the artery to the liver.

HEPATIC VENO-OCCLUSIVE DISEASE. Liver failure caused by chemotherapy that may benefit from glutamine supplementation.

HEPATITIS. Inflammation of the liver caused by a virus, chemical, or drug.

HEPATITIS B VIRUS (HBV). A virus that attacks the liver and that can be reactivated by obinutuzumab or ofatumumab treatment.

HEPATOBLASTOMA. A cancerous tumor of the liver. Individuals with FAP are at increased risk for developing this type of tumor at a young age.

HEPATOCELLULAR CARCINOMA. Malignant cancer of the liver that may arise in the liver or metastasize from elsewhere in the body.

HER2. Human epidermal growth factor receptor 2, which is overproduced in HER2-positive breast cancers.

HERD IMMUNITY. Community immunity; disease protection for nonimmune or unvaccinated individuals that is conferred by the prevailing immunity within a population due to widespread vaccination coverage.

HEREDITARY NONPOLYPOSIS COLORECTAL CANCER (HNPCC). Lynch syndrome; the most common familial cancer syndrome that increases the risk of colorectal cancer, especially at a younger age; caused by inherited mutations in any of several genes, most of which are involved in DNA repair.

HEREDITARY SPHEROCYTOSIS. A hereditary disorder that leads to a chronic form of anemia (too few red blood cells) due to an abnormality in the red blood cell membrane.

HERPES SIMPLEX. Either of two viral diseases marked by clusters of small watery blisters, one affecting the area of the mouth and lips (HSV-1) and the other the genitals (HSV-2).

HERPES ZOSTER. An acute infectious viral disease characterized by painful, fluid-filled lesions. It is also known as shingles. Herpes zoster is caused by the varicella zoster virus (VZV), which causes chickenpox. The skin blisters of herpes zoster typically erupt months or even years after the initial episode of chickenpox.

HETEROCYCLIC AMINES (HCAS). Chemicals that form in meat cooked at high temperatures and that can damage DNA and may increase the risk of cancer.

HIGHLY ACTIVE ANTIRETROVIRAL THERAPY (HAART). A form of drug-combination treatment for HIV infection introduced in 1998. Most HAART regimens are combinations of three or four drugs, usually nucleoside analogs and protease inhibitors.

HISTOLOGY. The study of tissues.

HISTOPATHOLOGY. The study of diseased tissues on the microscopic level.

HIV/AIDS. Human immunodeficiency virus/acquired immune deficiency syndrome.

HLA TYPE. Refers to the unique set of proteins called human leukocyte antigens. These proteins are present on each individual's cell and allow the immune system to recognize 'self' from 'foreign.' HLA type is particularly important in organ and tissue transplantation.

HODGKIN LYMPHOMA. Cancer of the lymphatic system, characterized by lymph node enlargement and the presence of large polyploid cells called Reed-Sternberg cells; also called Hodgkin disease.

HOLISTIC. Any approach to health care that emphasizes the patient's total well-being, including psychological and spiritual, as well as physical aspects.

HOME PARENTERAL NUTRITION (HPN). Liquid nutrition via infusion for patients who are malnourished, or who have had surgery altering the usual process of chewing, swallowing, or digesting food.

HOMEOSTASIS. A state of the human body when self-regulating mechanisms are working, the body is in equilibrium, and there is no uncontrolled cell growth.

HOMOGRAFT. A graft made from tissue taken from a genetically nonidentical donor of the same species. It is also called an allograft.

HORMONE. A substance, such as cortisol or estrogen, that causes specific effects on target organs in the body. Hormones may be required for tumor growth or survival. Hormones usually travel in the bloodstream from the organ where they originate to a different organ where they have their effect.

HORMONE RECEPTORS. Proteins on the surfaces of cells that bind the female hormones estrogen and/or progesterone; hormone-positive breast cancers have less risk of recurrence because the hormones or the receptors that promote their growth can be blocked.

HORMONE REPLACEMENT THERAPY (HRT). Treatment of menopausal symptoms with the female hormones estrogen and/or progesterone.

HORMONE THERAPY. Cancer treatment that affects the hormone balance of the body, such as by blocking estrogen receptors or preventing estrogen production.

HOSPICE. A program that provides specialized medical and spiritual care for patients at the end of life. Hospice care may be delivered in the patient's home, in hospitals, or in separate facilities.

HUMAN CHORIONIC GONADOTROPIN (HCG). A hormone secreted by the placenta in early pregnancy and produced by some tumors; beta-hCG is a tumor marker for some germ-cell cancers.

HUMAN DEVELOPMENT INDEX (HDI). A population assessment ranging from low to very high and based on life expectancy at birth, educational attainment, and per capita income.

HUMAN GENOME PROJECT. An international project begun in 1990 and completed in 2003 that sequenced the three billion bases of DNA in the human genome.

HUMAN HERPESVIRUS-8 (HHV-8). Also called Kaposi sarcoma herpesvirus (KSHV); a virus that can cause Kaposi sarcoma in people with immune deficiency and that is present in the lymph nodes of many patients with multicentric Castleman disease, especially those with HIV/AIDS.

HUMAN IMMUNODEFICIENCY VIRUS (HIV). The virus that causes acquired immune deficiency syndrome (AIDS).

HUMAN LEUKOCYTE ANTIGEN (HLA). A group of protein molecules located on bone marrow cells that can provoke an immune response. A donor's and a recipient's HLA types should match as closely as possible to prevent the recipient's immune system from attacking the donor's marrow as a foreign material that does not belong in the body.

HUMAN PAPILLOMAVIRUSES (HPV). A family of viruses that cause common warts of the hands and feet, as well as lesions and warts in the genital and vaginal area. More than 50 types of HPV have been identified, some of which are linked to cancerous and precancerous conditions, including cancer of the cervix. A vaccine is now available against some of these viruses.

HUMANIZATION. The process of replacing the animal portions of a protein, such as an antibody produced in an animal, with human portions so that the human immune system does not recognize the protein as foreign.

HUMANIZED MONOCLONAL ANTIBODY. Human-like antibodies usually genetically engineered in mice and used in a therapeutic manner.

HYDATIDIFORM MOLE. Multiple cysts arising from the degeneration of chorionic villi—early fetal tissue that is imbedded into the uterine lining—and characterized by an enlarged uterus and vaginal bleeding.

HYDROCELE. A benign condition in which fluid collects around a testicle, causing enlargement. Hydroceles are usually painless unless they grow very large.

HYDROCEPHALUS. A condition marked by the buildup of cerebrospinal fluid within the skull, causing increased pressure on the brain and a variety of neurologic symptoms. Stereotactic surgery can be used to place a catheter within the brain in order to drain the excess fluid.

HYDROGEN. The simplest, most common element known in the universe. It is composed of a single electron (negatively charged particle) circling a nucleus consisting of a single proton (positively charged particle).

HYDRONEPHROSIS. Severe swelling of the kidney due to backup of urine. It may occur because of an obstruction, calculi, tumor, or other pathological conditions.

HYPERALIMENTATION. The administration of a nutrient solution into a large, central vein near the heart. It is sometimes used to supplement eating, but can also provide complete nourishment.

HYPERCALCEMIA. Abnormally high levels of calcium in the blood, causing muscle pain, weakness, and loss of appetite. Severe cases can result in kidney failure.

HYPERCALCEMIA OF MALIGNANCY. Also called tumor-induced hypercalcemia; high levels of calcium in the blood from the dissolving of bone, either directly by cancer cells or indirectly by chemicals released from cancer cells.

HYPERCELLULAR. Bone marrow is described as being hypercellular if the number of cells present in the bone marrow is unusually great.

HYPERGLYCEMIA. An abnormally increased level of glucose (sugar) in the blood.

HYPERICIN. A chemical derived from plants that kills cells after being activated by visible light.

HYPERKALEMIA. Excess potassium in the blood.

HYPERPHOSPHATEMIA. Excess phosphate in the blood.

HYPERPLASIA. Generalized overgrowth of body tissues or organs due to excessive increases in the number of cells.

HYPERSENSITIVITY. An abnormally sensitive reaction to a stimulus, similar to an allergic reaction.

HYPERURICEMIA. Excess uric acid in the blood.

HYPERVISCOSITY. Thick, viscous blood, caused by the accumulation of large proteins, such as immunoglobulins, in the serum.

HYPERVISCOSITY SYNDROME. Overly viscous blood that cannot flow easily.

HYPOGEUSIA. Decreased taste sensitivity.

HYPOGLYCEMIA. An abnormally low blood glucose level.

HYPONATREMIA. A condition in which the serum sodium concentration falls to less than 135 milliequivalents per liter (mEq/L), caused by too little excretion of water or by too much water in the bloodstream; in severe cases, hyponatremia leads to water intoxication, characterized by confusion, lethargy, muscle spasms, convulsions, and coma.

HYPOPHARYNX. The lowermost part of the throat or the pharynx.

HYPOTHALAMIC-PITUITARY-ADRENAL (HPA) AXIS. A set of influences and feedback interactions among three endocrine glands, the hypothalamus, the pituitary, and the two adrenal glands. The HPA axis governs the body's response to stress and regulates many other body functions, including digestion, moods and feelings, the immune system, and the person's general level of energy.

HYPOVOLEMIA. A condition in which the volume of the blood in the body is decreased, due either to a loss of blood itself or a loss of blood plasma (the liquid portion of blood).

HYPOVOLEMIC SHOCK. Shock caused by a lack of circulating blood.

HYPOXIA. Lack of oxygen supply to cells that may lead to cell injury and ultimately cell death.

HYSTERECTOMY. Surgical removal of part or all of the uterus.

I

IATROGENIC. Caused unintentionally by medical treatment.

IDIOPATHIC THROMBOCYTOPENIA PURPURA (ITP). A rare autoimmune disorder characterized by an acute shortage of platelets with resultant bruising and spontaneous bleeding.

ILEOANAL RESERVOIR. Also known as ileoanal anastomosis or ileoanal pull through; a colon like pouch created from the last few inches of the ileum to collect stool and allow for normal bowel movements through the intact anus after removal of the large intestine.

ILEOSTOMY. Surgical connection of the ileum to an opening in the abdominal wall to create an artificial anus.

ILEUM. The last division of the small intestine between the jejunum and the large intestine.

IMMUNE RESPONSE. The body's natural protective reaction against disease and infection.

IMMUNE SYSTEM. The body's mechanism to fight infections, toxic substances, and to recognize and neutralize or eliminate foreign material (for example, a body organ transplanted from another person).

IMMUNITY. Ability to resist the effects of agents, such as bacteria and viruses, that cause disease.

IMMUNOCYTOCHEMISTRY. Method for staining cells or tissues using antibodies so that the location of a target molecule can be determined.

IMMUNODEFICIENCY. A disorder in which the immune system is ineffective or disabled due either to acquired or inherited disease.

IMMUNOELECTROPHORESIS. Use of an electrical field to separate proteins in a mixture (such as blood or urine), on the basis of the size and electrical charge of the proteins; followed by the detection of an antigen (such as IgM), using a specific antibody.

IMMUNOGLOBULIN (IG). Antibody; large protein produced by B cells that recognizes and binds to a specific antigen.

IMMUNOHISTOCHEMICAL TECHNIQUE. Scientific laboratory technique in which proteins present in or on a cell are identified using antibodies.

IMMUNOMODULATING. Affecting the immune response or immune-system functioning.

IMMUNOPHENOTYPING. Immunohistochemistry or flow cytometry to identify cell types using antibodies.

IMMUNOSUPPRESSANT. An agent that decreases activity of the immune system (for example, radiation or drugs).

IMMUNOSUPPRESSIVE. Any form of treatment that inhibits the body's normal immune response.

IMMUNOTHERAPY. Therapy that stimulates, enhances, or suppresses the body's immune response;

includes products such as monoclonal antibodies, vaccines, and growth factors.

IMMUNOTOXINS. Antibodies produced in the laboratory that recognize specific substances that are more abundant in cancer cells than in normal cells; immunotoxins identify cancer cells and deliver a powerful toxin that kills the cells.

IMPLANT. A device inserted into the body to either treat cancer or to replace or substitute for a lost part or ability.

IN VIVO. Gene therapy in which a vector is used to introduce genetic material into cells within the body.

INCISION. A surgical cut or gash.

INCOMPLETE FREUD'S ADJUVANT (IFA). A mineral oil-emulsifying agent adjuvant that is often used in cancer vaccines.

INCONTINENCE. The inability to retain urine or bowel movements until a person is ready to expel them voluntarily.

INDICATION. A valid reason for prescribing a certain medication.

INDOLE-3-CARBINOL (I3C). A metabolite of glucosinolates that may have cancer-preventing activity.

INDOLENT. Relatively inactive or slow-spreading.

INDUCTION THERAPY. Initial intensive course of chemotherapy designed to wipe out abnormal cells and allow regrowth of normal cells.

INFECTIOUS MONONUCLEOSIS. A common viral infection caused by Epstein-Barr virus (EBV) with symptoms of sore throat, fever, and fatigue.

INFERIOR VENA CAVA. The large vein that returns blood from the lower body to the heart.

INFERTILITY. The inability to become pregnant or carry a pregnancy to term.

INFILTRATING LOBULAR CARCINOMA. A type of cancer that accounts for 8% to 10% of breast cancers. In breasts that are especially dense, ultrasound can be useful in identifying these masses.

INFLAMMATION. A response to injury, irritation, or illness characterized by redness, pain, swelling, and heat.

INFLAMMATORY BOWEL DISEASE (IBD). A disease that can be divided into two types: Crohn's disease and ulcerative colitis. Patients with Crohn's disease can have inflammation of the full thickness of the walls of the entire gastrointestinal tract. In patients with ulcerative colitis, the inflammation is limited to the surface of the walls of the large intestine and rectum.

INFORMED CONSENT. A process for obtaining a patient's permission before a medical intervention, or obtaining a research subject's permission prior to enrollment in a clinical trial.

INFUSION THERAPY. Administration of a medication as a liquid through an intravenous (IV) device.

INGUINAL. Referring to the groin area.

INHERITED DISORDER. A disease that tends to occur within a family. A disease or disorder may be inherited when a specific gene or gene mutation is passed from parent to child, predisposing the individual to developing the disease or disorder.

INNATE IMMUNE SYSTEM. The subsystem of the immune system comprised of cells and mechanisms that defend the body against infection in an immediate but nonspecific fashion.

INOSITOL HEXAPHOSPHATE (IP6). Phytic acid; a phytochemical in high-fiber foods that may have cancer-preventing properties.

INSTILLATION. Dropping a liquid into a body part such as the bladder.

INSUFFLATION. Inflation of the abdominal cavity using carbon dioxide; performed prior to laparoscopy to give the surgeon space to maneuver surgical equipment.

INSULIN. A hormone required for the metabolism of carbohydrates, lipids, and proteins, and regulation of blood sugar levels; lack of insulin or insulin insensitivity results in high blood sugar levels and diabetes.

INSULIN-LIKE GROWTH FACTOR-1 (IGF-1). An insulin-like growth factor that normally declines after puberty, but that is produced by fat cells and may be associated with increased cancer risk.

INSULINOMA. Tumor that arises from the insulin-producing cells in the pancreas.

INTEGRATIVE. An approach to cancer treatment that combines mainstream therapies with one or more complementary therapies.

INTERFERON. A potent immune-defense protein produced by viral-infected cells; used as an anti-cancer and anti-viral drug.

INTERFERON ALPHA. A chemical made naturally by the immune system and also manufactured as a drug.

INTERLEUKIN-6 (IL-6). A small molecule produced by immune-system and other cells that has a variety of activities including inducing the maturation of B cells, the growth and proliferation of T cells and myeloma cells, and the synthesis of plasma proteins.

INTERLEUKIN-11 (IL-11). A growth factor that stimulates platelet production in the bone marrow; oprelvekin is a recombinant form of IL-11 that is used to prevent or treat thrombocytopenia.

INTERLEUKINS. A family of potent immune-defense molecules; used in various clinical therapies.

INTERNATIONAL PROGNOSTIC INDEX (IPI). A system for predicting the prognosis of lymphoma patients on the basis of five factors.

INTERSTITIAL CYSTITIS. A chronic inflammatory condition of the bladder involving symptoms of bladder pain, frequent urination, and burning during urination.

INTERSTITIAL PNEUMONITIS. Type of lung disease caused by inflammation of the tissue and space around the air sacs of the lungs.

INTERSTITIAL RADIATION THERAPY. The process of placing radioactive sources directly into a tumor. These radioactive sources can be temporary (removed after the proper dose is reached) or permanent.

INTERVENTIONAL RADIOGRAPHY. Diagnostic and therapeutic x-ray procedures that are invasive or surgical in nature but do not require the use of general anesthesia.

INTESTINE. Commonly called the bowels, divided into the small and large intestine. They extend from the stomach to the anus. The small intestine is about 20 ft. (6 m) long. The large intestine is about 5 ft. (1.5 m) long.

INTRA-ARTERIAL. Regional chemotherapy delivered into an artery that leads to the tumor.

INTRACAVITARY. Regional chemotherapy delivered into a body cavity.

INTRACAVITARY RADIATION. Radiation therapy for vaginal cancer in which a cylindrical container holding a radioactive substance is placed into the vagina for one or two days.

INTRACRANIAL HYPERTENSION. A higher than normal pressure of the fluid in the skull.

INTRACRANIAL PRESSURE (ICP). Pressure inside the skull.

INTRAMUSCULAR (IM). Injected into a muscle.

INTRAMUSCULAR ADMINISTRATION. An injection, usually in the hip or arm, in which medication is delivered into a muscle.

INTRAOCULAR RETINOBLASTOMA. Cancer that is confined to the eye and has not spread to other parts of the body.

INTRAPERITONEAL (IP). Within the abdominal cavity.

INTRAPLEURAL. Infused into the chest cavity.

INTRATHECAL. Administered into the cerebrospinal fluid.

INTRATHECAL CHEMOTHERAPY. Chemotherapeutic drugs instilled directly into the spinal fluid, either by spinal tap or through a special reservoir.

INTRATHECAL THERAPY. Injection of a drug directly into the CSF using lumbar puncture.

INTRAVASATION. The entrance of cancer cells from a tumor into a vessel.

INTRAVENOUS. Administered into the body through a vein.

INTRAVENOUS ADMINISTRATION. Introduction of medication straight into a vein (commonly called IV).

INTRAVENOUS INJECTION. Injection directly into the vein.

INTRAVENOUS LINE. A tube that is inserted directly into a vein to carry medicine directly to the bloodstream, bypassing the stomach and other digestive organs that might alter the medicine.

INTRAVENOUS PYELOGRAM (IVP). A procedure in which dye injected into a vein in the arm travels through the body and concentrates in the urine for discharge. When an x-ray is taken, the dye highlights the kidneys, ureters, and urinary bladder, which reveals any abnormalities of the urinary tract.

INTRAVESICAL. Referring to any drug or treatment injected or instilled directly into the bladder.

INTUSSUSCEPTION. The folding of one segment of the intestine into another segment of the intestine.

INVASIVE. A descriptive term for tumors that spread to nearby structures.

INVERSION. A piece of a chromosome that is removed from the chromosome, inverted, and reinserted into the same location on the chromosome.

INVESTIGATIONAL DRUG. A drug that has not been approved for marketing by the FDA. These drugs are generally available to patients through participation in clinical trials/research studies.

IONIZING RADIATION. Electromagnetic radiation with enough energy to remove electrons from atoms, causing those atoms to become ionized or charged; high-frequency radiation including x-rays and gamma rays.

ISCHEMIA. A lack of normal blood supply to an organ or body part because of blockages or constriction of the blood vessels.

ISLETS OF LANGERHANS. Clusters of cells in the pancreas that make up the endocrine tissue.

ISOFLAVONES. Common phytonutrients with antioxidant and estrogenic activities.

ISOTOPES. Forms of a chemical element that have the same number of protons (atomic number) but different numbers of neutrons and different atomic weights.

J

JAUNDICE. Also termed icterus; an increase in blood bile pigments that are deposited in the skin, eyes, deeper tissue, and excretions. The skin and whites of the eyes will appear yellow.

JEJUNOSTOMY TUBE. J-tube; a feeding tube that goes directly into the small intestine.

JUGULAR VEINS. Large veins located on each side of the neck that return the blood from the head to the heart into two branches (external and internal).

K

KAPOSI SARCOMA. A rare connective tissue cancer that causes painless purplish-red (in light skin) or brown (in dark skin) blotches and is a diagnostic marker for HIV/AIDS.

KARYOTYPE. The specific chromosomal makeup of a particular cell.

KEGEL EXERCISES. Repetitive contractions of the muscles used to halt urinary flow, in order to enhance sexual responsiveness and control incontinence.

KERATINOCYTE. The most common type of skin cell; keratinocytes produce the protein keratin that provides strength for skin, hair, and nails.

KERATOCONJUNCTIVITIS. Inflammation of the conjunctiva and cornea of the eye.

KIDNEY FAILURE. Inability of the kidneys to excrete waste and maintain a proper chemical balance. Also called renal failure.

KIDNEY STONE. A concretion in the kidney made of various materials, such as uric acid crystals, calcium, or lipids. These concretions, or stones, cause severe pain when they are transported from the kidney into the bladder and out of the body.

KILOGRAM (KG). Metric measure that equals 2.2 pounds.

KINASE INHIBITOR. A drug that inhibits an enzyme called a kinase that adds phosphate to a protein in a signaling pathway.

KINASES. Proteins that add phosphates to other proteins in cell-signaling pathways.

KLATSKIN'S TUMORS. A name that is sometimes used to describe extrahepatic bile duct cancers located in the upper half of the bile duct. Klatskin's tumors are also known as perihilar bile duct tumors.

KLINEFELTER'S SYNDROME. A genetic disorder in which a man has at least one extra X chromosome in addition to the normal XY karyotype. Some men with Klinefelter's may have three or even four X chromosomes. In addition to gynecomastia, men with Klinefelter's have smaller-than-normal testicles and are sterile.

KNUDSON HYPOTHESIS. The hypothesis that cancer results from two (or more) mutations to a cell's DNA. It is sometimes called the two-hit hypothesis. The hypothesis was first suggested by Carl Nordling in 1953 and later reformulated by Alfred Knudson in 1971.

KRAS. A gene that is mutated in 30%–40% of colorectal tumors.

L

LACTATE DEHYDROGENASE (LDH). An enzyme that can be a tumor marker in the blood for some cancers.

LANDMARK. An anatomical structure that is easy to recognize and suitable as a reference point in locating other structures or making measurements.

LAPAROSCOPE. An instrument used to examine body cavities during certain types of surgery.

LAPAROSCOPIC SURGERY. Minimally invasive surgery in which a camera and surgical instruments are inserted through a small incision.

LAPAROSCOPY. The examination of the inside of the abdomen through a lighted tube (endoscope) inserted through a small incision, sometimes accompanied by surgery.

LAPAROTOMY. A surgical procedure in which the surgeon makes a large incision through the wall of the abdomen in order to gain access to the organs inside the abdominal cavity.

LARGE INTESTINE. Also called the colon, this structure has six major divisions: cecum, ascending colon, transverse colon, descending colon, sigmoid colon, and rectum.

LARYNGECTOMY. Surgical removal of the larynx.

LARYNGOPHARYNGECTOMY. Surgical removal of both the larynx and the pharynx.

LARYNGOSCOPY. The visualization of the larynx and vocal cords. This may be done directly with a fiber-optic scope (laryngoscope) or indirectly with mirrors.

LARYNX. Also known as the voice box, the larynx is composed of cartilage that contains the apparatus for voice production. This includes the vocal cords and the muscles and ligaments that move the cords.

LASER-CAPTURE MICRODISSECTION MICROSCOPE. An instrument that uses low-energy laser beams and special transfer film to lift single cells from a tissue.

LATE EFFECT. A condition or symptom that appears after the acute phase of a disease has run its course. The late effect may be caused directly by the original disease or indirectly by treatments for the disease.

LATISSIMUS DORSI. In Latin, this muscle literally means "widest of the back." This is a large fan-shaped muscle that covers a wide area of the back.

LAVAGE. Washing out.

LEIOMYOSARCOMA. A cancerous tumor of smooth (involuntary) muscle tissue.

LEPTIN. A peptide hormone produced by fat cells that acts on the hypothalamus to suppress appetite and burn stored fat.

LESION. An injured, diseased, or damaged area of tissue.

LEUCOVORIN. A drug that is sometimes used as the antidote for high dose treatments of the chemotherapy drug methotrexate.

LEUCOVORIN RESCUE. A cancer therapy where the drug leucovorin protects healthy cells from toxic chemotherapy.

LEUKAPHERESIS. A technique that uses a machine to remove stem cells from the blood; the cells are frozen and then returned to the patient following treatment that has destroyed the bone marrow.

LEUKEMIA. Group of cancers of the blood or bone marrow characterized by an abnormal multiplication of white blood cells.

LEUKOCORIA. An abnormal red reflex; a pupil that reflects white instead of black or red on a flash photograph; indicative of retinoblastoma.

LEUKOCYTES. Also called white blood cells, leukocytes fight infection and boost the immune system.

LEUKOCYTOSIS. Increased numbers of circulating white blood cells; an indication of infection.

LEUKOPENIA. A reduction in the normal number of white blood cells in the blood.

LEUKOPLAKIA. A flat whitish-colored area of the oral mucosa that is not caused by thrush or any other specific disease.

LHRH AGONISTS. Luteinizing hormone-releasing hormone (LHRH) drugs that initially cause the testes to make and release testosterone. With time, as the amount of testosterone in the blood rises, LHRH agonists stop the production of luteinizing hormone, which results in stopping overall production of testosterone.

LICHEN SCLEROSUS. A condition in which the skin of the vulva develops white patches and becomes thinner. It may be characterized by itching or have no symptoms. It is also known as kraurosis vulvae.

LI-FRAUMENI SYNDROME. A hereditary cancer predisposition syndrome that increases a person's risk of breast cancer, brain cancer, and osteosarcoma.

LIGNANS. A class of plant phenolic compounds with antioxidant and estrogenic activities.

LINDANE. Gamma-hexachlorocyclohexane; a neurotoxic insecticide that was widely used on crops in the 1960s and 1970s and is still used to treat lice and scabies.

LIPIDS. Any of a group of organic compounds consisting of fats, oils, and related substances that, along with proteins and carbohydrates, are the structural components of living cells.

LIPOSARCOMA. A cancer arising from immature fat cells of the bone marrow.

LIPOSOMES. An artificially produced, microscopic sphere, consisting of a drug surrounded by a cell membrane, used to help drugs get into target cells.

LIVER FUNCTION TESTS (LFTS). Blood tests that measure the blood serum levels of several enzymes produced by the liver.

LOBULAR CARCINOMA. Breast cancer that originates in the milk-producing glands.

LOBULAR CARCINOMA-IN-SITU (LCIS). Breast cancer that is confined to the milk-producing glands.

LOBULE. A small lobe or subdivision of a lobe (often on a gland) that may be seen on the surface of the gland as a bump or bulge.

LOCAL ANESTHETIC. A liquid used to numb a small area of the skin.

LOCALIZED. Confined to a small area.

LOOP ELECTROSURGICAL EXCISION PROCEDURE (LEEP). Cone biopsy performed with a wire that is heated by electrical current.

LUMBAR PUNCTURE. Also called a spinal tap, a procedure for the withdrawal of spinal fluid from the lumbar region of the spinal cord for diagnosis, or for injection of a dye for imaging, or for administering medication or an anesthetic.

LUMEN. The cavity or channel within a tube or tubular organ, such as a blood vessel or the intestine.

LUMPECTOMY. Breast-conserving surgery that removes only the cancerous tumor and a limited amount of normal surrounding tissue.

LUNASIN. A peptide in soy and some cereal grains that may have anticancer properties.

LUPUS ERYTHEMATOSUS. A long-term disease that affects women four times more often than men, characterized by severe swelling of the blood vessels giving rise to arthritis, kidney disorders, red rash over the nose and cheeks, weakness, fatigue, weight loss, photosensitivity, fever, and skin sores that may spread to the mucous membranes and other tissues of the body; also called systemic or disseminated lupus erythematosus.

LUTEAL PHASE. The part of the menstrual cycle that begins after ovulation and ends at menstruation.

LUTEINIZING HORMONE. A hormone that comes from part of the brain known as the pituitary gland. The testes will only produce testosterone if adequate levels of luteinizing hormone are present.

LUTEINIZING HORMONE-RELEASING HORMONE (LHRH) AGONIST. A substance that blocks the action of LHRH, a hormone that stimulates the production of testosterone (a male hormone) in men and women. Used to treat prostate cancers that require testosterone for growth.

LYCOPENE. A red plant pigment with antioxidant properties.

LYMPH. The almost colorless fluid that bathes body tissues. Lymph is found in the lymphatic vessels and carries lymphocytes that have entered the lymph glands from the blood.

LYMPH GLAND. A small bean-shaped organ consisting of a loose meshwork of tissue in which large numbers of white blood cells are embedded.

LYMPH NODE. A small mass of bean-shaped tissue that produces cells and proteins that fight infection. As an important part of the body's lymphatic system, these nodes clean and filter foreign or toxic cells, such as bacteria or cancer cells, out of the lymph fluid.

LYMPH NODE DISSECTION. Surgical removal of a group of lymph nodes.

LYMPHATIC. Pertaining to lymph, the clear fluid that is collected from tissues, flows through special vessels, and joins the venous circulation.

LYMPHATIC SYSTEM. The tissues and organs (including the bone marrow, spleen, thymus, and lymph nodes) that produce and store cells that fight infection, together with the network of vessels that carry lymph throughout the body.

LYMPHATICS. Channels that are conduits for lymph.

LYMPHEDEMA. Retention of lymph fluid in an affected (by surgery or disease) area.

LYMPHOBLASTS. The cancerous cells of ALL; immature forms of lymphocytes, white blood cells that fight infection.

LYMPHOCELE. A mass surrounded by an abnormal sac that contains lymph (fluid that is collected from tissues throughout the body) from diseased or injured lymphatic channels.

LYMPHOCYTE. A type of white blood cell that defends the body against infection and disease. Lymphocytes are found in the bloodstream, the lymphatic system, and lymphoid organs. The two main types of lymphocytes are the B cells (produced in the bone marrow) and the T cells (produced in the thymus).

LYMPHOCYTIC LEUKEMIA. An acute form of childhood leukemia characterized by the development of abnormal cells in the bone marrow and lymph cells found in blood-forming tissues.

LYMPHOMA. A type of cancer that affects lymph cells and tissues, including certain white blood cells (T cells and B cells), lymph nodes, bone marrow, and the spleen. Abnormal cells (lymphocyte/leukocyte) multiply uncontrollably.

M

MACROBIOTIC DIET. A diet based primarily on whole grains, vegetables, and beans, and avoiding refined or processed foods. It is sometimes recommended by practitioners of alternative medicine as a preventive for cancer.

MACROCYTIC ANEMIA. Anemia where blood cells are much larger than normal.

MACROPHAGE. A type of phagocyte that engulfs and digests cancer cells as well as bacteria and other microbes.

MAGNETIC FIELD. The three-dimensional area surrounding a magnet, in which its force is active. During an MRI, the patient's body is permeated by the force field of a superconducting magnet.

MAGNETIC RESONANCE IMAGING (MRI). A diagnostic imaging examination that uses magnetic fields and radiowaves to reconstruct detailed images of the body, especially soft tissue.

MAINSTREAM SMOKE. The tobacco smoke exhaled by a smoker.

MAINTENANCE THERAPY. The last stage in treatment of ALL. The purpose of this stage is to provide long-term exposure to lower doses of drugs and to give the immune system time to kill the leukemia cells.

MALIGNANCY. The presence of tumor-causing cancer cells in organ tissue.

MALIGNANT. Cancerous.

MALIGNANT FIBROUS HISTIOCYTOMA (MFH). A former designation for 40% of all soft tissue sarcomas.

MALIGNANT PLEURAL MESOTHELIOMA (MPM). A cancer of the mesothelium that lines the chest cavity; caused by exposure to asbestos.

MALIGNANT TUMOR. Cancer; an abnormal proliferation of cells that can spread to other sites.

MAMMOGRAM. A screening test that uses x-rays to look at a woman's breasts for any abnormalities, such as cancer.

MAMMOGRAPHY. An imaging technique that produces x-ray pictures of the breast called mammograms.

MAMMOTOME. Also known as a vacuum-assisted biopsy; a method for performing breast biopsies using suction to draw tissue into an opening in the side of a cylinder inserted into the breast tissue. A rotating knife then cuts tissue samples from the rest of the breast.

MANDIBLE. The medical term for the lower jaw or jawbone.

MANIA. The phase of bipolar disorder in which the patient is easily excited, hyperactive, agitated, and unrealistically cheerful.

MANOMETER. A device used to measure fluid pressure.

MANTLE CELL LYMPHOMA. Type of cancer that originates in the white blood cells of the immune system, specifically the lymphocytes.

MANTRA. A sacred word or phrase, used in some forms of meditation to deepen the meditative state.

MARGIN OF RESECTION. The area between the cancerous tumor and the edges of the removed tissue.

MASS SPECTROSCOPY (MS). A technique that separates mixtures of substances, such as proteins, on the basis of molecular weight and electrical charge.

MASS-TO-CHARGE RATIO (M/Z). The ratio of the molecular mass of a substance to its electrical charge; used for protein separation by mass spectroscopy.

MASTECTOMY. Surgical removal of breast tissue. Mastectomy may be partial, when only some tissue is removed, or radical, when all breast tissue and adjacent tissues are removed.

MASTOPEXY. Surgical procedure to lift up a breast; may be used on opposite breast to achieve symmetrical appearance with a reconstructed breast.

MATERIAL SAFETY DATA SHEET (MSDS). A document that provides workers and emergency personnel with information about chemicals in the workplace, including physical data, safe handling, storage and disposal, toxicity, health effects, and first aid.

MATRIX METALLOPROTEINASES (MMPS). Enzymes that break down the extracellular matrix between cells.

MATURATION. The process by which stem cells transform from immature cells without a specific function into a particular type of blood cell with defined functions.

MAXILLA. The medical term for the upper jaw, which is formed by the fusion of two bones at the center of the roof of the mouth.

MAXIMUM TOLERATED DOSE (MTD). The highest dose of an investigational drug that patients can tolerate without life-threatening or fatal side effects.

MCCUNE-ALBRIGHT SYNDROME. A genetic disorder that includes bone, endocrine, and skin abnormalities. Some individuals with this syndrome show the effects of excessive secretion of pituitary growth hormone.

MEDIAN. A type of middle or average value. The median is the number in the middle of a sequence of numbers.

MEDIASTINOSCOPE. A thin hollow tube for performing mediastinoscopy.

MEDIASTINOSCOPY. A minimally invasive procedure in which a lighted fiberoptic instrument with a tiny video camera is passed through a small incision in the mediastinum, about one inch above the breast bone. It is performed to assess the lymph nodes in the pleural cavity and obtain a biopsy of mediastinal tissue.

MEDIASTINOTOMY. Surgical incision into the mediastinum.

MEDIASTINUM. The area between the lungs, bounded by the spine, breastbone, and diaphragm.

MEDITATION. A practice of inward focus that is known to reduce stress and anxiety. Many meditation methods are practiced, some in which the individual focuses on a word or phrase to the exclusion of other thoughts. Other methods follow the breath, and some follow a guided message.

MEDULLARY OSTEOSARCOMA. An osteosarcoma located within the bone. It is also called a central osteosarcoma.

MEDULLARY THYROID CANCER (MTC). A slow-growing tumor associated with multiple endocrine neoplasia (MEN).

MEDULLOBLASTOMA. A malignant tumor of the cerebellum that occurs mostly in children and is considered a type of primitive neuroectodermal tumor. Medulloblastomas are sometimes classified as infratentorial primitive neuroectodermal tumors because they develop underneath the tentorium.

MEGACOLON. Abnormally large colon associated with some chronic intestine disorders.

MEGAKARYOCYTES. Platelet precursor cells in the bone marrow.

MEK. Mitogen-activated protein kinase; mitogen/extracellular signal-regulated kinase; an enzyme that adds a phosphate to the enzyme mitogen-activated protein kinase in a cell-signaling pathway controlled by B-raf; the target of trametinib.

MELANIN. Skin pigment that causes tanning.

MELANOCYTE. A specialized skin cell that makes pigment. Tanning of the skin results from an increase in the number and activity level of melanocytes.

MELANOMA. A malignant skin tumor that originates in melanocytes (pigmented cells) of normal skin or moles.

MELATONIN. A hormone that regulates moods and the sleep-wake cycle in humans. It is produced by the pineal body.

MENARCHE. The medical term for a girl's first menstrual period.

MENGHINI NEEDLE/JAMSHEDI NEEDLE. Special needles used to obtain a sample of liver tissue by aspiration.

MENINGES. The three layers of tissue that cover the brain and spinal cord.

MENINGIOMA. A tumor that occurs in the meninges, the membranes that cover the brain and spinal cord. Meningiomas usually grow slowly and primarily affect adults.

MENINGITIS. An infection or inflammation which is caused by bacteria or a virus and affects the membranes or tissues that cover the brain and spinal cord.

MENOPAUSAL HORMONE THERAPY (MHT). Treatment of menopausal symptoms with estrogen or estrogen and progesterone.

MENOPAUSE. The female developmental stage at which menstruation ceases.

MENORRHAGIA. Excessive menstrual bleeding.

MERKEL CELLS. Specialized cells of the skin that are located at the base of some hairs. These cells are believed to function as touch receptors. They are named for a nineteenth-century German professor of anatomy.

MESODERM. The middle layer of embryonic cells that gives rise to skin, connective tissue, blood and lymph vessels, the urogenital system, and most muscles.

MESOTHELIOMA. A rare form of cancer that develops in the mesothelium, the membrane that forms the lining of several body cavities including the chest cavity and the peritoneum. It is most commonly caused by exposure to asbestos.

METASTASIS (PLURAL, METASTASES). The spread of cancer cells from the primary site of a malignant tumor or lesion to a nearby or distant location in the body.

METASTASIZE. The process by which cancer spreads from its original site to other parts of the body.

METASTASIZED. Cancer that has spread from its site of origin to other parts of the body.

METASTATIC. Referring to a cancer that has spread to an organ or tissue from a primary cancer located elsewhere in the body.

METASTATIC CANCER. A cancer that has spread to an organ or tissue from a primary cancer located elsewhere in the body.

METHADONE. A synthetic opioid used as an anti-addictive treatment in patients who are dependent on or addicted to opioids.

MICROARRAY. A glass or plastic slide with attached proteins that specifically bind to other proteins in a mixture for identification and proteomic analysis.

MICROCALCIFICATIONS. Tiny flecks that are too small to be felt. They are important markers of cancer that show up on ultrasounds and mammograms.

MICROCEPHALY. A congenital anomaly in which the head is small in proportion to the body, the brain is underdeveloped, and there is some degree of mental retardation.

MICROMETASTASIS (PLURAL, MICROMETASTASES). Small tumors formed by cancer cells that have broken off from a primary tumor and traveled through blood or lymph vessels to different sites in the body where they have begun to grow and multiply.

MICROSATELLITE INSTABILITY (MSI). A condition of genetic instability that indicates that DNA mismatch repair (MMR) is not working properly. When MMR fails, correct gene sequences are not preserved and random fragments called microsatellites are formed. Cells with MSI tend to accumulate genetic errors rather than correcting them.

MICROTUBLES. A tubular structure located in cells that helps them to replicate.

MICROWAVES. Relatively low-frequency electromagnetic radiation of wavelengths ranging from about one millimeter to one meter.

MILIARY TUMOR. A very small tumor, sometimes described as the size of a small seed or grain of sand. The English word "miliary" comes from the Latin word for millet seed.

MILLICURIE. Unit for measuring radioactivity.

MILLIGRAM (MG). One-thousandth of a gram. A gram is the metric measure that equals about 0.035 ounces.

MILLIMETER-WAVE SCANNERS. The technology used in full-body security scanners, such as in airports, that directs millimeter-length radiofrequency energy that penetrates clothing and bounces off the skin and concealed objects.

MITOCHONDRIA. A small round or rod-shaped body that is found within most cells and produces enzymes for the metabolic conversion of food to energy.

MITOSIS. The process of cell division.

MITOTIC. Relating to mitosis, or the process by which a cell divides into two cells, each with identical sets of chromosomes.

MITOTIC INHIBITOR. A chemotherapy drug that prevents cells from dividing.

MODIFIED RADICAL MASTECTOMY. Total mastectomy with axillary lymph node dissection, but with preservation of the chest muscles.

MOHS SURGERY. A form of microscopically controlled surgery that allows for the precise removal of cancerous tissue. It is commonly used to treat various types of skin cancer, particularly in areas of the body where preserving as much tissue as possible is essential. Mohs surgery is also known as micrographic surgery.

MOLAR PREGNANCY. A complete or partial hydatidiform mole, in which the ovum is fertilized but lacks genetic material or the fetus has multiple anomalies and eventually dies; complete evacuation of the uterus is necessary to avoid the development of choriocarcinoma.

MOLE. A pigmented spot, mark, or permanent protrusion on the skin.

MOLECULAR OXYGEN. The most common form of oxygen in the atmosphere and in living tissues, consisting of two oxygen atoms in a stable bond (O_2). It is also called dioxygen.

MONOCLONAL. Genetically engineered antibodies specific for one antigen.

MONOCLONAL ANTIBODIES. Identical antibodies that recognize and bind to a specific protein; often used as targeted drugs.

MONOCLONAL GAMMOPATHY OF UNDETERMINED SIGNIFICANCE (MGUS). Common condition in which M-protein is present, but there are no tumors or other symptoms of disease.

MONOCYTE. A specialized type of white blood cell that attacks other cells, and acts as a phagocyte.

MONOTHERAPY. Treatment of a disease or disorder with the use of a single drug.

MORCELLATION. The division of tissue or tumors into smaller pieces.

M-PROTEIN. Monoclonal or myeloma protein; paraprotein; abnormal antibody found in large amounts in the blood and urine of individuals with multiple myeloma.

MRI. Magnetic resonance imaging.

MUCINOUS (COLLOID) CARCINOMA. A type of cancer that accounts for 1% to 2% of breast cancers. Resembles medullary carcinoma in ultrasound and mammogram, but usually affects older women.

MUCOSA. The smooth moist inner lining of some body organs, including the stomach; also referred to as a mucous membrane.

MUCOSITIS. An inflammation of the lining of the digestive tract, often accompanied by mouth and throat lesions.

MÜLLERIAN DUCTS. Paired ducts in the human embryo that give rise to the fallopian tubes, uterus, cervix, and the upper one-third of the vagina in females. The Müllerian ducts disappear in males.

MULTICENTRIC. Primary cancers that develop at two or more sites simultaneously.

MULTICENTRIC CASTLEMAN DISEASE (MCD). Castleman disease affecting multiple lymph nodes and possibly other lymphatic tissue throughout the body, especially in patients infected with HIV.

MULTIFOCAL. More than one independent tumor.

MULTIPLE ENDOCRINE NEOPLASIA SYNDROME TYPE I. An inherited disorder that affects the endocrine glands. The pituitary gland becomes overactive in about one-sixth of the individuals with this syndrome.

MULTIPLE MYELOMA. Type of cancer that originates in the white blood cells of the immune system, specifically the plasma cells.

MULTIPLE SCLEROSIS. Autoimmune disease where the immune system attacks the nervous system, causing scars in the brain and spinal cord and physical and cognitive difficulty.

MULTITARGETED ANTI-FOLATE (MTA). A drug that targets various folate-dependent enzymes.

MUTAGEN. A physical or chemical agent that changes the DNA of an organism and thus increases the number of its mutations above the normal level. Many mutagens are also carcinogens.

MUTANT. Altered, not normal.

MUTATION. A change in the genetic makeup of a cell that may occur spontaneously or be environmentally induced.

MYCOBACTERIA. Rod-shaped bacteria, some of which cause human diseases such as tuberculosis.

MYCOSIS FUNGOIDES. A well-defined subset of cutaneous T-cell llymphoma (CTCL) in which mushroom-shaped tumors form on the skin.

MYELIN SHEATH. The cover that surrounds many nerve cells and helps to increase the speed by which information travels along the nerve.

MYELODYSPLASIA. Also called myelodysplastic syndrome, it is a condition in which the bone marrow does not function normally and can affect the various types of blood cells produced in the bone marrow. Often referred to as a preleukemia and may progress and become acute leukemia.

MYELODYSPLASTIC SYNDROME (MDS). A disease where the bone marrow stops producing healthy blood cells and the cells that are produced function poorly. This syndrome sometimes develops into leukemia.

MYELOFIBROSIS. An anemic condition in which bone marrow cells are abnormal or defective and become fibrotic.

MYELOGRAM. X-ray examination of the spinal cord after injection of a contrast substance or dye that shows up on x-rays.

MYELOID BLAST CELL. Type of cancer cell originating in the bone marrow.

MYELOID PROGENITOR CELL. A stem cell normally found in the bone marrow that is responsible for making red blood cells, platelets, and some white blood cells (granulocytes and monocytes).

MYELOMA. Cancer of the bone marrow.

MYELOSUPPRESSION. A condition in which bone marrow activity is diminished, resulting in decreased platelet, red blood cell, and white blood cell counts.

MYOCARDIAL INFARCTION. Heart attack.

MYOCLONUS. Brief involuntary jerking or twitching of a muscle or group of muscles.

N

NANOMETER. A measurement of length equal to 10^{-9} meters, or one billionth of a meter, used as the unit of measurement for light waves.

NARCOTIC. A drug that dulls senses and relieves pain but that in excessive use causes stupor, coma, or convulsions.

NARCOTIC ANALGESIC. A classification of medications that relieves pain by temporarily depressing the central nervous system.

NARROW-ANGLE GLAUCOMA. Glaucoma is a disease where increased pressure in the eye causes damage and changes to the field of vision. Narrow-angle refers to a specific type of damage.

NASAL CAVITY. The cavity between the floor of the cranium and the roof of the mouth.

NASAL POLYP. A noncancerous teardrop-shaped mass that grows out from the inner lining of the nasal cavity.

NASOSCOPE. A type of endoscope designed specifically to be inserted through the nose and used for examination of the nasal cavity.

NATURAL KILLER (NK) CELL. A type of lymphocyte that kills cancer cells and certain microorganisms.

NAUSEA. The subjective feeling of abdominal discomfort associated with the urge to vomit.

NECROSIS. Cellular or tissue death.

NEEDLE BIOPSY. The procedure of using a large hollow needle to obtain a sample of intact tissue.

NELSON'S SYNDROME. An endocrine disorder characterized by increased secretion of ACTH and melanocyte stimulating hormone by the pituitary gland.

NEOADJUVANT CHEMOTHERAPY. Chemotherapy that is given before the main or primary treatment, usually surgery.

NEOADJUVANT THERAPY. The administration of chemotherapy or other treatment prior to surgery to shrink the tumor and improve the chances of successful treatment.

NEOBLADDER. An artificial bladder constructed out of a section of intestine to replace a cancerous bladder. The neobladder is connected to the patient's urethra as well as ureters, thus allowing normal urination.

NEOPLASIA. Abnormal growth of cells, which may lead to a neoplasm, or tumor.

NEOPLASM. A new growth or tumor.

NEOVASCULARIZATION. Abnormal or overabundant blood vessel formation, as in a cancerous tumor.

NEPHRECTOMY. A surgical procedure performed to remove a kidney.

NEPHROGENIC DIABETES INSIPIDUS. A condition in which the kidneys do not retain urine, resulting in excess urination and thirst, and very watered-down urine.

NERVOUS SYSTEM. The network of nerve tissue of the body. It includes the brain, the spinal cord and the ganglia (group of nerve cells).

NEUROBLAST CELLS. Cells produced by the fetus that mature into nerve cells and adrenal medulla cells.

NEUROENDOCRINE. Relating to nerves and glands that produce hormones.

NEUROFIBROMA. A fibrous tumor of nerve tissue.

NEUROFIBROMATOSIS. A rare, genetic disease that causes tumors to grow in the nervous system.

NEUROFIBROMATOSIS TYPE 2 (NF2). A hereditary condition associated with an increased risk of bilateral acoustic neuromas, other nerve cell tumors, and cataracts.

NEUROHORMONE. A hormone produced by specialized neurons or neuroendocrine cells.

NEUROLOGIC. Involving the nervous system.

NEUROLOGICAL EXAM. A physical examination that focuses on the patient's nerves, reflexes, motor and sensory functions, and muscle strength and tone.

NEURON. Specialized cell of the nervous system that transmits nervous system signals. It consists of a cell body linked to a long branch (axon) and to several short ones (dendrites).

NEURON-SPECIFIC ENOLASE (NSE). An enzyme that may be elevated in tumors originating in neuroendocrine cells.

NEUROPATHIC. Referring to nerve pain.

NEUROPATHIC PAIN. Pain that is felt near the surface of the skin, along nerve pathways.

NEUROTOXIC. A substance that is harmful to the nervous system.

NEUROTRANSMITTERS. Nervous system chemicals that transmit information between nerve cells.

NEUTROPENIA. A condition in which the blood contains an abnormally low level of neutrophils (white blood cells).

NEUTROPHIL. The most common type of white blood cell in humans, responsible for protecting the body against infection.

NEVUS (PLURAL, NEVI). The medical term for a common skin mole.

NIACIN. Nicotinic acid; vitamin B3.

NICOTINE. A colorless, oily chemical found in tobacco that makes smokers physically dependent on smoking. Nicotine is a stimulant to the central nervous system and is poisonous in large doses.

NITRITES. Meat preservatives that may increase cancer risk if converted to nitrosamines.

NITROSAMINES. Naturally occurring compounds, some of which are known to be carcinogenic; nitrosamines are sometimes found in cured meats such as bacon.

NOCICEPTOR. A nerve cell that senses pain and transmits pain signals.

NON-HODGKIN LYMPHOMA. A cancer of the lymph system that causes the accumulation of large numbers of defective (cancerous) immune system cells.

NONINVASIVE TUMORS. Tumors that have not penetrated the muscle wall and/or spread to other parts of the body.

NON-IONIZING RADIATION. Low-frequency electromagnetic radiation with insufficient energy to ionize atoms, including radio waves, microwaves, and radio-frequency energy from cell phones.

NONMELANOMA SKIN CANCER. A squamous cell carcinoma or basal cell carcinoma.

NON-MYELOABLATIVE ALLOGENEIC BONE MARROW TRANSPLANT. Also called a "mini" bone marrow transplant. This type of bone marrow transplant involves receiving low-doses of chemotherapy and radiation therapy, followed by the infusion of a donor's bone marrow or peripheral stem cells. The goal is to suppress the patient's own bone marrow with low-dose chemotherapy and radiation therapy to allow the donor's cells to engraft.

NONPALPABLE. Cannot be felt by hand. In cancer, growths that are nonpalpable are too small to be felt, but may be seen on ultrasounds or mammograms.

NON-PHARMACOLOGICAL. Therapy that does not involve drugs.

NON-RMS. All soft tissue sarcomas in children that are not rhabdomyosarcoma.

NON-SEMINOMA. Any germ-cell cancer of the testicle that is not a pure seminoma.

NON-SMALL CELL LUNG CANCER (NSCLC). The most common type of lung cancer; includes squamous cell carcinoma, adenocarcinoma, and large cell carcinoma.

NONSTEROIDAL ANTI-INFLAMMATORY DRUGS (NSAIDS). Over-the-counter and prescription medications for reducing pain and inflammation.

NONTOXIC. Does not cause harm.

NUCLEAR MEDICINE. A subspecialty of radiology used to show the function and anatomy of body organs. Very small amounts of radioactive substances, or tracers, are detected with a special camera as they accumulate in certain organs and tissues.

NUCLEOTIDES. The subunits or building blocks of nucleic acids like DNA and RNA.

NUCLEUS. The part of the cell containing chromosomes.

O

OBESITY. Excessive weight due to accumulation of fat, usually defined as a body mass index (BMI) of 30 or above or body weight greater than 30% above normal on standard height-weight tables.

OCCULT. Not visible or easily detected.

OCCULT BLOOD. Presence of blood that cannot be seen with the naked eye.

OCULAR ORBIT. Bony cavity containing the eyeball.

OFATUMUMAB. A monoclonal antibody used to treat chronic lymphocytic leukemia.

OLIGOASTROCYTOMA. A type of brain tumor that is a mixture of oligodendroglioma and astrocytoma. Also called a mixed glioma.

OLIGONUCLEOTIDE. A relatively short single-stranded nucleic acid chain, either RNA or DNA.

OMEGA-3 FATTY ACIDS. Polyunsaturated fatty acids that are beneficial for the heart.

OMENTUM. The layer of peritoneal tissue that covers the abdominal organs. Its name comes from the Latin word for apron.

OMMAYA RESERVOIR. A special device surgically placed under the scalp with a direct connection to spinal fluid. Medications to treat central nervous system disease are injected into the reservoir.

ONCOGENE. A gene that has the potential, if mutated, to transform a cell into cancer; proto-oncogenes promote normal cell growth and division.

ONCOLOGIST. A physician who specializes in the diagnosis and treatment of cancer.

ONCOLOGY. The branch of medicine that deals with the diagnosis and treatment of cancer.

ONCOLYTIC. Pertaining to or characterized by the destruction (lysis) of tumor cells.

ONCOLYTIC VIRUS. A viral vector that can destroy cancer cells by infecting them and either bursting the cell directly or carrying a gene that destroys the cell.

OOPHORECTOMY. Surgical removal of the ovaries; often performed laparoscopically.

OPHTHALMOLOGIST. A physician who specializes in diseases of the eye.

OPIOID. A synthetic analgesic that has narcotic properties similar to opiates but is not derived from opium.

OPPORTUNISTIC INFECTIONS (OI). Diseases caused by organisms that multiply to the point of producing symptoms only when the body's immune system is impaired.

OPTIC NERVE. The nerve fibers that transmit signals from the eye to the brain.

ORAL MUCOSITIS. Inflammation of the mucous membranes of the mouth.

ORCHIECTOMY. Surgical removal of the testicles. It is sometimes performed to lower androgen levels in patients with metastatic male breast cancer.

ORGANOCHLORINES. A large class of pesticides that includes 2,4-D and the discontinued insecticides DDT, chlordane, and aldrin.

ORGANOPHOSPHATES. A large class of pesticides including the neurotoxic insecticides malathion and naled and glyphosate (N-[phosphonomethyl]glycine), the most widely used herbicide in the United States.

OROPHARYNX. A set of structures behind the oral cavity that lies between the upper portion of the pharynx and the lower portion of the throat. The oropharynx contains the tonsils, the base of the tongue, and the soft palate.

ORPHAN DRUG. A one-of-a-kind drug that treats a rare disease—"rare disease" defined by the Food and Drug Association as one affecting fewer than 200,000 Americans. The category of orphan drug includes experimental as well as approved medications. Certain photosensitizing drugs used in Europe are considered orphan drugs in the United States.

ORTHOTICS. Supports for the bracing of weak or ineffectual muscles or joints.

OSMOTIC PRESSURE. The pressure in a liquid exerted by chemicals dissolved in it. It forces a balancing of water in proportion to the amount of dissolved chemicals in two compartments separated by a semi-permeable membrane.

OSTEOBLAST. Bone-forming cell.

OSTEOBLASTOMA. A benign tumor that most frequently occurs in the vertebrae, leg bones, or arm bones of children and young adults.

OSTEOCHONDROMAS. Small benign tumors that develop in the bone and cartilage in people with a hereditary form of this disorder. Osteochondromas are a risk factor for later osteosarcoma.

OSTEOCLAST. Cell that absorbs bone tissue.

OSTEOGENIC. Creating bone.

OSTEOGENIC SARCOMA. Another name for osteosarcoma.

OSTEOLYTIC LESION. Soft spot or hole in bone caused by cancer cells.

OSTEOMA. A usually benign tumor of bone tissue.

OSTEOPOROSIS. Condition in which the bones become weak and porous, due to loss of calcium and destruction of cells.

OSTEOSARCOMA. A tumor of the bone. The most common childhood cancer.

OSTOMY. General term meaning a surgical procedure in which an artificial opening is formed to either allow waste (stool or urine) to pass from the body, or to allow food into the GI tract. An ostomy can be permanent or temporary, as well as single-barreled, double-barreled, or a loop.

OTOLARYNGOLOGIST. A physician who diagnoses and treats disorders of the head and neck; sometimes called an ear, nose, and throat specialist or ENT.

OUTCOMES RESEARCH. Public health research that measures and evaluates the end result of the structures and processes of health care on the well-being of the patients. Outcomes research typically measures the efficiency, effectiveness, safety, and patient-centeredness of medical care.

OVARIAN FOLLICLE. Several layers of cells that surround a maturing egg in the ovary.

OVARY (PLURAL, OVARIES). One of two small oval-shaped organs located on either side of the uterus. They are female reproductive glands in which the ova (eggs) are formed.

OVER-THE-COUNTER (OTC). A drug that can be purchased without a doctor's prescription.

OXIDANTS. Molecules such as free radicals that can cause oxidative damage to cellular components including DNA.

OXIDATIVE STRESS. A condition in which the body is producing an excess of oxygen-free radicals.

OZONE. A type of oxygen gas that occurs in a layer about 15 miles (24 kilometers) above Earth's surface and that helps protect living organisms from the damaging effects of the sun's ultraviolet rays.

P

P53. A tumor suppressor gene that, when mutated, is associated with a high risk for certain cancers.

PACKED RED BLOOD CELLS. Blood obtained from a donor that has had the fluid portion (plasma) removed so that only red cells are transfused.

PAGET DISEASE. Chronic inflammation of the bone, with the bones becoming thinner and softer.

PAGET DISEASE OF THE BREAST. Cancer of breast nipples that occurs in both men and women. Paget's is characterized by oozy and crusty skin inflammation (dermatitis).

PALLIATION. Care and treatment given to relieve or lessen pain without attempting to cure.

PALLIATIVE. Referring to treatments that are intended to relieve pain and other symptoms of a disease but not to cure.

PALPATE. To examine by means of touch.

PALPATION. A simple technique in which a doctor presses lightly on the surface of the body to feel the organs or tissues underneath.

PANCREAS. A large gland located on the back wall of the abdomen, extending from the duodenum (first part of the small intestine) to the spleen. The pancreas produces enzymes essential for digestion and the hormones insulin and glucagon, which play a role in diabetes.

PANCREATECTOMY. Partial or total surgical removal of the pancreas.

PANCREATICODUODENECTOMY. Removal of all or part of the pancreas along with the duodenum. Also known as "Whipple's procedure" or "Whipple's operation."

PANCREATITIS. An inflammation of the pancreas diagnosed on the basis of severe pain that begins in the abdomen and moves to the back, fever, loss of appetite, nausea, vomiting, and jaundice.

PANCYTOPENIA. Disorder in which all blood elements are deficient (red blood cells, white blood cells, and platelets).

PAP (PAPANICOLAOU) TEST. Removal of cervical cells to screen for cancer. The test was invented by and named for a Greek physician, George Papanicolaou, who was an early pioneer in cancer detection; it is also called a Pap smear.

PAPILLARY THYROID CARCINOMA. The most common type of thyroid cancer, which develops in follicular cells and is well-differentiated.

PAPILLEDEMA. Swelling of the optic disc due to increased intracranial pressure.

PAPILLOMA. A wart-like growth with a bumpy surface that can grow inside the nasal cavity and destroy healthy tissue. Papillomas are not themselves cancerous, but can give rise to squamous cell carcinomas.

PARACENTESIS. A procedure in which a needle is inserted into the peritoneal cavity to withdraw peritoneal fluid, either as a treatment for ascites or to obtain a sample of the fluid to diagnose metastatic cancer.

PARALYTIC ILEUS. Disruption of normal muscle contraction within the intestines.

PARAPROTEIN. M-protein; abnormal immunoglobulin produced in multiple myeloma.

PARASITE. An organism that lives by taking its nourishment from another organism.

PARENTERAL. Medications administered through intravenous, subcutaneous, or intramuscular injection.

PARENTERAL NUTRITION (PN). Feeding administered most often by an infusion into a vein. It can be used if the gut is not functioning properly or due to other reasons that prevent normal or enteral feeding.

PARENTERAL NUTRITIONAL SUPPORT. Intravenous nutrition that bypasses the intestines and its contribution to digestion.

PARIETAL CELLS. Stomach cells that secrete gastric acid to aid in digestion.

PAROXYSM. A sudden attack of symptoms.

PARTIAL CYSTECTOMY. A surgical procedure where cancerous tissue is removed by cutting out a small piece of the bladder.

PARTIAL MASTECTOMY. Segmental mastectomy; removal of only the cancerous breast tissue and some of the surrounding normal tissue.

PATENT. Open.

PATHOGEN. Any disease-causing microorganism.

PATHOGNOMONIC. Characteristic of a disease; a pattern of symptoms not found in any other condition.

PATHOLOGIC. Characterized by disease or the structural and functional changes due to disease.

PATHOLOGIST. A person who specializes in studying diseases. In particular, this person examines the structural and functional changes in the tissues and organs of the body that are caused by disease or that cause disease themselves.

PATHOPHYSIOLOGY. The functional changes in the body that occur in response to disease or injury.

PATIENT CONTROLLED ANALGESIC (PCA). A device resembling an intravenous pump that allows patients to self-medicate within pre-established dosage parameters for pain control.

PECTORALIS MINOR. A triangular-shaped muscle in front of (anterior) the axilla.

PEDICLE FLAP. Also called an attached flap; this is a section of tissue, with its blood supply intact, which is maneuvered to another part of the body.

PEDIGREE. A family tree. Often used by a genetic counselor to determine whether a disease may be passed from a parent to a child.

PELVIC EXENTERATION. Extensive surgery to remove the uterus, ovaries, pelvic lymph nodes, part or all of the vagina, and the bladder, rectum, and/or part of the colon.

PELVIS. Basin-shaped body cavity containing and protecting the bladder, the rectum, and the reproductive organs.

PENECTOMY. Surgical removal of the penis.

PENETRANCE. The likelihood that a person will develop a disease (such as cancer), if they have a mutation in a gene that increases their risk of developing that disorder.

PENILE REHABILITATION. Frequent use of erectile dysfunction drugs, penile injections, or a vacuum constriction device to achieve erections to keep the tissue healthy, and low-dose ED drugs to improve blood flow to healing nerves following cancer surgery.

PEPTIC ULCER. Distinct erosions of the inner layer of the stomach or small intestine.

PERCUTANEOUS. Performed through the skin.

PERCUTANEOUS BIOPSY. A biopsy in which the needle is inserted and the sample removed through the skin.

PERFORATION. Puncture or tear.

PERICARDIAL EFFUSION. Escape of fluid into the pericardium—the sac that encloses the heart.

PERICARDITIS. An inflammation of the pericardium, the membrane covering the heart, marked by pain that begins in the chest and moves to the shoulder or neck, fever, difficulty breathing, and a dry cough.

PERICARDIUM. The thin membrane that surrounds the heart.

PERIOSTEUM. A membrane that covers the outer surfaces of all bones except for the joints of the long bones.

PERIPHERAL BLOOD STEM CELL TRANSPLANT (PBSCT). A procedure that collects and stores healthy young and non-developed blood stem cells. These are then given back to a patient to help them recover from high doses of chemotherapy that they received to destroy their cancer.

PERIPHERAL NERVOUS SYSTEM (PNS). Nerves outside of the brain and spinal cord.

PERIPHERAL NEUROPATHY. Symptoms resulting from damage to the peripheral nerves, that is, nerves not found in the spinal cord or brain.

PERIPHERAL OSTEOSARCOMA. An osteosarcoma that develops on the surface of the bone.

PERIPHERAL STEM CELLS. Stem cells that are taken directly from the circulating blood and used for transplantation. Stem cells are more concentrated in the bone marrow, but they can also be extracted from the bloodstream.

PERIPHERALLY INSERTED CENTRAL CATHETER (PICC). A vascular access device that is inserted through an arm or leg vein to the inferior or superior vena cava near the heart.

PERISTALSIS. Wave-like movement of the colon to pass feces along.

PERITONEUM. Smooth membrane that lines the cavity of the abdomen and surrounds the viscera (large interior organs) forming a nearly closed bag.

PERITONITIS. Inflammation of the peritoneum. It may be accompanied by abdominal pain and tenderness, constipation, vomiting, and moderate fever.

PERMETHRIN. A common neurotoxic insecticide and insect repellent.

PERSONALIZED MEDICINE. Medical care based on the specific genome and proteome of an individual patient's cancer cells.

PET. Positron emission tomography; highly specialized nuclear medicine imaging technique using radioactive substances to identify active tumors.

PETECHIAE. Pinpoint red spots seen on the skin of individuals with low platelet counts.

PEUTZ-JEGHERS SYNDROME. A rare inherited disorder characterized by pigmented discoloration of the lips, polyps in the digestive tract and urinary bladder, and an increased risk of breast cancer.

PHAGOCYTE. A specialized white blood cell that protects the body by ingesting bacteria, foreign particles, and dead or dying cells.

PHARMACOLOGICAL. Therapy that relies on drugs.

PHARYNX. The passageway for air from the nasal cavity to the larynx and for food from the mouth to the esophagus.

PHENOLIC ACIDS. Common plant metabolites that can function as phytonutrients.

PHENYLKETONURIA. Disorder of metabolism involving a deficiency in liver enzymes that metabolize the amino acid phenylalanine, causing it to accumulate and resulting in severe medical problems.

PHEOCHROMOCYTOMA. A tumor of the adrenal gland.

PHILADELPHIA (PH) CHROMOSOME. An abnormal chromosome found in 20% of adults and 5% of children with ALL, the presence of which indicates a somewhat worse prognosis.

PHIMOSIS. A medical condition in which the foreskin cannot be completely retracted over the glans.

PHLEBOTOMY. The removal of blood, usually through a vein.

PHOSPHOPROTEOMICS. The study of the subset of proteins in a cell or blood or tissue that are phosphorylated.

PHOSPHORYLATION. The addition of a phosphate molecule to a protein, usually to regulate its activity; dephosphorylation is the removal of a phosphate molecule.

PHOTOCOAGULATION. Cancer treatment that destroys a tumor with an intense beam of laser light.

PHOTODYNAMIC THERAPY. A combination of special light rays and drugs that are used to destroy cancerous cells.

PHOTOMULTIPLIER. A device that is designed to be extremely sensitive to electromagnetic radiation, especially within the ultraviolet, visible, and near-infrared ranges of the electromagnetic spectrum.

PHOTON. A quantum of electromagnetic radiation with no mass and no charge.

PHOTOSENSITIVITY. An abnormal sensitivity of the skin to ultraviolet light, often resulting from use of an oral or topical drug, that leads to accelerated and severe burning and blistering of the skin.

PHOTOSENSITIZING AGENTS. Ultraviolet or sunlight-activated drugs used in the treatment of certain cancer types.

PHTHALATES. Chemicals used in a wide variety of plastics and food packaging that may increase cancer risk.

PHYTOCHEMICAL. A nonnutritive bioactive plant substance, such as a flavonoid or carotenoid, considered to have a beneficial effect on human health.

PHYTOESTROGENS. Plant compounds that have activities of the human hormone estrogen.

PHYTONUTRIENTS. Phytochemicals; micronutrients in plant foods.

PINEAL GLAND. A small cone-shaped endocrine gland attached to the roof of the third ventricle of the brain. The pineal body, which is also known as the pineal gland or epiphysis, secretes melatonin.

PINEOCYTOMA. A slower-growing tumor of the pineal body found more commonly in adults.

PITUITARY GLAND. A tissue located at the base of the brain that is divided into two parts (anterior and posterior). The pituitary gland produces many different hormones that regulate body metabolism or control the production of other hormones.

PLACEBO. A pill or liquid given during the study of a drug or dietary supplement that contains no medication or active ingredient. Usually study participants do not know if they are receiving a pill containing the drug or an identical–appearing placebo.

PLACENTA. The organ that develops in the uterus during pregnancy and connects the mother's blood supply with that of the fetus.

PLAQUE. Fatty material that is deposited on the inside of the arterial wall.

PLASMA. The liquid part of blood.

PLASMA CELL. Type of white blood cell that produces antibodies; derived from an antigen-specific B cell.

PLASMAPHERESIS. Plasma exchange transfusion; the separation of serum from blood cells to treat hyperviscosity of the blood.

PLASTIC SURGERY. A type of surgery that is performed to alter the physical characteristics of a patient. This medical discipline is subdivided into cosmetic surgery and reconstructive surgery.

PLATELET. A type of blood cell responsible for blood coagulation and for the repair of damaged blood vessels.

PLATELETPHERESIS. A procedure in which platelets are removed from whole blood.

PLEURA. The membrane that covers the outer layer of the lungs and adjoining structures and the inner chest wall.

PLEURAL CAVITY. The space between the lungs and the chest wall.

PLEURAL EFFUSION. The abnormal buildup of fluid within the pleural space.

PLEURAL SPACE. The small space between the two layers of the membrane that covers the lungs and lines the inner surface of the chest.

PLEURODESIS. A procedure that attaches the outside of the lung to the inside of the chest wall to help prevent the lung from collapsing. This may be a surgical procedure or it can be accomplished by instilling a chemical irritant such as talc into the lung, which causes the pleura to adhere to the chest wall.

PLOIDY. The number of sets of 23 chromosomes found in a human cell.

PNEUMOCYSTIS CARINII PNEUMONIA (PCP). Serious type of pneumonia caused by the protozoan *Pneumocystis carinii*.

PNEUMONITIS. Lung inflammation.

PNEUMOPERITONEUM. The presence of air or gas in a cavity.

PNEUMOTHORAX. A collapse of the lung due to a sudden change of pressure within the chest cavity.

POINT MUTATION. A type of mutation that causes a single nucleotide in DNA or RNA to be replaced by another nucleotide.

POLYCHLORINATED BIPHENYLS (PCBS). Industrial chemicals and environmental pollutants that are toxic and carcinogenic and accumulate in animal tissues.

POLYCYCLIC AROMATIC HYDROCARBONS (PAHS). Chemicals that may increase the risk of cancer.

POLYCYSTIC KIDNEY DISEASE. A hereditary kidney disease that causes fluid- or blood-filled pouches of tissue called cysts to form on the tubules of the kidneys. These cysts impair normal kidney function.

POLYCYTHEMIA VERA. A blood disease in which too many red blood cells exist in the body.

POLYMERASE CHAIN REACTION (PCR). A method used to directly detect and quantify specific DNA or RNA in blood or tissue.

POLYP. A lump of tissue protruding from the lining of an organ, such as the nose, bladder, or intestine.

POLYPECTOMY. The removal of polyps in the colon, usually during colonoscopy or flexible sigmoidoscopy.

POLYPHENOLS. Antioxidant phytochemicals that prevent or neutralize the effects of free radicals and may have cancer-preventing activity.

PORCELAIN GALLBLADDER. A condition in which calcium is deposited in the walls of the gallbladder, causing the organ to become whitish or bluish-white in appearance and brittle. It is a risk factor for gallbladder cancer.

PORPHYRINS. Pigments found in the body that have an active affinity for metals.

PORTAL HYPERTENSION. A condition caused by cirrhosis of the liver. It is characterized by impaired or reversed blood flow from the portal vein to the liver, an enlarged spleen, and dilated veins in the esophagus and stomach.

PORTAL VEIN THROMBOSIS. The development of a blood clot in the vein that brings blood into the liver. Untreated portal vein thrombosis causes portal hypertension.

POSITRON. A positively charged particle; also called an "antielectron," the antimatter counterpart of the electron.

POSITRON EMISSION TOMOGRAPHY (PET) SCAN. An imaging system that creates a picture showing the location of tumor cells in the body. A substance called radionuclide dye is injected into a vein, and the PET scanner rotates around the body to create the picture. Malignant tumor cells show up brighter in the picture because they are more active and take up more dye than normal cells.

POSTERIOR COMMISSURE. A bundle of fibers that connects the two cerebral hemispheres near the third ventricle of the brain.

POSTMENOPAUSAL. Women who have stopped menstruating, usually due to their age.

PRECANCEROUS. Abnormal and with a high probability of turning into cancer, but not yet a cancer.

PRECANCEROUS DERMATOSIS. Another name for Bowen disease.

PRECURSOR B CELL. An immature lymphocyte (white blood cell).

PREDICTIVE FACTORS. Factors that predict the likelihood that a particular cancer will respond to adjuvant chemotherapy.

PREDISPOSING MUTATION. A germline mutation that increases an individual's susceptibility or predisposition to a disease or disorder, including cancer. It is also called a susceptibility gene.

PREGNANCY CATEGORY. A system of classifying drugs according to their established risks for use during pregnancy. Category A: Controlled human studies have demonstrated no fetal risk. Category B: Animal studies indicate no fetal risk, but no human studies; or adverse effects in animals, but not in well-controlled human studies. Category C: No adequate human or animal studies; or adverse fetal effects in animal studies, but no available human data. Category D: Evidence of fetal risk, but benefits outweigh risks. Category X: Evidence of fetal risk. Risks outweigh any benefits.

PRENATAL TESTING. Testing for a disease, such as a genetic condition, in an unborn baby.

PRESACRAL AREA. The lowest part of the back.

PREVALENCE. The number of people in a population diagnosed with a particular cancer and alive at the end of a given year.

PRIMARY BRAIN TUMOR. A tumor that starts in the brain, as distinct from a metastatic tumor that begins elsewhere in the body and spreads to the brain. A pineoblastoma is one type of primary brain tumor.

PRIMARY SCLEROSING CHOLANGITIS (PSC). A chronic disease that causes inflammation and scarring of the bile ducts. It is a risk factor for bile duct cancer.

PRIMARY TUMOR. A cancer's origin or initial growth.

PRIMITIVE. Simple or undifferentiated. Some tumors are classified as primitive tumors because they arise from cells that have not yet separated into groups of more specialized cells.

PRIMITIVE NEUROECTODERMAL TUMOR (PNET). A type of Ewing tumor in soft tissue with some characteristics of embryonic nerve tissue.

PROCOAGULANTS. Inducing the blood to clot.

PROCTOSIGMOIDOSCOPY. A visual examination of the rectum and sigmoid colon using a sigmoidoscope, also known as sigmoidoscopy.

PRODRUG. An inactive drug that is enzymatically converted to its active form within a target cell.

PROGESTERONE. A steroid hormone produced in the ovaries and involved in the menstrual cycle and pregnancy. Its levels rise during pregnancy, when it is produced by the placenta instead of the ovaries.

PROGESTERONE RECEPTOR (PR). A protein on the surface of cells that binds the female hormone progesterone; a marker on PR-positive breast cancer cells.

PROGESTINS. Synthetic hormones resembling progesterone and used in the treatment of advanced endometrial cancer.

PROGNOSTIC FACTORS. Factors that predict the likelihood that a particular cancer will recur.

PROGRESSION-FREE SURVIVAL (PFS). The length of time patients survive without their cancer progressing; used in clinical trials to measure the effectiveness of a drug.

PROGRESSIVE MULTIFOCAL LEUKOENCEPHALOPATHY (PML). A life-threatening brain infection that is a rare side effect of obinutuzumab and ofatumumab.

PROLIA. Denosumab for preventing bone weakness in patients on hormone therapy for prostate or breast cancer and for treating osteoporosis.

PROLIFERATION. Reproduction of a cell. It differs from growth in that it is a change in number rather than size.

PROPHYLACTIC. Referring to a medication given or procedure performed to prevent or reduce the risk of disease rather than treat disease.

PROPHYLACTIC MASTECTOMY. Removal of a healthy breast to prevent possible future breast cancer.

PROPHYLACTIC SURGERY. The preventive removal of an organ or tissue before a disease such as cancer develops.

PROSPECTIVE COHORT STUDY. A research study in which a large group of research subjects that differ in regard to the factor being studied is recruited and followed over time (typically many years) to determine whether and to what extent the factor has affected their health outcomes.

PROSTAGLANDINS. Hormones that cause pain and swelling in the body.

PROSTATE. Gland in males that surrounds the urine tube (urethra) at the base of the bladder.

PROSTATE GLAND. A small gland in the male genitals that contributes to the production of seminal fluid.

PROSTATECTOMY. Surgical removal of the prostate gland to treat prostate cancer.

PROSTATE-SPECIFIC ANTIGEN (PSA). A protein produced by the prostate gland that may be found in elevated levels in the blood when a person develops certain diseases of the prostate, notably prostate cancer.

PROSTATE-SPECIFIC ANTIGEN TEST. Measures the level of prostate antigen in the blood to identify the presence of prostate cancer.

PROSTATIC ACID PHOSPHATASE (PAP). An antigen on the surface of most prostate cancer cells that is used in the sipuleucel-T vaccine.

PROSTHESIS. An artificial device that replaces or augments a body part.

PROSTHODONTIST. A dentist with specialized training in restoring dental function after surgery and making dental prostheses.

PROTEASOME. Protein complexes inside cells that are responsible for degrading unneeded cellular proteins, thereby allowing the cell to remain alive.

PROTEASOME INHIBITORS. Drugs that halt or alter the function of proteasomes.

PROTEIN. A substance produced by a gene that is involved in creating the traits of the human body, such as hair and eye color, or is involved in controlling the basic functions of the human body.

PROTEIN ARRAY. The pattern of proteins in blood, tissue, or a cell as determined by mass spectrometry.

PROTEIN-CALORIE MALNUTRITION. A lack of sufficient protein and calories to sustain the body's composition, resulting in weight loss and muscle wasting.

PROTEOME. The collection of all of the proteins in a cell, tissue, or organism.

PROTEOMICS. The large-scale study of proteins, particularly their structure and functions.

PROTHROMBIN. A plasma protein, produced by the liver and converted to thrombin by activation factors in the plasma, involved in blood coagulation; also called factor II.

PROTHROMBIN TEST. A common test to measure the amount of time it takes for a patient's blood to clot; measurements are in seconds.

PROTOCOL. A written, scientific guideline used for treatment planning in clinical trials.

PROTO-ONCOGENE. A gene that can become an oncogene due to mutations or increased expression.

PROTOZOA. Single-celled organisms.

PSORIASIS. Chronic autoimmune disease affecting skin and joints that causes red scaly patches on the skin.

PSYCHOSIS. A loss of contact with reality.

PSYCHOTOMIMETIC. Capable of producing psychotic effects.

PULMONARY. Pertaining to the lungs.

PULMONARY EDEMA. A disease characterized by excessive fluid in the lungs and difficulty breathing.

PULMONARY EMBOLISM. Formation in a blood vessel of a clot (thrombus) that breaks loose (embolus), is carried by the blood stream, and blocks a vessel in the lungs; also called a pulmonary thromboembolism.

PULMONARY FIBROSIS. Disease in which there are deposits of fibrous tissue in the tissue and space around the air sacs of the lungs.

PULMONARY NODULE. Also called a lung nodule; a lesion surrounded by normal lung tissue. Nodules may be caused by bacteria, fungi, or a tumor (benign or cancerous).

PULMONARY REHABILITATION. A program to treat COPD, which generally includes education and counseling, exercise, nutritional guidance, techniques to improve breathing, and emotional support.

PURINE. A substance that is part of the structure of guanine and adenine, molecules that combine to form DNA.

PYELOGRAPHY. A type of x-ray procedure applied to a portion of the urinary tract, of which the kidneys form part.

PYLORUS. The opening from the stomach into the small intestine.

PYRETHROIDS. Synthetic insecticides that resemble pyrethrins from chrysanthemums.

PYRIMIDINE. Class of molecules that includes gemcitabine and deoxycytidine.

Q

QT PROLONGATION. Potentially dangerous heart condition that affects the rhythm of the heartbeat and alters the ECG reading of the heart.

QUACKERY. A fraudulent form of treatment or therapy.

QUALITATIVE RESEARCH. Research that involves in-depth understanding of human behavior and the factors that govern that behavior. In cancer research, qualitative approaches are often used in such fields as survivorship research, psychosocial research, and palliative care research.

QUANTITATIVE RESEARCH. Research that measures objective data by statistical, mathematical, or numerical data and various computational techniques.

QUERCETIN. A yellow plant pigment with antioxidant activity.

R

RADIATION. Cancer treatment with x-rays or other sources of ionizing radiation.

RADIATION THERAPY. The use of high-energy radiation from x-rays, cobalt, radium, and other sources to kill cancer cells and shrink tumors. Radiation may come from a machine outside the body (external beam radiation therapy) or from materials called radioisotopes. Radioisotopes produce radiation and are placed in or near the tumor or in the area near the cancer cells. This type of radiation treatment is called internal radiation therapy, implant radiation, interstitial radiation, or brachytherapy. Systemic radiation therapy uses a radioactive substance, such as a radio-labeled monoclonal antibody that circulates throughout the body.

RADICAL CYSTECTOMY. A surgical procedure that removes the entire bladder and occasionally other adjoining organs.

RADICAL MASTECTOMY. Removal of the breast, chest muscles, axillary lymph nodes, and associated skin and subcutaneous tissue.

RADICAL PROSTATECTOMY. Surgical removal of the entire prostate, a common method of treating prostate cancer.

RADICAL RESECTION. Surgical resection that removes the blood supply and lymph system supplying the organ along with the organ.

RADIO WAVES. Electromagnetic energy of the frequency range corresponding to that used in radio communications, usually 10,000–300 billion cycles per second. Radio waves are the same as visible light, x-rays, and all other types of electromagnetic radiation, but are of a higher frequency.

RADIOACTIVE. Relating to radiation emitted by certain substances.

RADIOFREQUENCY ABLATION. A technique for removing a tumor by heating it with a radiofrequency current passed through a needle electrode.

RADIOGRAPHICALLY DENSE. Having an abundance of glandular tissue that results in diminished anatomic detail on a mammogram.

RADIOIMMUNOTHERAPY. A treatment in which a radioactive material is delivered to specific cells by using a protein that binds to the surface of the target cells.

RADIOLOGIC PROCEDURE. A medical procedure, such as an x-ray, that uses radiation or other sources to create images useful in diagnosis.

RADIOLOGICALLY OCCULT. Radiologically unapparent or undefined.

RADIOLOGIST. A medical doctor who specializes in interpreting radiologic (imaging) studies. Imaging studies include x-ray, computed tomography (CT), and magnetic resonance imaging (MRI).

RADIONUCLIDE. A chemical substance, called an isotope, that exhibits radioactivity. A gamma camera, used in nuclear medicine procedures, will pick up the radioactive signals as the substance gathers in an organ or tissue. They are sometimes referred to as tracers.

RADIONUCLIDE IMAGING. An imaging technique in which a radionuclide is injected through tissue and a display is obtained from a scanner device.

RADIOPHARMACEUTICAL. A radioactive drug.

RADIOSURGERY. A form of radiation therapy in which tissue is destroyed by external beam radiation. In spite of its name, radiosurgery is not actually surgery and no incision is made.

RADIOTHERAPY. Disease treatment involving exposure to x-rays or other types of radiation.

RADON. An radioactive gaseous element that is present in soils, including those under buildings.

RALOXIFENE. A selective estrogen receptor modulator (SERM) approved for the chemoprevention of breast cancer.

RANK. Receptor activator of nuclear factor kappa B; the receptor on osteoclasts that is activated by RANK ligand and inhibited by denosumab.

RANK LIGAND (RANKL). The protein that activates osteoclasts to break down bone; denosumab binding to RANKL prevents this activation.

RAS. A member of a family of genes that can mutate to oncogenes that are linked to common human cancers.

RATE. The number of new cancer cases or cancer deaths per 100,000 people per year.

RAYNAUD'S PHENOMENON. A condition that affects the fingers and toes and may involve pain, pale color, and abnormal sensation (e.g., burning or prickling).

RB1. A cell-cycle control and tumor-suppressor gene; deletion or mutation of RB1 can lead to retinoblastoma.

REACTIVE OXYGEN SPECIES (ROS). Highly reactive molecules containing oxygen that are normal byproducts of metabolism, including alcohol metabolism, and that have important roles in cells, but that can contribute to damage from cancer.

RECEPTOR. A molecule, usually a protein, inside or on the surface of a cell that binds a specific chemical group or molecule, such as a hormone or growth factor, to initiate a sequence of events.

RECEPTOR TYROSINE KINASE (RTK). Cell surface receptors that interact with growth factors and hormones to affect the normal life cycle of a cell.

RECEPTORS. Molecules, usually found on the surface of a cell, that are required for cells to be influenced by hormones and other growth factors.

RECIPIENT. The person on the receiving end of a transplant or blood transfusion.

RECOMBINANT PROTEIN. A manipulated or modified form of a protein that results in the ability to produce the modified protein on a large scale.

RECOMMENDED DIETARY ALLOWANCE (RDA). Recommended daily allowance; the approximate amount of a nutrient that should be ingested daily.

RECONSTRUCTIVE SURGERY. A form of plastic surgery that is performed to repair or reshape abnormally formed tissue to improve the form and/or function of that tissue.

RECTAL. Pertaining to the rectum, which is the last portion of the large intestine.

RECTAL PROLAPSE. Protrusion of the rectal mucous membrane through the anus.

RECTUM. The portion of the large intestine where feces is stored before leaving the body.

RECUR, RECURRENCE. Referring to cancer that reappears after initial treatment and the passage of time.

RED BLOOD CELLS (RBCS). Cells that carry hemoglobin (the molecule that transports oxygen) and help remove wastes from tissues throughout the body.

REED-STERNBERG CELLS. An abnormal binuclear lymphocyte that is characteristic of Hodgkin disease.

REFRACTORY CANCER. Cancer that is not responding to treatment.

REINFUSION. The transfer through a vein of healthy stem cells or bone marrow to a patient that has received large doses of chemotherapy.

REMISSION. Disappearance of the signs and symptoms of cancer. When this happens, the disease is said to be "in remission." A remission can be temporary or permanent.

RENAL. Having to do with the kidneys.

RENAL CELL CARCINOMA. Cancer of the kidney that originates in the very small tubes in the kidney that filter the blood and remove waste products.

RENAL PAPILLARY NECROSIS. A medical condition affecting the kidney that increases a person's risk of developing a tumor of the renal pelvis.

RENAL PELVIS. That portion of the collecting system of the kidney that empties into the ureter.

RENAL ULTRASOUND. A painless and non-invasive diagnostic imaging procedure that bounces high frequency sound waves off the kidneys to produce precise images of areas inside the kidney (sonograms).

REPETITIVE STRESS INJURY (RSI). Any of various musculoskeletal disorders—such as tendinitis or carpal tunnel syndrome—that are caused by cumulative damage to muscles, tendons, ligaments, nerves, or joints from highly repetitive movements, such as of the hand, wrist, arm, or shoulder; also referred to as a repetitive strain injury.

RESECT. To remove surgically.

RESECTABLE CANCER. A tumor that can be surgically removed.

RESECTION. Surgical removal of a portion of an organ or body part.

RESORPTION. Dissolving of bone, as with multiple myeloma or bone metastases from other cancers.

RESPITE CARE. Temporary care provided to a patient so that the regular caregiver(s) can be relieved for a short time. Respite care may be given in the patient's home, in a nursing home, or in an adult day care facility.

RESVERATROL. An antioxidant found in grapes that is thought to inhibit cell proliferation and may help prevent cancer.

RET (REARRANGED DURING TRANSFECTION) GENE. Located on chromosome 10q11.2, mutations in this gene are associated with two very different disorders, the multiple endocrine neoplasia (MEN) syndromes and Hirschsprung disease.

RETINA. The light-sensitive layer of the eye that receives images and sends them to the brain.

RETINOBLASTOMA. A type of eye cancer that usually develops in children. There is some evidence that retinoblastoma is a risk factor for nasal cancer.

RETINOIDS. A group of natural and synthetic compounds that resemble vitamin A in their activity.

RETROGRADE PYELOGRAM. A pyelography or x-ray technique in which a dye is injected into the kidneys through the ureters.

RETROGRADE PYELOGRAPHY. A test in which dye is injected through a catheter placed with a cystoscope into the ureter to make the lining of the bladder, ureters, and kidneys easier to see on x-rays.

RETROPERITONEUM. The space between the peritoneum and the back abdominal wall that contains the kidneys and pancreas.

RHABDOMYOSARCOMA (RMS). A cancerous tumor of skeletal muscle; the most common soft tissue sarcoma in children.

RISK-REDUCING SALPINGO-OOPHORECTOMY (RRSO). Preventive or prophylactic surgical removal of the fallopian tubes and ovaries to reduce the risk of ovarian or breast cancers.

RITUXIMAB/CHLORAMBUCIL (RCLB). A combination monoclonal antibody/chlorambucil treatment for chronic lymphocytic leukemia.

RNA (RIBONUCLEIC ACID). A molecule found in all living cells that plays a role in transmitting information from the DNA to the protein-forming system of the cell.

ROLE STRAIN. The experience of someone who is filling a specific role (for example, the role of caregiver) that is frustrated by excessive obligations or multiple demands on time, energy or availability.

ROTHMUND-THOMSON SYNDROME. A rare disorder characterized by short stature, early hair loss, skin rashes, and noncancerous abnormalities of the bones. It is a risk factor for osteosarcoma.

S

S PHASE. The part of the cell division cycle during which the genetic material, DNA, is duplicated.

SACRUM. The last five vertebrae (bones) of the spinal column, which are fused into a single mass commonly called the tail bone.

SALIVARY GLANDS. Structures in the mouth that make and release (secrete) saliva that helps with digestion.

SALPINGO-OOPHORECTOMY. Surgical removal of the fallopian tubes and the ovaries.

SALVAGE THERAPY. Treatment measures taken late in the course of a disease after other therapies have failed. It is also known as rescue therapy.

SANCTUARY SITES. Areas within the body which are relatively impermeable to medications such as chemotherapy but which can harbor cancerous cells. Some of these sites are the central nervous system, the testicles, and the eyes.

SAPONINS. Mostly toxic plant glucosides that produce a soapy lather.

SARCOIDOSIS. A chronic disease characterized by nodules in the lungs, skin, lymph nodes, and bones, although any tissue or organ in the body may be affected.

SARCOMA. Any cancer that develops in bone, fat, muscle, cartilage, or soft tissue.

SATIATION. A feeling of fullness or satisfaction during or after food intake.

SATURATED FAT. Hydrogenated fat; fat molecules that contain only single bonds, especially animal fats.

SCAR REVISION. A surgical procedure that attempts to diminish the physical appearance of a scar. This procedure is also used to add flexibility and range of motion to joints and muscles that were previously restricted by a particular scar.

SCHWANNOMA. Tumor that grows from the cells that line the nerves of the body (Schwann cells).

SCINTIGRAPHY. A test used in nuclear medicine to detect abnormalities in the process of bone remodeling. Also called a bone scan, the test involves injecting the patient with radioactive technetium and then scanning the body with a gamma camera. Scintigraphy should not be confused with bone density tests.

SCINTILLATOR. A material that exhibits the property of luminescence (also called "scintillation") when it is excited by ionizing radiation.

SCLEROSANT. A chemical that causes the membranes of the pleural space to stick together.

SCLEROSING AGENTS. Drugs that are instilled into parts of the body to deliberately induce scarring.

SCOTOMA. An area of lost or depressed vision within the visual field that is surrounded by an area of normal vision.

SCROTUM. The pouch of skin on the outside of the male body that holds the testes.

SECOND CANCER. A different primary cancer that occurs at least two months after cancer treatment ends. Second cancers may occur months or years after treatment for a first cancer has concluded.

SECONDARY DIABETES. Form of diabetes resulting from damage to the pancreas.

SECONDHAND SMOKE. Passive smoke; tobacco smoke given off by a cigarette or exhaled by a smoker and inhaled by others.

SEIZURE. Sudden, uncontrolled electrical activity in the brain resulting in characteristic twitching, or spastic, movements that may be accompanied by loss of consciousness.

SELECTIVE ESTROGEN RECEPTOR MODULATOR (SERM). A drug that has estrogenic effects in some body tissues and antiestrogenic effects in other tissues.

SELENIUM. An essential trace element in meat and grains that may reduce the risk of cancer.

SELENOPROTEIN. Enzymes and other proteins containing the element selenium.

SELF-ANTIGEN. An antigen that is recognized by the immune system as a normal component of the human body.

SEMINOMA. A type of testicular germ-cell cancer.

SENTINEL LYMPH NODE. The first lymph node to receive lymph fluid from a tumor. If the sentinel node is cancer-free, then it is likely that the cancerous cells have not metastasized.

SEPSIS. An infection that has spread into the blood.

SEPTIC BLOOD. Blood that is infected with bacteria to the point of illness, may be fatal.

SEPTICEMIA. Systemic disease associated with the presence and persistence of pathogenic microorganisms or their toxins in the blood.

SEQUENCING. A method of performing genetic testing in which the chemical order of a patient's DNA is compared to that of normal DNA.

SEQUESTRATION. A process in which the spleen withdraws blood cells from circulation and stores them.

SERINE/THREONINE KINASE. An enzyme that adds phosphate to the amino acids serine and threonine in a protein.

SERUM ASCITES ALBUMIN GRADIENT (SAAG). A measurement of the concentration of albumin in the ascites fluid compared to the concentration of albumin in the blood. Ascites caused by portal hypertension usually has a SAAG above 1.1; ascites caused by cancer usually has a SAAG lower than 1.1.

SERUM SICKNESS. A type of allergic reaction against blood proteins. Serum sickness develops when the immune system makes antibodies against proteins that are not normally found in the body.

SEXUALLY TRANSMITTED INFECTION (STI). An infection transmitted through sexual activity.

SÉZARY SYNDROME. A leukemic variant of CTCL that is characterized by the spread of abnormal T cells into the blood circulation and by erythroderma.

SHINGLES. A disease caused by the Herpes zoster virus—the same virus that causes chickenpox. Symptoms of shingles include pain and blisters along one nerve, usually on the face, chest, stomach, or back.

SHORT BOWEL SYNDROME. A condition that occurs after a large segment of the small intestine has been removed; it is treated with glutamine.

SHUNT. A tube that is inserted surgically beneath the skin to drain excess fluid from the brain or the abdomen and carry it elsewhere in the body or into the venous circulation.

SIALOGOGUE. A medication given to increase the flow of saliva.

SICKLE CELL DISEASE (SCD). Any of a group of inherited disorders characterized by a genetic flaw in hemoglobin production. Hemoglobin is the substance within red blood cells that enables them to transport oxygen. The hemoglobin produced in patients with SCD has a kink in its structure that forces the red blood cells to take on a sickle shape, inhibiting their circulation and causing pain. This disorder primarily affects people of African descent.

SIDESTREAM SMOKE. The smoke emitted from burning tobacco (not exhaled by a smoker).

SIGMOID COLON. The last third of the intestinal tract that joins the rectum.

SIGMOIDOSCOPY. Examination of the rectum and lower colon with a flexible instrument passed through the anus.

SINGLET OXYGEN. A highly reactive form of the oxygen molecule (O_2) formed during PDT that helps to destroy cancer cells by attacking the cell membranes.

SIPULEUCEL-T. The first approved therapeutic cancer vaccine; used for certain metastatic prostate cancers.

SKELETAL-RELATED EVENTS (SRES). Bone fractures and other damage occurring in weakened bones.

SKIN TAG. A small outgrowth of skin tissue that may be smooth or irregular, flesh-colored, and benign.

SKIN TEST. A test used to diagnose allergies.

SKIN-SPARING MASTECTOMY. Removal of the breast tissue, leaving the skin intact for breast reconstruction.

SMALL INTESTINE. The part of the digestive tract located between the stomach and the large intestine.

SMEGMA. A whitish, waxy substance that accumulates under the foreskin in uncircumcised males. It is formed from dead skin cells, oils secreted by the skin, and moisture.

SOLID TUMOR. A tumor that consists of tissue.

SOMATIC CELLS. All the cells of the body except for the egg and sperm cells.

SOMATIC MUTATION. A mutation that is not inherited from a parent or passed on to offspring. Somatic mutations are also called acquired mutations.

SOMATIC PAIN. Localized pain such as bone pain from cancer metastases.

SONOGRAM. A computer picture of areas inside the body created by bouncing sound waves off organs and other tissues. Also called ultrasonogram or ultrasound.

SORAFENIB. A drug used to treat several types of cancer that differs in only one atom from regorafenib.

SPERMATIC CORD. A tube-like structure that extends from the testicle to the groin area. It contains blood vessels, nerves, and a duct to carry spermatic fluid.

SPF. Sun protection factor; a number assigned to sunscreens that indicates the amount of UV-B radiation that is required to produce sunburn in the presence of the sunscreen, relative to the amount of UV-B radiation required to burn unprotected skin.

SPHINCTER. A circular band of muscle fibers that constricts or closes a passageway in the body. The esophagus has sphincters at its upper and lower ends.

SPINA BIFIDA. A congenital defect in the spinal column, characterized by the absence of the vertebral arches through which the spinal membranes and spinal cord may protrude.

SPINAL CANAL. The cavity or hollow space within the spine that contains cerebrospinal fluid (CSF).

SPINAL CORD. The bundle of nerves that runs inside the backbone.

SPINAL FLUID SHUNT. A small tube that is surgically implanted to allow excess spinal fluid to drain directly into the abdominal cavity.

SPINDLE CELLS. Spindle-shaped cells typically found in connective tissue.

SPIRAL CT. Also referred to as helical CT, this method allows for continuous 360-degree x-ray image capture.

SPIRITUALITY. In general, a subjective experience of or interest in the transcendent, connection with the universe, or a search for ultimate meaning. There is, however, no universally agreed-upon definition of spirituality.

SPLEEN. An organ of the lymphatic system, on the left side of the abdomen near the stomach; it produces and stores lymphocytes, filters the blood, and destroys old blood cells.

SPLENECTOMY. Surgical removal of the spleen.

SPLENOMEGALY. Enlargement of the spleen.

SPORADIC. Occurring in isolated or scattered instances.

SPORADIC CANCERS. Cancers caused by acquired rather than germline mutations.

SPUTUM. Matter ejected from the lungs, bronchi, and trachea through the mouth.

SPUTUM CYTOLOGY. A lab test in which a microscope is used to check for cancer cells in the sputum.

SQUAMOUS CELL. A flat, scale-like cell found in epithelial tissue. Squamous cells are polygon-shaped when viewed from above.

SQUAMOUS CELL CARCINOMA (SCC). Cancer that originates in the squamous cells of the skin or linings of various organs.

SQUAMOUS INTRAEPITHELIAL LESION (SIL). Abnormal growth of squamous cells on the surface of the cervix.

STAGE. The extent to which a cancer has spread from its original site to other parts of the body. A Stage 1 cancer is less advanced than a Stage 4 cancer.

STAGING. The use of various diagnostic methods to accurately determine the extent of a disease; used to select the appropriate type and amount of treatment and to predict the outcome of treatment.

STAGING SYSTEM. A system that describes a cancer based on how far it has spread from its original site.

STEM CELL. Cell that gives rise to a lineage of cells. Particularly used to describe the most primitive cells in the bone marrow from which all the various types of blood cell are derived.

STEM CELL TRANSPLANT. Treatment procedure by which young blood stem cells are collected from the patient (autologous) or another matched donor (allogeneic). High-dose chemotherapy and/or radiation is given, and the stem cells are reinserted into the patient to rebuild his or her immune system.

STENOSIS. Narrowing of a duct or canal.

STENT. A thin rod-like or tube-like device made of wire mesh, inserted into a blood vessel or duct to keep it open.

STEREOTACTIC. Characterized by precise positioning in space. When applied to radiosurgery, stereotactic refers to a system of three-dimensional coordinates for locating the target site.

STEREOTACTIC BIOPSY. A biopsy performed by precisely locating areas of abnormal growth through the use of delicate instruments.

STEREOTACTIC RADIOSURGERY. A very precise form of radiation therapy used to treat brain tumors with targeted radiation doses and three-dimensional imaging.

STEREOTACTIC SURGERY. Surgery that uses sophisticated methods of imaging internal organs in order to make the most precise surgical incisions.

STERILE. Procedures carried out with instruments that have been sterilized, meaning that they are completely free from microorganisms (germs) that could cause infection.

STERILITY. Inability to have children.

STEROIDS. Corticosteroids; a large class of naturally occurring and synthetic hormones and medications, including anti-inflammatory drugs.

STOMA. An artificial opening between two cavities or between a cavity and the surface of the body.

STRICTURE. An abnormal narrowing of a duct or canal.

STRICTUREPLASTY. A procedure that shortens and widens strictures in the intestine without removing sections of the intestine; used to treat Crohn's disease.

STROKE. Medical condition in which blood flow to a part of the brain is compromised due to blockage of the blood vessel or blood vessel hemorrhage.

STROMA. The supporting connective tissue of the breast or other organ.

SUBCAPSULAR. Inside the outer tissue covering of the testicle.

SUBCUTANEOUS. Under the skin.

SUBCUTANEOUS EMPHYSEMA. A pathologic accumulation of air underneath the skin resulting from improper insufflation technique.

SUICIDE GENE. A gene that produces an enzyme that converts a prodrug to its active toxic form that kills the cell.

SULFORAPHANE. An anticarcinogenic isothiocyanate in cruciferous vegetables that is thought to stimulate the production of enzymes that detoxify carcinogens.

SUNBLOCK. A skin preparation containing an active ingredient, such as titanium oxide, that prevents sunburn by physically blocking out ultraviolet radiation.

SUNSCREEN. A skin preparation containing an active ingredient, such as benzophenone, that prevents sunburn by chemically absorbing ultraviolet radiation.

SUPERINFECTION. An overgrowth, during antimicrobial treatment for another infection, of a microorganism not affected by the treatment.

SUPERIOR VENA CAVA (SVC) SYNDROME. Obstruction or compression of the superior vena cava, the second largest vein in the body that returns blood from the upper part of the body to the atrium of the heart.

SUPPORTIVE CARE. In regard to cancer, the prevention or management of the adverse effects of cancer and cancer treatment.

SUPRATENTORIAL. Located above the tentorium, the tentlike membrane that covers the cerebellum.

SURGICAL ONCOLOGY. The branch of surgery that specializes in the surgical management of cancer.

SURVIVAL. The probability of survival one, three, or five years after cancer diagnosis.

SURVIVAL GUILT. A feeling of guilt about having done something wrong by surviving some event or experience when others did not. It is also called survivor's guilt or survival syndrome.

SURVIVORSHIP. Cancer survivorship refers to the life of a person with cancer after treatment is complete. It encompasses physical, emotional, and financial issues, such as late effects of cancer treatment, follow-up care, and family and caregiver relationships.

SURVIVORSHIP CARE PLAN (SCP). The record of a patient's cancer history and recommendations for follow-up care. It details the responsibilities of all care providers, whether cancer-related, primary care, or psychosocial. The SCP is intended to improve the survivor's care coordination and avoid duplication of resources.

SYNDROME. A series of symptoms or medical events occurring together and pointing to a single disease as the cause.

SYNDROME OF INAPPROPRIATE ANTIDIURETIC HORMONE (SIADH). Overproduction of an antidiuretic hormone by cancer cells or a side effect of chemotherapy.

SYNERGISTIC. Effects in which the combined action of two or more processes or entities is greater than the sum of either acting alone.

SYNOSTOSIS. Union of two or more bones to form a single bone.

SYNTHETIC. Artificially made; not occurring naturally or being developed from a natural source.

SYSTEMIC. Affecting the entire body in general instead of being confined to a local area or organ.

SYSTEMIC CHEMOTHERAPY. Cancer treatment with powerful drugs that are administered throughout the body, usually by injection, or an intravenous needle, and sometimes orally.

T

T CELLS. Immune-system cells that originate in the thymus gland. Killer or cytotoxic T cells can destroy cancer cells; T helper cells recognize antigens and coordinate immune responses.

T'AI CHI. An Asian practice of breathing and slow physical movements that develops strength and reduces stress.

TAMOXIFEN. A drug used to treat breast cancer and help prevent breast cancer in women at high risk of the disease.

TAMPONADE. A medical emergency in which fluid or other substances between the pericardium and heart muscle compress the heart muscle and interfere with the normal pumping of blood.

TARDIVE DYSKINESIA. A disorder brought on by the use of certain antipsychotic medications, characterized by uncontrollable muscle spasms.

TARGETED IMMUNOTHERAPY. An immunological drug, such as a monoclonal antibody, that interferes with specific molecules involved in cancer cell growth and/or survival.

TARGETED THERAPY. In cancer treatment, a type of drug therapy that blocks tumors by interfering with signaling pathways or specific molecules that the cancer cells need for growth. Also called biologic therapy, targeted therapy is less harmful to normal cells than traditional chemotherapy.

TAXANE. An inhibitor of breast cancer cell division, such as paclitaxel (Taxol) or docetaxel.

TAXOIDS. A complex molecule that is chemically similar to paclitaxel.

TELEHEALTH. The use of the telephone, Internet, and other forms of telecommunication to support long-distance health care, education of health care professionals, and public health concerns.

TEMPORAL LOBES. The two lobes of the cerebrum of the brain that are responsible for coordination, speech, hearing, memory, and awareness of time.

TENDON. Connective tissue that attaches muscle to bone.

TENTORIUM. The membrane that separates the cerebrum from the cerebellum.

TERATOGEN. Drug or chemical agent that has the potential to cause birth defects in a developing fetus.

TERATOGENIC. Affecting normal fetal development, leading to congenital malformations; teratogens include alcohol, certain medications, and radiation.

TERATOMA. A tumor consisting of different types of tissue, as of skin, hair, and muscle, caused by the development of independent germ cells.

TERMINAL BLASTIC PHASE. The final stage of CML.

TESTES (SINGULAR, TESTIS). Male reproductive organs that produce sperm and the hormone testosterone.

TESTICLE. The testis and its enclosing structures.

TESTOSTERONE. The main male hormone. It is produced in the testes and is responsible for the development of primary and secondary male sexual traits.

TETANY. Muscle spasms that can be life-threatening.

TETRACYCLINE. A broad-spectrum antibiotic.

TETRAPLOID. Four sets of chromosomes. The normal amount in a human cell that is about to divide to form two new cells.

THALASSEMIA. A group of inherited disorders that affects hemoglobin production. Because hemoglobin production is impaired, a person with this disorder may suffer mild to severe anemia. Certain types of thalassemia can be fatal.

THALIDOMIDE. A drug similar to pomalidomide that was widely prescribed in the 1950s and caused severe fetal malformations and death.

T-HELPER CELLS. Immune system cells that are critical in coordinating the immune response that directs other immune system components, including killer T-cells and antibodies, to destroy bacteria and viruses in the body.

THERAPEUTIC INDEX. A ratio of the maximum tolerated dose of a drug divided by the dose used in treatment.

THORACENTESIS. Removal of fluid from the pleural cavity.

THORACIC. Refers to the chest area. The thorax runs between the abdomen and neck and is encased in the ribs.

THORACOSCOPY. Examination of the contents of the chest through a thin, lighted fiberoptic instrument with a camera that is passed through a small incision.

THROMBOCYTOPENIA. The medical term for low levels of platelets in the blood (below 50,000 platelets per microliter).

THROMBOEMBOLIC DISEASE. A condition in which a blood vessel is obstructed by an embolus carried in the bloodstream from the site of formation.

THROMBOEMBOLIC EVENT. Formation in a blood vessel of a clot (thrombus) that breaks loose (embolus), is carried by the blood stream, and blocks another vessel, such as in a stroke.

THROMBOEMBOLISM. A blood clot that blocks a blood vessel in the cardiovascular system, most often in a lung.

THROMBOPENIA. Decreased number of platelets in the blood.

THROMBOPHLEBITIS. Inflammation of veins, associated with the formation of blood clots.

THROMBOSIS. The formation of a blood clot in an artery or vein that may be accompanied by inflammation. If untreated in arteries, thrombosis can lead to death of the nearby tissue.

THRUSH. A yeast infection of the mouth and throat caused by *Candida*. It is also known as oropharyngeal candidiasis.

THYMUS. An organ of the lymphatic system, located behind the breast bone, that produces the T lymphocytes of the immune system.

THYROID. A gland in the throat that produces hormones that regulate growth and metabolism.

THYROID GLANDS. Small glands on each side of the trachea (windpipe) that secrete hormones to regulate metabolism and growth.

THYROIDECTOMY. Surgical removal of the thyroid gland.

THYROID-STIMULATING HORMONE (TSH). A hormone secreted by the pituitary gland that regulates the production and secretion of thyroid hormones.

TILT TABLE. An apparatus for rotating a person from horizontal to an oblique or vertical position; also referred to as a tiltboard.

TINNITUS. A sensation of ringing or other similar sound in the ears.

TISSUE-FLAP SURGERY. Breast reconstruction using tissues from elsewhere in the body.

TNM. A cancer staging system, in which T indicates the size and location of the primary tumor, N signifies lymph node involvement, and M is metastasis to distant parts of the body.

TOLERANCE. Decreased susceptibility to the effects of a drug as a result of its continued administration.

TONSILS. Small masses of tissue at the back of the throat. They are components of the lymphatic system that function in immunity by removing the excess fluid around cells.

TOPICAL. Referring to a treatment that is applied directly to the exterior of the body (skin, hair, eyes, nails).

TOPOISOMERASE INHIBITORS. Chemotherapy drugs that prevent DNA strands from copying themselves (replicating).

TOTAL MASTECTOMY. Simple mastectomy; removal of the breast tissue, nipple and a small portion of the overlying skin.

TOTAL-SKIN ELECTRON BEAM THERAPY. A method of radiation therapy used to treat CTCL by bombarding the entire body surface with high energy electrons.

TOXIC. Poisonous.

TOXICOLOGY. The branch of medicine concerned with the effects of poisonous or toxic substances and treatment of these effects. Toxicologists are often involved in investigations of cancer clusters to help investigate possible causes.

TOXOPLASMOSIS. Infection caused by the protozoan parasite *Toxoplasma gondii*, affecting animals and humans with suppressed immune systems.

TRACER. A radioactive, or radiation-emitting, substance used in a nuclear medicine scan.

TRACHEA. Windpipe; the tube made of cartilage that carries air from the nose and mouth to the lungs.

TRACHELECTOMY. A surgical procedure in which the cervix and upper portion of the vagina are removed, but the uterus is left intact with an artificial purse-string opening. This procedure allows a woman to conceive after removal of a cancerous cervix.

TRACHEOBRONCHIAL. Pertaining both to the tracheal and bronchial tubes or to their junction.

TRACHEOTOMY. A surgical procedure in which an artificial opening is made in the trachea (windpipe) to allow air into the lungs.

TRACTION. Pulling force exerted on a skeletal structure by a special device or piece of equipment.

TRAMETINIB. Mekinist; a drug that may be used in combination with dabrafenib to treat certain melanomas.

TRANSCUTANEOUS ELECTRICAL NERVE STIMULATION (TENS). A mild electric current passed through the skin to relieve pain.

TRANSFORMATION ZONE. The boundary between the ectocervix and the endocervix. It is where most cervical cancers begin.

TRANSFUSION. An infusion of blood or blood products from a donor to another person.

TRANSFUSION REACTION. An allergic reaction of the recipient of donated blood to some of the cells or proteins in donor blood.

TRANSFUSION-RELATED ACUTE LUNG INJURY (TRALI). A life-threatening transfusion reaction, especially to antigens in transfused plasma.

TRANSIENT ISCHEMIC ATTACK. Changes in the blood supply to a particular area of the brain, resulting in brief neurologic dysfunction that persists less than 24 hours.

TRANSLATIONAL RESEARCH. Research that aims to "translate" laboratory findings to practical applications. In medicine, translational research involves finding clinical applications for the results of basic research.

TRANSLOCATION. The transfer of one part of a chromosome to another chromosome during cell division. A balanced translocation occurs when pieces from two different chromosomes exchange places without loss or gain of any chromosome material. An unbalanced translocation involves the unequal loss or gain of genetic information between two chromosomes.

TRANSPLANT. Referring to the removal of tissue from one part of the body for implantation to another part of the body, or the removal of tissue or an organ from one individual and its implantation into another individual.

TRANSRECTAL ULTRASONOGRAPHY. Test that uses a small rectal probe to create an image of the prostate gland.

TRANSURETHRAL RESECTION. A surgical procedure to remove abnormal tissue from the bladder using an instrument called a cystoscope.

TRANSURETHRAL RESECTION OF THE PROSTATE (TURP). Surgical removal of a portion of the prostate through the urethra, a method of treating the symptoms of an enlarged prostate, whether from BPH or cancer.

TRASTUZUMAB. A monoclonal antibody that binds HER2 and is commonly used as targeted therapy for HER2-positive breast cancer.

TRAUMATIC BRAIN INJURY (TBI). Traumatic injury to the brain. Injury may occur either as a closed head injury, such as the head hitting a car's windshield, or as a penetrating head injury, as when a bullet pierces the skull. Both may cause damage that ranges from mild to profound. Very severe injury can be fatal because of profound brain damage.

TRICHOMONIASIS. Infection caused by a protozoan of the genus *Trichomonas*, especially vaginitis caused by *Trichomonas vaginalis*.

TRIGEMINAL NEURALGIA. A nerve problem associated with pain.

TRIGLYCERIDES. Blood component measured with cholesterol to make up the lipid profile, which helps determine the likelihood of an individual to develop heart disease.

TRILATERAL RETINOBLASTOMA. Retinoblastomas in both eyes and an independent brain tumor.

TRIPLE-NEGATIVE BREAST CANCER. Aggressive and difficult-to-treat breast cancer, in which the cells do not express estrogen and progesterone receptors and do not overexpress HER2.

TROCAR. A small sharp instrument used to puncture the abdomen at the beginning of the laparoscopic procedure.

TRYPTOPHAN. An essential amino acid that is sometimes used in combination with glutamine supplementation.

TUBE FEEDING. Feeding or nutrition through a tube placed into the body through the esophagus, nose, stomach, intestines, or via a surgically constructed artificial orifice called a stoma.

TUBERCULOSIS. Potentially fatal infectious disease that commonly affects the lungs, is highly contagious, and is caused by an organism known as mycobacterium.

TUBULAR CARCINOMA. A type of cancer that accounts for approximately 1% to 2% of breast cancers. Can appear small on ultrasound or mammogram.

TUBULE. Small tubular part of an animal.

TUMOR. An abnormal mass of tissue. Tumors may be either benign (noncancerous) or malignant (cancerous).

TUMOR GRADING. The degree of abnormality of cancer cells compared with normal cells. Establishing a grade allows the physician to determine further courses of treatment.

TUMOR LYSIS SYNDROME (TLS). Excess uric acid, potassium, and phosphate in the blood due to the rapid destruction of large numbers of cancer cells from radiation or chemotherapy.

TUMOR MARKER. A type of protein found in blood, urine, or body tissues that can be measured and used to detect the presence of cancer.

TUMOR NECROSIS FACTOR (TNF). A protein that destroys cells showing abnormally rapid growth; used in immunotherapy to shrink tumors.

TUMOR STAGING. The method used by oncologists to determine the risk from a cancerous tumor. A number—ranging from 1A–4B—is assigned to predict the level of invasion by a tumor, and offer a prognosis for morbidity and mortality.

TUMOR SUPPRESSOR. A protein such as p53 that helps prevent cancer; mutations that cause familial cancer syndromes are often in genes encoding tumor suppressors.

TUMOR SUPPRESSOR GENE. Gene involved in controlling normal cell growth. A mutation can turn off the gene, resulting in cell growth and tumor formation.

TURCOT SYNDROME. A childhood cancer syndrome associated with mutations in the *MLH1*, *MSH2*, *MSH6*, and *PMS2* genes.

TYROSINE. A non-essential amino acid. Amino acids are the building blocks of protein. They are the raw materials used by the body to make protein. Tyrosine is labeled "non-essential" because when the amino acids are lacking in the diet, they can be manufactured by the body.

TYROSINE KINASE. An enzyme that adds a phosphate to the amino acid tyrosine in a protein.

U

ULCERATIVE COLITIS. A chronic condition in which recurrent ulcers are found in the colon. It is manifested clinically by abdominal cramping and rectal bleeding.

ULTRASONOGRAM. A procedure where high-frequency sound waves that cannot be heard by human ears are bounced off internal organs and tissues. These sound waves produce a pattern of echoes that are then used by a computer to create sonograms, or pictures of areas inside the body.

ULTRASOUND. A diagnostic imaging technique that uses sound waves to form images of organs and blood vessels inside the body.

ULTRAVIOLET (UV) LIGHT. Light waves that have a shorter wavelength than visible light, but a longer wavelength than x-rays. Exposure to UV rays can cause sunburns, skin cancers, and cataract formation.

UMBILICAL CORD BLOOD (UBC). Blood collected from the umbilical cord after birth and used as a source of hematopoietic progenitor or stem cells.

UNCOATING. The stage in the life cycle of a virus in which it sheds its protein coat or envelope after it has gained entry to a host cell. Some antiviral drugs work by targeting the protein coat, thus preventing the virus from reproducing inside the cell.

UNICENTRIC CASTLEMAN DISEASE. Localized Castleman disease; the most common type of the disease, affecting only a single lymph node or group of nodes.

UNIFOCAL RETINOBLASTOMA. A single tumor in one eye.

UNILATERAL RETINOBLASTOMA. Tumor or tumors affecting only one eye.

UNRESECTABLE CANCER. A tumor that cannot be completely removed by surgery.

UNSATURATED FAT. Fat molecules with one or more double bonds, as in vegetable oils.

UREMIA. The buildup of toxic nitrogenous substances in the blood that are usually excreted by the kidneys.

URETER. The fibromuscular tube that transports the urine from the kidney to the bladder.

URETEROSCOPY. A diagnostic procedure that increases the diagnostic accuracy of the examination of possible renal pelvis tumors. Ureteroscopy may cause damage to some portion of the urinary tract. Therefore, ureteroscopy is usually reserved for those patients for whom unanswered questions remain after conventional diagnostic approaches have been completed.

URETHRA. The tube that carries urine from the bladder to outside the body. In females, the urethral opening is between the vagina and clitoris; in males, the urethra travels through the penis, opening at the tip.

URETHRAL. Relating to the urethra, a passageway from the bladder to outside the body.

URIC ACID. White, poorly soluble crystals found in the urine. Sometimes uric acid forms small solid stones or crystals that are deposited in different organs in the body, such as the kidney. High levels of uric acid can be seen in patients with gout or cancer.

URINARY CONTINENT DIVERSION. A surgical procedure that restores urinary continence by diverting urinary function around the bladder and into the intestines, thereby allowing for natural evacuation through the rectum or an implanted artificial sphincter.

URINE CULTURE. A test performed on urine samples in the lab to see if bacteria are present.

URINE CYTOLOGY. The examination of the urine under a microscope to look for cancerous or precancerous cells.

UROGRAPHY. A type of x-ray procedure applied to a portion of the urinary tract, of which the kidneys form part.

UROGYNECOLOGIST. A physician that specializes in female medical conditions concerning the urinary and reproductive systems.

UROLOGY. The branch of medicine that deals with disorders of the urinary tract in both males and females, and with the genital organs in males.

URORADIOLOGIST. A radiologist that specializes in diagnostic imaging of the urinary tract and kidneys.

UROSTOMY. A surgical procedure in which the ureters are disconnected from the bladder and connected to an opening (see stoma) on the abdomen, allowing urine to flow into a collection bag.

UROTHELIUM. The innermost layer of tissue in the human bladder. Most cancers of the bladder begin in this layer. The urothelium is also called the transitional epithelium.

U.S. FOOD AND DRUG ADMINISTRATION. A government agency that oversees public safety in relation to drugs and medical devices.

UTERINE FIBROID. A noncancerous tumor of the uterus that can range from the size of a pea to the size of a grapefruit. Small fibroids require no treatment, but those causing serious symptoms may need to be removed.

V

VACUUM CONSTRICTION DEVICE (VCD). A cylinder placed over the penis that creates a vacuum to achieve and maintain an erection.

VAGINAL DILATOR. A rubber or plastic tube used to stretch the vagina following radiation or surgery to treat cancer.

VAGINAL SPECULUM. An instrument inserted into the vagina that expands and allows for examination of the vagina and cervix.

VAGINAL STENOSIS. Narrowing of the vagina due to a buildup of scar tissue.

VAGINECTOMY. Surgical removal of the vagina. An artificial vagina can be constructed using grafts of skin or intestinal tissue.

VAGINISMUS. Painful spasmodic contractions of the vagina.

VARICOCELE. A benign condition in which the veins in the scrotum dilate, causing swelling and lumpiness around the testicle. Varicoceles are usually painless but may cause the scrotum to feel heavy or to feel like "a bag of worms" when the scrotum is examined.

VAS DEFERENS (PLURAL, VASA DEFERENTIA). A tube that is a continuation of the epididymis. This tube transports sperm from the testis to the prostatic urethra.

VASCULAR ACCESS DEVICE (VAD). A catheter that remains in place for the administration of drugs, fluids, or nutrition and/or blood withdrawal.

VASCULAR ENDOTHELIAL CELLS. Cells that form blood vessels.

VASCULAR ENDOTHELIAL GROWTH FACTOR (VEGF). A chemical compound in the body that contributes to the growth of new blood vessels.

VASCULAR ENDOTHELIAL GROWTH FACTOR RECEPTOR-2 (VEGFR-2). The receptor that binds vascular endothelial growth factors to initiate angiogenesis; the target of ramucirumab.

VASCULITIS (PLURAL, VASCULITIDES). Inflammation of blood or lymphatic vessels.

VECTOR. In gene therapy, a virus or other DNA molecule used to convey foreign genetic material into another cell where it can be replicated.

VEGAN. A vegetarian who omits all animal products, including eggs and milk, from the diet.

VEIN THROMBOSIS. A condition characterized by a blood clot in a vein.

VENA CAVA. Very large veins. There are two vena cava in the body. The superior vena cava returns blood from the upper limbs, head, and neck to the heart and the inferior vena cava returns blood from the lower limbs to the heart.

VENOGRAPHY. Technique used for examining veins for blockage, using a dye to make the vein visible with scans similar to x-rays.

VENTRICLES. Small cavities within the brain filled with cerebrospinal fluid.

VERMILION BORDER. The thin line that divides the vermilion (reddish or reddish-orange)-colored portion of the upper or lower lip from the surrounding skin.

VERTEBRAE. The bones of the spinal column; there are 33 along the spine, with five (called L1–L5) making up the lower lumbar region.

VERTIGO. A feeling of spinning or whirling.

VESTIBULOCOCHLEAR NERVE. Eighth cranial nerve; nerve that transmits information about hearing and balance from the ear to the brain.

VINBLASTINE. A chemotherapy drug that is a vinca alkaloid.

VINCA ALKALOID. A class of chemotherapy drugs that includes vinblastine, vincristine, vindesine, and vinorelbine.

VIRTUAL COLONOSCOPY. Technique that provides views of the colon to screen for colon polyps and cancer. The images are produced by computerized manipulations rather than direct observation through the colonoscope; one technique uses the x-ray images from a CT scan, and the other uses magnetic images from an MRI scan.

VIRTUAL REALITY. The creation of a convincing visual and auditory environment by computer technology for pain management in patients.

VIRUS-LIKE PARTICLE (VLP). Viral proteins used in preventive vaccines against human papillomavirus and hepatitis B virus.

VISCERAL PAIN. Pain caused by activation of nociceptors in internal organs, such as those of the chest, abdomen, or pelvis.

VISUALIZATION. A technique for forming mental images or pictures of the healing process as a means of strengthening the immune system and/or fighting disease agents such as cancer cells.

VITAMIN A. Any of several fat-soluble vitamins with antioxidant activities.

VITAMIN B_{12}. Cobalamin; a protein complex of animal origin that is required for the formation of red blood cells.

VITAMIN D. Any of several fat-soluble vitamins that are required for normal bone and teeth structure and various other physiological functions. Vitamin D is obtained from some foods and is produced in the body through the action of ultraviolet radiation.

VITAMIN E. Alpha-tocopherol; an essential fat-soluble vitamin with antioxidant activity.

VOLUME EXPANDER. Any of several solutions that can be transfused when fluid (but not blood components) is required, as for preventing or treating shock.

VULVA. The outer part of the female genitals.

W

WASTING. Weight loss in tissues such as skeletal muscle and adipose tissue (fat).

WELL-DIFFERENTIATED TUMOR. A tumor that grows relatively slowly and in a well-defined shape.

WHIPPLE PROCEDURE. Surgical removal of the head of the pancreas, part of the small intestine, and some surrounding tissue.

WHITE BLOOD CELLS (WBCS). Blood cells, including lymphocytes, neutrophils, eosinophils, macrophages, and mast cells, that are produced in the bone marrow and help the body fight infection and disease.

WILMS TUMOR. A malignant tumor of the kidney; occurs most frequently in children.

WITHDRAWAL SYNDROME. A group of physical and psychological symptoms experienced by opioid addicts when the drug is abruptly discontinued. It lasts for two to seven days and includes chills, nausea, muscle pain, flu-like symptoms, restlessness, anxiety, panic attacks, depression, and mood swings. Withdrawal syndrome can also occur with sudden discontinuation of benzodiazepine tranquilizers.

X

XENOGRAFT. A graft made from tissue taken from a donor of another species.

XERODERMA PIGMENTOSUM (XP). A rare inherited skin disorder in which skin cells lack an enzyme needed to repair damage to the cells' DNA caused by sunlight.

XEROSTOMIA. The medical term for dry mouth.

X-LINKED TRAITS. Genetic conditions associated with mutations in genes on the X chromosome. A male carrying such a mutation will contract the disorder associated with it because he carries only one X chromosome. A female carrying a mutation on just one X chromosome, with a normal gene on the other chromosome, will not be affected by the disease.

Y

YOLK SAC. A membranous sac attached to an embryo, which functions as the circulatory system of the human embryo before internal circulation begins.

Z

Z-PLASTY. A technique used in plastic surgery to elongate a scar as part of scar revision surgery. The name comes from the Z shape of the incision made by the surgeon.

INDEX

The index is alphabetized using a word-by-word system. References to individual volumes are listed before colons; numbers following a colon refer to specific page numbers within that particular volume. **Boldface** references indicate main topical essays. Photographs and illustration references are highlighted with an italicized page number. Tables and figures are indicated with the page number followed by a lowercase, italicized *t* or *f*, respectively.

A

AARP, 1:51–52

Abarelix, 1:**1–2**

ABCD mole check system, 3:1601*t*, 1606, 1615–1616, 1868

Abdominal dropsy. *See* Ascites

Abdominal fat, 2:1257

Abdominal surgery, 2:1019–1020, 3:1572–1573

Abdominal swelling, 1:276, 277

Abdominal tap. *See* Paracentesis

Abdominoperineal resection, 1:379, 476, 3:1584

Abscesses, 3:1645

Abusive families, 2:706

Accelerated FDA approval, 2:927

Accelerated partial breast irradiation, 1:**2–4**

Accolate. *See* Zafirlukast

Acetylcholine, 2:945–946

Achalasia, 1:665, 670

Acid reflux. *See* Gastroesophageal reflux disease; Heartburn

Acinar cell carcinoma, 3:1349

Acitretin, 1:241

Aclasta. *See* Zoledronate

Acoustic neuromas, 1:*4,* **4–8**

Acquired immune system, 2:891–893

Acquired mutations. *See* Somatic mutations

Acral lentiginous melanoma, 2:1102

Acromegaly, 2:1166, 3:1423, 1424

ACTH. *See* Adrenocorticotropic hormone

Actinic cheilitis, 3:1605

Actinic keratosis

 non-melanoma skin cancer, 3:1611

 skin cancer, 3:1604, 1605

 skin checks, 3:1615, 1616

squamous cell carcinoma of the skin, 3:1649

Actinomycin-D. *See* Dactinomycin

Active surveillance. *See* Watchful waiting

Actonel. *See* Risedronate

Acupuncture and acupressure

 acute lymphocytic leukemia, 1:16

 breast cancer, 1:256

 complementary cancer therapies, 1:503

 for gastrointestinal complications, 2:766

 for nausea and vomiting, 2:1222

 neuropathy, 2:1236

 pain management, 3:1334

 pericardial effusion, 3:1386

 pneumonia, 3:1442

 smoking cessation, 3:1623

Acute erythroblastic leukemia, 1:*8,* **8–10**

Acute immune hemolytic reaction, 3:1771

Acute leukemias. *See* Leukemias, acute

Acute lymphoblastic leukemia

 acute leukemias, 2:978–981

 childhood cancers, 1:435–436

 dasatinib, 1:569

 gene therapy, 2:774

 rituximab, 3:1552

 second cancers, 3:1566–1568

 teniposide, 3:1711

Acute lymphocytic leukemia, 1:*11,* **11–18**

 acute myelocytic leukemia compared to, 1:19

 amsacrine, 1:88–89

 asparaginase, 1:154

 BCR-ABL inhibitors, 1:180

 cytogenetic analysis, 1:556

 daunorubicin, 1:572

 idarubicin, 2:881

 mercaptopurine, 2:1118–1119

 with myelofibrosis, 2:1191

pegaspargase, 3:1373–1375

staging system, 3:1815

vindesine, 3:1850

Acute myeloblastic leukemia, 2:978–981

Acute myelocytic leukemia, 1:*19,* **19–24**

 acute erythroblastic leukemia, 1:8–10

 childhood cancers, 1:435–436

 gemtuzumab, 2:770–771

 idarubicin, 2:881–882

 mercaptopurine, 2:1118–1119

 myeloproliferative disease progression, 2:1197

 occupational exposure, 2:1267

 second cancers, 3:1565–1566, 1568

 as secondary cancer, 2:853

 staging system, 3:1816

 tumor markers, 3:1807

Acute myelogenous leukemia. *See* Acute myelocytic leukemia

Acute myeloid leukemia. *See* Acute myelocytic leukemia

Acute non-lymphocytic leukemia, 2:1152

Acute promyelocytic leukemia, 1:149–150, 3:1786–1787

Acute radiation dermatitis, 3:1489, 1491

Acute respiratory distress, 3:1762

Acyclovir, 1:144–146, 2:842, 844

Adalimumab, 1:200

Adaptogens, 1:36

Adcetris. *See* Brentuximab vedotin

Addiction. *See* Drug dependence; Substance abuse

Addison's disease, 1:34

Adenocarcinoma, 1:**24–25**

 Barrett's esophagus, 1:171–174

 bile duct cancer, 1:193

 bronchoalveolar lung cancer, 1:269–272

Index

Colorectal cancer *(continued)*
  obesity association, 2:1258
  panitumumab, 3:1354–1356
  pregnancy and cancer, 3:1456
  regorafenib, 3:1533
  screening, 1:334–336, 335*t*, 339, 340–342, 3:1527*t*
  sexuality issues, 3:1583, 1584
  sigmoidoscopy, 3:1589–1592
  trimetrexate, 3:1789
  tumor markers, 3:1805, 1807
  vitamins and the prevention of, 3:1855
Colorectal surgery, 1:**491–496**, *492*
Colostomy, 1:*492*, **496–500**, *497*
  aftercare, 1:477
  carcinoid tumors, gastrointestinal, 1:379
  colectomy *vs.*, 1:475
  colon cancer, 1:483
  colorectal surgery, 1:492–493
  exenteration, 1:689, 690
  rectal cancer, 3:1528
  sexuality issues, 3:1584
Colposcopy, 2:864, 3:1455
Combination therapy
  cancer vaccines, 1:355
  chemotherapy types, 1:425
  for drug resistance, 1:623
  exocrine pancreatic cancer, 3:1352
  leucovorin, 2:977
  lung cancer, small cell, 2:1042
  ovarian cancer, 2:1320
  pancreatic cancer, 3:1343
  pegaspargase, 3:1373
  pemetrexed, 3:1376
  prostate cancer, 3:1466
  rhabdomyosarcoma, 3:1549
  rituximab, 3:1553
  stomach cancer, 3:1667
  thiotepa, 3:1728
  triple negative breast cancer, 3:1792
  tumor necrosis factor, 3:1809
  vindesine, 3:1850
  Wilms tumor, 3:1887
Combretastatin A-4, 1:98
Comfort measures, 2:766
Communication
  cancer pain prevention, 1:49
  family and caregiver issues, 2:705
Complementary cancer therapies. *See* Alternative and complementary therapies
Complete blood count
  acute leukemias, 2:980

acute lymphocytic leukemia, 1:13
acute myelocytic leukemia, 1:21
chronic leukemias, 2:984
hemolytic anemia, 2:832
Compliance issues, 2:705
Complications. *See* specific procedures/substances
Computed tomography, 1:**508–512**, *509, 510*
  angiography, 1:104
  cancer in pregnant women, 3:1457
  cervical cancer, 1:408
  colonography, 1:336, 341
  cutaneous ureterostomy, 3:1829
  endocrine pancreatic cancer, 3:1346
  endoscopic retrograde cholangiopancreatography after, 1:641
  exocrine pancreatic cancer, 3:1350
  extragonadal germ cell tumors, 1:695
  gallbladder cancer, 2:747
  head and neck cancers, 2:824
  hemoptysis, 2:835
  Hodgkin lymphoma, 2:850
  imaging study types, 2:884
  intravenous urography, 2:925
  kidney cancer, 2:942
  laryngeal cancer, 2:957
  lung cancer, non-small cell, 2:1036
  lymphography, 3:1577
  mediastinal tumors, 2:1088
  before mediastinoscopy, 2:1092
  medulloblastomas, 2:1096
  meningiomas, 2:1114–1115
  nasopharyngeal cancer, 2:1211
  oral cancers, 2:1298
  oropharyngeal cancer, 2:1308
  ovarian cancer, 2:1318
  ovarian epithelial cancer, 2:1325–1326
  pancreatic cancer, 3:1342
  paranasal sinus cancer, 3:1363, 1364
  parathyroid cancer, 3:1370
  pharyngectomy, 3:1398
  pheochromocytoma, 3:1404
  positron emission tomography compared to, 3:1451, 1452
  radiation exposure risks, 1:326
  salivary gland tumors, 3:1556
  small intestine cancer, 3:1618
  stomach cancer, 2:758, 3:1666
  testicular cancer, 3:1715
  thoracentesis, 3:1731
  transitional cell carcinoma, 3:1775
  von Hippel-Lindau disease, 3:1857

  von Recklinghausen neurofibromatosis, 3:1859–1860
  Wilms tumor, 3:1887
  x-rays, 3:1890–1891
  See also CT-guided biopsy
Computer-aided diagnosis, 1:267–268
Conception issues. *See* Fertility and reproductive issues
Concerta. *See* Methylphenidate
Cone biopsy, 1:**513–515**, *514*
Congenital disorders
  craniosynostosis, 1:521–523
  extracranial germ cell tumors, 1:692
  Fanconi anemia with, 2:708
  herpes simplex, 2:841
  Horner syndrome, 2:857
  ifosfamide, 2:883
  melphalan, 2:1111
  pemetrexed, 3:1376
  pentostatin, 3:1382
  phenytoin, 3:1401
  pomalidomide, 3:1446
  raloxifene, 3:1513
  streptozocin, 3:1672
  sunitinib, 3:1677
  thalidomide, 3:1723, 1724
  thioguanine, 3:1727
  tositumomab, 3:1761
  valrubicin, 3:1842
  Wilms tumor with, 3:1885
Consolidated Omnibus Budget Reconciliation Act, 2:828
Consolidation phase, 1:15–16, 22, 23
Constipation
  gastrointestinal complications, 2:764–766
  incontinence, cancer-related, 2:904, 905–906
  laxatives, 2:970–973
  oncologic emergencies, 2:1284
  opioids, 2:1292
Consumptive coagulopathy. *See* Disseminated intravascular coagulation
Continent diversion, 1:546–547, 3:1826–1827, 1835
Continent ileostomy, 1:493
Continuous hyperthermic peritoneal perfusion, 2:872
Contraception
  amenorrhea, 1:78
  lomustine, 2:1015
  pomalidomide, 3:1446
  sunitinib, 3:1677
  thalidomide, 3:1724
  toremifene, 3:1760

Eye surgery, 2:1150
eyeGENE program, 3:1542

F

Facial tumors, 1:276
Failure to thrive, 1:106–107
Fairness, 3:1640
Fallopian tube cancers, 2:811
False test results
    cancer screening risks, 1:342
    fecal occult blood tests, 2:714
    genetic testing, 1:311–312
    mammography, 2:1073
    Pap tests, 3:1358
    pheochromocytoma, 3:1404
    prostate cancer, 3:1461
    screening tests, 3:1565
    sentinel lymph node biopsy, 3:1578
    sentinel lymph node mapping, 3:1581
FAM regimen, 2:1149–1150
Familial adenomatous polyposis
    cancer biology, 1:298
    cancer predisposition, 1:319
    childhood liver cancer, 1:439
    colon cancer causes, 1:480
    familial cancer syndromes, 2:700
    genetic testing, 2:781
    rectal cancer, 3:1525
    small intestine cancer, 3:1618
    soft tissue sarcoma, 3:1627
    stomach cancer, 3:1665
    thyroid cancer, 3:1752, 1753
Familial cancer syndromes, 2:**699–703,**
    699t
    cancer genetics, 1:310
    cancer predisposition, 1:317–323
    Cowden syndrome, 3:1788
    head and neck cancers, 2:822
    medulloblastomas, 2:1096, 1098
    osteosarcoma, 2:1312, 1314
    pancreatic cancer, 3:1341, 1346
    parathyroid cancer, 3:1369
    Peutz-Jeghers syndrome,
        3:1395–1397
    pheochromocytoma, 3:1402–1403
    pituitary tumors, 3:1423
    rectal cancer, 3:1525, 1526, 1529
    rhabdomyosarcoma, 3:1547,
        1549–1550
    second cancers, 3:1567
    soft tissue sarcoma, 3:1626–1627
    stomach cancer, 3:1664

thyroid cancer, 3:1752, 1753
von Hippel-Lindau disease,
    3:1856–1857
Familial erythroleukemia, 1:9
Familial melanoma, 2:1104–1105
Familial multiple endocrine neoplasia.
    See Multiple endocrine neoplasia
Familial nonmedullary thyroid
    carcinoma, 3:1752
Family and caregiver issues, 2:**703–707**
    cancer survivorship, 1:346
    childhood cancers, 1:434–435
    home health services, 2:855
    hyperthermia, 2:873
    intrathecal chemotherapy, 2:923
    pineoblastomas, 3:1421
    supratentorial primitive
        neuroectodermal tumors, 3:1684
Family Caregiver Alliance, 2:703, 705,
    706
Family history
    bile duct cancer, 1:195
    BRCA1 and *BRCA2* genes, 1:245,
        247
    breast cancer, 1:252
    cancer biology, 1:298–299
    cancer causes, 1:289
    cancer predisposition, 1:320
    cancer screening guidelines,
        1:341–342
    chronic leukemias, 2:983
    chronic lymphocytic leukemia, 1:458
    colon cancer, 1:480
    colorectal cancer, 1:336–337, 3:1589
    endometrial cancer, 1:633
    exocrine pancreatic cancer, 3:1353
    lung cancer, small cell, 2:1040
    malignant melanoma, 3:1604
    multiple endocrine neoplasia, 1:378
    non-melanoma skin cancer, 3:1610
    pancreatic cancer, 3:1340, 1344,
        1880
    retinoblastoma, 3:1542
    Richter syndrome, 3:1550
    simple mastectomy, 3:1593
    skin cancer, 3:1614
    skin cancer risk factors, 3:1605
    triple negative breast cancer,
        3:1790–1791
    See also Cancer predisposition;
        Familial cancer syndromes
Famotidine, 2:845
FAMP. *See* Fludarabine
Fanconi anemia, 2:**707–709**
    cancer predisposition, 1:320

familial cancer syndromes, 2:700
oral cancers, 2:1297
Fareston. *See* Toremifene
Farmed fish, 2:1277
Farmers, 2:1267, 3:1391–1394
Fasting, 1:504
Fat grafting, 3:1520
Fat tissue sarcomas, 3:1624
Fatigue, 2:**709–712**
    adrenal fatigue, 1:34–38
    hairy cell leukemia, 2:815–816, 818
    hemolytic anemia, 2:833
    hypercalcemia, 2:869
    intensity-modulated radiation
        therapy, 2:914
    Lambert-Eaton myasthenic
        syndrome, 2:945
    leiomyosarcoma treatment, 2:975
    leukoencephalopathy, 2:987
    mantle cell lymphoma, 2:1077
    nasal cancer, 2:1207
    radiation therapy side effects, 1:520
Fats and cancer risk. *See* High-fat diet
Febrile neutropenia, 2:1199, 1200, 1282
Febrile reaction with transfusion
    therapy, 3:1771
Fecal immunochemical testing, 1:335,
    341
Fecal impaction, 2:764
Fecal incontinence. *See* Incontinence,
    cancer-related
Fecal occult blood tests, 2:**713–714**
    colon cancer screening, 1:481
    colorectal cancer screening
        guidelines, 1:341
    sigmoidoscopy alternatives, 3:1592
Federal Communications Commission,
    U.S., 3:1507
Federal Trade Commission, U.S., 1:676
Fee-for-service health insurance, 2:828
Feeding tubes. *See* Tube enterostomy
Feminization. *See* Secondary sex
    characteristics
Fentanyl, 2:1291
Fertility and reproductive issues,
    2:**714–717,** 715t
    aldesleukin, 1:64
    amenorrhea, 1:78
    bladder cancer, 1:216
    cancer in pregnant women, 3:1458
    cervical cancer, 1:409–410
    childhood cancer treatment effects,
        1:440
    chlorambucil, 1:444
    cisplatin, 1:469

Fertility and reproductive issues
(continued)
  cladribine, 1:471
  cyclophosphamide, 1:542
  cystectomy, 1:546
  endometrial cancer risk factors, 1:633
  environmental factors in cancer
    development, 1:646
  exenteration, 1:690
  fludarabine, 2:736
  germ cell tumor treatment, 2:787
  goserelin acetate, 2:804
  gynecologic cancers, 2:812
  Hodgkin lymphoma treatment, 2:852
  hydroxyurea, 2:867
  ifosfamide, 2:883
  late effects of cancer treatment, 2:966
  lomustine, 2:1015
  mechlorethamine, 2:1084
  ovarian cancer, 2:1319
  ovarian epithelial cancer, 2:1326
  pomalidomide, 3:1446
  regorafenib, 3:1535
  tamoxifen, 3:1699
  testicular cancer, 3:1715–1717
  vindesine, 3:1851
Fetal and embryonic development
  chordomas, 1:448–449
  extracranial germ cell tumors, 1:691
  extragonadal germ cell tumors, 1:694
  germ cell tumors, 2:783
  myasthenia gravis, 2:1177
  pregnancy and cancer, 3:1456–1457
Fetal exposure. *See* Pregnancy
Fetal tissues, 3:1653
Fever, 1:561, 2:**717–722**
Fiberoptics
  brochoscopy, 2:1032
  oropharyngeal cancer diagnosis,
    2:1308
  photodynamic therapy, 3:1410
Fibrin and fibrogen tumor markers,
  3:1806
Fibroadenoma, 2:724
Fibroblasts, 2:726
Fibrocystic condition of the breast,
  1:252, 567, 568, 2:722, **722–725**
Fibrohistiocytic tumors, 3:1624
Fibrosarcoma, 2:726, **726–729,**
  3:1624–1625, 1631
Fibrosis, 2:724, 1197
Fight or flight response, 1:34, 35
FIGO staging system. *See* International
  Federation of Gynecology and
  Obstetrics staging system

Figs, 1:359
Filgrastim, 2:**729–731**
  immunotherapy types, 2:899
  for neutropenia, 2:1243–1244
  topotecan interactions, 3:1759
Financial issues, 1:346
Finasteride, 1:421–422
Fine-needle aspiration, 1:*206*
  biopsy types, 1:205–207
  breast cancer, 2:1155
  cytology samples, 1:557
  exocrine pancreatic cancer, 3:1350
  Hodgkin lymphoma, 2:850
  laryngeal cancer, 2:957
  liver biopsy, 2:1004–1007
  lymph node biopsy, 2:1044
  male breast cancer, 2:1062
  mediastinoscopy alternatives,
    2:1092–1093
  pancreatic cancer, 3:1342
  soft tissue sarcomas, 3:1627
Finland, 2:1257
Firmagon. *See* Degarelix
Fish and fish oil
  adrenal fatigue, 1:37
  cancer risk, 1:603–604
  omega-3 fatty acids, 2:1276–1278
Fistulas, 1:191, 2:800
Fistulography, 2:887
5-alpha reductase inhibitors, 1:625–626
5-Azacitidine. *See* Azacitidine
5-Fluorouracil. *See* Fluorouracil
5-HT$_3$ receptor antagonists, 2:1221
Five-year survival rates. *See* Survival
  rates
FK506. *See* Tacrolimus
Flagyl. *See* Metronidazole
Flap surgery, 2:1079–1080, 3:1399,
  1519–1522
Flavonoids, 2:1109, 1142, 1143
Flax, 1:359–360
Flaxseed, 2:1277
Flexible sigmoidoscopy. *See*
  Sigmoidoscopy
Flow cytometry, 2:*732,* **732–733**
  cancer of unknown primary, 1:314
  multiple myeloma, 2:1174
  myelodysplastic syndromes, 2:1186
  soft tissue sarcomas, 3:1628
  See also DNA flow cytometry
Floxuridine, 2:**733–735**
Fluconazole, 1:136, 137
Fludara. *See* Fludarabine
Fludarabine, 2:**735–737**

Fluid intake
  cisplatin, 1:468, 469
  diarrhea, 1:598
  gastrointestinal complications, 2:765
  hypercalcemia, 2:869
Fluid retention. *See* Edema
Fluorescein angiography, 1:103
Fluorescence bronchoscopy, 1:273
Fluorescent *in situ* hybridization, 3:1628
Fluorescent-activated cell sorting
  analysis. *See* Flow cytometry
Fluorodeoxyuridine. *See* Floxuridine
Fluoroquinolones, 1:184
Fluoroscopy
  imaging study types, 2:887
  lymphangiography, 2:1050
  radiation dermatitis, 3:1490
  upper gastrointestinal series,
    3:1823–1825
  x-rays, 3:1890–1891
Fluorouracil, 2:*737,* **737–738**
  basal cell carcinoma, 1:178
  cardiomyopathy, 1:390
  folic acid for the effects of,
    2:740–741
  hand-foot syndrome, 2:819–820
  laryngeal cancer, 2:959
  leucovorin with, 2:976–977
  levamisole with, 2:993
  mucositis, 2:1162
  squamous cell carcinoma of the skin,
    3:1650
Fluoxymesterone, 2:**738–740,** 3:1720,
  1721, 1877
Flurazepam, 1:187
Folate. *See* Folic acid
Folic acid, 2:**740–741**
  alcohol consumption and cancer,
    1:60, 62
  cancer prevention, 2:1143, 1144,
    1146
  for hemolytic anemia, 2:833
  leucovorin, 2:976–977
  methotrexate, 2:1135–1136
  risks, 2:1146
  role, 3:1854
Folinic acid. *See* Leucovorin
Folkman, Judah, 1:96, 394
Follicular carcinoma, 3:1751, 1754,
  1755
Follow-up
  Burkitt lymphoma, 1:280
  carcinoid tumors, gastrointestinal,
    1:380–381
  esophageal cancer, 1:667

G

O

Index

Index

Stomach acid blockers. *See* Gastric acid blockers
Stomach cancer, 3:*1663*, **1663–1669**
   cigarettes, 1:466
   Epstein-Barr virus association, 1:656
   gastrectomy, 2:753–756
   gastroduodenostomy, 2:757–759
   gastrointestinal cancer types, 2:760–761
   global rates, 2:797
   mitomycin-C, 2:1149–1150
   paraneoplastic syndromes, 3:1367
   ramucirumab, 3:1514–1516
   trastuzumab, 3:1784, 1785
   tube enterostomy, 3:1797
   tumor markers, 3:1806
Stomatitis, 3:*1669*, **1669–1671**
Stool tests
   cancer screening, 1:335, 341
   diarrhea, 1:597
   fecal occult blood tests, 2:713–714
Streptococcus pneumoniae, 1:623
Streptozocin, 3:**1671–1673**
Stress
   adrenal fatigue, 1:34–38
   amenorrhea, 1:78
   environmental factors in cancer development, 1:646
   family and caregiver issues, 2:705
   gastrointestinal complications, 2:765
   nasal cancer, 2:1207
   occupational exposures, 2:1269
   smoking cessation, 3:1622
Stroke, 3:1414, 1415
Stromal cell tumors, ovarian, 2:1316
Stromal tumors, gastrointestinal. *See* Gastrointestinal stromal tumors
Strontium-89, 3:1508–1511
Stunt. *See* Sunitinib
Subcapsular orchiectomy, 2:1303
Subcutaneous mastectomy, 3:1595
Subglottis, 2:955
Substance abuse, 2:1011, 3:**1673–1676**
   See also Drug dependence
Substance P neurokinin receptor antagonists, 1:130–132
Sudden death, 2:1138
Suicide, 3:1641
"Suicide genes," 2:772
Sulfadiazine, 1:113–114, 116
Sulfamethoxazole-trimehoprim, 1:113–116
Sulfatrim. *See* Sulfamethoxazole-trimehoprim
Sulfonamides, 1:115

Sulforaphane, 1:359, 2:1143, 1144
Sulfur-containing phytochemicals, 2:1142
Sulindac, 3:1630
Sun exposure
   alcohol consumption, 1:62
   basal cell carcinoma, 1:175, 176, 178–179
   Bowen disease, 1:241
   cancer prevention, 1:326
   dacarbazine, 1:564
   environmental factors in cancer development, 1:646
   head and neck cancers, 2:822, 826
   lip cancer, 2:1000
   melanoma, 2:1102, 1104, 1108–1109
   Merkel cell carcinoma, 2:1120, 1121, 1122
   nasal cancer treatment, 2:1207
   non-melanoma skin cancer, 1:161, 3:1610, 1612
   occupational exposures, 2:1266, 1267
   oral cancers, 2:1297, 1302
   panitumumab precautions, 3:1355
   photodynamic therapy, 3:1411
   porfimer sodium precautions, 3:1449
   skin cancer, 3:1605–1608
   squamous cell carcinoma of the skin, 3:1649, 1651
   tanning, 3:1700–1703
Sunitinib, 3:**1676–1679**
   angiogenesis, 1:98
   carcinoid tumors, lung, 1:385
   epidermal growth factor receptor antagonists, 1:652
   soft tissue sarcomas, 3:1630
Sunlamps. *See* Tanning
Sunless tanning products, 3:1702
Sunscreen, 2:1108, 3:1607, 1612, 1651, 1703
Superficial spreading melanoma, 2:1102
Superior vena cava syndrome, 2:1040, 1281–1283, 1285, 1286, 3:**1679–1680**
Supplemental health insurance, 2:829
Support groups
   body image/self image, 1:219–220
   cancer survivorship issues, 1:347
   endocrine pancreatic cancer, 3:1348
   exocrine pancreatic cancer, 3:1353
   Kaposi sarcoma, 2:938
   laryngeal cancer, 2:960
   late effects of cancer treatment, 2:968
   modified radical mastectomy, 2:1156
   orchiectomy, 2:1306

   ovarian cancer, 2:1321
   ovarian epithelial cancer, 2:1327
   pineoblastomas, 3:1421
   psycho-oncology, 3:1481
   rectal cancer, 3:1530
   salivary gland tumors, 3:1557
   simple mastectomy, 3:1596
   smoking cessation, 3:1623
   urethral cancer, 3:1834
Supportive care
   myelodysplastic syndromes, 2:1186–1187
   myelosuppression, treatment-induced, 2:1200
   oprelvekin, 2:1294–1295
   pleural effusion, 3:1432
Supraglottis, 2:955, 956
Suprasellar cyst. *See* Craniopharyngioma
Supratentorial primitive neurectodermal tumors, 3:**1680–1684**
Suprefact. *See* Buserelin
Suramin, 3:**1684–1686**
Surgeon experience, 2:951, 3:1880
Surgery
   acoustic neuromas, 1:7
   adenomas, 1:27
   adrenal tumors, 1:41
   adrenocortical carcinoma, 1:44
   adult cancer pain, 1:46, 47
   astrocytomas, 1:157, 158
   Barrett's esophagus, 1:173
   basal cell carcinoma, 1:177–178
   bile duct cancer, 1:196, 197–198
   bladder cancer, 1:214
   body image/self image, 1:219
   bone pain, 1:235
   Bowen disease, 1:241
   BRCA1 and *BRCA2* genes, 1:249
   breast cancer, 1:254–255
   Burkitt lymphoma, 1:278
   cancer, 1:291–292
   cancer biology, 1:299
   cancer in pregnant women, 3:1456
   carcinoid tumors, gastrointestinal, 1:379–380
   carcinoid tumors, lung, 1:384
   Castleman disease, 1:397, 398
   central nervous system carcinoma, 1:401
   central nervous system lymphoma, 1:403
   cervical cancer, 1:409–410, 3:1359
   childhood cancers, 1:438
   chondrosarcoma, 1:447

T

Tumor markers *(continued)*
    testicular cancer, 3:1714–1715
Tumor necrosis factor, 2:1134, 3:1434, **1809**
Tumor removal, 3:**1809–1813,** *1810*
    See also Surgery
Tumor size
    adjuvant chemotherapy, 1:28
    TNM staging system, 3:1814–1815
Tumor staging, 3:**1813–1817,** 1813*t*
    acute myelocytic leukemia, 1:21
    adrenocortical carcinoma, 1:44
    American Joint Committee on Cancer, 1:79
    anal cancer, 1:91
    astrocytomas, 1:157
    Barrett's esophagus, 1:173
    basal cell carcinoma, 1:177
    bile duct cancer, 1:196–197
    bladder cancer, 1:213–214
    breast cancer, 1:162, 254, 2:1155
    bronchoalveolar lung cancer, 1:270–271
    Burkitt lymphoma, 1:278
    cancer biology, 1:297
    cancer genetics, 1:311
    cancer in pregnant women, 3:1457
    cancer of unknown primary, 1:315
    carcinoid tumors, gastrointestinal, 1:379
    carcinoid tumors, lung, 1:384
    cervical cancer, 1:408–409
    chondrosarcoma, 1:447
    choroid plexus tumors, 1:452
    chronic lymphocytic leukemia, 1:459, 461
    chronic myelocytic leukemia, 1:464
    colon cancer, 1:482–483
    cutaneous T-cell lymphoma, 1:537
    endocrine pancreatic cancer, 3:1347
    endometrial cancer, 1:635
    esophageal cancer, 1:666, 670, 672
    Ewing sarcoma, 1:686
    exocrine pancreatic cancer, 3:1351
    extracranial germ cell tumors, 1:693
    fibrosarcomas, 2:727
    gallbladder cancer, 2:748
    germ cell tumors, 2:785
    gestational trophoblastic tumors, 2:789–791
    giant cell tumors, 2:793
    hairy cell leukemia, 2:816–817
    Hodgkin lymphoma, 2:849, 850–851
    Kaposi sarcoma, 2:936
    kidney cancer, 2:942

laparosocpy, 2:948
laryngeal cancer, 2:958
leiomyosarcoma, 2:975
lip cancer, 2:1001–1002
liver cancer, 2:1010
lumpectomy, 2:1026
lung cancer, non-small cell, 2:1036
lung cancer, small cell, 2:1041–1042
male breast cancer, 2:1062–1063
malignant fibrous histiocytoma, 2:1066
mediastinoscopy, 2:1090
medulloblastomas, 2:1096–1097
melanoma, 2:1106–1107
meningiomas, 2:1115
Merkel cell carcinoma, 2:1121
mesothelioma, 2:1126
multiple endocrine neoplasia, 2:1167
multiple myeloma, 2:1174, 1174*t*
mycosis fungoides, 2:1181
myelodysplastic syndromes, 2:1186
myeloproliferative diseases, 2:1195
nasal cancer, 2:1205–1206
nasopharyngeal cancer, 2:1211
neuroblastomas, 2:1230
neuroendocrine tumors, 2:1234
oligodendrogliomas, 2:1275
oral cancers, 2:1299
oropharyngeal cancer, 2:1309
ovarian cancer, 2:1319
ovarian epithelial cancer, 2:1326
pancreatic cancer, 3:1342–1343
paranasal sinus cancer, 3:1364
parathyroid cancer, 3:1370
pheochromocytoma, 3:1404
pituitary tumors, 3:1424
prostate cancer, 3:1462–1463
rectal cancer, 3:1527–1528
renal pelvis tumors, 3:1538–1539
retinoblastoma, 3:1543–1544
rhabdomyosarcoma, 3:1548
salivary gland tumors, 3:1557
Sézary syndrome, 3:1588
skin cancer, 3:1606
small intestine cancer, 3:1618–1619
soft tissue sarcomas, 3:1628–1629
squamous cell carcinoma of the skin, 3:1650
stomach cancer, 3:1666–1667
supratentorial primitive neuroectodermal tumors, 3:1682–1683
surgical oncology, 3:1688
testicular cancer, 3:1715

thymic cancer, 3:1745
thymomas, 3:1749
thyroid cancer, 3:1754
transitional cell carcinoma, 3:1776
triple negative breast cancer, 3:1792
tumor removal, 3:1810
urethral cancer, 3:1832–1833
vaginal cancer, 3:1838
vulvar cancer, 3:1865
Wilms tumor, 3:1887
Tumor suppressor genes
    cancer biology, 1:295–296
    cancer genetics, 1:308–309
    cancer predisposition, 1:317
    carcinogenesis, 1:373
    chromosome rearrangements, 1:455
    genetic testing, 2:776–777
    medulloblastomas, 2:1096
    melanoma, 2:1105
    metastasis, 2:1130
    multiple myeloma, 2:1172
    von Hippel-Lindau disease, 3:1856–1857
Tumor suppressor proteins, 2:897, 3:1541
Tumor-induced hypercalcemia, 3:1893
Tumor-infiltrating lymphocytes, 2:902
Tumors
    adenocarcinomas, 1:24–25
    adrenal insufficiency, 1:35
    adrenal tumors, 1:38–41
    adult cancer pain, 1:46
    angiogenesis, 1:96–97
    angiogenesis inhibitors, 1:101
    astrocytomas, 1:156–160
    basal cell carcinoma, 1:175–179
    bile duct cancer, 1:193–194
    bone pain, 1:234
    brain and central nervous system tumors, 1:242–244
    Burkitt lymphoma, 1:276, 277
    cancer biology, 1:297
    carcinoid tumors, gastrointestinal, 1:376–381
    carcinoid tumors, lung, 1:382–386
    carcinoma, 1:386
    central nervous system carcinoma, 1:399–402
    chemoembolization, 1:416–418
    chondrosarcoma, 1:445–448
    chondrosarcomas, 1:445–448
    chordomas, 1:448–450
    choroid plexus tumors, 1:450–453
    Cushing syndrome, 1:533
    cystosarcoma phyllodes, 1:548–551

V

V600E *BRAF* mutation, 1:559–560
Vaccine interactions
  carmustine, 1:393
  everolimus, 1:683
  gemcitabine, 2:769
  ibritumomab, 2:880
  immune globulin, 2:891
  methotrexate, 2:1136
  obinutuzumab, 2:1263
  pemetrexed, 3:1377
Vaccines, cancer. *See* Cancer vaccines;
  Immunotherapy
Vacuum scraping, 1:612
Vagal-sparing esophagectomy, 1:671
Vaginal adenosis, 3:1840
Vaginal atrophy, 3:1586
Vaginal cancer, 2:807–813,
  3:1356–1359, **1837–1841**
Vaginectomy, 3:1839
Vagotomy, 2:755
Vagus nerve, 2:961
Valaxona. *See* Diazepam
Valdecoxib, 1:540–541
Valganciclovir, 1:145, 146
Valium. *See* Diazepam
Valrubicin, 3:**1841–1842**
Valstar. *See* Valrubicin
Vancocin. *See* Vancomycin
Vancomycin, 1:113–114, 115
Varenicline tartrate, 3:1623
Varicella zoster virus, 2:843
Varmus, Harold, 2:1214
Vascular access, 3:**1842–1847,** *1843,*
  1845
Vascular endothelial growth factor
  angiogenesis, 1:96–100
  antibiotics, 1:113
  colon cancer, 1:484
  human growth factors, 2:861
  ramucirumab, 3:1514
Vascularization. *See* Angiogenesis
Vasculitis, 2:770
Vasomotor symptoms, 2:1245–1246
Vasopressors, 2:910
Vattikuti Urology Institute, 3:1469
VDS. *See* Vindesine
Vectibix. *See* Panitumumab
Vector vaccines, 2:903
Vectors, gene therapy, 2:773, 774
Vegan diet, 1:504
Velban. *See* Vinblastine
Velcade. *See* Bortezomib

Velsar. *See* Vinblastine
Venoglobulin. *See* Immune globulin
Venography, 1:44
Ventilators, 1:51–52
Vepesid. *See* Etoposide
Versed. *See* Midazolam
Verteporfin, 3:1411
Vertigo, 1:5–7
Vestibular schwannomas. *See* Acoustic
  neuromas
Vestibulocochlear nerve, 1:4–5
Vi-Atro. *See* Atropine and
  diphenoxylate
Vidarabine, 3:1444
Vidaza. *See* Azacitidine
Video-assisted thoracoscopic surgery,
  2:1030–1032, 3:1733, 1737–1738,
  1745
Villous adenoma, 3:1530
Vinblastine, 2:936, 3:1694, **1847–1848,**
  1852
Vinca alkaloids
  syndrome of inappropriate
    antidiuretic hormone, 3:1694
  vinblastine, 3:1847–1848
  vincristine, 3:1848–1850
  vindesine, 3:1850–1852
  vinorelbine, 3:1852–1853
Vincaleukoblastine. *See* Vinblastine
Vincasar. *See* Vincristine
Vincrex. *See* Vincristine
Vincristine, 3:**1848–1850,** *1849,* 1852
  Kaposi sarcoma, 2:936
  pegaspargase interactions, 3:1374
  soft tissue sarcomas, 3:1630
  syndrome of inappropriate
    antidiuretic hormone, 3:1694
Vindesine, 3:**1850–1852**
Vinorelbine, 3:1694, 1851, **1852–1853**
Vinyl chloride
  cancer clusters, 1:301
  occupational exposures, 2:1266,
    1267
  soft tissue sarcoma, 3:1626
Vioxx. *See* Cyclooxygenase 2 inhibitors
Vipoma, 3:1346
ViraferonPeg, 2:917
Viral vectors, 1:355
Virilization. *See* Secondary sex
  characteristics
Virtual colonoscopy, 1:481–482, 488
Virtual reality, 3:1334
Virus therapies, 1:201
Virus vaccines, 2:880
Viruses

acute leukemia risk factors, 2:979
AIDS-related cancer risk factors,
  1:57
antiviral therapy, 1:143–146
Burkitt lymphoma, 1:277
cancer causes, 1:288–289
cancer genetics, 1:309
cancer prevention, 1:326
cervical cancer prevention,
  1:411–412
drug resistance, 1:622
gene therapy, 2:772
gene vectors, 2:773, 774
hemolytic anemia, 2:831
interferons, 2:916
lip cancer risk factors, 2:1001
nasal cancer, 2:1203, 1204, 1208
nasopharyngeal cancer, 2:1210
oncologic emergencies, 2:1284, 1286
oropharyngeal cancer, 2:1308
paranasal sinus cancer, 3:1363
See also Specific types
Visceral pain, 3:1333
Vision
  chemotherapy, 1:431
  childhood cancer treatment effects,
    1:439
  denileukin diftitox precautions, 1:582
  retinoblastoma, 3:1545
  tamoxifen, 3:1700
Visiting Nurses Association, 2:854
Vismodegib, 1:178, 3:1607
Visual inspection with acetic acid, 1:411
Visudyne. *See* Verteporfin
Vitamin A
  risks, 2:1146
  role, 3:1854
  smoking, 3:1855
Vitamin B$_6$, 3:1854
Vitamin C
  adrenal fatigue, 1:37
  interactions, 3:1855
  role, 3:1854
Vitamin D
  cancer prevention, 2:1146, 3:1855
  hypocalcemia, 2:876
  multiple endocrine neoplasia, 2:1168
  multiple myeloma, 2:1175
  sun exposure, 3:1701
Vitamin deficiencies. *See* Malnutrition
Vitamin E
  ado-trastuzumab emtansine
    interactions, 1:33
  antioxidants, 1:142